KIDNEY STONES

MEDICAL AND SURGICAL MANAGEMENT

KIDNEY STONES

MEDICAL AND SURGICAL MANAGEMENT

SECOND EDITION

Editors

Fredric L Coe MD
Professor
Department of Medicine, Nephrology
University of Chicago
Chicago, Illinois, USA

Elaine M Worcester MD
Professor
Department of Medicine, Nephrology
University of Chicago
Chicago, Illinois, USA

Andrew P Evan PhD
Professor Emeritus
Department of Anatomy and Cell Biology
Indiana University School of Medicine
Indianapolis, Indiana, USA

James E Lingeman MD FACS
Professor
Department of Urology
Indiana University School of Medicine
Indianapolis, Indiana, USA

JAYPEE

JAYPEE BROTHERS MEDICAL PUBLISHERS
The Health Sciences Publisher
New Delhi | London | Panama

Jaypee Brothers Medical Publishers (P) Ltd

Headquarters
Jaypee Brothers Medical Publishers (P) Ltd.
4838/24, Ansari Road, Daryaganj
New Delhi 110 002, India
Phone: +91-11-43574357
Fax: +91-11-43574314
E-mail: jaypee@jaypeebrothers.com

Overseas Offices
JP Medical Ltd.
83, Victoria Street, London
SW1H 0HW (UK)
Phone: +44-20 3170 8910
Fax: +44(0)20 3008 6180
E-mail: info@jpmedpub.com

Jaypee-Highlights Medical Publishers Inc.
City of Knowledge, Bld. 235, 2nd Floor, Clayton
Panama City, Panama
Phone: +1 507-301-0496
Fax: +1 507-301-0499
E-mail: cservice@jphmedical.com

Jaypee Brothers Medical Publishers (P) Ltd.
Bhotahity, Kathmandu, Nepal
Phone: +977-9741283608
E-mail: kathmandu@jaypeebrothers.com

Website: www.jaypeebrothers.com
Website: www.jaypeedigital.com

Inquiries for bulk sales may be solicited at: jaypee@jaypeebrothers.com

Kidney Stones: Medical and Surgical Management

First Edition: **1996**

Second Edition: **2020**

ISBN: 978-93-5152-942-2

Printed at: Samrat Offset Pvt. Ltd.

Dedicated to

All patients that suffer from the stone, that what we have accomplished might comfort them and better their lives.

Contributors

Megan K Applewhite MD
Assistant Professor of Surgery
Albany Medical Center
Albany, New York, USA

John R Asplin MD FASN
Medical Director
Lintholink Corporation
Chicago, Illinois, USA

Dean G Assimos MD
Professor and Chair
Anton J Bueschen MD Endowed Chair in Urologic Surgery and Research
Department of Urology
University of Alabama at Birmingham
Birmingham, Alabama, USA

Aaron D Benson MD
OSF Healthcare
Peoria, Illinois, USA

Kristin J Bergsland PhD
Research Associate
(Assistant Professor)
Department of Medicine
Nephrology Section
University of Chicago
Chicago, Illinois, USA

Amit Bhattu MD
Urologist
Department of Urology
Muljibhai Patel Urological Hospital
Nadiad, Gujarat, India

René JM Bindels PhD
Professor
Department of Physiology
Radboud University Medical Center
Nijmegen, The Netherlands

Marc E De Broe MD PhD
Emeritus Professor of Medicine
Laboratory of Pathophysiology
University of Antwerp
Antwerp, Belgium

David A Bushinsky MD
Professor of Medicine Pharmacology and Physiology
University of Rochester School of Medicine and Dentistry
Rochester, New York, USA

Fernando Cabrera MD
Urologist
Section of Endourology and Minimally Invasive Urology
Department of Urology
Cleveland Clinic Florida
Weston, Florida, USA

Aluizio Barbosa Carvalho MD PhD
Bone Disease Unit Coordinator
Affiliate Professor
Nephrology Division
Federal University of São Paulo
São Paulo, Brazil

Yew-Lam Chong
MBBS MMed (Surgery) FAMS (Urology)
Chairman, Division of Surgery
Head, Department of Urology
Tan Tock Seng Hospital
Singapore

Fredric L Coe MD
Professor
Department of Medicine, Nephrology
University of Chicago
Chicago, Illinois, USA

William A Critchlow MD
Urologist
Department of Urology
Mayo Clinic Arizona
Phoenix, Arizona, USA

Gary C Curhan MD ScD FASN
Professor of Medicine
Harvard Medical School
Professor of Epidemiology
Harvard School of Public Health
Channing Division of Network Medicine/Renal Division
Brigham and Women's Hospital
Boston, Massachusetts, USA

Mitra R de Cógáin MD
Kaiser Permanente
San Diego, California, USA

Michel Daudon PhD
AP-HP
Department of Biochemistry
A Necker-Entants Malades Hospital
Paris, France

Mahesh Desai MS FRCS FACS
Medical Director
Muljibhai Patel Urological Hospital
Nadiad, Gujarat, India

Mihir M Desai MD
Professor of Clinical Urology
Health Sciences Campus
Los Angeles, California, USA

Patrick C D'Haese PhD
Professor
Department of Biomedical Sciences
Laboratory of Pathophysiology
University of Antwerp
Wilrijk, Belgium

Andrew P Evan PhD
Professor Emeritus
Department of Anatomy and Cell Biology
Indiana University School of Medicine
Indianapolis, Indiana, USA

Murray J Favus MD
Professor
Department of Urology
Department of Medicine
Endocrinology Section
University of Chicago
Chicago, Illinois, USA

Kevin K Frick PhD
Research Assistant Professor
University of Rochester
School of Medicine and Dentistry
Rochester, New York, USA

Daniel G Fuster MD
Associate Professor of Nephrology
University of Bern
Bern, Switzerland

Giovanni Gambaro MD PhD
Professor of Nephrology
Department of Internal Medicine
Division of Nephrology
Catholic University of the Sacred Heart
Rome, Italy

Arvind P Ganpule MS MNANS
Consultant and Chief
Division of Laparoscopy
Muljibhai Patel Urological Hospital
Nadiad, Gujarat, India

David S Goldfarb MD FACP FASN FNKF
Professor of Medicine and Physiology
New York Harbor VA Healthcare System
New York University School of Medicine
New York, USA

Laurie B Gower PhD
Professor
Department of Materials Science and Engineering
University of Florida
Gainesville, Florida, USA

Joshua H Grimes PhD
Clinical Medical Physics Resident
Department of Radiology
Mayo Clinic
Rochester, Minnesota, USA

Raymon H Grogan MD
Professor of Surgery
University of Chicago Medicine
Chicago, Illinois, USA

Mitchell L Halperin
MDCM FRCP(C) FRS (Canada)
Professor Emeritus
Department of Medicine/Nephrology
University of Toronto School of Medicine
Toronto, Ontario, Canada

Lee Hamm MD
Senior Vice President and Dean
James R Doty Distinguished Professor and Chair
Tulane University School of Medicine
New Orleans, Louisiana, USA

Joe Harris PhD
Post-doctoral Researcher
Department of Materials Science and Engineering
Friedrich-Alexander-University Erlangen-Nürnberg
Erlangen, Germany

Ita Pfeferman Heilberg Md PhD
Kidney Stone Unit Coordinator
Associate Professor
Nephrology Division
Federal University of São Paulo
São Paulo, Brazil

Kathleen S Hering-Smith MS PhD
Associate Professor
Department of Medicine
Section of Nephrology
Tulane University School of Medicine
New Orleans, Louisiana, USA

Joost GJ Hoenderop PhD
Professor
Department of Physiology
Radboud University Medical Center
Nijmegen, Netherlands

Mitchell R Humphreys MD
Professor and Fellowship Director
Department of Urology
Mayo Clinic Arizona
Phoenix, Arizona, USA

Edwin L Kaplan MD
Professor
Department of Surgery
University of Chicago
Chicago, Illinois, USA

Amy E Krambeck MD
Michael O Koch Professor of Urology
Indiana University School of Medicine
Indianapolis, Indiana, USA

Nancy S Krieger PhD
Research Associate Professor
Department of Medicine
University of Rochester School of Medicine
Rochester, New York, USA

Mohan Kumar MD
Consultant Urologist
Muljibhai Patel Urological Hospital
Nadiad, Gujarat, India

Anke L Lameris PhD
Physiologist
Radboud University Medical Center
Nijmegen, Netherlands

John C Lieske MD
Professor of Medicine
Division of Nephrology and Hypertension
Mayo Clinic
Rochester, Minnesota, USA

James E Lingeman MD FACS
Professor
Department of Urology
Indiana University School of Medicine
Indianapolis, Indiana, USA

Michael Lipkin MD MBA
Associate Professor of Urology
Duke University Medical Center
Durham, North Carolina, USA

Archana Lovett BS PhD
Graduate Assistant
Department of Materials Science and Engineering
University of Florida
Gainesville, Florida, USA

Brian R Matlaga MD MPH
Professor of Urology
Johns Hopkins University School of Medicine
Director
Stone Disease
The James Buchanan Brady Urological Institute
Baltimore, Maryland, USA

Jane S Matsumoto MD
Assistant Professor
Department of Radiology
Mayo Clinic
Rochester, Minnesota, USA

Cynthia H McCollough PhD
Professor
Department of Radiology
Mayo Clinic
Rochester, Minnesota, USA

Nicole L Miller MD
Associate Professor
Department of Urologic Surgery
Vanderbilt University
Nashville, Tennessee, USA

Dawn S Milliner MD
Professor of Medicine and Pediatrics
Mayo Clinic
Rochester, Minnesota, USA

Orson W Moe MD
Professor of Medicine
Director, Charles and Jane Pak Center of Mineral Metabolism and Clinical Research
Director
O'Brien Kidney Research Core
University of Texas Southwestern Medical Center
Dallas, Texas, USA

Lama Nazzal MD
Assistant Professor of Medicine
New York University School of Medicine
New York City, New York, USA

Craig A Peters MD
Chief, Pediatric Urology
Children's Health System Texas
Professor of Urology
University of Texas Southwestern
Dallas, Texas, USA

Keng-Siang Png MD FRCS (Urol)
Consultant, Department of Urology
Tan Tan Tock Seng Hospital
Singapore

Glenn M Preminger MD
Professor of Urology
Duke University School of Medicine
Durham, North Carolina, USA

Andrew D Rule MD
Professor of Medicine
Division of Nephrology and Hypertension
Mayo Clinic
Rochester, Minnesota, USA

Khashayar Sakhaee MD
Professor and Clinical Director
Charles and Jane Pak Center for Mineral Metabolism and Clinical Research
University of Texas Southwestern Medical Center
Dallas, Texas, USA

David J Sas DO
Assistant Professor of Medicine
Mayo Clinic
Rochester, Minnesota, USA

Daniel Schneider MD
Urology Specialist
Department of Urology
Mayo Clinic Arizona
Scottsdale, Arizona, USA

Michelle Jo Semins MD
Assistant Professor
Department of Urology
University of Pittsburgh
Pittsburgh, Pennsylvania, USA

Stephen Scott Sparks MD
Assistant Professor
Department of Urology
Children's Hospital Los Angeles
University of Southern California
Los Angeles, California, USA

Jubilee Tan MD
Urologist
Department of Urology
University of Alabama
Birmingham, Alabama, USA

Yung-khan Tan MD
Senior Consultant
Department of Urology
Tan Tan Tock Seng Hospital
Singapore

Eric N Taylor MD
Associate Professor of Medicine
Tufts University School of Medicine
Boston, Massachusetts
Division of Nephrology and Transplantation
Maine Medical Center
Portland, Maine, USA

Anja Verhulst PhD
Post-Doctoral Fellow
Laboratory of Pathophysiology
University of Antwerp
Antwerp, Belgium

Benjamin A Vervaet PhD
Department of Biomedical Sciences
University of Antwerp
Antwerp, Belgium

James C Williams Jr PhD
Department of Anatomy and Cell Biology
Indiana University School of Medicine
Indianapolis, Indiana, USA

Stephan E Wolf PhD
Professor
Department of Materials Science and Engineering
Freidrich-Alexander University Erlangen-Nürnberg
Erlangen, Germany

Michael YC Wong MD
Medical Director
Urology and Fertility Center
Mount Elizabeth Hospital
Singapore

Elaine M Worcester MD
Professor
Department of Medicine, Nephrology
University of Chicago
Chicago, Illinois, USA

Preface

The Plough and the Star

Fifty years have gone since I first came, and many who worked this field with me are gone. I have read or heard some say nothing alters, we are where we were before, have learned little we did not know. I say that is wrong, and they who have said it are wrong. Here is my evidence, this ample book filled with new knowledge, knowledge of what our senses show us and reasonable visions of how things came to be the way they are.

This field of mine—I lay some claims being an elder, though it is ours, of course—this field is like everywhere we do science. But, may be being so present, so undeniable, the stones themselves can make their causes seem, by contrast, gauzy dreamy things, and those who seek them dreamers. That is not new. The causes of stones have always been uncertain. But we care because of ancient distinctions, treatment by cause or treatment empiric, medicine of remedies or medicine of science.

This is a book for physicians and we all know how things are. Patients are ill and we seek in them a disease that causes their illness. Stones are a disease and their illnesses obvious. As if one satisfaction were not enough, surgeons can cure the disease. It is for them a kind of perfection: the stones so evident, and the result so much a cure, for a time.

But, what next? Stones recur. Surgeons tire of repetition, patients more so. Inevitably comes the question. We must treat by cause or by empirics, by science or by remedy, and as we do so judge this field of ours as to its fitness and maturity. Judge the work that came before us, and the work done now.

It is strange but true that a field matures by causes, by understanding things as they are in terms of things that made them be as they are. Yet those causes, those things that make the evident diseases be as they are, they are themselves impossibly distant gleaming brilliant things beyond our common ken. We can know what is there, but only imagine why.

So it is for stones. We observe them, catalog their crystals, perhaps the proteins of their matrix, study the patients who form them, and imagine. The word for our imaginings saves us from seeming dreamers. It means where we push off from. But hypotheses arise from dreams, from images, from imaginings. There is no other way, and we all know it.

Physicians have imagined the causes of disease forever. What changed things, perhaps five hundred years ago, was the deduction, the demand for the necessary prediction which would prove the imaginings false or not false as if each prophetess were tested by the happening.

Have we all not done this? Have we all not tested visions? Even in the microcosm of our practices, we imagine–illness comes from this disease, or that one, and we test if we are right, or wrong.

Surgeons, perhaps, least suffer from the enigma of imagination. Stones, as I have said, are remarkably present, and the purpose of the surgeon their extirpation—the success of which is rarely doubtful. They do research. But surgical research itself is not usually about causes. It is about remedy: better ways, better instruments. And the test gives a clear answer: better, no better, worse.

The rest of us, cognitive, and physically less inclined, care about remedies too, and test them with results, perhaps less clear, for we end up counting stones and bickering among ourselves about bias and sufficiency. Did this remedy slow their recurrence? Did we repeat the trials often enough to be done with them and simply use what we have?

Both enterprises, the hunt for better surgery, the hunt for better medicines, are often called technology research, practical research, pragmatic research, and the answers are more or less what one would find in testing refrigerators, or dishwashers, or automobiles: better, worse, no different, not good, good.

That is to say medicine is about the remedy. It is humble that way. Ultimately, we serve people who are ill because of disease, who want health and for us to restore it: rightly so. But we dream, sometimes, about the invisible causes of things and say with some reasons that treatment by cause is ultimately a grace because ultimately better than treatment by empirics, treatment by remedy.

We have examples.

Do you remember peptic ulcer?

It was the corrosive acid caused it, how could things be otherwise? Antacids helped them heal. When industry produced the acid blockers, they worked, they helped the ulcers heal. What more could we desire? What more should we desire? The remedy was workable, and based on an evident cause—a cause afloat on oceans of measurement, shielded by mountains of published papers, central to a universe of understanding.

The silly dream that bacteria could live in stomach acid and cause the ulcers was just that, silly and a dream, silk and gossamer in the stern winter of finished science, of working technology, but true even so. Those who dreamed were scorned and slighted, hardly thought of by working scientists who ruled the field—until the proof came, and everything altered. The remedy from the dream is more enduring and more efficient than any that had been before. Even more, somehow those bacteria cause cancer that can, one hopes, be avoided.

Do you want another?

Remember, then, when rising systolic blood pressure was natural, part of how we age, the way nature contrived to force blood through old and narrowed vessels. Lower it, and cause great harm. When that was first tried those who tried it feared. But they were right. To lower it staves off strokes, and heart attacks, and heart failure, and death. No one anymore thinks grandma should have her high systolic pressure as a defense against stroke, as a way to perfuse her brain. It would be as wrong as it was wrong, once, to think the opposite.

There is a power that cause confers, not always channeled into remedy, at least not right away, but a power of vision, of prophecy, of understanding. I would like to say we pursue the causes of things because of that power, but the truth may be otherwise.

The world our senses show us came to be the way it is, somehow, and how is present never to our senses, only to our imaginings, our dreaming selves. Bacteria living in our stomachs, an idle trait of age a lurking killer, how odd to imagine this. But those who did conceived a change of kind, of type, of truth as we can know it.

Such time as we spend in dreaming, howsoever profitable, is time not spent in more pragmatic, workmanlike pursuits. Thus, the unavoidable tension, the inevitable dispute. If false dreams issue from the gates of ivory, the time for them is lost time, the money spent for them lost money while the world waits for us, expecting something better for our pay. So it is, the dreamer lives in hopes of vindication, while the rest content themselves to do the work of the world.

This book depicts, whose preface I am writing, all we have, our field in full abundance and, as best we know, what made it so, and what might come of knowing.

As every book of medicine portrays some field caught up in time, like smiling pictured children age long since has swept away, we are here upon a moment, knowledge and uncertainties, wisdom and silliness mixed together as in all of medicine. Those experts who wrote here made of what they think is true a grand and royal portrait time will prove false howsoever beautiful its colors and its shapes. They made a book of certainties. They made a book of dreams.

Who worked this field before us, were as fine as we, but we have worked as they, and taken things beyond their time. I have heard some say nothing alters, and we are where we were a generation past. This book is our rebuke, our argument, and our disdain in trade for theirs.

Science is forever moving, not toward eternal truth, for that is silliness, but toward a greater richness. Scientists measure, and what they measure an enduring legacy to whom their field will pass. Tests of remedy or a dream, all dreams that fail and those not failed enrich the treasury. What's false is burned away. The rest, like jeweled crowns and diadems, remains the kingdom's riches. Thus it is that science is forever growing, and forever new.

As for me, I have long worked this amiable soil and offered up to the judgments of time what it has yielded me. I have had my dreams proved false, some hopeful yet, in seeming true. And I delight to look upon this thing, this work of those I work with, those I know and prize for their accomplishments. Here are their offerings, the gorgeous artifacts of labor spent, the brilliancies of cultivated minds. Strangers come, someday, to work our field will gaze upon this portrait at a time we cannot know, and say: 'Who worked this field before us were as fine as we, but we shall carry things beyond their time.'

Fredric L Coe

Acknowledgments

I wish to thank Mr Jitendar P Vij (Group Chairman), Mr Ankit Vij (Group President) and the editorial team at Jaypee Brothers Medical Publishers, New Delhi, India for their dedicated guidance and expertise with special mention of Ms Chetna Malhotra Vohra (Associate Director—Content Strategy) and Ms Anamika Talukdar (Development Editor) to help me complete the chapters. It was a pleasure working with all the publishing team at Jaypee Brothers Medical Publishers, New Delhi, India for the book proofs and editing, etc.

Contents

SECTION 3: Surgical Management of Kidney Stones

Section Editor: *James E Lingeman*

Section 1

Characteristics and Formation of Kidney Stones

—Andrew P Evan

CHAPTER 1

Epidemiology of Kidney Stones

Eric N Taylor, Gary C Curhan

OVERVIEW

Kidney stones are highly prevalent, are a major cause of morbidity, and inflict a large cost on the healthcare system. Epidemiologic studies have quantified the increasing incidence and prevalence of nephrolithiasis and have delineated a wide variety of dietary, nondietary, and urinary risk factors for kidney stone formation.

At least four considerations should be kept in mind in any review of kidney stones. First, it is necessary to prioritize studies that focus on actual kidney stones as an outcome, rather than urine composition. The difficulties of using urine composition as a proxy for kidney stone risk are manifest by the wide array of well-established nonurinary kidney stone risk factors and data implicating the renal interstitium as the site of initial stone formation.[1-3] Second, the importance of many kidney stone risk factors vary by individual characteristics such as age, sex, and BMI. Third, there is a relative scarcity of randomized controlled trials (RCTs) in the field of kidney stone prevention. Thus, data from well-performed observational studies can be considered in the clinical setting when devising treatment plans to reduce kidney stone recurrence. Finally, RCTs and large observational studies that help inform current understanding of kidney stone risk factors consist of participants with known calcium oxalate nephrolithiasis or populations who likely have a predominance of calcium oxalate stone disease. Thus, some conclusions from studies of calcium kidney stone disease (e.g. RCT data for water intake and stone prevention) are by necessity applied, albeit carefully and with attention to renal physiology, to less common stone types.

PREVALENCE, INCIDENCE, AND RECURRENCE

Prevalence

The prevalence of nephrolithiasis, defined as a history of stone disease, varies by age, sex, race, and geography. The prevalence in the United States increases with age and is approximately 11% for men and 7% for women: kidney stones occur in about 1 in 11 people in the United States.[4] Kidney stone prevalence has increased steadily over the last 35 years for men and women, whether black, Hispanic, or white (Fig. 1.1).[4,5] Although the prevalence is consistently lower in blacks and Hispanics than in whites, increases in prevalence over time have been higher for blacks and Hispanics.[4] Increased detection of asymptomatic stones resulting from the increasing use and sensitivity of radiologic studies may explain in part the rise in prevalence.

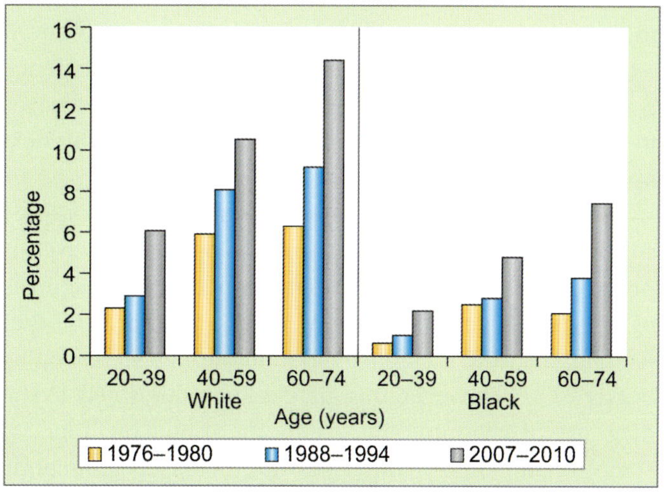

Fig. 1.1: Prevalence of history of kidney stones by age and race.[4,5]

Relatively few population-based studies of the prevalence of nephrolithiasis have been conducted outside of the United States. Prevalence of stone disease has increased in Japan[6] and Germany.[7]

A study of over 1 million individuals in the United States found geographic variability with a north-south and west-east gradient; the highest prevalence of self-reported nephrolithiasis was in the southeastern United States.[8]

Although the prevalence of nephrolithiasis has been consistently found to be higher in men than women, a decrease in the male-to-female ratio was suggested by a study of hospital discharges.[9] Data from the Nationwide Inpatient Survey between 1997 and 2002 found a male-to-female ratio 1.3:1. Similarly, the male-to-female prevalence ratio in the most recent NHANES data was ~1.5, substantially lower than the commonly reported ratio of 2–3:1.

Incidence

The incidence of nephrolithiasis, defined as the first stone event, also varies by age, sex, and race. White males have the highest incidence rates. In men, the incidence begins to rise after age 20, peaks between 40 and 60 years at ~3/1,000/y and then declines.[10-12] In women, the incidence is higher in the late 20s at 2.5/1,000/y and then decreases to 1/1,000/y by age 50, remaining at this rate for the next several decades.[11-14]

As with prevalence, attempts to compare kidney stone incidence rates over time are complicated by trends toward more frequent imaging and concomitant diagnosis of asymptomatic kidney stones. Over a 24-year period in Iceland, the total incidence of kidney stones increased by nearly 28%.[15] However, this increase was due solely to the diagnosis of asymptomatic stones; the annual incidence of symptomatic kidney stones did not increase significantly in either men or women.

A study in Rochester, Minnesota raised the possibility that incidence rates may be decreasing. Using the same methodology as a study performed 30 years earlier, the recent study reported incidence rates since 1990 may be falling in men and have leveled off in women.[16] Because there were only 157 cases in men and 91 in women, additional larger studies are needed.

Recurrence Rates

Case series suggest 30–40% of untreated individuals will form another stone within 5 years after the initial episode.[12] The recurrence rates in the control arms of RCTs and an observational study from Olmstead County[17] are lower. The risk of recurrence is influenced by stone type and urinary composition. Features associated with higher rates of recurrence include younger age, male sex, a family history of kidney stones, and uric acid stones.[17] Fortunately, randomized trials demonstrated that interventions can reduce the likelihood of recurrence by >50%.[18-21]

KIDNEY STONE TYPE

Calcium containing kidney stones are the most common, accounting for >80% of incident and recurrent kidney stones (Figs. 1.2 and 1.3).[22-25] The majority (>80%) of calcium stones have calcium oxalate as their major constituent; predominantly calcium phosphate stones are less common.[26] Uric acid stones represent between 5% and 10% of stones, followed by cystine, struvite, and other less common stone types.[22-25] Analysis of stone composition in developing countries[27,28] confirms the preponderance of calcium oxalate nephrolithiasis worldwide.

Stone composition can vary by country. Although the majority of kidney stones in one Japanese series were

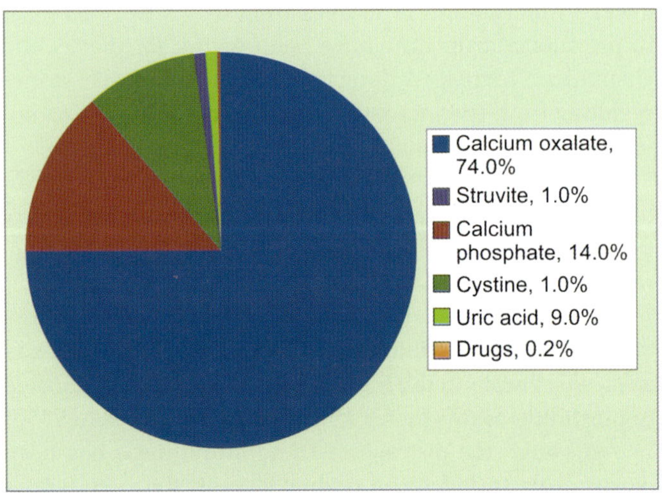

Fig. 1.2: Proportion of types of kidney stones in first-time stone formers (N = 11,666).
Courtesy: Professor Michel Daudon is from Paris, France.

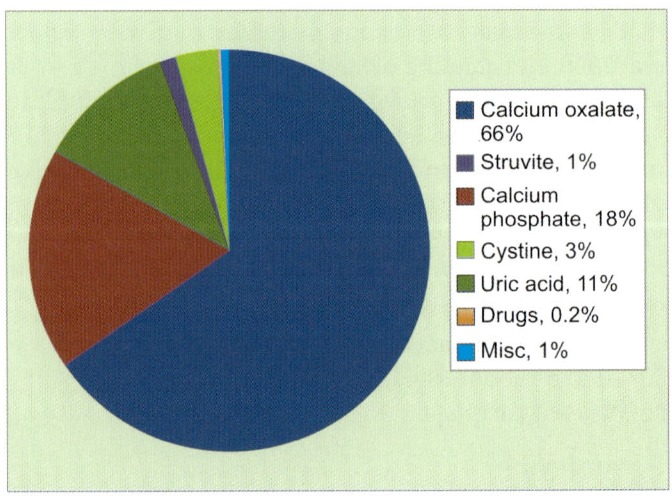

Fig. 1.3: Proportion of types of kidney stones in recurrent stone formers (N = 8,671).
Courtesy: Professor Michel Daudon is from Paris, France.

calcium oxalate, the proportion of uric acid stones was 16%,[29] higher than reported in many other countries. A high prevalence of struvite stones still occurs in some non-industrialized countries: women in Sub-Saharan Africa had struvite present in 43% of kidney stones.[30]

Kidney stone composition also may have changed over time. For example, the proportion of struvite stones in Australia decreased from 14% in the 1970s to <7% 40 years later,[31] presumably reflecting improvement in management of urinary tract infections in the Australian population. Some[26] but not all[32] series suggest that the proportion of calcium phosphate in calcium stones may have increased over time. The reason for a potential increase in calcium phosphate temporally is unknown; there has been speculation that preventive or therapeutic maneuvers (such as potassium citrate administration or extracorporeal shock wave lithotripsy [ESWL]) may contribute.[26]

Finally, kidney stone composition varies by sex, body size, and a variety of comorbidities. Women with calcium stones tend to have a greater proportion of calcium phosphate in kidney stones compared to men,[22,26,32] and uric acid stones are more common in men than women.[33] Independent of age and gender, higher BMI and diabetes mellitus are both associated with uric acid as compared with calcium kidney stones,[33,34] a phenomena presumably due to the lower urine pH associated with insulin resistance.[35]

COST

The financial burden of nephrolithiasis in the United States is difficult to quantify but is in the billions of dollars. In the year 2000, estimates for the annual healthcare expenditure associated directly with kidney stones ranged between $2.1 billion[36] and $4.5 billion[37] (or about $5.75 billion in year 2010 dollars). Indirect annual costs of stones in 2000 (due to lost days of work) were estimated to be $775 million[37] (about $995 million in 2010 dollars).

Relatively few studies outside the United States have examined the costs of kidney stone disease. In 2010, the annual budget impact for stone disease in France was estimated to be about 590 million Euros[38] (about $775 million dollars using average 2010 exchange rates). If France had the same population as the United States in 2010, the cost would have been about $3.7 billion.

Costs due to stone disease in the United States appear to have increased substantially over time. In 2000, the cost of treating and diagnosing stones in the emergency department in the United States was estimated at just under $500 million.[36] In a recent study, hospital emergency department charges (which are often higher than actual costs) for stone disease increased annually by 10% over a 4-year period and by 2009 totaled $5 billion[39] (about $4 billon in year 2000). Reasons for these increased hospital charges are unclear, but may be due in part to higher utilization of computed tomography.

NONDIETARY RISK FACTORS

Family History

Studies of twins and populations have demonstrated that the common forms of stone disease are heritable.[40] A family history of stone disease more than doubles the risk of incident kidney stone formation[41] and increases the risk of stone recurrence by 60%.[17] The increased risk is likely due to both genetic predisposition and similar environmental exposures. Numerous genetic causes of rare forms of nephrolithiasis (e.g. cystinuria and dent disease) have been identified, but information is still limited on genes that contribute to risk of the common forms of stone disease.

Race/Ethnicity

In a cross-sectional Canadian study, individuals of Arabic, west Indian, west Asian, and Latin American descent were more likely to be stone formers than those of European descent.[42] Overall, African Americans have a lower frequency of stones.[4,5]

Systemic Disorders

There is substantial evidence that nephrolithiasis is a systemic disorder. Well-known conditions that lead to calcium kidney stone formation include primary hyperparathyroidism, renal tubular acidosis, and Crohn's disease. A wide variety of other common conditions including obesity, diabetes mellitus, gout, and gallstones have been linked to the development of kidney stones, and a history of kidney stones is a potential risk factor for the development of systemic diseases such as osteoporosis, chronic kidney disease, coronary heart disease, and hypertension (Table 1.1).

Increasing body size, assessed by weight, body mass index or waist circumference, increases the risk of stone formation independent of other risk factors including diet;[43] for unexplained reasons, the impact is greater in

Table 1.1: Common conditions associated with nephrolithiasis.

Systemic conditions that are risk factors for nephrolithiasis	*Systemic conditions for which nephrolithiasis may be a risk factor*
Obesity	Osteoporosis/bone fracture
Diabetes	Hypertension
Primary hyperparathyroidism	Coronary heart disease
Gout	Chronic kidney disease
Inflammatory bowel disease	
Gallstones	

women than in men. For example, the risk of stone formation for individuals with a BMI $\geq$ 30 kg/m^2 compared with those with a BMI 21–23 was 30% higher among men but nearly twofold higher among women. Although individuals with higher BMI have markedly different 24-hour urine composition than those with lower BMI, including higher urine oxalate and uric acid and lower urine pH,[44,45] the calculated relative supersaturation was significantly higher only for uric acid. Additional research is needed to explore further why obesity, independent of diet, may increase the risk of calcium kidney stone formation.

Diabetes mellitus has also been associated with an increased risk of stone formation, independent of diet and body size.[46] Cross-sectionally, individuals with a history of diabetes were >30% more likely also to have a history of nephrolithiasis. Prospectively, a history of DM increased the risk of stone formation by 30–50% in women but not in men. In support of these findings, a study based on NHANES III data found that the risk of being a stone former increased with an increasing number of metabolic syndrome traits.[47]

The association between hypertension and nephrolithiasis is complex. Some prospective studies reported that individuals with hypertension were more likely to develop kidney stones,[48,49] but large-scale prospective cohort studies to date have not identified hypertension as an independent risk factor for kidney stone formation.[50,51] However, a history of kidney stones is clearly associated with an increased risk of developing hypertension.[50-52] In large-scale prospective studies that accounted for differences in age, diet, body size, and other comorbidities, individuals with kidney stones were about 25% more likely to develop hypertension than their nonstone forming counterparts.[50,51]

Other common diseases such as gout and cholelithiasis are associated with higher risk of kidney stones. In a cross-sectional study, individuals with gout were 50% more likely to have a history of stones.[53] When examined prospectively, individuals with a history of gout had a twofold higher risk of incident nephrolithiasis, independent of diet, weight, and medications.[54] Large-scale prospective cohort studies report that participants with a history of gallstones are about 30% more likely to develop incident symptomatic kidney stones after adjusting for differences in diet, body size, and other comorbidities.[55]

The identification of kidney stone disease as a risk factor for other conditions provides additional evidence that nephrolithiasis is a systemic disorder. For example, a number of studies report lower bone mineral density in individuals with a history of nephrolithiasis compared with those who do not.[56] The potential mechanism(s) of bone loss in stone formers is unknown, but it is possible that higher urine calcium may result in a negative calcium balance. In a study of 46 stone formers and their first-degree relatives followed for 3 years, the correlation between higher baseline 24-hour calcium excretion and subsequent decrease in femoral neck z-score was –0.37.[57] This relation was independent of calcium intake and 24-hour urine markers of dietary acid load such as ammonium and sulfate. Previous reports suggest that individuals with nephrolithiasis may have higher risk of bone fracture.[58,59] In a longitudinal study of 624 individuals with history of kidney stones living in Rochester, Minnesota, the risk of an incident vertebral fracture was > 4 times that expected for Rochester individuals of comparable age.[59] A recent study utilizing electronic medical record data from the United Kingdom compared > 50,000 individuals with diagnostic codes for urolithiasis to over 500,000 participants without such codes matched on age and sex. The risk of incident bone fracture in individuals with a history of kidney stones was 10% higher in men and also was higher in women between the ages of 30 and 79 (the highest hazards ratio in women was 1.52 for those aged 30–39 years).[60]

Recent data also implicate kidney stone disease as an independent risk factor for the development of coronary heart disease. In a case-control study including over 15,000 participants with a mean follow-up of 9 years, participants with a history of kidney stones were 31% more likely to have an incident myocardial infarction after adjustment for a wide variety of comorbidities.[61] In large prospective cohort studies, a history of kidney stones was associated with an increased risk of incident coronary heart disease in women (but not men) that was independent of age, body size, dietary intakes, and comorbid conditions.[62] A prospective study of over 3 million individuals in Alberta, Canada, found a history of nephrolithiasis was associated with an increased risk of coronary heart disease and

Table 1.2: Dietary factors that may increase or decrease the risk of calcium oxalate kidney stones.

Dietary factor	*Proposed mechanism(s)*
Increase risk	
Sodium	Increased urinary calcium excretion
Oxalate	Increased urinary oxalate excretion
Animal protein	Increased urinary calcium excretion; reduced urinary citrate excretion
Vitamin C	Increased oxalate generation and excretion
Carbohydrates	Increased urinary calcium
Decrease risk	
Dietary calcium	Binding of dietary oxalate in gut
Potassium-rich foods	Increased urinary citrate excretion; reduced urinary calcium excretion
Phytate	Inhibition of calcium oxalate crystal formation
Magnesium	Reduced dietary oxalate absorption; inhibition of calcium oxalate crystal formation

stroke; the risks were higher in women than in men and in younger than older individuals.[63]

Cross-sectional data from NHANES III[64] as well as case-control studies[65,66] and a cohort study[67] suggest that kidney stones may represent an independent risk factor for chronic kidney disease. Using the same database mentioned above, investigators performed a prospective study of nearly 2 million individuals in Alberta, Canada, and found a history of nephrolithiasis was associated with an increased risk of developing chronic kidney disease (CKD) or end-stage renal disease (ESRD); however, the absolute risks were small.

Environmental Factors

Occupations or settings with higher insensible fluid losses, such as a hot environment, increase risk of stone formation by reducing urine volume.[68] The risk will also be higher when individuals have restricted access to water or bathroom facilities, leading to lower fluid intake and lower urine volume. It is possible that global warming and continued urbanization may increase the world wide burden of nephrolithiasis in the future.[69]

DIET AND STONE DISEASE

Because most data on the relation between diet and stone disease come from observational and physiologic studies, care must be taken when interpreting studies of diet and risk. Retrospective assessments of diet may be biased because individuals who develop stones may subsequently change their diet. Results from studies that use change in urine composition as a surrogate for actual stone formation should viewed with caution because the composition of the urine does not completely predict risk and not all the components that modify risk are included in the calculation of supersaturation (e.g. urine phytate). Thus, prospective studies that assess a variety of nutrients are best suited for examining the associations between dietary factors and risk of actual stone formation. Finally, associations between specific dietary factors and risk may vary by age, sex, and body size.

Dietary Risk Factors: Calcium Oxalate Stones

More than 80% of kidney stones contain calcium, and the majority of calcium stones consist primarily of calcium oxalate[70] (*see* Fig. 1.2). Because calcium oxalate is most common, the majority of studies have focused on risk factors for this stone type. Dietary factors associated with increased or decreased risk are listed in Table 1.2.

Calcium

In the past, higher calcium intake was believed to increase the risk of stone formation. However, there is now substantial evidence demonstrating that a higher calcium diet is associated with a *reduced* risk of stone formation. One potential mechanism to explain this apparent paradox is that the higher calcium intake will bind dietary oxalate in the gut, thereby reducing oxalate absorption and urinary excretion.[71]

Several large prospective observational studies in men and women consistently support a reduced risk of stone formation with increasing dietary calcium intake. Compared to individuals in the lowest quintile of dietary calcium intake, those in the highest quintile had more than a 30% lower risk of forming a stone.[10,13,14] These results were adjusted for multiple factors, including age, body mass index, total fluid intake, the use of thiazide diuretics, and the intake of nutrients such as animal protein, magnesium, phosphorous, sodium, and potassium. In the Women's Health Initiative Observational Study, higher dietary calcium also was associated with a lower risk of incident kidney stones.[72] Calcium intake is an example of how the impact of a risk factor may vary by age: there was an inverse association between dietary calcium and stone formation in men younger than 60 years of age, but no significant association was found for men 60 years or older.[73]

These observational findings have been confirmed by a 5-year randomized controlled clinical trial that compared stone recurrence in 120 men with a history of calcium oxalate nephrolithiasis and idiopathic hypercalciuria assigned to a diet low in calcium (400 mg/d) or to a diet with "normal" calcium content (1,200 mg/d) and lower amounts of animal protein and sodium.[18] Of note, 1,200 mg/d would represent a "high" calcium diet for many free-living individuals (in one prospective cohort study, men who subsequently developed an incident symptomatic kidney stone had mean dietary calcium of about 800 mg/d[10]). In addition, participants in both arms of the RCT were advised to avoid consuming a variety of specific foods high in oxalate. The risk of developing a recurrent stone on the higher calcium diet was 51% lower than for the low-calcium diet (Fig. 1.4).[18]

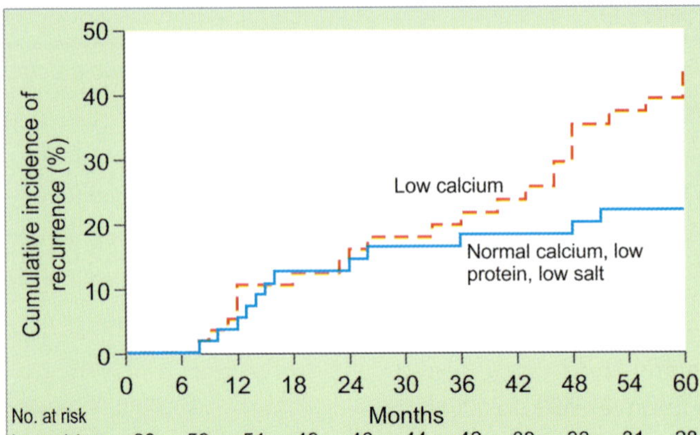

No. at risk											
Low calcium	60	59	51	49	46	44	42	39	33	31	28
Normal calcium, low protein, low salt	60	57	53	47	46	45	44	43	41	40	40

Fig. 1.4: Comparison of low versus normal calcium diets for kidney stone prevention.[18]

Unlike their counterparts consuming the low-calcium diet, the men in the "normal" calcium diet arm of the trial had significant decreases in 24-hour urine oxalate compared with baseline, suggesting that intestinal oxalate binding by calcium may have played a role in the study results. The "normal" calcium diet also resulted in a 49% decrease in urine calcium excretion compared to baseline, likely due to the concomitant restriction of sodium and animal protein intakes. Because dietary sodium and animal protein may influence calcium stone formation, this trial, although suggestive, did not directly address the independent role of dietary calcium in the pathogenesis of kidney stones.

It is possible that dairy products (the major source of dietary calcium) may contain as yet unidentified factors that inhibit calcium kidney stones. The men in the low-calcium diet arm in the RCT displayed in Figure 1.2 decreased calcium intake by limiting intake of milk, yogurt, and cheese. However, large-scale prospective cohort studies have reported that dietary calcium from nondairy sources (in addition to dietary calcium from dairy) also is independently associated with a reduced risk of kidney stones.[74]

The impact of supplemental calcium on stone risk may be different from dietary calcium. In an observational study of older women, calcium supplement users were 20% more likely to form a stone than women who did not take supplements.[13] The Women's Health Initiative randomized trial also found an increased risk with calcium supplementation (1,000 mg/d), though the supplements also contained 400 IU/d of vitamin D3.[75] In younger women and men, there was no association between calcium supplement use and risk of stone formation.[10,14] The discrepancy between the risks from dietary calcium and calcium supplements, at least in the observational study, may be due to the timing of calcium intake. Calcium supplements are not typically taken with meals, which would diminish binding of dietary oxalate.

Because the absolute risk of forming the first kidney stone by a supplement user is only slightly increased (1.2 cases/1,000 women per year compared to 1.0/1,000 per year), supplement use is not a major contributor to stone risk. However, individuals with a history of calcium nephrolithiasis should be encouraged to obtain calcium from dietary rather than supplemental sources.

Oxalate

Although urine oxalate is a well-established and important risk factor for calcium oxalate stone formation, the role of dietary oxalate in the pathogenesis of calcium oxalate nephrolithiasis remains unclear.[76] First, the proportion of urinary oxalate derived from dietary oxalate is controversial; estimates range from 10% to 50%.[76] Thus, a substantial proportion of urinary oxalate is derived from the endogenous production such as the metabolism of glycine, glycolate, and hydroxyproline. Second, other dietary factors influence urine oxalate. For example, vitamin C supplementation may be an important contributor[77-79] because it can be metabolized to oxalate. Third, much of the oxalate in food may not be readily absorbed due to low bioavailability. Finally, there is variation between individuals with respect to the GI absorption of dietary oxalate. For instance, up to one-third of patients with calcium oxalate nephrolithiasis may have higher absorption of dietary oxalate.[80] The reasons for the higher absorption are unclear but likely candidates include genetic predisposition and the intestinal microbiota. One study found individuals with a history of calcium oxalate nephrolithiasis were less likely to be colonized with *Oxalobacter formigenes*, an intestinal bacterium that degrades oxalate.[81]

Older reports of the oxalate content in food may be unreliable due to measurement issues, related to the quality of the assay procedure as well as the variability in oxalate content of the same food items. More recently, however, reliable assays for the direct determination of the oxalate content of food, including ion chromatography and capillary electrophoresis, have been developed. One study used these new methods to measure the oxalate content of >200 food items, measuring several different samples for each food and also performing each measure in triplicate (the values can be found at https://regepi.bwh.harvard.edu/health/Oxalate/files). Some representative foods from this list are shown in Table 1.3. Although they are sometimes grouped into "very high" or "high" oxalate categories, this distinction is arbitrary. An individual can consume large amounts of oxalate by eating individual foods that are very high in oxalate or by eating larger quantities of foods that are more moderate in oxalate content.

Large-scale prospective studies of the relation between dietary oxalate and kidney stone formation have been completed. Surprisingly, the impact of dietary oxalate, even when comparing substantial differences in intake, was modest in men and older women and not associated with stone formation in younger women.[82] These population-based data should not be interpreted to mean that dietary oxalate restriction is ineffective at preventing kidney stone recurrence in selected individuals, particularly those with higher urine oxalate excretion. There is likely a subgroup of patients who have increased oxalate absorption, which would result in an increased risk of calcium oxalate stone formation.

Table 1.3: Oxalate content of some foods.

Food	*Serving size*	*Oxalate content (mg) per serving*
Spinach	½ cup cooked	755
Rhubarb	½ cup	541
Buckwheat	1 cup	133
Almonds	1 oz	124
Potato	1 medium	97
Corn meal/grits	1 cup	97
Beets	½ cup	76
Cashews	1 oz	49
Peanuts	1 oz	27
Raspberries	½ cup	24
Tea	1 cup	14
Milk chocolate	1 oz	5
Coffee	1 cup	2
Blueberries	½ cup	2
Kale	1 cup	2

A comprehensive list of the oxalate content of individual food items (expressed as mg/serving) can be found at https://regepi.bwh.harvard.edu/health/Oxalate/files.

Sodium

Higher sodium intake results in decreased renal tubule sodium reabsorption with a subsequent reduction in calcium reabsorption. Restriction of sodium intake is a highly effective means of lowering urine calcium and therefore represents a mainstay in the dietary treatment of calcium nephrolithiasis. A RCT of dietary salt restriction in calcium oxalate stone formers with idiopathic hypercalciuria demonstrated that for every 100 mmol decrease in urine sodium, urine calcium decreased by about 100 mg/d.[83]

Previous prospective cohort studies found a positive, independent association between sodium consumption and new kidney stone formation in women but not men.[10,13] In the Women's Health Initiative Observational Study, women in the highest compared with lowest quintile of sodium intake had a 61% increased risk of incident nephrolithiasis.[72]

Animal Protein

Higher animal protein intake may increase urinary calcium and decrease urinary citrate,[84] thereby increasing the risk of stone formation. However, when studied prospectively, animal protein was associated with an increased risk in men but not women.[10,13,14,72] Further, the increased risk in men was only found among men with BMI < 25 kg/m^2.[73]

Potassium

Higher dietary potassium intake was associated with a lower risk of incident stone formation in men and older women[10,13,73] possibly by reducing urine calcium excretion[85] or increasing urine citrate. Recent data also shows that higher dietary potassium was associated with lower risk of incident stones in younger women.[115]

Sugars

Higher intake of sucrose increases urinary calcium excretion independent of calcium intake.[86] In prospective studies, sucrose was associated with an increased risk in women and fructose was associated with an increased risk in men and women.[13,14,87]

Magnesium

Although higher magnesium intake may reduce dietary oxalate absorption, randomized trials of magnesium supplements did not find a protective effect on stone recurrence, though the dropout rates in these studies were high. In prospective observational studies, higher dietary magnesium was associated with a lower risk of stone formation in men[73] but not women.[13,14]

Vitamin C

Vitamin C (ascorbic acid) can be metabolized to oxalate and may increase the risk of calcium kidney stone formation. Consumption of 1,000 mg of supplemental vitamin C twice daily increased mean urinary oxalate excretion by 22%, but there was notable between-person variability.[78] In a prospective observational study, men who consumed 1,000 mg or more per day of vitamin C had a 40% higher risk of stone formation compared to men who consumed <90 mg/d (the recommended dietary allowance).[73] In a prospective cohort study of Swedish men, supplemental vitamin C use was associated with a near doubling of the risk of incident kidney stones.[88] While these data do not support the restriction of dietary vitamin C (because many foods high in vitamin C contain alkali, which could raise urine citrate and thereby inhibit calcium oxalate crystal formation), calcium oxalate stone formers should avoid high-dose vitamin C supplements.

More research is needed to elucidate the relation between vitamin C intake, oxalate metabolism, and kidney stone risk. First, it is uncertain whether vitamin C intake is associated with risk in women. Second, feeding studies of vitamin C and urine composition may be substantially complicated by ex vivo nonenzymatic conversion of urinary vitamin C to oxalate in the collection vessel during storage and/or analysis.[89]

Vitamin B6

Although high-dose vitamin B6 (pyridoxine) reduces oxalate production in selected patients with type 1 primary hyperoxaluria,[90,91] it is unclear if there would be benefit from the use of vitamin B6 supplements to prevent common stone disease. In an observational study, higher intake of vitamin B6 was not associated with a reduced risk of kidney stone formation in men.[92,93]

Phytate

Phytate, found in whole grains and beans, was observed to reduce risk of stone formation in younger women,[14] possibly by directly inhibiting calcium oxalate crystal formation.

Dietary Patterns

Although the examination of individual nutrients provides valuable insights, it may be easier for patients to follow certain types of dietary patterns than modifying individual nutrients. Relatively few studies have examined the impact of overall diet or dietary patterns on risk of stone formation. The Dietary Approaches to Stop Hypertension (DASH) diet, which is high in fruits and vegetables, moderate in low-fat dairy products, and low in red and processed meats, represents a novel potential means of kidney stone prevention. In a large, prospective observational study of three distinct cohorts, a higher dietary DASH score (meaning a diet more similar to the DASH diet) was associated with a 40–45% reduction in the risk of incident kidney stone formation.[94] Although participants in the highest compared with lowest quintile of dietary DASH score in this study had a marked reduction in risk of kidney stones, their dietary oxalate intake was about 60% higher. The association between higher DASH score and lower stone risk was independent of age, body size, hypertension, diabetes, thiazide use, and intakes of total calories, fluid, caffeine, and alcohol.

The potential mechanism(s) underlying the impact of a DASH diet on kidney stone risk require elucidation. Intakes of fruit and vegetables have a major effect on urine composition. In a metabolic study of 12 adults, the complete elimination of fruits and vegetables from the diet lowered urine oxalate by 31% but also decreased urine citrate and increased urine calcium.[95] The net effect was an increase in urinary supersaturation with respect to calcium oxalate. In a cross-sectional study of nearly 3,500 individuals with and without nephrolithiasis, higher dietary DASH scores were associated with slightly higher 24-hour urine oxalate excretions but lower 24-hour urine citrate and higher 24-hour urine volume.[96] Recently, a randomized trial compared the effects of a DASH-style diet versus a low-oxalate diet on urine composition in 57 individuals with recurrent nephrolithiasis and urine oxalate > 40 mg/d.[97] Although limited by small size and a high drop-out rate, the results were provocative. The DASH diet resulted in urine citrate that was > 220 mg/d higher compared with the low-oxalate diet. Although other differences were not statistically significant compared with the low-oxalate diet, the DASH diet resulted in higher urine oxalate, higher urine volume, and lower urine supersaturation with respect to calcium oxalate.

Dietary Risk Factors for Other Stone Types

For the less common stone types, little data exist to support the role of specific dietary factors in kidney stone formation. It is possible to speculate about the impact of diet based on urine composition and our current understanding of pathophysiology, but it should be remembered that the many of the older recommendations for calcium oxalate stone prevention based on urine composition or pathophysiologic considerations were later found not to be supported by prospective studies of actual stone formation.

Uric Acid Stones

Although higher urine uric acid also contributes, the major determinant of uric acid crystal formation is low urine pH (the solubility of uric acid increases markedly as the urine pH increases from 5.0 to 6.5). Decreasing consumption of meat, chicken, and seafood will decrease purine intake and, therefore, reduce uric acid production; this may also increase urinary pH by reducing acid production. Higher intakes of fruits and vegetables raise the urine pH and should reduce the risk of uric acid crystal formation.

Given the well-documented association between greater weight and higher uric acid production and excretion and lower urine pH,[44,45] it would be reasonable to encourage dietary intakes designed to maintain a healthy weight in individuals with recurrent uric acid stones.

Cystine Stones

Restricting sodium intake may reduce the urinary excretion of cystine.[98] The solubility of cystine increases as urinary pH rises,[99] thus higher fruit and vegetable consumption may be beneficial. There is little evidence to support the dietary restriction of proteins high in cystine, though reducing animal protein intake may be beneficial by increasing urine pH.

Calcium Phosphate Stones

Because patients with type 1 (distal) renal tubular acidosis and stone disease may benefit from alkali supplementation, they may also benefit from a diet high in fruits and vegetables. It should be noted, however, that an increase in urinary pH can increase the risk of calcium phosphate crystal formation. Dietary maneuvers directed at decreasing urinary calcium excretion (such as sodium and animal protein restriction) would also be expected to decrease calcium phosphate stone recurrence. It is unknown whether dietary phosphorus restriction would decrease calcium phosphate stone risk.

BEVERAGES AND CALCIUM STONES

Total Fluid

Nephrolithiasis is a disease driven by the urinary concentration of lithogenic factors. Thus, fluid intake, the main determinant of urine volume plays a critical role in kidney stone formation. Prospective observational data consistently demonstrate that higher fluid intake is associated with lower risk of incident kidney stones.[10,13,14] In a 5-year RCT of first time calcium stone formers, higher water intake resulted in a marked reduction in kidney stone recurrence.[100] In this trial, 99 participants were assigned higher water intake with a 24-hour urine volume goal of 2 L, whereas no specific intervention was employed for the 100 participants in the control arm. At baseline, 24-hour urine volume was about 1 L in both groups. Individuals in the high water intake group were instructed to measure their

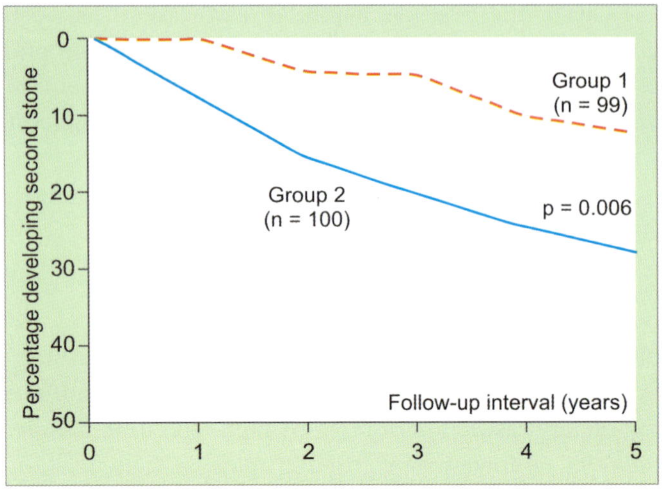

Fig. 1.5: Water intake and recurrent stone events in individuals with calcium nephrolithiasis. Group 1 randomized to high water intake and Group 2 without intervention.
Source: Reproduced with permission from Borghi L, Meschi T, Amato F, et al. Urinary volume, water and recurrences in idiopathic calcium nephrolithiasis: a 5-year randomized prospective study. J Urol. 1996;155:839-43.

urine volume at home every 2–3 months. Participants in the high water intake group (Group 1 in Fig. 1.5) had a mean 24-hour urine volume just over 2.5 L/d at years 3, 4, and 5 of the trial and had more than a 50% reduction in stone recurrence compared to the control group (Group 2).

Individual Beverages

While total fluid intake is most commonly discussed, the type of beverage consumed may influence risk beyond just the volume of the beverage consumed.[101] The associations between specific beverages, accounting for fluid intake, with kidney stone formation are presented in Table 1.4.

Despite previous beliefs to the contrary, alcoholic beverages, coffee, and tea are not associated with an increased risk of kidney stone formation. In fact, observational studies have consistently found that coffee, tea, beer, and wine are associated with a *reduced* risk of stone formation.[101-103] The mechanisms for these protective associations may be related to inhibition of antidiuretic hormone action in the kidney by caffeine and inhibition of antidiuretic hormone secretion by alcohol. In large-scale prospective studies, caffeine intake is independently associated with a lower risk of incident stones.[104] The role of tea deserves special mention. There is a widespread belief that tea is high in oxalate and should be avoided. A cup of tea contains 14 mg of oxalate. Although this is

Table 1.4: Select beverages and risk of incident stone formation[101] with possible mechanism.

Beverage	*Proposed mechanisms*
Types associated with lower risk	
Coffee Tea	Caffeine induced diuresis, leading to decreased urinary concentration
Beer Wine	Alcohol induced diuresis, leading to decreased urinary concentration
Orange juice	Increased urine citrate excretion
Types associated with higher risk	
Sugar-sweetened soda Punch	High-fructose content possibly leading to increased urinary excretion of calcium, oxalate, and uric acid

not insignificant, the bioavailability does not appear to be high. A feeding study of tea demonstrated a negligible impact on urinary oxalate.[105]

Citrus juices, such as orange and grapefruit juice, theoretically could reduce the risk of calcium stone formation by increasing urine citrate. The prospective studies found that compared with participants who consumed less than one serving per week of orange juice, participants who consumed one serving per day or more had a 12% lower risk of incident kidney stone formation.[101] This association was independent of differences in age, race, body size, comorbidities, dietary intakes, and consumption of other beverages. Grapefruit juice intake was not associated with risk. One feeding study found that grapefruit consumption increased not only urine citrate but also urine oxalate.[106]

The relation between citrate-containing beverages and urine citrate is complex. A major determinant of urine citrate excretion is acid-base status: alkalosis decreases renal tubule reabsorption of filtered citrate and increases urinary citrate excretion.[107] Thus, the effect of an orally administered citrate-containing fluid on urine citrate depends in part on fluid pH. Beverages with lower pH will have a predominance of hydrogen ion as the accompanying citrate cation, whereas beverages with higher pH have potassium as the accompanying cation. Unlike potassium citrate, intestinally absorbed citrate in the protonated form is neutral from an acid-base standpoint and would be expected (in the absence of very large quantities that overwhelm the liver's capacity to metabolize citrate to bicarbonate) to have minimal impact on urinary citrate. This principle was illustrated in a crossover metabolic study of 13 volunteers on standardized diets who consumed the same volume of water, lemonade, or orange juice with meals.[108] Although participants consumed identical quantities of citrate in lemonade and orange juice, only orange juice resulted in higher urine citrate excretion.

An early report about the increase in urine citrate by homemade lemonade[109] generated substantial enthusiasm about this beverage for preventing stone recurrence. However, subsequent studies did not consistently replicate the findings. The citrate and malate content of lemonade and several diet sodas were measured,[110] with most beverages containing <8 meq of alkali per liter. Thus, it would take consumption of at least several liters per day to have an expected increase in urine citrate.

The consumption of sugar-sweetened sodas ("soft drinks") is clearly associated with a higher risk of incident kidney stones,[101-103] but the exact mechanism is uncertain. Sugar-sweetened sodas contain fructose, which has been associated with an increased the risk of kidney stones.[87] Dietary patterns associated with sweetened soda consumption were found to increase the risk of stone formation.[94] Intakes of other sugar-sweetened beverages, such as punch, also are associated with higher risk of kidney stones.[101]

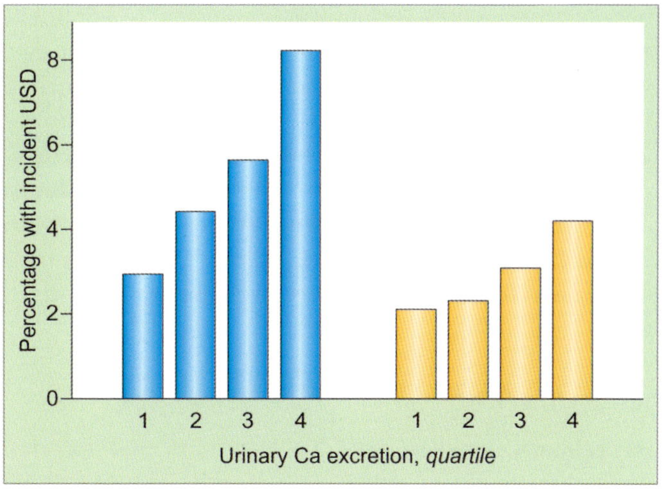

Fig. 1.6: Percentage of individuals without a history of nephrolithiasis who subsequently developed incident urinary stone disease (USD) by quartile of baseline urinary calcium (Ca) excretion.[112] Blue bars are men; Orange bars are women.

URINARY FACTORS

The 24-hour urine collection provides important prognostic information and guides preventive recommendations. Like many laboratory tests, urine results have traditionally been categorized into "normal" and "abnormal." However, this grouping is unsatisfactory. Substantial differences in kidney stone risk associated with higher or lower 24-hour urine values occur within ranges considered "normal."[77] Urine values are continuous so the dichotomization into "normal" and "abnormal" is arbitrary and potentially misleading. Thus, while terms of abnormal excretion such as "hypercalciuria," "hyperoxaluria," or "hypocitraturia" are often used clinically and in the scientific literature, the limitations of these terms should be acknowledged.

Urine Calcium

Hypercalciuria had traditionally been defined as urine calcium excretion > 300 mg/d in men and > 250 mg/d in women[111] on a 1,000-mg/d calcium diet, but more commonly used definitions have lower thresholds and no dietary requirement. Using the traditional definitions, ~20–40% of patients with calcium stone disease will be classified as having hypercalciuria. Although possibly reasonable from a calcium balance perspective, there is insufficient justification with respect to stone formation to use different thresholds for males and females.

Higher urine calcium is an established, major risk factor for calcium kidney stone formation. In a large cross-sectional study of over 2,200 stone formers and 1,100 non-stone formers, participants with 24-hour urine calcium >350 mg were between 5 and 6 times as likely to have a history of kidney stones compared with participants with 24-hour urine calcium <100 mg.[77] The higher kidney stone risk associated with higher 24-hour urine calcium started well below usual cutoffs for "hypercalciuria" and was independent of age, 24-hour urine creatinine, and other urinary factors. In a 9 year prospective cohort study that included over 3,000 men and women without a history of nephrolithiasis at baseline, higher urine calcium was strongly associated with an increased risk of developing an incident kidney stone (Fig. 1.6).[112] For each ~100 mg/d higher urine calcium at baseline, the risk was 20% higher for incident kidney stone formation.

Urine Oxalate

Hyperoxaluria is often defined as urinary oxalate excretion >45 mg/d, though here too a variety of thresholds are in use. Elevated urinary oxalate excretion is 3–4 times more common among men (~40%) than in women (~10%).[77] Mean urinary oxalate levels are only slightly higher in kidney stone cases than in controls, but in multivariate models urine oxalate is clearly an important independent risk factor for stone formation.[77] Depending on their age, women with 24-hour urine oxalate >40 mg were between 2.5 and 3.5 times as likely to have a history of kidney stones compared with women with 24-hour urine oxalate <20 mg.[77] Men with 24-hour urine oxalate >50 mg were over 3 times as likely to have a history of kidney stones compared with men with 24-hour urine oxalate <25 mg.[77] Of note, in men and women the risk begins to rise well below the 45 mg/d level.

Urine Uric Acid

The relation between uric acid excretion and calcium stone disease is unsettled. Some early cross-sectional studies reported that hyperuricosuria (typically defined as >800 mg/d in men or 750 mg/d in women) was more frequent in patients who form calcium stones than controls.[113] However, in the cross-sectional study of over 2,200 stone formers and 1,100 nonstone formers, a higher urine uric acid was associated with a lower likelihood of being a stone former in men, and there was no higher risk in women.[77] A double-blind trial of allopurinol successfully decreased recurrence rates of calcium stones in patients with hyperuricosuria suggesting that uric acid is important,[19] but it is possible that the beneficial effect of allopurinol was through a mechanism unrelated to lowering of urine uric acid.

Urine Citrate

Hypocitraturia, often defined as 24-hour excretion < 320 mg/d, increases risk of calcium stone formation[114] and is found in 5–11% of first time stone formers.[77] There is suggestive evidence that increasing urinary citrate into the high-normal range could provide additional protection.[77] Individuals with 24-hour urine citrate <300 mg were between 3 and 4 times as likely to have a history of kidney stones compared with those with 24-hour urine citrate >800 mg.[77] As with other urinary factors, the risk varied by urine citrate level even within the "normal" range.

SUMMARY

Epidemiologic studies have greatly expanded our understanding of risk factors for stone disease. A variety of dietary, nondietary, and urinary risk factors contribute to the risk of kidney stone formation and the importance of these varies by age, sex ,and BMI. There is a paucity of randomized trials in the field, and more interventional studies are needed to further our understanding of risk factors for the "hard" outcome of kidney stone formation.

REFERENCES

1. Evan A, Lingeman J, Coe FL, et al. Randall's plaque: pathogenesis and role in calcium oxalate nephrolithiasis. Kidney Int. 2006;69(8):1313-8.
2. Evan AP, Lingeman JE, Coe FL, et al. Randall's plaque of patients with nephrolithiasis begins in basement membranes of thin loops of Henle. J Clin Invest. 2003;111(5):607-16.
3. Miller NL, Gillen DL, Williams JC, Jr, et al. A formal test of the hypothesis that idiopathic calcium oxalate stones grow on Randall's plaque. BJU Int. 2009;103(7):966-71.
4. Scales CD, Jr, Smith AC, Hanley JM, Saigal CS. Prevalence of kidney stones in the United States. Eur Urol. 2012;62(1):160-5.
5. Stamatelou KK, Francis ME, Jones CA, et al. Time trends in reported prevalence of kidney stones in the United States: 1976-1994. Kidney Int. 2003;63(5):1817-23.
6. Yoshida O, Okada Y. Epidemiology of urolithiasis in Japan: a chronological and geographical study. Urol Int. 1990;45: 104-11.
7. Hesse A, Brandle E, Wilbert D, et al. Study on the prevalence and incidence of urolithiasis in Germany comparing the years 1979 vs. 2000. Eur Urol. 2003;44(6):709-13.
8. Soucie J, Coates R, McClellan W, et al. Relation between geographic variability in kidney stones prevalence and risk factors for stones. Am J Epidemiol. 1996;143:487-95.
9. Scales CD, Jr, Curtis LH, Norris RD, et al. Changing gender prevalence of stone disease. J Urol. 2007;177(3):979-82.
10. Curhan GC, Willett WC, Rimm EB, et al. A prospective study of dietary calcium and other nutrients and the risk of symptomatic kidney stones. N Engl J Med. 1993;328(12):833-8.
11. Hiatt RA, Dales LG, Friedman GD, et al. Frequency of urolithiasis in a prepaid medical care program. Am J Epidemiol. 1982;115:255-65.
12. Johnson CM, Wilson DM, O'Fallon WM, et al. Renal stone epidemiology: a 25-year study in Rochester, Minnesota. Kidney Int. 1979;16(5):624-31.
13. Curhan G, Willett W, Speizer F,et al. Comparison of dietary calcium with supplemental calcium and other nutrients as factors affecting the risk for kidney stones in women. Ann Intern Med. 1997;126:497-504.
14. Curhan GC, Willett WC, Knight EL,et al. Dietary factors and the risk of incident kidney stones in younger women (Nurses' Health Study II). Arch Intern Med. 2004;164:885-91.
15. Edvardsson VO, Indridason OS, Haraldsson G,et al. Temporal trends in the incidence of kidney stone disease. Kidney Int. 2013;83(1):146-52.
16. Lieske JC, Pena de la Vega LS, Slezak JM, et al. Renal stone epidemiology in Rochester, Minnesota: an update. Kidney Int. 2006;69(4):760-4.
17. Rule AD, Lieske JC, Li X, et al. The ROKS nomogram for predicting a second symptomatic stone episode. J Am Soc Nephrol. 2014;25(12):2878-86.

18. Borghi L, Schianchi T, Meschi T, et al. Comparison of two diets for the prevention of recurrent stones in idiopathic hypercalciuria. N Engl J Med. 2002;346(2):77-84.
19. Ettinger B, Tang A, Citron JT, et al. Randomized trial of allopurinol in the prevention of calcium oxalate calculi. N Engl J Med. 198627;315(22):1386-9.
20. Ettinger B, Pak CY, Citron JT, et al. Potassium-magnesium citrate is an effective prophylaxis against recurrent calcium oxalate nephrolithiasis. J Urol. 1997;158(6):2069-73.
21. Ettinger B, Citron JT, Livermore B, et al. Chlorthalidone reduces calcium oxalate calculous recurrence but magnesium hydroxide does not. J Urol. 1988;139(4):679-84.
22. Daudon M, Donsimoni R, Hennequin C, et al. Sex- and age-related composition of 10 617 calculi analyzed by infrared spectroscopy. Urol Res. 1995;23(5):319-26.
23. Herring LC. Observations on the analysis of ten thousand urinary calculi. J Urol. 1962;88:545-62.
24. Mandel NS, Mandel GS. Urinary tract stone disease in the United States veteran population. II. Geographical analysis of variations in composition. J Urol. 1989;142(6):1516-21.
25. Pak CY, Poindexter JR, Adams-Huet B, et al. Predictive value of kidney stone composition in the detection of metabolic abnormalities. Am J Med. 2003;115(1):26-32.
26. Parks JH, Worcester EM, Coe FL, et al. Clinical implications of abundant calcium phosphate in routinely analyzed kidney stones. Kidney Int. 2004;66(2):777-85.
27. Alaya A, Nouri A, Belgith M, et al. Changes in urinary stone composition in the Tunisian population: a retrospective study of 1,301 cases. Ann Lab Med. 2012;32(3):177-83.
28. Ansari MS, Gupta NP, Hemal AK, et al. Spectrum of stone composition: structural analysis of 1050 upper urinary tract calculi from northern India. Int J Urol. 2005;12(1):12-6.
29. Hossain RZ, Ogawa Y, Hokama S, et al. Urolithiasis in Okinawa, Japan: a relatively high prevalence of uric acid stones. Int J Urol. 2003;10(8):411-5.
30. Daudon M, Bounxouei B, Santa Cruz F, et al. Composition of renal stones currently observed in non-industrialized countries. Prog Urol. 2004;14(6):1151-61.
31. Lee MC, Bariol SV. Changes in upper urinary tract stone composition in Australia over the past 30 years. BJU Int. 2013;112 (Suppl 2):65-8.
32. Gault MH, Chafe L. Relationship of frequency, age, sex, stone weight and composition in 15,624 stones: comparison of resutls for 1980 to 1983 and 1995 to 1998. J Urol. 2000;164(2):302-7.
33. Daudon M, Traxer O, Conort P, et al. Type 2 diabetes increases the risk for uric acid stones. J Am Soc Nephrol. 2006;17(7):2026-33.
34. Daudon M, Lacour B, Jungers P. Influence of body size on urinary stone composition in men and women. Urol Res. 2006;34(3):193-9.
35. Abate N, Chandalia M, Cabo-Chan AV, Jr, et al. The metabolic syndrome and uric acid nephrolithiasis: novel features of renal manifestation of insulin resistance. Kidney Int. 2004;65(2):386-92.
36. Pearle MS, Calhoun EA, Curhan GC. Urologic diseases in America project: urolithiasis. J Urol. 2005;173(3):848-57.
37. Saigal CS, Joyce G, Timilsina AR. Direct and indirect costs of nephrolithiasis in an employed population: opportunity for disease management? Kidney Int. 2005;68(4):1808-14.
38. Lotan Y, Buendia Jimenez I, Lenoir-Wijnkoop I, et al. Primary prevention of nephrolithiasis is cost-effective for a national healthcare system. BJU Int. 2012;110(11 Pt C):E1060-7.
39. Ghani KR, Roghmann F, Sammon JD, et al. Emergency department visits in the United States for upper urinary tract stones: trends in hospitalization and charges. J Urol. 2014;191(1):90-6.
40. Goldfarb DS, Fischer ME, Keich Y, et al. A twin study of genetic and dietary influences on nephrolithiasis: a report from the Vietnam Era Twin (VET) Registry. Kidney Int. 2005;67(3):1053-61.
41. Curhan G, Willett W, Rimm E, et al. Family history and risk of kidney stones. J Am Soc Nephrol. 1997;8:1568-73.
42. Mente A, Honey RJ, McLaughlin JR, et al. Ethnic differences in relative risk of idiopathic calcium nephrolithiasis in North America. J Urol. 2007;178(5):1992-7; discussion 7.
43. Taylor EN, Stampfer MJ, Curhan GC. Obesity, weight gain, and the risk of kidney stones. JAMA. 2005;293(4):455-62.
44. Maalouf NM, Sakhaee K, Parks JH, et al. Association of urinary pH with body weight in nephrolithiasis. Kidney Int. 2004;65(4):1422-5.
45. Taylor EN, Curhan GC. Body size and 24-hour urine composition. Am J Kidney Dis. 2006;48(6):905-15.
46. Taylor EN, Stampfer MJ, Curhan GC. Diabetes mellitus and the risk of nephrolithiasis. Kidney Int. 2005;68(3):1230-5.
47. West B, Luke A, Durazo-Arvizu RA, et al. Metabolic syndrome and self-reported history of kidney stones: the National Health and Nutrition Examination Survey (NHANES III) 1988-1994. Am J Kidney Dis. 2008;51(5):741-7.
48. Borghi L, Meschi T, Guerra A, et al. Essential arterial hypertension and stone disease. Kidney Int. 1999;55(6):2397-406.
49. Cappuccio FP, Siani A, Barba G, et al. A prospective study of hypertension and the incidence of kidney stones in men. J Hypertens. 1999;17(7):1017-22.
50. Madore F, Stampfer MJ, Rimm EB, et al. Nephrolithiasis and risk of hypertension. Am J Hypertens. 1998;11(1 Pt 1):46-53.
51. Madore F, Stampfer MJ, Willett WC, et al. Nephrolithiasis and risk of hypertension in women. Am J Kidney Dis. 1998;32(5):802-7.
52. Strazzullo P, Barba G, Vuotto P, et al. Past history of nephrolithiasis and incidence of hypertension in men: a reappraisal based on the results of the Olivetti Prospective Heart Study. Nephrol Dial Transplant. 2001;16(11):2232-5.
53. Kramer HM, Curhan G. The association between gout and nephrolithiasis: the National Health and Nutrition Examination Survey III, 1988-1994. Am J Kidney Dis. 2002;40(1):37-42.
54. Kramer HJ, Choi HK, Atkinson K, et al. The association between gout and nephrolithiasis in men: The Health Professionals' Follow-Up Study. Kidney Int. 2003;64(3):1022-6.
55. Taylor EN, Chan AT, Giovannucci EL, et al. Cholelithiasis and the risk of nephrolithiasis. J Urol. 2011;186(5):1882-7.
56. Sakhaee K, Maalouf NM, Kumar R, et al. Nephrolithiasis-associated bone disease: pathogenesis and treatment options. Kidney Int. 2011;79(4):393-403.

57. Asplin JR, Donahue S, Kinder J, et al. Urine calcium excretion predicts bone loss in idiopathic hypercalciuria. Kidney Int. 2006;70(8):1463-7.
58. Lauderdale DS, Thisted RA, Wen M, et al. Bone mineral density and fracture among prevalent kidney stone cases in the Third National Health and Nutrition Examination Survey. J Bone Miner Res. 2001;16(10):1893-8.
59. Melton LJ, 3rd, Crowson CS, Khosla S, et al. Fracture risk among patients with urolithiasis: a population-based cohort study. Kidney Int. 1998;53(2):459-64.
60. Denburg MR, Leonard MB, Haynes K, et al. Risk of fracture in urolithiasis: a population-based cohort study using the health improvement network. Clin J Am Soc Nephrol (In Press). 2014;9(12):2133-40.
61. Rule AD, Roger VL, Melton LJ, 3rd, et al. Kidney stones associate with increased risk for myocardial infarction. J Am Soc Nephrol. 2010;21(10):1641-4.
62. Ferraro PM, Taylor EN, Eisner BH, et al. History of kidney stones and the risk of coronary heart disease. JAMA. 2013;310(4):408-15.
63. Alexander RT, Hemmelgarn BR, Wiebe N, et al. Kidney stones and cardiovascular events: a cohort study. Clin J Am Soc Nephrol. [Research Support, Non-U.S. Gov't]. 2014;9(3):506-12.
64. Gillen DL, Worcester EM, Coe FL. Decreased renal function among adults with a history of nephrolithiasis: A study of NHANES III. Kidney Int. 2005;67(2):685-90.
65. Rule AD, Bergstralh EJ, Melton LJ, 3rd, et al. Kidney stones and the risk for chronic kidney disease. Clin J Am Soc Nephrol. 2009;4(4):804-11.
66. Vupputuri S, Soucie JM, McClellan W, et al. History of kidney stones as a possible risk factor for chronic kidney disease. Ann Epidemiol. 2004;14(3):222-8.
67. Alexander RT, Hemmelgarn BR, Wiebe N, et al. Kidney stones and kidney function loss: a cohort study. [Research Support, N.I.H., Extramural Research Support, Non-U.S. Gov't]. BMJ. 2012;345:e5287.
68. Atan L, Andreoni C, Ortiz V, et al. High kidney stone risk in men working in steel industry at hot temperatures. Urology. 2005;65(5):858-61.
69. Fakheri RJ, Goldfarb DS. Ambient temperature as a contributor to kidney stone formation: implications of global warming. Kidney Int. 2011;79(11):1178-85.
70. Coe FL, Parks JH, Asplin JR. The pathogenesis and treatment of kidney stones. N Engl J Med. 1992;327(16):1141-52.
71. Hess B, Jost C, Zipperle L, et al. High-calcium intake abolishes hyperoxaluria and reduces urinary crystallization during a 20-fold normal oxalate load in humans. Nephrol Dial Transplant. 1998;13:2241-7.
72. Sorensen MD, Kahn AJ, Reiner AP, et al. Impact of nutritional factors on incident kidney stone formation: a report from the WHI OS. J Urol. 2012;187(5):1645-9.
73. Taylor EN, Stampfer MJ, Curhan GC. Dietary factors and the risk of incident kidney stones in men: new insights after 14 years of follow-up. J Am Soc Nephrol. 2004;15(12):3225-32.
74. Taylor EN, Curhan GC. Dietary calcium from dairy and non-dairy sources, and risk of symptomatic kidney stones. J Urol. 2013;190(4):1255-9.
75. Jackson RD, LaCroix AZ, Gass M, et al. Calcium plus vitamin D supplementation and the risk of fractures. N Engl J Med. 2006;354(7):669-83.
76. Holmes RP, Assimos DG. The impact of dietary oxalate on kidney stone formation. Urol Res. 2004;32(5):311-6.
77. Curhan GC, Taylor EN. 24-h uric acid excretion and the risk of kidney stones. Kidney Int. 2008;73(4):489-96.
78. Traxer O, Huet B, Poindexter J, et al. Effect of ascorbic acid consumption on urinary stone risk factors. J Urol. 2003;170 (2 Pt 1):397-401.
79. Baxmann AC, De OGMC, Heilberg IP. Effect of vitamin C supplements on urinary oxalate and pH in calcium stone-forming patients. [Clinical Trial Controlled Clinical Trial Research Support, Non-U.S. Gov't]. Kidney Int. 2003;63(3):1066-71.
80. Holmes RP, Goodman HO, Assimos DG. Contribution of dietary oxalate to urinary oxalate excretion. Kidney Int. 2001;59(1):270-6.
81. Kaufman DW, Kelly JP, Curhan GC, et al. Oxalobacter formigenes may reduce the risk of calcium oxalate kidney stones. J Am Soc Nephrol. 2008;19(6):1197-203.
82. Taylor EN, Curhan GC. Oxalate intake and the risk for nephrolithiasis. J Am Soc Nephrol. 2007;18(7):2198-204.
83. Nouvenne A, Meschi T, Prati B, et al. Effects of a low-salt diet on idiopathic hypercalciuria in calcium-oxalate stone formers: a 3-mo randomized controlled trial. Am J Clin Nutr. 2010;91(3):565-70.
84. Breslau N, Brinkely L, Hill K, Pak C. Relationship of animal protein-rich diet to kidney stone formation and calcium metabolism. J Clin Endocrinol Metab. 1988;66:140-6.
85. Lemann J, Jr, Pleuss JA, Gray RW, Hoffmann RG. Potassium administration reduces and potassium deprivation increases urinary calcium excretion in healthy adults [corrected]. Kidney Int. 1991;39(5):973-83.
86. Lemann J, Jr, Piering WF, Lennon EJ. Possible role of carbohydrate-induced calciuria in calcium oxalate kidney-stone formation. N Engl J Med. 1969;280(5):232-7.
87. Taylor EN, Curhan GC. Fructose consumption and the risk of kidney stones. Kidney Int. 2008;73(2):207-12.
88. Thomas LD, Elinder CG, et al. Ascorbic acid supplements and kidney stone incidence among men: a prospective study. JAMA Intern Med. 2013;173(5):386-8.
89. Robitaille L, Mamer OA, Miller WH, Jr, et al. Oxalic acid excretion after intravenous ascorbic acid administration. Metabolism. 2009;58(2):263-9.
90. Hoyer-Kuhn H, Kohbrok S, Volland R, et al. Vitamin b6 in primary hyperoxaluria I: first prospective trial after 40 years of practice. Clin J Am Soc Nephrol. 2014;9(3):468-77.
91. Monico CG, Rossetti S, Olson JB, et al. Pyridoxine effect in type I primary hyperoxaluria is associated with the most common mutant allele. Kidney Int. 2005;67(5):1704-9.
92. Curhan GC, Willett WC, Speizer FE, et al. Intake of vitamins B6 and C and the risk of kidney stones in women. J Am Soc Nephrol. 1999;10(4):840-5.
93. Curhan GC, Willett WC, Rimm EB, et al. A prospective study of the intake of vitamins C and B6, and the risk of kidney stones in men. J Urol. 1996;155(6):1847-51.

94. Taylor EN, Fung TT, Curhan GC. DASH-style diet associates with reduced risk for kidney stones. J Am Soc Nephrol. 2009;20(10):2253-9.
95. Meschi T, Maggiore U, Fiaccadori E, et al. The effect of fruits and vegetables on urinary stone risk factors. Kidney Int. 2004;66(6):2402-10.
96. Taylor EN, Stampfer MJ, Mount DB, et al. DASH-style diet and 24-hour urine composition. Clin J Am Soc Nephrol. 2010;5(12):2315-22.
97. Noori N, Honarkar E, Goldfarb DS, et al. Urinary lithogenic risk profile in recurrent stone formers with hyperoxaluria: a randomized controlled trial comparing DASH (Dietary Approaches to Stop Hypertension)-style and low-oxalate diets. Am J Kidney Dis. 2014;63(3):456-63.
98. Lindell A, Denneberg T, Edholm E, et al. The effect of sodium intake on cystinuria with and without tiopronin treatment. Nephron. 1995;71(4):407-15.
99. Nakagawa Y, Asplin JR, Goldfarb DS, et al. Clinical use of cystine supersaturation measurements. J Urol. 2000;164(5):1481-5.
100. Borghi L, Meschi T, Amato F, et al. Urinary volume, water and recurrences in idiopathic calcium nephrolithiasis: a 5-year randomized prospective study. J Urol. 1996;155:839-43.
101. Ferraro PM, Taylor EN, Gambaro G, et al. Soda and other beverages and the risk of kidney stones. Clin J Am Soc Nephrol. 2013;8(8):1389-95.
102. Curhan GC, Willett WC, Rimm EB, et al. Prospective study of beverage use and the risk of kidney stones. Am J Epidemiol. 1996;143(3):240-7.
103. Curhan GC, Willett WC, Speizer FE, et al. Beverage use and risk for kidney stones in women. Ann Intern Med. 1998;128(7):534-40.
104. Ferraro PM, Taylor EN, Gambaro G, et al. Caffeine intake and the risk of kidney stones. Am J Clin Nutr. 2014;100(6):1596-603.
105. Brinkley L, Gregory J, Pak C. A further study of oxalate bioavailability in foods. J Urol. 1990;144:94-6.
106. Goldfarb DS, Asplin JR. Effect of grapefruit juice on urinary lithogenicity. J Urol. 2001;166(1):263-7.
107. Simpson DP. Citrate excretion: a window on renal metabolism. Am J Physiol. 1983;244(3):F223-34.
108. Odvina CV. Comparative value of orange juice versus lemonade in reducing stone-forming risk. Clin J Am Soc Nephrol. 2006;1(6):1269-74.
109. Seltzer M, Low R, McDonald M, et al. Dietary manipulation with lemonade to treat hypocitraturic calcium nephrolithiasis. J Urol. 1996;156:907-9.
110. Eisner BH, Asplin JR, Goldfarb DS, et al. Citrate, malate and alkali content in commonly consumed diet sodas: implications for nephrolithiasis treatment. J Urol. 2010;183(6):2419-23.
111. Hodgkinson A, Pyrah LN. The urinary excretion of calcium and inorganic phosphate in 344 patients with calcium stone of renal origin. Br J Surg. 1958;46(195):10-8.
112. Cirillo M, Stellato D, Panarelli P, et al. Cross-sectional and prospective data on urinary calcium and urinary stone disease. Kidney Int. 2003;63(6):2200-6.
113. Coe FL. Hyperuricosuric calcium oxalate nephrolithiasis. Kidney Int. 1978;13(5):418-26.
114. Pak CY. Citrate and renal calculi: an update. Miner Electrolyte Metab. 1994;20(6):371-7.
115. Ferraro PM, Mandel EI, Curhan GC, et al. Dietary protein and potassium, diet-dependent net acid load, and risk of incident kidney stones. Clin J Am Soc Nephrol. 2016;11(10):1834-44.

CHAPTER

2

Nonclassical Crystallization Processes: Potential Relevance to Stone Formation

Stephan E Wolf, Joe Harris, Archana Lovett, Laurie B Gower

PROLOG

This chapter is subdivided into two parts. In the first part we give the reader an overview of both the classical and nonclassical theories of crystal growth in order to explain the fundamental principles implicit in mineralization processes. In the second part we discuss idiopathic stone formation, with particular attention placed on how nonclassical crystal growth can explain some of the mechanisms involved in nephrolithiasis. For those readers who have a good grounding in the modes of crystal growth (see Section "From idealized to real crystallization systems: classical versus nonclassical crystallization processes"), and classical concepts of stone formation (see Section "General considerations of stone formation"), we recommend moving directly to Section "Overview of nonclassical crystallization concepts involved in stone formation," which begins with the discussion on the relevance on nonclassical mechanisms to stone formation, followed by Section "Mineralogical signatures of nonclassical mineralization processes occurring in stone formation" which focuses on mineralization signatures that we have found to support the hypothesis that nonclassical crystallization mechanisms are involved in stone formation.

FROM IDEALIZED TO REAL CRYSTALLIZATION SYSTEMS: CLASSICAL VERSUS NONCLASSICAL CRYSTALLIZATION PROCESSES

Concepts of Classical Crystallization

In the 1920s, the foundations for our traditional understanding of crystal formation and growth were laid by Becker, Döring, Volmer, and other pioneers.[1-3] Since then this model has found its place in textbooks and is often referred to as classical nucleation theory (CNT). When considering crystallization of ionic salts from solution—as it occurs in stone formation—the driving force for nucleation is related to the solution's supersaturation, which arises from an ion concentration that exceeds saturation, and is quantified as the ion activity product divided by the equilibrium solubility product (K_{sp}). Classical nucleation theory describes the genesis of a new phase within a supersaturated mother phase by stochastic formation of small nascent clusters by an ion-by-ion attachment process. Nucleation of a new phase occurs when the radius of randomly forming unstable clusters reaches a critical cluster size (r_c), at which point the energetic cost of forming the new phase (the interfacial, or surface energy ΔG_S) is outbalanced by the energy released by formation of bonds within the bulk phase (the bulk energy ΔG_V) (Fig. 2.1A). Below the critical radius, the nascent clusters redissolve, whereas clusters that are larger than the critical radius become stable and form the new crystalline phase. These clusters will grow, further reducing the Gibbs free energy of the system as long as supersaturation prevails. In other words, the stochastically forming density fluctuations, the unstable clusters, have to overcome an energetic barrier to nucleation (ΔG^*) raised by the creation of new interfaces (the positive change in ΔG_s curve in Fig. 2.1A). Beyond this barrier the favorable bulk energy (negative ΔG_v curve) overcomes the unfavorable energetic contribution from the formation of new surfaces such that the overall free energy of the nucleus, $\Delta G_{N,}$ decreases, allowing for further spontaneous growth of the nucleus, until the supersaturation (the driving force for the reaction) is reduced to the point of saturation. The nucleation event is considered to occur when the cluster size surpasses r_c, and can be considered a nucleus as it has become a new and stable phase. The height of the nucleation barrier (ΔG_N^* at $\partial\Delta G_N(r^*)/\partial r=0$) is a function of the supersaturation of the mother solution and also of the interfacial energy of the newly forming phase. The formation rate of the nuclei (J_N) is described by an Arrhenius relationship, analogous to chemical kinetics, $J_N \propto \exp(\Delta G_N^*/k_BT)$. It is strongly dependent on the height of the barrier, and therefore parameters such as interfacial energy affect the rate of nucleation. As the interfacial and bulk energy rests on structural aspects, these important

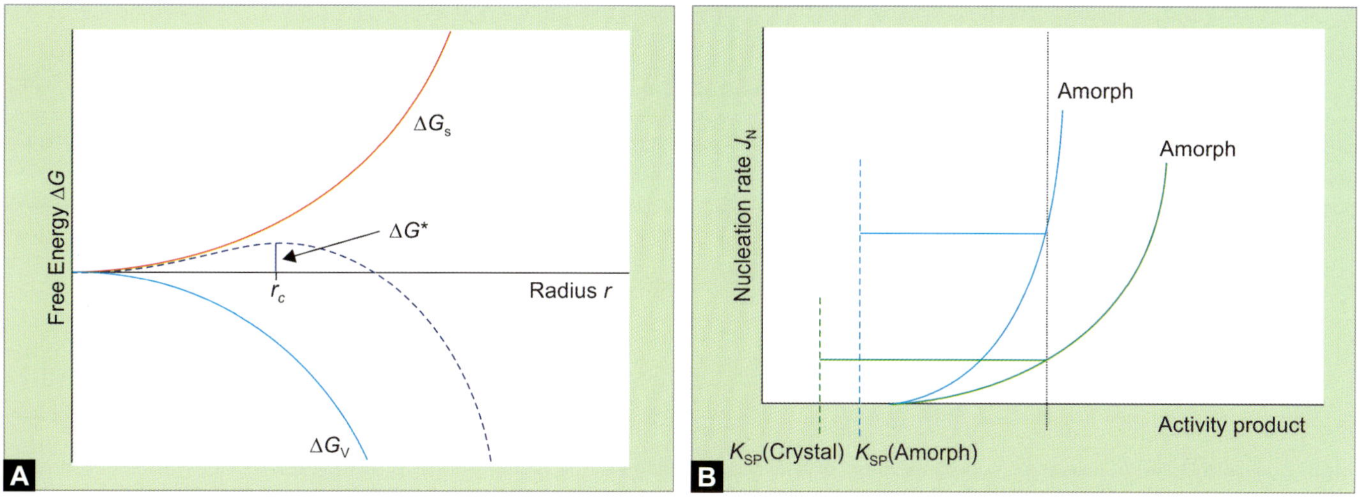

Figs. 2.1A and B: (A) The formation of a nucleus with the radius *r* leads to an overall free energy as indicated by the dashed line. The cross-over point at which bulk energy (blue curve) compensates the penalty of creating a new surface (green curve) is given by the critical radius r_c. (B) The rate of nucleation, J_N, is a function of supersaturation, naturally, but also strongly depends on the interfacial energy of the respective phase. Phases with low interfacial energy have a higher rate of nucleation at identical supersaturation for the given phase.

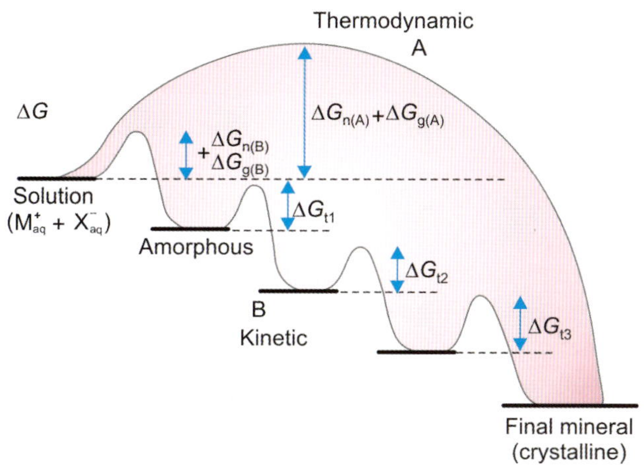

Fig. 2.2: The empirical Ostwald-Lussac rule of stages states that crystallization often occurs in steps, where the thermodynamically metastable phases form first and then transform successively to more stable phases. The less stable phases are often more hydrated and may be amorphous, so that the interfacial energy of these phases is lower and, therefore, their nucleation rates are higher.
Source: Reprinted with permission from Cölfen H, Mann S. Higher-order organization by mesoscale self-assembly and transformation of hybrid nanostructures. Angew Chemie Int Ed. 2003;42: 2350-65.

values can, and do, vary for different forming phases (Fig. 2.1B). The well-known Ostwald-Lussac law of stages, which dates back to 1897,[4] can be seen as a paraphrase of this. It states that in a crystallizing system with multiple phases possible (as the system is above their solubility limit), the most thermodynamically stable crystal phase does not directly form, and instead the more soluble, least dense phase is often precipitated first. After this, the metastable precipitated phase can undergo a series of phase transformations, even passing through other metastable phases if the energy barriers for such a multistep pathway are more easily overcome, before the most thermodynamically stable phase is finally reached (Fig. 2.2).[5] Through the years, the predictions of the Ostwald-Lussac law of stages have stood the test of time and have shown to hold true for numerous crystallizing systems.[6-9] Although such a crystallization reaction passes through one or more precursors before reaching the most thermodynamically stable crystal phase, it is still considered a classical crystallization pathway, but may be referred to as a multistep pathway.

It is the energetic cost of creating a new interface that is the source of the barrier to nucleation; therefore, the presence of heterogeneous interfaces or foreign bodies can dramatically lower this barrier, providing a lower energy route to nucleation, and allowing it to occur at lower supersaturation. Therefore, homogenous nucleation is often, and correctly, described as a rare phenomenon. In supersaturated solutions under realistic conditions, competition between homogeneous and heterogeneous nucleation processes virtually always occurs; only in select cases are nucleating interfaces fully absent. The surface of reaction vessels, biological membranes, dispersed impurities, functionalized surfaces (e.g. self-assembled monolayers or Langmuir films), protein aggregates,[10] or even the interface of two intermixing educt solutions[11] are common

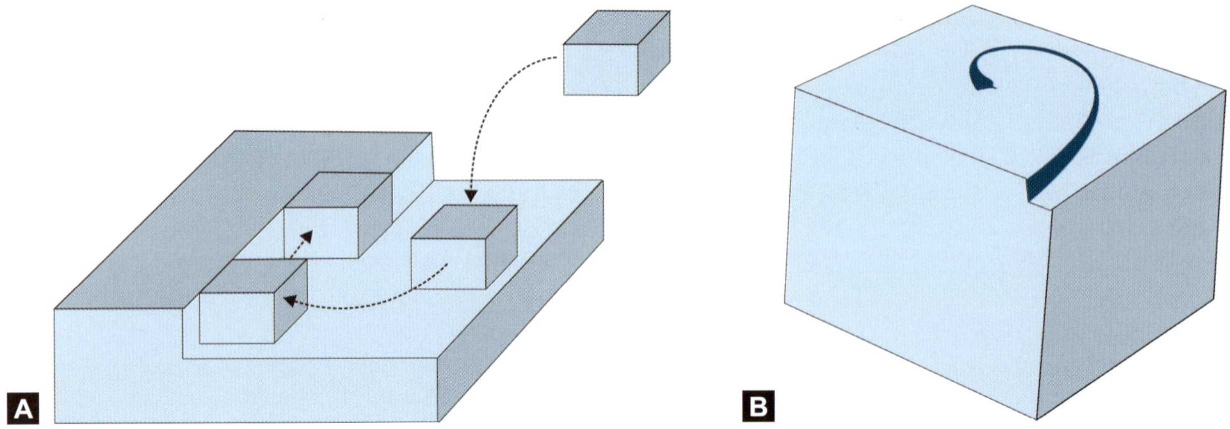

Figs. 2.3A and B: (A) At moderate supersaturation, crystal growth occurs at the higher energy growth steps by step-wise incorporation of monomers (ions or molecules). (B) Schematic representation of a screw dislocation, which provides a perpetual step edge as incoming monomers attach at the edge and continue to build up the terrace.

elicitors for heterogeneous nucleation. The interface can have a templating effect favoring the nucleation of certain crystal planes on the substrate whose two-dimensional symmetry is commensurate to the arrangement of the functional groups at the interface. This is not only widely employed in crystal engineering,[12] but also observed in biomineralizing systems as a means to allow for control of the crystallographic orientation of biominerals.[13,14] One aspect that is commonly neglected in classical nucleation models is the occurrence of the Gibbs–Thomson effect: small nuclei with high curvature have a higher solubility compared to those of small curvature. Ostwald ripening,[15,16] i.e. the growth of larger particles at the expense of smaller ones, is a phenomenological description of the consequence on the postnucleation stage caused by this effect.[16] This occurs because the local supersaturation becomes depleted in the vicinity of large growing particles, to the point that nearby smaller particles (with a higher K_{sp}) are no longer surrounded by solution that is supersaturated relative to their K_{sp}. The Gibbs–Thomson effect is not only active on larger length scales, it also strongly impacts the early and, probably, prenucleation stages of phase separation. However, how strongly it affects the structure of nucleation clusters and their critical radius is hard to assess and therefore commonly ignored.[17]

Once stable crystals of the new phase have been formed, be it by homogeneous or heterogeneous nucleation, their further growth is classically outlined by the Terrace Step Kink model introduced by Frank, Kossel, and Stranski.[18-21]parts III and IV with the form (on the atomic scale In this model, the crystal growth is described by attachment of individual monomers, be it atoms, ions, or molecules (Fig. 2.3A). For the formation of a new growth layer on a flat crystal region—the latter is called a crystal terrace—a process has to occur that is similar to the nucleation process outlined above. In this two-dimensional nucleation process, the barrier for nucleation of a new island is raised not by interfacial energy but by the Gibbs–Thomson effect. The initially high curvature of the new island increases its solubility, so that a sufficiently high supersaturation is needed for formation of a stable terrace. Once such an island has reached a critical radius, it becomes a new stable and further growing terrace. At low supersaturations (low driving force), the critical size for formation of a new and stable island increases so that the probability for its formation is very small, and growth of the crystal cannot proceed by this mechanism. Nevertheless, in real systems crystal growth still occurs as crystals always contain a certain number of imperfections, such as dislocations. These dislocations represent a constant source of growth steps so that crystal growth can even occur at low concentrations by spiral growth (Fig. 2.3B), as described below.

As in the case of nucleation, the growth of a terrace occurs by ion- or monomer-wise attachment processes. New building blocks are incorporated at the border of crystal terraces, which do not yet fully cover the crystal surface (Fig. 2.3A). These steps are also not complete and contain kinks. The process of attachment of a new monomer to the crystal is a multistep process: a monomer has to achieve bulk diffusion through the solution, adsorption to the crystal surface, dehydration, surface diffusion to the actual growth site and, finally, incorporation into the crystal lattice at the active site. The highest amount of energy is released if the new monomer attaches to the kink ("half crystal") site (Fig. 2.3A, last stage). It then shares the highest number of bonds with the existing crystal; this is therefore the predominating site of crystal growth. One has to bear in mind that in real systems, spiral growth and formation of new kinks or islands also occur if sufficient supersaturation prevails.

The process of crystal growth is not nonreversible. Quite the contrary, it is in fact a very dynamic process even at equilibrium; the monomers can detach from the crystal surface by thermally activated processes. Steps are not static but move constantly back and forth, and monomers are constantly attaching and leaving the site of crystal growth. In equilibrium, the incoming and the outgoing flux of monomers are equal. However, the amount of free energy that is released upon attachment of a monomer to each kink site is different because the atomic arrangement differs along different crystallographic planes; therefore, some kinks and steps grow faster than others during prevailing supersaturation. The final, and facetted, equilibrium morphology of a growing crystal is dominated by the slowest-growing crystal faces because they express the lowest energy surfaces; the higher-energy planes favor rapid adsorption of species to lower their energy, and are thus the fastest growing, with the result that these faces become smaller or even fully grow themselves out of existence, becoming the edges and corners that delineate the lowest energy faces of the final crystal.

Influence of Additives on Classical Crystallization

In biological systems, the formation and growth of a new crystalline phase is strongly influenced by the (often highly concentrated) additives and impurities present in the respective body fluid. The presence of various inorganic ions, such as Mg^{2+} or Sr^{2+}, can severely affect the nucleation and growth processes; moreover, the interaction of bioorganic molecules and solutes with the mineralizing system is even greater than that of the inorganic ions.[10,22] In the classical model, the interaction of the growing crystal with additives in the solution is typically expressed by a changing growth rate of the various crystal faces, as discussed in the preceding paragraphs. The change of growth rates gives the forming crystal a different equilibrium morphology; the crystal expresses different faces ("trachts") and/or aspect-ratio, resulting in a crystal shape ("habit") that can distinctly differ from the observed equilibrium crystal morphology in the absence of additives. This effect is based on attachment of additives to the sites of active crystal growth, i.e. growth spirals, kinks, and steps. Depending on the interaction of the additive with the crystal interface, the additive will change the growth rate of the individual growth steps. Currently, four different mechanisms of growth step inhibition are well documented.

1. *Reduction of interfacial energy:* Additives that lower the interfacial energy of surfaces or growth steps can distinctly change a crystal's appearance since the directional growth rate and dissolution rate are a sensitive function of the interfacial energy. The final equilibrium shape expresses only the interface exhibiting the lowest interfacial energy.
2. *Incorporation*: Impurities, such as strontium or magnesium ions incorporated in a crystal in lieu of calcium ions, not only distort the local symmetry and structure of the crystal, but consequently they increase the free energy of the crystal by an enthalpic contribution from the lattice strain, which in turn increases the solubility (K_{sp}) of the crystal. This results in a lower local supersaturation and, therefore, a lower rate of crystal growth.
3. *Kink blocking*: Additives that selectively attach to the kink site can lead to a distinct decrease in kink site density, and thus crystal growth. To achieve this, they do not need to bind permanently to the kink site; it is sufficient if they block kink propagation by attachment for a relatively short residence time.
4. *Step pinning*: If an impurity attaches firmly to growth steps and cannot be replaced by monomers due to its strong binding energy, the only way for crystal growth to continue is for the steps to grow around the blocking agent. If the distance between two blocked sites is larger than the critical radius of a new terrace island, then the growth of the crystal proceeds without disturbance. But if the distance is smaller, the Gibbs–Thomson effect intervenes and the step moves slowly or is halted because it faces an apparently lower supersaturation due to its increased curvature.

An exact understanding and study of the interaction of additives with growth steps of minerals can lead to new therapies preventing pathological biomineral formation. Standard treatment of stones often involves increasing dietary magnesium or citric acid uptake as they act as crystal growth inhibitors. In the case of cystinuria, which is a rare but high-morbidity stone resulting from the build-up of cysteine, a treatment was developed based on inhibition studies using in situ atomic force microscopy (AFM). In these studies, *L*-cystine dimethylester and *L*-cystine methylester were identified as efficient crystal growth inhibitors because they specifically bind to the set of {100} steps.[23] This suggests that high-throughput techniques can be employed to identify potential candidates who may be able to block classical nucleation and growth of calcium oxalate (CaOx) in vivo.[24] However, when considering the influence of crystallization inhibitors, one must be cautious because nonclassical crystallization processes can also result from such inhibitory species, and this can lead to an assortment of outcomes.

Nonclassical Crystallization Processes Challenge the Traditional Concepts

The classical models of crystal nucleation and crystal growth, as outlined above, work relatively well in well-controlled or near-ideal model systems.[14,25] However, the limitations of the classical theoretical framework become apparent when systems are studied that experience non-ideal or realistic conditions. Such a situation is prevalent in biomineralization systems in vivo, which can entail high supersaturation, strong interaction of the growing mineral phase with additives, impurities, water, and/or the presence of interfaces inducing heterogeneous nucleation. Crystallization processes that occur under such nonideal conditions are often unpredictable and inexplicable using classical models. They are beyond the scope of the traditional textbook theories and are therefore perceived as examples of "nonclassical crystallization." They of course must still follow the basic rules of thermodynamics, but the molecular level mechanisms deviate substantially from the CNT described above.

The main deficiency in the picture of crystal formation drawn by the classical theories is the shared postulate that the fundamental processes occur only by addition of monomers to the growing nucleus/crystal. Recent research has, however, revealed a myriad of examples in which the mineralization proceeds by aggregation of a colloidal intermediate in lieu of the postulated monomer-by-monomer growth. Mineralization pathways that follow pathways outside of the classical framework typically proceed by an alternative, particle-mediated growth mechanism, in lieu of the ion-by-ion growth envisioned by classical models, and are thus subsumed under the notion of nonclassical crystallization.[26,27] Recent research revealed a triumvirate of three important nonclassical pathways: (1) the process of oriented attachment, (2) the occurrence of a liquid-condensed phase of mineral precursor that can be stabilized during the polymer-induced liquid-precursor (PILP) process, and (3) the existence of prenucleation clusters (PNCs).

The latter phenomenon, the existence of PNCs, reveals a major shortcoming of the CNT. Gebauer et al. recently provided evidence for the existence of stable clusters, with a remarkable size of up to 70 ions at pH 9, before the nucleation event, in aqueous solutions of calcium carbonate ($CaCO_3$).[28] This finding shook the confidence of the scientific community in the notions and concepts of the classical models of crystal growth, and its full ramifications for various disciplines are yet to be fathomed. Shortly after this disputed contribution,[29] the existence of PNCs was further corroborated with cryogenic transmission microscopy of $CaCO_3$ formation under heterogeneous conditions;[30] Kellermeier et al. later provided further evidence by stabilization and imaging of PNCs by means of silicate as a capping agent.[31] A first insight into their structural composition was given by Wolf et al. employing electrospray ionization mass spectroscopy (ESI-MS) and X-ray absorption near edge structure (XANES) on the Ca-K edge of a saturated calcium bicarbonate solution:[32] the clusters have a typical cation to anion ratio of 1:1 and contain a non-negligible amount of water. These findings fit well with computer simulations that have described PNCs as a dynamically ordered liquid-like oxyanion polymer that consists of chains, branches, and rings with a 1:1 ratio of ions.[33] Moreover, PNCs have additionally been detected in systems other than $CaCO_3$: Wolf et al. showed their existence in different bivalent metal carbonates systems (M = Sr, Ba, Cd, Mn, and Pb),[32] and others have provided evidence of their existence in solutions of CaOx,[28] amino acids,[34] and calcium phosphate (CaP).[35]

For the CaP system, the formation of apparently discrete clusters in solutions was postulated by Posner in the mid-1970s. Amorphous calcium phosphate (ACP) typically represents the first solid mineral phase that forms in supersaturated solutions. Structural analyses of the near-range order of ACP led Posner and Betts to the conclusion that ACP is formed by the aggregation of clusters with a discrete composition of $Ca_9(PO_4)_6$.[36] The existence of these so-called Posner's clusters with a particle size of up to 1 nm was demonstrated by Onuma et al. in simulated body fluid under conditions that were supersaturated with respect to hydroxyapatite (HA) and undersaturated with respect to ACP and octacalcium phosphate ($Ca_8H_2(PO_4)_6 \cdot 5H_2O$).[37] The existence of Posner's clusters in simulated body fluid, the formation of ACP by their aggregation, and the subsequent solid-state transformation to crystalline apatite, have been further corroborated by cryogenic transmission electron microscopy (cryo-TEM) under heterogeneous conditions.[35] It is still a matter of debate[38] whether Posner's clusters represent a true solute species and can consequently be seen as valid prenucleation species—as proposed by Dey et al.[35]—or whether they are characterized by nanoparticulate quality and therefore represent a new and dispersed phase that follows a cluster-growth mechanism.[37] Posner's clusters have typically been considered to be of particulate character with a discrete particle diameter of 9.5 Å detectable by X-rays[36]; however, recently they were described as "two deprotonated prenucleation complexes in which all negative charges are compensated by complexing calcium ions."[39] It was concluded that the previously reported PNCs generated under heterogeneous conditions were actually soluble ion-association complexes $[Ca(HPO_4)_3]^{4-}$ that are able to form insoluble "aggregates" of $[Ca_2(HPO_4)_3]^{2-}$ by uptake of calcium. Although the stoichiometry of this reaction remains unclear, it seems that trisphosphate calcium complexes serve as a fundamental building block for the formation of ACP, which does not follow the proposed model of cluster growth of Onuma et al.[37] Interestingly, this returns the concept of prenucleation clusters to the realm of inorganic complex chemistry and underlines that classical nucleation theories neglect the solution chemistry of inorganic salt components.[40] These contributions, and the ongoing discussions on the ramifications of these findings, clearly demonstrate the shortcomings of the classical picture, which oversimplifies crystal growth in both the early and late stages. A simple bottom line emerges: crystals may also accrete larger entities than single ions or molecules.

In addition to this small but fundamental insight, in recent years much has been learned about the complexity of mineralization occurring under nonideal conditions. There is an ever-expanding number of contributions that report mineralization pathways in which an intermediate colloidal precursor occurs whose presence alters the character of the crystallization process fundamentally. This transient and colloidal agent replaces the solvated ions/molecules in their role as the fundamental building block driving mineralization: The bulk mineral phase does not grow by ion-attachment but instead by aggregation and attachment of colloidal entities that are much larger than the classical ionic/molecular units or even nonclassical PNCs. These building blocks consist of colloidal entities, be they nanocrystallites, solid-amorphous, or liquid colloids of the precipitating mineral. The mineralization is driven by the aggregation (and/or coalescence) of these colloids, followed potentially by several steps of maturation. These maturation steps may involve Ostwald coarsening and compaction, dehydration and solidification, or phase transformation to a crystalline phase of higher stability. Mineralization by colloid attachment and eventual phase transformation seems to be ubiquitous in biological mineralization as a large number of biominerals show the nanogranular structure indicative of growth by a colloid-mediated process. They all consist of fused nanogranules that are 50–150 nm in diameter, rather than featuring the smooth facets observed in crystals grown in the "classical" ion-by-ion manner. It is not only calcareous biominerals such as mollusk shells or the spines and exoskeleton of sea urchins that share this nanogranular unity[41-45] brachiopods,[41] calcisponges,[46] glass sponges,[47,48] coccoliths,[49] and even bone[50] are also granular at the nanoscale. The nanogranules within biominerals typically feature exceptional crystallographic ordering and often appear as a single crystal under X-ray diffraction. This phenomenon is commonly subsumed under the term "mesocrystal." The hallmark of mesocrystal is an apparent single-crystallinity, although they feature a mesoscopic structural organization, i.e. they are composed of nanocrystallites in a common crystallographic register.[26,51]

Two different pathways leading to the formation of mesocrystals have been identified. The first such pathway for efficient generation of mesocrystals is oriented attachment.[52-54] It involves initial formation of nanocrystallites[55] that subsequently rotate to orient their lattice to match that of the neighboring crystal before finally attaching, leading to self-assembly into mosaic crystals[56] with a negligible angle spread by attachment under lattice-matching.[54,57] Due to the small angle spread and their particle-mediated growth, the apparently single-crystalline mineral bodies can adopt exceptional and nonfaceted crystal morphologies.[26,51,53-55,58] The co-oriented particles can, in a later stage of the reaction, fuse to give a single crystal with nonequilibrium morphology, or the particles can remain distinguishable when stabilized by adsorbates.[26,52,59] The nanoscale and mesocrystalline organization of biominerals,[43,45] notably similar to those observed in synthetic mesocrystals, triggered speculation that the process of oriented attachment could occur in biomineralization.[60,61] However, this assumption is in clear conflict with the well-established finding that the formation of biominerals typically occurs via a transient, metastable amorphous mineral precursor.[43,62-67] As the fundamental building blocks fueling the growth of biominerals are amorphous and, therefore, strictly isotropic in their properties, oriented attachment has clearly to be excluded as a probable formation mechanism for most biogenic mesocrystals. Moreover, recent studies have shown that biominerals have a space-filling character, which further excludes formation via oriented attachment as an aggregational growth of solid particles would lead to a body interspersed with voids.[68]

Biomimetic approaches imitating biomineralization processes with conceptualized, and thus simplified model systems, have clearly evidenced the occurrence of an intermediate amorphous phase in mineralization processes under near-biological conditions.[40,64,69,70] The characteristic formation of the amorphous phase in the presence of certain additives can be simplistically explained by the fact that these additives efficiently suppress nucleation or growth of crystalline mineral phases by attaching to the nuclei and growth steps of crystals, thereby blocking or slowing down the advancement of the growth steps. The supersaturated system can then only lower its free energy by formation of an amorphous phase that, due to its higher solubility, necessitates a higher supersaturation. If the amorphous phase is stabilized sufficiently, a nonclassical pathway opens up in which the amorphous intermediate drives the subsequent steps, mineralization by aggregation to an amorphous body that, in a later stage, can transform into a crystalline state by a quasi solid-to-solid transformation.[69,71,72] Because the final transformation proceeds pseudomorphically—i.e. under preservation of the external morphology, as well as the nanoscopic colloidal texture—mesocrystalline bodies with nonequilibrium morphologies can be achieved that were inaccessible and inexplicable by classical crystallization processes.

The first observation and characterization of a truly pseudomorphic mineralization process was reported by Gower et al. in 2000.[73] Polyelectrolytes, such as polyaspartate (polyAsp) or polyacrylic acid, were employed as additives in order to mimic the action of highly acidic biomacromolecules that are commonly associated with biominerals. These efficiently suppress classical nucleation of a solid crystalline phase, and give rise to the separation of a highly-hydrated and thus liquid-condensed mineral precursor phase (Figs. 2.4A to E). Colloidal droplets of this so-called PILP phase become the crucial mineralization agents forming amorphous mineral bodies by aggregation and coalescence processes. Over the course of time, and in parallel to the accretion processes, the highly hydrated liquid phase dehydrates and consecutively solidifies. The final solid amorphous mineral body eventually undergoes a pseudomorphic phase transformation, i.e. it crystallizes with retention of its nonequilibrium morphology by a quasi-solid/solid phase transformation. In addition to forming single crystals with nonequilibrium morphologies, the phase transformation can occur by spherulitic mechanisms and lead to complex crystallographic features such as lattice tilting, as observed in biominerals.[74] As the mineral remains in its initial shape, even during phase transformation, the PILP pathway is able to generate an impressive multitude of nonfaceted, nonequilibrium mineral morphologies inexplicable by classical theories.[75-78] The liquid-like character of this transient liquid-condensed mineral phase was observed by Gower et al. using optical microscopy, but then further evidenced by its capability to infiltrate pores under the action of capillary forces,[75] and by recent transmission electron microscopy (TEM) studies that showed that the liquid-condensed mineral phase initially behaves as a typical emulsion, and undergoes coalescence to large smears of liquid when exposed to shear stress.[32,40] Furthermore, the remnant colloidal texture of the bulk materials formed by the PILP process is a strong indication that the mineralization process occurs by colloid aggregation (Fig. 2.4E).

The physicochemical formation mechanisms underlying the PILP process remain enigmatic; several questions are today still unsolved. As the PILP process can be triggered in vitro by employing acidic polymers as a process-directing agent, the PILP phenomenon was mainly attributed to the polyanionic polymeric additive. It was assumed that the main action of the polymer comprises induction and stabilization of the liquid precursor by sequestering ions and water, thereby triggering the unusual liquid/liquid phase separation. However, Wolf et al. subsequently showed that the formation of a liquid-amorphous mineral precursor phase is also possible in the absence of any additives, albeit under near-ideal conditions.[32,40] Experiments were conducted in which a droplet of reaction solution was acoustically levitated to almost entirely circumvent heterogeneous nucleation. With this approach, they were able to evidence for the first time that the formation of the liquid-condensed mineral precursor phase is not solely induced by polymers; the capability

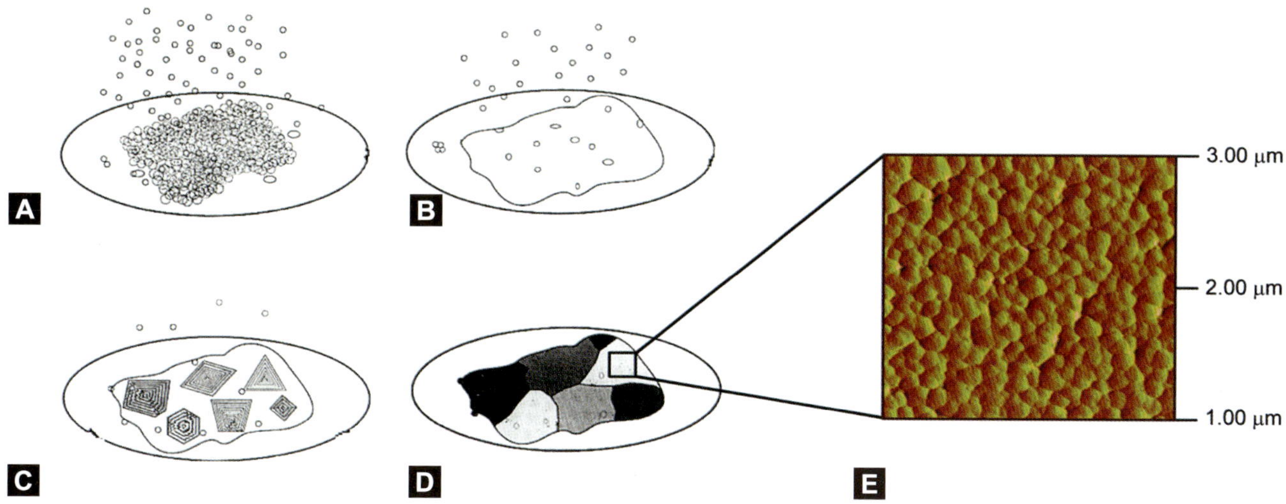

Figs. 2.4A to E: (A to D) Sketch of a typical polymer-induced liquid-precursor (PILP) process. (A) Liquid–liquid phase separation occurs as the negatively charged polymer sequesters calcium and carbonate ions (or clusters, or condensed phases), along with entrapped water, to form ion-enriched nanodroplets. (B) These droplets are so highly hydrated that the amorphous precursor has fluidic character, which allows coalescence into a continuous film. (C) The film solidifies and undergoes an amorphous to crystalline transformation, sometimes exhibiting transition bars from excluded polymeric impurity, which ultimately fill in, (D) creating a continuous crystalline film. Each step occurs in the aqueous crystallizing solution; the object on which the products accumulate represents a round glass coverslip that is placed in the crystallizing dish, although other substrates have been found to have a pronounced impact on the transformation kinetics. (E) Atomic forced micrographs of a mineral film generated by a PILP process. Although the colloidal texture is evident at the nanoscale, this same calcite film appeared very smooth at the microscale (inset: polarized light microscopy using a gypsum waveplate, where the birefringent calcite film exhibits a smooth texture).
Source (for Parts A to D): Reprinted with permission from Gower LB and Odom DJ. Deposition of calcium carbonate films by a polymer-induced liquid-precursor (PILP) process. J Cryst Growth. 2000;210(4):719-34.
Source (for Part E): Reprinted with permission from Kim YY, Douglas EP and Gower LB. Patterning inorganic ($CaCO_3$) thin films via a polymer-induced liquid-precursor process. Langmuir. 2007;23:4862-70.

to form a liquid-condensed mineral precursor phase is a trait of the mineral itself if crystallized under homogeneous conditions. Bewernitz et al. further corroborated the presence of a liquid condensed phase (LCP) through a variety of analytical techniques,[79] but also showed that when the polyAsp additive is included, the phase accumulates to a far greater extent, and importantly, this phase, which we call the PILP phase, is sufficiently stabilized to generate the multistep precursor mechanism. In other words, without polymer additive, the LCP apparently redissolves and precipitates into classical faceted crystals, but polymer stabilization of the LCP creates a PILP amorphous precursor that undergoes pseudomorphic transformation. It is this latter process that leaves mineralogical signatures of the crystallization pathway, such as crystals with nonequilibrium morphologies and nanocolloidal textures.

Currently, we do not have a comprehensive understanding of all the crucial actions of the polymer during the PILP process. The most apparent action of the polymer is to sequester cations,[80] PNCs, or LCP, all of which will reduce the supersaturation of the mother solution, which reduces the system's thermodynamic tendency to undergo phase separation in general. Counterintuitively, this can kinetically favor the formation of an amorphous phase with higher solubility in lieu of a crystalline phase with lower solubility, but this is because the key parameter that determines the height of the nucleation barrier is the interfacial energy. Compared to a crystalline phase, the penalty for creation of a new interface is low for amorphous phases, and presumably much lower for liquid-like and highly hydrated phases. Therefore, the formation of the liquid-amorphous phase can precede that of a crystalline phase as it is kinetically favored (Fig. 2.2); consequently, far more of the liquid-condensed mineral precursor phase is produced in the presence of the polymer. The PILP phase could be envisioned as an additional level (prior to the amorphous stage) in the reaction coordinate diagram of Figure 2.2. It is of importance to stress to the stone community that the fundamental insight here is that an "inhibitory" additive, which suppresses classical nucleation of a crystalline phase, can ultimately give rise to the formation of an amorphous phase; hence the reason Gower referred to this as a "process-directing agent" is because it transforms the reaction into a multistep crystallization mechanism. However, the presence of the process-directing agent not only drastically reduces the nucleation rate of a crystalline phase, it also prolongs the lifetime of the amorphous phase from a short-lived, transient species to the principal building blocks of what we refer to as a colloidal assembly to transformation (CAT) mineralization reaction.[80] It is this CAT mechanism that takes the crystallization into the nonclassical regime.

The process-directing action of the polymer therefore fundamentally rests on kinetically hampering the classical formation of the thermodynamically stable product. This leads to the formation of liquid-amorphous colloids, which then further undergo the process of mineralization. The next steps of the CAT mineralization pathway are the key steps of assembly, which consists of aggregation and coalescence to an amorphous mineral body (Fig. 2.4B). Although this is a nonclassical crystallization pathway, the aspects related to aggregation of colloids are governed by the classical model of DLVO (on the names of Derjaguin, Landau, Vervey, and Overbeek) theory. The DLVO theory describes the interaction potential between dispersed colloids as a result of a superposition of attractive van-der-Waals forces and repulsive electrostatic interactions. The latter arises from the diffuse ionic layers around the charged colloids. The interaction potentials between charged entities in solutions—be it colloids, polymers, proteins, etc.—are strongly dependent on the electrolyte concentration in the continuous medium, i.e. the ionic strength, as salts quite efficiently screen the Coulombic interactions. The Debye screening length $1/\kappa$ is a commonly employed measure for this because it describes the size of the diffusive double layer around charged dispersed colloids and represents the distance at which the electric potential drops to 1/e of its initial value. The screening length is quite large in essentially pure water (500 nm at 10 mmol/L), but rapidly decreases with increasing ionic strength (i.e. electrolyte content); e.g. increasing the electrolyte to 0.1 mol/L shrinks the double layer to no >5 nm. Below a critical ionic strength, electrostatic repulsion prevails and the emulsion experiences electrostatic stabilization. Above the critical ionic strength, the diffusive layer becomes too small to withstand van-der-Waals forces; the colloids can therefore move to within such close proximity that coagulation/coalescence can occur. The repulsive barrier can also be overcome by mere shear forces, i.e. by hydrodynamic forces pushing the colloids together, across the potential barrier. Wolf et al. showed recently that the liquid-condensed mineral precursor phase behaves initially like a classical, electrostatically stabilized (nano) emulsion during the early stages of mineralization: shear stress leads to coalescence, and an increase in the ionic strength of the mother solution induces strong aggregation of the nanodroplets.[32,40,80]

The behavior of colloids dispersed in a liquid continuous phase becomes much more complicated when polyelectrolytes are present in the dispersion. In accordance with DLVO, the polyelectrolytes interact with each other and with the dispersed phase. In the somewhat simpler case of oppositely charged colloids (e.g. negatively stabilized droplets and positively charged polymer), the polymer will accumulate and adsorb on the surface of the colloids, which leads to flocculation by charge neutralization and/or particle bridging. Incomplete annihilation of the colloid surface charge can lead to patchy particles that will also flocculate. In the case of like-charged colloids (or, more generally, in the case of nonadsorbing polymers), more complex scenarios can take place. In these instances, the conformational free energy of the polymer has to be taken into account when assessing the stability of dispersion. In colloid science, these effects are known as depletion effects (Fig. 2.5). The driving force of depletion effects arises from the tendency of polymers to adopt the energetically most favored random coil conformation in solution, i.e. the minimization of the solution's free energy. Under confinement, e.g. when in close proximity with an interface, the polymer's conformational freedom may be reduced as it becomes squeezed into tighter space, which in turn increases the free energy of the system. The system therefore changes to maximize the conformational freedom of the polymeric additive as far as it is possible. At elevated concentration of polymer, the conformational freedom of the additive is reduced by the interaction between individual polymers. If the colloids were to move within close proximity of each other, they would confine polymer molecules residing in the intercolloidal space, thereby further reducing the conformational freedom of the polymers. This leads to an additional repulsive force between the colloids; the emulsion is stabilized by so-called depletion stabilization. If the concentration of the polymers is so low that the interaction between the colloids and the polymer dominates, it is energetically favorable for the two solutes to be separated, and the system

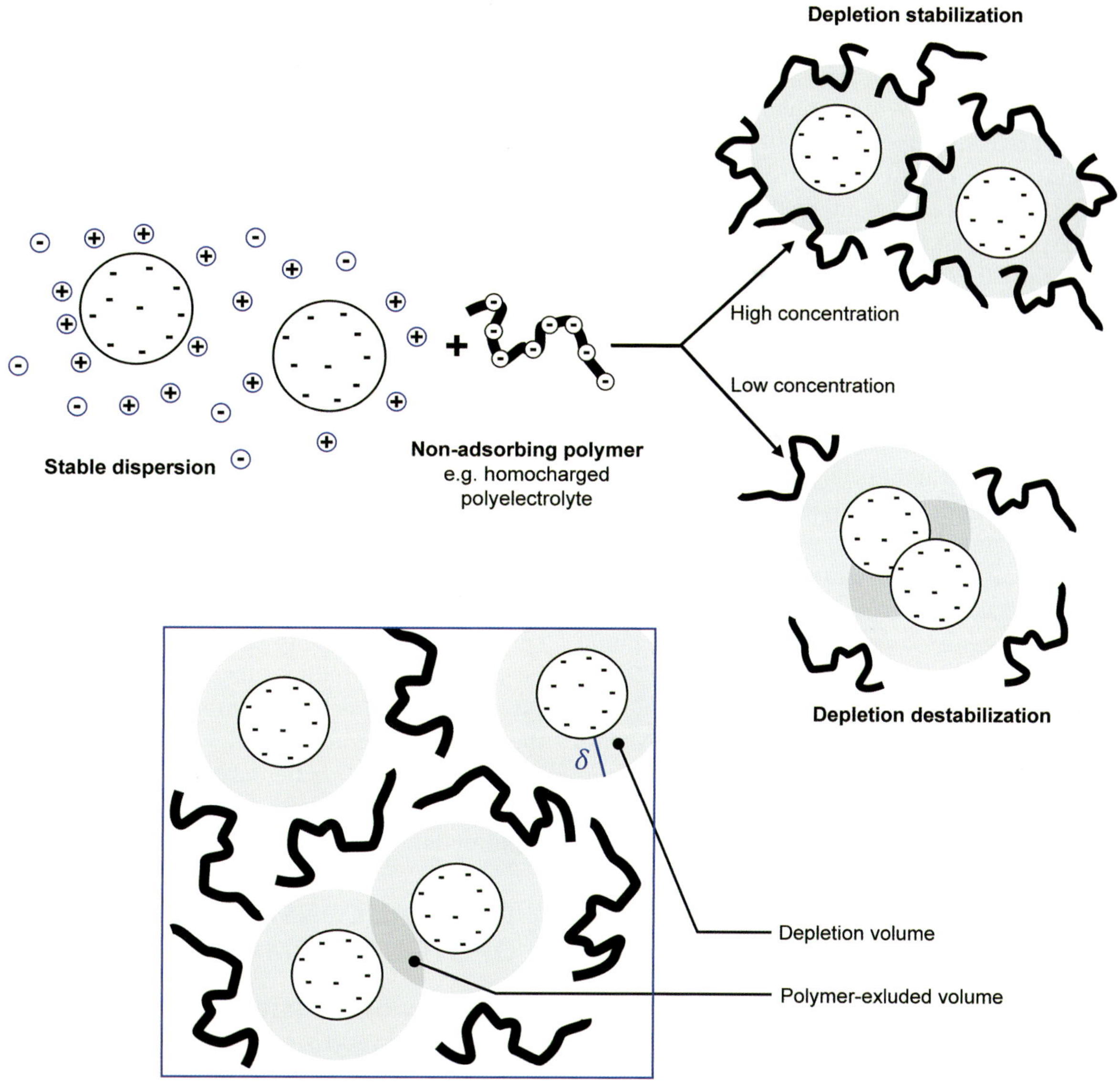

Fig. 2.5: Nonadsorbing polymers (e.g. noncharged or homocharged) can give rise to depletion effects that destabilize emulsified systems. The driving force of this effect is the maximization of the conformational freedom of the polymers. In the depletion volume, which surrounds every droplet, the conformational freedom of the nonadsorbing polymers is restricted by interaction with the colloid. A demulsification, i.e. a breaking of the dispersion, leads then to an increase in conformational freedom because no polymer-colloid interaction takes place anymore. If the concentration of polymer is too high so that the conformational freedom of the polymers is already restricted by polymer–polymer interactions, demulsification will not lead to increased conformational freedom. The dispersion is stabilized because demulsification would require that the polymers leave the interparticle space that would involve diffusion of polymers against their concentration gradient.

consequently undergoes phase separation; the system experiences depletion destabilization. Wolf et al. showed in a series of experiments that the impact of differently charged polymers on the liquid-condensed mineral precursor emulsion exactly fits this description.[32,40,80] They showed that positively charged polymers in general destabilize the liquid-condensed phase leading to mineral films and nonequilibrium morphologies characteristic of the PILP process (i.e. destabilization by charge neutralization); negatively charged polymers destabilize the LCP phase at low concentrations, but stabilize the LCP phase and enhance its lifetime considerably at high concentrations (i.e. depletion destabilization and stabilization, respectively).[43,80] In the light of these results, a core role of the polymer during the PILP process is to break the initially electrostabilized nanoemulsion of the liquid-condensed mineral precursor. This allows for the aggregation and coalescence of the nanosized droplets to form a mineral body with nanocolloidal texture (Fig. 2.4E).

If a substrate or template is presented to a PILP-mineralizing system, it is not only the interaction of the additive with the PILP phase that plays a central role, but also the interaction of the PILP phase and/or of the additive with the substrate. The capability of the PILP process to infiltrate porous and nanosized compartments is most impressively demonstrated by intrafibrillar mineralization of collagen fibers with CaP under PILP conditions, i.e. in presence of a process-directing polymer such as polyaspartate. The mineralized fibers show remarkable similarities to native bone: Intrafibrillar and uniaxially-oriented crystals are formed that are oriented roughly parallel to the fibril axis, generating identical diffraction patterns to native bone.[81,82] Standard mineralization processes are not capable of generating similar results as extrafibrillar mineralization occurs instead. The current model first proposed by Olszta and Gower proposes that the liquid PILP phase infiltrates the collagen fibrils via the gap regions, possibly driven by capillary forces. The adsorption of amorphous precursor colloids to the gap zones of collagen fibrils was later corroborated by a cryo-TEM study by Nudelman et al.,[83] although the mechanism proposed by them was based more on diffusion of colloids into the fibrils due to electrostatic attractions. In another recent contribution, Berg et al. showed that Mg ions, used as an additive during a PILP process, can distinctly influence the wetting behavior of the PILP phase on electrospun fiber meshes functionalized with biomimetic peptides. Coating of the fibers was successfully accomplished in the presence of Mg, whereas no mineral coverage of the fibers was achieved in the absence of Mg. If the fibers were functionalized with hydroxyl groups, wetting was only possible in the absence of Mg.[84] These contributions exemplify another key action of the process-directing additive: It can control the interaction of the mineral precursor with substrates and matrices present in the mineralization compartment. This is achieved by either altering the templating action and/or changing the wettability of the liquid-condensed mineral precursor phase with the substrate.

Summarizing the first part of this chapter, we have revisited the classical concepts of crystallization and reviewed recent findings that have challenged this traditional perspective. We have drawn particular attention to the PILP process, which starkly contrasts the classical scheme in which the final morphology of the crystal is governed by the slowest growing crystal faces. This biomimetic mineralization process is induced by the presence of small amounts of "nonspecific" acidic and basic polymers, and therefore might be suspected in crystallization systems that involve (bio)polymeric additives and crystallization inhibitors. The PILP process is a nonclassical mineralization process that proceeds by accretion of colloidal entities to form a nonequilibrium shaped body, which later pseudomorphically transforms into a crystalline material. The polymeric additive that acts as a process-directing agent circumvents the fundamental pathway of classical crystallization. Numerous studies evidence the existence of nonclassical pathways of mineralization by CAT, both in biological and biomimetic mineralization systems, although in the biological systems it still remains to be determined if the amorphous precursor colloids have fluidic character. Nevertheless, an impressive number of features long considered enigmatic in the biomineral world have now been duplicated in the beaker using this relatively simple PILP process.[64] The large number of publications suggests that mineralization by CAT, whether by solid or liquid colloids, is the fundamental growth mode that underlies the formation of a large number of calcareous and CaP biominerals.[63,85-87]

GENERAL CONSIDERATIONS OF STONE FORMATION

Overview of Classical Crystallization Concepts Involved in Idiopathic Stone Formation

This chapter will be mainly focused on idiopathic stone formation, which is the most prevalent yet least understood mechanism of nephrolithiasis.[88,89] This is not to say that nonclassical mechanisms are not relevant to other stones types; it only means that the authors are more familiar with the literature in this area, and have developed model systems to provide insight. We hope that the discussion will be sufficient for providing the reader with the ability to make such judgments on their own as they encounter other stone types.

Idiopathic stone formation leads to stones that are predominantly calcium oxalate (CaOx), yet are often found to have a calcium phosphate core. This suggests that the CaOx overgrew on a CaP mineral core that likely had previously formed from Randall's plaques (RP).[89-97] The formation of the two different minerals in these composite stones—CaP within the renal tissue and CaOx in the urine—is thought to be due to the different pH and ionic constituents present in those respective environments.[89,92,98-100] Randall's plaques are typically comprised of the carbonated apatite phase of CaP.[92,94,101-103] In the loop of Henle, the pH ranges from 6.5 to 7.3,[104-106] which favors apatite formation (pH > 6.2).[107-109] In the urine, the pH can fluctuate between 4.5 and 8 throughout the day so that the average value tends to be acidic (around pH 6).[100-111] These conditions favor CaOx formation, which tends to occur at pH values <7.[100,105,109] While both calcium oxalate monohydrate (COM) and calcium oxalate dihydrate (COD) are found in stones, COM is the primary phase. The calcium oxalate trihydrate phase (COT) is rarely seen in CaOx stones.[92,101,111-113] These observations correlate well with the relative stabilities of the CaOx phases. In the CaOx system, hydrated mineral phases are generally the more soluble phases. However, if metastable phases are involved in early stages of stone formation or growth, they might not be detected. Stone extraction typically occurs well after its initial formation, and in the meantime, the thermodynamic driving force pushes them to transform to the most stable phase. This would be particularly strong for the least stable COT phase. On the other hand, the noticeable presence of the metastable COD phase may result from organic materials that either promote its formation (e.g. by altering the energy barriers to nucleation, *see* Figs. 2.1A and B) or that stabilize the intermediate phase by preventing its phase transformation (*see* Fig. 2.2). The latter case might occur if the mineral is coated by an organic matric that prevents its dissolution and reprecipitation into a more stable phase.

Naturally, sufficient supersaturation of the respective ions is necessary for Randall's plaques and stone formation.[88,89,114,115] In the loop of Henle, there is evidence of supersaturation with respect to CaP.[98,99,107,116] Calcium oxalate however, does not tend to form in the renal tissue since it is not likely that there is a sufficiently high CaOx supersaturation at normal levels in the nephron above the distal part of the collecting duct.[99,107,117] Calcium oxalate crystals are generally metastable at the supersaturation levels found in the urine of idiopathic stone formers,[118] yet crystals are found in both stone formers and nonstone formers,[119,120] suggesting that its nucleation must occur heterogeneously, or that promoters lower the energy barrier to homogenous nucleation. While Randall's plaques appear to be more common in patients with stone disease, the kidneys of many nonstone formers also have these deposits,[121] so it seems that there are multiple factors at work. For example, nonstone formers could have more effective inhibitory proteins that prohibit overgrowth of CaOx on exposed Randall's plaques.

Additives can also play a role in modulating aggregation of crystals, as shown by Wesson and coworkers for CaOx.[122] Calcium oxalate, constituting about three quarters of all kidney stones, can crystallize both in a monohydrate (COM, whewellite) and a dihydrate mineral phase (COD, weddellite), whereas more than two thirds of all stones (partially) contain COM. Recent contributions suggested an even stronger prevalence of COM in stones formed by primary hyperoxaluria under treatment with crystallization inhibitors such as citrate or magnesium.[123] Calcium oxalate monohydrate is also known to exhibit an affinity to cell surfaces of renal tubules exceeding that of COD,[124,125] which indicates that heterogeneous interaction or templating effects may play a central role in retention of crystals, providing time for crystal growth and/or aggregation in stone formation.[126] Interestingly, certain biopolymers, such as osteopontin or nephrocalcin, were found to preferentially induce formation of COD; other biopolymers did not show this phase selection activity, e.g. chondroitin.[122] In recent contributions, it was shown that the Tamm–Horsfall protein is an efficient inhibitor of COM aggregation and therefore a protective agent against COM stone formation. This antiaggregational behavior rests on the post-translational glycosylation of this protein; desialylation of THP leads to protein aggregation, which then acts as a promoter of COM aggregation—an impressive demonstration of the crucial role additives such as biopolymers play during classical crystallization processes in vivo.[127]

Solution conditions are not the only factors in the formation of Randall's plaques and stones. The thermodynamics and kinetics of the processes that control crystal formation and phase are also heavily influenced by the wide variety of renal and urinary molecules present in these environments. Randall's plaques and stones also contain various organics such as proteins, lipids, and polysaccharides that constitute 1–5 wt%, which no doubt have some influence on the process of stone formation.[93,128-131] There are many hypotheses regarding the roles of these various macromolecules, but they typically consider them from the simple perspective of either acting as promoters or inhibitors of crystal nucleation/growth or aggregation. While these functions can depend on the state of the protein (e.g. glycosylation, phosphorylation, cleavage, etc.), or under differing urinary conditions,[112,128-130,132-138] we feel such descriptions still fail to provide a satisfactory explanation of how the mineral phase is actually formed.

To date, the general view of the stone community regarding idiopathic stones has only considered aspects that have long been deliberated because they fall under the category of classical crystallization, such as the issues discussed in this section. However, from a materials science and crystal growth perspective, renal stones become even more interesting in that the individual crystals typically have unusual morphologies and textures. We propose that these features might serve as "mineralogical signatures" that can be useful in deciphering the mechanism(s) by which the crystals may have formed, and by understanding the mechanism of formation, one might be able to better elucidate the role that various urinary species play in influencing these processes.

Overview of Nonclassical Crystallization Concepts Involved in Stone Formation

The crystallogenesis of CaOx and other stone-forming minerals in nephrolithiasis is not yet well understood despite this phenomenon being central to ectopic mineral formation. A better understanding of the fundamental growth processes and identification of the fundamental building blocks of stones is therefore urgently needed, and would hold great importance for drug development and treatment. The relevance of nonclassical growth processes becomes apparent if one compares the typical urine transit times with the crystal growth rate of COM, a typical stone former; COM stone formation seems to be only possible in vivo by aggregational processes because the classical growth rates of COM are so slow that a single crystal grown by classical processes cannot reach a sufficient diameter to be caught in the terminal collecting duct of the kidney.[139-141]

Furthermore, we have clear indication that solutions of the minerals that occur in stone formation, i.e. CaOx,[28] CaP,[35] and cysteine,[34] all feature PNCs. As of yet, it is still unclear how they impact on the mineralization processes—do they serve as fundamental building blocks? This question, tied up with the issue of their exact structural composition, is of special importance when designing efficient crystallization inhibitors: Not only do they have to block the growth of crystals by classical, ionic growth modes, but they also have to block accretion processes involving PNCs. For the CaP system, it is now clear that the formation of ACP is governed by aggregation and densification of Posner's clusters. Consequently, if we want to block growth of a CaP crystal, not only do we have to block ion-wise growth of the system, but we also have to suppress the nonclassical growth pathway, i.e. aggregation of Posner's clusters to larger entities that can eventually crystallize. For these mineralization processes by colloid aggregation and transformation, an amorphous intermediate is of importance and has not only been identified for the CaP system, but also recently in the CaOx system.[142]

In the first part of the chapter, we saw that the development of classical growth inhibitors may be a double-edged sword: The PILP process demonstrates that an efficient classical crystal growth inhibitor can be a potent promoter of nonclassical growth processes. There is a large body of literature in the stone community that has defined various proteins as "inhibitors" or "promoters" of crystal nucleation and growth. In light of the other potential outcomes that can result from inhibitory macromolecules, the role of such species may need to be re-examined.

Adhesion processes, involving both epithelial cell surfaces and mineral surfaces of already settled microcrystal aggregates, seem to play an important role in nephrolithiasis. It is worth mentioning that proteins, such as osteopontin, used as an additive during sample-probe interaction studies by AFM, can dramatically change the interaction behavior of mineral surfaces with carboxylate-functionalized probes.[139-141] This bears remarkable similarities to recent findings that wettability of interfaces by PILP phases can be tuned by the selection of crystallization additives. Biopolymers may not only play a key role in controlling crystallization but also a distinct and perhaps critical role in controlling aggregation processes of the fundamental mineral colloids during nephrolithiasis, as described in detail in Section "Nonclassical crystallization processes challenge the traditional concepts".

MINERALOGICAL SIGNATURES OF NONCLASSICAL MINERALIZATION PROCESSES OCCURRING IN STONE FORMATION

Most of the following discussion on nonclassical processes will be focused on the CAT mechanism. This is justified because it leads to significant changes in the micro- and nanostructure of the mineral that can be readily identified. Prenucleation clusters are most likely present in the urine and somehow involved in the process of crystallization but, so far, their impact on the overall crystallization process is unclear. As to crystal formation by oriented attachment, mineralogical signatures can be produced by this formation mechanism (such as a mesocrystalline texture, and uniformly oriented microfacets on the surface resulting from the attachment of pre-existing nanocrystals); however, one has to be careful because both of these features can also be produced by transformation of an amorphous phase. For example, a mesocrystalline texture is an inherent aspect of crystals formed via the CAT mechanism, given that the crystal forms via colloid assembly; and amorphous materials, or even crystalline materials with curved surfaces (formed pseudomorphically into such a nonequilibrium morphology), will ultimately try to lower their surface energy over time. So given sufficient mobility (i.e. if they remain in solution long enough), the surface will reorganize to form microfacets that express lower energy planes. Given that oriented attachment has mainly been demonstrated for thin anisotropic constructs at the nanoscale, with little evidence of bulk scale crystals being formed by this mechanism, it seems unlikely to be relevant to stone formation. Nevertheless, we will point out features from our observations that could relate to this mechanism, as well as the CAT mechanism.

It is our hypothesis that amorphous phases from the CAT mechanism may be involved in some stages of stone formation. This is based on comparison of the mineralogical signatures found in stones with those produced in vitro using model systems. Although these model systems are vastly oversimplified relative to the highly complex urinary environment, they have allowed researchers to better understand the physicochemical mechanisms that can occur during crystallization of ionic salts, and particularly in the presence of additives. For example, in Gower's model system of the PILP process (see part 1 of this chapter),[64,82,90,93,94,103,109,130,143-145] a variety of features have been found in various calcium-based mineral products that bear a striking resemblance to features found in biominerals,[64] including both biologically controlled biominerals, as well as the pathological biominerals found in Randall's plaques and CaOx stones.[130,143,146] Because the PILP droplets are highly hydrated, this amorphous precursor has fluidic character, at least in the early stages.[130,145,147] This allows the droplets to coalesce into smooth coatings and films prior to crystallization, which upon pseudomorphic transformation produces nonequilibrium morphologies and textures in the mineral products, unlike crystals produced by the classical crystallization mechanism.[64,73,82,130,143,145] Though the PILP process was first identified with $CaCO_3$,[73] given that the CaP and CaOx minerals can also form amorphous phases,[83,142,148-150] Gower's group expanded their in vitro model system to demonstrate that PILP features can be produced in these mineral systems as well.[64,82,144]

Our hypothesis that Randall's plaques and stones may involve an amorphous or PILP precursor is based on the fact that the renal and urinary environment contains many different acidic macromolecular species, and polyelectrolytes in general are known to induce or promote nonclassical crystallization pathways under the right conditions.[64] It was even found that many of the proteins incorporated within stones are generally acidic,[128] and thus one might predict that they became entrapped within an amorphous or PILP-like phase during their formation.[151-153] Therefore, given this distinct possibility, we decided to examine some stones ourselves (kindly provided by Saeed Khan), as well as inspect images shown in the literature, to see if there is any evidence to suggest they formed via a nonclassical pathway.

Spherulites and Spherules

Figures 2.6A and B show a typical CaP/CaOx composite stone from the literature.[109] The outer region is composed of CaOx, and radial growth of the polycrystals indicates that it has formed via a spherulitic growth mechanism (Fig. 2.6A). In this case, the spherulite also contains concentric layers of defects, and those have been shown in many reports to contain organic impurities. The core of the stone is made of ACP, and at a higher magnification one can see that it is formed by aggregation of partially coalesced globules (Fig. 2.6B).[109] These melded morphologies are sometimes referred to as agglomerates as opposed to aggregates.[154] Gower's in vitro model system has been able to produce similar nonequilibrium structures of partially coalesced ACP spherules (Fig. 2.6C). It was proposed that this morphology results from the accumulation of PILP droplets that have partially fused into larger assemblies due to their partially fluidic character. In other words, because the PILP droplets densify with time as they transform into a more stable state, they do not always stay fluidic long enough to coalescence into smooth films, and instead become gel-like spherules before ultimately solidifying into whatever nonequilibrium morphology they had previously adopted.[130,144] Note that spherules are not the same as spherulites, the latter of which are defined as being formed by the radial growth of polycrystals from a central nidus. We use the term spherule to refer to the smaller, micron-sized entities that have a rounded morphology, which suggests they are/were amorphous "particles" (either solid ACP or PILP droplets) prior to crystallization. Amorphous materials are isotropic, and thus their surface energy is minimized by creating a sphere (or filling space in a compartment); in the case of crystals, their surface energy is minimized by expressing the lowest energy crystallographic planes as facets. The PILP spherules were identified as initially being amorphous through in situ observations under polarized light microscopy, where they lacked birefringence in the early stages of the reaction, before they then transformed and crystallized to become brightly birefringent (Fig. 2.11B).[73]

Some CaP agglomerates have also been seen in our own high-resolution analysis of stones (Figs. 2.7A to D). The agglomerates seen here have a rough and more granular texture, and at higher magnification some of the individual units seem to be less spherical; this may be because they are starting to form facets as they transform into the crystalline state (which can occur through dissolution and recrystallization, rather than retention of shape through pseudomorphic transformation). The more granular texture within individual spherules seems to suggest that the precursor nanoparticles were more solid-like in this example.

Calcium oxalate formed via the PILP process can also form such spherule morphologies, and notably, these have a tendency to aggregate and partially coalesce into agglomerates (Fig. 2.6D), or to form more organized assemblies into larger scale spherulites (Fig. 2.11B, central Maltese cross). Calcium oxalate spherulites are prevalent in stones, which will be discussed further in Sections "Aggregation versus spherulitic growth mechanisms" and "Concentric laminations."

Nanogranular and Colloidal Textures

A related feature derived from the CAT mechanism is the nanogranular or colloidal texture of bulk crystals, and this provides another mineralogical signature that appears to be present in some CaOx crystals in stones (Figs. 2.8A and B). In the PILP model system, the mineral films of calcite, which appear smooth at low magnification, also have this colloidal texture when viewed at high magnification via AFM (Fig. 2.8C).[76,155] The dimensions of the colloidal substituents range from approximately 50 to 100 nm for early stage precipitates, but can grow to a few microns in size, becoming the globules mentioned above (where they seem to become more gel-like as they increase in size). The mechanism for how and why this colloidal texture remains is not fully understood. It may be that the precursor is not purely liquid at this stage; and we have observed that the PILP droplets appear to rapidly solidify upon attaching to a surface. Alternatively, there may be remnants of the polymer that had surrounded the colloids, making them remain distinguishable. In any case, the high density of the CAT materials seems unlikely to have formed by simple aggregation of solid particles, which would be expected to lead to far more pore space between particles (unless the nanoparticles partly dissolve and fuse together, which may have been the case in the example of Figure 2.7). Clearly this issue needs further study, but one thing that can be said is that these colloidal textures are not seen in conventionally formed crystals, so this texture is suggestive that some type of CAT mechanism is involved.[64]

Atomic force microscopy of some of the PILP-formed calcite films also showed a layered structure (Fig. 2.8D), and layered textures are often seen in the crystals of stones (Fig. 2.8). In addition, we have found other colloidal textures in the COM crystals of stones (Figs. 2.9A to F), which in these cases appear to be more organized in their assembly (as opposed to the randomly organized globules of CaP core (Fig. 2.6B), or the CaOx structures in Fig. 2.8B). The higher degree of organization could be suggestive of oriented attachment, but given that the colloidal remnants do not appear faceted (thus were not nanocrystals), we believe that they were amorphous and partially fluidic colloids that led to the organized assemblies via other mechanisms. For example, the PILP system has led to highly anisotropic nanofibers of carbonate-based minerals, which were first proposed to arise from an solution-precursor-solid (SPS) mechanism,[156] before the hypothesis was modified to suggest an autocatalytic selective adsorption of PILP droplets at high energy curved protrusions.[157] Kim et al. formed similar nanofibers,[77] but proposed two different mechanisms for the directional assemblies, where they suggested that nanocrystals might assemble by oriented attachment, while the amorphous colloids might assemble by polarization of the copolymer-rich particles. Given that Gower's system did not use copolymers yet produced similar nanofibers, this latter hypothesis seems unlikely. In any case, the nanofibers do not really resemble anything seen in stones, and serve only to demonstrate that directional growth can occur without an oriented attachment mechanism. Perhaps a more pertinent example is the directionality seen on the surface pattern of the layered PILP film

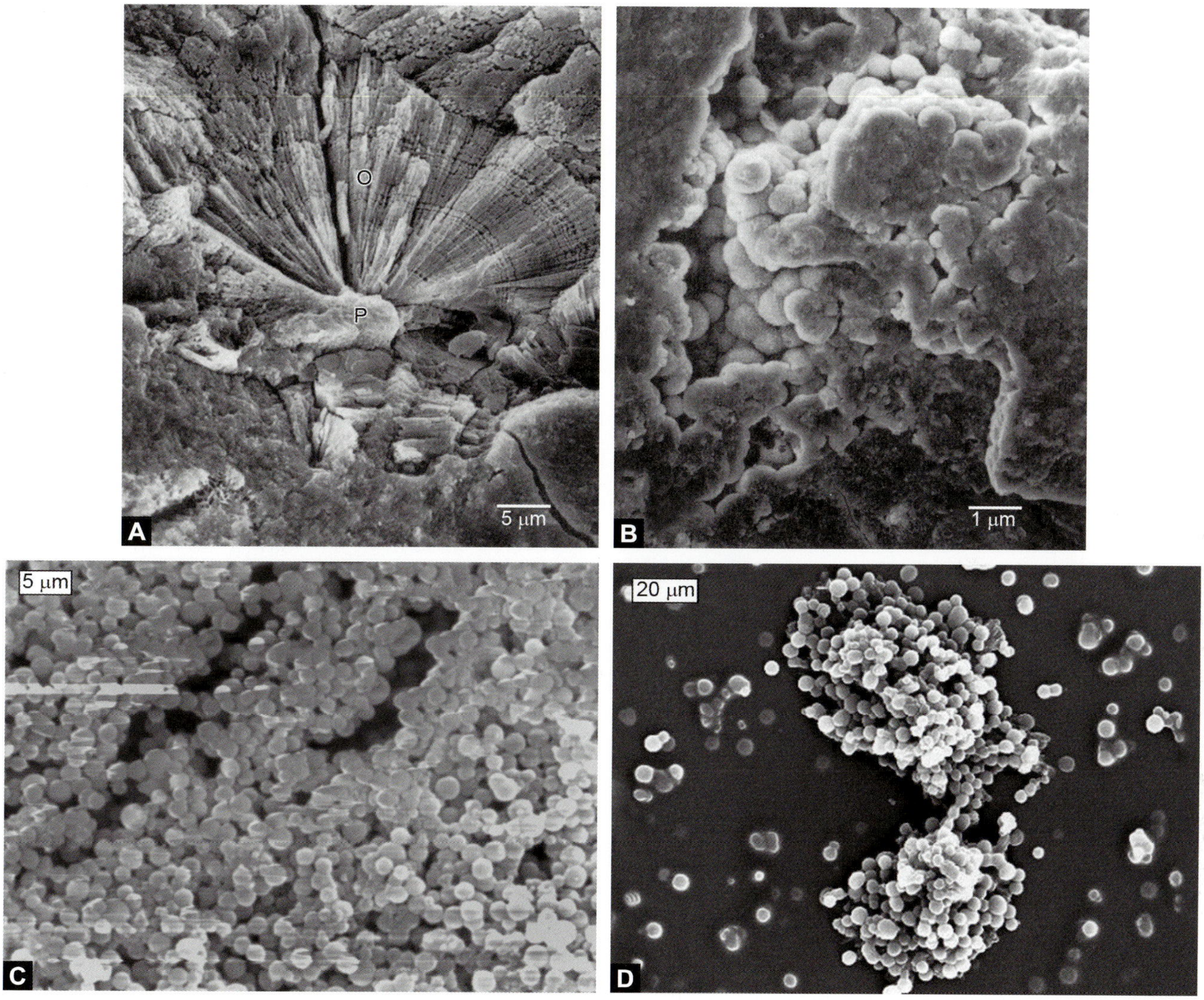

Figs. 2.6A to D: Comparison of textures within a calcium oxalate–calcium phosphate (CaOx-CaP) composite renal stone to polymer-induced liquid precursor-formed spherules. (A) Scanning electron microscopy of the stone shows an outer layer (O) that is composed of CaOx mineral that grew in a radial growth pattern (as a spherulite). Concentric laminations are also seen in the spherulitic region of the stone. The core of the stone is made of CaP mineral (P). (B) When the core is examined at a higher magnification, it appears to be made up of agglomerates of partially coalesced amorphous calcium phosphate (ACP) globules. (C and D) Agglomerated morphologies produced in vitro in the PILP model system using polyaspartate additive. (C) Melded ACP spherules that have partially coalesced (top right) resemble the core of the stone. (D) Aggregation and fusion of CaOx particles that are cemented to a mostly smooth CaOx film, where in the latter case, the PILP droplets were apparently more fluidic.
Source (for Parts A and B): Reprinted with permission from Khan SR. Calcium phosphate/calcium oxalate crystal association in urinary stones: implications for heterogeneous nucleation of calcium oxalate. J Urol. 2015;157(1):376-83.
Source (for Parts C and D): Reprinted with permission from Amos FF, Olszta MJ, Khan SR, et al. Relevance of a polymer-induced liquid-precursor (PILP) mineralization process to normal and pathological biomineralization. Biomineralization—Medical Aspects of Solubility. John Wiley & Sons, Ltd; 2006. Pp. 125-217. doi:10.1002/0470092122.ch4. .

shown in Figure 2.8D. In conclusion, while the actual mechanism of directional assembly remains controversial, this colloidal texture nevertheless appears to be quite common in stones, given that it was observed in all four composite stones that were randomly selected—noting however, that this was not a comprehensive study.

Colloidal surface texture was also observed in pure CaOx stones, but was removed with bleach treatment, indicating that it was comprised of mostly organic matter. The presence of a relatively large amount of organic matter in stones certainly presents some challenges in examining textures that appear to have been once fluidic.

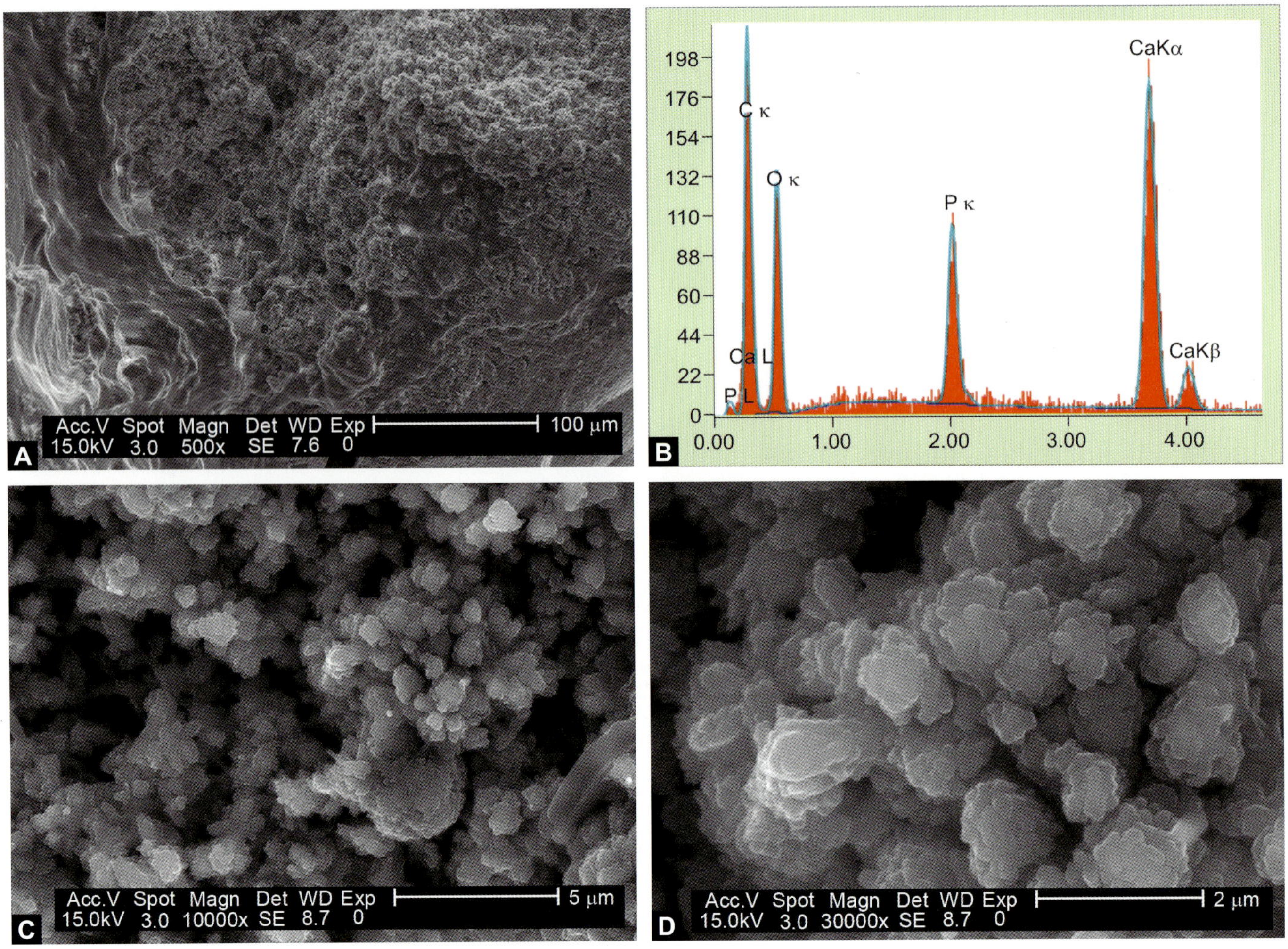

Figs. 2.7A to D: High-resolution scanning electron microscopy of plaque deposits within a calcium oxalate renal stone. At low magnification (A), the energy-dispersive X-ray spectroscopy (EDS) (B) confirms the mineral is calcium phosphate. When examined at a higher magnifications (C and D), the plaque has a similar agglomerated morphology comprised of what appears to be amorphous globules. While many appear to be spherules, they have a rather granular subtexture, and some appear to have flattened surfaces and may be transforming into faceted crystals.

Aggregation versus Spherulitic Growth Mechanisms

There are different mechanisms by which aggregates can form. Aggregates can be formed when many nuclei are formed simultaneously and grow into one another, or mobile crystals may aggregate and attach when they encounter one another.[154] In the latter case, the aggregation of preformed crystals can be exacerbated in the presence of polyelectrolytes, particularly when the polymers have opposite charge. Studies by Wesson et al. demonstrate this type of mechanism in vitro, and then further show that urinary macromolecules from stone formers either did not prevent aggregation, or actually promoted further aggregation of crystals.[158] In these types of aggregation scenarios, there is usually considerable space trapped between crystallites, and the individual crystals exhibit a more faceted crystal habit as their formation follows the classical pathway (Figs. 2.10A and B).[64,130] In the case of HA, spherulitic growth is common, although radial growth of the platelets is not as clearly seen because the platelets themselves are often irregular in shape (Figs. 2.10C and D). These low-density spherulites may even form from an amorphous phase, which typically undergoes dissolution and recrystallization, and thus would still be considered a classical, albeit two-step crystallization. These "classical" types of aggregation mechanism are not the focus of our discussion here. However, it is useful for comparison to the

PILP process, where the space surrounding the forming crystallites is already filled with the fluidic or amorphous precursor, which also crystallizes, so the pseudomorphic transformation type of crystallization tends to produce densely filled mineral structures. This is particularly evident in dense spherulites formed from an amorphous precursor.

It should be noted that spherulites are also called polycrystalline aggregates, but this terminology is misleading given that they do not form by aggregation of preformed crystals.[159] They are instead formed by a growth mechanism where the polycrystals grow radially from a central nidus, producing an overall spherical structure, but with an internal texture revealing the radial polycrystals. Many CaOx stones exhibit this radial texture and are clearly formed by spherulitic growth, which is distinctly different than the aggregation of preformed crystals, described previously. The question is not whether or not these types of stone are formed via spherulitic growth (it is clear that they are); the question is whether the spherulitic growth proceeds via a classical or nonclassical process. We have observed that spherulites formed via the PILP process (Figs. 2.11A to E) differ from spherulites formed via a classical crystallization process because they tend to be fully dense spheres for the reason mentioned above. In contrast, if the polycrystals are grown from solution rather than from within an amorphous globule, the resulting spherulites are not usually as compact because radial growth of needles or lamellae will inherently lead to more space between crystallites as they proceed further and further away from the central core.[130] The exception to this occurs if there is a lot of secondary nucleation (growth of the primary crystals), which can lead to infilling via branches (which occurs in polymer spherulites), or twinning in the case of inorganics; but this situation of secondary nucleation generally requires relatively high supersaturation, which is then also more prone to formation of an amorphous precursor. When examining spherulitic minerals in polarized light microscopy, the radial growth pattern leads to a "Maltese cross" pattern when viewed between crossed polars (Figs. 2.11B and E). This is helpful for examining the dense spherulites, where it would be difficult to identify the individual crystallites in an optical microscope. The CaOx spherulites found in stones typically are densely packed spherulites, as shown in Figure 2.6A, thus it seems likely that they are growing within some type of amorphous precursor. In the PILP model system, it was observed that CaP spherulites were formed from preformed amorphous globules that were relatively soft and gel-like in the early stages (Fig. 2.11E), as evidenced by their weak birefringence and collapse upon drying.[130,143]

Concentric Laminations

As for the concentric laminations seen in stones (*see* Fig. 2.6A), these are usually attributed to daily or dietary growth rings that may occur when the urine becomes intermittently more supersaturated. While this seems reasonable for the layers that are visually seen at the macroscale, we propose an alternative hypothesis for the concentric layers that occur at the nano- to microscale.[130] The banded appearance could be due to a diffusion-limited exclusion of the proteins or other impurities as the precursor phase solidifies. During crystallization, impurities are often excluded, but in this case, they can only be excluded a short distance because the crystallization is taking place in a densifying amorphous phase; thus, one might expect it to lead to entrapped layers of organics.[64] Such a diffusion-limited mechanism has been demonstrated in a 2D system using a combination of polarized light microscopy (Fig. 2.12A) and a fluorescently tagged polymer (Fig. 2.12B), while observing in situ the transformation of PILP-formed $CaCO_3$ films.[130,144] The fluorescein (FITC)-labeled polyAsp gets accumulated in the transition bars. The transition bars are linear (bars) in single crystals because the impurity is excluded along specific crystallographic growth planes, but in the case of radially growing spherulites, the exclusion path leads to transition bars in the form of concentric laminations. The bulk, three-dimensional CaP spherulites formed with the PILP mechanism also exhibit this concentrically laminated structure (*see* Fig. 2.11E).[130,144]

It is intriguing that concentric laminations are also observed at the nanoscale in the CaP nodules of Randall's plaque (Figs. 2.13A to D). The early stage Randall's plaques mineral deposits in the basement membrane appear as electron dense, spherical objects, around 50 nm in diameter, while the later stage, larger deposits show similar alternating rings of mineral (apatite) and organic matrix.[90,93,94,103,109] There is no evidence of crystallites in the early stage, and their round spherule form (without radial polycrystals) suggests that they may form via an amorphous precursor,[146] as already postulated. The early stage PILP droplets form at a similar size scale (50–100 nm), so it is feasible that if a critical supersaturation of CaP ions forms in the renal tissue, and in the presence of various "inhibitory" proteins (to crystallization), the system might

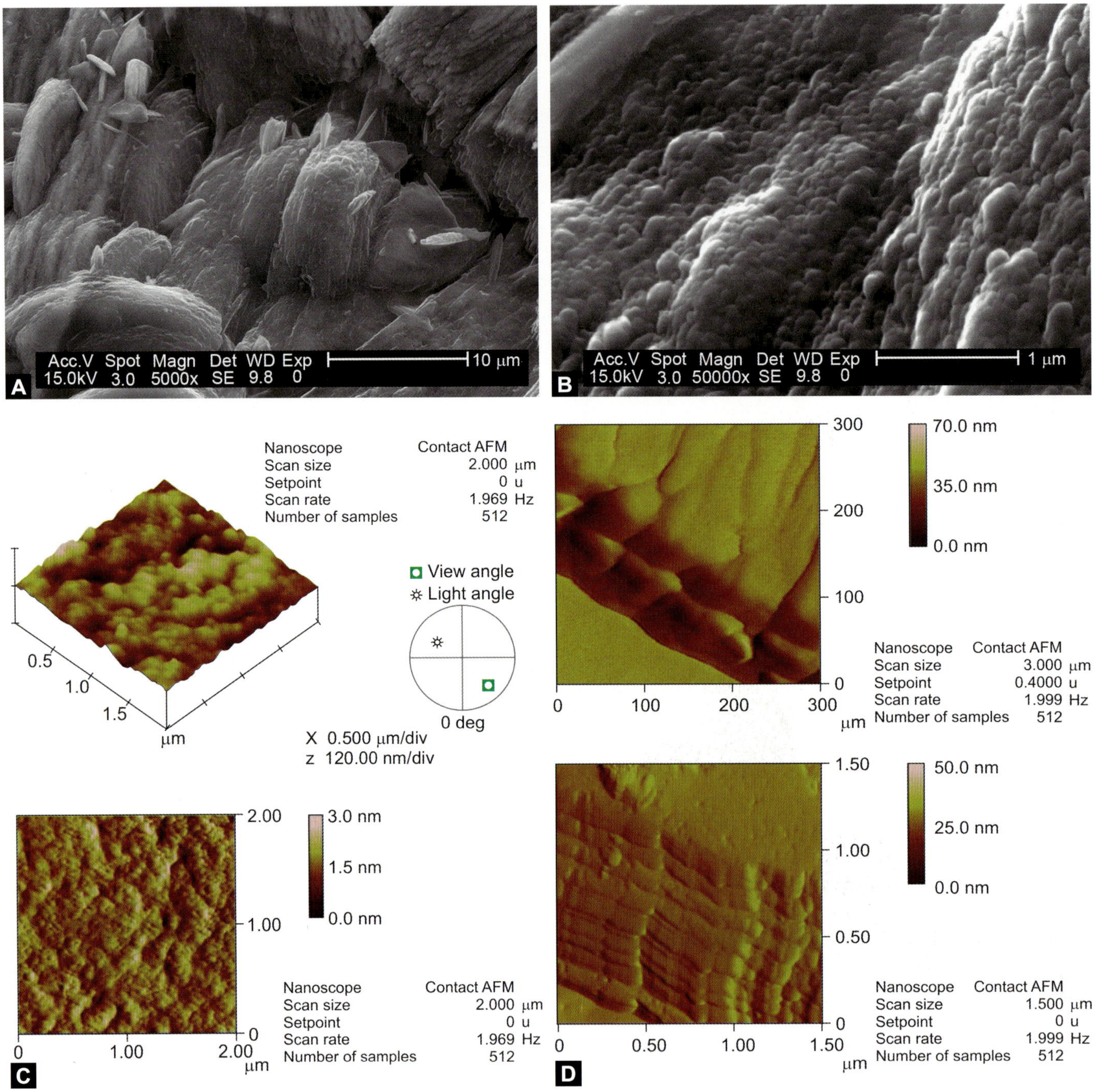

Figs. 2.8A to D: Comparison of the colloidal nanotexture in stones and polymer-induced liquid precursor (PILP)-formed films. To note, this sample was first treated with sodium hypochlorite (active chlorine 13%) for 60 minutes to remove organics, and thus verify that the colloidal structures present are indeed mineral and not organics. (A) Low magnification scanning electron microscopy of some oblong calcium oxalate monohydrate (COM) crystals in a native kidney stone. The fin-like outgrowths are likely from dissolution and recrystallization of some of the underlying amorphous material. (B) At higher magnification, the crystals exhibit a colloidal texture on their surfaces. Nearly all COM crystals of this type in the stones we examined displayed this texture. (C) PILP-formed calcite films also exhibit this colloidal texture, in this case imaged by atomic force microscopy (height mode and defection mode are shown on the top and bottom, respectively). The top surface of this film (which faced the air–water interface in a Langmuir trough) was relatively rough, while the bottom surface that faced the solution was smoother, similar to that shown in Figure 2.4. (D) These calcite films sometimes also develop an internal layered nanostructure.

Source (for Parts C and D): Reprinted with permission from Amos FF. Template-Assisted Mineral Formation via an Amorphous Liquid Phase Precursor Route. Gainesville, University of Florida, 2005.

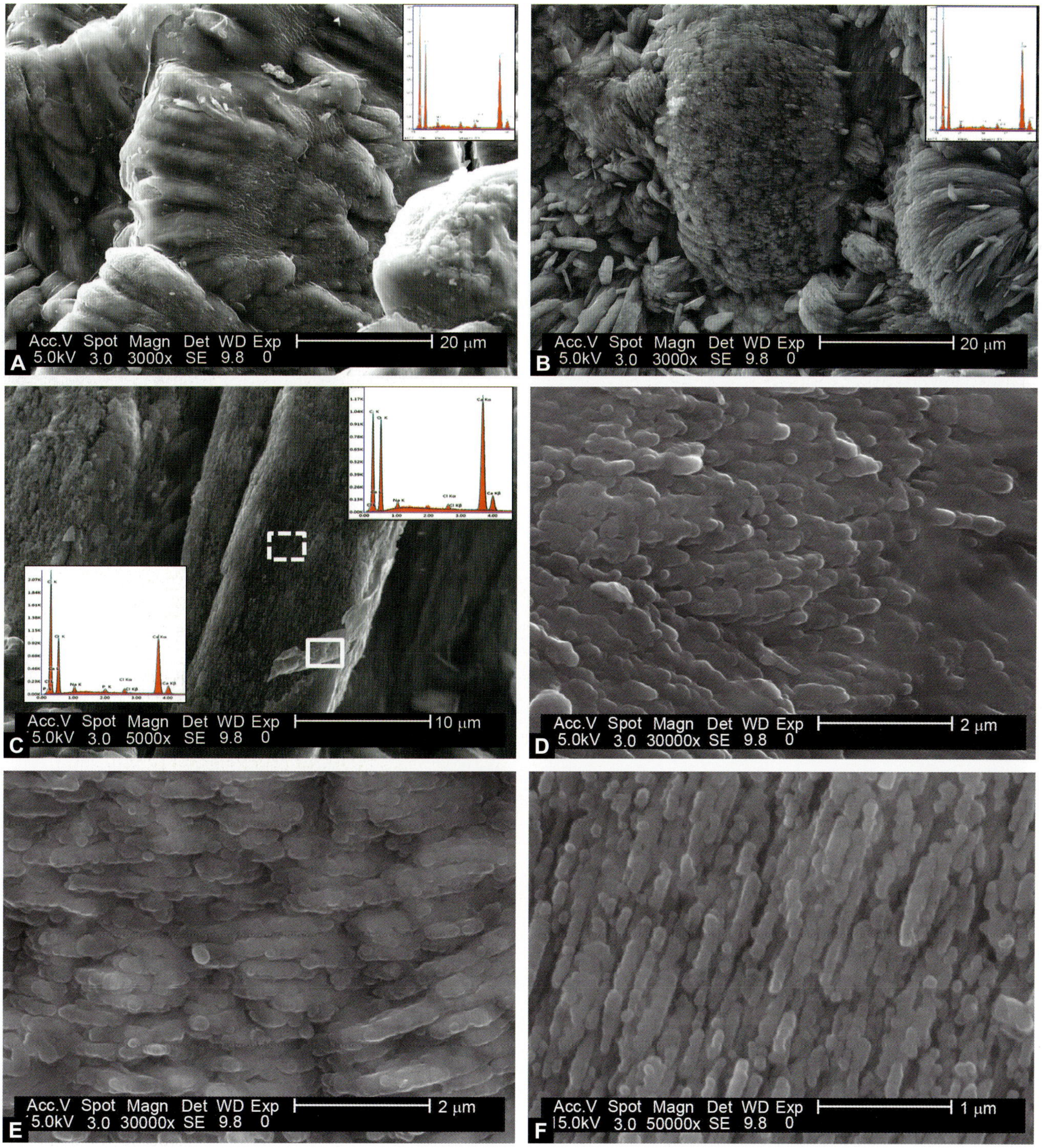

Figs. 2.9A to F: Scanning electron microscopy of calcium oxalate (CaOx) deposits on and within a CaOx renal stone, demonstrating the directional assemblies of some colloidal precursor particles. To note, the stones shown here were also treated with sodium hypochlorite (active chlorine 13%) for 60 minutes to remove organics. At lower magnification (A, C, and E), energy-dispersive X-ray spectroscopy (EDS) confirms the mineral is CaOx, and based on the plate-like, tabular morphology, the phase is likely calcium oxalate monohydrate. (D to F) When examined at higher magnifications, the crystals exhibit a colloidal texture, but the more organized structures appear to have formed from a directional accumulation of the precursor nanoparticles/droplets, leading to structures stacked into sheets or plates of mineral. Note in (D), there appears to be some organic material remaining, which was fairly thick and appears to be peeling off the crystal that it coated. The organic matter correlates to the larger carbon peak seen in the EDS spectrum (bottom left inset) taken of the region in the dashed box, in comparison to the more pure mineral phase (dashed box), which shows a lower amount of carbon in its EDS spectrum (top right inset).

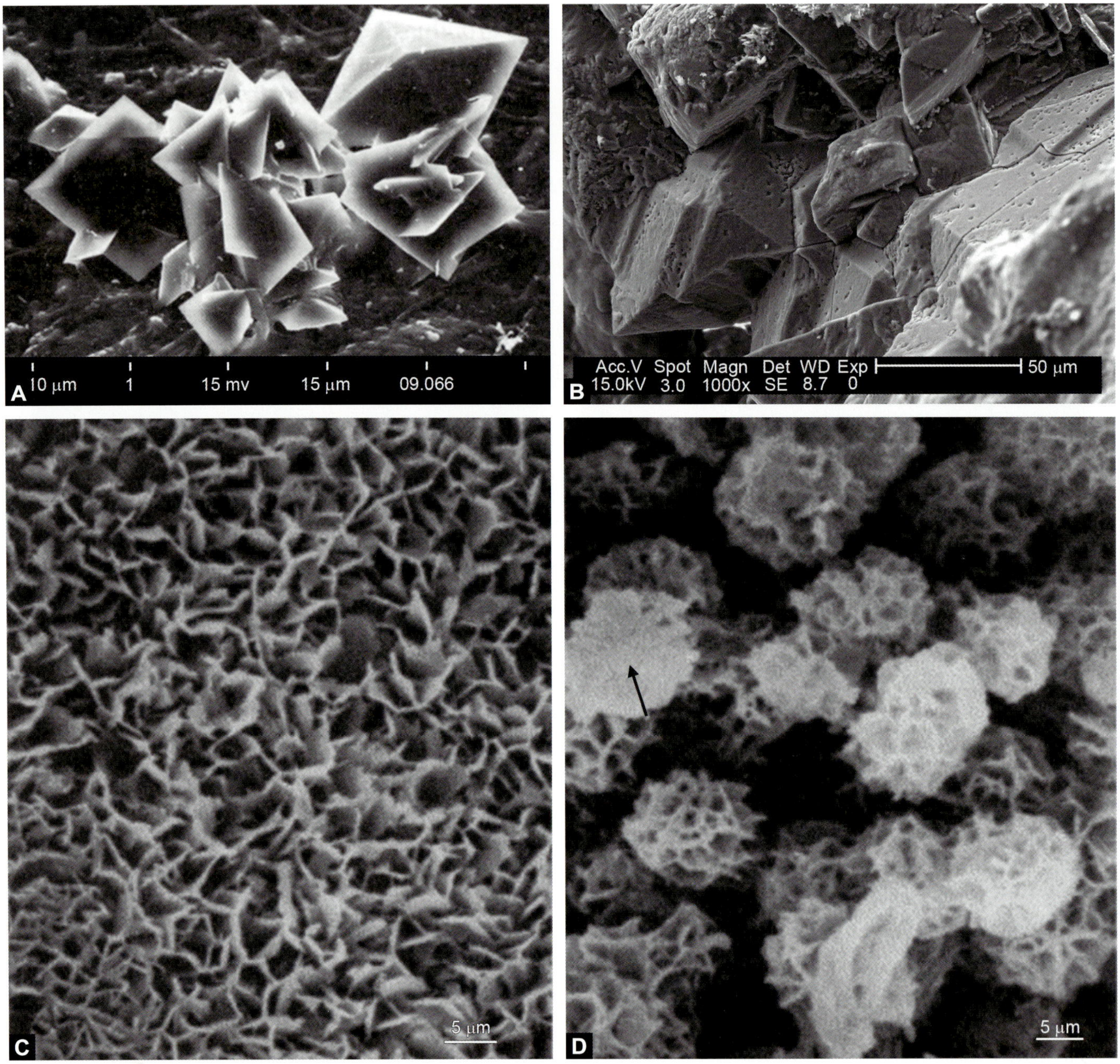

Figs. 2.10A to D: Aggregates in stones that appear to have formed from a more classical growth mechanism. (A and B) Aggregates of calcium oxalate crystals in stones with preformed and intergrown crystals with a faceted habit. Based on the bipyramid morphology, the phase is likely calcium oxalate dihydrate. (B) If one zooms in on the single crystals, numerous pores can be seen. The prevalence of pores is often an indication that the single crystals had entrapped organic impurities during their formation; but they still appear to have formed via a classical crystallization. (C and D) Scanning electron microscope of calcium phosphate stones that were experimentally induced in male rats. Individual hydroxyapatite crystals have an irregular platy shape, and if there is a high nucleation density, can either form an entire coating of mineral crust; or can form more clearly as spherical aggregates (spherulites) if the precipitates are more isolated. The growth texture may not appear to be radial, and this may be because these structures often form from an amorphous precursor.
Source (for Part A): Reprinted with permission from Amos FF, Olszta MJ, Khan SR, et al. Relevance of a polymer-induced liquid-precursor (PILP) mineralization process to normal and pathological biomineralization. Biomineralization—Medical Aspects of Solubility. John Wiley & Sons, Ltd; 2006. pp. 125-217.
Source (for Parts C and D): Reprinted with permission from Khan SR. Calcium phosphate/calcium oxalate crystal association in urinary stones: implications for heterogeneous nucleation of calcium oxalate. J Urol. 2015;157(1):376-83.

"crash out" with either liquid-liquid phase separation of PILP type droplets, or amorphous solid particles. The formation of ACP is common place, even without polymer additive, given its low solubility. Grases et al.,[160] who used AFM to study the in vitro formation of ACP spherules, found that the spherules (on the order of 50–200 mm) were formed via assembly of Posner clusters to nanoparticles to microparticles. It would be reasonable to predict that, given the various organics present in the physiological tissue, if they become entrapped in the mineral precursor, they would hinder crystallization until they were excluded, which might thereby lead to such layering. However, this layering phenomenon has not yet been demonstrated in vitro at the nanoscale.

To note, the calcium-based mineral and the size of the RP spherules differ substantially from the PILP products, which are comprised of $CaCO_3$ and CaP spherulites on the order of tens of microns in size,[130,144] while the CaP spherules in RP are on the order of tens of nanometers in size.[93] Thus this feature deserves further study to determine if it is due to the same formation mechanism. Nevertheless, it seems unlikely that the layering at the nanoscale in RP could be caused by intermittent mineral-organic deposition, so we believe that exclusion of the impurity as the phase solidifies may be a more reasonable explanation. However, given the very different length scales for the RP nodule layers (nanoscale layering) versus those in the $CaCO_3$ and CaP PILP systems (micron scale layering), the shorter diffusion distances in the nodules suggest that the precursor in the tissue becomes solid-like more quickly. On the other hand, the layering seen in the CaOx spherulitic regions of stones is quite consistent with the micron scale layering in the PILP model system. We are currently developing a plaque model system to determine if this nanoscale feature can be reproduced in vitro, along with the microscale features.

Layered Crystalline Aggregates and Single Crystals

One intriguing "aggregate" pattern seen in stones is the stacks of tablets, as seen in Figures 2.14A to D. It is difficult to imagine that such densely packed and well-organized layers could arise from aggregation of preformed crystals, where they would have had to match themselves with tablets of the same size, and then align themselves into such a registry. Therefore, we offer some other possible mechanisms based on observations of similar structures in the literature. In the case of uric acid stones, sometimes stacks of crystals form because the first formed precipitates of uric acid dihydrate transform into the more stable anhydrous form.[161] By analogy, such a transformation might be expected for the COT or COD metastable forms of CaOx, which in time should transform into the more stable COM phase. The loss of water leads to the volume contraction that sometimes causes cracks to form or a breakup of the overall crystal morphology.

In addition to the CaOx stacked superstructures discussed above, comparable morphologies of adjacently situated platelets of calcite have been generated in vitro. In one example, analogous stacked superstructures of pseudohexagonal calcite platelets were synthesized in vitro within water-in-oil microemulsions (Figs. 2.15A and B).[162] In this system, single hexagonal calcite platelets 20 nm in thickness are formed, on the surfaces of which spiral steps produce a propagating helical stacked outgrowth. Recurrence of this process over time results in the formation of crystallographically aligned stacks of interlocked platelets oriented in the {001} plane, interspaced with the surfactant molecules used in synthesis. These stacked tabular structures appear similar in morphology to those observed in Figure 2.14A. Interestingly, the width of the platelets along the growth axis was variable, whereas the thickness of approximately 20 nm remained constant. However, while the morphology appears similar to the stacked tablets in stones, the reaction conditions differ substantially given that there is no organic solvent present within the urine to facilitate the microemulsion synthesis of stacks. Nevertheless, one could imagine other factors leading to spiral outgrowths and formation of stacked superstructures. Indeed, in the PILP system spiral growth of PILP films that coated vaterite spherulites produced large helical structures of vaterite (a metastable phase of $CaCO_3$). While this is not helical stacks of thin tablets, it demonstrates the propensity for forming spiral or screw type defects.

Another group has shown similar superstructures, but in aqueous-based conditions, where stacks of calcite platelets assemble into pillars when using the polyelectrolyte poly (acrylic acid) (Figs. 2.15C and D).[163] Notably, this polymer is commonly used to generate a PILP precursor, so it is possible that the nanoparticles are PILP-like droplets.[64] In their system, the stacks of plates were grown on a variety of calcite substrates, and interestingly, regardless of the crystallographic orientation of the face on which the stacks were grown, the platelets were always aligned parallel to the {104} plane (the most stable plane of calcite). This could arise from microfaceting,[163] which often occurs in crystals with nonequilibrium morphologies

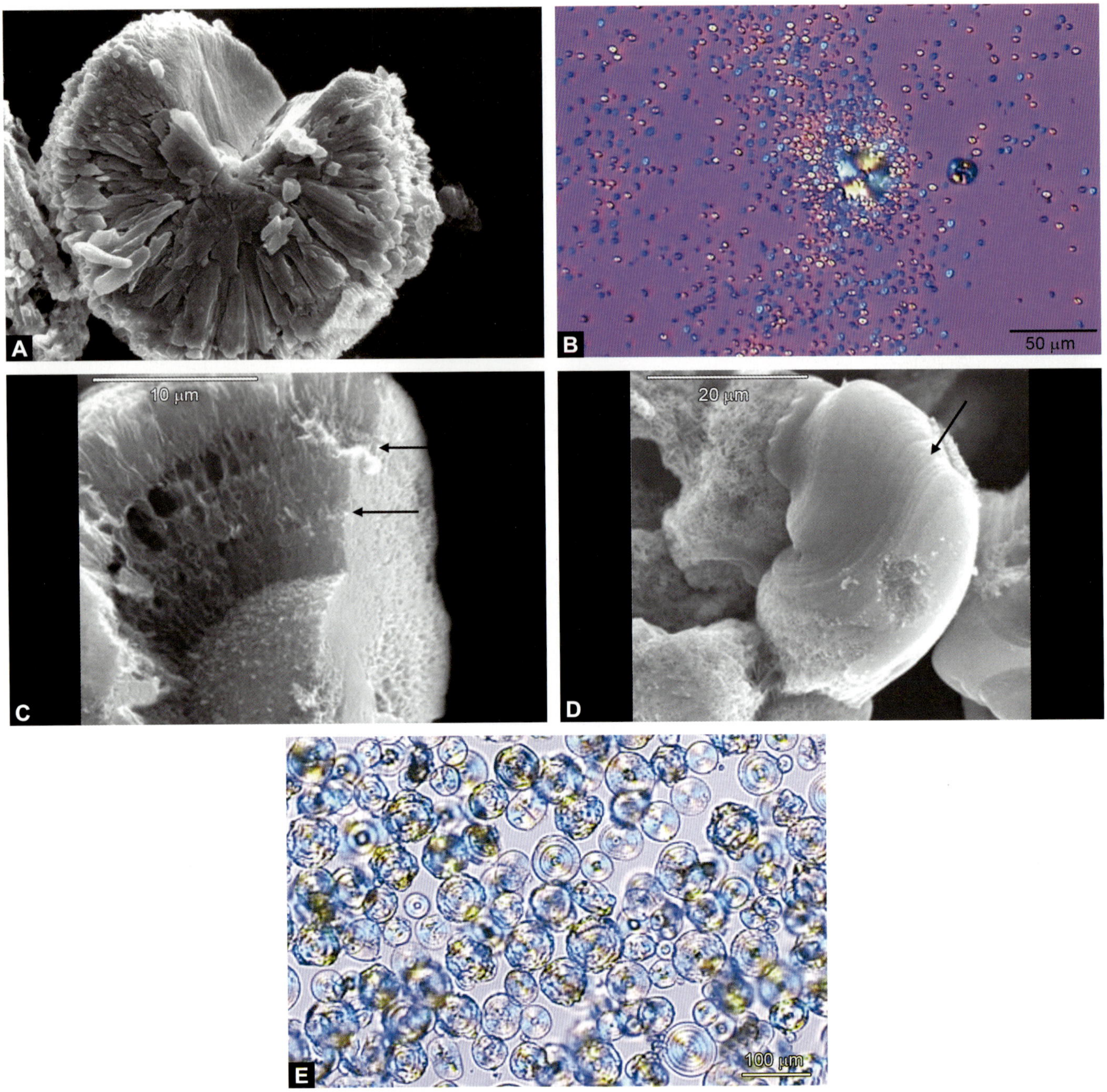

Figs. 2.11A to E: Dense spherulites produced via the polymer-induced liquid precursor (PILP) process in both (A and B) calcium oxalate (CaOx) and (C and D) calcium phosphate (CaP) mineral. (A) The CaOx spherulite has a radial texture and appears to be a relatively dense polycrystalline aggregate. (B) During formation, the precursor droplets (which are now crystalline spherules, and therefore birefringent) can be seen as having aggregated into a spherulite in the middle, as evidenced by the Maltese cross (the cross is magenta in color when using the first-order red waveplate). The tiny spherules do not have a Maltese cross, and are therefore not spherulites; they are instead single crystals with a nonequilibrium morphology created by pseudomorphic transformation. (C and D) The CaP spherulites are also densely packed, and the laminated textures can be seen both in (C and D, arrows) scanning electron microscopy and (E) with polarized light microscopy. Their faint birefringence is because they have not yet fully crystallized.

Source (for Parts A, B and E): Reprinted with permission from Amos FF, Olszta MJ, Khan SR, et al. Relevance of a polymer-induced liquid-precursor (PILP) mineralization process to normal and pathological biomineralization. Biomineralization—Medical Aspects of Solubility. John Wiley & Sons, Ltd.; 2006. pp. 125-217.

Source (for Parts C and D): Reprinted with permission from Amos FF, Dai L, Kumar R, et al. Mechanism of formation of concentrically laminated spherules: implication to Randall's plaque and stone formation. Urol Res. 2009;37:11-7.

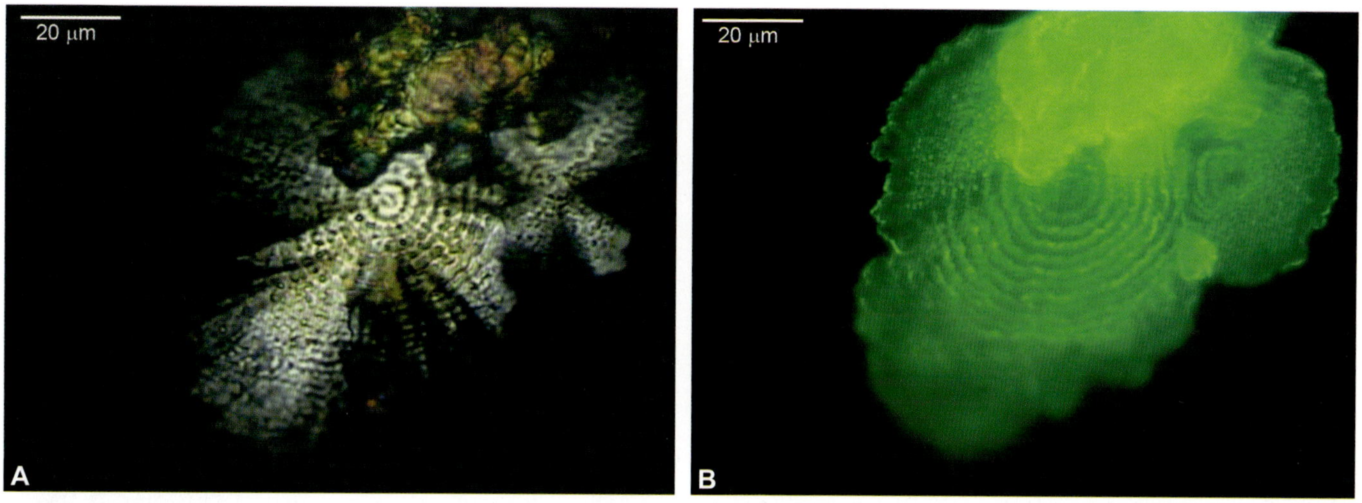

Figs. 2.12A and B: Concentric laminations seen in polymer-induced liquid precursor (PILP)-formed calcium carbonate films. (A) Polarized light microscopy shows concentric rings that occur during the amorphous to crystalline transformation as radial growth proceeds outward during the growth of the spherulite. (B) When viewing the same sample in fluorescence microscopy, the fluorescein (FITC)-labeled polyaspartate demonstrates that the "transition bars" are created by diffusion-limited exclusion of the polymer, which occurs because it is an impurity to the crystallization. Note, these laminations are spaced at about a couple of microns.
Source: Reprinted with permission from Amos FF, Olszta MJ, Khan SR, et al. Relevance of a polymer-induced liquid-precursor (PILP) mineralization process to normal and pathological biomineralization. Biomineralization—Medical Aspects of Solubility. John Wiley & Sons, Ltd; 2006. pp. 125-217.

(which transformed from an amorphous phase) to reduce the energetically unfavorable curved surfaces of a crystal fiber.[156] Atomic force microscopy studies during growth of the pillars show that unlike the microemulsion system, the stacks of plates are formed from anisotropic assembly of small amorphous or liquid-like nanoparticles stabilized by the polyelectrolyte. So while both methods generate morphologies similar to that seen in Figure 2.14, the possible growth modes for genesis of such structures are merely suggested and not fully elucidated. In the stone examples we have examined, there is not any evidence thus far to suggest that the screw type growth has occurred. For example, in Figure 2.14C and D (crystal on the left), the stacks appear to be within single crystals of COM. In Figures 2.14A and B, the stacks appear to be more like partial spherulites whose growth in all directions is stunted by growth in confinement (crowding from a high nucleation density restricts outward growth). So we have searched for other possibilities to consider.

The layered crystals, particularly those that are single-crystalline (Figs. 2.14C and D), bear some resemblance to crystals grown in hydrogels. As shown by Estroff et al. in their hydrogel model system,[164] depending on the strength of the gel, the organic fibers can become overgrown by the crystal in strong gels, leading to homogeneous incorporation of organic throughout the crystal, while in weaker gels, the struts of the gel can get pushed outward from the crystallization pressure, leading to a more heterogeneous incorporation of fibrils throughout the crystal, resulting in a breakdown of the crystal structure that sometimes forms layers. An assortment of morphologies was produced in their gel-grown crystals, ranging from distorted crystals with some layering, to dense spherulitic structures (but none that fully resemble these stacks). The growth in gels mechanism might be thought of as an extreme example of the transition bars shown in the PILP system, where there is a much larger amount of organic material to deal with in crystallization in gels. In this case, however, the organic chains are crosslinked, thereby restricting themselves from being fully excluded, rather than the densifying precursor limiting diffusion in the PILP system. Both of these processes lead to the occlusion of organic impurities. This is seen in some stone samples, where one can see numerous small pores where the entrapped organics reside and lead to such defects, even in the well-faceted single crystals that presumably formed by the classical mechanism (*see* Fig. 2.10B). In the stacked tablets example, the large space between layers may also be from entrapped organics that disrupted the crystal growth. It should be noted that crystals grown in gels have been shown to sometimes first form an amorphous phase, so these processes may not be

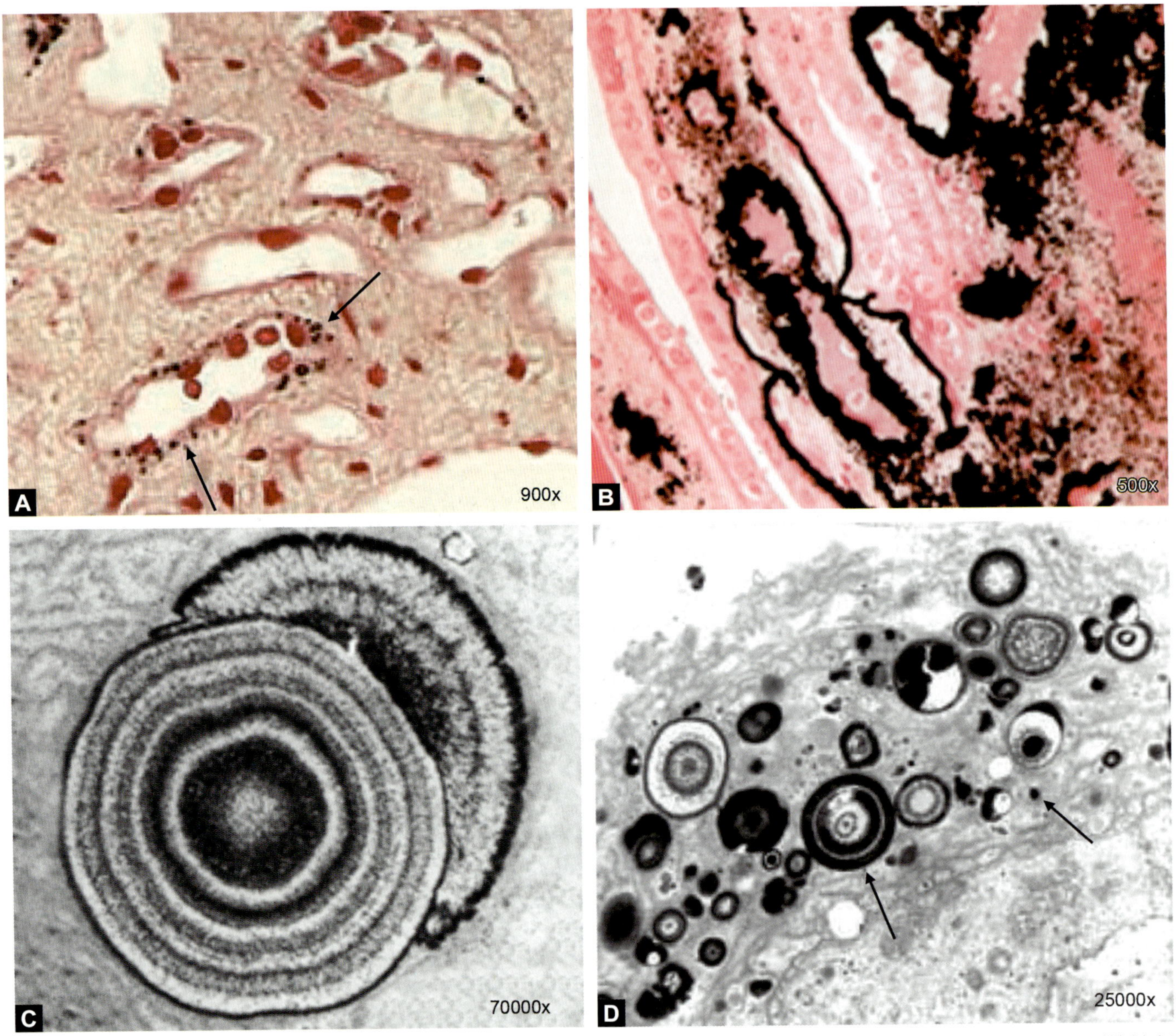

Figs. 2.13A to D: Histology and transmission electron microscopy (TEM) images of the earliest stages of Randall's plaques. (A) Light micrographs of stained sections show that spherules first appear in the basement membrane of the thin loops of Henle (arrows). (B) Accumulation of mineral as it spreads throughout the interstitium in the early stages of Randall's plaques. (C) Closer examination using TEM shows early stage calcium phosphate (CaP) spherules with alternating light (mineral) and electron dense (stained organic) rings. Individual spherules are found to be ~50 nm in diameter. (D) As the spherules grow, one can see that the location of organic material is quite variable, yet there does appear to be a central dark core in many of these, suggesting that the precursor phase may nucleate on some organic nidus, such as accumulated protein or cellular debris.
Source: Reprinted with permission from Evan A, Lingeman J, Coe FL, et al. Randall's plaque: pathogenesis and role in calcium oxalate nephrolithiasis. Kidney Int. 2006;69:1313-8.

mutually exclusive. Given the prevalence of this texture in stones, further studies are warranted.

Mineral Cement

The amorphous phase, depending on its degree of fluidity, can also seep into cracks and crevices between preformed crystals by capillary action, and then solidify, acting as a mineral cement by fastening the crystals together. This has been frequently observed in the $CaCO_3$ PILP system, where the precursor seeps in between crystals and cements them together (*see* Fig. 45 in Gower's Chemical Reviews paper).[64] This may occur in stone formation,

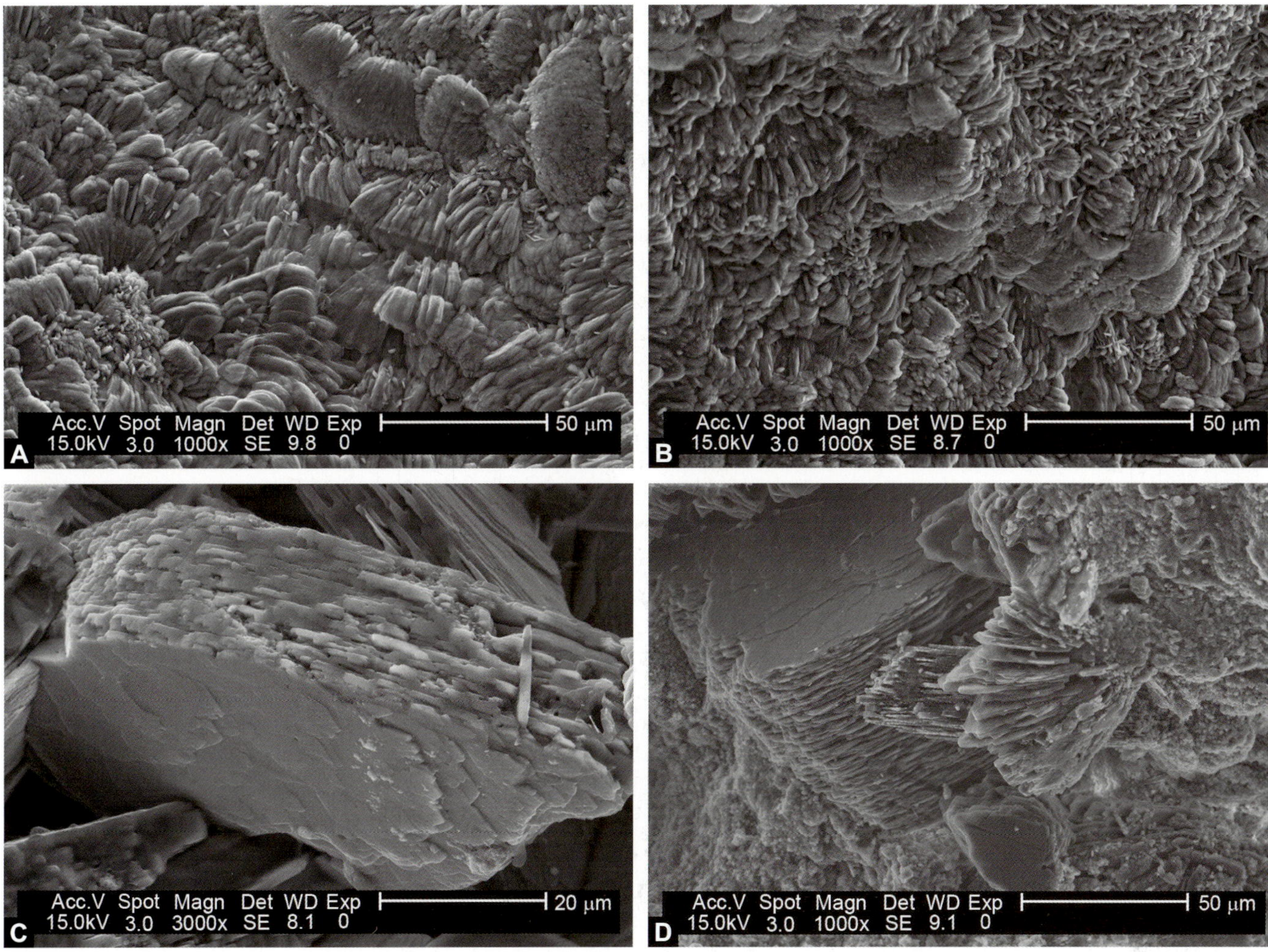

Figs. 2.14A to D: Layered aggregates and crystals in stones. (A) Aggregates consisting of densely packed stacks of tabular crystals were prevalent in this stone. The formation mechanism is an enigma, but may be related to growth in gels, and/or a high nucleation density. Some stacks even appear to be partial spherulites that could not grow radially due to the confined space. (B) Similar region with a high density of polycrystals, but with more rod-like bundles, rather than stacks of parallel tablets. This example also gives the impression that there is a high density of nucleation sites. (C) This individual crystal has layering, but it is most likely a single crystal, and not an aggregate, but exhibits this mesocrystalline texture once the organic matter has been removed by the bleach treatment. Note, jagged microfacets have formed on the bottom surface, which likely occurred to lower its surface energy since it had a somewhat curved surface initially. (D) In this example, a similar layering pattern is seen in what appears to be a large mesocrystal on the left. Microfaceting is seen on its surface where it appears to be transforming into a single crystal. There is another entity in the middle right that is growing platelets that splay outward and are not stacked in parallel, resembling part of a spherulite. All of these strange stacked crystals are surrounded by what appears to be a whole mesh of amorphous granules. Thus, we infer that these layered crystals are transforming from an amorphous phase, but not in a pseudomorphic transformation. There may be localized dissolution and recrystallization that leads to these layers.

leaving to very cohesive, densely packed monoliths. It can be difficult to define a mineralogical signature for this, but one might expect nonequilibrium morphologies, perhaps with a fluidic appearance from the seeping precursor phase (Figs. 2.16A and B). In our limited analysis of stones, the evidence for this was not as straightforward. For example, the CaOx bundles shown in Figure. 2.9A appear to be cemented together; however, we are not certain if that is a mineral cement or organic coating. Although the sample was bleached, a very thick organic layer may not have been fully removed. Given the smoother texture and stretchy appearance in some regions, as well as somewhat lighter contrast than surrounding mineral, we suspect this is an organic coating. In comparison, the interconnections

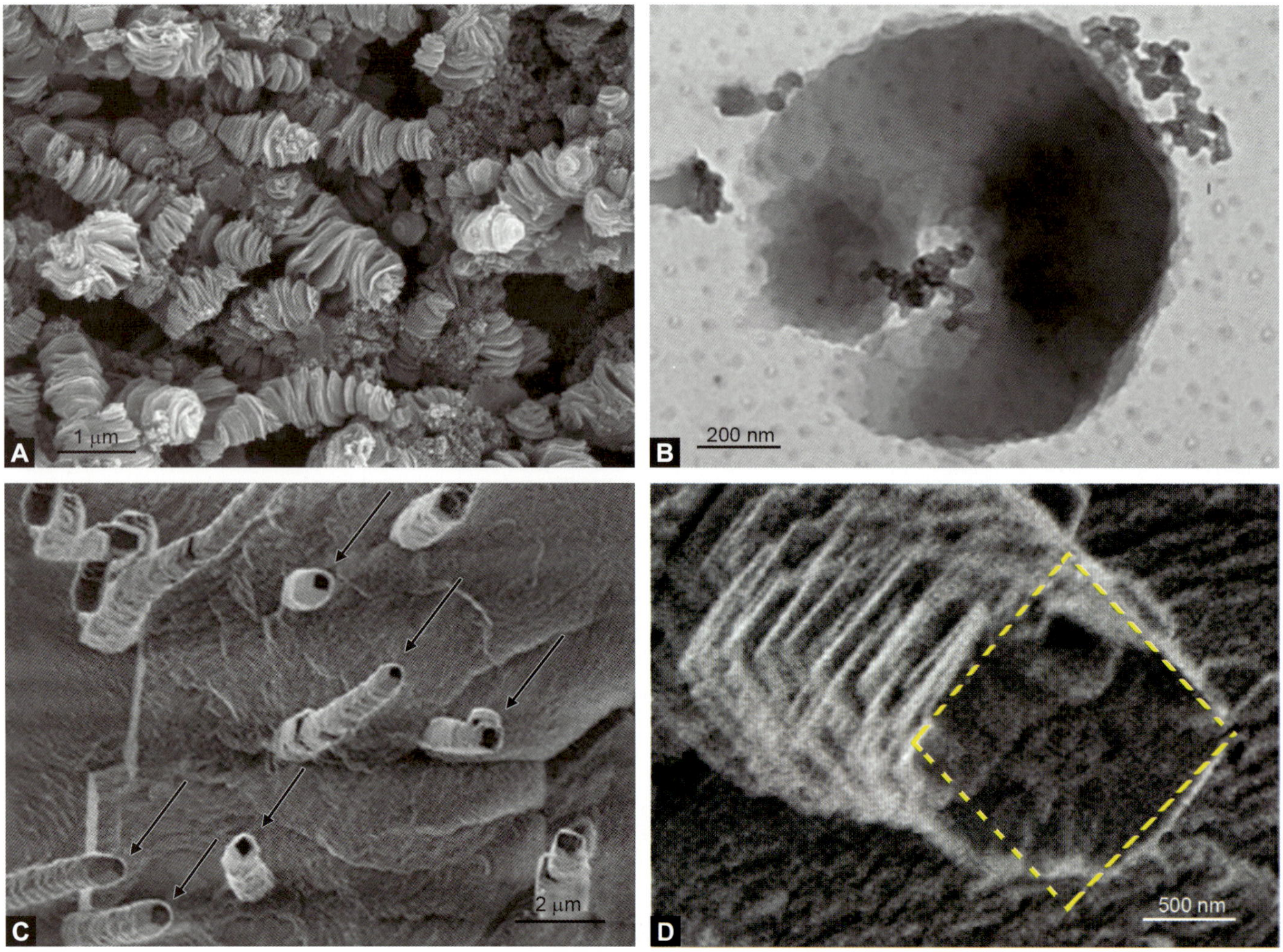

Figs. 2.15A to D: Comparative stacked superstructures observed in the calcium carbonate literature from Viravaidya et al. and Long et al., respectively. (A) Scanning electron microscopic image showing stacked lamellar calcite superstructures, (B) transmission electron microscope of a primary plate-like crystal showing spiral outgrowth that produces such stacks by helical propagation. Although not discussed in the paper, there does appear to be aggregation of colloidal precursors (with dark contrast expected for mineral phase) surrounding this growing crystal. The waviness of some of the "tablets" is also suggestive of a polymer-induced liquid precursor-like precursor. (C and D) Low and high magnification SEM micrographs, respectively, show stacked calcite micropillars that were observed via AFM to form from rounded precursor nanoparticles that aggregated in an anistropic (1D) fashion, and upon fusion and growth, they reorganized into the microfaceted pillars. In this case, the microfaceting appears to result from iso epitaxy with the underlying (104) calcite template during the amorphous to crystalline transformation.

Source (for Parts A and B): Reprinted with permission from Viravaidya C, Li M and Mann S. Microemulsion-based synthesis of stacked calcium carbonate (calcite) superstructures. Chem Commun. 2004;(19):2182-3.

Source (for Parts C and D): Reprinted with permission from Long X, Ma Y, Cho KR, et al. Oriented calcite micropillars and prisms formed through aggregation and recrystallization of poly(acrylic acid) stabilized nanoparticles. Cryst Growth Des. 2013;13:3856-63.

between tablets in Figure 2.16B appear to be of the same consistency and contrast as the crystallites (scanning electron microscope contrast is influenced by atomic number), so we believe that this is an example of mineral cement.[64,130] These crystals are less space filling because the tabular crystals likely grew from solution or a gel before they infilled with mineral. Lastly, all of this discussion is assuming the precursor has not changed its morphology, which as discussed in Section "Intermediate Textures" is not always the case.

Collagen Mineralization

While it has been theorized that RP mineral first forms as spherules in the basement membrane, which then spreads into the interstitium (*see* Figs. 2.13A and B),[93,94] some evidence shows early stage mineral starting within collagen fibrils and/or on matrix vesicles present in the interstitium.[103,165] Collagen is generally a poor nucleator of HA, and requires relatively high supersaturations and, even then, HA crystals nucleate predominantly as extrafibrillar spherulites on the surface of the scaffold (Fig. 2.17A). At very high concentrations, the spherulites merge and grow into a thick crust of platelets that coat the surface of the scaffold (analogous to the crust shown in Fig. 2.10C). However, using acidic (anionic) polymer additives, Gower's group has been able to promote intrafibrillar mineralization of type-I collagen via the PILP process (Fig. 2.17B), as discussed in part 1 of this chapter. To recap, the hypothesis is that the fluidic properties of the amorphous precursor droplets enable them to be drawn into the gaps and grooves of the collagen fibrils by capillary forces (Fig. 2.17C).[82,145,147] Others have suggested that solid amorphous precursor nanoparticles diffuse into the gap zones of the collagen fibrils.[83] In either case, the collagen fibrils become infiltrated with the amorphous mineral precursor, which then crystallizes into nano-sized HA crystals embedded within the interstices of the collagen fibril.[82,145] Notably, a dark banding pattern is seen in the TEM images of collagen found in the interstitial plaque, and this contrast pattern created by mineral (without stain) is usually indicative of intrafibrillar mineral.[90,103] Thus, it is possible that the collagen in the interstitial plaque helps stimulate the mineral formation, as we have observed in our model system. In the latter case, while the acidic polymer is highly inhibitory to crystallization (the solution remains clear and free of precipitates), when a collagen matrix is added, the mineral precursor nanodroplets are sequestered directly into the fibrils, which can be observed as a whitening and stiffening of the matrix as it becomes infiltrated with mineral. This ability of collagen to "promote" mineralization (in a solution stabilized with precursor) is particularly relevant to stone formation, because various cells may be secreting "inhibitory" proteins to keep the mineral phase from nucleating, but if the supersaturation becomes high enough, precursor nanodroplets may crash out of the solution, and with collagen fibrils nearby, the nanodroplets would be able to infiltrate and crystallize. For example, osteopontin is a multifunctional protein secreted by renal epithelial cells as well as macrophages (which may be present if the kidney tissue is inflamed), and although osteopontin (OPN) is a well-known "inhibitor" of crystal nucleation, Gower's group has shown that it leads to rapid mineralization of collagen (Fig. 2.17B), while the surrounding solution stays clear (stabilized) for several days. This even occurs when using biogenic tissue, as seen in decellularized porcine kidneys mineralized with OPN (Fig. 2.17D).

Interestingly, intrafibrillar mineral often occurs before any mineral is found on the surface of the fibrils, which is the opposite of the conventional crystallization (without polymer), where the mineral spherulites form predominantly on the surface of the fibrils.[145,151,152] Both types of CaP mineral seem to be present in stones, where some images in the literature show spherulitic clusters of platy HA crystallites (Figs. 2.10C and D),[113,119] while others are more suggestive of collagen associated intrafibrillar mineral.[90,103]

Intermediate Textures

It was shown in an ex situ study by Khan that just underneath or at the surface of the papillary epithelium where the plaque had broken across, spherulites with fine, radial crystallites appear to be embedded underneath the mineralized fibrous collagen layer.[113] This extrafibrillar crystal crust (not shown here) resembles the spherulites shown in Figure 2.17A, and may have occurred where the mineral was not confined by the collagen at the papillary tip where the matrix terminates, or when the collagen had already been completely filled with mineral.[146] These deposits appear somewhat denser than the CaP spherulites produced in a classical crystallization (*see* Fig. 2.10C). As described previously, the spherulites produced in the conventional mineralization are usually porous due to the separate nature of the platy polycrystals, but some of the spherulites found in Randall's plaques appear more dense.[103] It is likely that spherulites with this intermediate texture originated as an amorphous phase, which ultimately broke down into faceted crystals. In our CaP PILP system, the driving force to form faceted crystals appears to be quite strong, and it is therefore far less common to have a pseudomorphic transformation of ACP. For example, the oddly-shaped twisting mineral precursor shown in Figure 2.18A was clearly formed from a dense amorphous phase, but is now transforming into platelets (Fig. 2.18B). Interestingly, this seems to be occurring from the inside out, rather than via dissolution and recrystallization, which one would think would start at the surface. In contrast, the CaOx mesocrystal shown in Figure 2.14C appears

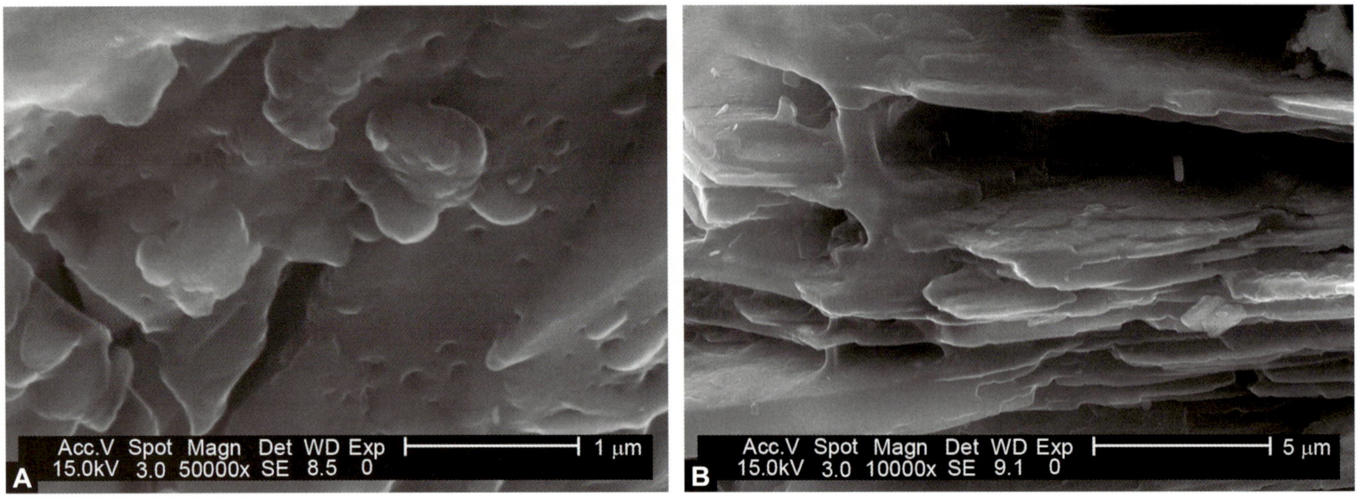

Figs. 2.16A and B: High magnification scanning electron microscopy zoomed into some stone regions showing cementitious mineral. The samples were first treated with bleach to remove organics, which can look similar. (A) The nondescript and globby morphology suggests that a liquid-like or gel precursor had coated the crystal. (B) The layers in this aggregate appear to be cemented together with mineral struts. There is no evidence of a discontinuity with the crystals, and the uniform contrast with the mineral layers suggests that the struts are also mineral.

to be undergoing some dissolution/recrystallization, as judging from the microfacets present on bottom surface. Microfacets are also seen on the top surface of the layered crystal in Figure 2.14D.

The various transformation mechanisms of precursor phases are not yet well understood. Given that we first stated that facets and equilibrium morphologies tend to be indicators of classical crystallization, it becomes painfully clear that it can become difficult to decipher the original formation mechanism, particularly if the precursor transforms by a dissolution and recrystallization process. At this point, we consider the colloidal nanotexture resulting from the CAT mechanism to be the most reliable mineralogical signature of a nonclassical crystallization, and this texture does in fact seem to be prevalent in stones. Therefore, we conclude that there is a strong likelihood that nonclassical crystallization processes are involved in various aspects of idiopathic stone formation.

RENAL AND URINARY CONSTITUENTS THAT MIGHT BE POTENTIAL CANDIDATES IN PROMOTING NONCLASSICAL PROCESSES

As we continue with our model system studies, there are certain urinary species that we predict might be most likely to act as a process-directing agent (i.e. transform the reaction to a nonclassical process).

A protein of great interest is osteopontin (or uropontin, the urinary form of osteopontin). This multifunctional phosphorylated glycoprotein contains a high content of aspartic and glutamic residues and has been known to play a role in a wide range of biological processes, including inflammation and mineralization.[112,115,132,135,166] Osteopontin has been shown to be important in the pathogenesis of renal stones,[89,128,129,132-134] and has been identified as one of the most prevalent proteins in the matrix layer.[92,93,103,128] It also has been shown to be present in the concentric laminations found in RP (where it was identified with immunostaining).[93] Osteopontin is involved in the chemotaxis of multinucleate giant cells, monocytes, and macrophages to the sites of Randall's plaques due to an inflammatory response caused by the CaP crystals.[115,167] This can result in crystal migration to the papillary surface, and its erosion causes the nidus to be exposed to urine where CaOx stone deposition can occur.[115] Exposure of renal epithelial cells to CaOx (and CaP) causes several urinary molecules to be upregulated, including osteopontin. While this is usually believed to be inhibitory to nucleation,[135,168-171] with high supersaturations (or other conditions), osteopontin could conceivably induce crystallization by the PILP process, as it has been shown to do so in vitro.[64,146,151] In addition, osteopontin undergoes significant post-translational modification; the degree of phosphorylation, glycosylation, or both could change it from an inhibitor to a promoter of crystallization.[133,135,136,172] Our prior studies with osteopontin (extracted from bovine milk) were performed to see if

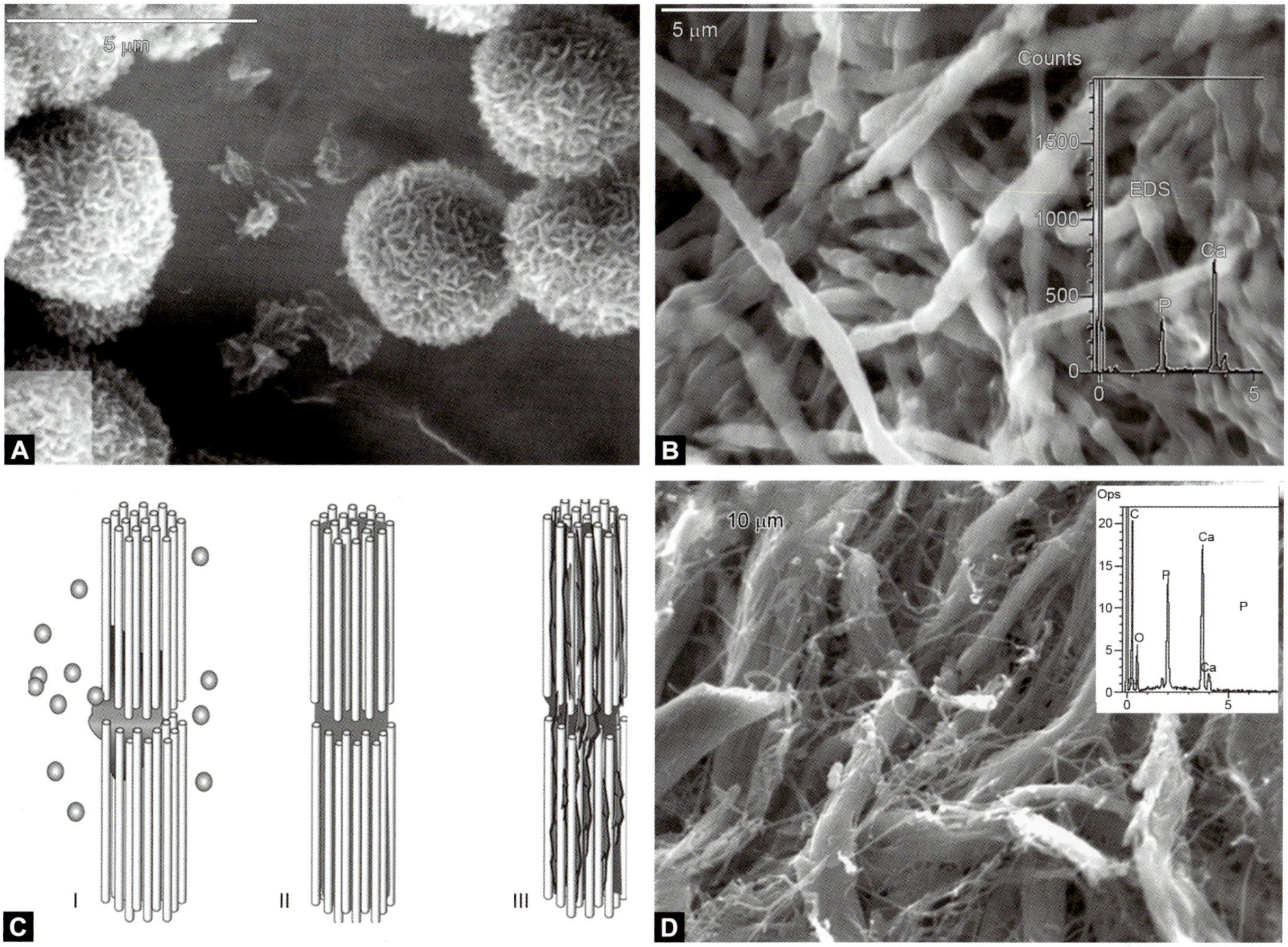

Figs. 2.17A to D: Mineral formation in the presence of organic substrates. (A) Scanning electron microscopy (SEM) of a type-I collagen sponge mineralized by the classical crystallization process (without a process-directing agent), which results in extrafibrillar spherulitic clusters of Hap that nucleate heterogeneously on the surface of the scaffold. (B) SEM of a type-I collagen sponge mineralized by the polymer-induced liquid precursor (PILP) process using osteopontin (OPN) as the PILP-inducing acidic macromolecule, which leads to a high degree of intrafibrillar mineral. Inset shows an energy-dispersive X-ray spectroscopy (EDS) spectrum of the same region, demonstrating that the collagen fibrils contain calcium phosphate, even though it is not apparent on the surface. (C) Proposed mechanism of intrafibrillar mineralization of collagen via the PILP process: (i) PILP nanodroplets adsorb to and infiltrate into the gap zones of a collagen fibril. (ii) Precursor solidifies into amorphous calcium phosphate and crystallizes, (iii) resulting in the fibrils being embedded with nanocrystals of hydroxyapatite. (D) Polymer-induced liquid precursor mineralization of the collagen within the interstitium of a decellularized porcine kidney. Intrafibrillar mineralization occurs just as readily in biologically-derived tissues as it does in reconstituted collagen scaffolds.

Source (for Parts A and B): Reprinted with permission Rodriguez DE, Thula-Mata T, Toro EJ, et al. Multifunctional role of osteopontin in directing intrafibrillar mineralization of collagen and activation of osteoclasts. Acta Biomater. 2014;10:494-507.

Source (for Part C): Olszta MJ, et al. Bone structure and formation: a new perspective. Mater Sci Eng R Reports. 2007;58:77-116.

osteopontin would behave similarly to polyAsp since it is an intrinsically disordered and acidic protein. We found that even though this protein is inhibitory to crystal formation via the classical nucleation and growth pathway, it can induce the PILP process and form an amorphous precursor, and that this pathway can actually promote the intrafibrillar mineralization of collagen fibrils (Figs. 2.17B and D).[151]

As mentioned, many of the other proteins found in stones, as well as in urine, are acidic.[132,133,173] Interestingly,

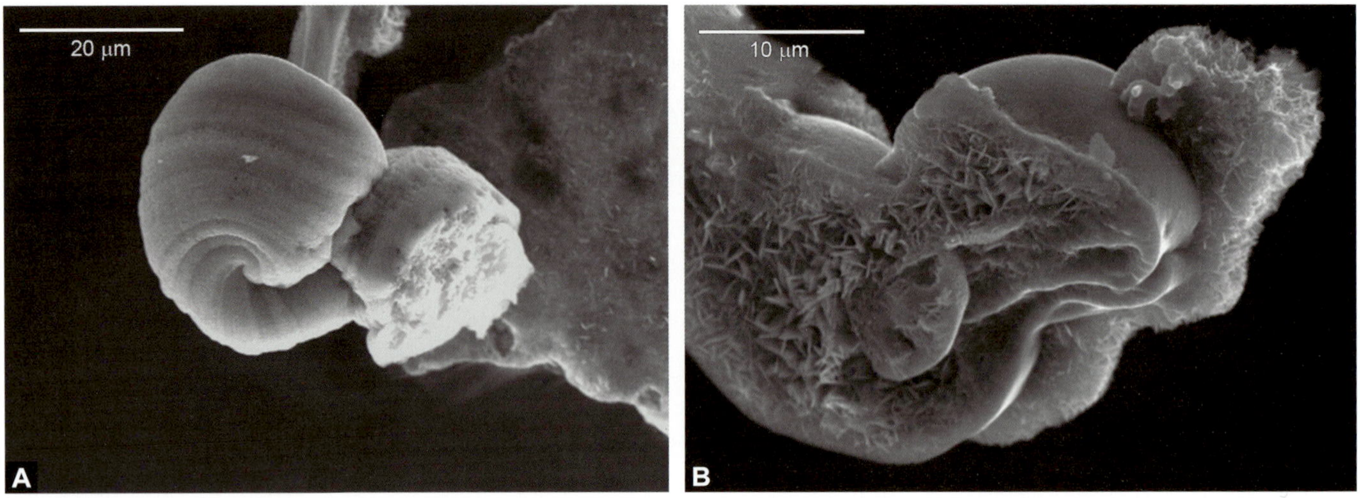

Figs. 2.18A and B: Scanning electron microscope of polymer-induced liquid precursor-formed calcium phosphate phase with unusual morphology and diffuse layering. (A) The twisting shape and surface curvature indicate the mineral was amorphous, but in (B), the interior appears to be transforming into crystalline platelets. In general, the amorphous calcium phosphate precursor does not undergo pseudomorphic transformation as readily, and tends to break down and reorganize into its favored platelet morphology. This, however, will depend on the additive that is used to induce and stabilize the amorphous phase. Stabilization might also be achieved with an organic coating that prevents access to water, which can aid in the dissolution and recrystallization.
Source: Reprinted with permission from Amos FF, Dai L, Kumar R, et al. Mechanism of formation of concentrically laminated spherules: implication to Randall's plaque and stone formation. Urol Res. 2009;37:11-7.

however, in several studies stone formers were found to actually contain less acidic forms of these molecules, or less of the protein in general. For instance, CaOx stone formers had lower levels of the highly charged Fetuin-A in both renal tissue and urine. The Tamm–Horsfall protein, the most abundant protein in urine,[173] has been shown to contain less sialic acid in stone formers, making it less negatively charged,[174] and that desialylated Tamm–Horsfall protein causes COM aggregation.[127] Even with osteopontin, it is suggested that stone formers have a relatively less acidic isoform compared to nonstone formers,[133] and compared to milk osteopontin, the urinary form is much less phosphorylated and thus less acidic. [175] Thus, further studies need to be conducted to determine if these proteins can still form an amorphous phase, especially in conditions favorable for crystallization.

Finally, it is worth mentioning that transformation into a more stable crystalline phase and microfaceting on nonequilibrium morphologies of the stable phase may result in a loss of signatures in the final crystal product. In the first case of phase transformations, sometimes films formed using the PILP process will dissolve before they can crystallize. Crystal aggregates can grow, causing a local depletion of ions, and the metastable amorphous phase is more likely to dissolve due to its higher solubility.[64,73] For the second case of micofaceting, one has to keep in mind that almost all morphologies that can be generated by the PILP process, are not thermodynamically favored, they represent nonequilibrium morphologies. Therefore, surface reorganization into a more stable structure is likely to occur and microfacets can form.[64,156] We are convinced that these mechanisms are also involved in stone aggregate formation or in formation of faceted crystals in kidney stones.[64]

CONCLUSION

It is obvious that many factors influence stone formation. While classical crystallization pathways certainly do play a role in this disease, classical models are incapable of explaining the unusual morphologies and textures seen in stones and Randall's plaques. Consequently, we propose that some parts of stone formation may also occur via nonclassical mechanisms. Obviously, this overview has not provided hard evidence to prove our various hypotheses. Our goal was to explore the possibility of alternative mechanisms in stone formation and to review the evidence for nonclassical mechanisms that stem from a variety of characteristic mineralogical signatures in stones. Of course one would not expect the body to secrete proteins that would deliberately lead to stones, but we believe that they are secreted due to their inhibitory activity, or as an inflammatory response. This may be successful at preventing crystal nucleation in most cases, but if the protein is defective, or becomes overwhelmed under conditions of higher supersaturations (or other factors), the system could then crash-out with mineral precursors via the nonclassical pathway(s). It is our hope that by understanding the crystallization mechanisms at play, therapeutic treatments or cures can be developed for treating this painful and recurring disease. To meet this goal, further studies of nonclassical crystallization mechanisms, and their relevance to stone formation, are warranted.

ACKNOWLEDGMENTS

This material is based upon work supported by the National Institutes of Health (NIH) from the National Institute of Diabetes and Digestive and Kidney Diseases (NIDDK) of under Award Number R01DK092311, the National Institute of Dental & Craniofacial Research (NIDCR) Award Number 5R01DE016849-07, and the National Science Foundation (NSF) under Grant Number DMR-1309657. Any opinions, findings, and conclusions or recommendations expressed in this material are those of the authors and do not necessarily reflect the views of the National Institutes of Health or the National Science Foundation. SEW gratefully acknowledges financial support by an Emmy Noether research grant issued by the German Research Foundation (DFG, N° WO1712/3-1). JH would like to acknowledge the Erlangen DFG cluster of excellence (EAM) for financial support.

REFERENCES

1. Becker R, Döring W. Kinetische Behandlung der Keimbildung in übersättigten Dämpfen. Ann Phys. 1935;416(8):719-52.
2. Volmer M, Weber A. Tröpfchenbildung in Dämpfen/ Germ-formation in oversaturated figures. Z Phys Chem. 1926;119:277.
3. Volmer M. Die chemische Reaktion. Kinetik der Phasenbildung, Bd IV. Verlag Th. Steinkopff, Dresden and Leipzig; 1939. P. 416.
4. Ostwald W. Studien über die Bildung und Umwandlung fester Körper. Z Phys Chem. 1897;22:495-503.
5. Navrotsky A. Energetic clues to pathways to biomineralization: precursors, clusters, and nanoparticles. Proc Natl Acad Sci USA. 2004;101:12096-101.
6. Chung SY, Kim YM, Kim JG, et al. Multiphase transformation and Ostwald's rule of stages during crystallization of a metal phosphate. Nat Phys. 2009;5:68-73.
7. Baumgartner J, Dey A, Bomans PH, et al. Nucleation and growth of magnetite from solution. Nat Mater. 2013;12:310-4.
8. Navrotsky A, Dooley D, Reeder R, et al. Calorimetric studies of the energetics of order-disorder in the system Mg1-xFexCa$(CO_3)_2$. Am Mineral. 1999;84:1622-6.
9. Carpenter MA, Putnis A, Navrotsky A, et al. Enthalpy effects associated with Al/Si ordering in anhydrous Mg-cordierite. Geochim Cosmochim Acta. 1983;47:899-906.
10. Pipich V, Balz M, Wolf SE, et al. Nucleation and growth of $CaCO_3$ mediated by the egg-white protein ovalbumin: a time-resolved in situ study using small-angle neutron scattering. J Am Chem Soc. 2008;130:1098-105.
11. Haberkorn H, Franke D, Frechen T, et al. Early stages of particle formation in precipitation reactions—quinacridone and boehmite as generic examples. J Colloid Interface Sci. 2003;259:112-26.
12. Tremel W, Küther J, Balz M, et al. In: Bäuerlein (ed). Handbook of Biomineralization. Berlin: Wiley-VCH Verlag GmbH; 2007. Pp. 209-32. doi:10.1002/9783527619443.ch36
13. Hu Q, Nielsen MH, Freeman CL, Hamm LM, Tao J, et al. The thermodynamics of calcite nucleation at organic interfaces: classical vs. non-classical pathways. Faraday Discuss. 2012;159:509.
14. Giuffre AJ, Hamm LM, Han N, et al. Polysaccharide chemistry regulates kinetics of calcite nucleation through competition of interfacial energies. Proc Natl Acad Sci USA. 2013;110:9261-6.
15. Ostwald W. Über die Vermeintliche Isomerie des Roten und Gelben Quecksilberoxyds und die Oberflächenspannung Fester Körper. Z Phys Chem. 1900;34:495-503.
16. Wagner C. Theorie Der Alterung Von Niederschlagen Durch Umlosen (Ostwald-Reifung). Zeitschrift Fur Elektrochemie. 1961;65:581-91.
17. Perez M. Gibbs-Thomson effects in phase transformations. Scr Mater. 2005;52:709-12.
18. Burton WK, Cabrera N, Frank FC. The growth of crystals and the equilibrium structure of their surfaces. Philos. Trans R Soc A Math Phys Eng Sci. 1951;243;299-358.
19. Stranski IN. The theory of crystal growth. Z Phys Chem. 1928;136:259-78.
20. Kossel W. The theory of crystal growth. Nachr Ges Wiss Göttingen, Math Klasse. 1927;136:135-43.
21. Frank FC. The influence of dislocations on crystal growth. Discuss Faraday Soc. 1949;5:48.
22. Wolf SE, Loges N, Mathiasch B, et al. Phase selection of calcium carbonate through the chirality of adsorbed amino acids. Angew Chemie Int Ed. 2007;46:5618-23.
23. Rimer JD, An Z, Zhu Z, et al. Crystal growth inhibitors for the prevention of L-cystine kidney stones through molecular design. Science. 2010;330:337-41.
24. Farmanesh S, et al. High-throughput platform for design and screening of peptides as inhibitors of calcium oxalate monohydrate crystallization. J Cryst Growth. 2013;373:13-9.
25. Petsev DN, Chen K, Gliko O, Vekilov P. Diffusion-limited kinetics of the solution-solid phase transition of molecular substances. Proc Nat Acad Sci USA. 2003;100:792-6.

26. Cölfen H, Antonietti M. Mesocrystals and Nonclassical Crystallization. Berlin: Wiley-VCH Verlag GmbH, 2008.
27. De Yoreo JJ, Gilbert PU, Sommerdijk NA, et al. Crystallization by particle attachment in synthetic, biogenic, and geologic environments. Science. 2015;349:aaa6760-aaa6760.
28. Gebauer D, Völkel A, Cölfen H. Stable prenucleation calcium carbonate clusters. Science. 2008;322:1819-22.
29. General Discussion. Faraday Discuss. 2012;136:103.
30. Pouget EM, Bomans PH, Goos JA, et al. The initial stages of template-controlled $CaCO_3$ formation revealed by cryo-TEM. Science. 2009;323:1455-8.
31. Kellermeier M, Gebauer D, Melero-García E, Drechsler M, Talmon Y, et al. Colloidal stabilization of calcium carbonate prenucleation clusters with silica. Adv Funct Mater. 2012;22:4301-11.
32. Wolf SE, Müller L, Barrea R, et al. Carbonate-coordinated metal complexes precede the formation of liquid amorphous mineral emulsions of divalent metal carbonates. Nanoscale. 2011;3:1158-65.
33. Demichelis R, Raiteri P, Gale JD, et al. Stable prenucleation mineral clusters are liquid-like ionic polymers. Nat Commun. 2011;2:590.
34. Kellermeier M, Rosenberg R, Moise A, Anders U, Przybylski M, et al. Amino acids form prenucleation clusters: ESI-MS as a fast detection method in comparison to analytical ultracentrifugation. Faraday Discuss. 2012;159:23.
35. Dey A, Bomans PH, Müller FA, Will J, Frederik PM, et al. The role of prenucleation clusters in surface-induced calcium phosphate crystallization. Nat Mater. 2010;9:1010-4.
36. Posner AS, Betts F. Synthetic amorphous calcium phosphate and its relation to bone mineral structure. Acc Chem Res. 1975;8:273-81.
37. Onuma K, Ito A. Cluster growth model for hydroxyapatite. Chem Mater. 1998;10:3346-51.
38. Gebauer D, Kellermeier M, Gale JD, et al. Pre-nucleation clusters as solute precursors in crystallisation. Chem Soc Rev. 2014;43:2348-71.
39. Habraken WJ, Tao J, Brylka LJ, Friedrich H, et al. Ion-association complexes unite classical and non-classical theories for the biomimetic nucleation of calcium phosphate. Nat Commun. 2013;4:1507.
40. Wolf SE, Leiterer J, Kappl M, et al. Early homogenous amorphous precursor stages of calcium carbonate and subsequent crystal growth in levitated droplets. J Am Chem Soc. 2008;130:12342-7.
41. Dauphin Y. The nanostructural unity of Mollusc shells. Mineral Mag. 2008;72:243-6.
42. Wolf SE, Böhm CF, Harris J, Hajir M, Mondeshki M, et al. Single nanogranules preserve intracrystalline amorphicity in biominerals. in Key Engineering Materials 2015;672:47-59.
43. Wolf SE, Lieberwirth I, Natalio F, Bardeau JF, Delorme N, et al. Merging models of biomineralisation with concepts of nonclassical crystallisation: is a liquid amorphous precursor involved in the formation of the prismatic layer of the Mediterranean Fan Mussel Pinna nobilis? Faraday Discuss. 2012;159:433.
44. Rousseau M, Lopez E, Stempflé P, et al. Multiscale structure of sheet nacre. Biomaterials. 2005;26:6254-62.
45. Seto J, Ma Y, Davis SA, et al. Structure-property relationships of a biological mesocrystal in the adult sea urchin spine. Proc Nat Acad Sci USA. 2011;109:1-6.
46. Sethmann I, Putnis A, Grassmann O, et al. Observation of nano-clustered calcite growth via a transient phase mediated by organic polyanions: a close match for biomineralization. Am Mineral. 2005;90:1213-7.
47. Aizenberg J, Weaver JC, Thanawala MS, et al. Skeleton of Euplectella sp.: structural hierarchy from the nanoscale to the macroscale. Science. 2005;309:275-8.
48. Weaver JC, Aizenberg J, Fantner GE, et al. Hierarchical assembly of the siliceous skeletal lattice of the hexactinellid sponge Euplectella aspergillum. J Struct Biol. 2007;158:93-106.
49. Henriksen K, Young JR, Bown PR, et al. Coccolith biomineralisation studied with atomic force microscopy. Palaeontology. 2004;47:725-43.
50. Tai K, Ulm FJ, Ortiz C. Nanogranular origins of the strength of bone. Nano Lett. 2006;6:2520-5.
51. Cölfen H, Mann S. Higher-order organization by mesoscale self-assembly and transformation of hybrid nanostructures. Angew Chemie Int Ed. 2003;42:2350-65.
52. Cölfen H, Antonietti M. Mesocrystals: inorganic superstructures made by highly parallel crystallization and controlled alignment. Angew Chemie Int Ed. 2005;44:5576-91.
53. Penn RL, Banfield JF. Oriented attachment and growth, twinning, polytypism, and formation of metastable phases: insights from nanocrystalline TiO_2. Am Mineral. 1998;83:1077-82.
54. Penn RL. Imperfect oriented attachment: dislocation generation in defect-free nanocrystals. Science. 1998;281:969-71.
55. Penn RL, Soltis JA. Characterizing crystal growth by oriented aggregation. Cryst Eng Comm. 2014;16:1409-18.
56. Darwin CG XCII. The reflexion of X-rays from imperfect crystals. Philos Mag Ser. 1922;6(43):800-29.
57. Li D, Nielsen MH, Lee JR, et al. Direction-specific interactions control crystal growth by oriented attachment. Science. 2012;336:1014-8.
58. Wang T, Cölfen H, Antonietti M. Nonclassical crystallization: mesocrystals and morphology change of $CaCO_3$ crystals in the presence of a polyelectrolyte additive. J Am Chem Soc. 2005;127:3246-7.
59. Niederberger M, Cölfen H. Oriented attachment and mesocrystals: non-classical crystallization mechanisms based on nanoparticle assembly. Phys Chem Chem Phys. 2006;8:3271-87.
60. Oaki Y, Imai H. Nanoengineering in echinoderms: the emergence of morphology from nanobricks. Small. 2006;2:66-70.
61. Oaki Y, Imai H. The hierarchical architecture of nacre and its mimetic materials. Angew Chemie Int Ed. 2005;44:6571-5.
62. Gong YU, Killian CE, Olson IC, et al. Phase transitions in biogenic amorphous calcium carbonate. Proc Natl Acad Sci USA. 2012;109:6088-93.
63. Killian CE, Metzler RA, Gong YU, et al. Mechanism of calcite co-orientation in the sea urchin tooth. J Am Chem Soc. 2009;131:18404-09.

64. Gower LB. Biomimetic model systems for investigating the amorphous precursor pathway and its role in biomineralization. Chem Rev. 2008;108:4551-627.
65. Addadi L, Raz S, Weiner S. Taking advantage of disorder: amorphous calcium carbonate and its roles in biomineralization. Adv Mater. 2003;15:959-70.
66. Politi Y, Levi-Kalisman Y, Raz S, Wilt F, Addadi L, et al. Structural characterization of the transient amorphous calcium carbonate precursor phase in sea urchin embryos. Adv Funct Mater. 2006;16:1289-98.
67. Levi-Kalisman Y, Raz S, Weiner S, et al. Structural differences between biogenic amorphous calcium carbonate phases using X-ray absorption spectroscopy. Adv Funct Mater. 2002;12:43.
68. Yang L, Killian CE, Kunz M, et al. Biomineral nanoparticles are space-filling. Nanoscale. 2011;3:603-09.
69. Gal A, Weiner S, Addadi L. A perspective on underlying crystal growth mechanisms in biomineralization: solution mediated growth versus nanosphere particle accretion. Cryst Eng Comm. 2015;17:2606-15.
70. Meldrum FC, Cölfen H. Controlling mineral morphologies and structures in biological and synthetic systems. Chem Rev. 2008;108:4332–432.
71. Gal A, Kahil K, Vidavsky V, DeVol RT, Gilbert PUPA, et al. Particle accretion mechanism underlies biological crystal growth from an amorphous precursor phase. Adv Funct Mater. 2014;24:5420-6.
72. Ihli J, Wong WC, Noel EH, et al. Dehydration and crystallization of amorphous calcium carbonate in solution and in air. Nat Commun. 2014;5:3169.
73. Gower LB, Odom DDJ. Deposition of calcium carbonate films by a polymer-induced liquid-precursor (PILP) process. J Cryst Growth. 2000;210:719-34.
74. Harris J, Mey I, Hajir M, et al. Pseudomorphic transformation of amorphous calcium carbonate films follows spherulitic growth mechanisms and can give rise to crystal lattice tilting. Cryst Eng Comm. 2015;17:6831-7.
75. Kim YY, Hetherington NB, Noel EH, et al. Capillarity creates single-crystal calcite nanowires from amorphous calcium carbonate. Angew Chemie Int Ed. 2011;50:12572-7.
76. Kim YY, Douglas EP, Gower LB. Patterning inorganic ($CaCO_3$) thin films via a polymer-induced liquid-precursor process. Langmuir. 2007;23:4862-70.
77. Kim YY, Kulak AN, Li Y, Batten T, Kuball M, et al. Substrate-directed formation of calcium carbonate fibres. J Mater Chem. 2009;19:387.
78. Han JT, Xu X, Kim DH, et al. Mosaic, single-crystal $CaCO_3$ thin films fabricated on modified polymer templates. Adv Funct Mater. 2005;15:475-80.
79. Bewernitz MA, Gebauer D, Long J, et al. A metastable liquid precursor phase of calcium carbonate and its interactions with polyaspartate. Faraday Discuss. 2012;159:291.
80. Wolf SE, Leiterer J, Pipich V, et al. Strong stabilization of amorphous calcium carbonate emulsion by ovalbumin: gaining insight into the mechanism of 'polymer-induced liquid precursor' processes. J Am Chem Soc. 2011;133:12642-9.
81. Jee SS, Culver L, Li Y, et al. Biomimetic mineralization of collagen via an enzyme-aided PILP process. J Cryst Growth. 2010;312:1249-56.
82. Olszta MJ, Cheng X, Jee SS, Kumar R, Kim YY, et al. Bone structure and formation: a new perspective. Mater Sci Eng R Reports. 2007;58:77-116.
83. Nudelman F, Pieterse K, George A, et al. The role of collagen in bone apatite formation in the presence of hydroxyapatite nucleation inhibitors. Nat Mater. 2010;9:1004-09.
84. Berg JK, Jordan T, Binder Y, et al. Mg^{2+} tunes the wettability of liquid precursors of $CaCO_3$: toward controlling mineralization sites in hybrid materials. J Am Chem Soc. 2013;135:12512-5.
85. Politi Y, Arad T, Klein E, et al. Sea urchin spine calcite forms via a transient amorphous calcium carbonate phase. Science. 2004;306:1161-4.
86. Beniash E, Metzler RA, Lam RSK, et al. Transient amorphous calcium phosphate in forming enamel. J Struct Biol. 2009;166:133-43.
87. Mahamid J, Sharir A, Addadi L, et al. Amorphous calcium phosphate is a major component of the forming fin bones of zebrafish: Indications for an amorphous precursor phase. Proc Natl Acad Sci USA. 2008;105:12748-53.
88. Evan AP, Worcester EM, Coe FL, et al. Mechanisms of human kidney stone formation. Urolithiasis. 2015;43 Suppl 1:19-32.
89. Coe FL, Evan AP, Worcester EM, et al. Three pathways for human kidney stone formation. Urol. Res. 2010;38:147-60.
90. Evan A, Lingeman J, Coe FL, et al. Randall's plaque: pathogenesis and role in calcium oxalate nephrolithiasis. Kidney Int. 2006;69:1313-8.
91. Evan AP. Physiopathology and etiology of stone formation in the kidney and the urinary tract. Pediatr. Nephrol. 2010;25:831-41.
92. Evan AP, Coe FL, Lingeman JE, et al. Mechanism of formation of human calcium oxalate renal stones on Randall's plaque. Anat Rec Adv Integr Anat Evol Biol. 2007;290:1315-23.
93. Evan AP, Coe FL, Rittling SR, et al. Apatite plaque particles in inner medulla of kidneys of calcium oxalate stone formers: osteopontin localization. Kidney Int. 2005;68:145-54.
94. Evan AP, Lingeman JE, Coe FL, et al. Randall's plaque of patients with nephrolithiasis begins in basement membranes of thin loops of Henle. J Clin Invest. 2003;111:607-16.
95. Bagga HS, Chi T, Miller J, et al. New insights into the pathogenesis of renal calculi. Urol Clin North Am. 2013;40:1-12.
96. Sayer JA, Carr G, Simmons NL. Nephrocalcinosis: molecular insights into calcium precipitation within the kidney. Clin Sci (Lond). 2004;106:549-61.
97. Tiselius HG. A hypothesis of calcium stone formation: an interpretation of stone research during the past decades. Urol Res. 2011;39:231-43.
98. Kok DJ, Schell-Feith EA. Risk factors for crystallization in the nephron: the role of renal development. J Am Soc Nephrol. 1999;10 (Suppl) 1:S364-70.
99. Luptak J, Bek-Jensen H, Fornander AM, Hojgaard I, Nilsson MA, et al. Crystallization of calcium oxalate and calcium phosphate at supersaturation levels corresponding to

those in different parts of the nephron. Scanning Microsc. 1994;8:47-62.

100. Wagner CA, Mohebbi N. Urinary pH and stone formation. J Nephrol. 2010;23 (S16):S165-S169.
101. Daudon M, Traxer O, Jungers P, et al. Stone morphology suggestive of Randall's plaque. AIP Conf Proc. 2007;900:26-34.
102. Grases F, Costa-Bauzá A, Prieto RM, et al. Renal papillary calcification and the development of calcium oxalate monohydrate papillary renal calculi: a case series study. BMC Urol. 2013;13:14.
103. Khan SR, Rodriguez DE, Gower LB, et al. Association of Randall's plaques with collagen fibers and membrane vesicles. J Urol. 2012;187:1094-100.
104. Højgaard I, Tiselius HG. Crystallization in the nephron. Urol Res. 1999;27:397-403.
105. Rodgers AL, Allie-Hamdulay S, Jackson G, et al. Simulating calcium salt precipitation in the nephron using chemical speciation. Urol Res. 2011;39:245-51.
106. Fasano JM, Khan SR. Intratubular crystallization of calcium oxalate in the presence of membrane vesicles: an in vitro study. Kidney Int. 2001;59:169-78.
107. Deganello S, Asplin J, Coe FL. Evidence that tubule fluid in the thin segment of the loop of Henle normally is supersaturated and forms a poorly crystallized hydroxyapatite that can initiate renal stones. Kidney Int. 1990;37(1):472.
108. Nancollas GH, Henneman ZJ. Calcium oxalate: calcium phosphate transformations. Urol Res. 2010;38:277-80.
109. Khan SR. Calcium phosphate/calcium oxalate crystal association in urinary stones: implications for heterogeneous nucleation of calcium oxalate. J Urol. 2015;157:376-83.
110. Worcester EM, Coe FL. Does idiopathic hypercalciuria trigger calcium-sensing receptor–mediated protection from urinary supersaturation ? J Am Soc Nephrol. 2009;20:1657-9.
111. Thomas A, Rosseeva E, Hochrein O, et al. Mimicking the growth of a pathologic biomineral: shape development and structures of calcium oxalate dihydrate in the presence of polyacrylic acid. Chem—A Eur J. 2012;18:4000-09.
112. Christmas KG, Gower LB, Khan SR, et al. Aggregation and dispersion characteristics of calcium oxalate monohydrate: effect of urinary species. J Colloid Interface Sci. 2002;256: 168-74.
113. Zhang D, Qi L, Ma J, et al. Morphological control of calcium oxalate dihydrate by a double-hydrophilic block copolymer. Chem Mater. 2002;14:2450-7.
114. El-Shall H, Jeon J, Abdel-Aal EA, Khan S, Gower L, et al. A study of primary nucleation of calcium oxalate monohydrate: I-effect of supersaturation. Cryst Res Technol. 2004;39:214-21.
115. Khan SR. Renal tubular damage/dysfunction: key to the formation of kidney stones. Urol Res. 2006;34:86-91.
116. Pak CY, Hayashi Y, Arnold LH. Heterogeneous nucleation with urate, calcium phosphate and calcium oxalate. Proc Soc Exp Biol Med. 1976;153:83-7.
117. Tiselius HG, Lindbäck B, Fornander AM, et al. Studies on the role of calcium phosphate in the process of calcium oxalate crystal formation. Urol Res. 2009;37:181-92.
118. Khan SR, Canales BK. Unified theory on the pathogenesis of Randall's plaques and plugs. Urolithiasis. 2014;43:109-23.
119. Robertson WG, Peacock M. Calcium oxalate crystalluria and inhibitors of crystallization in recurrent renal stone-formers. Clin Sci. 1972;43:499-506.
120. Rodgers AL, De Klerk DP. Crystalluria and urolithiasis in a relatively stone-free population. Scan. Electron Microsc. 1986;(Pt 3):1157-67.
121. Weller RO, Nester B, Cooke SA. Calcification in the human renal papilla: an electron-microscope study. J Pathol. 1972;107:211-6.
122. Wesson JA, Worcester EM, Wiessner JH, et al. Control of calcium oxalate crystal structure and cell adherence by urinary macromolecules. Kidney Int. 1998;53:952-7.
123. Jacob DE, Grohe B, Geßner M, et al. Kidney stones in primary hyperoxaluria: new lessons learnt. PLoS One. 2013;8:e70617.
124. Lieske JC, Leonard R, Toback FG. Adhesion of calcium oxalate monohydrate crystals to renal epithelial cells is inhibited by specific anions. Am J Physiol. 1995;268:F604–F612.
125. Mandel N. Crystal-membrane interaction in kidney stone disease. J Am Soc Nephrol. 1994;5:S37-45.
126. Wesson J, Worcester EM. Formation of hydrated calcium oxalates in the presence of poly-L-aspartic acid. Scanning Microsc. 1996;10:415-24.
127. Viswanathan P, Rimer JD, Kolbach AM, et al. Calcium oxalate monohydrate aggregation induced by aggregation of desialylated Tamm-Horsfall protein. Urol Res. 2011;39:269-82.
128. Thurgood LA, Wang T, Chataway TK, et al. Comparison of the specific incorporation of intracrystalline proteins into urinary calcium oxalate monohydrate and dihydrate crystals. J Proteome Res. 2010;9:4745–57.
129. Canales BK, Anderson L, Higgins L, et al. Second prize: comprehensive proteomic analysis of human calcium oxalate monohydrate kidney stone matrix. J Endourol. 2008;22: 1161-7.
130. Gower LB, Amos FF, Khan SR. Mineralogical signatures of stone formation mechanisms. Urol Res. 2010;38:281-92.
131. Khan SR, Atmani F, Glenton P, et al. Lipids and membranes in the organic matrix of urinary calcific crystals and stones. Calcif Tissue Int. 1996;59:357-65.
132. Khan SR, Kok DJ. Modulators of urinary stone formation. Front Biosci. 2004;9:1450-82.
133. Kolbach AM, Afzal O, Halligan B, et al. Relative deficiency of acidic isoforms of osteopontin from stone former urine. Urol Res. 2012;40:447-54.
134. Mo L, Liaw L, Evan AP, et al. Renal calcinosis and stone formation in mice lacking osteopontin, Tamm-Horsfall protein, or both. Am J Physiol Renal Physiol. 2007;293:F1935-43.
135. Gericke, A, Qin C, Spevak L, et al. Importance of phosphorylation for osteopontin regulation of biomineralization. Calcif Tissue Int. 2005;77:45-54.
136. Boskey AL, Christensen B, Taleb H, et al. Post-translational modification of osteopontin: effects on in vitro hydroxyapatite formation and growth. Biochem Biophys Res Commun. 2012;419:333-8.
137. Ebrahimpour A, Perez L, Nancollas GH. Induced crystal growth of calcium oxalate monohydrate at hydroxyapatite surfaces. The influence of human serum albumin, citrate, and magnesium. Langmuir. 1991;7:577-83.

138. Konya E, Umekawa T, Iguchi M, et al. The role of osteopontin on calcium oxalate crystal formation. Eur Urol. 2003;43: 564-71.
139. Sheng X, Jung T, Wesson JA, et al. Adhesion at calcium oxalate crystal surfaces and the effect of urinary constituents. Proc Natl Acad Sci USA. 2005;102:267-72.
140. Kok DJ, Khan SR. Calcium oxalate nephrolithiasis, a free or fixed particle disease. Kidney Int. 1994;46:847-54.
141. Finlayson B, Reid F. The expectation of free and fixed particles in urinary stone. Invest Urol. 1978;15:442-8.
142. Ihli J, Wang YW, Cantaert B, et al. Precipitation of amorphous calcium oxalate in aqueous solution. Chem Mater. 2015;27:3999-4007.
143. Amos FF, Dai L, Kumar R, et al. Mechanism of formation of concentrically laminated spherules: implication to Randall's plaque and stone formation. Urol Res. 2009;37:11-7.
144. Amos FF, Olszta MJ, Khan SR, et al. Relevance of a polymer-induced liquid-precursor (PILP) mineralization process to normal and pathological biomineralization. Biomineralization—Medical Aspects of Solubility. John Wiley & Sons, Ltd, Chichester, UK; 2006. Pp. 125-217. doi:10.1002/0470092122.ch4
145. Jee SS, Thula TT, Gower LB. Development of bone-like composites via the polymer-induced liquid-precursor (PILP) process. Part 1: influence of polymer molecular weight. Acta Biomater. 2010;6:3676-86.
146. Chidambaram A, Rodriguez D, Khan S, et al. Biomimetic Randall's plaque as an in vitro model system for studying the role of acidic biopolymers in idiopathic stone formation. Urolithiasis. 2015;43 (Suppl 1):77-92.
147. Olszta MJ, Douglas EP, Gower LB. Scanning electron microscopic analysis of the mineralization of type I collagen via a polymer-induced liquid-precursor (PILP) process. Calcif Tissue Int. 2003;72:583-91.
148. Hajir M, Graf R, Tremel W. Stable amorphous calcium oxalate: synthesis and potential intermediate in biomineralization. Chem Commun. 2014;50:6534.
149. Christoffersen J, Christoffersen MR, Kibalczyz W, et al. A contribution to the understanding of the formation of calcium phosphates. J Cryst Growth. 1989;94:767-77.
150. Mahamid J, Aichmayer B, Shimoni E, et al. Mapping amorphous calcium phosphate transformation into crystalline mineral from the cell to the bone in zebrafish fin rays. Proc Natl Acad Sci USA. 2010;107:6316-21.
151. Rodriguez DE, Thula-Mata T, Toro EJ, et al. Multifunctional role of osteopontin in directing intrafibrillar mineralization of collagen and activation of osteoclasts. Acta Biomater. 2014;10:494-507.
152. Thula TT, Svedlund F, Rodriguez DE, et al. Mimicking the nanostructure of bone: comparison of polymeric process-directing agents. Polymers (Basel). 2011;3:10-35.
153. Kim YK, Gu LS, Bryan TE, et al. Mineralisation of reconstituted collagen using polyvinylphosphonic acid/polyacrylic acid templating matrix protein analogues in the presence of calcium, phosphate and hydroxyl ions. Biomaterials. 2010;31:6618-27.
154. Borchardt-Ott W. Crystallography: an Introduction. Springer-Verlag Berlin Heidelberg, 2012.
155. Amos FF. Template-Assisted Mineral Formation via an Amorphous Liquid Phase Precursor Route. Gainesville, University of Florida, 2005.
156. Olszta MJ, Gajjeraman S, Kaufman M, et al. Nanofibrous calcite synthesized via a solution-precursor-solid mechanism. Chem Mater. 2004;16:2355-62.
157. Homeijer SJ, Barrett RA, Gower LB. Polymer-induced liquid-precursor (PILP) process in the non-calcium based systems of barium and strontium carbonate. Cryst Growth Des. 2010;10:1040-52.
158. Wesson JA, Ganne V, Beshensky AM, et al. Regulation by macromolecules of calcium oxalate crystal aggregation in stone formers. Urol Res. 2005;33:206-12.
159. Shtukenberg AG, Punin YO, Gunn E, et al. Spherulites. Chem Rev. 2012;112:1805-38.
160. Grases F, Zelenkova M, Sohnel O. Structure and formation mechanism of calcium phosphate concretions formed in simulated body fluid. Urolithiasis. 2014;42:9-16.
161. Grases F, Villacampa AI, Costa-Bauzá A, et al. Uric acid calculi: types, etiology and mechanisms of formation. Clin Chim Acta. 2000;302:89-104.
162. Viravaidya C, Li M, Mann S. Microemulsion-based synthesis of stacked calcium carbonate (calcite) superstructures. Chem Commun. 2004;(19):2182-3.
163. Long X, Ma Y, Cho KR, Li D, De Yoreo JJ, et al. Oriented calcite micropillars and prisms formed through aggregation and recrystallization of poly (acrylic acid) stabilized nanoparticles. Cryst Growth Des. 2013;13:3856-63.
164. Asenath-Smith E, Li H, Keene EC, et al. Crystal growth of calcium carbonate in hydrogels as a model of biomineralization. Adv Funct Mater. 2012;22:2891-914.
165. Golub EE. Biomineralization and matrix vesicles in biology and pathology. Semin Immunopathol. 2011;33:409-17.
166. Xie Y, Sakatsume M, Nishi S, et al. Expression, roles, receptors, and regulation of osteopontin in the kidney. Kidney Int. 2001;60:1645-57.
167. Xie AJ, Zhang L, Zhu J, Shen YH, Xu Z, et al. Formation of calcium oxalate concentric precipitate rings in two-dimensional agar gel systems containing Ca^{2+}–RE^{3+} (RE=Er, Gd and La)–C2O42–. Colloids Surfaces A Physicochem Eng Asp. 2009;332:192-9.
168. Wesson JA, Johnson RJ, Mazzali M, et al. Osteopontin is a critical inhibitor of calcium oxalate crystal formation and retention in renal tubules. J Am Soc Nephrol. 2003;14:139-47.
169. Kleinman JG, Beshensky A, Worcester EM, et al. Expression of osteopontin, a urinary inhibitor of stone mineral crystal growth, in rat kidney. Kidney Int. 1995;47:1585-96.
170. Shiraga H, Min W, VanDusen WJ, et al. Inhibition of calcium oxalate crystal growth in vitro by uropontin: another member of the aspartic acid-rich protein superfamily. Proc Natl Acad Sci USA. 1992;89:426-30.
171. Worcester EM, Beshensky AM. Osteopontin inhibits nucleation of calcium oxalate crystals. Ann N Y Acad Sci. 1995;760:375-7.

172. Hug S, Grohe B, Jalkanen J, Chan B, Galarreta B, et al. Mechanism of inhibition of calcium oxalate crystal growth by an osteopontin phosphopeptide. Soft Matter. 2012;8:1226.
173. Jahnen-Dechent W, Heiss A, Schäfer C, et al. Fetuin-A regulation of calcified matrix metabolism. Circ Res. 2011;108: 1494-509.
174. Knorle R, Schnierle P, Koch A, et al. Tamm-Horsfall glycoprotein: role in inhibition and promotion of renal calcium oxalate stone formation studied with Fourier-transform infrared spectroscopy. Clin Chem. 1994;40:1739-43.
175. Christensen B, Petersen TE, Sorensen ES. Post-translational modification and proteolytic processing of urinary osteopontin. Biochem J. 2008;411:53-61.

CHAPTER

3 Biology and Clinical Relevance of Urine Crystallization Inhibitors

Kristin J Bergsland

INTRODUCTION

Supersaturation (SS), the presence of a substance in solution at a concentration above its solubility, is the driving force for crystallization.[1] In urine, SS for calcium oxalate (CaOx), calcium phosphate (CaP) and uric acid (UA) are the most relevant contributors to the formation of the majority of human kidney stones.[2] Stone-forming patients generally have elevated SS values compared to healthy people; these SS values are effective in identifying causes of stones and are used to guide treatment.[3] However, even normal human urine is frequently supersaturated for stone-forming salts, yet most people do not form stones. This is due to the well-known ability of urine to inhibit the nucleation, growth and aggregation of crystals.[4] This ability is widely considered an essential defense against stones that is indeed abnormal among male and female stone formers.[5,6] Crystallization inhibition is mediated by molecules in urine that slow the formation of crystals. It is possible that some molecules may exhibit abnormalities, which result in reduced inhibition effectiveness in a stone-forming population. Many molecules, large and small, in urine are involved in controlling crystal nucleation, growth and aggregation, as well as crystal interaction with the renal tubular epithelial cells and crystal retention within the kidney. Aggarwal et al. have provided a comprehensive review of molecules found in urine and stone matrix, and how they modulate stone formation.[7] To date, no individual defects have been shown to be a sole cause of stones. In this chapter, urinary molecules that are thought to contribute the most to the overall crystallization-inhibitory effect of urine on calcium stone-forming salts will be discussed. Since calcium-containing stones represent the vast majority of human stones (>80%) and urinary inhibitors are not so important in preventing the formation of other types such as UA, only inhibitors of calcium crystallization will be considered.[8]

SMALL MOLECULES

Part of the capacity of urine to inhibit calcium crystallization is found in low-molecular-weight (LMW), dialyzable substances that are known to reduce SS of calcium salts.[1]

Citrate

Citrate is an established kinetic retardant of calcium crystallization.[9] Citrate creates soluble complexes with calcium in urine, thereby inhibiting the nucleation, growth and aggregation of CaOx and CaP crystals.[10–14] Citrate has generally been found to be present at reduced levels in the urine of adult stone formers, a deficiency that is thought to facilitate stone formation.[15,16] Two randomized controlled trials have shown citrate supplementation to be effective in reducing recurrence of calcium stones.[17,18] Consequently, citrate is often prescribed as a treatment to decrease risk of urine crystallization in calcium stone-forming patients.[19,20]

However, the effective clinical use of citrate is complicated since urinary citrate levels are influenced by many factors, including age, sex and metabolism. Miyake et al. found that the urinary excretion rate of citrate in healthy children is two- to threefold higher than in adults, when adjusted for body size,[21] supporting a role for citrate in the reduced incidence of nephrolithiasis in children compared to adults. We and others have found sex-dependent differences in citrate excretion starting around puberty, with citrate excretion in boys declining with age and girls having significantly higher urinary citrate than boys after about the age of 12 years (Figs. 3.1A and B).[22,23] Likewise, among healthy adults, citrate excretion is higher in females than males.[24] Thus female sex hormones may play an important role in maintaining elevated urinary citrate levels. However, citrate excretion has been found to be increased among overweight and obese stone formers of both sexes compared to nonobese stone formers.[25,26] Changes in urinary citrate level can also be affected by the acid–base

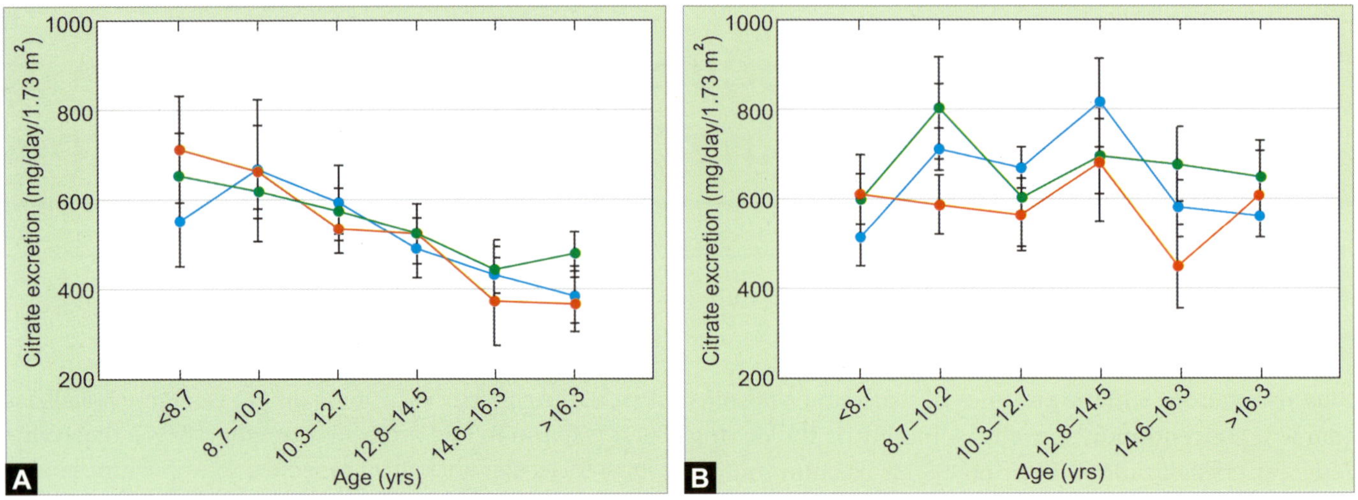

Figs. 3.1A and B: Urine citrate by sex and age. Daily excretions of citrate are expressed per 1.73 m^2 body surface area in boys (A) and girls (B) by age sextile. Values are mean ± standard error of the mean. Citrate declines with age in boys, $p < 0.001$ for the regression.[22] (Blue: Stone formers; Red: Non-stone forming siblings of stone formers; Green: Unrelated non-stone forming children).

status, with citrate excretion being decreased under conditions of systemic or intracellular acidosis.[23,27] The physiological mechanisms governing urine citrate excretion are not completely understood, but may involve differential regulation of the Na^+-dependent dicarboxylate co-transporter, NaDC-1, which facilitates citrate reabsorption in the proximal tubule.[28] Administration of citrate can raise urine pH, and therefore CaP SS, in addition to urine citrate concentration, which may increase risk of crystallization, although this effect may be offset by its ability to chelate and lower urine calcium.[29-31] Altogether, more research is needed to determine which patients may benefit most from treatment with citrate, with age, sex, weight and urine pH potentially affecting the risk-to-benefit ratio for stone prevention. The reader is referred to a series of excellent articles by Fredric Coe on the subject of the relationship of citrate to the formation and prevention of kidney stones.[32]

Magnesium

Magnesium (Mg) is present at millimolar concentrations in urine where it competes with calcium for binding of oxalate.[33] Magnesium ions destabilize calcium oxalate ion pairs and reduce the size of their aggregates.[34] Magnesium oxalate is two orders of magnitude more soluble than calcium oxalate; therefore, urine Mg reduces the risk of crystallization of insoluble calcium salts and subsequent stone formation.[35] The incidence of hypomagnesiuria, defined as <3 mmol per day for men and <2.2 mmol per day for women, has been reported to be 19–60% in calcium stone formers.[36,37] As such, there has been much interest in the use of Mg supplements as therapy for CaOx nephrolithiasis. However, evidence from clinical trials has not justified the use of Mg as a sole therapy for stones, possibly due to poor gastrointestinal (GI) absorption.[33] In a double-blind, randomized, placebo-controlled trial, Ettinger et al. were not able to show a difference between the recurrence rates of the Mg and placebo groups in 51 patients with a history of at least two stones.[38] However, the addition of Mg to potassium citrate therapy seems to improve outcomes; providing Mg as a mixed salt (Mg potassium citrate) reduced calcium stone recurrence by 90%, similar to potassium citrate, but with better GI tolerance.[17]

Pyrophosphate

Pyrophosphate inhibits crystallization of CaOx and CaP in vitro.[39,40] At normal urinary concentrations, pyrophosphate is a more potent inhibitor of hydroxyapatite crystal growth than either citrate or Mg.[41] Studies comparing pyrophosphate levels in the urine of stone formers versus healthy controls have produced mixed results, with some studies showing reduced pyrophosphate excretion in stone formers[42,43] and others showing no difference.[44,45] Pyrophosphate excretion varies with age and sex, with a tendency toward higher excretion with increasing age and higher excretion in men than in women.[43] Urinary pyrophosphate is presumably of endogenous origin and is likely a reflection of bone metabolism.[44] Interestingly, in a study of the effect of chronic stress on urine composition of CaOx stone patients, measures of stress were positively correlated with blood cortisol and urinary pyrophosphate levels.[46] Cortisol triggers bone mineral resorption and increases urine calcium excretion,[47] so pyrophosphate excretion may be correspondingly elevated to protect against urine crystallization.[46] Men have been found to have a higher cortisol response to stress compared with women,[48] which is in accord with the sex difference in pyrophosphate excretion. All in all, urine pyrophosphate levels may have more to do with demographic and lifestyle factors than with stone-forming status.

Phytate

Phytate, or inositol hexaphosphate, is a natural compound that is found in abundance in plants, especially in whole grains, seeds and nuts.[49] Phytate contains six phosphate groups, each with two hydroxyl moieties, which allow chelation of divalent metal ions including Fe^{2+}, Zn^{2+}, Mg^{2+} and Ca^{2+}.[50] In vitro studies have shown phytate to be a powerful inhibitor of CaOx and CaP crystallization due to the multiple negatively charged phosphate groups that bind calcium in solution.[35,49,51] Phytate is normally found in urine at levels that are directly related to dietary intake,[52] and urinary phytate has been found to be reduced in calcium stone formers relative to healthy controls.[53] A large epidemiologic study of >96,000 women in the United States showed that phytate intake was associated with a reduced risk of stone formation.[54] The major potential drawback for phytate as a treatment to reduce stone risk is that it forms insoluble metal ion complexes that are poorly absorbed by the GI tract.[55] Excretion of insoluble complexes of phytate with essential minerals such as iron and zinc can lead to reduced bioavailability and mineral deficiency.[56] In fact, micronutrient malnutrition due to phytate consumption from plants is a recognized problem worldwide, and breeding low-phytate crop varieties is an active area of agricultural research.[57] There is also evidence that CaOx stone formers who consume vegetarian diets should avoid foods that are high in phytate, as chelation of calcium by phytate in the GI tract results in an increase in intestinal absorption and urinary excretion of oxalate.[58] Thus, the potent ion-chelating ability of phytate represents a potential benefit to stone patients in inhibiting urine crystallization that is countered by the disadvantage of depleting essential minerals and increasing oxalate excretion.

MACROMOLECULES

Most of the capacity of urine to inhibit crystallization appears to reside not in the ionic milieu of urine but in the larger molecules that cannot be removed by dialysis.[59,60] One such class of molecules is glycosaminoglycans (GAGs) such as chondroitin sulfate, heparan sulfate and hyaluronic acid.[61] Another class is urine proteins with crystallization inhibitory properties, including prothrombin fragment 1 (PF1),[62] osteopontin (OPN; uropontin),[63] inter-alpha-trypsin inhibitor (ITI),[64] bikunin (BK, a portion of the ITI),[65] Tamm–Horsfall protein (THP),[66] albumin[67] and calgranulin.[68] These macromolecules are all expressed in the kidney, and may contribute to the overall crystallization inhibitory effect of urine. Because of their ability to bind calcium, many so-called inhibitors can also act as promoters of crystal formation and deposition depending upon experimental conditions and whether the molecules are fixed to a substrate.[69] Organic macromolecules, including GAGs and proteins, form the matrix of calcium stones and comprise 2–3% of the weight of the stone.[50] In addition to their effects on crystallization, all of these molecules have other normal biological functions including, but not limited to, modulation of tubule and transporter functions, mediation of inflammation and the innate immune response, formation and stabilization of extracellular matrix, facilitation of wound healing and tissue repair, and antimicrobial protection.[70–75] Thus, the clinical relevance of these molecules to kidney stone disease may not be solely due to their effects on calcium crystallization inhibition but also to their other functions in the kidney and urinary tract. Here, the clinical relevance of these proteins to the pathophysiology of calcium nephrolithiasis will be examined.

Glycosaminoglycans

Glycosaminoglycans are long unbranched polysaccharides consisting of a repeating disaccharide unit.[76] They are synthesized by epithelial cells lining the urinary tract where they serve to form a water-tight barrier to shield the cell surface from urinary solutes, proteins, bacteria and crystals.[77] The most abundant GAGs in urine are chondroitin sulfates A and C and heparan sulfate; also present at lower levels are hyaluronic acid, dermatan sulfate and keratan sulfate.[78] Glycosaminoglycans are highly negatively charged and have been shown to be potent inhibitors of growth and aggregation of CaOx and CaP crystals in vitro.[40,79-81] These inhibitory properties are largely due to the effects of chondroitin sulfate and, to a lesser extent, heparan sulfate.[50] Altered abundance of urinary GAGs has been shown to be associated with interstitial cystitis,[82,83] but a plethora of studies examining the relationship between urine GAG concentration or excretion and stone formation has failed to demonstrate any conclusive association.[50] Urinary GAGs are increased in interstitial cystitis as a result of chronic bladder epithelial damage and neurogenic inflammation.[84] Urinary GAG levels are more likely to be a reflection of inflammatory processes in the kidney and urinary tract than to be related to a marker of stone formation.

Urine Proteins

Prothrombin Fragment 1

Prothrombin fragment 1 is a potent inhibitor of CaOx crystal growth and aggregation[62] and also the most prominent protein in the organic matrix of CaOx crystals precipitated from fresh human urine.[85] Urinary PF1 also inhibits CaOx crystal attachment to cultured cells.[86] Prothrombin fragment 1 comprises the first 155 amino acids of prothrombin, including a 10-residue γ-carboxyglutamic acid (Gla) domain that confers on PF1 a strong ability to bind calcium.[87] The potent inhibitory effect of PF1 on CaOx crystallization has been ascribed to this Gla domain, which is absent from other prothrombin activation fragments including thrombin and the F2 fragment.[88] Liu et al. showed that the Gla composition of urinary PF1 as well as its ability to inhibit CaOx crystal growth was significantly decreased in patients with CaOx stones.[89] However, Buchholz et al. found no difference in the ability of urine from patients taking warfarin to inhibit CaOx crystal growth compared to urine from healthy individuals.[90] Gamma carboxylation is a vitamin-K-dependent process that is inhibited by the drug warfarin, so the absence of increased crystal growth in the presence of warfarin does not support a substantial role for vitamin-K-dependent proteins such as PF1 in inhibiting urine crystallization.

Prothrombin fragment 1 is also highly glycosylated[91] and the level of sialylation may contribute to its effectiveness in inhibiting CaOx crystallization. Webber et al. found a correlation between the genetically determined levels of PF1 sialylation and the incidence of CaOx stone disease in racial groups among the South African population.[92] Glycosylation of PF1 was also found to govern CaOx crystal nucleation and aggregation, but it does not play a role in inhibiting crystal growth.[93]

Prothrombin fragment 1 is produced by thrombin cleavage of a precursor protein, prothrombin, and is associated with activation of blood coagulation.[87] It is primarily produced by the liver, but the prothrombin gene is also expressed in the kidneys of humans and animals.[94,95] Prothrombin conversion to thrombin and prothrombin fragments is the last step in the coagulation cascade, and there is evidence that this can occur at sites of renal injury.[96] Acting via protease-activated receptors in the kidney, thrombin mediates several intracellular-signaling pathways and plays a role in the inflammatory response to tissue damage, stimulation of epithelial cell proliferation and extracellular matrix deposition.[97,98] Immunohistochemical analysis of human kidneys has shown that PF1 is synthesized in tubular epithelial cells of the thick ascending limb of the loop of Henle (TALH) and the distal convoluted tubule, and is more abundant in the kidneys of stone formers than in healthy individuals.[99] It is unclear whether urinary PF1 derives from serum prothrombin or is the product of renal prothrombin gene expression. In a study of first-degree family members of calcium stone formers, we found that prothrombin fragments in urine (mainly larger PF1-containing activation peptides of prothrombin such as PF1+2) were strong predictors of stone formation in men.[100] However, others have found no differences in the relative abundance of PF1 in the urine of CaOx stone formers compared to healthy people.[101]

A genetic link between a prothrombin gene variant and increased kidney stone risk has been identified in female calcium stone-forming patients in Thailand.[102] A nonsynonymous change leading to a threonine (T)-to-methionine (M) substitution at amino acid 165 (T165M) was located in the kringle 1 domain of PF1.[103] Structural modeling of PF1 suggests that the T165M substitution may affect the function of PF1 by blocking hydrogen bond formation with glutamic acid at position 180. The PF1 kringle 1 domain is thought to be important in mediating interactions with other proteins within the blood coagulation cascade such as cofactor Va,[104] and it is believed to play a role in inducing migration and activation of human neutrophils.[105] How this mutation affects the risk of stone formation is yet to be understood. The prevalence of stone disease in the Thai population shows a typical male predominance, with a male-to-female ratio of about 2:1; the reason why this variant plays a role only in females is also unclear.[103]

Osteopontin

Osteopontin is a member of the SIBLING family of proteins (*S*mall *I*ntegrin-*B*inding *Li*ga*n*d, *N*-linked *G*lycoprotein), which plays a role in matrix mineralization, most commonly in bone and dentin.[106] OPN has been found to be expressed in several tissues and cell types, including the mineralized bone matrix, macrophages, dendritic cells, endothelial cells, smooth muscle cells and epithelial cells.[107] It is also expressed in the kidney in glomerular mesangial cells, podocytes, collecting duct, thin loop of Henle and urothelial cells.[108-110] OPN is a chemokine that can modulate cell adhesion as well as autocrine and paracrine factors by interacting with cell surface receptors such as integrins.[111] OPN is rich in aspartic acid residues and is highly negatively charged, making it an avid calcium-binding protein.[112] OPN is abundantly found in the matrix of calcium stones[113,114] and is present in hydroxyapatite Randall's plaques in the renal medullary interstitium.[110,115] OPN is a potent inhibitor of CaOx crystal nucleation, growth and aggregation in vitro.[63,116] However, experiments using atomic force microscopy have shown that OPN may also promote aggregation of crystals and binding to cell surfaces by increasing the adhesiveness of crystals to which it is bound.[117] Similarly, Rodriguez et al. found that OPN can promote intrafibrillar mineralization of collagen with hydroxyapatite in an in vitro polymer-induced liquid-precursor biomineralization system.[118]

Osteopontin expression is induced by angiotensin II in different cell types, such as vascular smooth muscle cells, macrophages and epithelial cells of renal tubules.[107,132,133] Patients with nephrolithiasis have been found to have elevated urinary angiotensinogen,[134] which is a marker of intrarenal angiotensin II activity.[135] High dietary salt intake, which can increase the production of intrarenal angiotensin II, also increases renal OPN expression in rats.[136] Osteopontin expression is increased as well by hormones that regulate bone and mineral metabolism such as parathyroid hormone and vitamin D, which are often elevated in stone formers.[137,138] These results suggest that OPN expression would be expected to be increased in kidneys of stone formers compared to normal controls.

Osteopontin is difficult to measure in urine, likely because it is highly susceptible to cleavage by proteases in urine. There is evidence that urine from kidney stone patients has elevated serine protease activity that generates aberrant OPN species.[119] This may cause technical difficulties in OPN detection and quantification depending on the type of assay used. Most efforts to examine OPN abundance by enzyme-linked immunosorbent assay (ELISA) in urine from stone patients and normal controls have found decreased urinary OPN in stone formers.[120-122] However, other studies have found no difference, either by semiquantitative western blotting[101] or ELISA.[119] These disparities may be due to differences in the antibodies and methods used for detection of OPN; loss of an epitope in OPN due to proteolytic cleavage in urine could lead to failure of an antibody to detect certain fragments and overall underdetermination of OPN. In histopathology studies, Evan et al. found that OPN in renal medullary tissue was similarly expressed in normal and stone-forming subjects except for its localization in Randall's plaques of the stone formers.[110] Overall, whether there are differences in renal or urinary total OPN abundance between stone formers and healthy people is still an open question.

Proteolytic cleavage of OPN by thrombin and matrix metalloproteinases is a normal regulatory process that modulates the activity of OPN and its binding to integrin receptors in some tissues.[123] Thrombin cleavage of OPN produces three fragments that have different crystallization inhibitory properties in vitro, and it is the central fragment that has been found to effectively inhibit hydroxyapatite crystal formation and growth.[124] In urine, OPN may be cleaved by thrombin and/or other proteases that are present. Kolbach et al. have identified four isoforms of OPN in human urine and found that there is a relative deficiency of the two most acidic forms in urine from stone formers compared to that of normal individuals.[125] A decline in the most anionic of the OPN isoforms, that is, those that would interact most strongly with crystals to inhibit growth and aggregation, could be a factor promoting stone formation. Thus, proteolytic cleavage of OPN may affect the crystallization properties of urine and contribute to decreased crystal inhibition in stone formers.

Cleavage by thrombin exposes new epitopes in OPN that increase its capacity to bind and signal through integrin receptors to mediate functions such as cell cycle regulation and actin cytoskeleton dynamics.[126] In human kidneys, $\alpha_v\beta_3$ integrin is expressed in glomerular epithelial cells, Bowman's capsule, vascular endothelium and weakly in tubular epithelial cells; $\alpha_v\beta_5$ is similar, but also on the vascular endothelium, β1 expression is seen in glomerular epithelial cells, Bowman's capsule, the vascular epithelium and tubular epithelial cells.[109,127] In chronic inflammatory conditions with increased thrombin activity such as obesity, atherosclerosis and rheumatoid arthritis, production of thrombin-cleaved OPN fragments in urine is increased.[128] Some of these conditions, including obesity, diabetes and rheumatoid arthritis, are linked to a higher risk of kidney stones.[129,130] Antibodies have been developed to selectively target protease-cleaved OPN forms, which may have applications in treatment and prevention of various inflammatory diseases and cancer.[126] One such antibody against thrombin-cleaved OPN has been found to reduce renal crystal formation, tubular cell injury and crystal–cell attachment in mice with renal crystals induced by glyoxylate.[131] It is possible that differential protease cleavage of OPN in stone formers may alter its activities both in mediating crystallization and functioning as a chemokine in the kidney.

Mouse strains lacking the *Spp1* (secreted phosphoprotein 1) gene that encodes OPN have been generated.[139,140] Mo et al. found that 10% of the mice lacking OPN spontaneously form renal papillary interstitial deposits of CaP reminiscent of Randall's plaque, which are never seen in wild-type mice.[140] Paloian et al. found that OPN knockout (KO) mice on a high-phosphate diet developed nephrocalcinosis with substantial renal tubular and interstitial calcium deposition, and marked vascular calcification when compared with control mice.[141] In humans, the single nucleotide polymorphism (SNP) rs1126616 affecting Ala 250 in exon 7 of the *SPP1* gene has been linked with reduced OPN levels in serum and urine and increased susceptibility to nephrolithiasis.[142] Safarinejad et al. examined nine SNPs in the *SPP1* gene in CaOx stone formers and healthy individuals in Iran and found one SNP that was protective and three SNPs that were predisposing to CaOx stone formation.[143] Subjects with the protective polymorphism had increased levels of serum OPN and urinary calcium to OPN ratios, while those with the predisposing SNPs had lower serum and urine OPN. Others have found an association between SNPs in the promoter of the *SPP1* gene and risk of stone formation in Japanese and Turkish populations.[144,145] Together these suggest a role for OPN in preventing CaP crystallization and protection against nephrolithiasis that is as yet not clearly defined.

Osteopontin is a multifunctional protein that is upregulated in wound healing, fibrosis, autoimmune disease and atherosclerosis where it is highly expressed at sites of atherosclerotic plaques.[107] It is a potent activator of transcription factor NF-κB (nuclear factor-κB) that is involved in cellular responses to injury and stress; OPN is implicated in promoting epithelial–mesenchymal transition, which is a significant contributor to fibrotic phenotypes and cancer metastasis.[146] OPN expression is upregulated in renal epithelial cells in animal models of renal injury as well as in human renal allografts and diseases such as idiopathic membranous nephropathy, immunoglobulin A nephritis, lupus nephritis and essential hypertension with decompensated arteriolosclerosis.[109] OPN upregulation may mediate an early response to injury and promote regeneration and repair in the kidney. Mice with a disrupted *Spp1* gene exhibit significantly greater ischemia-induced renal dysfunction and structural damage than wild-type mice.[147] With regard to the role of OPN in stone formation, it is not clear whether OPN in the kidney serves to protect against stones by inhibiting crystallization or perhaps promotes interstitial crystal formation (Randall's plaque) and fibrosis seen in CaP stone formers.[148]

Inter-Alpha-Trypsin Inhibitor/Bikunin

Inter-alpha-trypsin inhibitor proteins are a group of serine protease inhibitors that are mainly synthesized in the liver but have also been detected in many other tissues, including intestine, kidney, stomach, placenta and brain.[149] At least four genes are involved in the synthesis of various members of the inter-alpha-trypsin family of proteins, three encoding heavy chains (H1, H2 and H3) of 75–85 kD, and one encoding the light chain, also known as bikunin, BK, with a molecular weight of 35–40 kD.[150,151] Bikunin can be linked covalently through its chondroitin-4-sulfate side chain to one or two heavy chains, forming the pre-alpha-inhibitor (H3 + BK, 125 kD) or ITI (H1 + H2 + BK, 180–220 kD), respectively.[152] All of these genes have been shown to be expressed in kidney cells.[153,154] ITI, pre-alpha-inhibitor, and all individual subunits have also been detected in urine[155,156] as well as in the matrix of calcium stones.[50,114] While the entire ITI molecule has been shown to inhibit CaOx crystallization,[157] the BK portion is itself a potent inhibitor.[65] The heavy chain components do not have inhibitory activity, and BK is thought to be responsible for the ability of ITI to inhibit CaOx crystallization.[158] To date, no polymorphisms in the genes encoding these proteins have been shown to be associated with nephrolithiasis. One study investigated the possible association between BK gene (*AMBP*) polymorphisms and urinary stone formation in a Turkish population, but found no significant differences in allele distribution between patients and controls.[159]

Inter-alpha-trypsin inhibitor expression is associated with response to inflammation or injury.[97] ITI proteins are thought to be part of the systemic innate immune system; they attenuate complement activation and play a role in limiting complement-dependent tissue injury.[149,160,161] Administration of exogenous BK and ITI proteins has been shown to reduce systemic inflammation in sepsis and systemic inflammatory disorders in mice and humans.[162,163] ITI proteins also play a role in extracellular matrix stabilization in a variety of tissues via binding to hyaluronan.[164] In rats, renal injury induced by hyperoxaluria and crystalluria has been shown to result in significant increases in the level of BK mRNA (messenger ribonucleic acid) expression in the kidney, and concomitant urinary excretion of high-molecular-weight (HMW) BK-containing proteins as well as heavy chains H1 and H3.[155,165,166] In humans, ITI and dimer of BK combined with H1 or H2 were found more often in urine in stone-forming males than in normal males.[156] We also found an increase of HMW (>50 kDa) immunoreactive ITI components in the urine of those who formed stones versus those who did not,[100] and another study confirmed increased urine ITI in stone formers versus normals of both sexes.[101]

Using immunohistochemistry in sections of human kidney tissue, Evan et al. explored the relationship between ITI, BK and calcium stone disease.[110] Heavy chain 3 (HC3) was found to be associated with hyaluronan in the interstitial matrix of the kidney. Widespread HC3 was only present in stone formers, and was found in collecting duct, thin loop and interstitial cells. HC3 colocalized with Randall's plaque (interstitial hydroxyapatite) and urothelial cells, and was also found in the matrix layer of individual plaque spherules. BK was present only in the collecting duct apical membranes and the loop cell cytoplasm of stone formers, colocalizing with HC3. The mechanism linking HC3 to stone disease is unclear but may involve a role for HC3 in stabilizing hyaluronan in the renal interstitial matrix. In the context of pulmonary epithelial cell injury, ITI interacts with hyaluronan and other extracellular matrix components and is an important regulator of cellular repair after injury.[167] Proteomic analysis of renal calculi indicates an important role for inflammatory processes in calcium stone formation.[113] Merchant et al. found that proteomic analysis of stones supports the hypothesis that stone formation induces a cellular inflammatory response and the protein components of this response contribute to the abundant stone matrix proteome. Perhaps ITI in kidney plays a similar role in a cellular inflammatory response in the kidney and in promoting repair of injured renal epithelial and interstitial cells.

Tamm–Horsfall Protein

Tamm–Horsfall protein, also known as uromodulin (UMOD), is a glycoprotein that is the most abundant protein excreted in urine under normal physiological conditions.[168] Made exclusively by epithelial cells in the TALH, THP enters the secretory pathway where it is glycosylphosphatidylinositol anchored, glycosylated, and sorted to the apical plasma membrane. Ultimately, THP is secreted into the urine via proteolytic cleavage by the plasma-membrane-bound serine protease hepsin.[169] In vitro crystallization experiments have shown that THP does not inhibit CaOx crystal nucleation or growth[170,171] but is a potent inhibitor of crystal aggregation.[172] Tamm–Horsfall protein from stone-forming patients inhibits CaOx crystal aggregation to a lesser degree than normal.[173] The high glycan content is important for the physicochemical properties and function of THP. Several studies have reported that stone formers produce THP with reduced levels of glycosylation, particularly sialic acid levels, which leads to reduced negative charge.[66,174] This reduced charge likely decreases the effectiveness of THP binding to Ca^{2+} or CaOx crystals in urine, thus limiting its aggregation-inhibitory activity.[175,176] Some studies have shown that desialylated and low sialic acid forms of THP actually promote crystal aggregation, a property that could ultimately contribute to stone formation.[177,178]

Whether kidney stone formers have defects in THP excretion remains unresolved. Some studies of recurrent calcium stone formers have observed decreased THP in the urine[179] while others have shown increased THP excretion.[180] People with extremely reduced urinary THP levels due to *UMOD* mutations do not show increased rates of renal stone formation.[168] These patients are more likely to have other uromodulin-associated kidney diseases such as medullary cystic kidney disease type 2 and familial juvenile hyperuricemic nephropathy, which, as opposed to calcium nephrolithiasis, are characterized by mild urine concentrating defects, reduced fractional excretion of UA, diffuse tubulointerstitial fibrosis with inflammatory cell infiltrates, cysts at the corticomedullary junction and chronic renal failure.[181,182] Thus, the relative importance of urine THP abundance in protection against stones is still an open question.

In a study of urinary excretion of THP in first-degree family members of calcium stone formers, we found that THP excretion differed by sex and by number of stones formed (K. Bergsland, unpublished). By western blotting, the major THP band (Fig. 3.2) migrated at about 85 kD, in agreement with the 80–90 kD molecular weight observed by others on sodium dodecyl sulfate polyacrylamide gel electrophoresis of

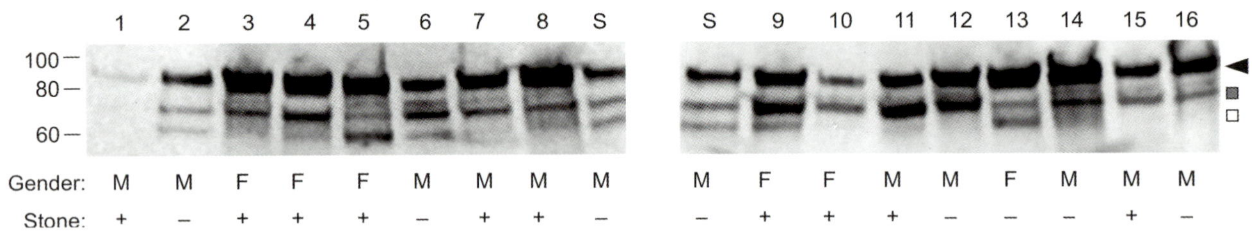

Fig. 3.2: Representative western blots of urinary Tamm–Horsfall protein (THP). Dialyzed urine protein samples were separated by sodium dodecyl sulfate polyacrylamide gel electrophoresis on 10% acrylamide gels under reducing conditions, blotted and immunodetected using an antibody to THP. Lanes 1–16 contain samples from different individuals. Lanes S contain a standard urine sample from a nonstone-forming male. Sizes of protein molecular weight standards (in kD) are indicated at left. The major THP band (arrowhead) migrated at about 85 kD; lower-molecular-weight forms likely represent THP precursors lacking glycosylation (57–60 kD, open square) or sialic acid modifications of glycan chains (69–71 kD, closed square). Semiquantitative abundances of various THP forms were calculated by dividing the optical density (OD) of each band by the total OD of lane S on the same blot. (F: Female; M: Male).

properly glycosylated, glycosylphosphatidylinositol-modified and membrane-anchored THP protein excreted in urine.[183] Lower-molecular-weight forms likely represent THP precursors lacking glycosylation (57–60 kD) or sialic acid modifications of glycan chains (69–71 kD).[184–186] When family members of stone formers (50 men, 50 women; half stone formers) were grouped within sex by the presence or absence of kidney stones, THP excretion in all men was the same (Fig. 3.3). Women stone formers tended to have less THP than those who had never had a stone but the difference was not significant. However, when subjects were stratified by the number of stones formed, THP excretion was greater in men with multiple stones compared to men who had formed one stone, a difference that was not observed in women (Fig. 3.3). These sex- and stone number-related differences may help explain the discrepant measurements of urine THP abundance seen in previously published studies, with one study finding less THP in stone formers and another finding more.[179,180] THP excretion in nonstone-forming men was intermediate between male single stone formers and multiple stone formers. Increased excretion of LMW THP was highly significant in men with multiple stones compared to male single stone formers and controls ($p < 0.0001$, both comparisons), but not in women (Fig. 3.4). Thus, increased excretion of both mature THP and LMW forms lacking post-translational modifications is strongly associated with having >1 stone in men. Low-molecular-weight forms of THP that lack post-translational modifications (glycosylation or sialic acid residues) are likely less effective in inhibiting crystal aggregation in urine; the increased proportion of LMW THP in the urine of male multiple stone formers may contribute to their higher rate of stone formation and perhaps to the increased prevalence of stones in men versus women.

Although THP is predominantly targeted to the apical membrane of TALH cells, there also is a lesser but significant basolateral release of THP by a mechanism that is not well understood.[187,188] Tamm–Horsfall protein can be detected in the blood of healthy individuals, suggesting that some degree of basolateral release of THP occurs normally.[187,189] Basolateral release is significantly increased during kidney injury; El-Achkar et al. found a major redirection of THP from the apical membrane toward the basolateral domain and interstitium during recovery from acute kidney injury.[190,191] This redirection corresponds with increased THP in the serum but not in the urine. Evidence suggests that basolateral THP plays an important role in halting intrarenal inflammatory signaling after ischemia reperfusion injury (IRI) by facilitating tubular cross-talk with the neighboring injured proximal tubule S3 segments.[187,191] Tamm–Horsfall protein is known to function as a "cytokine trap," forming in vivo complexes with renal and urinary cytokines, thus limiting their activation of inflammatory signaling pathways.[192] Mice deficient in THP show significantly more functional and histological renal damage after IRI, possibly due to reduced suppression by THP of proinflammatory cytokines and chemokines produced by S3.[193] These mice also have higher expression of toll-like receptor 4 (TLR4) in the basement membranes of injured tubular segments, indicating that THP may also normally act to limit renal injury by decreasing activation of innate immunity mediated by TLR4.

Studies in *Umod* gene KO mice have suggested a role for THP in protection against stone formation in the kidney. Lack of THP in KO mice leads to the formation of CaP (hydroxyapatite) crystals in the kidneys and progressive renal calcification.[140,194] In young mice, both intratubular and interstitial crystals are seen, but in older mice

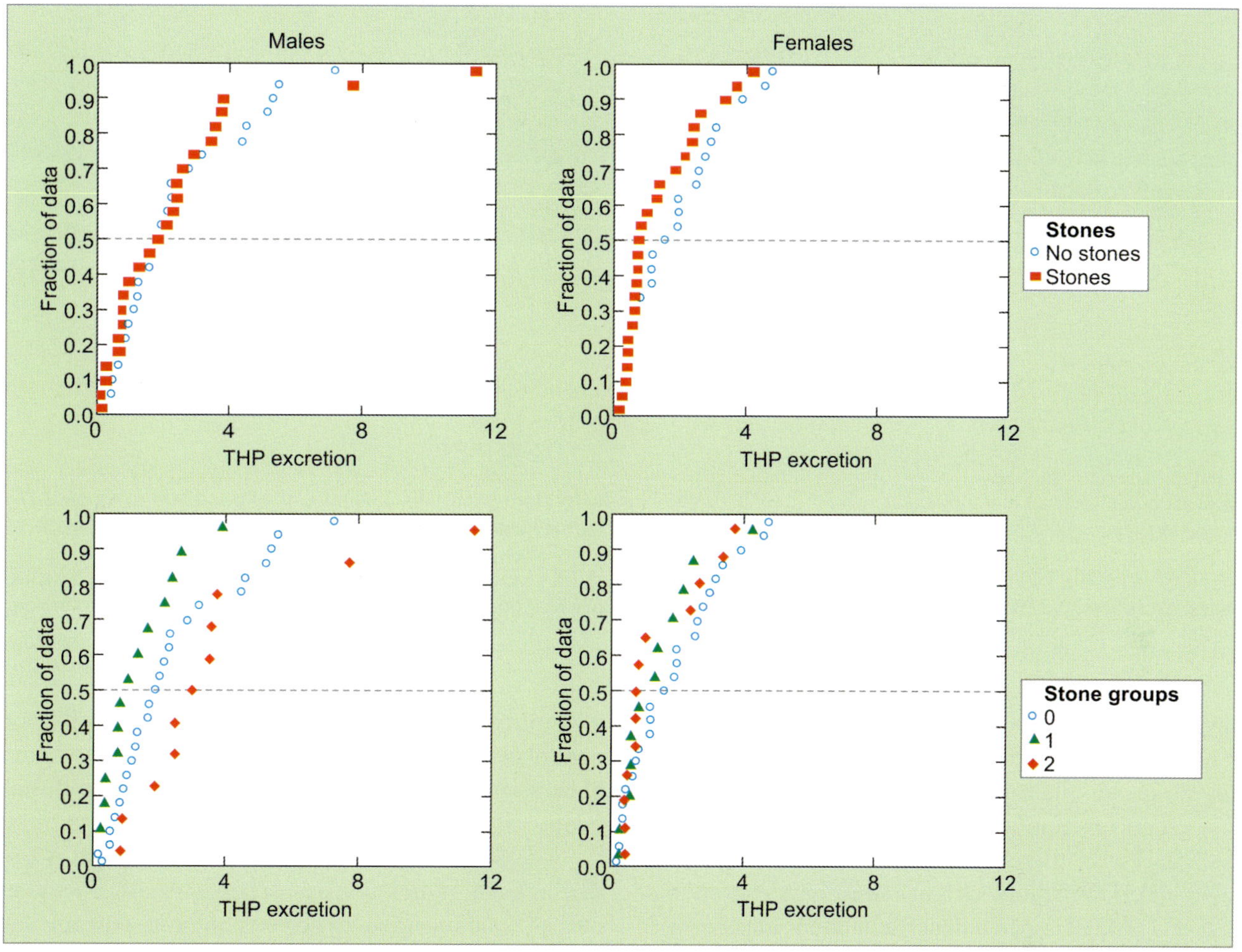

Fig. 3.3: Quantile plots of urine Tamm–Horsfall protein (THP) excretion. Estimations of excretion rates of mature THP were made by multiplying the semiquantitative measurements of each protein (Fig. 3.1) by the 24-hour urine volume. Males are at left and females are at right. In the top panels, subjects are grouped by stone status: nonstone formers (○) and stone formers (■). In the bottom panels, subjects are grouped by stone number: Nonstone formers (○), men with 1 stone, and women with 1–2 stones (▲), and men with ≥2 stones and women with ≥3 stones (♦). In subjects grouped by the presence or absence of kidney stones (top), THP excretion in all men was the same; female stone formers tended to have less THP than nonstone formers but the difference was not significant. In subjects grouped by the number of stones formed (bottom), THP excretion was greater in men with multiple stones compared to men who had formed one stone, a difference that was not observed in women.

interstitial crystals predominate. Tamm-Horsfall protein exerts its protective effect synergistically with OPN as seen in double KO mice.[140,168] The incidence of renal interstitial hydroxyapatite deposits is more than twice as high in the OPN + THP double KO than in either of the single-gene KOs alone. Crystals are mainly located in the renal papilla with the rest of the kidney devoid of any crystals. The pattern of interstitial crystallization in THP KO mice resembles Randall's plaques of human idiopathic CaOx stone formers with respect to histological location, chemical composition, ultrastructural features and lack of accompanying inflammation.[195,196] In humans, however, Randall's plaques also involve the basement membranes of the thin loops of Henle, and there is an overgrowth of CaOx stones atop regions of papillary crystallization, neither of which have been observed in THP KO mice.[197]

In humans, genome-wide association studies have linked a common variant in the *UMOD* gene on chromosome 16p12 to decreased risk of kidney stones.[198] The variant rs4293393-T, which is located in the promoter region of the *UMOD* gene about 550 bp upstream of the translational start, is present at high frequency in most modern populations (70–80% in Africans and Europeans and 92–95% in East Asians) and confers protection against calcium

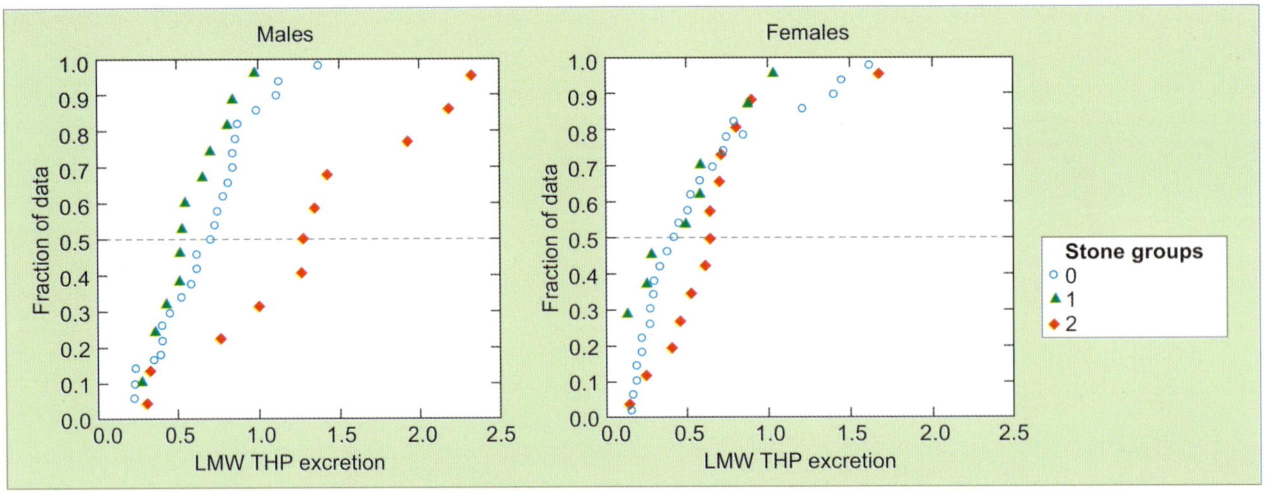

Fig. 3.4: Quantile plots of low molecular weight (LMW) Tamm–Horsfall protein excretion. Estimations of excretion rates of LMW THP forms lacking glycosylation or sialic acid modifications were made by multiplying the semiquantitative measurement of each protein band (Fig. 3.1) by the 24-hour urine volume. Males are at left, and females are at right. Subjects are grouped by stone number: Nonstone formers (○), men with 1 stone and women with 1–2 stones (▲), and men with ≥2 stones and women with ≥3 stones (♦). Increased excretion of LMW THP was highly significant in men with multiple stones compared to male single stone formers and controls ($p < 0.0001$, both comparisons), but not in women. (F: Female; M: Male).

kidney stones.[199] This variant has been shown to increase THP expression approximately twofold both in vivo in kidney tissue by quantitative reverse transcription polymerase chain reaction and in vitro in luciferase reporter assays.[200] Likewise, there is a strong association of this variant with an up to twofold increase in urinary excretion of THP; levels of THP rise in a dose-dependent manner with an increasing number of T alleles.[200,201]

A study of the frequency of the rs4293393-T allele in various modern and ancient human and nonhuman primate populations strongly suggests that this allele has been kept at high frequency through evolution because of its protective effect against urinary tract infections (UTIs).[199] The KO mice lacking THP have an increased susceptibility to UTI.[73,202] Tamm–Horsfall protein functions in defending the urinary tract against infections due to its ability to bind to pathogens and prevent their adherence to the urothelium.[203] There is evidence that, in a similar manner, THP coats CaOx crystals and helps prevent adhesion to cultured epithelial cells.[86,176] Perhaps the selective pressure to maintain the rs4293393-T allele because of its protective effect against UTI has had the fortuitous benefit over time of also protecting against stones. The minor rs4293393-C variant that is the risk allele for kidney stones also potentially increases susceptibility to UTIs.[199] It is interesting that, although a definitive study has not been done, there is evidence to suggest a correlation between the presence of UTI and stones. In several small single-center studies, a significantly higher incidence of UTI was observed in patients with stones, including not only struvite but metabolic stones composed of CaOx and CaP, than in healthy people.[204–206]

The same *UMOD* rs4293393-T variant that is protective against stones is also associated with an increased risk of salt-sensitive hypertension and chronic kidney disease.[198,200,207] Tamm–Horsfall protein is thought to play a role in water and electrolyte balance in the TALH. Evidence from THP KO mice suggests that THP facilitates the activation of the sodium-potassium-chloride transporter (NKCC2) and the renal outer medullary potassium channel (ROMK), the two main ion transporters involved in sodium chloride reabsorption by the TALH.[74,75] In mice lacking THP, both NKCC2 and ROMK accumulate in subapical intracellular vesicles resulting in decreased apical surface expression and reduced transporter activity. On the other hand, overexpression of wild-type THP in transgenic mice enhances NKCC2 activity and increases sodium reabsorption in the TALH, leading to salt-sensitive hypertension.[200] The *UMOD* rs4293393-C variant that is the risk allele for kidney stones would be expected to have the opposite effect, which is to decrease THP expression and NKCC2 activity and to reduce blood pressure. Trudu et al. investigated the role of *UMOD* variants in modulating blood pressure in humans and found that mean diastolic blood pressure was significantly lower in individuals that were heterozygous or homozygous for the rs4293393-

C allele relative to individuals that were homozygous for the T allele.[200] Interestingly, Ko et al. found that male patients with idiopathic hypercalciuria, a common trait among calcium stone formers, have lower systolic blood pressures than normal male patients.[208] Tamm–Horsfall protein also plays a role in modulating urine calcium excretion by stimulating calcium reabsorption in the distal nephron by decreasing endocytosis of the calcium channel TRPV5.[209] Tamm–Horsfall protein KO mice and mice carrying *UMOD* mutations found in human uromodulin-associated kidney diseases that severely reduce urinary THP levels exhibit hypercalciuria. Thus, *UMOD* genotypes that reduce expression of THP may link susceptibility to kidney stones and protection from hypertension via the effect of THP on calcium and salt reabsorption in the kidney.

Albumin

Human serum albumin is the second most abundant protein in urine, after THP. Albumin is primarily synthesized in the liver, functions as a carrier protein for fatty acids and hormones in the blood and plays a major role in stabilizing extracellular fluid volume by contributing to oncotic pressure of plasma. Albumin has an immunomodulatory and extracellular antioxidant defense functions mediated by its high capacity to bind lipopolysaccharide and other bacterial products (lipoteichoic acid and peptidoglycan), reactive oxygen species (ROS), nitric oxide and other nitrogen reactive species, and prostaglandins.[210,211] Albumin has also been found to have antimicrobial properties in exerting fungistatic activity.[212] Albumin is a large component of the matrix of calcium stones.[114,213,214] It does not inhibit CaOx crystal growth in vitro[170,171] and seems to promote nucleation of CaOx crystals, specifically the dihydrate form.[215] By contrast, albumin is an inhibitor of CaOx crystal aggregation in inorganic solutions[171,216] and urine.[170] Baumann and Affolter found that, somewhat paradoxically, when albumin was adsorbed onto CaP crystals it became a promoter of CaOx crystal aggregation rather than an inhibitor.[69] This was attributed to self-aggregation bridging zones of electrostatic repulsion between coated crystals with identical electrical surface charge. This effect was abolished when urine was diluted, arguing for the importance of stone formers maintaining adequate urine volume to diminish urinary SS and risk of crystal aggregation.

The gene encoding albumin may be expressed in kidney,[217] but it is more likely that albumin in urine is filtered from the blood. Pourmand et al. found increased albumin in the urine of recurrent calcium stone formers compared to normal controls.[218] Of 10 urine proteins measured, only albumin and transferrin (another blood protein) were different between the groups, suggesting renal bleeding or perhaps glomerular impairment as the source of these proteins in stone formers. All in all, the presence of albumin in stones is more likely due to its ubiquitous nature in blood, urine and tissue than to any specific role in regulation of crystallization or stone formation.

Calgranulins (S100A8 and S100A9)

S100A8 and S100A9, also known as calgranulin A and B or MRP8 and MRP14, are small, acidic, potent calcium-binding proteins that are abundantly present in the matrix of calcium stones.[114,219-222] S100A8 and S100A9 exist as monomers of about 10 and 14 kD, respectively, but preferentially form a S100A8/A9 heterodimer (also known as "calprotectin") in the presence of Zn^{2+} or Ca^{2+}.[223] S100A8/A9 exhibits antimicrobial activity by inhibiting bacterial adhesion to mucosal epithelia and sequestering essential trace elements such as Zn^{2+}.[224] Both S100A9 and S100A8/A9 can also form higher-order oligomers such as tetramers or even larger oligomers, and this multimer formation may regulate their function.[225-227] Calgranulin (likely S100A8) has been found to be a potent inhibitor of CaOx crystal growth and aggregation in the nanomolar range in vitro.[68] S100A8 and S100A9 are constitutively expressed in myeloid cells (monocytes, neutrophils and dendritic cells), but expression can also be induced in other cell types such as macrophages, vascular endothelial cells and fibroblasts.[219] In the kidney, S100A8 and S100A9 have also been found to be expressed in glomerulus, tubulointerstitial regions and collecting duct.[68,228,229] Polymorphisms in the genes for these proteins have been shown to be associated with periodontitis (S100A8)[230] and insulin resistance and type 2 diabetes (S100A9),[231] but not with nephrolithiasis thus far.[102]

Secreted S100A8 and S100A9 have been shown to be endogenous proinflammatory ligands that can activate cytokine signaling pathways and leukocyte recruitment via the receptor for advanced glycation endproducts and TLR4.[232,233] S100A8 and S100A9 are involved in acute response to injury and early inflammatory program initiation.[234] Circulating levels of S100A8 and S100A9 are increased in many disease conditions including cancer, neurodegenerative disorders, autoimmune and inflammatory diseases, including type 2 diabetes (T2DM) and obesity.[223,235–238] They are considered to be damage-associated molecular pattern molecules that are overexpressed at sites of local inflammation.[239] The genes for S100A8 and S100A9 are direct targets of NF-κB, which is stimulated downstream of TLR4 activation. Therefore, binding of these damage-associated molecular patterns to TLR4 can set up a positive feedback loop that contributes to perpetuation of the innate immune response.[240] TLR4 is expressed all along the nephron from Bowman's capsule to proximal convoluted tubule, TALH, distal tubule and collecting duct.[241] Continued stimulation of TLR4 in any of these locations could set off a "damage chain reaction" leading to chronic innate immune activation and enhanced tissue injury.[242]

However, these proteins also play anti-inflammatory roles in wound healing[243] and protection against oxidative tissue damage as a result of their extreme ability to scavenge oxidants.[227] Under conditions of oxidative stress, S100A8 and S100A9 may serve as sinks for reactive oxygen species (ROS) including HOCl, H_2O_2, and NO. Binding of ROS causes conformational changes and formation of covalent bonds in S100A8 and S100A9 homodimers and higher order homocomplexes.[227] S100A8 and S100A9 can self-assemble into a variety of amyloid complexes both in vitro and in vivo, and covalently-linked complexes of S100A9 have been identified in brain extracts of patients with familial Alzheimer's disease and in association with senile plaques.[244]

S100A8 and S100A9 may play roles in both normal and dystrophic calcification processes. Both are expressed in human bone and cartilage cells and may play a role in calcification of cartilage matrix and its replacement with trabecular bone.[245] S100A8 and S100A9 are abundant in osteoclasts and may contribute to regulation of the oxidative balance required for bone remodeling. S100A9 has been shown to be highly expressed in atherosclerotic plaque where it is associated with calcified areas.[246] Calcifying microvesicles from carotid artery isolates contain high levels of S100A9, with a lesser amount of S100A8. In addition, age-related protein amyloid structures in prostate, also called prostatic calculi or corpora amylacea, are primarily composed of amyloid forms of S100A8 and S100A9 in combination with hydroxyapatite.[247] To date, expression of these proteins in the kidney has not been investigated in the context of stone or Randall's plaque formation.

Whether the functional outcome of S100A8 and S100A9 expression is protective or injurious may depend on the types of cells expressing these proteins in particular microenvironments, their relative concentrations and post-translational modifications.[248] High circulating levels of S100A8/A9 are suggested to contribute to atherogenesis in patients suffering from acute and chronic inflammatory disorders such as periodontitis, rheumatoid arthritis, obesity and systemic lupus erythematosus.[235,249–251] However, it is possible that the high concentrations of S100A8 released following neutrophil and monocyte/macrophage accumulation in plaque may moderate oxidative damage and reduce inflammation by suppressing mast cell activation, thereby limiting atherogenesis.[248] In the kidney, glomerular and tubulointerstitial S100A8 expression was found to be increased in renal biopsy samples from obese or type 2 diabetic patients compared to controls.[228] Elevated S100A8 in injured tubular epithelial cells and surrounding macrophages was associated with tubulointerstitial fibrosis and progression of proteinuria in obese and type 2 diabetic patients. On the other hand, there is evidence that S100A8/A9 is protective against ischemia/reperfusion (IRI) injury. In a mouse model of IRI, renal abundances of S100A8 and S100A9, likely to be from infiltrating granulocytes, were normally increased in the corticomedullary region in wild-type mice.[252] However, S100A9 KO mice displayed defective tissue repair after I/R, increased renal damage, sustained inflammation, induction of fibrosis and increased expression of collagens, suggesting loss of a protective function of S100A9.

In a study of urinary excretion of S100A9 in first-degree family members of calcium kidney stone formers (same study as for THP, above), we found that S100A9 excretion differed by sex and by the number of stones formed (K. Bergsland, unpublished). Western blots showed a prominent immunoreactive band at 14 kD that is the major monomeric form of this protein (Fig. 3.5).[253] Monomeric S100A9 exists in two isoforms: full length (14 kD) and truncated S100A9* (~13.5 kD), which is translated from an alternate start site in the S100A9 gene and lacking four amino acids at the N-terminus.[225,227] In addition, HMW forms around 28, 42 and 56 kD were also apparent, which most likely represent dimers, trimers and tetramers of S100A9 induced by oxidative modification.[227] These complexes contain covalent bonds that are resistant to the reducing conditions of gel electrophoresis. Among men, but not women, excretion of HMW S100A9 (a sum of all forms ≥15 kD, i.e. larger than the monomer) was significantly increased in recurrent stone formers relative to single stone formers and nonstone-forming controls (Fig. 3.6). There were no differences between subject groups in the

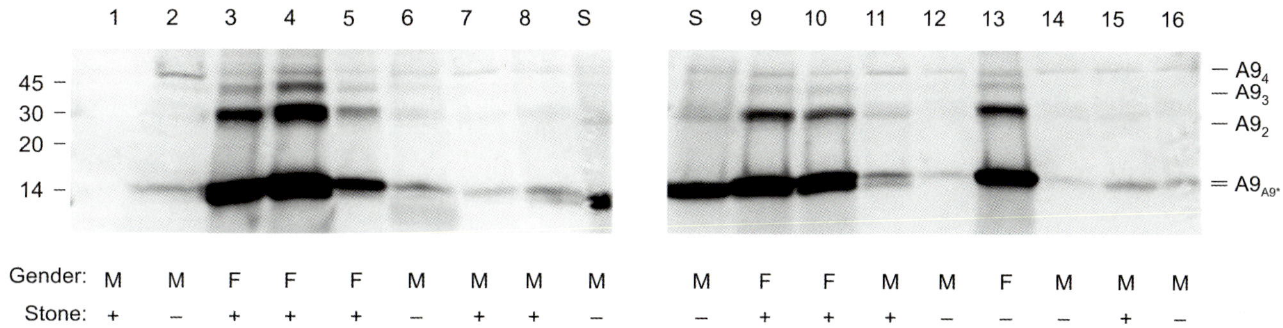

Fig. 3.5: Representative western blots of urinary S100A9. Lanes 1–16 contain samples from different individuals. Lanes S contain a standard urine sample from a nonstone-forming man. Sizes of protein molecular weight standards (in kD) are indicated at left. Positions of monomeric and multimeric forms are indicated at right. S100A9* (~13.5 kD) is a monomeric form which is translated from an alternate start site in the S100A9 gene and lacks four amino acids at the N-terminus.

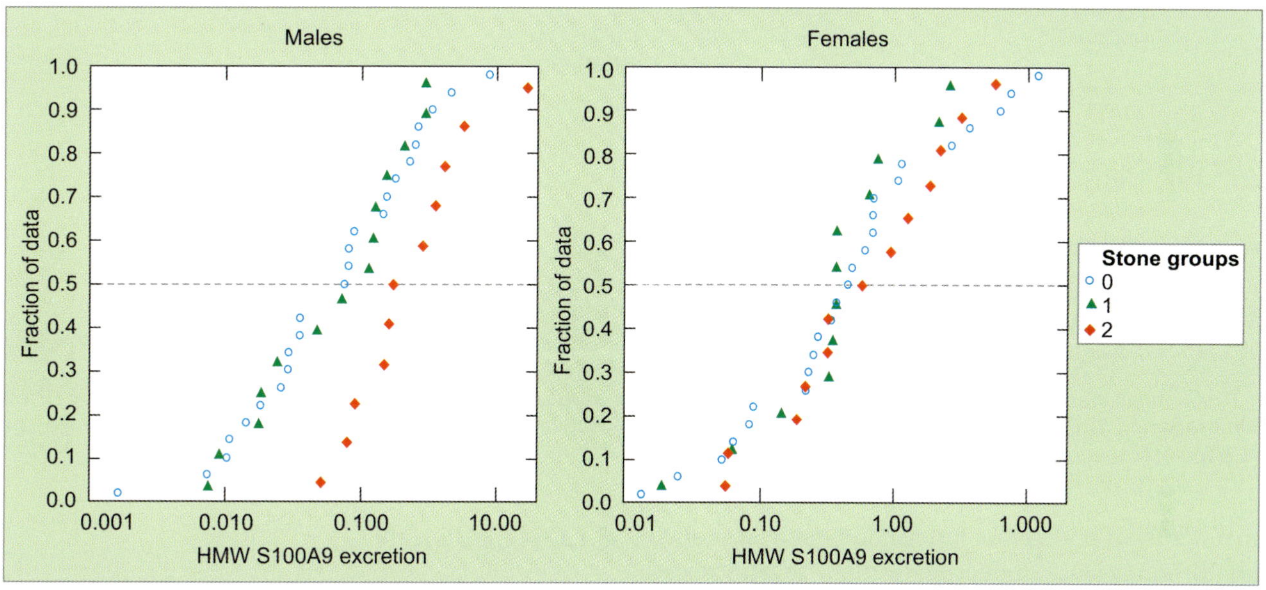

Fig. 3.6: Quantile plots of high-molecular-weight (HMW) S100A9 excretion. Estimations of excretion rates of HMW S100A9 forms (a sum of all forms ≥ 15 kD, i.e. larger than the monomer) were made by multiplying the semiquantitative measurement of each protein band (*see* Fig. 3.5) by the 24-hour urine volume. Males are at left and females are at right. Subjects are grouped by stone number: non-stone formers (○), men with 1 stone and women with 1–2 stones (▲), and men with ≥ 2 stones and women with ≥ 3 stones (♦). Increased excretion of HMW S100A9 was highly significant in men with multiple stones compared to male single stone formers and controls ($p < 0.05$, both comparisons), but not in women.

amount of monomer excreted, except that it was higher in females than males in general. Thus, elevated excretion of multimeric (HMW) forms of S100A9 is a particular feature of men who have had more than one stone.

It is not clear whether the S100A9 in urine from stone formers is coming from an intrarenal source or is filtered into the urine from the blood. Increased total urinary S100A8/A9 has been identified as a diagnostic marker of bladder cancer[254] and intrinsic acute kidney injury,[255] suggesting the urinary tract or kidney as the source. It has been found to be transiently elevated over a period of 48 hours in patients who have undergone renal ischemia during surgery.[256] Higher urinary S100A8/A9 is also a predictor of renal allograft injury and impaired function after kidney transplantation.[257] Other studies have suggested a systemic source for this protein. Ortega et al. found elevated levels of total urinary S100A8/A9 to be associated with chronic low-grade inflammation and insulin resistance in men.[258] By ELISA, urine S100A8/A9 was significantly increased in male patients with impaired glucose tolerance or T2DM

Table 3.1: Functions of crystallization inhibitor proteins in modulating innate immune response.

	Antimicrobial	*Cytokines*	*Antioxidant*	*Tissue repair*
PF1		Thrombin promotes cytokine and chemokine synthesis via PARs[97,98]; PF1 is a marker of thrombin generation		Thrombin interacts with PAR-1 to stimulate a regenerative response to tissue damage[98]
OPN		Potent chemoattractant for macrophages[146]	Repressor of inducible nitric oxide synthase [260]	Role in tissue remodeling and matrix reorganization after injury; promotes wound healing[260]
ITI/Bikunin		BK decreases binding of LPS to TLR4 and inhibits LPS-induced TNF α production[261]		Protease inhibitors, attenuate complement activation[160,161]; interact with hyaluronan to stabilize extracellular matrix after injury[167]
THP	Binds to microbes and prevents adhesion to epithelia[203]	"Cytokine trap" forms in vivo complexes with renal and urinary cytokines; limits activation of TLR4 and inflammatory signaling pathways[192]		
Albumin	Binds lipoteichoic acid and peptidoglycan[210]; antifungal[212]		Binds ROS, NO and other reactive nitrogen species[211]	
S100A8/A9	Inhibit adhesion to mucosal epithelia; potent Zn^{2+} binding limits micronutrient availability for microbes[224]	Endogenous ligand of RAGE and TLR4; promote expression of proinflammatory cytokines[233]	Avid oxidant scavengers; sink for ROS including HOCl, H_2O_2, and NO[227]	

(PF1: Prothrombin fragment 1; OPN: Osteopontin; ITI: Inter-alpha-trypsin inhibitor; THP: Tamm–Horsfall protein; PAR: Protease-activated receptor; TLR4: Toll-like receptor 4; RAGE: Receptor for advanced glycation endproducts; ROS: Reactive oxygen species; LPS: Lipopolysaccharide; TNFα: Tumor necrosis factor alpha).

independently of body mass index and positively associated with homeostasis model assessment–insulin resistance (HOMA-IR), inflammatory markers, and parameters of glucose and lipid metabolism. Diabetes and obesity are both associated with a risk of nephrolithiasis.[129] It is possible that S100A9 in urine from stone formers may be coming from both systemic and renal sources. Interestingly, we found that only higher-order forms of S100A9 were elevated in male recurrent stone formers, suggesting that an oxidative process is at play in these patients. Renal oxidative stress is higher in males compared to females,[259] which may explain this sex difference if urinary S100A9 is coming from the kidney. More research is needed to understand the association of S100A8 and S100A9 with nephrolithiasis and whether these urinary proteins are marking a cause or consequence of stone formation.

CONCLUSION

The overall capacity of urine to inhibit crystallization is determined by the actions and abundance of many molecules in this biological solution. There is much redundancy in the system, such that no one molecule is pre-eminent in this function. Making the situation more complicated is the fact that some molecules considered to be inhibitors of crystallization can, in fact, be promoters given the proper conditions. The sources of these proteins in urine are often unclear, being potentially derived from renal and/or systemic production. The proteins mentioned here all have other additional normal roles in mediating inflammation and the innate immune response, facilitating wound healing and tissue repair, managing oxidative stress or antimicrobial protection (Table 3.1). Observed differences in the context of stone formation may actually be related to alterations in their function in another system or process. Much more research will be required to untangle the complex interplay of pathways and determine the conditions that constitute optimal crystallization inhibition and factors that tip the balance toward stone formation.

REFERENCES

1. Tiselius H. Solution chemistry of supersaturation. In: Coe FL, Favus MJ, Pak CYC, Parks JH, Preminger GM (Eds). Kidney Stones: Medical and Surgical Management. Philadelphia, PA: Lippincott-Raven; 1996. pp. 33-64.
2. Parks JH, Coward M, Coe FL. Correspondence between stone composition and urine supersaturation in nephrolithiasis. Kidney Int. 1997;51(3):894-900.
3. Coe FL, Parks JH. Disorders of calcium stone formation. In: Seldin D, Giebisch G (Eds). The Kidney, 3rd edition. Philadelphia, PA: Lippincott, Williams and Wilkins; 2000. pp. 1841-67.
4. Coe FL, Parks JH. New insights into the pathophysiology and treatment of nephrolithiasis: new research venues. J Bone Miner Res. 1997;12(4):522-33.
5. Asplin JR, Parks JH, Chen MS, et al. Reduced crystallization inhibition by urine from men with nephrolithiasis. Kidney Int. 1999;56(4):1505-16.
6. Asplin JR, Parks JH, Nakagawa Y, et al. Reduced crystallization inhibition by urine from women with nephrolithiasis. Kidney Int. 2002;61(5):1821-9.
7. Aggarwal KP, Narula S, Kakkar M, et al. Nephrolithiasis: molecular mechanism of renal stone formation and the critical role played by modulators. Biomed Res Int. 2013;2013:292953.
8. Doizi S, Rodgers K, Poindexter J, et al. Assessment of urinary inhibitor or promoter activity in uric acid nephrolithiasis. J Urol. 2016;195(6):1799-804.
9. Tiselius HG, Berg C, Fornander AM, et al. Effects of citrate on the different phases of calcium oxalate crystallization. Scanning Microsc. 1993;7(1):381-9.
10. Berg C, Tiselius HG. The effects of citrate on hydroxyapatite induced calcium oxalate crystallization and on the formation of calcium phosphate crystals. Urol Res. 1989;17(3):167-72.
11. Pak CY. Citrate and renal calculi: an update. Miner Electrolyte Metab. 1994;20(6):371-7.
12. Hess B, Jordi S, Zipperle L, et al. Citrate determines calcium oxalate crystallization kinetics and crystal morphology-studies in the presence of Tamm–Horsfall protein of a healthy subject and a severely recurrent calcium stone former. Nephrol Dial Transplant. 2000;15(3):366-74.
13. Grohe B, O'Young J, Langdon A, et al. Citrate modulates calcium oxalate crystal growth by face-specific interactions. Cells Tissues Organs. 2011;194(2-4):176-81.
14. Greischar A, Nakagawa Y, Coe FL. Influence of urine pH and citrate concentration on the upper limit of metastability for calcium phosphate. J Urol. 2003;169(3):867-70.
15. Parks JH, Coe FL. A urinary calcium-citrate index for the evaluation of nephrolithiasis. Kidney Int. 1986;30(1):85-90.
16. Cupisti A, Morelli E, Lupetti S, et al. Low urine citrate excretion as main risk factor for recurrent calcium oxalate nephrolithiasis in males. Nephron. 1992;61(1):73-6.
17. Ettinger B, Pak CY, Citron JT, et al. Potassium-magnesium citrate is an effective prophylaxis against recurrent calcium oxalate nephrolithiasis. J Urol. 1997;158(6):2069-73.
18. Barcelo P, Wuhl O, Servitge E, et al. Randomized double-blind study of potassium citrate in idiopathic hypocitraturic calcium nephrolithiasis. J Urol. 1993;150(6):1761-4.
19. Phillips R, Hanchanale VS, Myatt A, et al. Citrate salts for preventing and treating calcium containing kidney stones in adults. Cochrane Database Syst Rev. 2015;(10):CD010057.
20. Coe FL, Evan A, Worcester E. Pathophysiology-based treatment of idiopathic calcium kidney stones. Clin J Am Soc Nephrol. 2011;6(8):2083-92.
21. Miyake O, Yoshimura K, Yoshioka T, et al. High urinary excretion level of citrate and magnesium in children: potential etiology for the reduced incidence of pediatric urolithiasis. Urol Res. 1998;26(3):209-13.
22. Bergsland KJ, Coe FL, White MD, et al. Urine risk factors in children with calcium kidney stones and their siblings. Kidney Int. 2012;81(11):1140-8.
23. Kirejczyk JK, Porowski T, Konstantynowicz J, et al. Urinary citrate excretion in healthy children depends on age and gender. Pediatr Nephrol. 2014;29(9):1575-82.
24. Hesse A, Classen A, Knoll M, et al. Dependence of urine composition on the age and sex of healthy subjects. Clin Chim Acta. 1986;160(2):79-86.
25. Powell CR, Stoller ML, Schwartz BF, et al. Impact of body weight on urinary electrolytes in urinary stone formers. Urology. 2000;55(6):825-30.
26. Shavit L, Ferraro PM, Johri N, et al. Effect of being overweight on urinary metabolic risk factors for kidney stone formation. Nephrol Dial Transplant. 2015;30(4):607-13.
27. Hamm LL. Renal handling of citrate. Kidney Int. 1990;38(4):728-35.
28. Ohana E, Shcheynikov N, Moe OW, et al. SLC26A6 and NaDC-1 transporters interact to regulate oxalate and citrate homeostasis. J Am Soc Nephrol. 2013;24(10):1617-26.
29. Pinheiro VB, Baxmann AC, Tiselius HG, et al. The effect of sodium bicarbonate upon urinary citrate excretion in calcium stone formers. Urology. 2013;82(1):33-7.
30. Sakhaee K, Alpern R, Jacobson HR, et al. Contrasting effects of various potassium salts on renal citrate excretion. J Clin Endocrinol Metab. 1991;72(2):396-400.
31. Caudarella R, Vescini F, Buffa A, et al. Citrate and mineral metabolism: kidney stones and bone disease. Front Biosci. 2003;8:s1084-106.
32. Coe FL. (2016). Citrate and the Ostwald limit. [online] Available from http://kidneystones.uchicago.edu/?s=citrate
33. Massey L. Magnesium therapy for nephrolithiasis. Magnes Res. 2005;18(2):123-6.
34. Riley JM, Kim H, Averch TD, et al. Effect of magnesium on calcium and oxalate ion binding. J Endourol. 2013;27(12):1487-92.

35. Grases F, Rodriguez A, Costa-Bauza A. Efficacy of mixtures of magnesium, citrate and phytate as calcium oxalate crystallization inhibitors in urine. J Urol. 2015;194(3):812-9.
36. Hess B, Hasler-Strub U, Ackermann D, et al. Metabolic evaluation of patients with recurrent idiopathic calcium nephrolithiasis. Nephrol Dial Transplant. 1997;12(7):1362-8.
37. Menditto VG, Lucci M, Polonara S. [The role of hypomagnesiuria in urolithiasis and renal colic: results from a prospective study of a metabolic evaluation protocola]. Minerva Med. 2012;103(5):377-82. [Article in Italian]
38. Ettinger B, Citron JT, Livermore B, et al. Chlorthalidone reduces calcium oxalate calculous recurrence but magnesium hydroxide does not. J Urol. 1988;139(4):679-84.
39. Sutor DJ. Growth studies of calcium oxalate in the presence of various ions and compounds. Br J Urol. 1969;41(2):171-8.
40. Ryall RL, Harnett RM, Marshall VR. The effect of urine, pyrophosphate, citrate, magnesium and glycosaminoglycans on the growth and aggregation of calcium oxalate crystals in vitro. Clin Chim Acta. 1981;112(3):349-56.
41. Wilson JW, Werness PG, Smith LH. Inhibitors of crystal growth of hydroxyapatite: a constant composition approach. J Urol. 1985;134(6):1255-8.
42. Roberts NB, Dutton J, Helliwell T, et al. Pyrophosphate in synovial fluid and urine and its relationship to urinary risk factors for stone disease. Ann Clin Biochem. 1992;29(Pt 5):529-34.
43. Schwille PO, Rumenapf G, Wolfel G, et al. Urinary pyrophosphate in patients with recurrent calcium urolithiasis and in healthy controls: a re-evaluation. J Urol. 1988;140(2):239-45.
44. O'Brien MM, Uhlemann I, McIntosh HW. Urinary pyrophosphate in normal subjects and in stone formers. Can Med Assoc J. 1967;96(2):100-3.
45. Robertson WG, Peacock M, Heyburn PJ, et al. Risk factors in calcium stone disease of the urinary tract. Br J Urol. 1978;50(7):449-54.
46. Arzoz-Fabregas M, Ibarz-Servio L, Fernandez-Castro J, et al. Chronic stress and calcium oxalate stone disease: influence on blood cortisol and urine composition. Urology. 2013;82(6):1246-52.
47. Mathis SL, Farley RS, Fuller DK, et al. The relationship between cortisol and bone mineral density in competitive male cyclists. J Sports Med (Hindawi Publ Corp). 2013;2013:896821.
48. Kirschbaum C, Wust S, Hellhammer D. Consistent sex differences in cortisol responses to psychological stress. Psychosom Med. 1992;54(6):648-57.
49. Saw NK, Chow K, Rao PN, et al. Effects of inositol hexaphosphate (phytate) on calcium binding, calcium oxalate crystallization and in vitro stone growth. J Urol. 2007;177(6):2366-70.
50. Ryall RL. The possible roles of inhibitors, promoters and macromolecules in the formation of calcium kidney stones. In: Rao PN, Preminger GM, Kavanagh JP (Eds). Urinary Tract Stone Disease. New York: Springer; 2011. pp. 31-60.
51. Grases F, Ramis M, Costa-Bauza A. Effects of phytate and pyrophosphate on brushite and hydroxyapatite crystallization. Comparison with the action of other polyphosphates. Urol Res. 2000;28(2):136-40.
52. Grases F, Simonet BM, March JG, et al. Inositol hexakisphosphate in urine: the relationship between oral intake and urinary excretion. BJU Int. 2000;85(1):138-42.
53. Grases F, March JG, Prieto RM, et al. Urinary phytate in calcium oxalate stone formers and healthy people—dietary effects on phytate excretion. Scand J Urol Nephrol. 2000;34(3):162-4.
54. Curhan GC, Willett WC, Knight EL, et al. Dietary factors and the risk of incident kidney stones in younger women: Nurses' Health Study II. Arch Intern Med. 2004;164(8):885-91.
55. Zhou JR, Erdman JW Jr. Phytic acid in health and disease. Crit Rev Food Sci Nutr. 1995;35(6):495-508.
56. Krebs NF. Update on zinc deficiency and excess in clinical pediatric practice. Ann Nutr Metab. 2013;62(Suppl 1):19-29.
57. Gupta RK, Gangoliya SS, Singh NK. Reduction of phytic acid and enhancement of bioavailable micronutrients in food grains. J Food Sci Technol. 2015;52(2):676-84.
58. Thomas E, von Unruh GE, Hesse A. Influence of a low- and a high-oxalate vegetarian diet on intestinal oxalate absorption and urinary excretion. Eur J Clin Nutr. 2008;62(9):1090-7.
59. Nakagawa Y, Abram V, Kezdy FJ, et al. Purification and characterization of the principal inhibitor of calcium oxalate monohydrate crystal growth in human urine. J Biol Chem. 1983;258(20):12594-600.
60. Worcester EM. Inhibitors of stone formation. Semin Nephrol. 1996;16(5):474-86.
61. Hurst RE. Structure, function, and pathology of proteoglycans and glycosaminoglycans in the urinary tract. World J Urol. 1994;12(1):3-10.
62. Ryall RL, Grover PK, Stapleton AM, et al. The urinary F1 activation peptide of human prothrombin is a potent inhibitor of calcium oxalate crystallization in undiluted human urine in vitro. Clin Sci (Lond). 1995;89(5):533-41.
63. Asplin JR, Arsenault D, Parks JH, et al. Contribution of human uropontin to inhibition of calcium oxalate crystallization. Kidney Int. 1998;53(1):194-9.
64. Atmani F, Mizon J, Khan SR. Inter-alpha-inhibitor: a protein family involved in the inhibition of calcium oxalate crystallization. Scanning Microsc. 1996;10(2):425-33.
65. Atmani F, Khan SR. Role of urinary bikunin in the inhibition of calcium oxalate crystallization. J Am Soc Nephrol. 1999;10(Suppl 14):S385-8.
66. Knorle R, Schnierle P, Koch A, et al. Tamm–Horsfall glycoprotein: role in inhibition and promotion of renal calcium oxalate stone formation studied with Fourier-transform infrared spectroscopy. Clin Chem. 1994;40(9):1739-43.
67. Rodgers AL, Mensah PD, Schwager SL, et al. Inhibition of calcium oxalate crystallization by commercial human serum albumin and human urinary albumin isolated from two different race groups: evidence for possible molecular differences. Urol Res. 2006;34(6):373-80.
68. Pillay SN, Asplin JR, Coe FL. Evidence that calgranulin is produced by kidney cells and is an inhibitor of calcium oxalate crystallization. Am J Physiol. 1998;275(2 Pt 2):F255-61.
69. Baumann JM, Affolter B. The paradoxical role of urinary macromolecules in the aggregation of calcium oxalate: a further plea to increase diuresis in stone metaphylaxis. Urolithiasis. 2016;44(4):311-7.

70. Doweiko JP, Nompleggi DJ. The role of albumin in human physiology and pathophysiology, Part III: Albumin and disease states. JPEN J Parenter Enteral Nutr. 1991;15(4):476-83.
71. Zhuo L, Kimata K. Structure and function of inter-alpha-trypsin inhibitor heavy chains. Connect Tissue Res. 2008;49(5):311-20.
72. Leanderson T, Liberg D, Ivars F. S100A9 as a pharmacological target molecule in inflammation and cancer. Endocr Metab Immune Disord Drug Targets. 2015;15(2):97-104.
73. Mo L, Zhu XH, Huang HY, et al. Ablation of the Tamm–Horsfall protein gene increases susceptibility of mice to bladder colonization by type 1-fimbriated *Escherichia coli*. Am J Physiol Renal Physiol. 2004;286(4):F795-802.
74. Mutig K, Kahl T, Saritas T, et al. Activation of the bumetanide-sensitive Na+,K+,2Cl- cotransporter (NKCC2) is facilitated by Tamm–Horsfall protein in a chloride-sensitive manner. J Biol Chem. 2011;286(34):30200-10.
75. Renigunta A, Renigunta V, Saritas T, et al. Tamm–Horsfall glycoprotein interacts with renal outer medullary potassium channel ROMK2 and regulates its function. J Biol Chem. 2011;286(3):2224-35.
76. Esko JD, Kimata K, Lindahl U. Proteoglycans and sulfated glycosaminoglycans. In: Varki A, Cummings RD, Esko JD, et al. (Eds). Essentials of Glycobiology, 2nd edition. Cold Spring Harbor, NY: Cold Spring Harbor Laboratory Press; 2009. 229-248
77. Parsons CL. The role of the urinary epithelium in the pathogenesis of interstitial cystitis/prostatitis/urethritis. Urology. 2007;69(4 Suppl):9-16.
78. Goldberg JM, Cotlier E. Specific isolation and analysis of mucopolysaccharides (glycosaminoglycans) from human urine. Clin Chim Acta. 1972;41:19-27.
79. Fleisch H. Inhibitors and promoters of stone formation. Kidney Int. 1978;13(5):361-71.
80. Kohri K, Garside J, Blacklock NJ. The effect of glycosaminoglycans on the crystallisation of calcium oxalate. Br J Urol. 1989;63(6):584-90.
81. Embery G, Rees S, Hall R, et al. Calcium- and hydroxyapatite-binding properties of glucuronic acid-rich and iduronic acid-rich glycosaminoglycans and proteoglycans. Eur J Oral Sci. 1998;106(Suppl 1):267-73.
82. Lokeshwar VB, Selzer MG, Cerwinka WH, et al. Urinary uronate and sulfated glycosaminoglycan levels: markers for interstitial cystitis severity. J Urol. 2005;174(1):344-9.
83. Hurst RE, Roy JB, Min KW, et al. A deficit of chondroitin sulfate proteoglycans on the bladder uroepithelium in interstitial cystitis. Urology. 1996;48(5):817-21.
84. Lazzeri M, Hurle R, Casale P, et al. Managing chronic bladder diseases with the administration of exogenous glycosaminoglycans: an update on the evidence. Ther Adv Urol. 2016;8(2):91-9.
85. Doyle IR, Ryall RL, Marshall VR. Inclusion of proteins into calcium oxalate crystals precipitated from human urine: a highly selective phenomenon. Clin Chem. 1991;37(9):1589-94.
86. Kumar V, Farell G, Lieske JC. Whole urinary proteins coat calcium oxalate monohydrate crystals to greatly decrease their adhesion to renal cells. J Urol. 2003;170(1):221-5.
87. Stapleton AM, Ryall RL. Blood coagulation proteins and urolithiasis are linked: crystal matrix protein is the F1 activation peptide of human prothrombin. Br J Urol. 1995;75(6):712-9.
88. Grover PK, Ryall RL. Effect of prothrombin and its activation fragments on calcium oxalate crystal growth and aggregation in undiluted human urine in vitro: relationship between protein structure and inhibitory activity. Clin Sci (Lond). 2002;102(4):425-34.
89. Liu J, Chen J, Wang T, et al. Effects of urinary prothrombin fragment 1 in the formation of calcium oxalate calculus. J Urol. 2005;173(1):113-6.
90. Buchholz NP, Kim DS, Grover PK, et al. The effect of warfarin therapy on the charge properties of urinary prothrombin fragment 1 and crystallization of calcium oxalate in undiluted human urine. J Bone Miner Res. 1999;14(6):1003-12.
91. Pletcher CH, Resnick RM, Wei GJ, et al. Deglycosylated prothrombin fragment 1. Calcium binding, phospholipid interaction, and self-assocation. J Biol Chem. 1980;255(15):7433-8.
92. Webber D, Radcliffe CM, Royle L, et al. Sialylation of urinary prothrombin fragment 1 is implicated as a contributory factor in the risk of calcium oxalate kidney stone formation. FEBS J. 2006;273(13):3024-37.
93. Webber D, Rodgers AL, Sturrock ED. Glycosylation of prothrombin fragment 1 governs calcium oxalate crystal nucleation and aggregation, but not crystal growth. Urol Res. 2007;35(6):277-85.
94. Grover PK, Dogra SC, Davidson BP, et al. The prothrombin gene is expressed in the rat kidney: Implications for urolithiasis research. Eur J Biochem. 2000;267(1):61-7.
95. Stapleton AM, Timme TL, Ryall RL. Gene expression of prothrombin in the human kidney and its potential relevance to kidney stone disease. Br J Urol. 1998;81(5):666-71.
96. Grandaliano G, Gesualdo L, Schena FP. Thrombin: a novel renal growth factor. Exp Nephrol. 1999;7(1):20-5.
97. Verkoelen CF, Schepers MS. Changing concepts in the aetiology of renal stones. Curr Opin Urol. 2000;10(6):539-44.
98. Grandaliano G, Monno R, Ranieri E, et al. Regenerative and proinflammatory effects of thrombin on human proximal tubular cells. J Am Soc Nephrol. 2000;11(6):1016-25.
99. Stapleton AM, Seymour AE, Brennan JS, et al. Immunohistochemical distribution and quantification of crystal matrix protein. Kidney Int. 1993;44(4):817-24.
100. Bergsland KJ, Kelly JK, Coe BJ, et al. Urine protein markers distinguish stone-forming from non-stone-forming relatives of calcium stone formers. Am J Physiol Renal Physiol. 2006;291(3):F530-6.
101. Hedgepeth RC, Yang L, Resnick MI, et al. Expression of proteins that inhibit calcium oxalate crystallization in vitro in the urine of normal and stone-forming individuals. Am J Kidney Dis. 2001;37(1):104-12.
102. Rungroj N, Sritippayawan S, Thongnoppakhun W, et al. Prothrombin haplotype associated with kidney stone disease in Northeastern Thai patients. Urology. 2011;77(1):249-23.
103. Rungroj N, Sudtachat N, Nettuwakul C, et al. Association between human prothrombin variant (T165M) and kidney stone disease. PLoS One. 2012;7(9):e45533.

104. Pozzi N, Chen Z, Pelc LA, et al. The linker connecting the two kringles plays a key role in prothrombin activation. Proc Natl Acad Sci USA. 2014;111(21):7630-5.
105. Mariano-Oliveira A, De Freitas MS, Monteiro RQ, et al. Prothrombin fragments containing kringle domains induce migration and activation of human neutrophils. Int J Biochem Cell Biol. 2008;40(3):517-29.
106. Staines KA, Macrae VE, Farquharson C. The importance of the SIBLING family of proteins on skeletal mineralisation and bone remodelling. J Endocrinol. 2012;214(3):241-55.
107. Ding Y, Chen J, Cui G, et al. Pathophysiological role of osteopontin and angiotensin II in atherosclerosis. Biochem Biophys Res Commun. 2016;471(1):5-9.
108. Endlich N, Sunohara M, Nietfeld W, et al. Analysis of differential gene expression in stretched podocytes: osteopontin enhances adaptation of podocytes to mechanical stress. FASEB J. 2002;16(13):1850-2.
109. Xie Y, Sakatsume M, Nishi S, et al. Expression, roles, receptors, and regulation of osteopontin in the kidney. Kidney Int. 2001;60(5):1645-57.
110. Evan AP, Bledsoe S, Worcester EM, et al. Renal inter-alpha-trypsin inhibitor heavy chain 3 increases in calcium oxalate stone-forming patients. Kidney Int. 2007;72(12):1503-11.
111. Inoue M, Shinohara ML. Intracellular osteopontin (iOPN) and immunity. Immunol Res. 2011;49(1-3):160-72.
112. Scatena M, Liaw L, Giachelli CM. Osteopontin: a multifunctional molecule regulating chronic inflammation and vascular disease. Arterioscler Thromb Vasc Biol. 2007;27(11):2302-9.
113. Merchant ML, Cummins TD, Wilkey DW, et al. Proteomic analysis of renal calculi indicates an important role for inflammatory processes in calcium stone formation. Am J Physiol Renal Physiol. 2008;295(4):F1254-8.
114. Witzmann FA, Evan AP, Coe FL, et al. Label-free proteomic methodology for the analysis of human kidney stone matrix composition. Proteome Sci. 2016;14:4.
115. Evan AP, Coe FL, Rittling SR, et al. Apatite plaque particles in inner medulla of kidneys of calcium oxalate stone formers: osteopontin localization. Kidney Int. 2005;68(1):145-54.
116. Nishio S, Iseda T, Takeda H, et al. Inhibitory effect of calcium phosphate-associated proteins on calcium oxalate crystallization: alpha2-HS-glycoprotein, prothrombin-F1 and osteopontin. BJU Int. 2000;86(4):543-8.
117. Sheng X, Jung T, Wesson JA, et al. Adhesion at calcium oxalate crystal surfaces and the effect of urinary constituents. Proc Natl Acad Sci USA. 2005;102(2):267-72.
118. Rodriguez DE, Thula-Mata T, Toro EJ, et al. Multifunctional role of osteopontin in directing intrafibrillar mineralization of collagen and activation of osteoclasts. Acta Biomater. 2014;10(1):494-507.
119. Bautista DS, Denstedt J, Chambers AF, et al. Low-molecular-weight variants of osteopontin generated by serine proteinases in urine of patients with kidney stones. J Cell Biochem. 1996;61(3):402-9.
120. Yasui T, Fujita K, Hayashi Y, et al. Quantification of osteopontin in the urine of healthy and stone-forming men. Urol Res. 1999;27(4):225-30.
121. Nishio S, Hatanaka M, Takeda H, et al. Calcium phosphate crystal-associated proteins: alpha-2-HS-glycoprotein, prothrombin fragment 1 and osteopontin. Int J Urol. 2001;8(8):S58-62.
122. Tsuji H, Tohru U, Hirotsugu U, et al. Urinary concentration of osteopontin and association with urinary supersaturation and crystal formation. Int J Urol. 2007;14(7):630-4.
123. Christensen B, Schack L, Klaning E, et al. Osteopontin is cleaved at multiple sites close to its integrin-binding motifs in milk and is a novel substrate for plasmin and cathepsin D. J Biol Chem. 2010;285(11):7929-37.
124. Boskey AL, Christensen B, Taleb H, et al. Post-translational modification of osteopontin: effects on in vitro hydroxyapatite formation and growth. Biochem Biophys Res Commun. 2012;419(2):333-8.
125. Kolbach AM, Afzal O, Halligan B, et al. Relative deficiency of acidic isoforms of osteopontin from stone former urine. Urol Res. 2012;40(5):447-54.
126. Jurets A, Le BM, Staffler G, et al. Inhibition of cellular adhesion by immunological targeting of osteopontin neoepitopes generated through matrix metalloproteinase and thrombin cleavage. PLoS One. 2016;11(2):e0148333.
127. Rabb H, Barroso-Vicens E, Adams R, et al. Alpha-V/beta-3 and alpha-V/beta-5 integrin distribution in neoplastic kidney. Am J Nephrol. 1996;16(5):402-8.
128. Shio K, Kobayashi H, Asano T, et al. Thrombin-cleaved osteopontin is increased in urine of patients with rheumatoid arthritis. J Rheumatol. 2010;37(4):704-10.
129. Lieske JC, de la Vega LS, Gettman MT, et al. Diabetes mellitus and the risk of urinary tract stones: a population-based case-control study. Am J Kidney Dis. 2006;48(6):897-904.
130. Ito S, Nozawa S, Ishikawa H, et al. Renal stones in patients with rheumatoid arthritis. J Rheumatol. 1997;24(11):2123-8.
131. Hamamoto S, Yasui T, Okada A, Hirose M, et al. Crucial role of the cryptic epitope SLAYGLR within osteopontin in renal crystal formation of mice. J Bone Miner Res. 2011;26(12):2967-77.
132. Giachelli CM, Pichler R, Lombardi D, et al. Osteopontin expression in angiotensin II-induced tubulointerstitial nephritis. Kidney Int. 1994;45(2):515-24.
133. Kupfahl C, Pink D, Friedrich K, et al. Angiotensin II directly increases transforming growth factor beta1 and osteopontin and indirectly affects collagen mRNA expression in the human heart. Cardiovasc Res. 2000;46(3):463-75.
134. Sun W, Feng Y, Yao XD, et al. Urinary angiotensinogen is elevated in patients with nephrolithiasis. Biomed Res Int. 2014;2014:349602.
135. Yamamoto T, Nakagawa T, Suzuki H, et al. Urinary angiotensinogen as a marker of intrarenal angiotensin II activity associated with deterioration of renal function in patients with chronic kidney disease. J Am Soc Nephrol. 2007;18(5):1558-65.
136. Cha JH, Ahn YH, Lim SW, et al. Decreased osteopontin expression in the rat kidney on a sodium deficient diet. Yonsei Med J. 2000;41(1):128-35.

137. Yasui T, Fujita K, Sasaki S, et al. Alendronate inhibits osteopontin expression enhanced by parathyroid hormone-related peptide (PTHrP) in the rat kidney. Urol Res. 1998;26(5):355-60.
138. Matkovits T, Christakos S. Variable in vivo regulation of rat vitamin D-dependent genes (osteopontin, Ca,Mg-adenosine triphosphatase, and 25-hydroxyvitamin D3 24-hydroxylase): implications for differing mechanisms of regulation and involvement of multiple factors. Endocrinology. 1995;136(9):3971-82.
139. Rittling SR, Matsumoto HN, McKee MD, et al. Mice lacking osteopontin show normal development and bone structure but display altered osteoclast formation in vitro. J Bone Miner Res. 1998;13(7):1101-11.
140. Mo L, Liaw L, Evan AP, et al. Renal calcinosis and stone formation in mice lacking osteopontin, Tamm–Horsfall protein, or both. Am J Physiol Renal Physiol. 2007;293(6):F1935-43.
141. Paloian NJ, Leaf EM, Giachelli CM. Osteopontin protects against high phosphate-induced nephrocalcinosis and vascular calcification. Kidney Int. 2016;89(5):1027-36.
142. Li X, Liu K, Pan Y, et al. Roles of osteopontin gene polymorphism (rs1126616), osteopontin levels in urine and serum, and the risk of urolithiasis: a meta-analysis. Biomed Res Int. 2015;2015:315043.
143. Safarinejad MR, Shafiei N, Safarinejad S. Association between polymorphisms in osteopontin gene (SPP1) and first episode calcium oxalate urolithiasis. Urolithiasis. 2013;41(4):303-13.
144. Gao B, Yasui T, Itoh Y, et al. Association of osteopontin gene haplotypes with nephrolithiasis. Kidney Int. 2007;72(5):592-8.
145. Gogebakan B, Igci YZ, Arslan A, et al. Association between the T-593A and C6982T polymorphisms of the osteopontin gene and risk of developing nephrolithiasis. Arch Med Res. 2010;41(6):442-8.
146. Kothari AN, Arffa ML, Chang V, et al. Osteopontin—a master regulator of epithelial–mesenchymal transition. J Clin Med. 2016;5(4):pii: E39.
147. Noiri E, Dickman K, Miller F, et al. Reduced tolerance to acute renal ischemia in mice with a targeted disruption of the osteopontin gene. Kidney Int. 1999;56(1):74-82.
148. Evan AP, Lingeman JE, Worcester EM, et al. Contrasting histopathology and crystal deposits in kidneys of idiopathic stone formers who produce hydroxy apatite, brushite, or calcium oxalate stones. Anat Rec (Hoboken). 2014;297(4):731-48.
149. Chen X, Rivard L, Naqvi S, et al. Expression and localization of Inter-alpha Inhibitors in rodent brain. Neuroscience. 2016;324:69-81.
150. Salier JP, Rouet P, Raguenez G, et al. The inter-alpha-inhibitor family: from structure to regulation. Biochem J. 1996;315 (Pt 1):1-9.
151. Sanchez D, Martinez S, Lindqvist A, et al. Expression of the AMBP gene transcript and its two protein products, alpha(1)-microglobulin and bikunin, in mouse embryogenesis. Mech Dev. 2002;117(1-2):293-8.
152. Enghild JJ, Thogersen IB, Pizzo SV, et al. Analysis of inter-alpha-trypsin inhibitor and a novel trypsin inhibitor, pre-alpha-trypsin inhibitor, from human plasma. Polypeptide chain stoichiometry and assembly by glycan. J Biol Chem. 1989;264(27):15975-81.
153. Mizushima S, Nii A, Kato K, et al. Gene expression of the two heavy chains and one light chain forming the inter-alpha-trypsin-inhibitor in human tissues. Biol Pharm Bull. 1998;21(2):167-9.
154. Janssen U, Thomas G, Glant T, et al. Expression of inter-alpha-trypsin inhibitor and tumor necrosis factor-stimulated gene 6 in renal proximal tubular epithelial cells. Kidney Int. 2001;60(1):126-36.
155. Iida S, Peck AB, Johnson-Tardieu J, et al. Temporal changes in mRNA expression for bikunin in the kidneys of rats during calcium oxalate nephrolithiasis. J Am Soc Nephrol. 1999;10(5):986-96.
156. Marengo SR, Resnick MI, Yang L, et al. Differential expression of urinary inter-alpha-trypsin inhibitor trimers and dimers in normal compared to active calcium oxalate stone forming men. J Urol. 1998;159(5):1444-50.
157. Dean C, Kanellos J, Pham H, et al. Effects of inter-alpha-inhibitor and several of its derivatives on calcium oxalate crystallization in vitro. Clin Sci (Lond). 2000;98(4):471-80.
158. Kobayashi H, Shibata K, Fujie M, et al. Identification of structural domains in inter-alpha-trypsin involved in calcium oxalate crystallization. Kidney Int. 1998;53(6):1727-35.
159. Igci M, Arslan A, Igci YZ, et al. Bikunin and alpha1-microglobulin/bikunin precursor (AMBP) gene mutational screening in patients with kidney stones: a case-control study. Scand J Urol Nephrol. 2010;44(6):413-9.
160. Garantziotis S, Hollingsworth JW, Ghanayem RB, et al. Inter-alpha-trypsin inhibitor attenuates complement activation and complement-induced lung injury. J Immunol. 2007;179(6):4187-92.
161. Okroj M, Holmquist E, Sjolander J, et al. Heavy chains of inter alpha inhibitor (IalphaI) inhibit the human complement system at early stages of the cascade. J Biol Chem. 2012;287(24):20100-10.
162. Singh K, Zhang LX, Bendelja K, et al. Inter-alpha inhibitor protein administration improves survival from neonatal sepsis in mice. Pediatr Res. 2010;68(3):242-7.
163. Lim YP, Bendelja K, Opal SM, et al. Correlation between mortality and the levels of inter-alpha inhibitors in the plasma of patients with severe sepsis. J Infect Dis. 2003;188(6):919-26.
164. Bost F, Diarra-Mehrpour M, Martin JP. Inter-alpha-trypsin inhibitor proteoglycan family--a group of proteins binding and stabilizing the extracellular matrix. Eur J Biochem. 1998;252(3):339-46.
165. Moriyama MT, Glenton PA, Khan SR. Expression of inter-alpha inhibitor related proteins in kidneys and urine of hyperoxaluric rats. J Urol. 2001;165(5):1687-92.
166. Eguchi Y, Inoue M, Iida S, et al. Heparan sulfate (HS)/heparan sulfate proteoglycan (HSPG) and bikunin are up-regulated during calcium oxalate nephrolithiasis in rat kidney. Kurume Med J. 2002;49(3):99-107.
167. Adair JE, Stober V, Sobhany M, et al. Inter-alpha-trypsin inhibitor promotes bronchial epithelial repair after injury through vitronectin binding. J Biol Chem. 2009;284(25):16922-30.
168. Rampoldi L, Scolari F, Amoroso A, et al. The rediscovery of uromodulin (Tamm–Horsfall protein): from tubulointerstitial

nephropathy to chronic kidney disease. Kidney Int. 2011;80(4):338-47.

169. Brunati M, Perucca S, Han L, et al. The serine protease hepsin mediates urinary secretion and polymerisation of Zona Pellucida domain protein uromodulin. Elife. 2015;4:e08887.
170. Ryall RL, Harnett RM, Hibberd CM, et al. Effects of chondroitin sulphate, human serum albumin and Tamm-Horsfall mucoprotein on calcium oxalate crystallization in undiluted human urine. Urol Res. 1991;19(3):181-8.
171. Worcester EM, Nakagawa Y, Wabner CL, et al. Crystal adsorption and growth slowing by nephrocalcin, albumin, and Tamm-Horsfall protein. Am J Physiol. 1988;255(6 Pt 2): F1197-205.
172. Hess B, Nakagawa Y, Coe FL. Inhibition of calcium oxalate monohydrate crystal aggregation by urine proteins. Am J Physiol. 1989;257(1 Pt 2):F99-106.
173. Hess B, Nakagawa Y, Parks JH, et al. Molecular abnormality of Tamm-Horsfall glycoprotein in calcium oxalate nephrolithiasis. Am J Physiol. 1991;260(4 Pt 2):F569-78.
174. Pragasam V, Kalaiselvi P, Subashini B, et al. Structural and functional modification of THP on nitration: comparison with stone formers THP. Nephron Physiol. 2005;99(1):28-34.
175. Konya E, Amasaki N, Umekawa T, et al. Influence of urinary sialic acid on calcium oxalate crystal formation. Urol Int. 2002;68(4):281-5.
176. Ratkalkar VN, Kleinman JG. Mechanisms of stone formation. Clin Rev Bone Miner Metab. 2011;9(3-4):187-97.
177. Hallson PC, Choong SK, Kasidas GP, et al. Effects of Tamm-Horsfall protein with normal and reduced sialic acid content upon the crystallization of calcium phosphate and calcium oxalate in human urine. Br J Urol. 1997;80(4):533-8.
178. Viswanathan P, Rimer JD, Kolbach AM, et al. Calcium oxalate monohydrate aggregation induced by aggregation of desialylated Tamm-Horsfall protein. Urol Res. 2011;39(4):269-82.
179. Romero MC, Nocera S, Nesse AB. Decreased Tamm-Horsfall protein in lithiasic patients. Clin Biochem. 1997;30(1):63-7.
180. Porile JL, Asplin JR, Parks JH, et al. Normal calcium oxalate crystal growth inhibition in severe calcium oxalate nephrolithiasis. J Am Soc Nephrol. 1996;7(4):602-7.
181. Devuyst O, Dahan K, Pirson Y. Tamm-Horsfall protein or uromodulin: new ideas about an old molecule. Nephrol Dial Transplant. 2005;20(7):1290-4.
182. Hart TC, Gorry MC, Hart PS, et al. Mutations of the UMOD gene are responsible for medullary cystic kidney disease 2 and familial juvenile hyperuricaemic nephropathy. J Med Genet. 2002;39(12):882-92.
183. Serafini-Cessi F, Malagolini N, Cavallone D. Tamm-Horsfall glycoprotein: biology and clinical relevance. Am J Kidney Dis. 2003;42(4):658-76.
184. Vylet'al P, Kublova M, Kalbacova M, et al. Alterations of uromodulin biology: a common denominator of the genetically heterogeneous FJHN/MCKD syndrome. Kidney Int. 2006;70(6):1155-69.
185. Youhanna S, Weber J, Beaujean V, et al. Determination of uromodulin in human urine: influence of storage and processing. Nephrol Dial Transplant. 2014;29(1):136-45.
186. Bernascone I, Vavassori S, Di PA, et al. Defective intracellular trafficking of uromodulin mutant isoforms. Traffic. 2006;7(11):1567-79.
187. El-Achkar TM, Wu XR. Uromodulin in kidney injury: an instigator, bystander, or protector? Am J Kidney Dis. 2012;59(3):452-61.
188. Jennings P, Aydin S, Kotanko P, et al. Membrane targeting and secretion of mutant uromodulin in familial juvenile hyperuricemic nephropathy. J Am Soc Nephrol. 2007;18(1):264-73.
189. Horton JK, Davies M, Woodhead JS, et al. A new and rapid immunochemiluminometric assay for the measurement of Tamm-Horsfall glycoprotein. Clin Chim Acta. 1988;174(2):225-37.
190. El-Achkar TM, McCracken R, Rauchman M, et al. Tamm-Horsfall protein-deficient thick ascending limbs promote injury to neighboring S3 segments in an MIP-2-dependent mechanism. Am J Physiol Renal Physiol. 2011;300(4): F999-1007.
191. El-Achkar TM, McCracken R, Liu Y, et al. Tamm-Horsfall protein translocates to the basolateral domain of thick ascending limbs, interstitium, and circulation during recovery from acute kidney injury. Am J Physiol Renal Physiol. 2013;304(8):F1066-75.
192. Liu Y, El-Achkar TM, Wu XR. Tamm-Horsfall protein regulates circulating and renal cytokines by affecting glomerular filtration rate and acting as a urinary cytokine trap. J Biol Chem. 2012;287(20):16365-78.
193. El-Achkar TM, Wu XR, Rauchman M, et al. Tamm-Horsfall protein protects the kidney from ischemic injury by decreasing inflammation and altering TLR4 expression. Am J Physiol Renal Physiol. 2008;295(2):F534-44.
194. Liu Y, Mo L, Goldfarb DS, et al. Progressive renal papillary calcification and ureteral stone formation in mice deficient for Tamm-Horsfall protein. Am J Physiol Renal Physiol. 2010;299(3):F469-78.
195. Evan AP, Lingeman JE, Coe FL, et al. Randall's plaque of patients with nephrolithiasis begins in basement membranes of thin loops of Henle. J Clin Invest. 2003;111(5):607-16.
196. Evan AP, Weinman EJ, Wu XR, et al. Comparison of the pathology of interstitial plaque in human ICSF stone patients to NHERF-1 and THP-null mice. Urol Res. 2010;38(6):439-52.
197. Wu XR. Interstitial calcinosis in renal papillae of genetically engineered mouse models: relation to Randall's plaques. Urolithiasis. 2015;43(Suppl 1):65-76.
198. Gudbjartsson DF, Holm H, Indridason OS, et al. Association of variants at UMOD with chronic kidney disease and kidney stones-role of age and comorbid diseases. PLoS Genet. 2010;6(7):e1001039.
199. Ghirotto S, Tassi F, Barbujani G, et al. The uromodulin gene locus shows evidence of pathogen adaptation through human evolution. J Am Soc Nephrol. 2016;27(10):2983-2996. pii: ASN.2015070830 (Epub ahead of print).
200. Trudu M, Janas S, Lanzani C, et al. Common noncoding UMOD gene variants induce salt-sensitive hypertension and kidney damage by increasing uromodulin expression. Nat Med. 2013;19(12):1655-60.

201. Olden M, Corre T, Hayward C, et al. Common variants in UMOD associate with urinary uromodulin levels: a meta-analysis. J Am Soc Nephrol. 2014;25(8):1869-82.
202. Bates JM, Raffi HM, Prasadan K, et al. Tamm–Horsfall protein knockout mice are more prone to urinary tract infection: rapid communication. Kidney Int. 2004;65(3):791-7.
203. Pak J, Pu Y, Zhang ZT, Hasty DL, Wu XR. Tamm–Horsfall protein binds to type 1 fimbriated *Escherichia coli* and prevents *E. coli* from binding to uroplakin Ia and Ib receptors. J Biol Chem. 2001;276(13):9924-30.
204. Holmgren K, Danielson BG, Fellstrom B, et al. The relation between urinary tract infections and stone composition in renal stone formers. Scand J Urol Nephrol. 1989;23(2):131-6.
205. Ohkawa M, Tokunaga S, Nakashima T, et al. Composition of urinary calculi related to urinary tract infection. J Urol. 1992;148(3 Pt 2):995-7.
206. Borghi L, Nouvenne A, Meschi T. Nephrolithiasis and urinary tract infections: "the chicken or the egg" dilemma? Nephrol Dial Transplant. 2012;27(11):3982-4.
207. Kottgen A, Glazer NL, Dehghan A, et al. Multiple loci associated with indices of renal function and chronic kidney disease. Nat Genet. 2009;41(6):712-7.
208. Ko B, Bergsland K, Gillen DL, et al. Sex differences in proximal and distal nephron function contribute to the mechanism of idiopathic hypercalcuria in calcium stone formers. Am J Physiol Regul Integr Comp Physiol. 2015;309(1):R85-R92.
209. Wolf MT, Wu XR, Huang CL. Uromodulin upregulates TRPV5 by impairing caveolin-mediated endocytosis. Kidney Int. 2013;84(1):130-7.
210. Arroyo V, Garcia-Martinez R, Salvatella X. Human serum albumin, systemic inflammation, and cirrhosis. J Hepatol. 2014;61(2):396-407.
211. Sitar ME, Aydin S, Cakatay U. Human serum albumin and its relation with oxidative stress. Clin Lab 2013;59(9-10):945-52.
212. Giles S, Czuprynski C. Novel role for albumin in innate immunity: serum albumin inhibits the growth of *Blastomyces dermatitidis* yeast form in vitro. Infect Immun 2003 Nov;71(11):6648-52.
213. Atmani F, Khan SR. Quantification of proteins extracted from calcium oxalate and calcium phosphate crystals induced in vitro in the urine of healthy controls and stone-forming patients. Urol Int. 2002;68(1):54-9.
214. Kaneko K, Kobayashi R, Yasuda M, et al. Comparison of matrix proteins in different types of urinary stone by proteomic analysis using liquid chromatography-tandem mass spectrometry. Int J Urol. 2012;19(8):765-72.
215. Cerini C, Geider S, Dussol B, et al. Nucleation of calcium oxalate crystals by albumin: involvement in the prevention of stone formation. Kidney Int. 1999;55(5):1776-86.
216. Grover PK, Moritz RL, Simpson RJ, et al. Inhibition of growth and aggregation of calcium oxalate crystals in vitro—a comparison of four human proteins. Eur J Biochem. 1998;253(3):637-44.
217. McLeod JF, Cooke NE. The vitamin D-binding protein, alpha-fetoprotein, albumin multigene family: detection of transcripts in multiple tissues. J Biol Chem. 1989 25;264(36):21760-9.
218. Pourmand G, Nasseh H, Sarrafnejad A, et al. Comparison of urinary proteins in calcium stone formers and healthy individuals: a case-control study. Urol Int 2006;76(2):163-8.
219. Schiopu A, Cotoi OS. S100A8 and S100A9: DAMPs at the crossroads between innate immunity, traditional risk factors, and cardiovascular disease. Mediators Inflamm 2013;2013:828354.
220. Okumura N, Tsujihata M, Momohara C, et al. Diversity in protein profiles of individual calcium oxalate kidney stones. PLoS One. 2013;8(7):e68624.
221. Thurgood LA, Ryall RL. Proteomic analysis of proteins selectively associated with hydroxyapatite, brushite, and uric acid crystals precipitated from human urine. J Proteome Res 2010.;9(10):5402-12.
222. Thurgood LA, Wang T, Chataway TK, et al. Comparison of the specific incorporation of intracrystalline proteins into urinary calcium oxalate monohydrate and dihydrate crystals. J Proteome Res. 2010;9(9):4745-57.
223. Vogl T, Gharibyan AL, Morozova-Roche LA. Pro-inflammatory S100A8 and S100A9 proteins: self-assembly into multifunctional native and amyloid complexes. Int J Mol Sci. 2012;13(3):2893-917.
224. Abtin A, Eckhart L, Glaser R, et al. The antimicrobial heterodimer S100A8/S100A9 (calprotectin) is upregulated by bacterial flagellin in human epidermal keratinocytes. J Invest Dermatol. 2010;130(10):2423-30.
225. Vogl T, Roth J, Sorg C, et al. Calcium-induced noncovalently linked tetramers of MRP8 and MRP14 detected by ultraviolet matrix-assisted laser desorption/ionization mass spectrometry. J Am Soc Mass Spectrom. 1999;10(11):1124-30.
226. Chakraborty P, Bjork P, Kallberg E, et al. Vesicular Location and Transport of S100A8 and S100A9 Proteins in Monocytoid Cells. PLoS One. 2015;10(12):e0145217.
227. Lim SY, Raftery MJ, Goyette J, et al. Oxidative modifications of S100 proteins: functional regulation by redox. J Leukoc Biol. 2009;86(3):577-87.
228. Kuwabara T, Mori K, Kasahara M, et al. Predictive significance of kidney myeloid-related protein 8 expression in patients with obesity or type 2 diabetes-associated kidney diseases. PLoS One. 2014;9(2):e88942.
229. Fujiu K, Manabe I, Nagai R. Renal collecting duct epithelial cells regulate inflammation in tubulointerstitial damage in mice. J Clin Invest. 2011;121(9):3425-41.
230. Sun X, Meng H, Shi D, et al. Analysis of plasma calprotectin and polymorphisms of S100A8 in patients with aggressive periodontitis. J Periodontal Res. 2011;46(3):354-60.
231. Ortega FJ, Mercader JM, Moreno-Navarrete JM, et al. Targeting the association of calgranulin B (S100A9) with insulin resistance and type 2 diabetes. J Mol Med (Berl). 2013;91(4):523-34.
232. Bjork P, Bjork A, Vogl T, et al. Identification of human S100A9 as a novel target for treatment of autoimmune disease via binding to quinoline-3-carboxamides. PLoS Biol. 2009;7(4):e97.
233. Vogl T, Tenbrock K, Ludwig S, et al. Mrp8 and Mrp14 are endogenous activators of toll-like receptor 4, promoting lethal, endotoxin-induced shock. Nat Med. 2007;13(9):1042-9.

234. Chernov AV, Dolkas J, Hoang K, et al. The calcium-binding proteins S100A8 and S100A9 initiate the early inflammatory program in injured peripheral nerves. J Biol Chem. 2015;290(18):11771-84.
235. Foell D, Frosch M, Sorg C, et al. Phagocyte-specific calcium-binding S100 proteins as clinical laboratory markers of inflammation. Clin Chim Acta. 2004;344(1-2):37-51.
236. Bouma G, Coppens JM, Lam-Tse WK, et al. An increased MRP8/14 expression and adhesion, but a decreased migration towards proinflammatory chemokines of type 1 diabetes monocytes. Clin Exp Immunol. 2005;141(3):509-17.
237. Frosch M, Ahlmann M, Vogl T, et al. The myeloid-related proteins 8 and 14 complex, a novel ligand of toll-like receptor 4, and interleukin-1beta form a positive feedback mechanism in systemic-onset juvenile idiopathic arthritis. Arthritis Rheum. 2009;60(3):883-91.
238. Mortensen OH, Nielsen AR, Erikstrup C, et al. Calprotectin—a novel marker of obesity. PLoS One 2009;4(10):e7419.
239. Foell D, Wittkowski H, Vogl T, et al. S100 proteins expressed in phagocytes: a novel group of damage-associated molecular pattern molecules. J Leukoc Biol. 2007;81(1):28-37.
240. Mellins ED, Macaubas C, Grom AA. Pathogenesis of systemic juvenile idiopathic arthritis: some answers, more questions. Nat Rev Rheumatol. 2011;7(7):416-26.
241. El-Achkar TM, Dagher PC. Renal toll-like receptors: recent advances and implications for disease. Nat Clin Pract Nephrol. 2006;2(10):568-81.
242. Piccinini AM, Midwood KS. DAMPening inflammation by modulating TLR signalling. Mediators Inflamm. 2010;2010: pii:672395.
243. Thorey IS, Roth J, Regenbogen J, et al. The Ca^{2+}-binding proteins S100A8 and S100A9 are encoded by novel injury-regulated genes. J Biol Chem. 2001;276(38):35818-25.
244. Shepherd CE, Goyette J, Utter V, et al. Inflammatory S100A9 and S100A12 proteins in Alzheimer's disease. Neurobiol Aging. 2006;27(11):1554-63.
245. Zreiqat H, Howlett CR, Gronthos S, et al. S100A8/S100A9 and their association with cartilage and bone. J Mol Histol. 2007; 38(5):381-91.
246. McCormick MM, Rahimi F, Bobryshev YV, et al. S100A8 and S100A9 in human arterial wall. Implications for atherogenesis. J Biol Chem. 2005;280(50):41521-9.
247. Yanamandra K, Alexeyev O, Zamotin V, et al. Amyloid formation by the pro-inflammatory S100A8/A9 proteins in the ageing prostate. PLoS One 2009;4(5):e5562.
248. Geczy CL, Chung YM, Hiroshima Y. Calgranulins may contribute vascular protection in atherogenesis. Circ J 2014;78(2):271-80.
249. Kido J, Kido R, Suryono, et al. Calprotectin release from human neutrophils is induced by *Porphyromonas gingivalis* lipopolysaccharide via the CD-14-Toll-like receptor-nuclear factor kappaB pathway. J Periodontal Res. 2003;38(6):557-63.
250. Tyden H, Lood C, Gullstrand B, et al. Increased serum levels of S100A8/A9 and S100A12 are associated with cardiovascular disease in patients with inactive systemic lupus erythematosus. Rheumatology (Oxford). 2013;52(11):2048-55.
251. Oesterle A, Bowman MA. S100A12 and the S100/calgranulins: Emerging biomarkers for atherosclerosis and possibly therapeutic targets. Arterioscler Thromb Vasc Biol. 2015;35(12):2496-507.
252. Dessing MC, Tammaro A, Pulskens WP, et al. The calcium-binding protein complex S100A8/A9 has a crucial role in controlling macrophage-mediated renal repair following ischemia/reperfusion. Kidney Int. 2015;87(1):85-94.
253. Nacken W, Roth J, Sorg C, et al. S100A9/S100A8: Myeloid representatives of the S100 protein family as prominent players in innate immunity. Microsc Res Tech. 2003;60(6):569-80.
254. Ebbing J, Mathia S, Seibert FS, et al. Urinary calprotectin: a new diagnostic marker in urothelial carcinoma of the bladder. World J Urol 2014 Dec;32(6):1485-92.
255. Heller F, Frischmann S, Grunbaum M, et al. Urinary calprotectin and the distinction between prerenal and intrinsic acute kidney injury. Clin J Am Soc Nephrol. 2011;6(10): 2347-55.
256. Ebbing J, Seibert FS, Pagonas N, et al. Dynamics of urinary calprotectin after renal ischaemia. PLoS One. 2016;11 (1):e0146395.
257. Tepel M, Borst C, Bistrup C, et al. Urinary calprotectin and posttransplant renal allograft injury. PLoS One. 2014;9 (11):e113006.
258. Ortega FJ, Sabater M, Moreno-Navarrete JM, et al. Serum and urinary concentrations of calprotectin as markers of insulin resistance and type 2 diabetes. Eur J Endocrinol. 2012;167(4):569-78.
259. Pechere-Bertschi A, Burnier M. Gonadal steroids, salt-sensitivity and renal function. Curr Opin Nephrol Hypertens. 2007;16(1):16-21.
260. Lund SA, Giachelli CM, Scatena M. The role of osteopontin in inflammatory processes. J Cell Commun Signal. 2009;3(3-4): 311-22.
261. Matsuzaki H, Kobayashi H, Yagyu T, et al. Bikunin inhibits lipopolysaccharide-induced tumor necrosis factor alpha induction in macrophages. Clin Diagn Lab Immunol. 2004; 11(6): 1140-7.

CHAPTER

4

Characteristics of Human Kidney Stones

Michel Daudon, James C Williams Jr

INTRODUCTION

Urinary stones are normally classified by their primary mineral content. At a minimum, the mineral content of the stone provides a therapeutic target for patient treatment. For example, if a stone is composed mainly of calcium oxalate, reduction of the level of supersaturation of calcium oxalate in the urine is a logical goal of any therapy to help prevent future stones.

However, stones do not become a clinical problem solely because the urine is supersaturated with regard to one or more minerals. Mineral precipitated within the urine normally is eliminated in the form of crystals or crystal aggregates without incident. In stone diseases, some other mechanism acts to retain the mineral within the urinary system so that a stone can grow large enough to elicit symptoms. Curing a stone disease would necessarily thus include the blocking of the active mechanism by which early, small stones are held within the kidney. These mechanisms of stone retention—such as growth on interstitial plaque, growth on ductal plugs, and urinary stasis—are still being described in the different kinds of stone formers, but clues as to these retention mechanisms are often found in the morphology of the stones.

Thus, the approach in this chapter is to describe the different morphologies of stones within compositional categories, but to also address when possible the mechanisms by which the stones were held in the urinary system long enough for them to grow into symptomatic calculi. In several of the commonest forms, the morphology of the stone provides definite clues as to the mechanism(s) of stone retention that were at work in the urinary system of the patient. Moreover, stone morphology may help to orient toward or confirm the diagnosis of specific pathologies such as primary hyperoxaluria type I, absorptive hyperoxaluria related to inflammatory bowel diseases, chronic diarrhea in the context of low phosphate and protein intake, or in inherited or acquired distal tubular acidosis.

CALCIUM OXALATE STONES

Calcium oxalate is the most common mineral found in urinary stones. Most human urine is supersaturated with respect to this compound throughout at least part of most every day,[1] and calcium oxalate is insoluble in urine at any pH,[2] so it is not surprising that this mineral could deposit—and remain permanently in place—on growing stones in many patients. When calcium oxalate is the majority mineral in stones, they appear in several morphological types.

Hard, Smooth, Dark, Calcium Oxalate Stones (Daudon Type Ia[3])

These stones are composed mainly of the monohydrate form of calcium oxalate [COM, or whewellite (pronounced "hew-əl-lite")]. They have a smooth surface, often with mammillary (or "mulberry") bumps, and a brown color that can be quite dark (Fig. 4.1). The interior of these stones consists of fine layers that are tightly apposed (Figs. 4.2A and B). Studies have shown that these concentric layers consist of radially aligned COM crystals that each are coated with a thin layer of protein;[3-5] the proteins that coat the crystals are presumably from the urine, but the nature of these proteins and the role that they play in cementing the stone together are not known. About 30% of all urinary stones are purely or partially formed of COM with this morphology.[6]

This type of stone is commonly found with a morphology suggestive of the stone having been retained in the kidney during its early growth by attachment to Randall's plaque on the renal papilla (Box 4.1). Of stones identified with the Randall's plaque morphology, about 80% are composed purely or partially of this hard, dark form of COM. Thus, the metabolic profile that leads to the formation of this morphology of calcium oxalate may also overlap with what gives rise to interstitial plaque.[7] However, it is also possible that the formation of Randall's plaque in

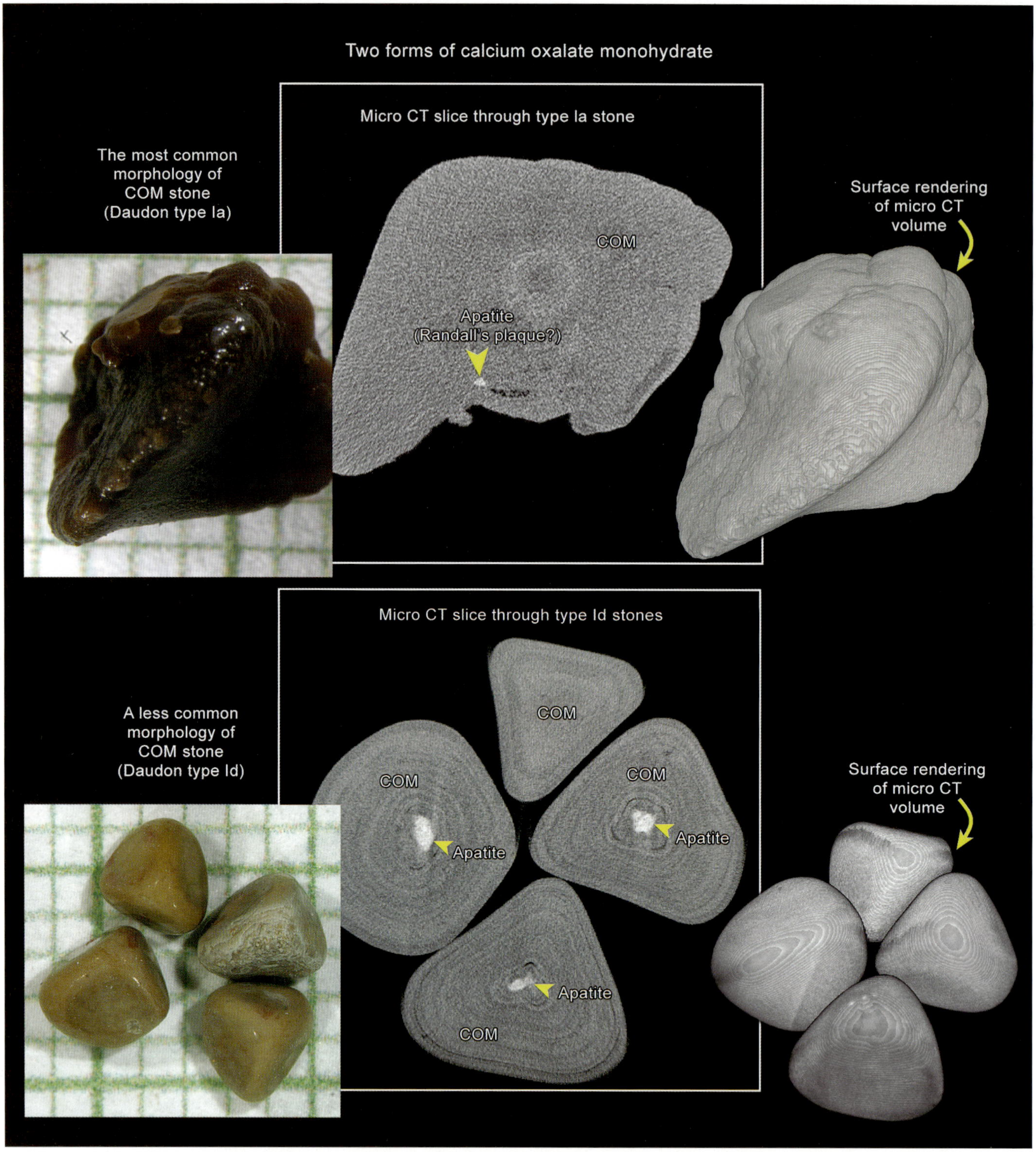

Fig. 4.1: Two of the morphological forms of calcium oxalate monohydrate (COM).

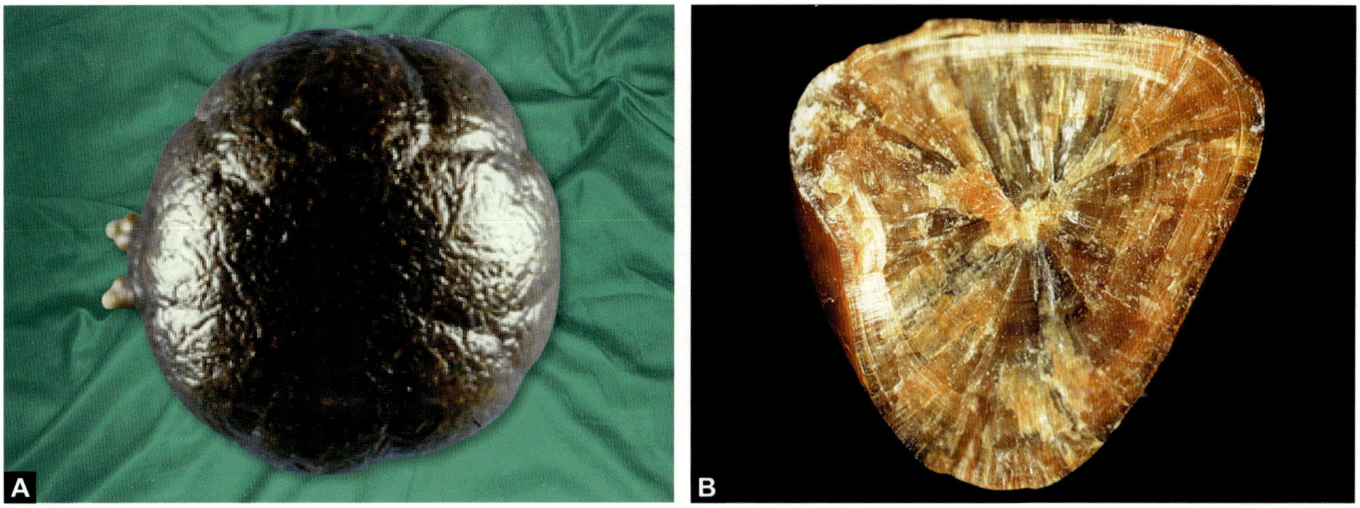

Figs. 4.2A and B: Another example of type Ia calcium oxalate monohydrate (COM). (A) Typical appearance of dark brown surface in this form of COM. This form of COM stone often correlates with low urine volume and moderately high levels of urine oxalate. (B) Sectioned stone shows internal layering. The origin of the colors in the layering is presumably alterations in nonmineral urine components, but this is not known. The packing of the mineral in this form of COM is quite dense, showing no sign of layers at the resolution of micro-CT (*see* Fig. 4.1).

Box 4.1: Randall's plaque: One mechanism for retaining stone within the kidney during early stages of stone growth.

- Interstitial apatite plaque forms within the tissue of the renal papilla; this mineral is not obviously inflammatory, and in itself seems to create no measureable effect on renal function.
- Interstitial plaque is somehow exposed to the calyceal urine; this certainly involves the breaching of the papillary epithelium, but the cause of this epithelial damage is not known.
- A tiny stone, composed of calcium oxalate, then grows on this exposed apatite plaque.
- The subsequent growth of the stone can be very slow, probably occurring in episodes stimulated by dietary events that result in high supersaturation of calcium oxalate; the stone cannot be expelled from the kidney when it is small, because it is firmly anchored to the interstitial tissue of the renal papilla.
- Stones growing on Randall's plaque may sometimes be released spontaneously,[9,10] but the mechanism by which the plaque region is separated from the surrounding papillary interstitium is unknown.

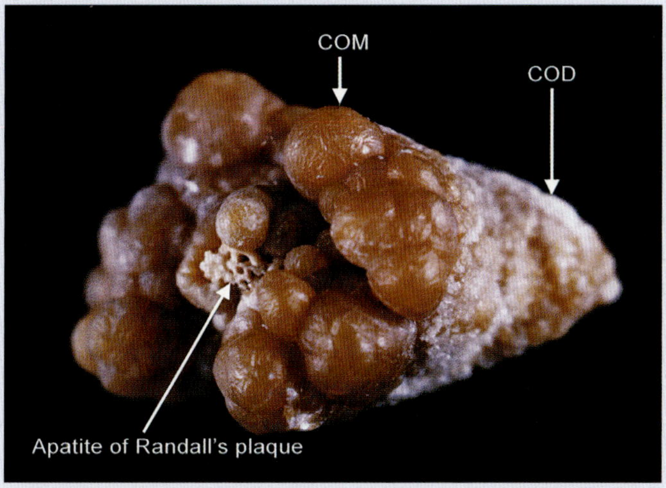

The figure shows the typical appearance of Randall's plaque on a small stone. The bulk of this stone consists of calcium oxalate monohydrate (COM) with some calcium oxalate dihydrate (COD) crystals on the surface to the right. Scanning electron microscopy has shown the presence of calcified tubules in the apatite of Randall's plaque on stone such as this,[10] confirming the hypothesis that this apatite region formed in renal tissue.

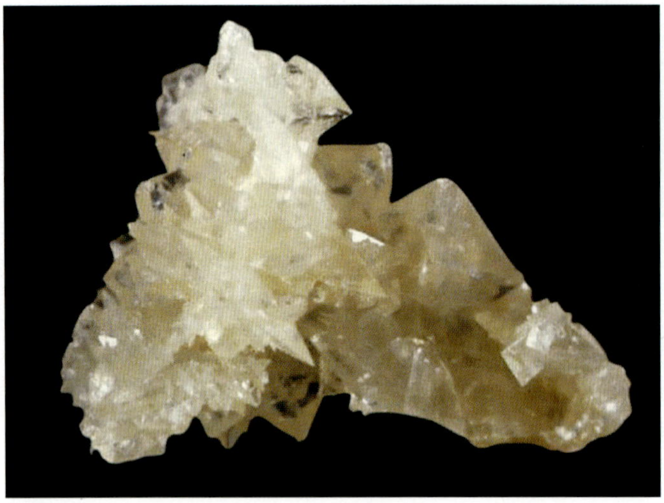

Fig. 4.3: Typical IIa stone made of nearly pure translucent and well-formed calcium oxalate dihydrate crystals in a patient suffering hypercalciuria.

the papillary interstitium may result from past metabolic factors—which could even be transient events, including perhaps injury to the papilla[8]—and that these factors may not be involved in the secondary crystallization of calcium oxalate onto the interstitial Randall's plaque.

Stones with Large, Polyhedral Shapes of Calcium Oxalate (Types IIA and IIB)

These stones are initially formed with the dihydrate form of calcium oxalate (COD, or weddellite; Figs. 4.3 and 4.4). In type IIa stones, COD crystals are apparently recently formed; the crystals are transparent, have sharp edges, and often are found to grow in a twinning pattern (Fig. 4.3 and upper part of Fig. 4.4).[11] Such freshly formed COD crystals are found in about a fourth of all urinary stones.[6] COD crystals are known to grow preferentially in environments in which the concentration of calcium greatly exceeds that of oxalate,[12] and there is some evidence that the prevalence of COD in a stone, rather than COM, correlates with hypercalciuria.[3,13]

However, the story of COD stones is complicated by the fact that COD, after it has formed, can undergo dehydration and convert to the monohydrate, COM. Thus, a stone can form initially as the dihydrate form of calcium oxalate, COD, and then later be transformed into COM, so that when the stone is analyzed it will be reported as being composed of the monohydrate form. The time that is required in the urinary system for COD to transform into COM is not known, and it appears that this transformation occurs in two very different ways.

It is not uncommon to see calcium oxalate stones—often those formed on Randall's plaque—as being composed of the hard, dark form of COM (type Ia) with fresh COD crystals (morphological type IIa) growing on the stone surface (Fig. 4.5). One hypothesis to explain this arrangement is that the bases of the COD crystals undergo dehydration into COM, with a transformation that is so thorough that the morphology of the calcium oxalate is altered from the large, transparent crystals of type IIa into the hard, brown COM of type Ia.[11,14] Thus, in such stones as shown in Figure 4.5, the primary mechanism of stone growth may be that of COD, but the bulk of the stone will be composed of type Ia COM, which has formed apparently by a slow and controlled transformation of COD to COM at the base of COD crystals. However, there is no evidence of COD crystals being primary in the overgrowth onto Randall's plaque,[15,16] and certainly type Ia COM can grow without any addition of COD crystals (*see* Figs. 4.1 and 4.2), so the importance of this COD-to-COM transformation in the formation of this type of stone is really not well described.

Such a controlled mechanism of transformation of COD to COM would involve a dramatic alteration in the crystal morphology, but the other mechanism of transformation is less altering, and quite prevalent. In this second kind of stone, initially composed of COD, the mineral undergoes dehydration into COM, but the initial shape of the COD crystals is largely retained (type IIb). However, these polyhedral shapes are no longer transparent, and the edges of the former COD crystals become blunt (*see* Fig. 4.4, lower). The nature of the COM within these stones is compact but not well organized.[3] This type-IIb form of calcium oxalate—in which the persisting morphology points to initial formation as COD, but which has transformed mostly or entirely into poorly organized COM—is found in about 20% of all urinary stones.[6] Note, however, that this morphological type is not reported by most laboratories, so that these stones will typically be reported as COM, without any comment on the morphology that points to initial formation as the dihydrate, COD.

Other Forms of Calcium Oxalate in Stones

About 6% of all stones contain COM in an unorganized form that shows no signs of having formed initially as COD (type Ib). These stones may be dark in color, and may have mammillary shapes on the surface, but unlike type

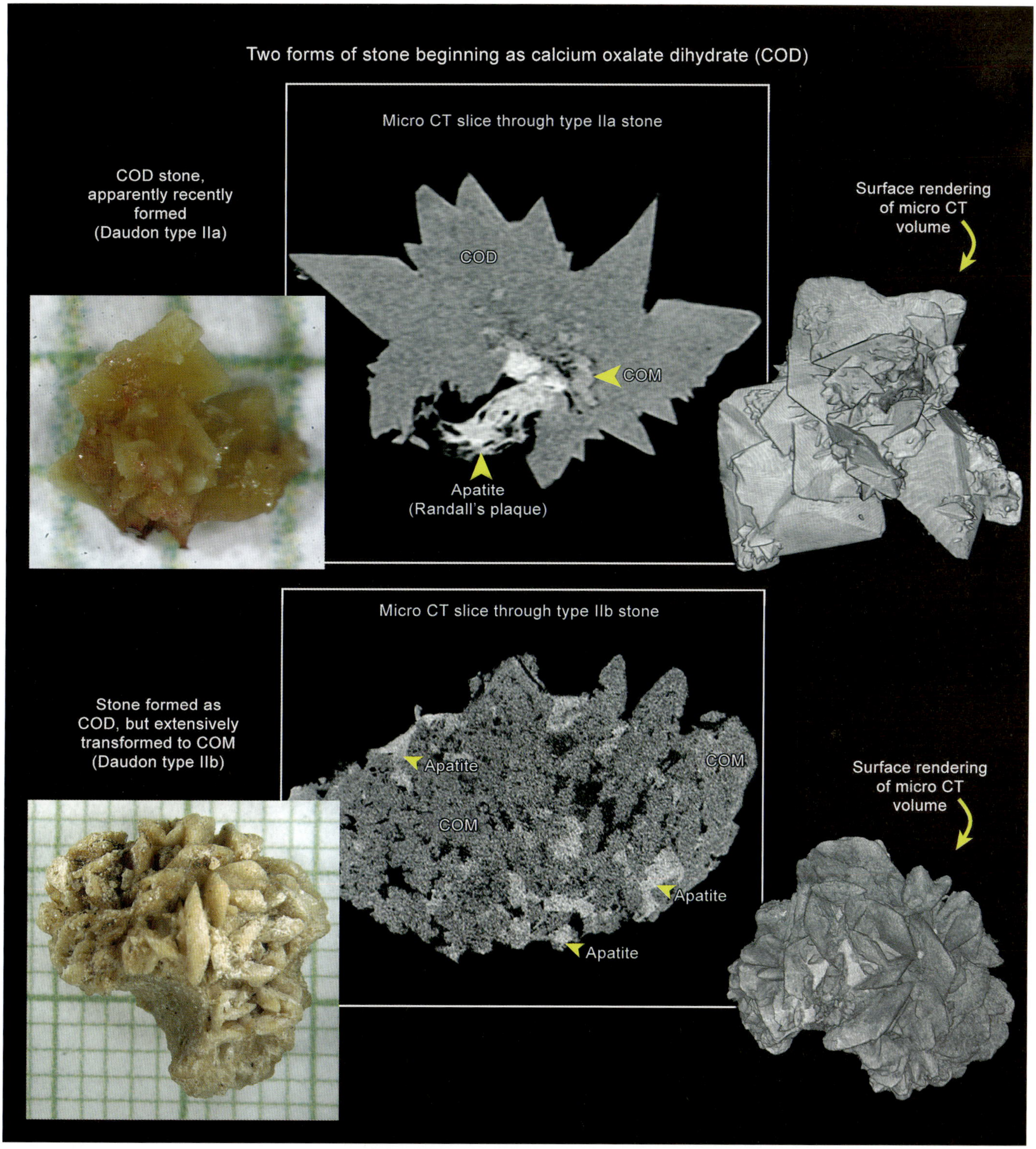

Fig. 4.4: Two forms of stones initially formed as calcium oxalate dihydrate (COD). (COM: Calcium oxalate monohydrate).

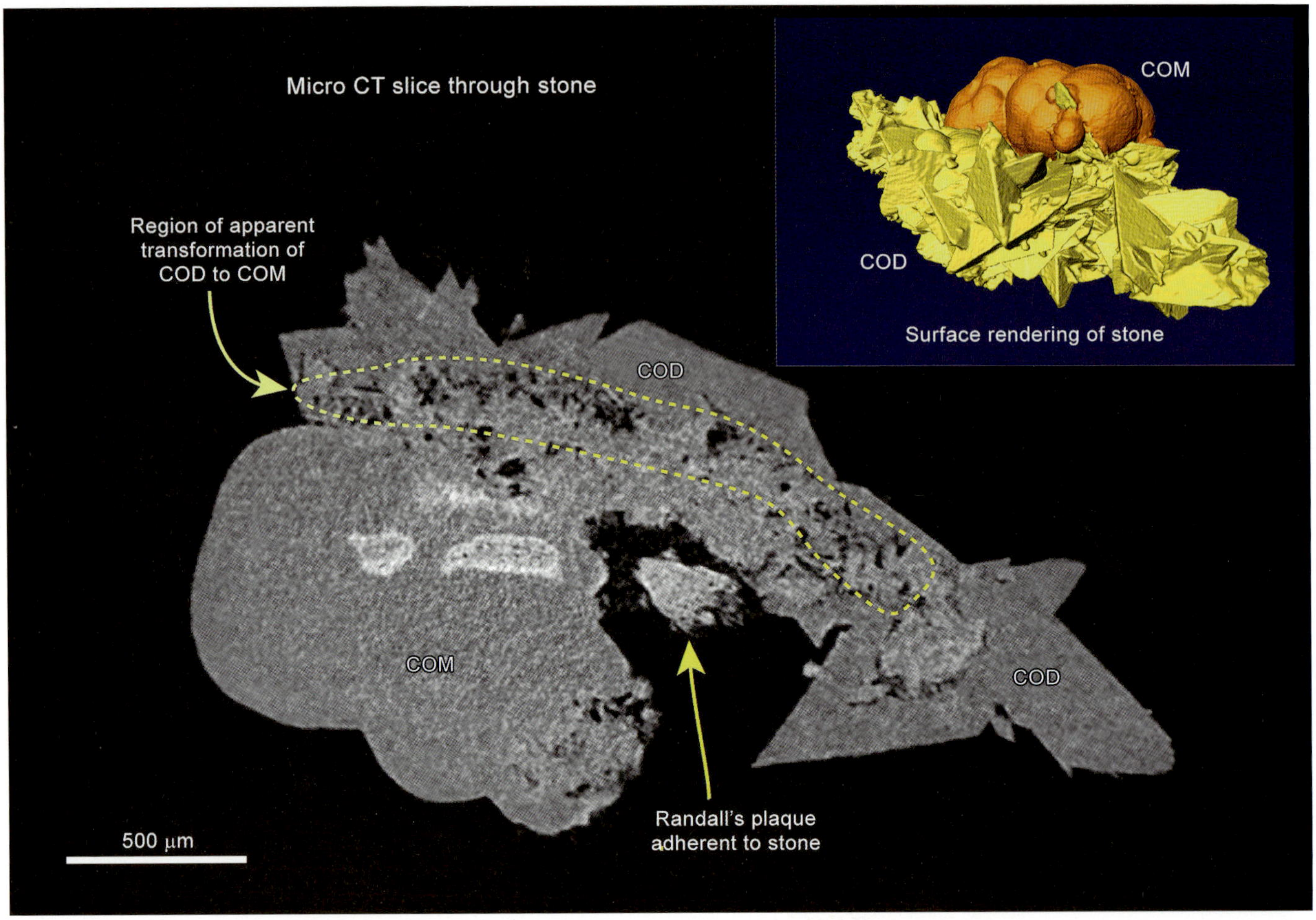

Fig. 4.5: Example of a calcium oxalate stone with dihydrate crystals on top of type Ia calcium oxalate monohydrate (COM). One hypothesis to describe this relatively common morphology is that the base of the calcium oxalate dihydrate (COD) crystals are transformed into COM in a controlled manner that leaves the COM crystals tightly packed within the body of the stone. This hypothesis would explain why this arrangement of COD-on-COM is common, but the hypothesis otherwise has little evidence to support it (*see* the text for details).

Ia stones, the COM is not organized into concentric layers of radially oriented crystals. Gaps are common within the stone mineral structure. This morphology of stone has been reported to be correlated with stasis in urine[3] (Box 4.2). Of note, this type of stone is especially susceptible to extracorporeal shockwave lithotripsy, but it is difficult to predict before treatment.[17]

In about 1% of all stone cases, calcium oxalate stones are found to be small and numerous, so that the stones pack the urinary space (types Id and IIc).[6] These are more commonly composed of the monohydrate (type Id, Figs. 4.6A and B), but multiple, packed stones composed of COD are also found (type IIc, Figs. 4.6A and B).[3] These stones (both types Id and IIc) have smooth surfaces, where they have rubbed up against one another (Figs. 4.6A and B). It would appear that confinement to a given region of the urinary system must be a requirement for the formation of this morphology of calcium oxalate stone, but the reason that the stones remain separate—rather than fusing into larger stones—is not apparent. The cause could be as simple as the forming stones being able to move; that is, it may be that small stones merge only when held together in a fixed manner, but this is only conjecture.

Calcium oxalate stones that form in severe types of hyperoxaluria tend to be formed of COM that is light in color (Figs. 4.7A and B). They are finely crystalline, but with an unorganized structure. Stones formed in cases of primary hyperoxaluria type I tend to be cream to light-brown in color, and the surfaces of the stones have the appearance of small bumps (or buds) in many places

Box 4.2: Urinary stasis: Another mechanism for retaining stone within the urinary system during early stages of stone growth.

- When urine flow is altered so that the dwell time of urine in any region of the urinary system is extended, the conditions can favor the growth of stone material into sizes that cannot be passed and that can eventually cause symptoms.
- The most obvious form of urinary stasis occurs in prostatic hyperplasia, when the emptying of the urinary bladder becomes incomplete. Urine thus can sit in the bladder for extended periods of time, allowing for growth of crystals or crystal aggregates into bladder stones.
- There is some evidence that abnormal peristalsis within the kidney could create functional stasis of urine, which could then favor the growth of renal stones.[18,19] Such stones could be symptomatic when passed, or could grow to such a size that they could not be passed, and result in renal symptoms.
- The existence of a stone within the renal collecting system probably increases the dwell time of urine in the vicinity of the stone,[20] so that a small stone formed by some mechanism of tissue attachment (such as Randall's plaque) could induce sufficient urinary stasis to allow the formation of other stones in free solution. If these stones are able to reach sufficient size, they could not be passed from the kidney. Moreover, any such stones would further alter urine flow within the kidney to allow more regions of functional urinary stasis within the collecting system.

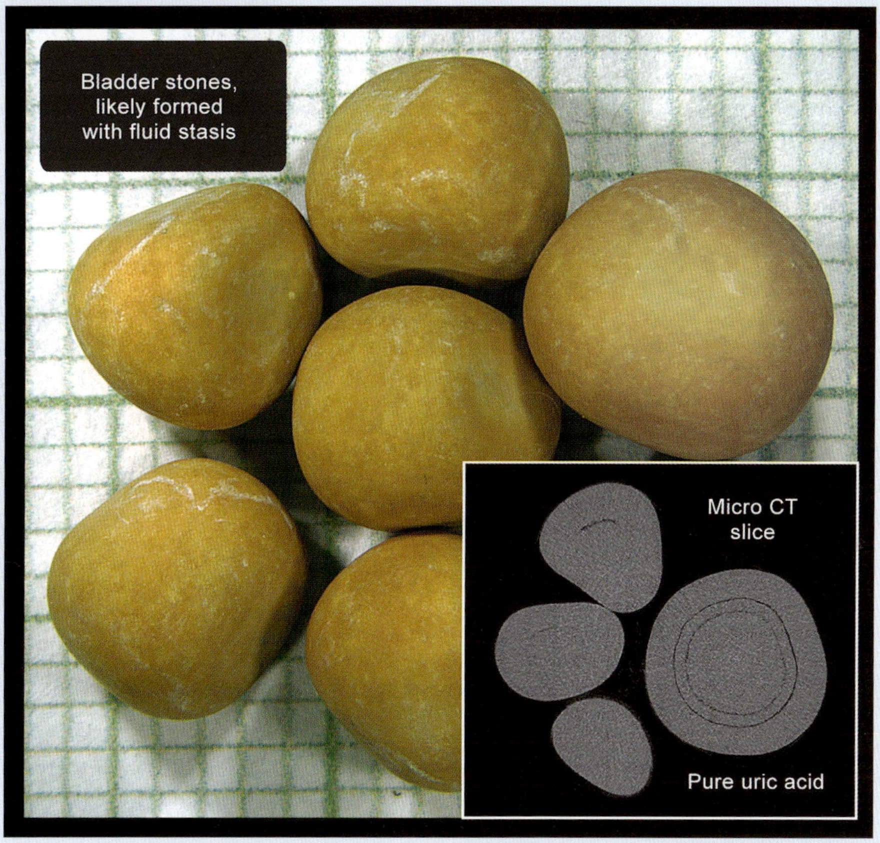
Bladder stones, likely formed with fluid stasis
Micro CT slice
Pure uric acid

The figure shows pure uric acid stones that were collected from urinary bladder. Such stones likely form under conditions of urinary stasis. Whether this mechanism of stone formation occurs within the kidney is still open to conjecture.

(type Ic).[3,6,21] Stones formed in patients with various forms of surgical removal of parts of the small intestine (extensive resection due, e.g. to Crohn's disease or radiation injury) can look very similar to those of primary hyperoxaluria, but tend to have an even more dramatically budded surface (type Ie, Figs. 4.7A and B).[6,22]

CALCIUM PHOSPHATE IN STONES

Apatite

The most common form of calcium phosphate in urinary stones occurs in the mineral form of apatite, which is found in some proportion in 80% of all stones.[23] Apatite

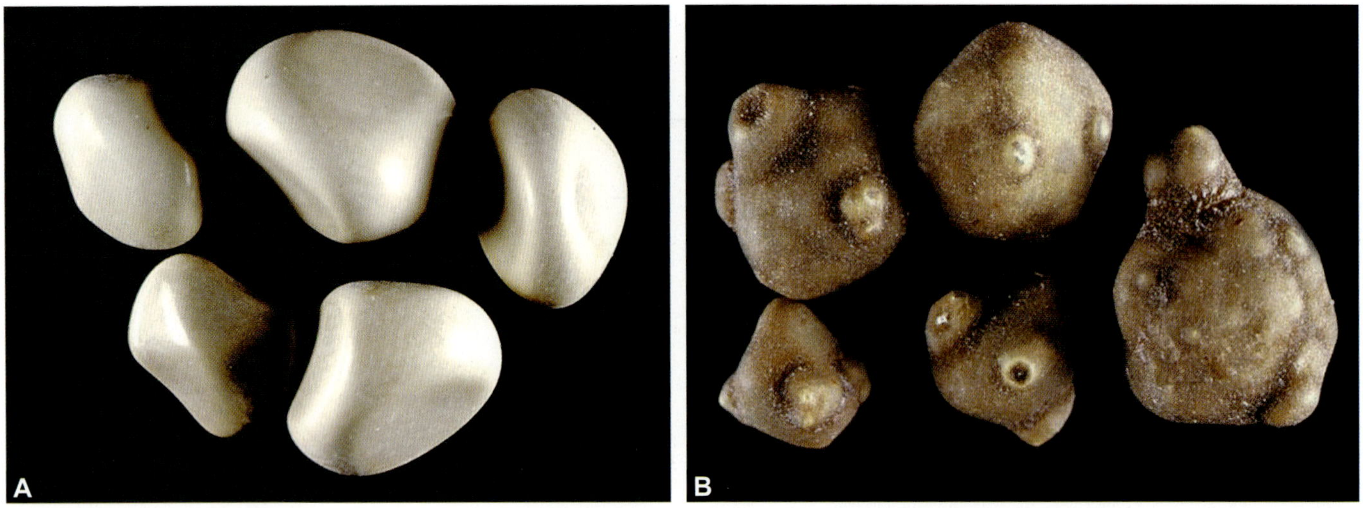

Figs. 4.6A and B: Morphological forms of calcium oxalate in which many, small stones are found packed together within the urinary space. (A) Calcium oxalate monohydrate, type Id (*see* also Fig. 4.1). (B) Calcium oxalate dihydrate, type IIc.

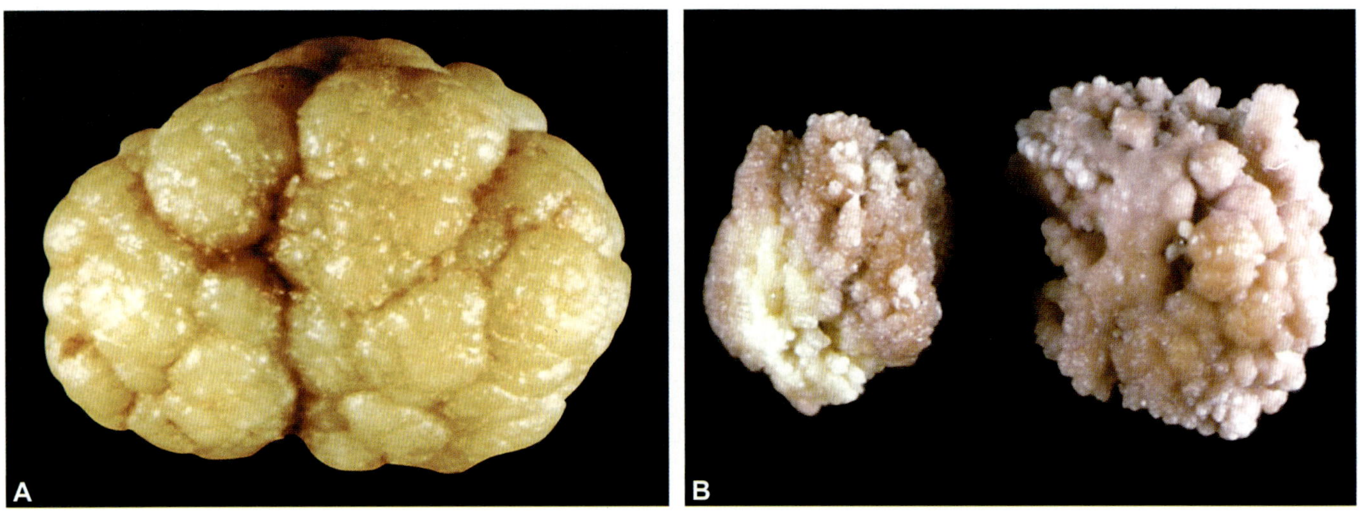

Figs. 4.7A and B: Morphological forms of calcium oxalate monohydrate associated with unusual levels of hyperoxaluria. (A) Type Ic, seen frequently with primary hyperoxaluria type 1. (B) Type Ie, seen frequently when stones occur following bowel resection.

in stones always contains some carbonate within its crystal structure, and so it is appropriate to call it carbapatite, but the amount of carbonate in the apatite varies (as is discussed more below). Some laboratories report all apatite as "hydroxyapatite"; others report all apatite as "carbonate apatite"; and still others report two forms of apatite: one low in carbonate (usually called "hydroxyapatite") and one high in carbonate ("carbonate apatite").[24] In fact, a continuum exists between apatite low and apatite high in carbonate.

Apatite as a Minor Component in Calcium Oxalate Stones

The most common secondary component in calcium oxalate stones is apatite. The proportion of apatite in calcium oxalate stones appears to increase with urine pH of the patient,[25] which makes sense from a physicochemical point of view, as apatite is quite soluble in urine at a pH below about 6.[26] However, the formation of apatite crystals is far from a simple process,[27] so that the addition of apatite to a stone is not merely a function of urine pH.

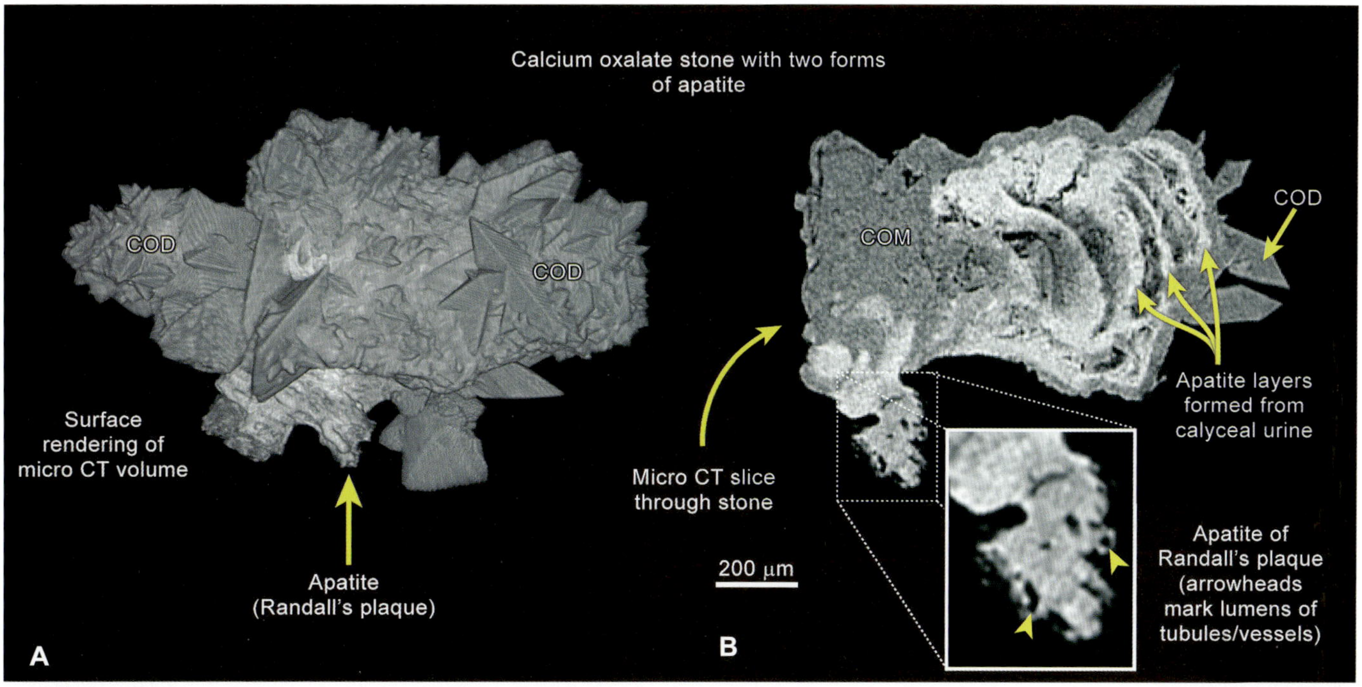

Figs. 4.8A and B: This stone shows the two forms of apatite commonly seen as a minor component of calcium oxalate stones. (A) The Randall's plaque, which formed within the papillary interstitium, shows a relatively even level of mineralization with cylindrical voids that show the lumens of tubules or vessels. (B) The apatite within the part of the stone that formed in the calyceal urine shows alternating layers of X-ray dense and lucent material. See the text for more details.

The morphology of apatite within calcium oxalate stones occurs in at least two distinct forms by micro-CT (Figs. 4.8A and B). The apatite within Randall's plaque appears typically as possessing a uniform X-ray attenuation, interrupted by voids that represent tubules and/or blood vessels that ran within the mineralized interstitium. Apatite that was laid onto the stone from the urine typically has a layered structure, with alternating X-ray dense and lucent layers. The physical cause of this alternation of X-ray appearance in layered apatite has not been studied, but in many cases infrared spectroscopy of the material suggests that the only mineral existing in such regions is apatite, with often a higher content of protein matrix than in calcium oxalate stones. Thus, the X-ray lucent regions within the layers must consist of apatite crystals that are suspended at low density within some kind of protein matrix.

The percentage of apatite in calcium oxalate stones has been observed in some patients to rise over time,[28] and this phenomenon correlates with urine pH.[25] The underlying reasons for such a transformation of stone mineral could reside in the fundamental etiology of this kind of stone former, but it also could be related to some kinds of treatments received after stones are initially diagnosed.[25] Future study of this problem would likely benefit from the use of micro-CT to measure the apatite content of stones, as this method can quantitate apatite volume percentage in a very sensitive manner that does not preclude other modes of analysis.[29]

Apatite as the Major Component of Stones

In about 15% of all stones, apatite is the primary mineral (about 10% counting only stones with no struvite).[23] The proportion of apatite stones is, however, much higher in women than in men (~30% of all stones in women, and ~17% counting only apatite stones with no struvite); the higher proportion of apatite stones in women than in men could be related in part to the higher incidence of urinary tract infection in women (Figs. 4.9A and B), but women also tend to have a higher amount of apatite in calcium oxalate stones,[6] which are not normally associated with infection, suggesting that there are other causes for the sex difference in apatite stone occurrence other than simply infection rates. One of the causes of this sex difference could be medullary sponge kidney, the prevalence of which being often found higher in women than in men as reported in several studies.[30,31]

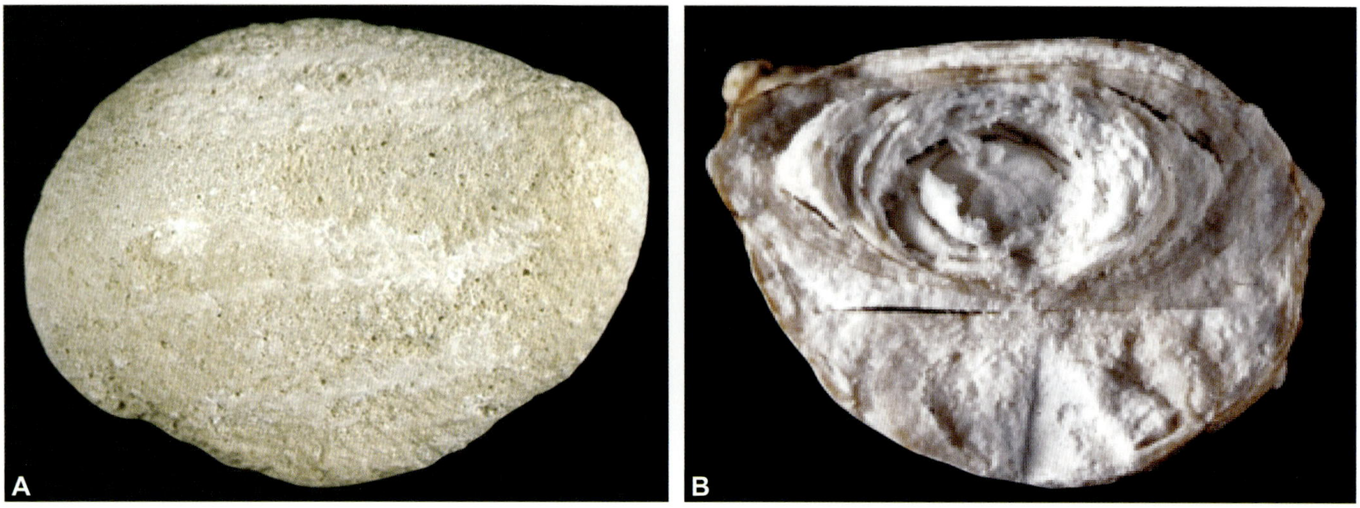

Figs. 4.9A and B: Surface (A) and section (B) of an infection-related IVa1 carbapatite stone also containing a high proportion of amorphous carbonated calcium phosphate. The carbonate rate is >15%, which is highly suggestive of urinary tract infection (UTI) by urea-splitting bacteria.

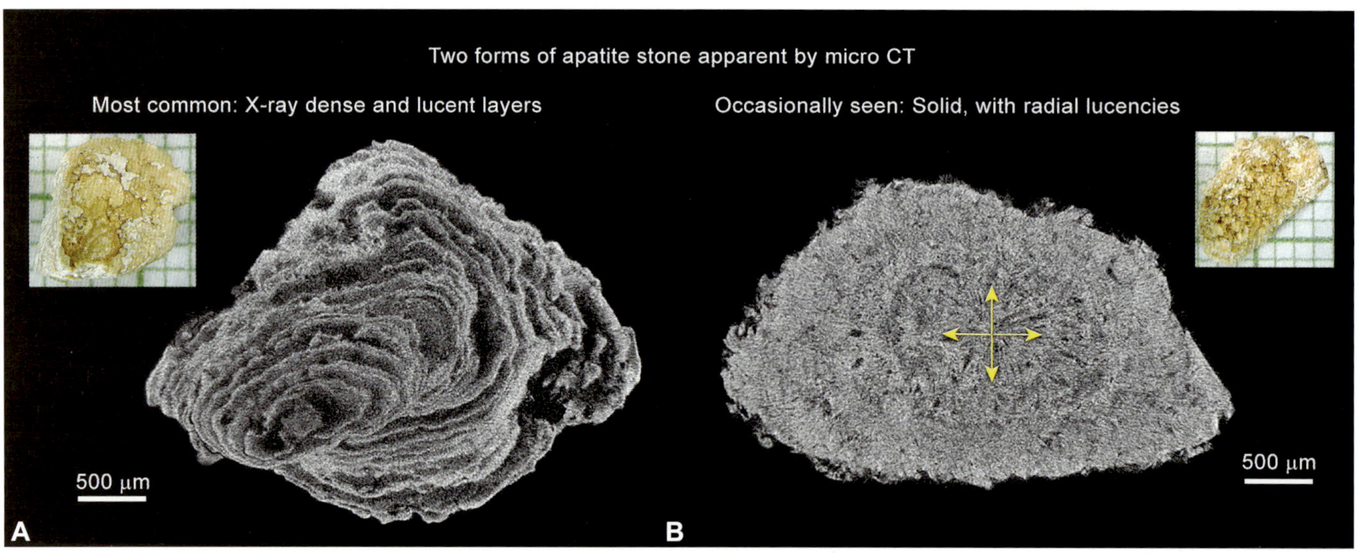

Figs. 4.10A and B: Several forms of pure apatite stone have been seen by micro-CT.[32] Shown here are the most common appearance (A) consisting of alternating layers of X-ray dense (white) and lucent (dark) material. Much less common are relatively solid stones (B), which have X-ray lucent regions radiating out from a single point within the stone. Apatite stones composed of multiple particles of apatite have also been described[32] (not shown).

By micro-CT, the majority of apatite stones usually have the same appearance of alternating bright and dark layers as mentioned above for the urine-formed apatite in calcium oxalate stones. However, the morphology of apatite can exhibit very different micro-CT characteristics in some stone formers (Figs. 4.10A and B); the reasons behind these different morphologies of apatite are not known.

One special morphology (type IVa2) of apatite stones that has been described is for apatite stones in patients with distal renal tubular acidosis (dRTA; Fig. 4.11). In this condition, the apatite stones typically have a glossy surface that often contains fine cracks. The predictive value of this morphology has not been tested, but one study found that this morphology of apatite stones was found in virtually all of 70 cases of dRTA.[23]

Patients with dRTA have been demonstrated to have plugging of their papillary collecting ducts with apatite, associated with loss of tubular epithelium and extensive fibrosis of the papillary interstitium.[33] Such plugging of papillary ducts with apatite has also been seen in patients making apatite stones but without dRTA, and in apatite stone formers at least some stones appear to be retained in the kidney during early growth by attachment to these ductal plugs (Box 4.3). Of note, these ductal plugs, though composed of apatite, do not have the same morphology as the same mineral growing in the urinary space (Box 4.3).

Concentric, alternating layers of apatite with COD (type IIa + IVa) have been reported to occur in as many as 50% of stones from patients with hyperparathyroidism,[35] and this morphology is quite common in any patient having hypercalciuria.[3,6] Most laboratories will not report this conformation, even though it is quite easy to recognize by visual inspection of a sectioned stone (Fig. 4.12).

Finally, there is some evidence that the amount of carbonate in apatite correlates with infection; as mentioned above, some analysis laboratories report the carbonate content of apatite stones, at least in terms of apatite having either low or high levels of carbonate.[24] However, it is not difficult to quantify the carbonate content in apatite using Fourier-transform infrared (FT-IR) spectroscopy to give a percentage value for carbonate content[36,37] (also see Box 4.4). Some studies have suggested that carbonate content of apatite above ~15% is a strong signal for past infection,[36,37] but this marker does not correlate perfectly with results from stone culture.[38] Clearly, more work needs to be done in describing the predictive value of apatite carbonation in understanding stone pathology, and this effort would be aided by standardization of nomenclature among clinical laboratories.[39]

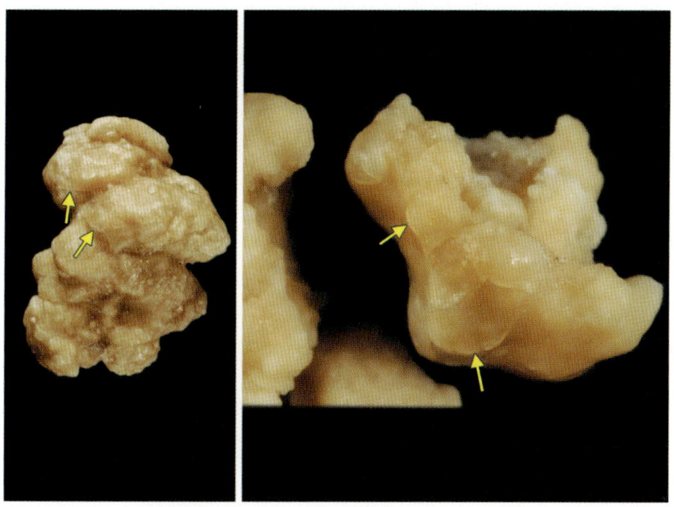

Fig. 4.11: Apatite stones formed in patients with distal renal tubular acidosis tend to have a shiny coat with tiny cracks visible by stereomicroscopy (arrows).

Brushite as the Major Component of Stones

Calcium phosphate in the mineral form of brushite (calcium hydrogen phosphate dihydrate, also called dicalcium phosphate; Daudon type IVd) marks a form of urinary stone disease that produces large stones that tend to recur quickly.[40] Brushite stones also tend to be physically hard, making their removal problematic.[41] More than one study has documented a substantial increase in brushite stones over the past few decades.[23,28] In France, the occurrence of brushite stones increased progressively from 0.9% in the years 1980–1984 up to 4.3% during the years 2005–2009.[23] The reasons for this increase in brushite stone disease are not known,[42,43] though it has been proposed that recurrent stone formers can convert from some other stone type (such as calcium oxalate) to the formation of brushite stones.[43] Because brushite stones are highly recurrent and difficult to manage clinically, understanding the causes of this growing problem may be especially important.[40]

But the formation of brushite as a stone mineral is enigmatic. On the one hand, it is known from in vitro studies that brushite is often the first form of calcium phosphate to crystallize out of solution[44] and that brushite is thought to be the precursor to the formation of apatite in many situations in vivo.[45] Thus, the absence of detectable brushite in most calcium stones is a bit surprising; if indeed

Box 4.3: Growth of stones on ductal plugs: Still another mechanism for retaining stone within the urinary system during early stages of stone growth.

- Several kinds of stone formation have been shown to result in mineral plugging of the papillary collecting ducts,[34] and some of these have been observed to have small stones growing in the calyceal urine, anchored to the papilla via the ductal plug.
- This thus represents yet another mechanism by which growing stones can be retained within the urinary space even when they are quite small.
- Although other causes may induce such nucleation and growth within ducts, renal distal tubular acidosis is typically an example of such stone formation. Another example is given with medullary sponge kidney.

Contd...

Contd...

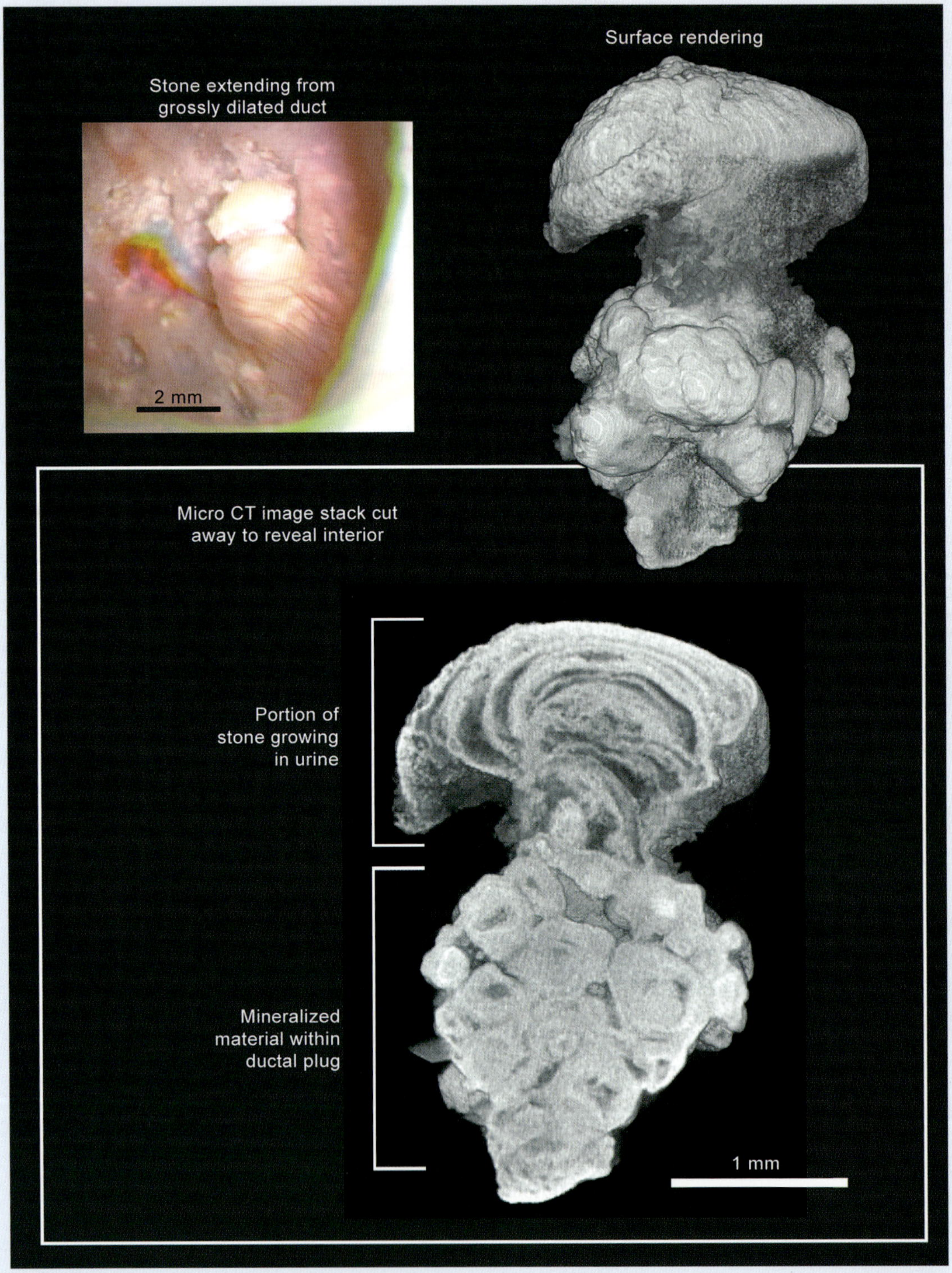

The figure illustrates a stone found in a hyperparathyroid patient, in which the portion growing in the calyceal urine was visibly distinct from the portion within the dilated duct of Bellini. The entire stone is composed of apatite, but notice the difference in morphology apparent in the micro-CT image, where the ductal portion of the stone appears as small spheres, fused together, while the urine portion of the stone has alternating X-ray dense and lucent layers, as is typical for apatite.

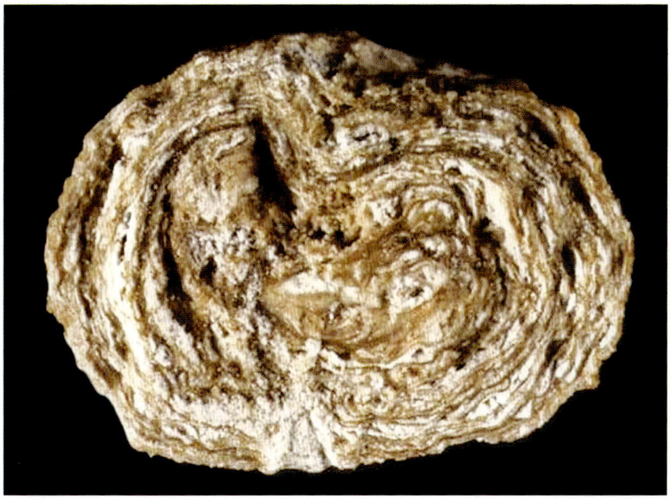

Fig. 4.12: Cross-section of a mixed stone exhibiting alternate layers of calcium oxalate dihydrate and apatite. Such a morphology corresponds to the type II+IV often found in cases of hypercalciuria and/or primary hyperparathyroidism.

brushite is a precursor for other crystals, conversion is evidently perfectly complete in most cases. On the other hand, the general absence of brushite in the vast majority of stones indicates that some aspects of urine physiology must be generally inhibitory to the formation of this form of calcium phosphate, so that brushite stone formers may have a unique pathology, which is still unexplained. That is, it is possible that brushite stone formers lack some inhibitor for brushite crystal formation, or alternately they may have urine factors that inhibit the normal conversion of brushite to apatite.[46] This concept of a unique pathology is supported by the finding that brushite crystals in urine are found as infrequently as are brushite stones, whereas other forms of calcium phosphate are much more common.[47] Brushite is also one of the mineral forms that *cannot* be detected by wet chemical analysis, an inexpensive but largely useless method of stone analysis that is still all-too-common throughout the world (*see* Box 4.4). This means that a lack of awareness of this form of stone disease in many countries may be simply because the stone analysis available there is not good enough to reveal it. However, stone morphology alone may help to recognize this important form of calcium phosphate stone (Figs. 4.13A and B).

Other Forms of Calcium Phosphate

Whitlockite is a complex crystal of calcium phosphate that includes minor amounts of magnesium and iron in the crystal lattice. It is found rarely in stones: Whitlockite is a minor component in about 5% of all stones,[48] but in only 0.2%, it is found as the major mineral.[23] The reasons for the formation of whitlockite are poorly studied, but there is some evidence that it occurs commonly in association with infection.[23]

Amorphous (noncrystalline) calcium phosphate is found in about 7% of all stones,[48] but in only ~0.2% of stones as the major component.[23] This form of calcium phosphate has been shown to be commonly associated with infection,[23] but no study of its predictive power for that condition has been done. It should be noted that amorphous materials cannot be detected by X-ray diffraction (*see* Box 4.4) so that laboratories in which that is the primary method of stone analysis will not be able to report the presence of amorphous calcium phosphate in a patient's stone.

Finally, octacalcium phosphate is a complex crystalline form that, like brushite, has been shown to be a probable precursor to apatite in many systems.[49] It is found, though, in only about 1% of all stones,[48] and it is the majority component in only about one-fifth of those.[23] It is found in about a quarter of apatite stones formed during pregnancy,[23,50] so something about the pregnant condition favors the formation of octacalcium phosphate. Octacalcium phosphate is known as an unstable form of calcium phosphate able to convert in apatite after few hours or days.[51] Thus, its presence within a stone could be a marker of a recent stone formation. However, in some cases, octacalcium phosphate may be found in the core of a stone and not in surrounding layers; the reason for the apparent stability of octacalcium phosphate in such stones remains to be clarified.

INFECTION STONES

Struvite

Magnesium ammonium phosphate hexahydrate—commonly designated by its mineral name, struvite—is universally considered to occur in human stones only in the context of infection, and most commonly in infection by an organism that can split urea. Using the enzyme urease, these organisms convert urine urea into carbon dioxide and ammonia; the ammonia raises the pH of the infected urine and contributes to the precipitation of struvite.[52]

Most commonly, struvite is seen mixed in with apatite, with the apatite being the major mineral component in the stones (type IVb, in about 6% of all stones[6]). Traditionally, this was the main type of stone that would be found to occupy most or all of the collecting system in a kidney—so-called staghorn stones (Fig. 4.14)—but a recent series reported that more than half of staghorn stones contained no struvite.[53] At the same time, it is also known that struvite

Box 4.4: Stone analysis.

- Best done using microdissection of the stone specimen, followed by either infrared spectroscopy or X-ray diffraction to identify mineral types.
- Specimen should be examined using a stereomicroscope, by a trained worker who can select regions of the specimen for mineral analysis.
- Infrared spectroscopy (usually called Fourier-transform infrared spectroscopy, FT-IR) provides conclusive identification of all major stone minerals; it also allows the quantification of carbonate content in apatite; disadvantages can include the time required for sample preparation and the lack of ability to distinguish some minerals when they are minor components of the stones.
- X-ray diffraction also provides conclusive identification of all major stone minerals; disadvantages include high cost of the instrument and the inability to detect noncrystalline substances.
- Wet chemical methods are NOT adequate for providing clinically relevant information.
- All methods of stone analysis can be affected by specimen selection errors (*see* Box 4.5).
- Stone analysis reports are not, at present, standardized such that the mineral types are named using the same descriptors, so physicians need to be aware that reports from different laboratories may use different terms for the same stone type.

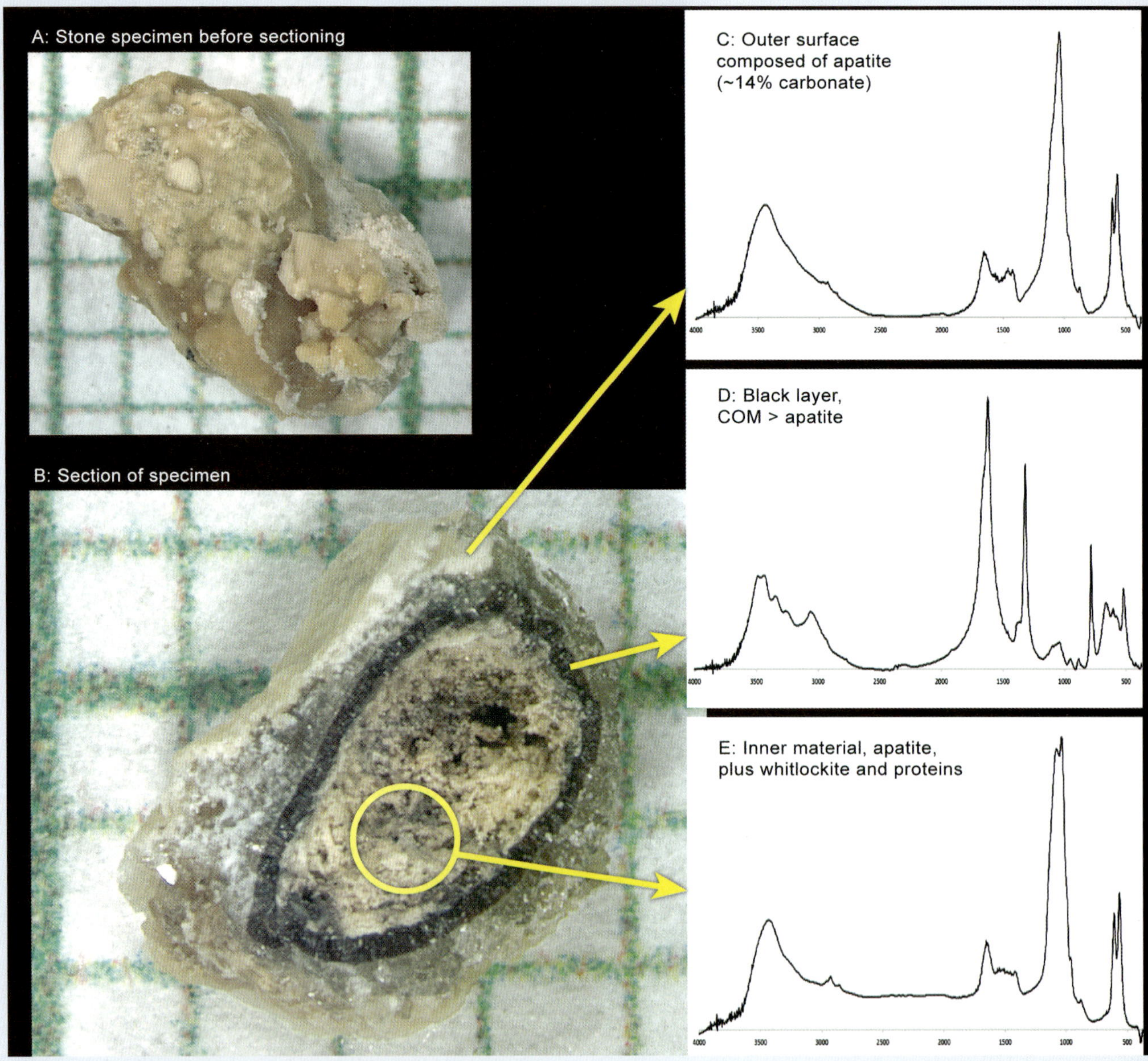

The figures show an example of stone analysis. Stone specimen (A) was cleaved (B) to allow dissection of layers, and FT-IR spectra for three of the five samples taken are shown at right (C to E).

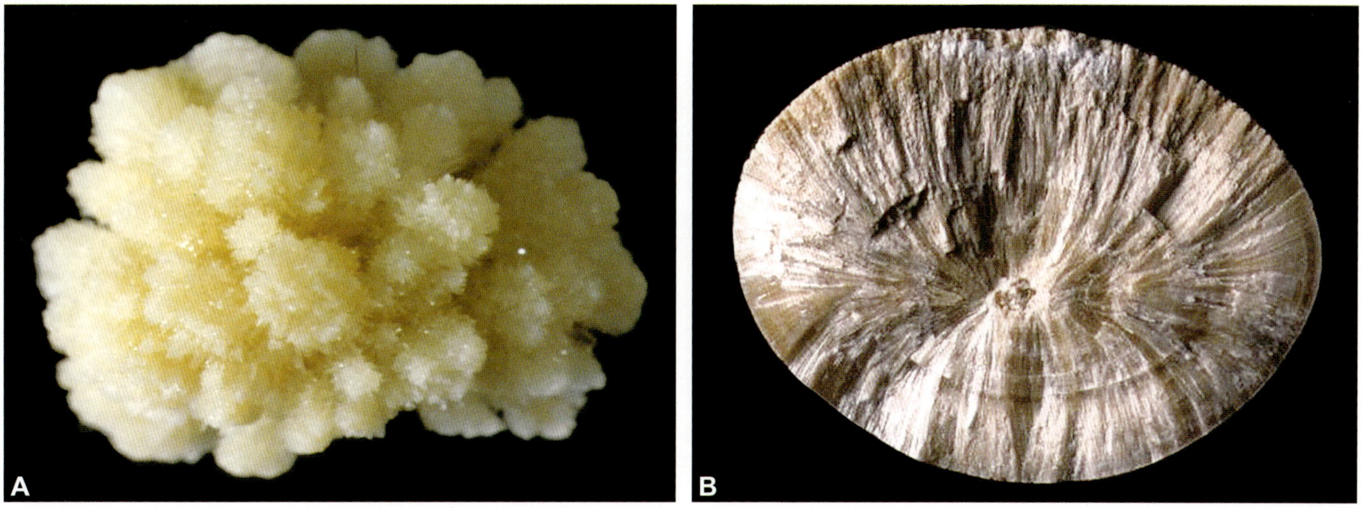

Figs. 4.13A and B: Brushite stones (type IVd). (A) Surface of a brushite stone with crystals that have the appearance of being recently formed. (B) Section of a brushite stone showing much more compact structure with concentric and radial organization.

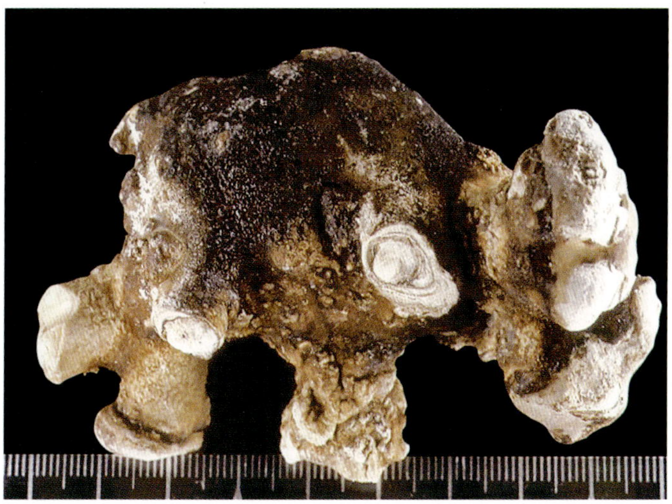

Fig. 4.14: Infection-related staghorn stone (type IVb) made of a mixture of apatite, amorphous carbonated calcium phosphate, and struvite. Scale at bottom is cm/mm.

may be the most unreliably reported stone mineral when it is present in mixed stones.[24] Struvite is also seen in relatively pure form in about 2% of all stones (type IVc).[6] Struvite is consistently found more often in stones from women than from men, a fact which is likely related to the higher frequency of urinary tract infections in females.[6]

PURINES IN STONES

Uric Acid

Stones composed wholly or in part of uric acid occur only when urine pH is sufficiently acidic, and several metabolic problems contribute to this rather common form of stones (types IIIa and IIIb, with one or the other present in about 10–20% of all stones[6,48]). These two morphologies of uric acid stones are very different (Fig. 4.15), suggesting that local conditions for their formation are distinctive in some way. Studies have identified diabetes mellitus, and especially the adult-onset form of diabetes, as correlating with a higher incidence of uric acid stones;[54,55] the morphology of uric acid stones in these patients is dominantly (85%) the less-organized form, type IIIb.[56] In addition, obesity in general is associated with a high percentage of stones containing uric acid.[57]

Uric acid stones can be treated by alkalizing the urine,[58,59] but published data on success rates with such medical therapy are few. Additionally, it is not known what proportion of uric acid stones are mixed with other minerals (Box 4.5) such that they cannot be dissolved by raising urine pH, nor is it known what the radiological characteristics might be for uric acid stones that are susceptible or resistant to medical treatment.

Urates

Stones composed wholly or in part of various forms of urate are relatively rare in developed countries, with the various species occurring in only about 5% of all stones.[48] All of the urates—ammonium acid urate (AAU), sodium urate, calcium urate, magnesium urate, potassium urate, sodium-potassium urate—can form only in an alkaline urine, but causes for the urinary environment that can form these minerals include infectious diarrhea, laxative abuse, and

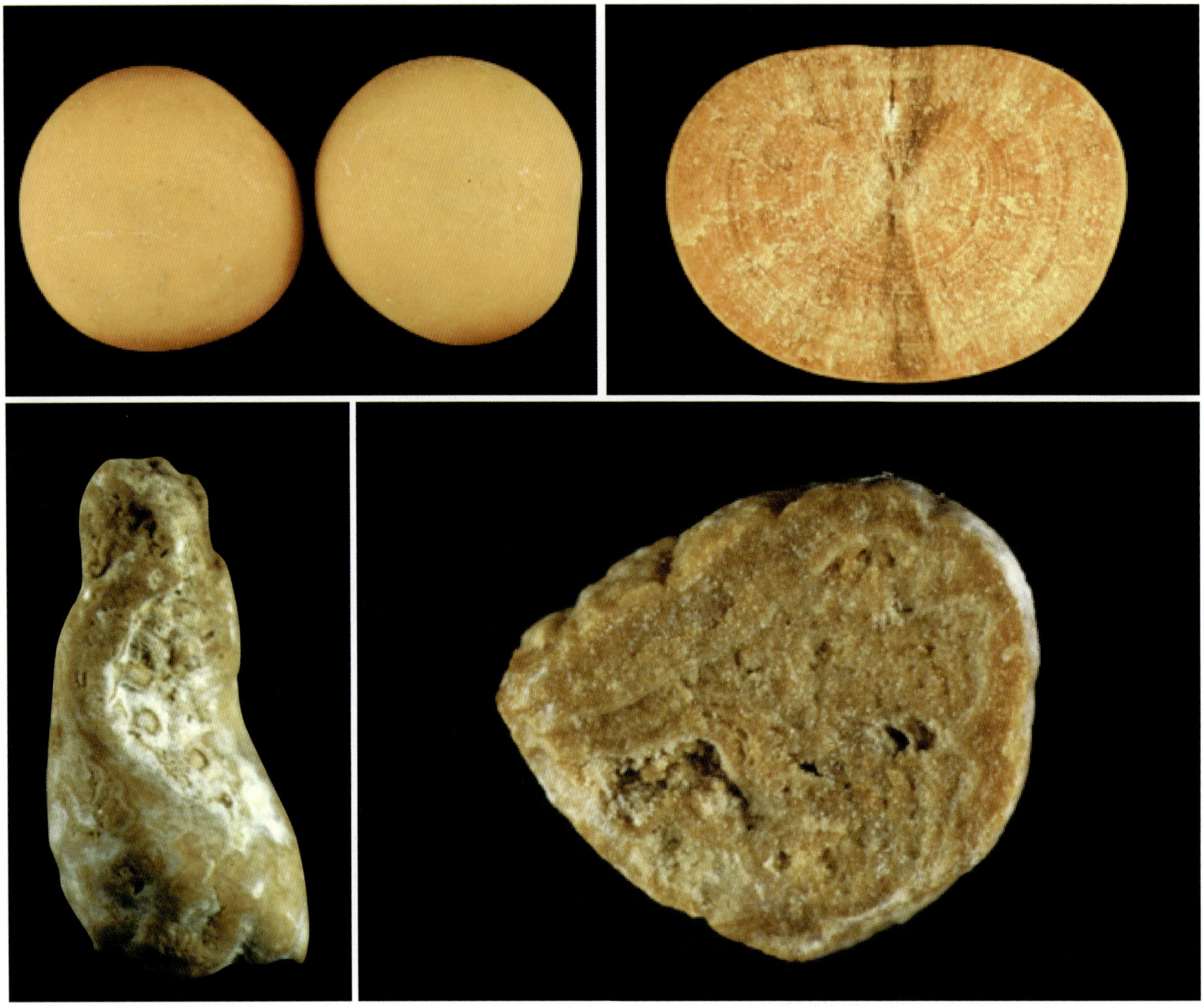

Fig. 4.15: Morphologies of uric acid stones. Upper: Typical surface (left) and section (right) of type IIIa stones. Note that surfaces are rather smooth, and interior of stone is quite organized. Lower: Typical surface (left) and section (right) of type IIIb stones. Note heterogeneous surface and porous, less-organized nature of the type IIIb stone.

malnutrition of various forms.[6] Among AAU stones, two different morphologies may be observed (types IIIc and IIId), the former being more often associated with excessive urinary alkalinization (infection by urea-splitting bacteria or excessive load of alkalinizing agents) and the latter commonly related to infectious diarrhea or laxative abuse. Thus, type IIIc stones have been identified more frequently in certain countries (specifically, in sub-Saharan Africa), while type IIId stones have been found more frequently in other parts of the world (especially in Southeast Asia).[65]

CYSTINE STONES

Cystine

Cystine stones occur only in cases of cystinuria, and this condition is caused by specific genetic defects.[61,66] Cystine stones are easily recognized by simple examination of their morphology (Fig. 4.16), and cystine crystals in urine are relatively easy to identify with simple microscopy,[66] but in spite of this, many patients are not identified properly

Box 4.5: Stones containing more than one mineral (mixed stones).

- Most stones (>90%) contain more than one mineral
- Minor stone components can often have clinical significance, even if the majority stone mineral is simply calcium oxalate. Examples:
  - Struvite[52]
  - Calcium phosphate in the form of apatite[25,26]
  - Calcium phosphate in the form of brushite[40]
  - Uric acid[60]
  - Ammonium acid urate[6]
  - Cystine[61]
  - Pharmaceuticals[62]
- Missing minor components during analysis can occur through at least three routes:
  - Physician selection of specimen to be sent to the laboratory. The specimen supplied for analysis ends up not being representative of the entire stone burden. If specimen for analysis contains only the major mineral in the stone burden, important minor constituents will not be identified. It is also possible to accidently select a stone specimen that misses the major mineral component, and contains only a minor component, so that the stone event is misclassified.
  - Technician selection of specimen(s) for analysis. The piece(s) of the stone taken for analysis (by FT-IR or X-ray diffraction) end up not being representative of all of the types of mineral in the stone specimen submitted to the laboratory. Stone examination before constitutional analysis may help to assess stone composition and heterogeneity.
  - Analytical protocol for stone analysis. Because an accurate stone analysis is time-consuming, in some laboratories stone composition is determined by grinding the whole stone sample. In such cases, the sensitivity of the method or the accuracy for reading analytical curves obtained from the sample is not sufficient to detect very minor components. Again, stone examination before analysis may help to detect and locate relevant minor components in the stone.
- Because minor components stones are under-reported (and underappreciated), the true clinical significance of many of these minor minerals is probably untested. For example, it may be that the apatite content in a calcium oxalate stone could provide important information about the acid-base pathophysiology in the patient,[25,42] but this minor constituent can be easily missed in standard analyses.[63,64]

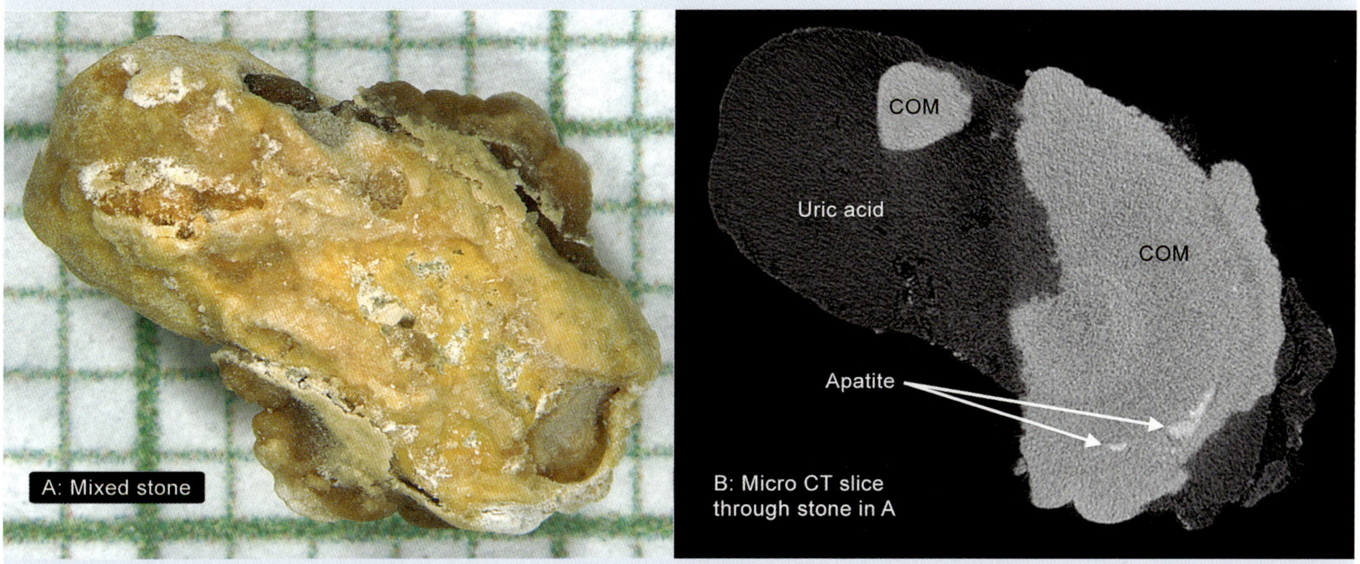

The figures show that the vast majority of stone are of mixed composition. This stone is easily seen to display two colors (A), and micro-CT imaging of the stone shows the uric acid and COM portions, as well as a small component of apatite that was buried within the COM. Most laboratories would likely correctly identify the uric acid and COM components of this obviously mixed stone, but few would detect the apatite that is present.[24]

early in their history of cystine nephrolithiasis. Cystinuria is also simple to identify using colorimetric tests in urine,[61] but the reagents critical for these tests do not have long shelf-lives, so that false-negative results for cystinuria may be more prevalent than is widely appreciated. Stone patients with cystinuria can produce stones rapidly, and they need to be managed in ways quite different from other stone patients,[61,66] so identification of this relatively rare form of stone needs to be accomplished on its first incidence, if possible.

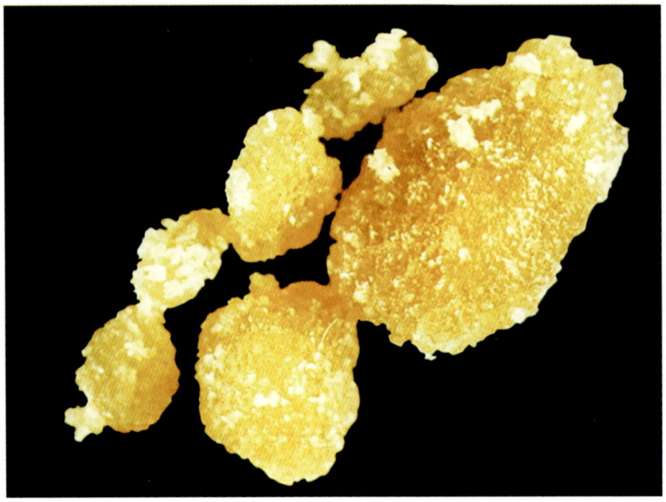

Fig. 4.16: Typical cystine stones (type Va).

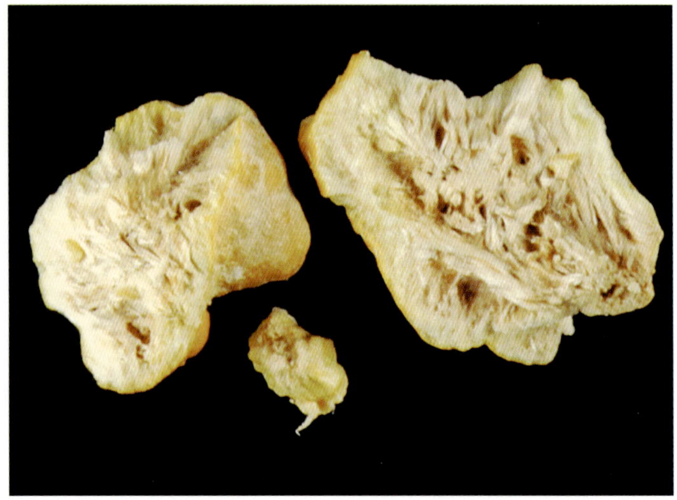

Fig. 4.17: Atazanavir calculi; note needle-like crystals distributed within the stones.

OTHER FORMS OF URINARY STONE

Stones Formed from Pharmaceuticals

Certain drugs can be excreted in the urine in sufficient concentrations that supersaturation is reached, and these drugs can then form stones. Among them, sulphonamides (e.g. sulfadiazine and sulfamethoxazole) and antiproteases (e.g. indinavir and atazanavir) are able to form pure or mixed stones easily diagnosed by infrared analysis.[62] Figure 4.17 shows a typical stone made of atazanavir. Such stones may be X-ray lucent,[67] but they also may be mixed with calcium salts, making their identification more problematic.[24] Drugs containing either ephedrine or guaifenesin, which can be abused as stimulants, may also form kidney stones.[68]

CONCLUDING COMMENTS

Need for Proper Stone Analysis in Understanding Stone Diseases

This chapter has reviewed the basics of the different kinds of human urinary stones that are likely to pass through any clinic that treats stone formers. We have emphasized some of the ways in which stone composition and morphology are linked to etiology, but this chapter is by no means an exhaustive treatment about what is known in this area.

Some practitioners have dismissed stone analysis as being irrelevant to patient treatment,[69] and it is likely that a great many physicians take little interest in stone analysis results in planning patient treatment. Part of the reason for this, frankly, is that good stone analysis can be difficult to do,[24] especially since the vast majority of stones are composed of more than one material,[48] so that the results that many physicians receive are not as useful as they could be (*see* Box 4.5). This is especially true for the many places around the world where stone analysis is still done using wet chemical methods; while these methods are relatively inexpensive, and produce a report that looks official, the content of the report is largely useless, and often also quite inaccurate.[70]

Because stone analysis is not uniformly good around the world—or even uniformly good within countries[24,70]—data on stone composition have not been correlated well with patient outcomes. That is, because of uncertainty and errors in stone analysis, most studies that have attempted to link clinical presentation with stone compositions are almost certain to find no significant correlations. This must be especially true for regions in which stone analysis is still done by wet chemical methods, where the errors inherent within such analyses[70] would certainly preclude any ability to identify relationships between stone components and patient characteristics.

But even with the use of modern spectroscopic methods of analyzing stone mineral, existing practice will not allow progress on some basic and important questions in understanding stone diseases. For example, there is substantial evidence to suggest that the formation of the dihydrate form of calcium oxalate is dependent on significant hypercalciuria.[12,13,37,71-73] However, most of the studies that found this correlation analyzed stones *using morphologic criteria*, in addition to spectroscopic analysis of mineral type; specifically, most of these studies were careful to take into account the fact that some calcium oxalate stones can form as COD, and then convert to COM over time (*see* Fig. 4.5). If the morphologic character of the stone is not identified, then those stones that formed as COD and later converted to COM (type IIb), will of course be classed as being composed of the monohydrate, thus losing the information about the original mineral formed.

Some suggestions of this correlation between hypercalciuria and the formation of the dihydrate of calcium oxalate have come in studies that did not utilize characterization of stones by morphology.[74,75] But these studies almost certainly had COD stones that converted to COM (type IIb) classed in with majority-COM stones, so that the observed correlations would be weaker than seen in the group above, which used stone morphology to class type IIb stones as originally forming as COD. Thus, this concept—that patients forming COD stones almost certainly experience chronic hypercalciuria, which could be an essential and treatable part of the etiology of their disease—has not been well established. Indeed, it would seem that a rigorous clinical study of the relationship between the mineral form of calcium oxalate and hypercalciuria could never be successful in establishing a strong correlation without the analysis of stone morphology being part of the patient workup.

This is just one example of the way in which improved stone analysis could benefit our studies of the different kinds of causes of urinary stones. Morphologic classification of stones is at least relatively inexpensive. All good stone laboratories already carry out examination of stone specimens by stereomicroscopy. If technicians were trained in morphologic identification, stones could easily be classed appropriately as part of the normal workflow in the laboratory. At first, physicians would not know how to utilize the data on stone morphology, but as clinical correlates emerged from such data, they could be incorporated into the analysis report in a way that would help to educate treating physicians about the information contained in the specimens from their patients. A detailed model for proper stone analysis already exists,[76] and this model could be emulated by other sites, which would also allow the power of recognizing stone morphology to be better tested and established. Of course, if such a model of employing stone morphology as part of stone analysis is not utilized in more places, it is less likely that recognition of the value of combined morphologic and spectroscopic analysis of stones will become widespread.

SUMMARY

Urinary stones occur in a wide range of compositions and morphologies, and many of these can be helpful in understanding etiology and planning patient treatment. Indeed, we argue that stone morphology and composition can be much more useful than it presently is, if proper methods were employed so that correlations could be made between stone type and patient pathology. The poor state of stone analysis, globally, is a barrier to better understanding of stone diseases. This, in combination with ignorance of the usefulness of stone analysis among medical professionals, means that many stone patients are not treated as effectively for their disorders as they could be.

Good stone analysis requires experience with the visual recognition of stone morphological types, combined with stone dissection and spectroscopic analysis of mineral components. Simple chemical analysis of urinary stones, though perceived to be inexpensive, is essentially a waste of time and money, and should be replaced with better practices. We are, frankly, in a state of catch-22 with stone analysis in its present forms. If stone analysis is not improved, few physicians will be able to recognize its benefits, and few good studies can be done to verify and extend the benefits already known. However, if the potential value for better stone analysis is not appreciated by medical communities, stone analysis methods will not be improved. It is our hope that this chapter will help to inform physicians of the essential benefit of good stone analysis in the optimal treatment of stone diseases.

REFERENCES

1. Abraham PA, Smith CL. Evaluation of factors involved in calcium stone formation. Miner Electrolyte Metab. 1987; 13:201-8.
2. Marshall RW, Robertson WG. Nomograms for the estimation of the saturation of urine with calcium oxalate, calcium phosphate, magnesium ammonium phosphate, uric acid, sodium acid urate, ammonium acid urate and cystine. Clin Chimica Acta. 1976;72:253-60.
3. Daudon M, Bader CA, Jungers P. Urinary calculi: review of classification methods and correlations with etiology. Scan Microsc. 1993;7:1081-106.
4. Kim KM. The stones. Scan Electron Microsc. 1982;Pt 4:1635-60.
5. Taller A, Grohe B, Rogers KA, et al. Specific adsorption of osteopontin and synthetic polypeptides to calcium oxalate monohydrate crystals. Biophys J. 2007;93:1768-77.
6. Daudon M. Analyse et classification des calculs: contribution à l'etiologie de la maladie lithiasique [Analysis and classification of calculi: contribution to the etiology of

calculous disease]. Revue medicale de la Suisse romande. 2004;124:445-53.
7. Kuo RL, Lingeman JE, Evan AP, et al. Urine calcium and volume predict coverage of renal papilla by Randall's plaque. Kidney Int. 2003;64:2150-54.
8. Stoller ML, Meng MV, Abrahams HM, et al. The primary stone event: a new hypothesis involving a vascular etiology. J Urol. 2004;171:1920-24.
9. Cifuentes Delatte L, Miñón Cifuentes J, Medina JA. New studies on papillary calculi. J Urol. 1987;137: 1024-9.
10. Cifuentes Delatte L, Miñón-Cifuentes JL, Medina JA. Papillary stones: calcified renal tubules in Randall's plaques. J Urol. 1985;133:490-94.
11. Hesse A, Berg W, Bothor C. Scanning electron microscopic investigations on the morphology and phase conversions of uroliths. Int Urol Nephrol. 1979;11:11-20.
12. Daudon M, Reveillaud RJ. Whewellite et weddellite: vers des étiopathogénies différentes. Intérêt du typage morphologique des calculs. Nephrologie. 1984;5:195-201.
13. Parent X, Boess G, Brignon P. Lithiase oxalocalcique. Relation entre facteurs de risque biochimiques et phase cristalline du calcul [Calcium oxalate stones. Relationship between biochemical risk factors and crystalline phase of the stone]. Progr Urol. 1999;9:1051-6.
14. Hesse A, Berg W, Schneider HJ, et al. A contribution to the formation mechanism of calcium oxalate urinary calculi. II. In Vitro Experiments Concerning the Theory of the Formation of Whewellite and Weddellite Urinary Calculi. Urol Res. 1976;4:157-60.
15. Evan AP, Coe FL, Lingeman JE, et al. Mechanism of formation of human calcium oxalate renal stones on Randall's plaque. Anat Rec. 2007;290:1315-23.
16. Daudon M, Traxer O, Williams JC, Jr, et al. Randall's plaques. In: Rao N, Kavanagh J, Preminger GM (Eds). Urinary Tract Stone Disease. New York: Springer; 2011. pp. 103-12.
17. Zarse CA, Hameed TA, Jackson ME, et al. CT visible internal stone structure—but not Hounsfield unit value—of calcium oxalate monohydrate (COM) calculi predicts lithotripsy fragility in vitro. Urol Res. 2007;35:201-6.
18. Schulz E. Studies on the influence of the flow field in the Pelvi-Calyceal System (PCS) on the formation of urinary calculi. Urol Res. 1987;15:281-6.
19. Schulz E, Hengst E, Brunding P, et al. Disturbed urinary transport in the pelvi-calyceal system in calcium-oxalate stone patients. Urol Res. 1987;15:109-13.
20. Williams JC, Jr, McAteer JA. Retention and growth of urinary stones—insights from imaging. J Nephrol. 2013;26:25-31.
21. Daudon M, Jungers P, Bazin D. Peculiar morphology of stones in primary hyperoxaluria. New Engl J Med. 2008;359:100-02.
22. Daudon M, Jungers P. Stone composition and morphology: a window on etiology. In: Talati JJ, Tiselius HG, Albala DM, Ye Z (Eds). Urolithiasis: Basic Science and Clinical Practice. London: Springer; 2012. pp. 113-40.
23. Daudon M, Bouzidi H, Bazin D. Composition and morphology of phosphate stones and their relation with etiology. Urol Res. 2010;38:459-67.
24. Krambeck AE, Khan NF, Jackson ME, et al. Inaccurate reporting of mineral composition by commercial stone analysis laboratories: implications for infection and metabolic stones. J Urol. 2010;184:1543-9.
25. Parks JH, Coe FL, Evan AP, et al. Urine pH in renal calcium stone formers who do and do not increase stone phosphate content with time. Nephrol Dial Transplant. 2009;24:130-36.
26. Hesse A, Heimbach D. Causes of phosphate stone formation and the importance of metaphylaxis by urinary acidification: a review. World J Urol. 1999;17:308-15.
27. Wang LJ, Nancollas GH. Calcium orthophosphates: crystallization and dissolution. Chem Rev. 2008;108:4628-69.
28. Mandel N, Mandel I, Fryjoff K, et al. Conversion of calcium oxalate to calcium phosphate with recurrent stone episodes. J Urol. 2003;169:2026-9.
29. Williams JC, Jr, Zarse CA, Jackson ME, et al. Variability of protein content in calcium oxalate monohydrate stones. J Endourol. 2006;20:560-64.
30. Parks JH, Coe FL, Strauss AL. Calcium nephrolithiasis and medullary sponge kidney in women. New Engl J Med. 1982;306:1088-91.
31. Thomas E, Witte Y, Thomas J, et al. Maladie de Cacchi et Ricci. Remarques radiologiques, épidémiologiques et biologiques. Progr Urol. 2000;10:29-35.
32. Pramanik R, Asplin JR, Jackson ME, et al. Protein content of human apatite and brushite kidney stones: significant correlation with morphologic measures. Urol Res. 2008;36:251-8.
33. Evan AP, Lingeman J, Coe F, et al. Renal histopathology of stone-forming patients with distal renal tubular acidosis. Kidney Int. 2007;71:795-801.
34. Coe FL, Evan AP, Lingeman JE, et al. Plaque and deposits in nine human stone diseases. Urol Res. 2010;38:239-47.
35. Daudon M, Cohen-Solal F, Lacour B. Apport de la morphologie des calculs au diagnostic étiologique des lithiases urinaires. Feuillets Biol. 2004;45:51-7.
36. Carpentier X, Daudon M, Traxer O, et al. Relationships between carbonation rate of carbapatite and morphologic characteristics of calcium phosphate stones and etiology. Urology. 2009;73:968-75.
37. Maurice-Estepa L, Levillain P, Lacour B, et al. Crystalline phase differentiation in urinary calcium phosphate and magnesium phosphate calculi. Scand J Urol Nephrol. 1999;33:299-305.
38. Englert KM, McAteer JA, Lingeman JE, et al. High carbonate level of apatite in kidney stones implies infection, but is it predictive? Urolithiasis. 2013;41:389-94.
39. Krambeck AE, Lingeman JE, McAteer JA, et al. Analysis of mixed stones is prone to error: a study with US laboratories using micro CT for verification of sample content. Urol Res. 2010;38:469-75.
40. Krambeck AE, Handa SE, Evan AP, et al. Profile of the brushite stone former. J Urol. 2010;184:1367-71.
41. Williams, Jr, JC, Daudon M, Traxer O, et al. Fragility of brushite stones in shock wave lithotripsy: absence of correlation with computerized tomography visible structure. J Urol. 2012;188:996-1001.

42. Parks JH, Worcester EM, Coe FL, et al. Clinical implications of abundant calcium phosphate in routinely analyzed kidney stones. Kidney Int. 2004;66:777-85.
43. Krambeck AE, Handa SE, Evan AP, et al. Brushite stone disease as a consequence of lithotripsy? Urol Res. 2010;38:293-9.
44. Pak CY, Eanes ED, Ruskin B. Spontaneous precipitation of brushite in urine: evidence that brushite is the nidus of renal stones originating as calcium phosphate. Proc Natl Acad Sci U S A. 1971;68:1456-60.
45. Nancollas GH. In vitro studies of calcium phosphate crystallization. In: Mann S, Webb J, Williams RJP (Eds). Biomineralization. Chemical and Biochemical Perspectives. Weinheim: VCH Verlagsgesellschaft; 1989. pp. 157-87.
46. Evan AP, Lingeman JE, Worcester EM, et al. Contrasting histopathology and crystal deposits in kidneys of idiopathic stone formers who produce hydroxy apatite, brushite, or calcium oxalate stones. Anat Rec. 2014;297:731-48.
47. Verdesca S, Fogazzi GB, Garigali G, et al. Crystalluria: prevalence, different types of crystals and the role of infrared spectroscopy. Clin Chem Lab Med. 2011;49:515-20.
48. Daudon M, Hennequin C, Lacour B, et al. Sex and age-related composition of 10617 calculi analyzed by infrared-spectroscopy. Urol Res. 1995;23:319-26.
49. Nancollas GH. The involvement of calcium phosphates in biological mineralization and demineralization processes. Pure Appl Chem. 1992;64:1673-8.
50. Meria P, Hadjadj H, Jungers P, et al. Stone formation and pregnancy: pathophysiological insights gained from morphoconstitutional stone analysis. J Urol. 2010;183:1412-6.
51. Iijima M, Kamemizu H, Wakamatsu N, et al. Transition of octacalcium phosphate to hydroxyapatite in solution at pH 7.4 and 37°C. J Cryst Growth. 1997;181:70-8.
52. Griffith DP. Infection-induced renal calculi. Kidney Int. 1982;21:422-30.
53. Viprakasit DP, Sawyer MD, Herrell SD, et al. Changing composition of staghorn calculi. J Urol. 2011;186:2285-90.
54. Cameron MA, Maalouf NM, Adams-Huet B, et al. Urine composition in type 2 diabetes: predisposition to uric acid nephrolithiasis. J Am Soc Nephrol. 2006;17:1422-8.
55. Daudon M, Traxer O, Conort P, et al. Type 2 diabetes increases the risk for uric acid stones. J Am Soc Nephrol. 2006;17:2026-33.
56. Daudon M. Lithiases uriques, lithiases radio-transparentes: place de la cristallurie et de l'analyse morpho-constitutionnelle des calculs. Sémin Univ Néphrol. 2012;38:142-51.
57. Ekeruo WO, Tan YH, Young MD, et al. Metabolic risk factors and the impact of medical therapy on the management of nephrolithiasis in obese patients. J Urol. 2004;172:159-63.
58. Cicerello E, Merlo F, Maccatrozzo L. Urinary alkalization for the treatment of uric acid nephrolithiasis. Arch Ital Urol Androl. 2010;82:145-8.
59. Mehta TH, Goldfarb DS. Uric acid stones and hyperuricosuria. Adv Chronic Kidney Dis. 2012;19:413-8.
60. Sakhaee K, Maalouf NM. Metabolic syndrome and uric acid nephrolithiasis. Semin Nephrol. 2008;28:174-80.
61. Mattoo A, Goldfarb DS. Cystinuria. Semin Nephrol. 2008;28:181-91.
62. Daudon M. Les nouveaux constituants des calculs urinaires. Feuillets de Biologie. 2007;48:19-24.
63. Hesse A, Kruse R, Geilenkeuser WJ, et al. Quality control in urinary stone analysis: results of 44 ring trials (1980-2001). Clin Chem Lab Med. 2005;43:298-303.
64. Pollack SS, Carlson GL. A comparison of x-ray diffraction and infrared technics for identifying kidney stones. Am J Clin Pathol. 1969;52:656-60.
65. Daudon M, Bounxouei B, Santa Cruz F, et al. Composition des calculs observés aujourd'hui dans les pays non industrialisés [Composition of renal stones currently observed in non-industrialized countries]. Progr Urol. 2004;14:1151-61.
66. Letavernier E, Traxer O, Haymann JP, et al. Cystinurie. Progr Urol. 2012;22:F119-23.
67. Schwartz BF, Schenkman N, Armenakas NA, et al. Imaging characteristics of indinavir calculi. J Urol. 1999;161:1085-7.
68. Assimos DG, Langestroer P, Leinbach RF, et al. Guaifenesin- and ephedrine-induced stones. J Endourol. 1999;13:665-7.
69. Henderson MJ. Stone analysis is not useful in the routine investigation of renal stone disease. Ann Clin Biochem. 1995;32(Pt 2):109-11.
70. Kasidas GP, Samuell CT, Weir TB. Renal stone analysis: why and how? Ann Clin Biochem. 2004;41:91-7.
71. Daudon M, Jungers P. Clinical value of crystalluria and quantitative morphoconstitutional analysis of urinary calculi. Nephron Physiol. 2004;98:31-6.
72. Daudon M, Reveillaud RJ. Typage morphologique des calculs oxalocalciques et données étiopathogéniques. Sem Hôp Paris. 1986;62:3159-68.
73. Normand M, Bergua D, Bouvet JP, et al. Corrélations entre la cause et la composition des calculs rénaux. Intérêt d'une analyse morphologique et infrarouge [Correlations between the cause and the composition of urinary stones—the interest of morphological and infrared-analysis]. Ann Biol Clin. 1989;47:29-34.
74. Asplin JR, Lingeman J, Kahnoski R, et al. Metabolic urinary correlates of calcium oxalate dihydrate in renal stones. J Urol. 1998;159:664-8.
75. Pierratos AE, Khalaff H, Cheng PT, et al. Clinical and biochemical differences in patients with pure calcium oxalate monohydrate and calcium oxalate dihydrate kidney stones. J Urol. 1994;151:571-4.
76. Daudon M. Pourquoi et comment analyser un calcul urinaire? [Why and how to analyze urinary calculus?] Progr Urol. 2007;17:2-6.

CHAPTER 5

Crystals in Human Kidneys

Andrew P Evan

The kidney stones themselves and their epidemiology ultimately arise from processes in the human kidney that somehow create the crystals and stones. The solution chemistry (Chapter 2) and modifying molecules (Chapter 3) all act on tubule fluid and urine but within the renal or perhaps calyceal or pelvic confines. Therefore, the renal epithelial and urothelial cells and the anatomical configurations of the calyces and tubule govern the process. The diseases, habits and possible genetic traits that lead to crystal formation are discussed elsewhere; here, we deal with where crystals are found, what they may be attached to, how they may interact with tissues or even with each other.

PATTERNS OF TISSUE MINERALIZATION

All stones share similar presenting symptoms, and urine supersaturation (SS) with respect to the mineral phase of the stone is essential for stone formation. However, recent studies using papillary biopsies of stone formers provide a view of the histology of renal crystal deposition, which suggests that the early sequence of events leading to stone formation differs greatly depending on the type of stone and on the urine chemistry leading to SS. Three general pathways for kidney stone formation (Fig. 5.1) are seen: (1) stones fixed to the surface of a renal papilla at sites of interstitial apatite (HA) plaque (termed Randall's plaque) as seen in idiopathic calcium oxalate (CaOx) stone formers (ICSF); (2) stones attached to plugs protruding from the openings of ducts of Bellini (BDs) as seen in primary hyperoxaluria, primary hyperparathyroidism (PHPT), ileostomy, small bowel resection, cystinuria, brushite, apatite and distal tubular acidosis; and (3) stones forming in free solution in the renal collecting system as in cystinuria. The presence of hydroxyapatite crystals in either the interstitial or tubular compartment (and sometimes both) of the renal medulla in stone formers is the rule, and has implications for the initial steps of stone formation and the potential for renal injury.

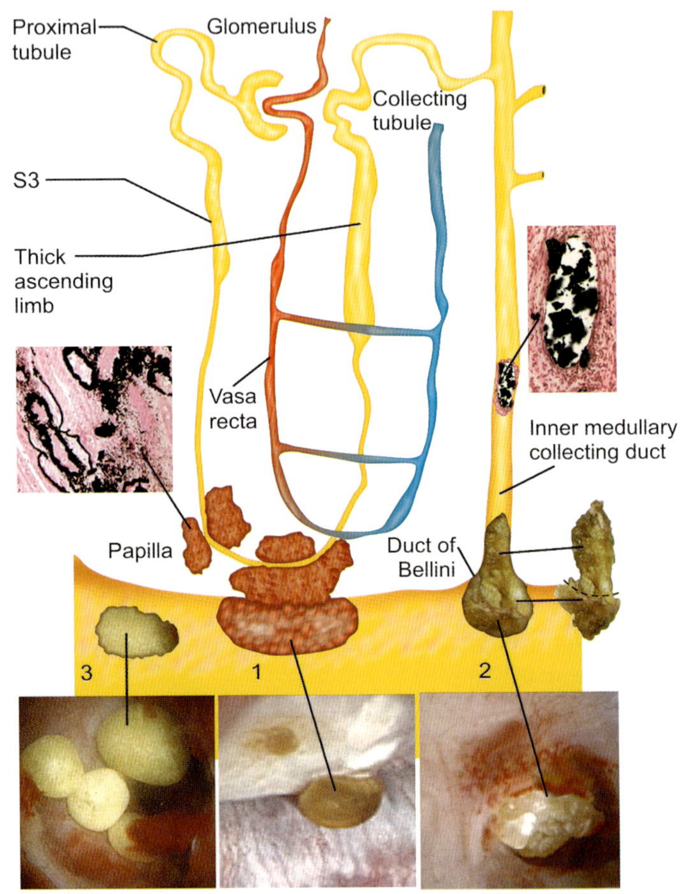

Fig. 5.1: Illustration of three pathways for kidney stone formation and growth. The first pathway (1) suggests that crystals in the urine can become attached to a site of exposed crystalline deposits of interstitial calcium phosphate following loss of the normal urothelial covering of the renal papilla. The second pathway (2) requires crystals nuclei to first form in the lumen of a nephron at sites of cell injury, which results in crystal attachment and growth that is called an intraluminal plug. In this illustration, crystal attachment occurred near the opening of a duct of Bellini and then a crystalline overgrowth formed on the end of the plug, forming a stone that projects into a minor calyx. The third pathway (3) represents "free particle" formation either in the collection system of the kidney or along the nephron.

PAPILLARY STONES FIXED TO SITES OF INTERSTITIAL (RANDALL'S) PLAQUE

Randall's Plaque Hypothesis

The first pathway to be considered suggests that crystals in the urine can become attached to a site of exposed crystalline deposits of interstitial calcium phosphate (CaP, termed Randall's plaque) following loss of the normal urothelial covering of the renal papilla (*see* Fig. 5.1).[1,2] An anchored nidus of urinary crystals could form as an overgrowth on the interstitial plaque, permitting a fixed stone to form and potentially grow over many years (Fig. 5.2). This theory is explicit in stating that sites of interstitial plaque are the initiating lesions. Randall examined 1,154 pairs of cadaveric kidneys by carefully opening the renal pelvis of each kidney and examining each accessible papilla with a hand lens. This examination revealed an "innocent"-appearing lesion that was a cream-colored area near the papillary tip and appeared to be subsurface or subepithelial in location, which Randall labeled as papillary lesion type 1. This lesion was seen in 20.5% of all the kidneys he studied. By light microscopy, the lesion was found to be a plaque of calcium salts deposited in the interstitial tissue and definitely not intraluminal in location, termed type I pattern. Evidence of inflammation was rarely found and deposits were localized initially to interstitial collagen material as well as tubular basement membranes. Subsequently, the deposits appeared to fill much of the intertubular space. Similar findings were published by Vermooten in 1942 and Cook in 1970.[3,4] Chemical analysis of the regions of plaque showed calcium, nitrogen, carbon dioxide and phosphorous. His next major observation was finding a small stone (2 mm) that projected into the lumen of the renal pelvis. It was firmly attached to an area of visible calcium plaque and found to be composed of calcium phosphate. Such stones were found attached to papilla in 65 kidneys. Randall was able to study several stones still attached to the papillary wall and concluded from these studies that (1) attached stones are growing from and are supported by interstitial calcium plaque; (2) the sites of interstitial plaque can lose their urothelial cell covering allowing the plaque to be exposed to the calyceal urine; and (3) that some detached stones have a concave surface with patches of phosphate material (possibly representing the attachment site to the interstitial plaque). Figure 5.3 shows a small laminated calculus attached by way of a narrow neck-like mineral stalk to a region of interstitial plaque published by Anderson in 1940 about the same time Randall was reporting his findings.[5] Anderson's observations strongly supported Randall's description of the pathogenesis of stone formation.

The observations Randall made from 1,154 pairs of postmortem kidneys were earth-shattering in their importance and originality. However, what Randall was not able to determine because of the techniques available to him in the 1930s was the composition of the mineral in the plaque, the type of crystalline material that formed right

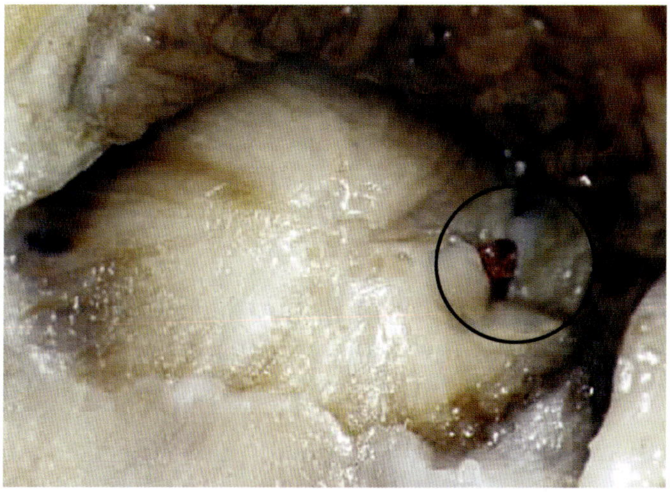

Fig. 5.2: A renal papilla from idiopathic calcium oxalate stone former patient. This dissecting microscopic image shows a small stone (dark object within circle) attached to the side of the papilla. This papilla is from the same kidney seen in Figure 5.4.

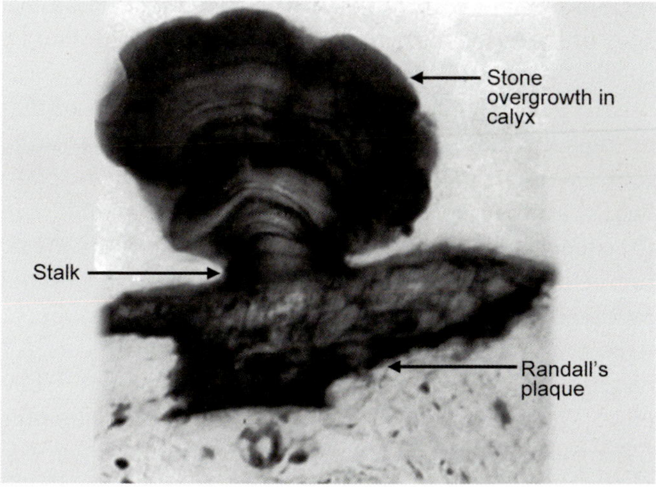

Fig. 5.3: Calcium plaque (Randall's) in tissue with attached early renal calculus. This micrograph shows a small laminated calculus attached by way of a narrow neck-like mineral stalk to a region of interstitial plaque published by Anderson in 1940, about the same time that Randall was reporting his findings.

at the site of overgrowth and the transition of mineral type (i.e. calcium oxalate, uric acid and calcium phosphate) from the site of attachment into the body of the stone. In addition, Randall lacked detailed clinical data on each of the patients for which he examined their kidneys and, therefore, suggested that all kidney stones formed according to his hypothesis. Consequently, his idea was easily challenged.

Endoscopic and Histologic Observations of Randall's Plaque

Low and Stoller were the first investigators to revisit kidney stone formers to document the presence of Randall's plaque using state-of-the-art endoscopic equipment, an approach that allowed these investigators to view individual renal papilla during stone removal by percutaneous nephrolithotomy (PNCL).[6] Their initial study revealed that plaque was more prevalent in stone formers as opposed to those undergoing endoscopy for conditions unrelated to stone disease. In particular, those with a history of calcium stones were found to have significantly more plaque. In a follow-up study, where the results of 24-hour urine metabolic studies were correlated with endoscopic, the authors concluded that patients with hypercalciuria trended toward increasing plaque density; however, no significant relationship was found. In our minds, these studies highlighted a possible association between calcium nephrolithiasis, especially in the setting of hypercalciuria and Randall's plaque, which led our group to hypothesize that regions of Randall's plaque develop in unique anatomical sites of the kidney and their formation is conditioned by specific stone-forming pathophysiologies.

To test this hypothesis, our team used state-of-the-art digital endoscopic equipment during PNCL for stone removal to (1) determine the surgical anatomy of the papilla, (2) obtain papillary biopsies of involved papilla and (3) collect detailed clinical histories and laboratory measurements of each patient.[7] The ICSF patients were selected as the primary group of stone formers; in that they appear to be a reasonably pure phenotype representing about 75% of all stone formers and do not have any systemic disease. Many, but not all of these ICSF, have idiopathic hypercalciuria (IH), a familial and presumably genetic trait. Digital images of all papillae were used to obtain papillary biopsies of regions with and without plaque for plaque surface determinations. During intraoperative endoscopy, sites of whitish material with irregular serpiginous borders were observed on or near the papillary tip

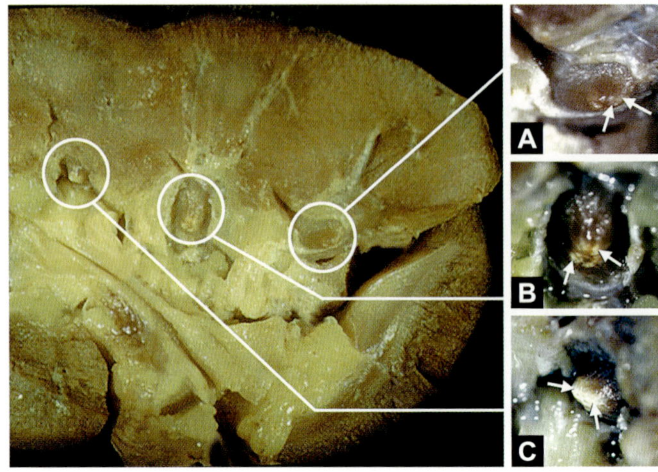

Figs. 5.4A to C: Examination of three separate papillae of an idiopathic calcium oxalate stone former (ICSF) patient using a dissecting microscope. Examination of three different papillae from the same kidney of an ICSF patient reveals a range of interstitial plaque coverage, with panel (B) showing dense plaque, modest coverage in panel (C) and minimal in panel (A). Arrows point to site of interstitial (Randall's, white) plaque.

in varying amounts and usually surrounding the openings of the BDs (Figs. 5.4A to C), the same plaque material described by Randall. The plaque is located deep in the urothelium (suburothelial) with a smooth outer surface except where it is pitted due to the removal of an attached stone. Light microscopic examination of Yasue-stained papillary biopsies revealed minute spherical deposits of mineral first laid down within the basement membrane of thin limbs of Henle in the inner medulla—close to where urine drips into the renal pelvis (Figs. 5.5A to H). Initially, these mineral deposits are seen as electron dense, spherically shaped objects of about 50 nm to multilayered spheres with alternating light (mineral layer) and dark (matrix layer) rings or bands (Figs. 5.5C and E). The individual deposits were then detected in the nearby interstitial space (Fig. 5.5B) and appeared to coalesce on the collagen bundles and become embedded in an electron dense matrix material, generating islands of plaque that surrounded several tubular segments (Fig. 5.5G).[7,8] Whether these deposits originated in the basement membrane of thin loops of Henle and migrated into the interstitial space or nucleated directly on the collagen bundles is not known (Fig. 5.6). These islands extended down to the basal side of the urothelium and encased the BDs (Fig. 5.5H). Using scanning electron microscopy, Khan revealed the spherical morphology of the individual interstitial deposit with their pin cushion-like external surface appearance mixed with numerous long, thin collagen

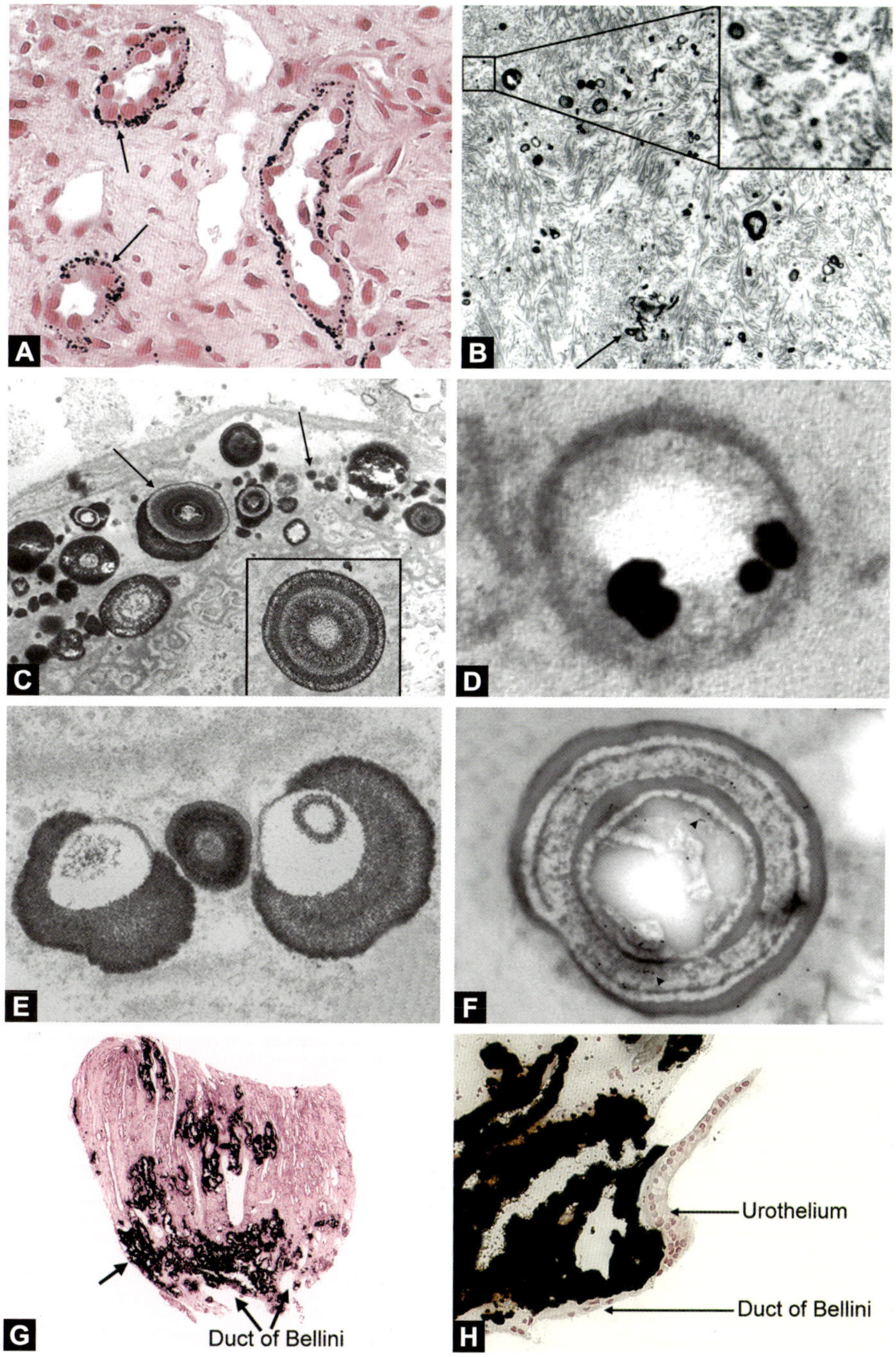

Figs. 5.5A to H: Histologic images of sites of interstitial (Randall's) plaque in an idiopathic calcium oxalate stone former patient. Panels (A) to (F) show details of the initial sites and sizes of crystalline deposits in the inner medulla as seen by light (A) and transmission electron microscopy (B to F). Sites of individual, spherical deposits (A, arrows) are first noted in the basement membranes of the thin loops of Henle forming dense rings or bands around these tubules. The deposits are also seen in the interstitial space (B, arrow) and tightly associated with collagen bundles (B, inset). Ultrastructural analysis of the deposits reveals these structures to be spherical in shape (C, arrows) and with an internal morphology of alternating light to electron-dense layers (one to nine layers) resembling a tree-ring pattern (C, inset). Immunoelectron microscopic studies localized osteopontin (D, dark circles) to the interface of the electron-dense organic layer and electron-lucent crystalline layer while heavy chain 3 of the inter-alpha-trypsin molecule was localized to the organic layer (F, arrowheads). Individual deposits varied in size from 50 nm in diameter with a single layer to nine alternating layers (C and E). With time the individual deposits accumulate in the interstitial space embedded in matrix filling the interstitial space (G, arrows) all the way down to the basal surface of the urothelium (H).

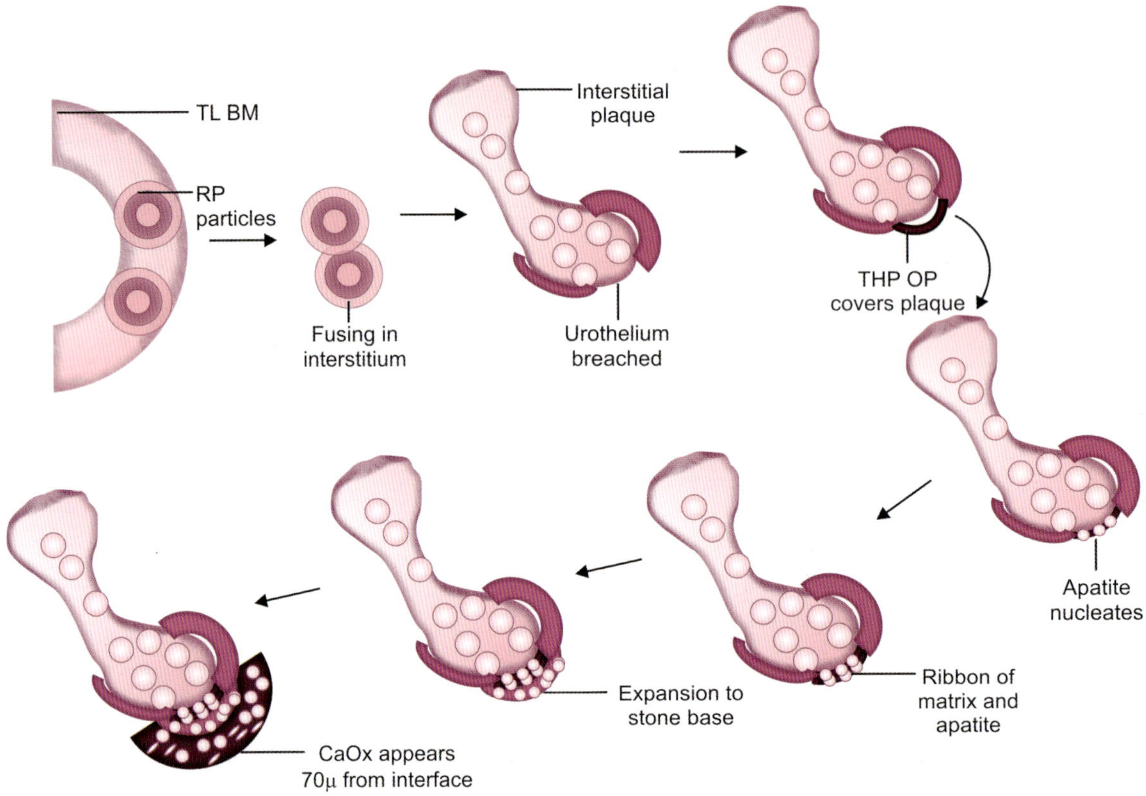

Fig. 5.6: Calcium oxalate stones grow on sites of interstitial (Randall's) plaque. The earliest nuclei of plaque appear in the basement membrane of the thin loops of Henle (leftmost figure) as multilayered spherulites of crystals and matrix material. Subsequently, interstitial plaque genesis (second figure, upper row) seems to occur on type 1 collagen in the interstitial space where individual spherulites appear to fuse. With time, islands of matrix and spherulites spread to the basal side of the urothelium and the plaque remains protected from the urine until the urothelium is breached (Fig. 5.3, upper row). At this point, the urine appears to create nucleations that form the base of an overgrowth (Figs 5.4 to 5.8). The urine proteins that form the immediate overlay include Tamm–Horsfall protein and osteopontin (OP), followed by amorphous hydroxyapatite. As the overgrowth region expands, there is a conversion of hydroxyapatite to calcium oxalate (CaOx), the primary mineral of the stone of an idiopathic calcium oxalate stone former stone patient. RP, Randall's plaque; TL: Thin loop; BM: Basement membrane.

fibers running between, and occasionally embedded within, the spherulites (Figs. 5.7A to F).[8] Another technique to visualize regions of interstitial plaque is to image a renal biopsy by micro-computed tomography (CT). In regions of moderate plaque deposition, micro-CT reveals a collar or sleeve of material surrounding tubular segments (thin loops of Henle) of the inner medulla with an obvious empty tubular lumen (Fig. 5.8A). In biopsies with denser regions of interstitial plaque, islands of material are seen completely surrounding the outer surface of individual tubular segments, again exposing an empty tubular lumen (Fig. 5.8B). No evidence of cell injury, inflammation, interstitial fibrosis or intratubular crystalline material was detected in any of the ICSF papillary biopsies.[7]

The mineral composition of the interstitial plaque was determined by micro-Fourier transform infrared (micro-FTIR) microspectroscopy and energy dispersive X-ray analysis (EDX) to always be biological apatite (calcium phosphate).[7,8] Further characterization of the plaque particles has identified osteopontin as one of the proteins forming the matrix layers (Fig. 5.5D) and heavy chain three (H3) of the inter-alpha-trypsin molecule at the matrix layer (Fig. 5.5F).[9,10] Both molecules have been previously identified as having inhibitory properties of crystal formation. Our understanding on how the interstitial spherulite might form in the renal interstitial space is limited to a study using an in vitro test system that generated agglomerates of coalesced mineral spherules with concentric laminations similar in morphology to Randall's plaque particles (Figs. 5.9A to D).[11] Acidic polypeptides (e.g. polyaspartic acid) were used to generate polymer-induced liquid-precursor phase droplets. The

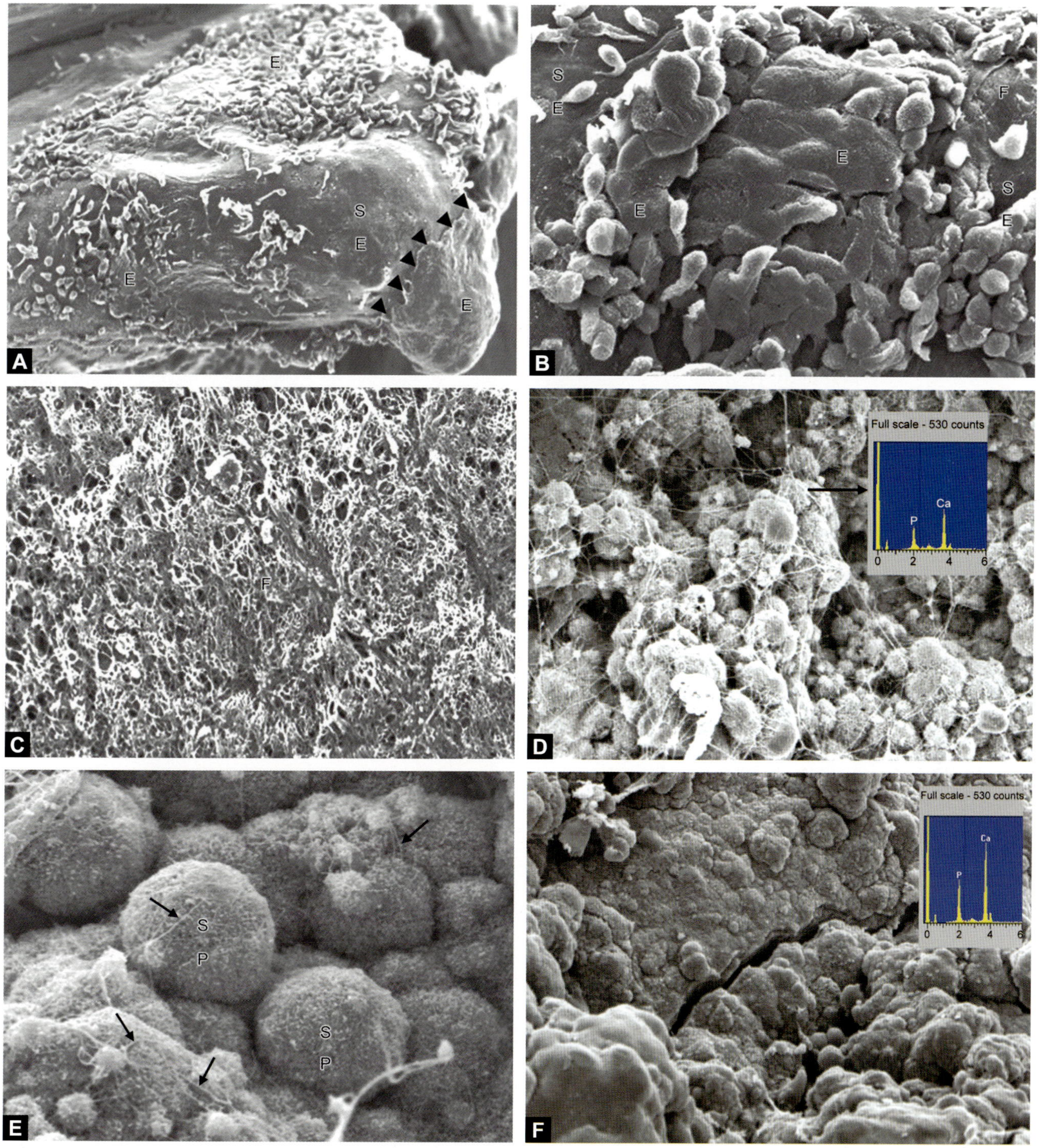

Figs. 5.7A to F: Scanning electron microscopy of Randall's plaque. Panel (A) shows plaque to appear as protrusion on papilla. Papillary surface epithelium (E) is sloughing, exposing subepithelial surface (SE). Panel (B) is a higher magnification at arrowheads of panel (A) demonstrating surface epithelium (E), subepithelial surface (SE) and area of exposed fibrous layer (F) beneath. Panel (C) is a higher magnification of the exposed fibrosis (F) layer. Panels (D) and (E) show numerous spherulites (SP) located under the fibrosis layer with needle-shaped crystallites on their surface and fibers (arrows) embedded inside. Panel (F) shows the surface of internal layer of fused spherulites. Insets in panels (D) and (F) show EDX of spherulites or fibers connecting spherulites, respectively.
Source: Reproduced from Khan SR, Rodriguez DE, Gower LB, et al. Association of Randall plaque with collagen fibers and membrane vesicles. J Urol. 2012;187:1094-100.

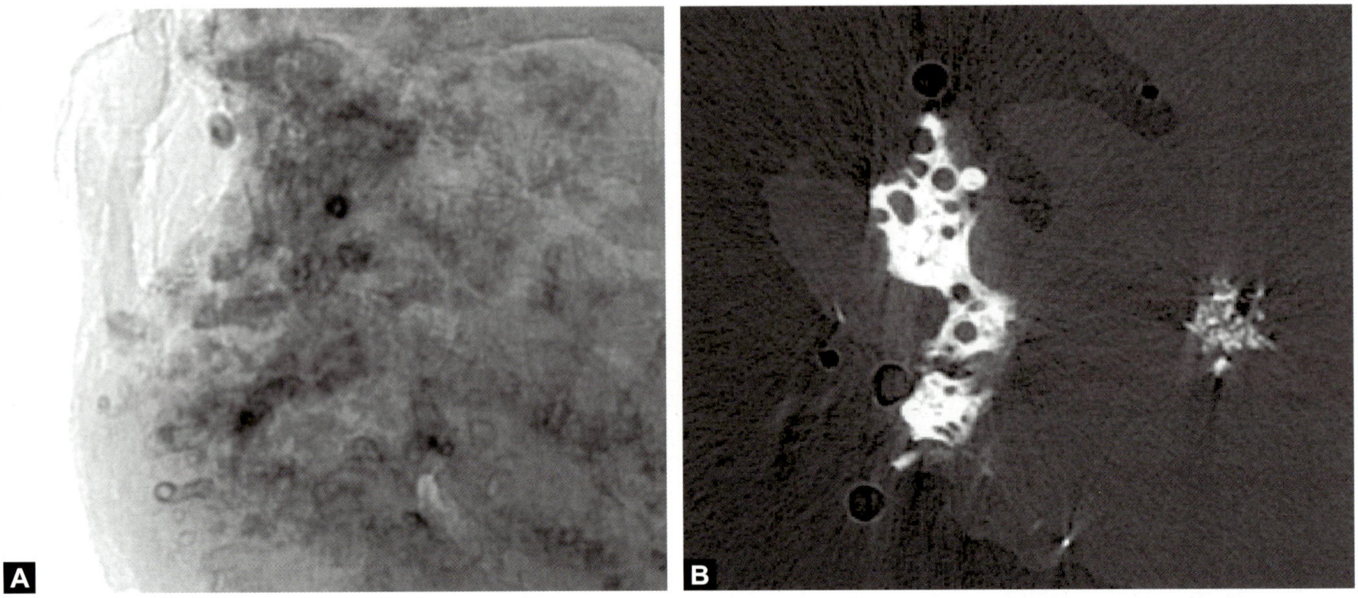

Figs. 5.8A and B: Sites of interstitial plaque in papillary biopsy of idiopathic calcium oxalate stone former patient viewed by micro-computed tomography (micro-CT). Panel (A) is a micro-CT shadow image of a whole papillary biopsy sample. It reveals early sites of interstitial plaque deposits as a sleeve surrounding nephron segments (see Fig. 5.2A) in the inner medulla. In this image the deposits are X-ray dense and thus appear black. Note that the tubular lumen is easily seen. Occasionally, a longitudinal view of a thin loop of Henle is seen with the plaque outlining the outer surface of the tubule but not in the lumen. Panel (B) is a slice from a tomogram that was generated from many shadow images. Here a large island of interstitial plaque (see Fig. 5.2G) is seen as a whitish material with dark circular profiles dotting it. The dark circles represent tubular segments passing through the interstitial plaque.

concentric laminations appear to result from diffusion-limited exclusion of the polymeric impurity, which leads to polymer-enriched layers and not by sequential deposition of mineral layers. Later in the chapter, a hypothesis will be described to explain why the plaque particles initially form in the basement membranes of thin loops of Henle deep in the inner medulla, the "vas washdown" theory.

Randall's Plaque Unique to ICSF

Since the original observations of Randall, several investigators have studied spontaneously passed stone and found a suggestive link between the development of an attached renal stone and Randall's plaque. Cifuentes found that 63 of 87 papillary stones, those stones with one smooth convex surface that faces the urine and a concave surface that faces the papilla, had a site of whitish Randall's plaque located in a depressed zone (umbilication) on the concave face.[12] Thirteen of the stones with Randall's plaque showed calcified renal tubules at the site of plaque, which demonstrated their intrapapillary origin. Others have verified these observations.[13,14] In a follow-up study, Cifuentes reported that of 142 spontaneously passed stones that had a convex–concave morphology, only 61 stones showed patches of calcium phosphate at the surface of the stone, suggesting that these stones could have developed on the site of interstitial plaque.[15] However, 81 stones lacked plaque on any surface.

In order to investigate events in stone formation that might distinguish different kinds of stone disease, Williams et al. have applied micro-CT with three-dimensional (3D) rendering software to inspect the interior and exterior crystalline structures of kidney stones with greater scrutiny than has previously been done.[16] With micro-CT, a structural map of a stone can be generated, which can then be used to guide further destructive forms of analysis (FTIR) as well as accurately determine stone mineral composition. To illustrate how valuable micro-CT analysis is in defining characteristics of an individual stone, a collection of stones retrieved from the same ICSF patient with IH at the time of surgery (Figs. 5.10A to I). Three different kinds of stones were analyzed: (1) attached stones removed from papillae at the time of surgery, (2) unattached stones found in the renal pelvis also removed at the time of surgery and (3) previously spontaneously passed stones that the patient had collected. Panel (A) shows the concave or papillary surface of an attached stone with a potential site of Randall's as seen by light microscopy. With

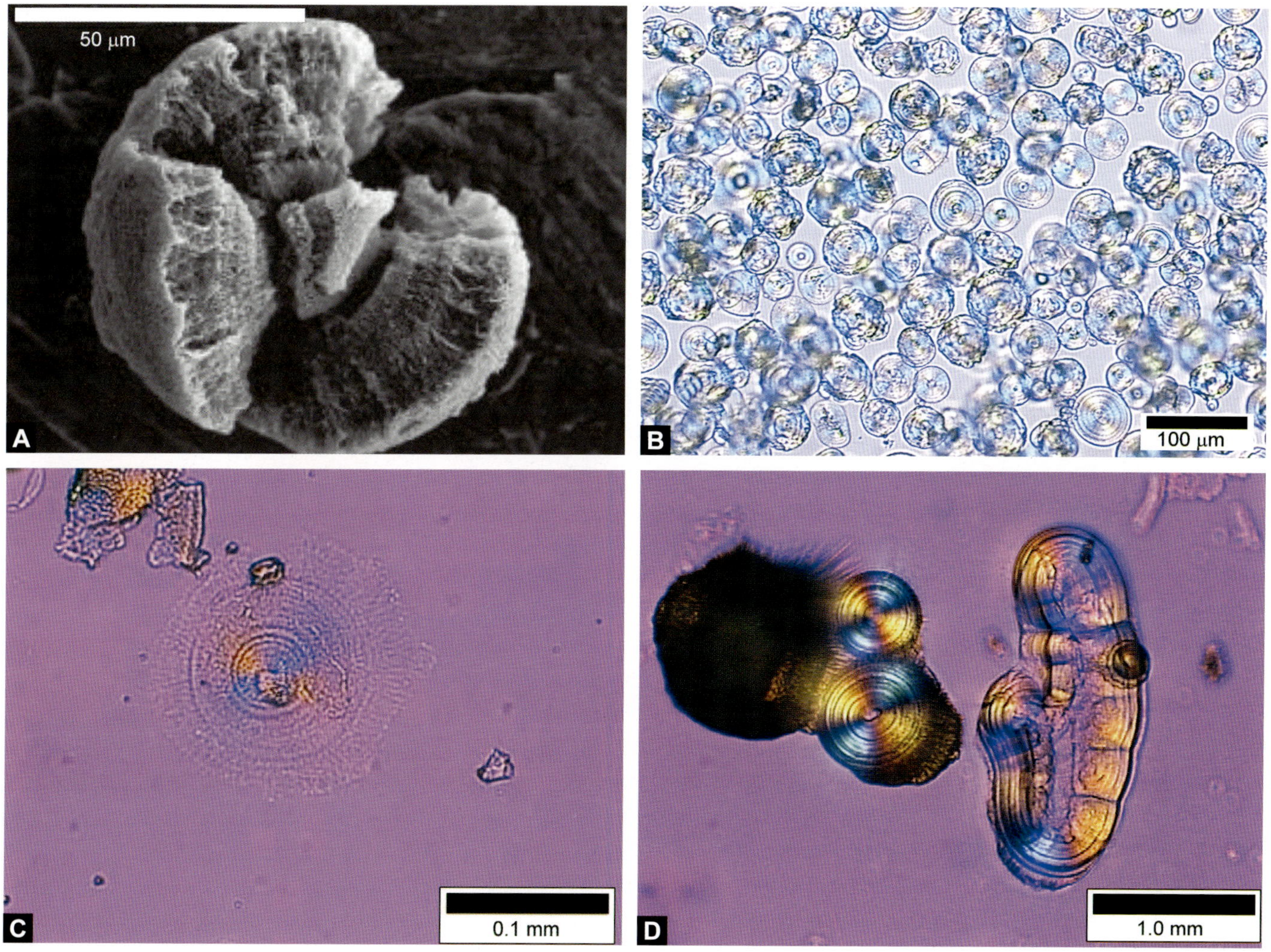

Figs. 5.9A to D: Formation of calcium phosphate spherulites from amorphous globules. Panel (A) is a scanning electron micrograph of a dense-packed spherulite with a denser shell and concentric laminations. Panel (B) is an image of early-stage globules showing a faint birefringence as they are just starting to crystallize. Panel (C) shows that some spherulites collapse upon drying and appear to be composed of a slightly rigid, gelatinous globule. Panel (D) shows maturing spherulites as they become highly birefringent and ultimately become brown as they densify and block light transmission. The particle on the right appears to be composed of coalesced globules of spherulites. The middle spherulite is starting to form a brown crust as it undergoes dissolution–recrystallization process. The spherulite to the left shows needles that grow from solution, as opposed to the dense-packed smooth-shelled spherulite in panel (A). All of the spherulites exhibit pronounced concentric lamination.

Source: Reproduced with permission from Amos FF, Olszta MJ, Khan SR, et al. Relevance of a polymer-induced liquid-precursor (PILP) mineralization process to normal and pathological biomineralization. In: Königsberger E, Königsberger L (Eds). Biomineralization-Medical Aspects of Solubility. West Sussex: Wiley; 2006. pp. 125-217.

micro-CT [panels (B) and (C)], the majority of the stone has a uniform X-ray attenuation value that is consistent with calcium oxalate monohydrate (COM), except for a small, focal region that has a higher attenuation value (appears white) consistent with apatite, a site of interstitial plaque (Randall's plaque). This stone was clearly attached to a renal papilla at a site of interstitial plaque, and during stone removal the stone was torn away from the papilla, leaving a region of plaque still on the stone and on the papilla.

The second group of stones was found free within the renal pelvis. A question arises: "Had these stones originally formed attached to the papilla at a site of interstitial plaque and then were dislodged"? If so, a small, focal site of apatite might still be found at the stone surface or within the stone. Panel (D) shows such a stone by light microscopy and a region of apatite could be identified. However, a micro-CT slice through the stone revealed an obvious small, focal site of apatite, presumably a site of interstitial

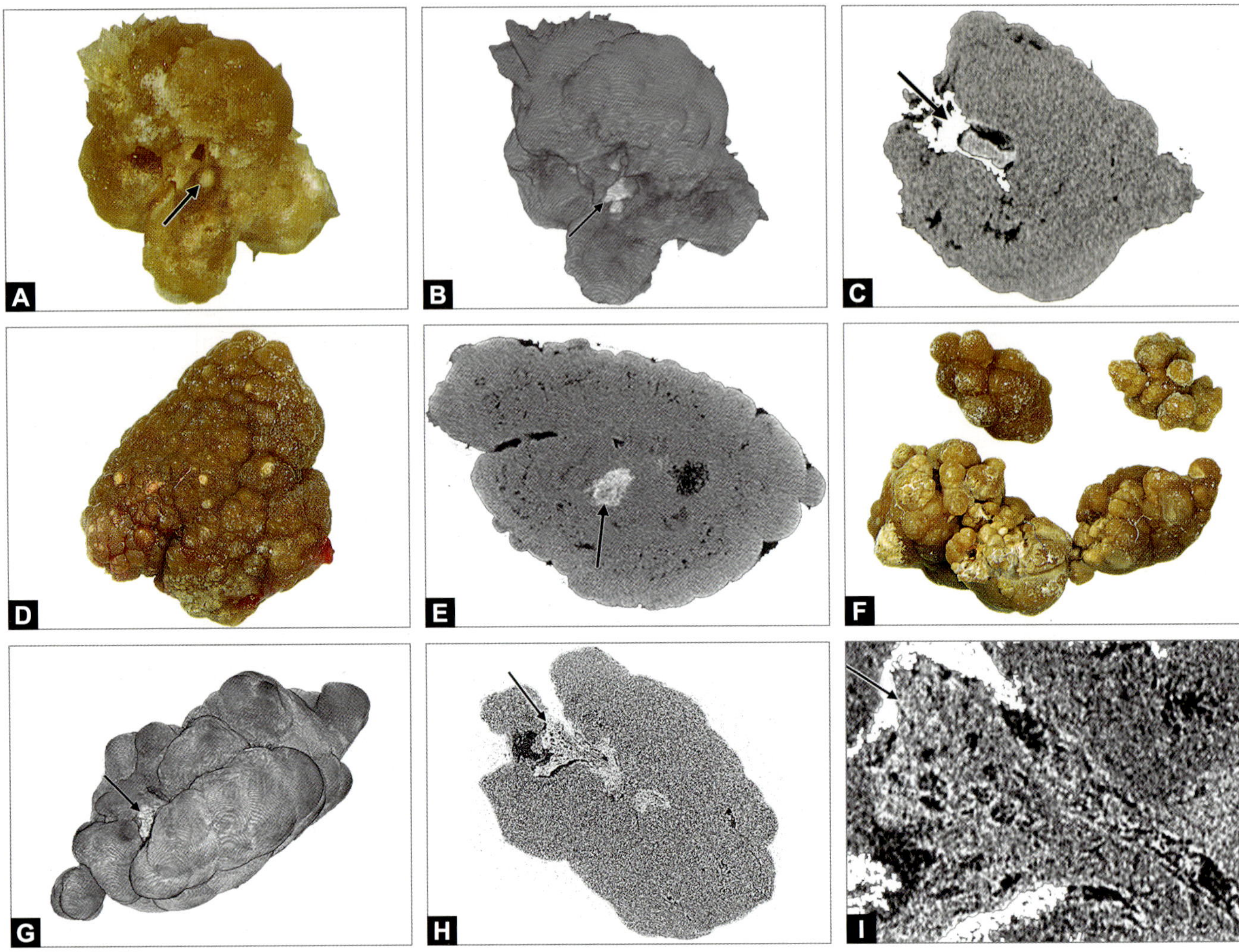

Figs. 5.10A to I: Set of attached stones, unattached stones and passed stone from the same idiopathic calcium oxalate stone former patient. Panel (A) shows the papillary surface of an attached stone with a site of Randall's (arrow) as seen by light microscopy. Panel (B) is a micro-CT surface reconstruction of the same stone in panel. Panel (C) is a single micro-CT slice showing the site of Randall's plaque (arrow). Panels (D) and (E) show a nonattached stone collected at the time of surgery from the same patient. While no visible site of Randall's plaqye is seen at the surface of the stone by light microscopy (D), micro-CT shows a small, focal region that has a higher attenuation value (arrow in panel (E) cinsistent with apatite in the interior of the stone. A set of passed stones from the same patient (Panels F-I) also do not show any apatite at the surface of the stone (Panel F) but micro-CT reveals apatite (arrow) in the interior with the appearance of Randall's plaque (Panel G to I)."

plaque [panel (E)], suggesting that after the stone fell free, additional mineral (COM) was deposited on the surfaces of the stone, burying the surface site of interstitial plaque deep within the stone. These observations support the early work by Feranadez, who reported a stone that showed no evidence of plaque at its surface but on breaking the stone open, the interior showed a region composed of calcium phosphate with calcified tubules; this suggested that the stone must have originated on plaque, was dislodged, and then grew layers of calcium oxalate over the plaque site.[17]

The third group of stones were spontaneously passed and brought in by the same patient on the day of surgery for analysis. Panels (G) to (I) show a few of these stones, and they are identical to the nonattached stones found in the renal pelvis on the day of surgery. Micro-CT imaging shows a region of Randall's plaque matrix [panel (I)] with luminal spaces suggestive of tubular profiles such as inner medullary collecting ducts (IMCD), a pattern previously seen by others. Thus, calcium oxalate stones in ICSF patients appear to grow like stalactites adherent to the tips of kidney papilla and typically are made of layers of calcium oxalate surrounding a core of apatite.

Testing the Hypothesis that Stones in ICSF Patients Grow on Interstitial Plaque

Building on Randall's finding and newer data suggesting that some CaOx stones do form attached to renal papilla, Matlaga et al. asked the question, "Does every calcium oxalate stone begin as an attached stone to a renal papilla or do only a minority of stones form in this way?"[18] To address this issue, they performed a retrospective study on a well-characterized population of common calcium oxalate stone formers, ICSF patients, whose stones were imaged with high-resolution, digital endoscopic equipment, and then removed for micro-CT analysis. Of 172 papillae inspected, 156 (91%) had plaque. Forty-nine papillae (28.5%) had attached stones and all of these papillae possessed sites of plaque. These observations confirmed Randall's original observations and showed a higher fraction of attached stones on plaque than he found. However, the investigators could not account for every stone these patients presented with at the time of surgery; thus, they could not determine the percentage of all stones that were attached compared to those unattached.

Therefore, Miller et al. employed a prospective design and a digital reconstruction protocol to document that CaOx stones grow attached to plaque in ICSF patients as the general rule, and that all attached stones are indeed directly connected to sites of interstitial plaque.[19] Nine ICSF patients were studied who had a total of 115 stones, of which 81 were verified to be directly attached to a site of interstitial (Randall's) plaque. Figures 5.11A to F illustrate the optical assessment steps used to determine the precise site on the papillary tip that an attached stone was anchored to and to identify the attachment site as Randall's plaque. Seven attached stones were processed through these steps and all were found attached to sites of plaque. In the 81 cases of attached stone, review of the video images postsurgery documented the presence of interstitial plaque in all cases. In addition, 25 unattached stones were found. Based on the observed data, the final point estimate for the number of stones attached to plaque was 0.754 (95% confidence interval: 0.575, 0.933), $p = 0.013$, which strongly suggests that in ICSF patients, stones develop attached to plaque as the general rule. Thus, growth on plaque appears to be a main mechanism of stone formation in ICSF, the most common type of patient encountered in clinical practice.

In a follow-up study, Miller et al. analyzed the 25 unattached stones collected from the original 9 ICSF patients using micro-CT.[19,20] Four of the 25 stones were lost during stone removal; 12 showed definite morphological evidence of having a site of Randall's plaque on the concave surface of the stone; and the remaining 9 stones had an internal structure consistent with a site of Randall's plaque composed of apatite that was covered in new layers of CaOx (a morphology identical to the spontaneously passed stones seen in Figs. 5.10G to I). Thus, this work, taken together with the prior study, strongly supports the idea of CaOx stones as papillary overgrowths on plaque.

Metabolic Correlates of Plaque Abundance in ICSF Patients

Risk Factors for Plaque Formation

One of our initial observations of the papilla tips of kidneys from ICSF patients using both light microscopic and endoscopic techniques was that interstitial plaque was common in these patients, whereas little to no plaque is seen in the kidneys of nonstone formers.[7] The next step in our understanding of the role of plaque in stone formation required an accurate determination of plaque abundance, which was accomplished using image analysis software applied to still images of papilla captured using digital video technology with advanced flexible endoscopy equipment to trace and quantitate plaque abundance. Plaque abundance was expressed as a percentage of coverage of the papillary surfaces. Our analysis of 14 ICSF patients and 4 nonstone formers showed that mean polar fractional plaque coverage was higher in the ICSF patients compared to the nonstone formers (7.4% vs 0.5%, $p = 0.012$), suggesting that interstitial plaque is unique to ICSF patients.

We reasoned next that because interstitial plaque first appears localized to the basement membrane of thin loops of Henle in the inner medulla, a select region of the nephron involved in water conservation and tubule fluid concentration, plaque abundance should be related to urine calcium excretion and urine volume in those stone patients with IH.[21] Plaque abundance and 24-hour risk factors were determined along with indices of crystallization inhibition, estimates of CaOx crystal growth inhibition and measurements of the upper limits of metastability in 14 ICSF patients and 4 nonstone formers who had previously undergone renal biopsy for plaque analysis.[7] This study found that the fraction of papillary surface covered by plaque was proportional to urine calcium and inversely proportional to urine volume and pH (Figs. 5.12A to E),

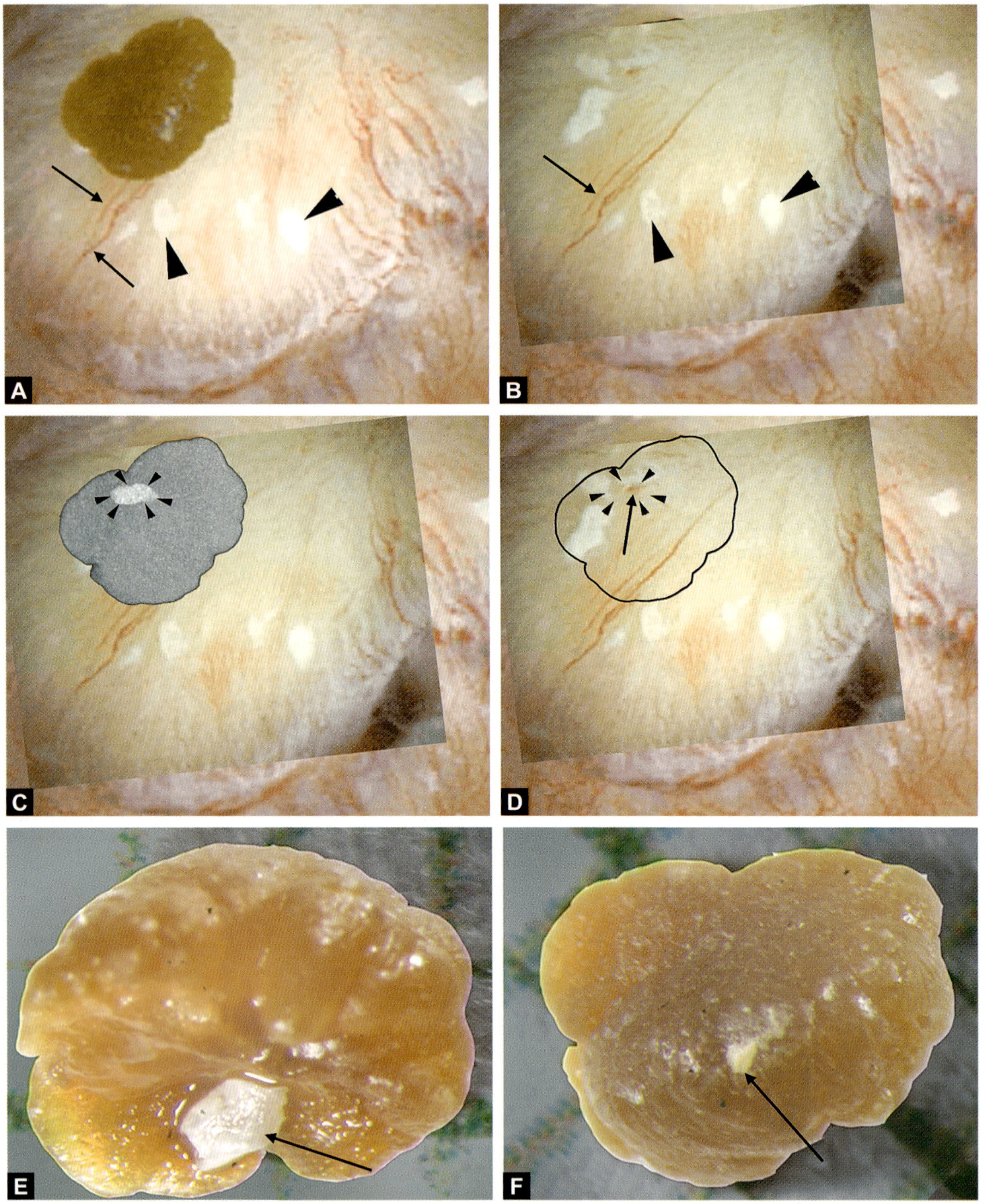

Figs. 5.11A to F: An attached stone before and after removal. A 3-mm stone (arrow) is visualized by a digital endoscope before removal (A) and after basket removal (B). In panel (A), regions of white plaque (arrowheads) and blood vessels (arrows) are seen near the attached stone and were used as markers for orientation purposes. The same regions of plaque and blood vessels are seen following removal of the attached stone (B). Panel (C) shows the same papillum as panel (A), but with a micro-computed tomography image of stone manipulated (ghosted) to show the position of the apatite region on the tissue side of the stone (arrowheads). In panel (D), an apatite region on the tissue side of the stone outlined by arrowheads is shown within the stone outline, against postremoval image of papillum; the apatite region on the stone aligns with a small area of hemorrhage on the plaque surface (arrow), presumably the site where the stone was attached to the papillum. Panel (E) shows that the removed stone has a white patch (arrow) on its tissue (attachment) surface, while the urinary surface (F) could be identified by the prominent area of discoloration (arrow) visible in panel (A).

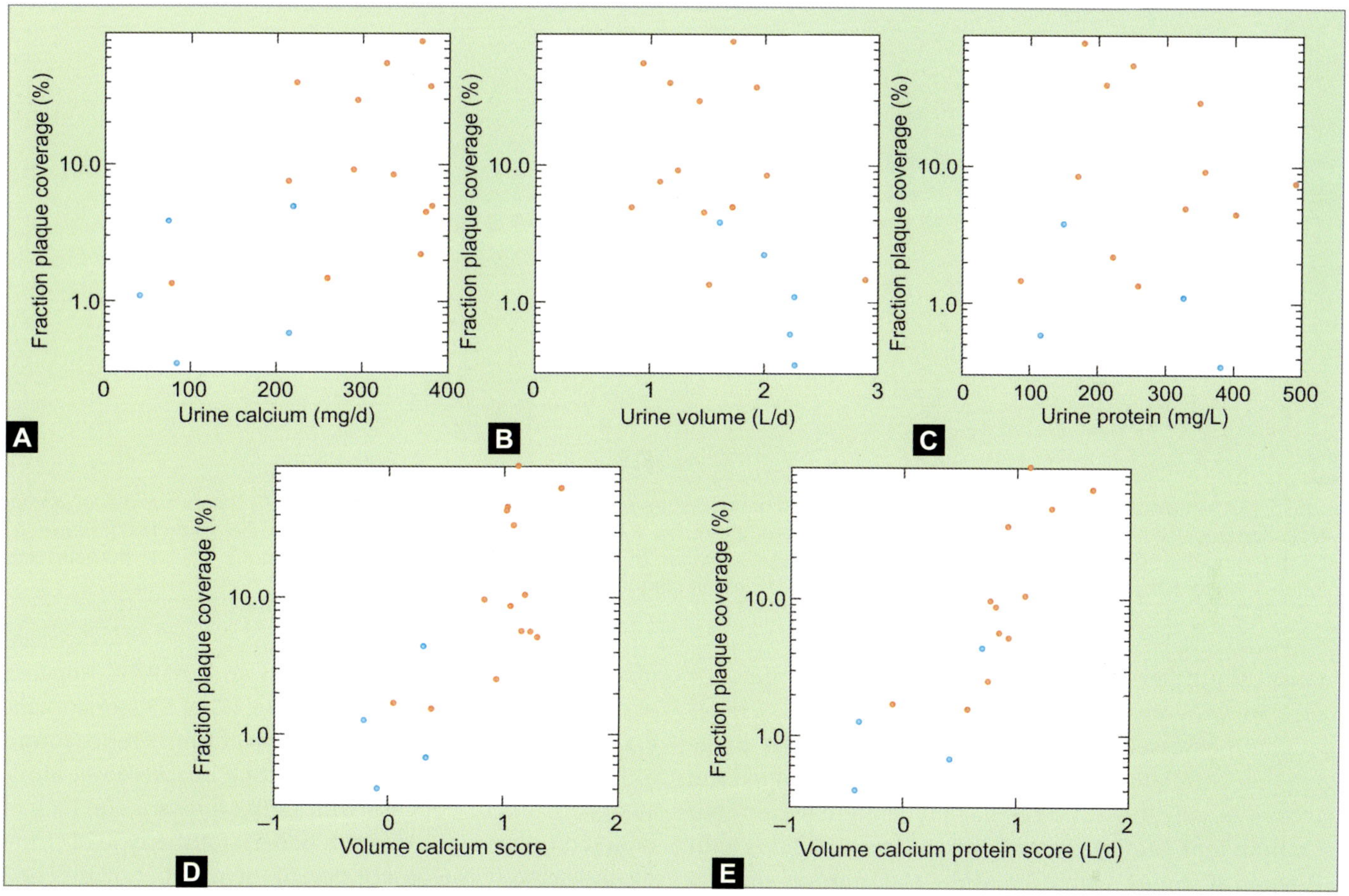

Figs. 5.12A to E: Urine correlates of papillary plaque. Fractional plaque coverage per papilla varies inversely with urine volume (A) among stone formers (dark circles) and nonstone-forming control subjects (open circles). Plaque coverage varies with urine calcium excretion (B) and is inverse to urine pH (C). A composite multivariate regression score using urine volume and calcium excretion (D) and one that includes urine pH (E) strongly correlate with plaque coverage.

suggesting that plaque formation arises from driving forces that are reflected in urine calcium excretion and urine volume.

Plaque abundance was noted to vary between ICSF patients with some having larger papillary areas of plaque (up to 10–28% plaque coverage).[21] Also, ICSF patients form differing number of stones, with some patients forming a few stones and others a larger number of stones. Therefore, we hypothesized that plaque coverage should increase proportionally with increasing stone number.[22] In 15 ICSF, who underwent percutaneous nephrolithotomy (PNL) for their stone burden with plaque mapping and biopsy and 4 control patients, we determined the number of kidney stones each patient generated up to the time of the study. Comparison of their plaque surface area to stone number was then performed using stepwise general linear modeling and simple regression. Figure 5.13A is a direct plot of stone number against log 10 mean plaque area, showing a strong correlation between these two variables. When the number of stones was plotted against plaque time score, the correlation was much stronger ($R2 = 0.592$; Fig. 5.13B). However, there was no correlation between plaque coverage and duration of stone disease ($p = 0.257$).

Plaque Abundance in ICSF Patients with Low Urine Calcium Levels

Two additional studies quantitated interstitial (Randall's) plaque area in a unique group of stone patients who were primarily female and with low to normal urinary calcium levels.[23,24] The first study examined 78 patients, 51 women and 27 men, comprising CaOx, CaP and uric acid stone formers. About 68% of patients had interstitial plaque with an average plaque coverage of 3.0%, which was not

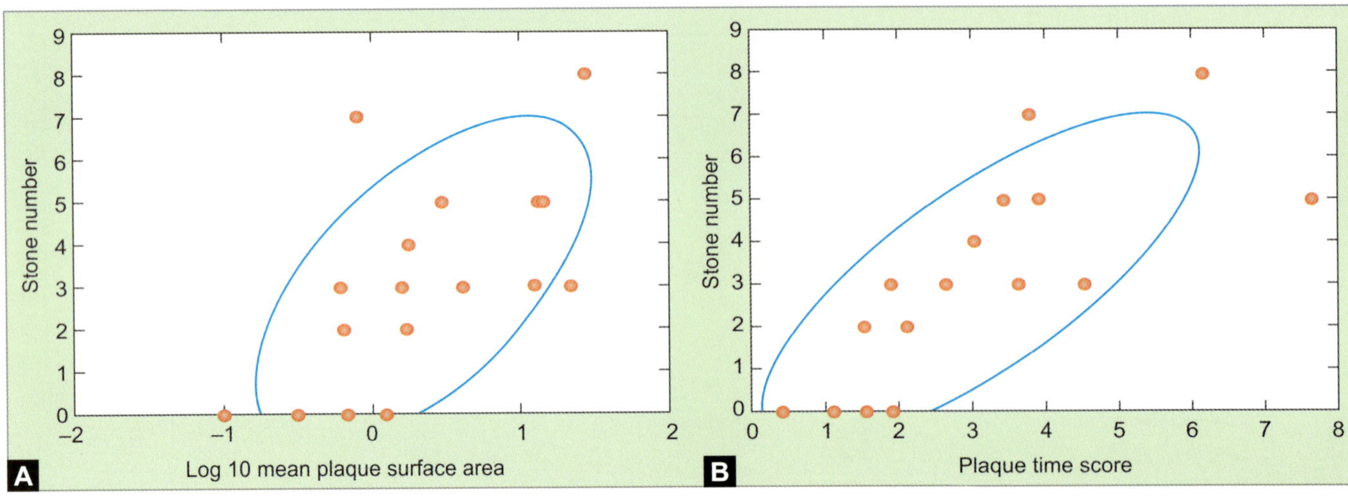

Figs. 5.13A and B: Stone number versus log transformed mean plaque surface or plaque time score. Panel (A) shows number of stones versus log transformed mean plaque surface area. Nonparametric ellipse of containment includes 2 standard deviation (SD). Panel (B) shows the number of stones versus multivariate regression equation from general linear model, including stone disease duration and plaque surface. Plaque time score × 1.788 + 1.386 × log 10 mean plaque surface area + 0.082 × time.

statistically different between stone types and did not correlate with any urinary analyte. In addition, 42% of all patients possessed histologic evidence of tubular plugging that correlated with pH and brushite SS, and led the authors to conclude that tubular plugging may be more common than previously recognized among patients with all types of stones. Only 10% of the CaOx group showed tubular plugging. These data clearly show that there were some ICSF patients who were female and with rather normal urinary calcium levels that possessed both white plaque and intraluminal plugs, a pattern not found in the predominantly male ICSF patients with high urine calcium level.[7] In a second study, 42 ICSF patients were divided into two groups, those with high amounts of Randall's plaque and those with low amounts of plaque.[24] Again the population was primarily female (27 of 42). The low plaque group (<5% plaque coverage) was usually obese, had a history of urinary tract infections, was less likely to have multiple prior stone events, had few sites of interstitial plaque particles, had a lower mean 24-hour urine calcium excretion and their stones lacked an apatite core (an apatite core correlates with attachment site). In contrast, those patients with a high amount of Randall's plaque (>5% plaque coverage) had evidence of attached stones, high urinary calcium levels and more prior stone events. A similar number of both the low- and high-plaque ICSF patients had tubular plugging.

Two recent reports from Europe have also attempted to determine the frequency of interstitial (Randall's) plaque during ureteroscopy (URS) and/or PNL. Ruggera et al. from Italy found plaque in 44.4% of 27 stone formers who were biopsied, whereas Traxer from France found 57% of 287 stone formers with plaque but were not biopsied.[25,26] A major concern with both studies is the lack of detailed phenotyping of each patient for the type of stone disease as well as a description of the number of attached versus unattached stones and their mineral composition.

As far as stone formation for those ICSF patients with high calcium levels, interstitial plaque would appear to be the key factor responsible for the initial site of stone formation and future growth. The ICSF group characterized by normal urinary calcium levels and primarily female is a unique group of stone formers that has not been studied carefully and therefore requires much more investigation. A question still remains: how do ICSF patients with low plaque and normal urinary calcium levels generate stones? These studies bring up another issue: How common is it for ICSF patients to possess attached stones and tubular plugging? Our group has identified a very small subset of ICSF patients that fit this description and will be presented later in this chapter.

Ultrastructural Features and Mineral Composition of Stone–Plaque Complex

Examination of an Intact Stone-Plaque Complex

The ICSF patients with IH form their stones attached to renal papilla as a rule and specifically to areas of interstitial plaque. As has been stated earlier in this chapter, the plaque is composed of spherical deposits of biological-hydroxyapatite that form initially in the basement membrane of the thin loops of Henle, then in the interstitial space and spreading down to the basal surface of the papillary urothelium. It is over these sites of Randall's plaque that CaOx stones grow. Normally, the interstitial plaque is separated from the urine by the urothelial layer, so for an attached stone to begin its formation on a region of plaque, the epithelial barrier has to be breached, allowing mineral deposition in the form of an overgrowth to be initiated.

In order to understand the events that may lead to attached stone formation, an en bloc biopsy of a 1-mm stone still attached to a site of interstitial plaque was obtained from an ICSF patient at the time of PNCL (Figs. 5.14A and B) for demineralization and examination by transmission electron microscopy (TEM).[27] Note that the biopsy included the entire stone still attached to visible zone of white plaque that was associated with a large chunk of papillary tissue, which is mostly interstitial plaque. By light microscopy (Fig. 5.14C) the old attachment surface of the stone (marked by an asterisk) and the matching region of exposed plaque on the renal tissue surface (marked in part by a rectangle) are easily identified even though they were separated during tissue preparation. Histologic analysis of the plaque-stone attachment site reveals a loss of urothelial cells over the interstitial plaque (Fig. 5.14C, arrows; Fig. 5.15A); above the tissue, in the old urinary space, rafts of crystals are embedded in a homogeneous gray matrix accompanied by cell debris (Fig. 5.15A, arrowheads). The exposed interstitial plaque is covered by a dark ribbon-like layer of alternating laminae of crystals—white in this figure—and black organic material (Fig. 5.15B) separating the region of plaque in the tissue from the urinary space. Masses of tiny crystals are seen growing

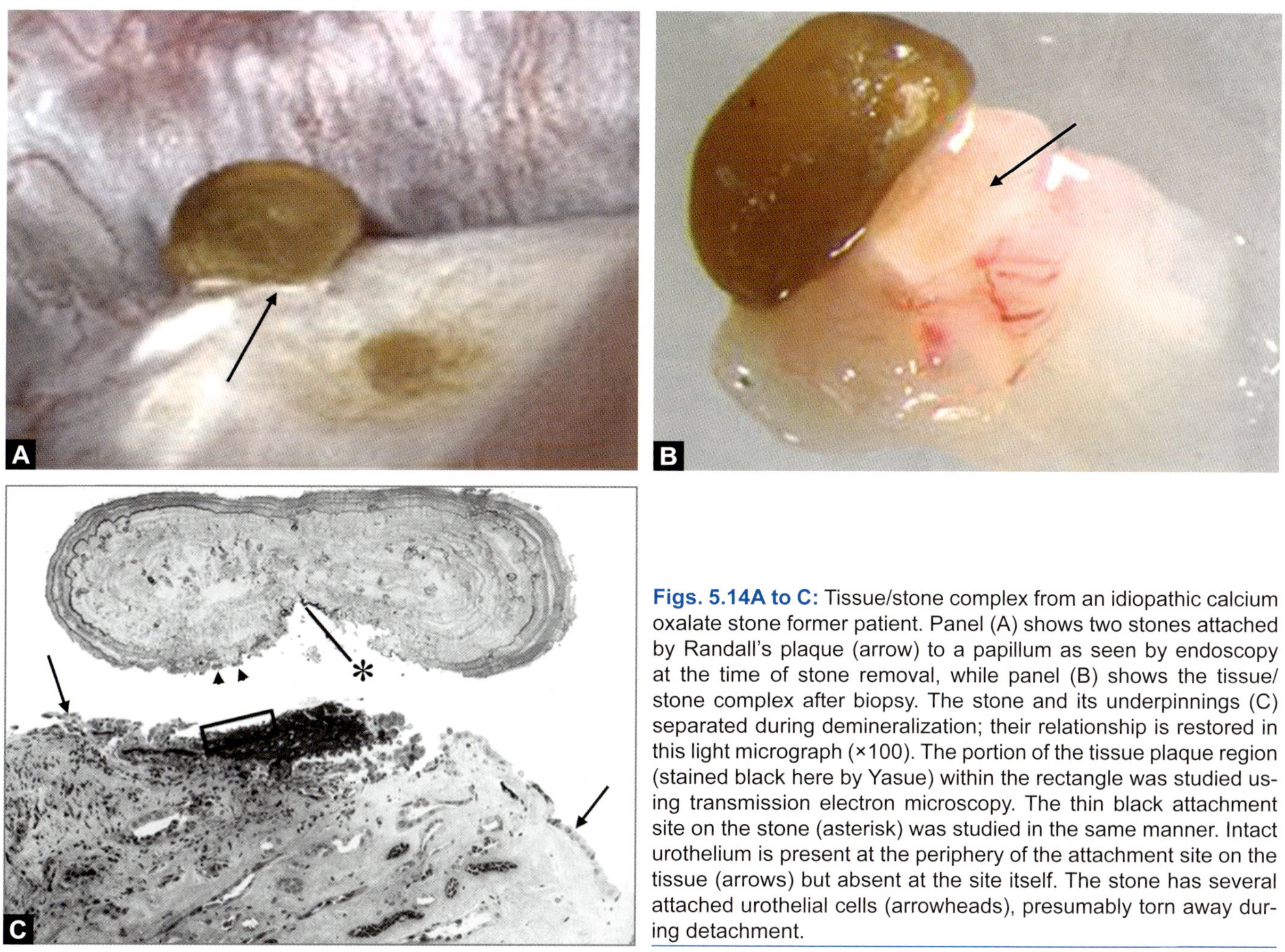

Figs. 5.14A to C: Tissue/stone complex from an idiopathic calcium oxalate stone former patient. Panel (A) shows two stones attached by Randall's plaque (arrow) to a papillum as seen by endoscopy at the time of stone removal, while panel (B) shows the tissue/stone complex after biopsy. The stone and its underpinnings (C) separated during demineralization; their relationship is restored in this light micrograph (×100). The portion of the tissue plaque region (stained black here by Yasue) within the rectangle was studied using transmission electron microscopy. The thin black attachment site on the stone (asterisk) was studied in the same manner. Intact urothelium is present at the periphery of the attachment site on the tissue (arrows) but absent at the site itself. The stone has several attached urothelial cells (arrowheads), presumably torn away during detachment.

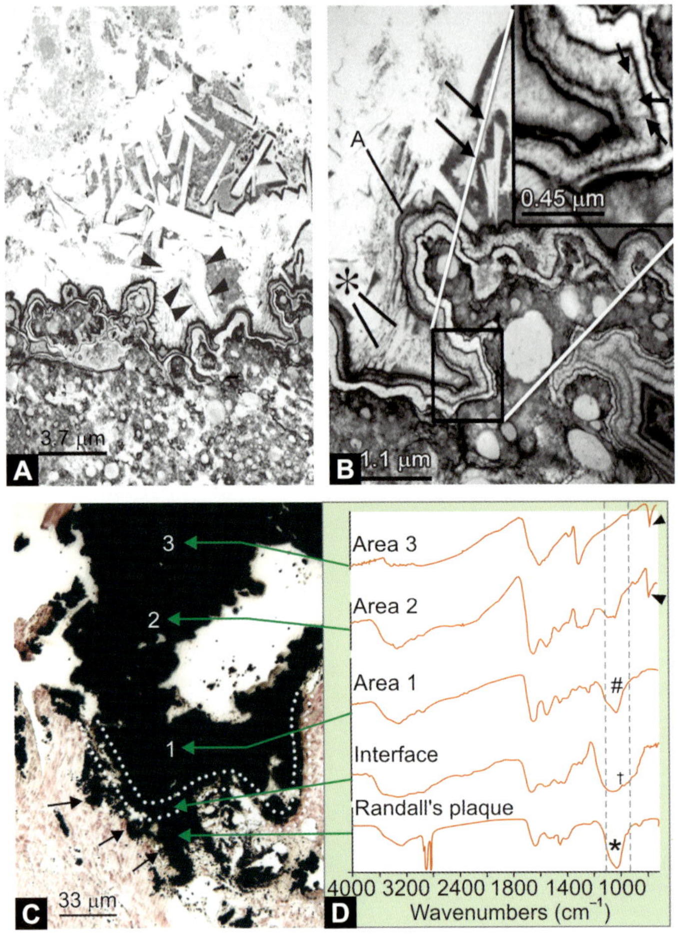

Figs. 5.15A to D: Ultrastructural and micro-Fourier transform infrared (micro-FTIR) features of attachment site of kidney stone from an idiopathic calcium oxalate stone former. Panel (A) is a high-magnification transmission electron micrograph of the tissue attachment site delineated by the rectangle. The region of Randall's plaque (lower third of the panel) is seen covered by a multilayer, ribbon-like structure (marked by arrow), which has several bundles of crystalline and matrix material inserting into it (arrowheads). The upper two-thirds represent the region of the developing stone or urine side. A region marked "A" is enlarged in panel (B). Note several small (asterisk) and large crystals (single arrow) embedded in the outer (urine) side of the ribbon. A small box area is enlarged to form the inset in the upper right corner of this panel to show the alternating layers (five thin black organic lamina and four white lamina) of the ribbon-like structure. Note that the white lamina is composed of tiny thin spicules that run perpendicular to the surface and have the appearance of multiple voids that contain tightly packed crystals (small arrows). By micro-FTIR (C and D), the mineral in the Randall's plaque [arrows in panel (C)] is apatite [asterisk in panel (D)], amorphous apatite [dagger in panel (D)] at the tissue–stone interface (outlined by dotted lines), back to apatite [pound sign in panel (D)] in the stone area closest to the interface and then progressing from mixture of apatite to just CaOx at area 3 [arrowheads in panel (D)].

directly in the outer surface of the ribbon (asterisk) facing the urinary space. Numerous microcrystals (Fig. 5.15B inset, small arrows) are seen within the inner lamina of the ribbon; one can count four white and five dark organic layers in this specimen. At the same resolution, but at another location, one again sees the large raft crystals imbedded in their homogeneous matrix (double arrow) and masses of crystals growing in the outer layer of the ribbon. Clearly, a unique set of events occurs once the urothelial layer is breached over a region of interstitial plaque.

When FTIR analysis was performed on intact tissue across the plaque–stone interface, a unique pattern of mineral composition was discovered (Figs. 5.15C and D). The tissue sites of Randall's plaque were composed of hydroxyapatite as has been shown previously.[7] However, the interface region, the site of the multilayered ribbon, was composed of amorphous apatite, while the overgrowth zone shows a transition from amorphous apatite to biological apatite. The actual stone showed a mineral composition that transitioned from apatite with some CaOx

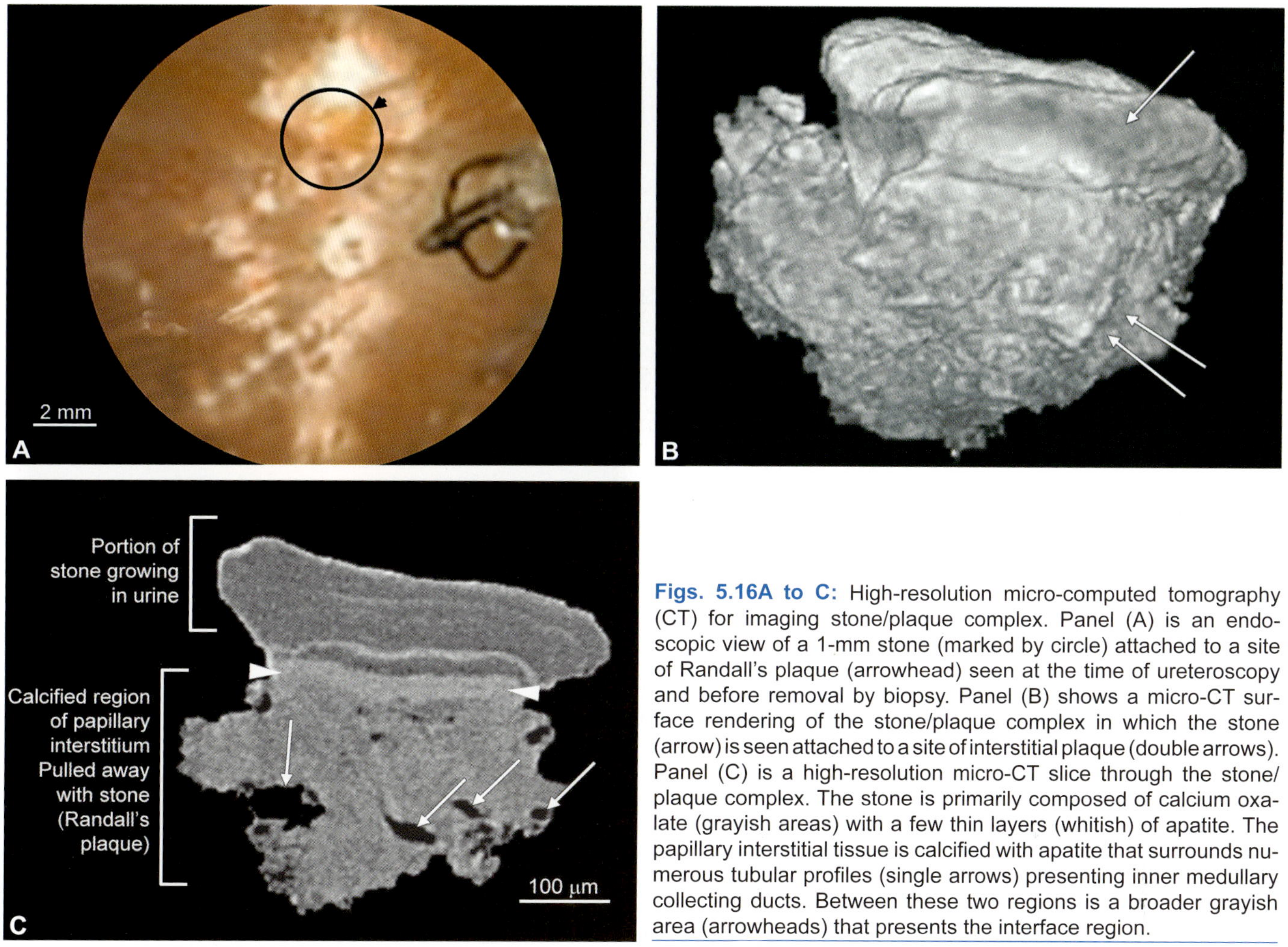

Figs. 5.16A to C: High-resolution micro-computed tomography (CT) for imaging stone/plaque complex. Panel (A) is an endoscopic view of a 1-mm stone (marked by circle) attached to a site of Randall's plaque (arrowhead) seen at the time of ureteroscopy and before removal by biopsy. Panel (B) shows a micro-CT surface rendering of the stone/plaque complex in which the stone (arrow) is seen attached to a site of interstitial plaque (double arrows). Panel (C) is a high-resolution micro-CT slice through the stone/plaque complex. The stone is primarily composed of calcium oxalate (grayish areas) with a few thin layers (whitish) of apatite. The papillary interstitial tissue is calcified with apatite that surrounds numerous tubular profiles (single arrows) presenting inner medullary collecting ducts. Between these two regions is a broader grayish area (arrowheads) that presents the interface region.

crystals to only CaOx crystals. Using ex vivo X-ray absorption spectroscopy, Daudon and Bazin also detected carbonated calcium phosphate and amorphous carbonated calcium phosphate in sites of Randall's plaque collected at the tip of the papilla.[28,29]

Obviously, this analysis has been done in only one sample because of the difficulty in obtaining the samples and processing, so the applicability of the findings as a general principle to stone formation is premature. In order to analyze more samples and in a more timely fashion, we are exploring the potential of high-resolution micro-CT as seen in Figures 5.16A to C. This approach not only allows us to accurately view the plaque–stone interface but by determining the Hounsfield values for this region the mineral composition can be defined. A unique feature of the stone/plaque complex seen in Figure 5.16 is the substantial amount of papillary interstitial tissue that was pulled off the papillary tip and remained attached to the stone. This tissue is primarily Randall's plaque noted by the apatite signature of the tissue by micro-CT and the presence of tubular profiles, the size of IMCD. A large amount of papillary interstitial tissue can remain adhered to the papillary surface of a stone removed at the time of surgery when the stone is found tightly attached to the papilla. When such a stone/plaque complex is removed, a blood spot is seen at the site of stone removal (*see* Fig. 5.11D). Stones that are loosely attached to the papilla may simply break off without extracting any papillary interstitial tissue.

Examination of the "Umbilication" Region of an Attached Stone

Another approach to understanding the early events of stone formation is to determine mineral composition of the "stalk" or nidus region (*see* Fig. 5.3) that anchors a site of exposed Randall's plaque located in the interstitial

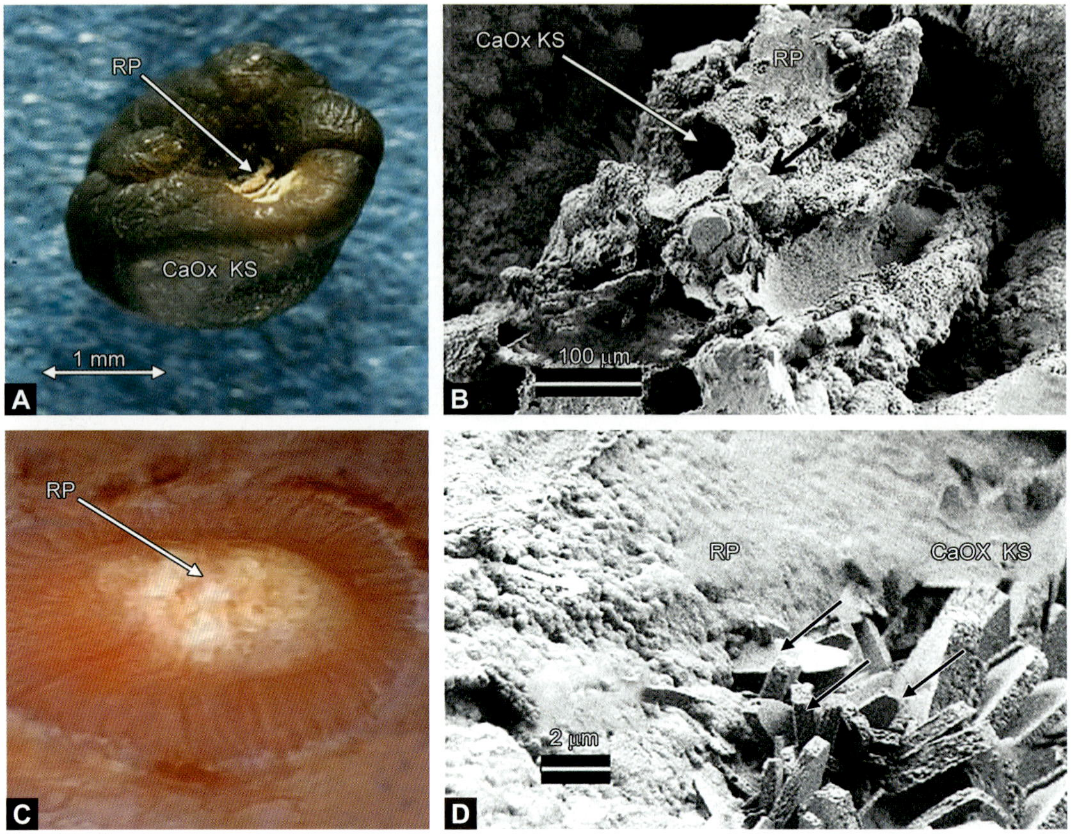

Figs. 5.17A to D: Morphology of the umbilication region of a human calcium oxalate (CaOx) renal stone. Panel (A) shows a site of Randall's plaque (RP) made of apatite at the umbilication on top of a kidney stone of whewellite (CaOx KS). Panel (B) shows a site of Randall's plaque at the surface of the papilla. Panel (C), a scanning electron micrograph, shows the complexity of a site of RP at the umbilication containing apatite crystals and calcified tubules and vessels (white arrow) and tubules filled by carbonated apatite plugs (black arrows). Panel (D) shows the interface area between RP and whewellite stone. Randall's plaque is made of carbonated apatite spherules (white arrow) surrounded by an unstructured glue-like material (black arrows).
Source: Reproduced from Bazin D, Daudon M, Combes C, et al. Characterization and some physiochemical aspects of pathological microcalcifications. Chem Rev. 2012;112:5092-120.

space to the developing stone. Daudon et al. collected the material found at a small depressed zone on the papillary stone surface termed an "umbilication" that corresponds to the stalk or nidus from 8,916 umbilicated kidney stones (Figs. 5.17A to D).[28,29] The primary mineral was carbapatite with smaller amounts of amorphous carbonated calcium phosphate and sodium hydrogen urate, and even smaller amounts of uric acid, brushite, whitlockite, glycosaminoglycans and lipids. Daudon et al. have now identified 15 different crystalline species in areas of Randall's plaque.[28,29] Of interest are the findings of a high carbonate content carbapatite and a low carbonate content carbapatite in sites of Randall's plaque. They suggested that the high carbonate content carbapatite correlates with the formation in the interstitium while the low carbonate content carbapatite correlates stronger with mechanisms associated with urine SS (BDs or urine). The small amounts of sodium hydrogen urate, whitlockite, uric acid and brushite strongly suggest that some of these umbilicated stones came from stone-forming phenotypes other than ICSF that also present with stones attached to the sites of Randall's plaque as well as BD plugs with overgrowths.[30-33] The brushite would have to be associated with brushite stone formers while sodium hydrogen urate, uric acid and whitlockite would be associated with those patients having bowel disease/surgery, such as ileostomy patients.[31-33] It is very likely that those stones with sodium hydrogen urate, uric acid, brushite and/or whitlockite were overgrowths on BD plugs and not on the stones attached to sites of Randall's plaque. In another study, this group detected high levels of the trace element zinc in the carbapatite of Randall's plaque compared to the carbapatite in a kidneys stone.[34]

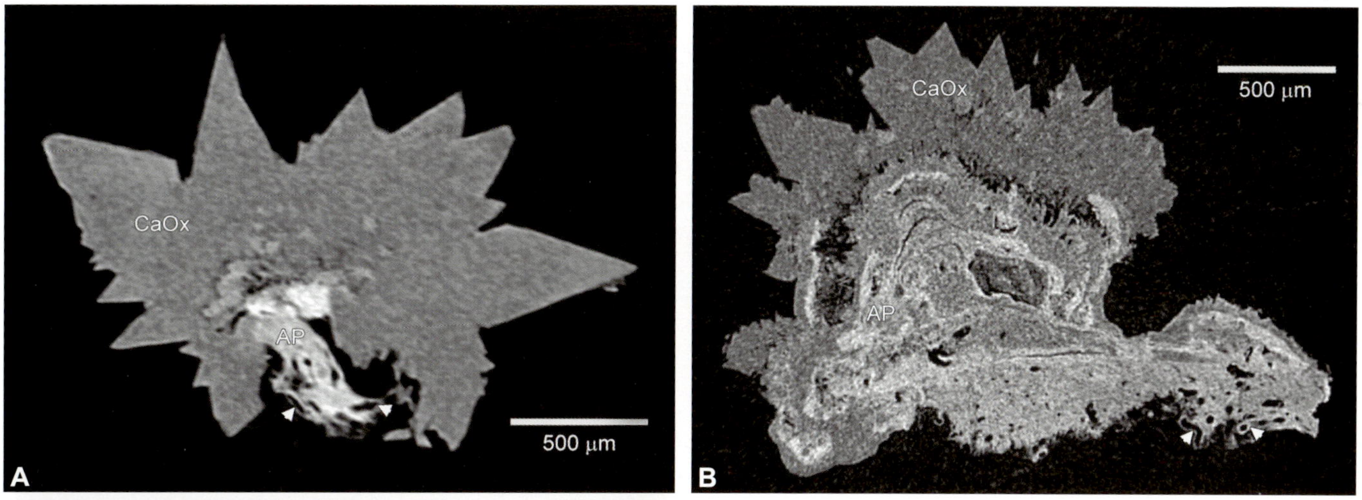

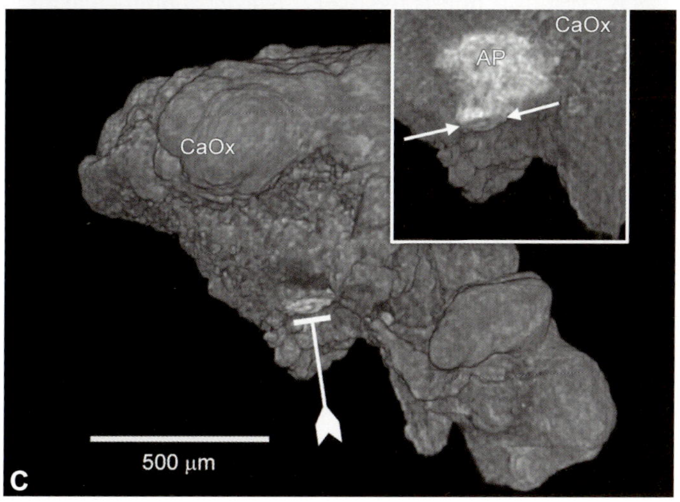

Figs. 5.18A to C: Morphological variations of the nidus region of an attached stone. Examples of the range of appearance of Randall's plaque as seen using micro-computed tomography (CT). (A) Typical attached stone pulled from papilla, with typical Randall's plaque. Stone is composed of calcium oxalate (CaOx) and apatite (AP). Examples of lumens of calcified tubule associated with the Randall's plaque are indicated by arrowheads. This piece of Randall's plaque, pulled away with the stone from the papillary interstitium, is about 150 μm wide at its site of connection to the calyceal stone. (B) Attached stone with unusually extensive region of Randall's plaque, which contains several tubular profiles indicated by arrowheads. This plaque region—stretching across the bottom of the image—is over 1,700 μm wide. (C) Surface rendering of a stone in which the Randall's plaque apparently broke during stone removal, leaving a stub, indicated by the blunt arrow. Stub region is 130 μm across. (inset) Higher-power cutaway view of the stub in panel (C), indicated by thin arrows.

There are several downsides to studying the umbilication region on a stone. First, one does not know where the stone separated from the nidus region because this breakage site varies greatly from stone to stone; the breakage point may be near the stone or, if lucky, near the plaque-stone interface or anywhere in between. Thus, it is difficult to know where along the length of the stalk the breakage occurred, which affects the interpretation of the data. This issue is linked to the detailed morphology of the nidus and how strong the stone is attached to the papillum. Daudon found the morphology of the umbilication region to be very diverse, varying from cylindrical to broad in shape, some with needle-shaped crystals and others with a tunnel covered by carbapatite and CaOx.[29] Our group has also noted the nidus to vary greatly in its morphology (Figs. 5.18A to C) where it can be seen as a single stalk or multiple stalks, narrow in width or broad, and with or without evidence of tubular profiles. The actual strength of the attachment varies with some stones tightly attached to the site of Randall's plaque while others barely hold on as observed by the surgeon at the time of stone removal. The morphology of the nidus most likely correlates with the strength of the attachment site. Second, the amount of mineral available at the umbilication for analysis can be extremely small, limiting the accuracy of the mineral determination.[34] A third issue relates to knowing if the umbilication is located on an overgrowth of a BD plug or if truly on an attached papillary stone. If one is studying a collection of passed stones, both types of stones (overgrowths on plugs or papillary stone) could be present. Daudon accurately defined those stones in his series with cylindrical deposits and/or tunnels as originating as tubular plugs/casts with or without overgrowths, not stones forming on sites of interstitial plaque.[29] This issue can be averted by studying only those stones retrieved at the time of surgery, where the surgeon can accurately determine the site of origin of each stone.

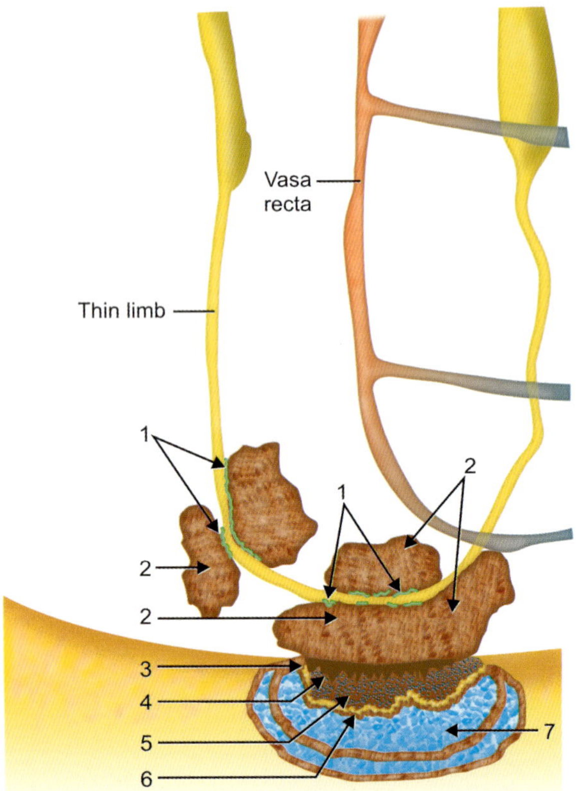

Fig. 5.19: Model of attached stone formation in idiopathic calcium oxalate stone former patients. 1: Interstitial plaque forms in the basement membranes of the thin loops of Henle; 2: interstitial plaque extends into the interstitial space as far down as the basal side of the urothelium; 3: select regions of plaque are exposed to the urine at sites of urothelial cell loss; 4: urinary molecules (proteins and ions) coat the exposed plaque, forming a continuous ribbon-like structure; 5: at some point in time, the rate and quantity of crystal formation permit explosive outward growth of large and small matrix-coated crystals of amorphous apatite, resulting in a heaping up of various-sized crystals into the urinary space; 6: a layer of biological apatite forms an overgrowth region as a result of the supersaturation levels of various ions in the urine— this is the first evidence of a newly forming attached calcium oxalate (CaOx) stone; and 7: a mixture of apatite and CaOx crystals is deposited over the layer of biological apatite. At this stage multiple alternating layers of apatite and CaOx may continue to be formed, or the process changes to only depositing CaOx.

A Model of Stone Formation in ICSF Patients

The numerous observations on Randall's plaque and the stone-plaque complex have resulted in a plausible sequence of events for stone formation and growth in the ICSF patient (Fig. 5.19). First, interstitial plaque is formed in the basement membranes of the thin loops of Henle. Second, the interstitial plaque extends into the interstitial space, forming islands of apatite deposits encased in a matrix material, which can extend to basal side of the urothelium. Third, select regions of plaque are exposed to the urine at sites of urothelial cell loss. Fourth, urinary molecules (proteins and ions) coat the exposed plaque, forming a continuous ribbon-like structure of alternating layers of matrix and crystals that covers the entire region of exposed plaque. Fifth, at some point in time the rate and quantity of crystal formation permit explosive outward growth of large and small matrix-coated crystals of amorphous apatite. This rapid formation of apatite crystals results in a heaping up of various-sized crystals into the urinary space. Sixth, a layer of biological apatite forms an overgrowth region as a result of the SS levels of various ions in the urine. This is the first evidence of a newly forming attached CaOx stone. Seventh, a mixture of apatite and CaOx crystals is deposited over the layer of biological apatite. At this stage, multiple alternating layers of apatite and CaOx may continue to be formed or the process changes to only depositing CaOx. Thus, it is our understanding that the growth of CaOx stones in ICSF patients requires a site of Randall's plaque, and when this site of plaque is exposed to the proteins and ions in the urine of a stone former, a new stone develops attached to the site of interstitial plaque.

Mechanisms of Plaque Formation in ICSF Patients

Since the discovery of Randall's plaque, a number of investigators have hypothesized on the mechanism of papillary calcification, which has included infection, vascular damage, aging processes, renal damage secondary to systemic disease or osteogenesis.[35-41] However, little insight into the pathogenesis of interstitial plaque formation has emerged until the discovery of a decrease in proximal tubule sodium reabsorption, primarily in stone-forming men with IH, resulting in an increased delivery of calcium to the distal nephron (see Chapter 8 for details).[42,43] Incorporating these data along with the detailed morphology of the vascular bundles of the renal medulla has led us to suggest the "vas washdown" hypothesis where the increased delivery of calcium to the distal nephron would raise the absolute rate of calcium reabsorption by the medullary thick ascending limbs above normal and thereby foster plaque formation via "vas washdown" of the extra calcium to the inner medulla by vas recta (Fig. 5.20). In principle, the thick ascending limb of the loops of Henle reabsorbs calcium without water into the interstitium of the outer medulla. The increased calcium reabsorbed by the thick ascending limb would then enter the vas recta blood

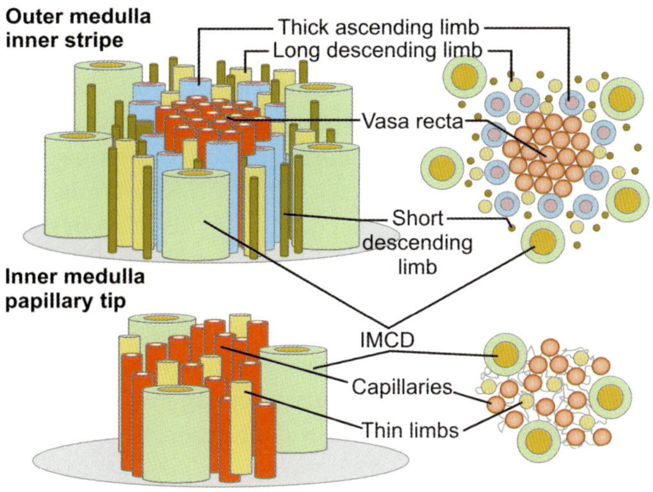

Fig. 5.20: Schematic drawing of outer medulla and papillary tip. Vasa recta descend in bundles through the inner stripe of the outer medulla (upper panels) surrounded by rings of thick ascending limbs. In the papillary tip, where Randall's plaque forms in the basement membranes of thin limbs (lower panels), thin limbs are each surrounded by three to four capillaries that derive from the descending vasa recta. IMCD, inner medullary collecting ducts.

located inside the ring of medullary thick ascending limbs. Countercurrent trapping will help retain the extra calcium there, allowing blood descending the vas recta along the long loops of juxtamedullary nephrons to be enriched with calcium as they descend into the inner medulla. As the calcium molarity increased in the inner medulla, crystalline deposits of apatite would first appear on the collagen fibers of the basement membranes of the thin loops by simple physicochemical mechanisms. Potentially the same thin loops would have a tubular fluid whose calcium molarity is higher than blood because of water extraction by the thin descending limbs of Henle. Thus, the basement membranes of the thin loops would be sandwiched in between two calcium-rich environments. As the calcium molarity increases in the interstitium of the inner medulla, apatite crystalline deposits would form on the type 1 collagen fibers all the way down to the basal side of the urothelium.

Characteristics of Intraluminal Deposits (Tubular Plugs)

General Features of Intraluminal Deposits

Randall, in his historic paper in 1940, described intraluminal calcifications which he termed papillary lesion type II in only 23 cases and compared it to the more common finding (204 cases) of interstitial plaque (papillary lesion type I).[1] The obvious difference in frequency between the type I and type II lesions suggests that they represent separate processes. Our biopsy and mapping studies have now examined 11 stone-forming phenotypes plus nonstone formers (Table 5.1) and intraluminal deposits or "tubular plugs" in 10 of these groups.[30-33,40,44-48] These observations are in great contrast to our original findings in ICSF patients and nonstone formers, where the only change noted was the presence of interstitial plaque.[7,47] Tubular plugs vary in number, size, mineral type, degree of luminal filling and location.[48] They are located primarily, but not exclusively, in IMCD and BDs and are associated with total destruction of those tubular lining cells adjacent to the crystals. Focal sites of interstitial fibrosis surround the plugged tubules. At the openings of BD, mineral plugs can protrude into the urinary space and present with a site of mineral overgrowth that is fixed to the distal end of intratubular plugs. Potentially, these overgrowths could develop into a clinical stone.

Table 5.1: Stone forming phenotypes studied.

1. Idiopathic CaOx stone former (idiopathic calcium oxalate stone former)
2. Obesity bypass (BP)
3. Ileostomy (ILEO)
4. Small bowel resection (SBR)
5. Primary hyperparathyroidism (PHPT)
6. Distal renal tubular acidosis (RTA)
7. Brushite (BR)
8. Cystinuria (Cys)
9. Primary hyperoxaluria (PH1) with and without ESRD
10. Calcium phosphate (apatite) (HA)
11. Medullary sponge kidney (MSK)
12. Normal people (N) nonstone formers

(ICSF: Idiopathic calcium oxalate stone formers; PH1: Primary hyperoxaluria type 1; HA, apatite; ESRD: End stage renal disease).

Intratubular crystalline deposits and renal tissue injury have been reported in patients with nephrolithiasis as early as 1933 as well as by others.[49-51] However, it was not until Finlayson and Reid proposed the "fixed particle" hypothesis in 1978, suggesting that smaller crystals can be retained in the tubular lumen by binding to the tubular epithelium, that a mechanistic concept linked crystal deposition and tubular injury.[52] Once the crystal-cell attachment step has occurred, the crystal nuclei would be fixed in position and exposed to a supersaturated ultrafiltrate that would facilitate further growth of these crystals, leading to extensive intratubular calcification termed "tubular nephrocalcinosis").[53] Extensive animal and cell culture work have been conducted on this topic and Vervaet has present a thorough examination of the cell biological evidence for the mechanisms involved in crystal retention in his thesis[54] as well as in this book Section 1. Chapter 6 entitled "CaOx and CaP crystal interactions with renal cells". Obviously, these issues have the potential to be vital to our understanding of the mechanisms of intratubular plug formation in kidney stone formers. Only those topics that directly relate to our human stone-forming groups will be discussed in detail in this chapter.

Initial Histopathologic Findings of Intratubular Plugs in Bypass Kidney Stone Patients

Our initial endoscopic and histopathologic study of papillary biopsies from 15 ICSF patients, 4 patients with stones due to intestinal bypass surgery for obesity and 4 non-stone formers, and a follow-up study detected intraluminal deposits/plugs only in the intestinal bypass patients.[7,54] Endoscopy revealed a few dilated BD with crystal deposits in the intestinal bypass patients, very few sites of Randall's plaque with otherwise normal papillary architecture. By histopathology, intraluminal crystals were detected in IMCD and BD of intestinal bypass patients as either partial or complete plugs in those tubular lumen (Figs. 5.21A to F), and the majority of crystals stained positive with the Yasue stain. Analysis of these intraluminal deposits by micro-FTIR found primarily hydroxyapatite and small traces of CaOx, a finding that was a surprise considering these bypass patients had hyperoxaluria.[7] A couple IMCD had crystals only attached to the apical cell surface appearing as a bright scrim outlining these cells as seen by light microscopic polarizing optics (Figs. 5.21A to F). At this early stage of plugging, the lining cells covered by the scrim appeared normal as well as the tubular cells nearby and the surrounding interstitial tissues.

To detect the presence of injured/regenerating cells in plugged as well as otherwise adjacent normal-appearing IMCD inner medullary papillary tissue from ICSF, intestinal bypass and controls were stained with hyaluronan.[54] While no tubular segments stained in the ICSF patients or controls, all intraluminal deposits and adjacent lining cells of plugged IMCD and BD found in on intestinal bypass tissue were positive for hyaluronan. In addition, many IMCD lining cells adjacent to sites of intraluminal deposits expressed focal hyaluronan staining of their apical cell membrane (Figs. 5.21A to F), suggesting that these cells were altered even though the cells appeared normal.[55] A distinct band of interstitial fibrosis of a varying thickness was noted completely surrounding the plugged tubules but not those with just hyaluronan positive staining. The apatite deposits do make sense if the IMCD lining cells were injured, possibly from crystalluria, resulting in a loss of pH control of the tubular fluid. Consequently, there would be a rise in the pH of the tubular fluid, which would favor apatite retention. With the formation of apatite crystals in the tubular lumen, crystal attachment would occur as a consequence of cell injury, creating a vicious circle leading to more cell damage and a further rise in tubular fluid pH.

Characteristics of Intraluminal Deposits/Plugs in Other Stone Phenotypes

- Endoscopic pattern of deposits: While limited evidence of plugging was seen in intestinal bypass papilla by high-resolution endoscopy, sites of IMCD and BD plugging were first noted in brushite patients by high-resolution endoscopy as two distinct patterns (Figs. 5.23A to D).[32] The first pattern appeared as large yellow deposits filling the dilated openings of BD, while other BD had mineral plugs protruding from the dilated openings into the urinary space with or without overgrowths attached to the distal end of BD plugs (termed "type 2" papillary lesion by Randall). The second pattern appeared as elongated suburothelial yellow deposits (termed "type 3") of variable size and length located on the sides of papillary tips, away from BD.[32] Some of these deposits in the brushite patients formed a spoke-and-wheel pattern around the circumference of the papilla extending the entire papilla. Histopathologic examination of papillary biopsies retrieved from sites containing the type 3 papillary lesion confirmed these deposits were confined to the lumens of primarily IMCD and a few BDs (Figs. 5.23A to D). The precise endoscopic pattern of intraluminal deposits for each stone phenotype will be described in the following section of this chapter.
- The other endoscopic findings associated with intraluminal plugs were pitting or depressions near the papillary tip along with flattening of the normal conical shape of the papilla. The pits were associated with a dilated opening of a BD that contained yellow crystalline material (Figs. 5.23A to D). In other words, pitting

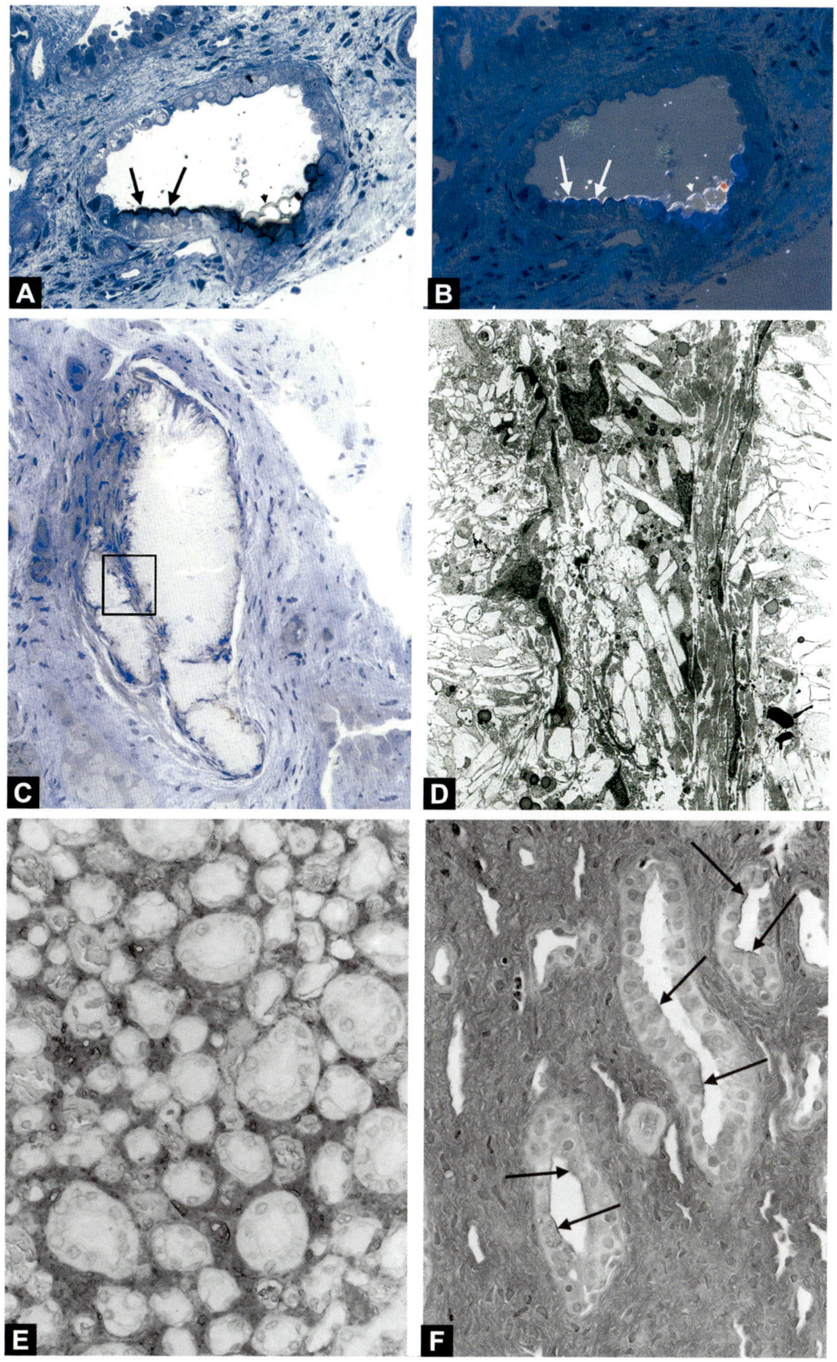

Figs. 5.21A to F: Inner medullary collecting ducts (IMCD) with intraluminal deposits from stone patients who underwent intestinal bypass surgery for obesity. Panels (A) and (B) show an IMCD section stained with Yasue and viewed with direct (A) and polarized (B) light. The IMCD cells are seen coated with a thin black layer (A, arrows) that represents areas of calcium deposit. Arrowheads highlight a thin region of staining at the apical cell surfaces noted at a branching point of an IMCD in which the black overlay on the cells is particularly clear. By polarized light (B) the overlay is birefringent and the birefringence faithfully follows the outlines of the Yasue-positive coating. The arrows and arrowhead point to the same structured marked by arrows and an arrowhead in A. Other IMCD that were completely plugged with mineral (C) showed a loss of all lining cells and extensive interstitial fibrosis surrounding the site of plugging. By transmission electron microscopy of a selected region of the tubule seen in panel (C) (outlined by a rectangle), no cellular detail could be detected; only crystalline material was identified (D). Selected regions of papillary biopsies from control and bypass patient were stained with hyaluronan to detect injured/regenerating IMCD cells that otherwise appear normal. No hyaluronan staining was seen in the control tissue (E), while focal sites of staining of apical membranes (F, arrows) of IMCD adjacent to site of intraluminal plugging were numerous.

appears to be part of type 2 deposits. A second type of pit was occasionally seen on the side of a papilla and did not appear to be associated with a dilated BD (Fig. 5.23). The genesis of such a pit is not clear. Flattening of the papillary is probably not the result of pitting but is linked to the degree of medullary interstitial fibrosis. Those stone phenotypes with diffuse interstitial fibrosis such as distal renal tubular acidosis and primary hyperoxaluria showed the highest degree of flattening, while stone patients with bypass surgery for obesity showed minimal change in the papillary shape.

- Tubular location of deposits: By histopathology, tubular plugging was found in IMCD and BD of all stone phenotypes we have examined to this date except ICSF with IH and no systemic diseases (Fig. 5.22). Additional tubular sites of plugging were noted in the outer medullary collecting ducts of brushite patients, in thick loops of Henle of ileostomy patients, in thick loops of Henle and distal convoluted tubules of cystine patients, and in outer medullary collecting ducts and cortical collecting ducts of patients with PHPT. Primary hyperoxaluric patients with end stage renal disease (ESRD) showed the largest number of involved tubular segments including thick loops of Henle, outer medullary collecting ducts, cortical collecting ducts, distal convoluted tubule and proximal tubules. A few ileostomy patients showed deposits in cortical collecting ducts.
- Mineral type of tubular deposits: The mineral type forming intraluminal deposits in IMCD analyzed by micro-FTIR has been noted to be primarily apatite intermixed with small amounts of CaOx for intestinal bypass patients with stones, distal renal tubular acidosis patients, medullary sponge kidneys (MSK) and patients with small bowel resection (Fig. 5.22).[7,33,40,46] Patients with PHPT, apatite stones or cystine stones had only apatite IMCD deposits, while primary hyperoxaluria patients had only CaOx IMCD deposits.[30,44,45,47] The BD plugs in cystine patients were composed of cystine, while the BD plugs found in ileostomy patients contained sodium or ammonium salts of uric acid.[37,45] The BD plugs analyzed in brushite patients contained varying admixtures of apatite, CaOx, and brushtie.[32] Plugs detected in the thick loops of Henle from ileostomy and cystine patients were apatite as were those located in distal convoluted tubules of cystine patients.[37,45,46] All plugs in primary hyperoxaluric patients with ESRD were calcium oxalate.[47]
- Size and number of tubular deposits: Using high-resolution micro-CT, the size and number/density of IMCD and BD deposits were determined in single papillary biopsies (Figs. 5.24A to F).[49] Brushite patients had the largest deposits (up to 4,000 mm in diameter), followed by ileostomy and primary hyperoxaluria, and medullary sponge. Cystine, bypass, small bowel resection, renal tubular acidosis, primary hyperparathyroid and apatite stone formers had small deposits (200 mm). Renal tubular acidosis, primary hyperoxaluria with ESRD and some apatite stone formers had extensive numbers of deposits (42 deposits per mm3), while all other stone phenotypes had moderate to low deposit number (4 deposits per mm^3).
- Cell injury and medullary interstitial fibrosis: As was stated earlier for stone patients with bypass surgery, the initial sites of intraluminal crystalline deposits were noted on the apical surface of IMCD lining cells, forming a scrim of crystals that are compatible with nucleation of crystals directly on cell membranes.[7] There appeared to be no evidence of cell injury to these cells as determined by routine light microscopy (*see* Figs. 5.21A to F). However, the use of hyaluronan staining, a tool to detect injured cell, revealed numerous IMCD tubules without crystals as well as all nearby tubules with deposits staining positive for hyaluronan. A similar pattern of crystal deposition and hyaluronan staining

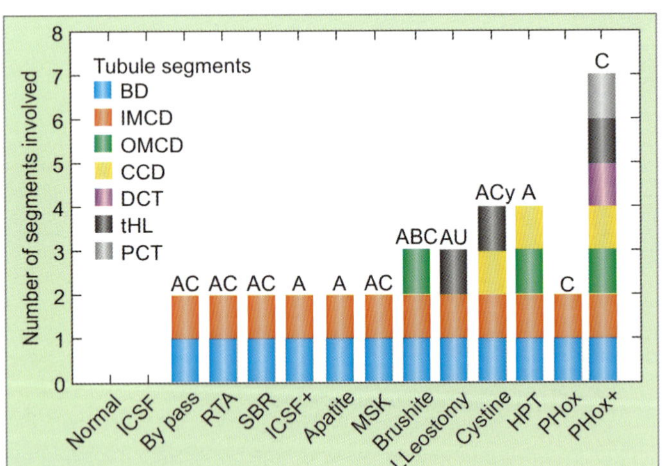

Fig. 5.22: Nephron segments containing deposits in 12 conditions. Nephron segments: BD: Duct of Bellini; IMCD, OMCD and CCD, inner and outer medullary and cortical collecting ducts; DCT, distal convoluted tubule; tHL, thin limbs of Henle's loop; PCT, proximal tubule. Mineral type in deposits: A, apatite; B, brushite; C, CaOx; Cy, cystine; AU, sodium or ammonium salts of uric acid. ICSF, idiopathic calcium oxalate stone formers; RTA, renal tubular acidosis; SBR, small bowel resection; MSK, medullary sponge kidney; HPT, hyperparathyroidism; PHox: Primary hyperoxaluria.

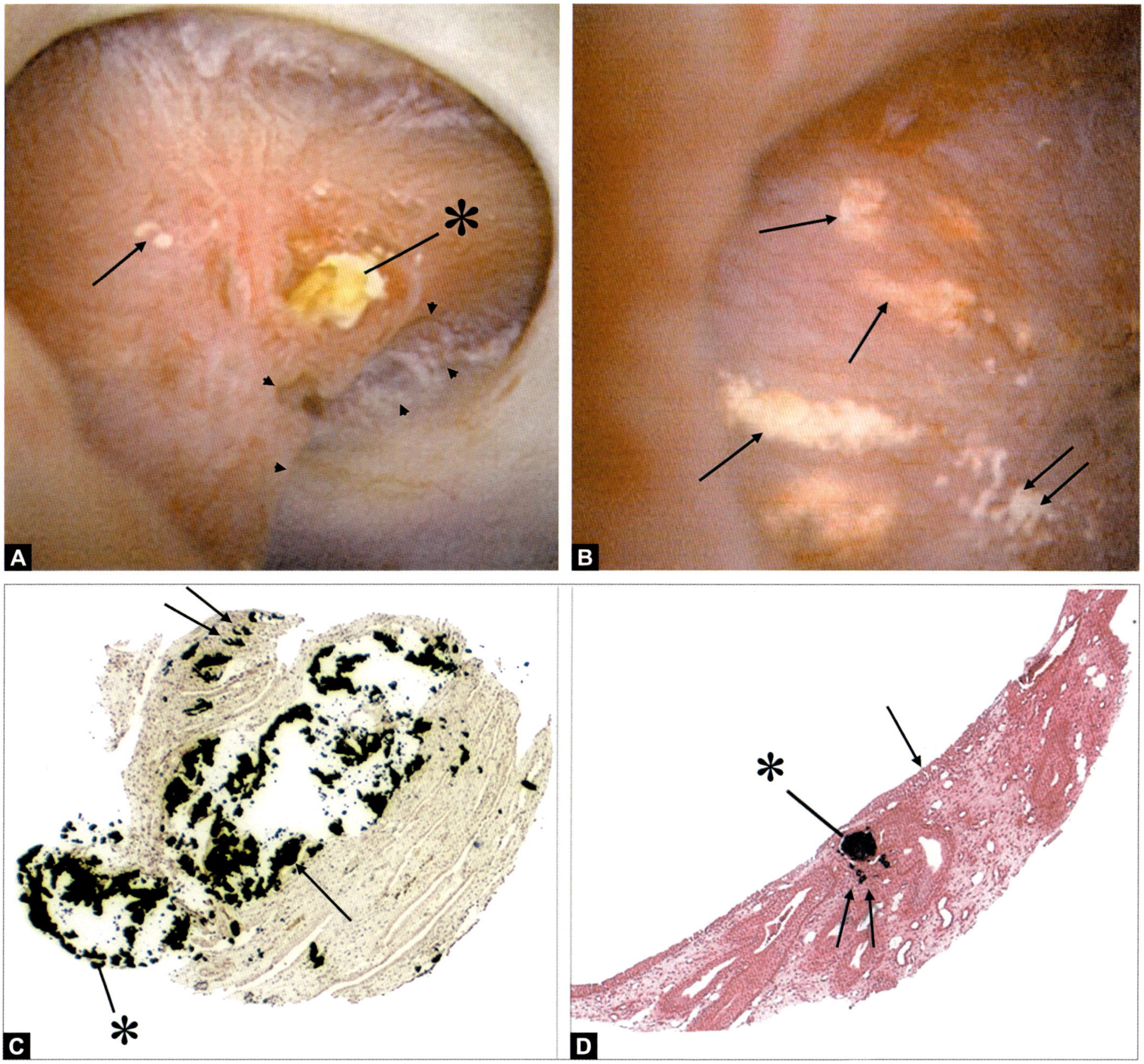

Figs. 5.23A to D: "Type 2" and "type 3" patterns of intraluminal deposits. Panel (A) is an example of a papilla from a brushite patient showing type 1 and type 2 patterns of deposits as seen by endoscopy. Irregular white (Randall's plaque) areas of crystalline deposits (arrow) represents the type 1 pattern while the asterisk denotes a site of yellowish deposits, the type 2 pattern, at the opening of a dilated duct of Bellini. A large pit (arrowheads) is seen on the side of the papilla near the dilated duct of Bellini (BD). Panel (B), also a papilla from a brushite patient, shows both type 1 and type 3 patterns of deposits. The arrows mark a series of elongated yellowish mineral deposits forming a spoke-and-wheel-like pattern around the circumference of the papilla. A double arrow marks a site of interstitial or Randall's plaque and illustrates the type 1 pattern of deposits. Panel (C) is a low-magnification light micrograph of a grossly dilated inner medullary collecting ducts (IMCD, arrow) filled with Yasue-positive material that has progressed distally to include a BD with mineral protruding (asterisk) through its dilated opening. A double arrow shows a site of interstitial plaque. Panel (D) documents that the yellowish deposits seen on the papillary surface (arrow) are indeed mineral filling IMCD (asterisk). Again the double arrow marks a site of Randall's plaque.

was detected in IMCD of a primary hyperoxaluric stone patient.[47] To date, we have not applied hyaluronan staining to papillary biopsies from all 11 of our stone phenotypes, so we do not know if this pattern of hyaluronan staining and plug formation occurs in all human stone formers with intraluminal deposits.

In general, as the intraluminal deposit enlarged to partially or completely fill the tubular lumen, lining cells of that nephron segment varied from irregular in shape, suggesting injury to complete loss (Figs. 5.21, 5.23 and 5.25). This pattern of injury was seen in all involved medullary segments (Fig. 5.22). Occasionally, denuded dead cells were seen mixed within the intraluminal mineral deposits. In those plugged tubules showing a complete loss of lining cells, the luminal crystals were embedded in the tubular basement membrane (Figs. 5.21A to F). The only exceptions to these observation were seen in the cystic IMCD tubules of MSKs that were filled with free-floating ductal stones and the loosely held BD plugs in cystinuric patients.[40,45]

The pattern of crystal deposition and cell injury was unique in cortical proximal tubules for primary hyperoxaluria patients with kidney stones (Figs. 5.25A to D).[47] Primary hyperoxaluria type 1 (PH1) patients with kidney stones and normal renal function possessed very small calcium oxalate crystals at the brush border of a few proximal tubules. No evidence of cell injury was noted at these crystalline sites. However, PH1 patients with ESRD showed extensive involvement of proximal tubular plugging. Regions of small intraluminal deposits positioned near lining cells induced extensive cell injury to frank necrosis. In response to the presence of these intraluminal deposits, the proximal tubular lining cells changed polarity, grew over these small deposits and thereby positioned the deposit outside of the tubules in order to maintain the health of the tubule. This process of isolating the crystals to the interstitial space is termed exotubulosis.

Interstitial fibrosis was always associated with site of intraluminal deposits regardless of location (cortical and medullary) and was consistently found in all stone phenotypes with plugs.[49] In general, these changes were noted as cuffing of fibrosis around isolated IMCD with deposits, thus focal. No chronic inflammatory changes were observed at these sites. Basement membrane thickening of the plugged IMCD was common. Because the sites of interstitial fibrosis appeared associated with only plugged tubules, the degree of interstitial fibrosis was minimal in stone patients with a few plugged tubules, such as bypass patients, and diffuse in stone patients where almost all IMCD are plugged, such as in distal renal tubular acidosis.

There were a few exceptions to the pattern of interstitial fibrosis just described in plugged stone patients. In brushite stone formers, extensive regions of focal interstitial fibrosis were noted as embedment of all nephron segments in dense fibrotic tissues that contained chronic inflammatory cells like giant cells.[32] Those tubules engulfed in the fibrotic tissue had extensively thickened basement membranes with narrowed tubular lumens and complete loss of lining cells. The unique nature of the fibrosis in brushite patients suggests that these changes are related additional factors than plugging. We have suggested that there may be an association of brushite stone disease with repeated shock wave lithotripsy (SWL) treatment inducing focal sites of injury in the renal medulla.[56,57]

A similar pattern of dense fibrosis was detected in primary hyperoxaluric patients with normal renal function; however, unlike brushite patients where the interstitial fibrosis is focal, in PH1 the change is diffuse, suggesting that there are other factors than plugging driving the fibrosis.[47] We have recently detected a high level of transforming growth factor receptor (TGFR) expression in the papillary biopsies of PH1 patients, indicating a potential pathway for crystal adhesion and cell injury.[58]

Overgrowths on BD plugs: Ducts of Bellini plugs present to the surgeon as dilated ducts filled with yellowish crystals. Occasionally, crystals from the urinary space grow over the distal ends of the intraluminal BD plugs and extend into the urinary space. The overgrowths are round in shape and are normally about 1–2 mm in diameter (Figs. 5.26A to G). At that size, they would not generate a clinical problem. One could imagine that those small overgrowths could detach and grow within a minor calyx to reach ≥3 mm and as such present a clinical episode on passage. Recently, a 4-mm overgrowth was found in a brushite stone former, indicating that these overgrowths can enlarge to a size large enough to potentially generate a clinical problem.

High-resolution micro-CT was used to identify the mineral content of plugs and their overgrowth regions in a variety of stone formers (Fig. 5.26 and Table 5.2). In Figure 5.26B, only apatite was found in the plug and overgrowth from an apatite stone former. The plug from a brushite stone former had a thin surface of CaOx over apatite while the plug had a mixture of CaOx, brushite and apatite (Fig. 5.26C). Ileostomy stone formers presented BD plugs composed of apatite and urate and the overgrowth is CaOx (Fig. 5.26D). Primary hyperparathyroid stone formers have BD plugs and overgrowths that are apatite (Fig. 5.26E). Figure 5.26F shows a long segment of a BD plug from an MSK that was mostly apatite with a small amount of CaOx while the overgrowth presented a ring-like pattern of concentric laminae of alternating apatite and COM. Plug and

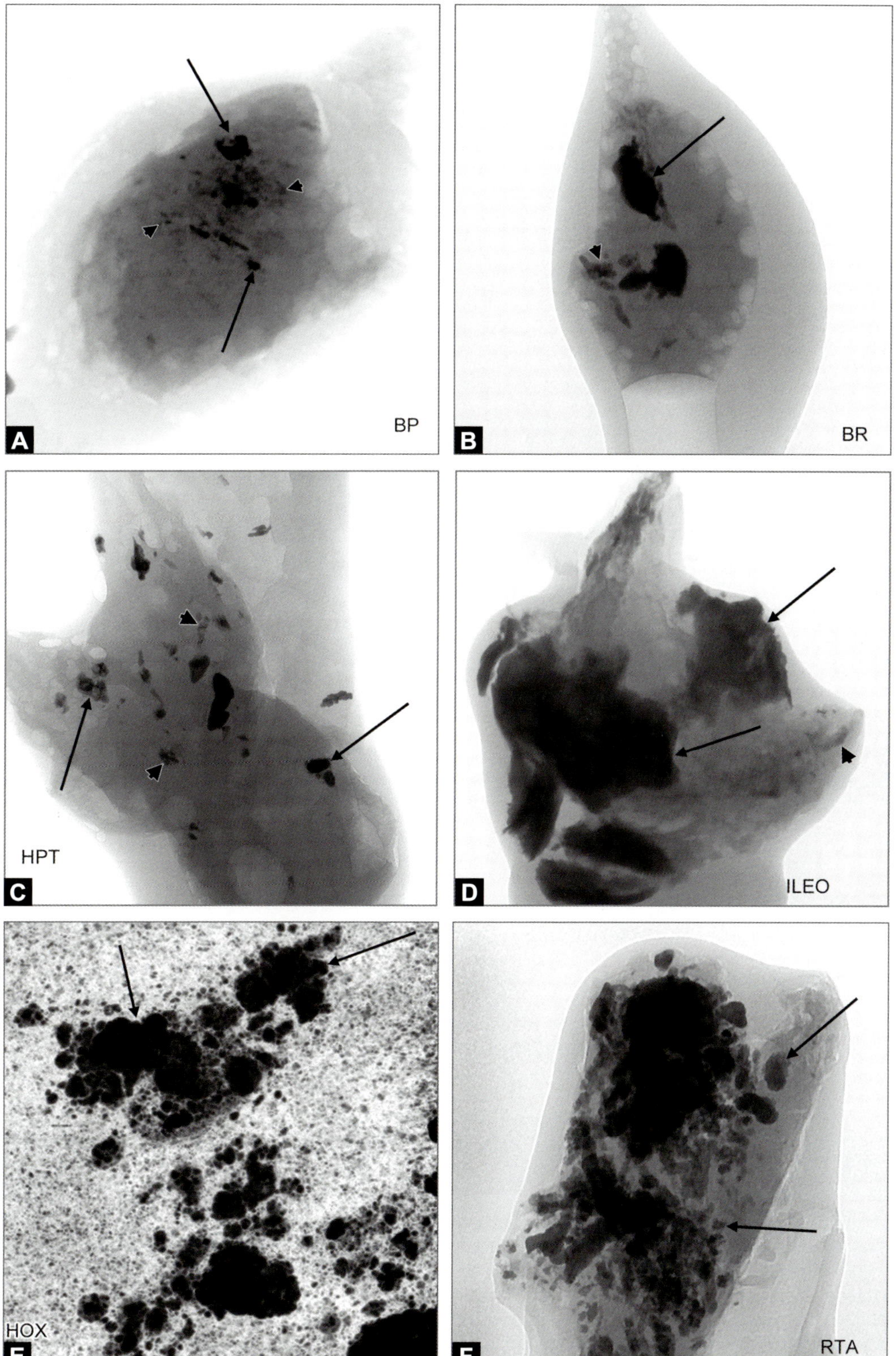

Figs. 5.24A to F: Micro-computed tomography (CT) analysis of deposits in six different stone disease. In all six panels, arrows point to intraluminal plugs and arrowheads to sites of Randall's plaque. From the micro-CT reconstructions, the density of deposits in cubic mm of tissue as well as the size of the deposits in mm was calculated. Panels (A to D, and F) are micro-CT shadow images, while panel (E) is a micro-CT cross-sectional image; see Table 5.1 for abbreviations.

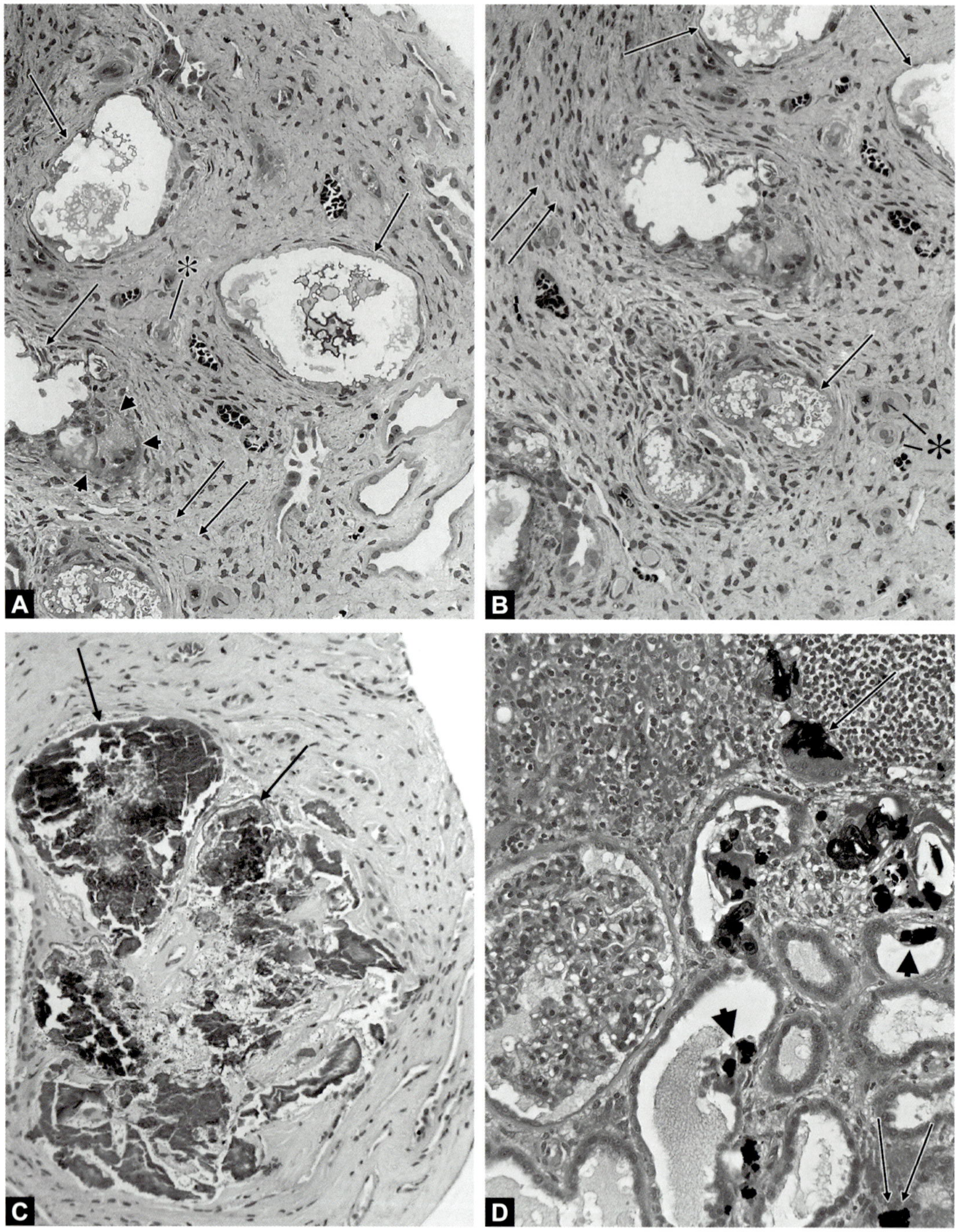

Figs. 5.25A to D: Interstitial changes associated with severely injured crystal filled inner medullary collecting ducts (IMCD) of the inner medulla and proximal tubules in the cortex. Panels (A to C) are light micrographs of papillary biopsies (from a brushite stone former) while panel D is a light micrograph of a cortical biopsy from a brushite stone former. The papillary biopsies were so heavily calcified that tissue needed decalcification with ethylenediaminetetraacetic acid prior to sectioning. Panels (A) and (B) show extensive cellular damage to several IMCD (arrows) where the mineral had been chemically removed. Extensive regions of interstitial fibrosis surround the injured IMCD (double arrows). Entrapped injured thin loops of Henle and vasa recta (asterisk) are noted in these fields of interstitial fibrosis. An occasional giant cell (arrowheads) suggestive of chronic inflammation was observed near damaged collecting ducts in panel (A). Panel (C) shows a biopsy that was not decalcified to reveal a series of crystalline-filled collecting ducts (arrows) embedded in a small ring of fibrotic tissue. (D) The cortex of brushite stone formers also showed extensive interstitial changes that included a loss of tubular profiles and sites of crystal deposits (double arrow). Some proximal tubular cells contained crystal deposits (arrowheads) while other crystal deposits were seen plugging a tubular lumen (single arrow).

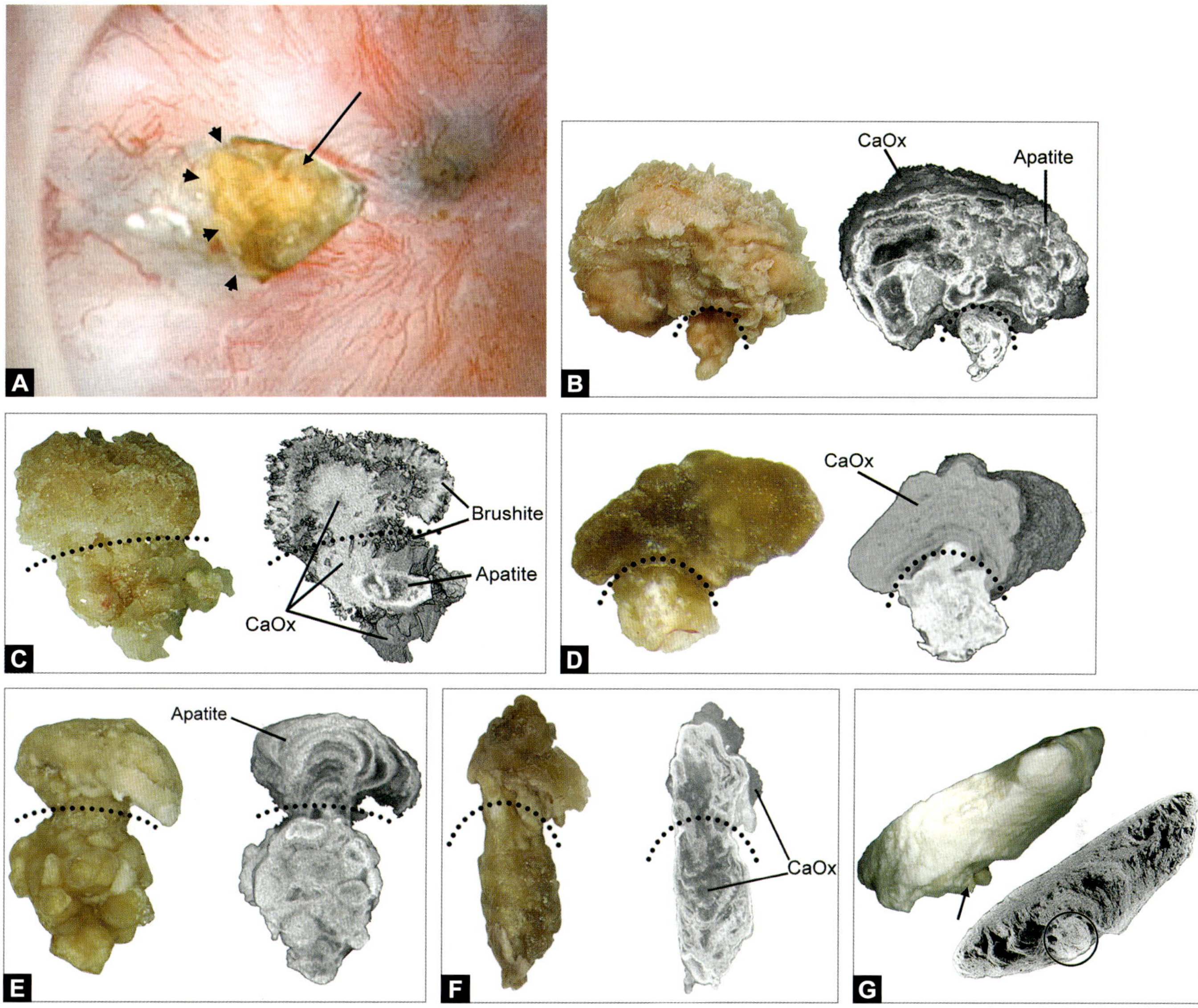

Figs. 5.26A to G: Endoscopic and high-resolution micro-computed tomography (CT) images of the duct of Bellini (BD) plugs with overgrowths. Panel (A) shows an overgrowth protruding into the urinary space through a dilated BD from a patient with distal renal tubular acidosis as viewed by high-resolution digital endoscopy at the time of stone removal. Panels (B) to (F) show a light micrograph of a BD plug with overgrowth region from an apatite, brushite, Ileostomy and primary hyperparathyroidism stones of patients, respectively, on the left and a corresponding micro-CT image generated from three-dimensional image stacks rendered for surface view and then sized for internal view from each of the plug/overgrowth structure on the right. A dotted line marks the region of the plug from the overgrowth that would occur at the opening of the BD. The mineral forming the plugs from apatite (B) and primary hyperparathyroid (E) is entirely apatite. The plug from the brushite patient (C) is a mixture of brushite, apatite and calcium oxalate (CaOx) while the plug from the ileostomy patient (D) is apatite and urates. The overgrowth regions from apatite (B) and primary hyperparathyroid patients (E) are primarily concentric layers of apatite, entirely CaOx for ileostomy patients (D) and a mixture of CaOx and BR for brushite patients (C). Panel (F) shows long segment of a BD plug from a medullary sponge kidney that was mostly apatite with a small amount of CaOx while the overgrowth presented a ring-like pattern of concentric laminae of alternating HA and COM. Panel (G) shows a long and slender pelvic stone removed from a patient with primary hyperparathyroidism that possibly started as an overgrowth on a BD plug. By micro-CT (lower image) the stone is seen as composed of apatite with a round inclusion region denoted by the ring and by an arrow in the light microscopic image. Possibly this inclusion region was the original plug because its layers of apatite are like those of plugs in being nodular as opposed to the concentric rings of most stones. HA, apatite.

Table 5.2: Composition of stones, ducts of Bellini plugs, overgrowths on plugs and ductal stones in 11 stone former phenotypes.

Pheno-type	*N*	*Stones on plaque*	*Ductal stones*	*Other stones*	*BD plugs*	*Over-Growth on plugs*
ICSF	30	CaOx/HA	-			?
HA	9	CaOx/HA	-	HA/CaOx	HA	HA
BR	23	CaOx/HA	-	BR/CaOx/HA	HA/CaOx/BR	BR
SBR	11	CaOx/HA	-	CaOx	HA	?
ILEO	7	CaOx/HA	-	Ua/CaOx	HA/NAU	?
PHPT	5	CaOx/HA	-	CaOx/HA/BR	HA	?
Bypass	5	-	-	CaOx	HA/CaOx (TRACE)	NONE
RTA	5	-	-	HA	HA/CaOx	HA
Cystine	7	-	Cystine/ha	CYSTINE	CYSTINE	CYSTINE
PH1	8	-	-	CaOx	CaOx	CaOx
MSK	12	CaOx	CaOx/HA	CaOx/HA/UA	CaOx/HA	CaOx

(N: Number of biopsied stone formers; BD: Duct of Bellini; SS: Supersaturation. Stone composition: HA, apatite; CaOx: Calcium oxalate; Br: Brushite; UA: Uric acid; NAU: Sodium acid urate, ICSF: Idiopathic calcium oxalate stone formers; SBR: Small bowel resection; ILEO: Ileostomy; PHPT: Primary hyperparathyroidism; RTA: Renal tubular acidosis; PH1: Primary hyperoxaluria type 1; MSK: Medullary sponge kidney; ? = Lack of data).

overgrowth compositions are detailed in Table 5.2 for all human stone-forming phenotypes we have studied.

If an overgrowth could detach from a BD plug, how might one know if a stone found free in the urinary collection system or ureter was an overgrowth, on Randall's plaque or a stone that formed freely in the collection system as is seen in cystinuric patients?[45] One possibility is that a stone attached to a papilla is found to be attached not on white plaque but to a BD plug. This situation should be evident to the surgeon at the time of intraoperative endoscopy. Also, the stone must have remnants of the plug at one border, the site where it was attached to a BD plug.

Another possibility is that an overgrowth has detached and is free in the collection system, grows into a clinically relevant stone and is removed. Within that stone, one might predict the ghost remnant of the plug or overgrowth buried in newly formed layers of mineral, creating a larger stone from the initially small overgrowth. On study of our collection of stones, we have found one example of such a ghost (Fig. 5.26G), a long and slender pelvic stone removed from a patient with PHPT that possibly started as an overgrowth on a BD plug. By micro-CT the stone is seen as composed of apatite with a round inclusion region denoted by the ring and by an arrow in the light microscopic image. Possibly, this inclusion region was the original plug because its layers of apatite are like those of plugs in being nodular as opposed to the concentric rings of most stones. Careful study of stones for heterogeneous inclusions may help clarify the question of whether BD plugs or overgrowths may be important stone nuclei.

- Mechanisms of plug formation: Crystal deposits in BD and IMCD plugs form in a tubular fluid close to the composition of urine. Thus, one would expect a general correspondence between urine SS and crystal composition. Normals appear to not form deposits and produce a urine with low CaOx SS and no CaP SS. They also have no uric acid. So the lack of deposits is compatible with their generally low or absent SS values. Bypass, renal tubular acidosis and primary hyperoxaluria stone formers have high CaOx SS and form deposits containing CaOx crystals. Brushite patients also have high CaOx SS, and in one deposit from one patient we have observed traces of CaOx. Brushite, cystine, primary hyperthyroidism and renal tubular acidosis stone formers have very high CaP SS and form deposits containing apatite. Thus, one can find a wide range of concordances supporting the notion that high SS promotes intraluminal deposit formation.
- However, small bowel resection, ileostomy and bypass patients have an acidic urine and low CaP SS, but still form abundant apatite BD deposits. Ileostomy stone formers form deposits that contain the sodium and ammonium salts of uric acid, which form at pH of 6 or more, but no detectable traces of uric acid. So in these three types of stone formers, deposits and urine SS are discordant and some additional mechanisms must be assumed to operate.
- Mechanisms of overgrowth formation: Overgrowth on plug surfaces has not been studied even though

Randall recognized the process.[1,2] Like overgrowth on plaque, the only factors that seem available to control overgrowth formation on BD plugs must be the composition, urine SS values and the urine molecules that deposit over plugs to generate the matrix of the overgrowth. The urine molecules that must cover the open face of the BD plug are unknown. Actual plugs with their overgrowth can be harvested and perhaps studied directly in their longitudinal dimension for matrix molecules and their relationship to crystals. Stones have never been studied for their matrix in such an oriented manner.

Supersaturation itself is not sufficient to explain the crystal composition of plugs and overgrowths. This is seen in both brushite and apatite stone formers who have high urine CaP SS with respect to brushite, but the plugs of the former are composed of brushite, CaOx and apatite, whereas those of the latter are pure apatite. Moreover, the overgrowth on plugs in brushite stone formers is BR while it is HA in the apatite stone formers.

Free Stones

- Calyces and pelvis: At surgery one commonly finds a myriad of unattached stones filling calyces and even the renal pelvis with no evidence on the stones of an attachment site. Examples are the CaOx stones in PH1 and obesity bypass, most brushite and apatite stones and all cystine stones. The real problem with determining if a stone formed in free solution is what scientific process would one use to test or falsify this hypothesis. To us this seems an ultimate challenge to the stone research community, and every effort is justified to work out new ways of testing mechanisms of clinical stone formation apart from growth on plaque and possibly as overgrowths on plugs.
- In the case of IMCD microliths, in cystinuria, stagnant urine is available as a breeding ground. But for the rest of stone formers, what would free solution formation mean? To us it would imply nucleation in urine, perhaps within a calyx, with some means for retention so that growth could occur. This theory is very close to the plugging overlay hypothesis; in that the latter holds that tiny overlays are retained and grow. A commonly held speculation is that cell debris is shed from the renal pelvis and serves as an anchor and nucleation site.[59]
- Ductal stones: The primary examples of ductal stones occur in MSKs and cystinuria. In both cases the stones are freely floating in the tubular fluid of IMCD and are round like marbles. In the case of MSK, the stones are composed of mixtures of apatite and CaOx, while the ductal stones in cystinuria are apatite and cystine. Also, in both phenotypes, the surgeon is able to detect these ductal stones and can use a laser to deroof the nephron segment they are located in and allow the stone to be released into the minor calyx.

The mechanism for their growth is not known. Like all supersaturated solutions, urine forms crystals over time. Simple retention within a dilated nephron segment may allow stagnant urine to create nuclei and eventually tiny stones. The numerous urine molecules that delay nucleation, growth, cell attachment and aggregation of crystals may coat the stones, minimizing attachment to epithelium. Both of these assertions are by way of hypotheses for future experimental tests.

PATTERNS OF MINERAL DEPOSIT IN SPECIFIC CLINICAL STONE PHENOTYPES

In this section of the chapter, 11 different stone phenotypes (*see* Table 5.1) will be characterized by their endoscopic and histopathologic changes detected in papillary and cortical biopsies obtained primarily at the time of PNL for stone removal and a few during URS.

IDIOPATHIC CALCIUM OXALATE STONE FORMS (ICSF)

About 75–85% of CaOx stone formers suffer from no systemic diseases like PHPT, sarcoidosis, vitamin D excess or renal tubular acidosis and as such were termed ICSF. In our studies of this group, we required each enrolled patient to be an active stone former (at least two stones) with no stones containing uric acid, struvite, cystine or over 50% calcium phosphate. In addition, all of the ICSF patients we studied presented with IH and were primarily male patients. All available medical records were collected and reviewed; two 24-hour urine samples were analyzed; a complete stone analysis including micro-CT analyses was performed; a recent serum sample was analyzed; and appropriate X-rays and CT scans were studied. These patients were undergoing surgery for their stone burden, usually by PNL until recently when the majority of patients have undergone URS. At the time of their stone removal, all papillae were video-recorded using a high-resolution endoscope followed by biopsies of selected papillae and outer cortex. These analytical protocols were performed on all stone formers studied for the 11 phenotypes.

In the earlier sections of this chapter, a detailed description was presented on the structural features of interstitial (white, Randall's) plaque; those observations will not be repeated here. However, the primary urologic and anatomic features of the ICSF kidney will be summarized. High-resolution endoscopy detected the unique feature of ICSF stone formers, individual stones attached to the papilla usually at its tip (Figs. 5.11, 5.14 and 5.27A to I) and focal sites of a whitish, subepithelial material (*see* Fig. 5.4).[7] When the attached stones were carefully detached from the papilla, we noted that they appeared to be attached to regions of white plaque. When regions of white plaque were biopsied and studied for histopathology, and those regions with the least amount of plaque were analyzed, individual deposits of alternating layers of matrix and mineral were noted in the basement membranes of the thin loops of Henle (*see* Fig. 5.4). Subsequently, these deposits were noted in the interstitial space adhered to collagen fibers and filling this space with a syncytium in which islands of crystals float in an organic sea as far down as the basal side of the urothelium covering the papilla (*see* Figs. 5.4 and 5.6). It is our hypothesis that under conditions we do not understand, there is a breach in the epithelial layer permitting exposure of the sites of interstitial plaque to the urine in the minor calyx resulting, sometimes, in the formation of an overgrowth region that can develop into a clinical stone (*see* Figs. 5.3, 5.14, 5.15 and 5.19).[27]

Histopathologic examination of papillary interstitial tissue and cortical biopsies revealed no intraluminal crystals in any tubular segments, no evidence of cell injury and no tissue inflammation, despite sites of interstitial plaque. Using papillary biopsy material, the mineral composition of the interstitial plaque was determined to be biological hydroxyapatite, that same mineral of bone. The nature of the interstitial plaque being like bone might explain the lack of pathologic tissue changes at sites of plaque. The resemblance of early sites of plaque to early bone formation suggested to us that plaque might have an osteogenic origin, so we tested for the presence of two critical translational factors in osteogenesis, Runx2 and Osterix. Neither factor was found expressed in the tissues of the inner medulla (Figs. 5.32A to L), strongly suggesting that interstitial plaque is not formed by mechanisms that control bone formation.[60]

Although several groups reported observing attached stones in ICSF patients, Miller et al. conducted a critical set of studies to test the hypothesis that CaOx stone detected in ICSF stone formers forms attached to sites of interstitial plaque.[19] This study and several additional studies testing this hypothesis were reviewed earlier in this chapter, so will not be repeated here. The consensus from these studies is that there is a general rule for stone growth in ICSF patients—i.e. growth on plaque appears to be a main mechanism of stone formation in ICSF stone formers, the most common type of patient encountered in clinical practice.

Other characteristics of ICSF stone formers are that their plaque abundance, measured from intraoperative images, varies directly with urine calcium excretion and inversely with urine volume and pH.[21] Also, the number of stone former by a stone former was found to be proportional to percent plaque coverage in those ICSF patients.[22] The link to higher urine calcium seems important because it mostly arises, in stone formers, from genetic so-called IH. These data suggest that IH patients with low urine volumes and urine of a mildly acidic level are mostly at risk for plaque and consequently kidney stones.

We recently obtained a group of five ICSF patients with numerous attached stones to Randall's plaque that also possessed intraluminal plugs in IMCD and BD seen as yellow plaque (Fig. 5.22, ICSF+). Preliminary observations suggest the plugs to contain apatite while an initial analysis of their clinical data suggests they might have a higher urinary pH.

Intestinal Bypass Surgery for Obesity

To contrast with findings in ICSF patients, we enrolled a group of patients with stones due to obesity-related bypass procedures. Endoscopy at the time of their PNL for stone removal found the papillary surface of all these patients to have a normal conical shape and no areas of Randall's plaque (Fig. 5.27B). However, a few openings of BD were dilated and surrounded by a few, small nodules. Histopathology detected Yasue-positive intraluminal deposits in a few IMCDs as far down as the BD with the mineral protruding into the urinary space (Fig. 5.27C). Crystal deposits were not found in the interstitial space or surrounding the thin loops of Henle.

Crystal deposition varied from partial or complete plugging IMCD and BD (Fig. 5.21). Areas of minimal crystal deposition formed a scrim over the apical surfaces of normal-appearing cells (*see* Fig. 5.21A). These initial crystals were CaOx (*see* Fig. 5.21B); however, the large

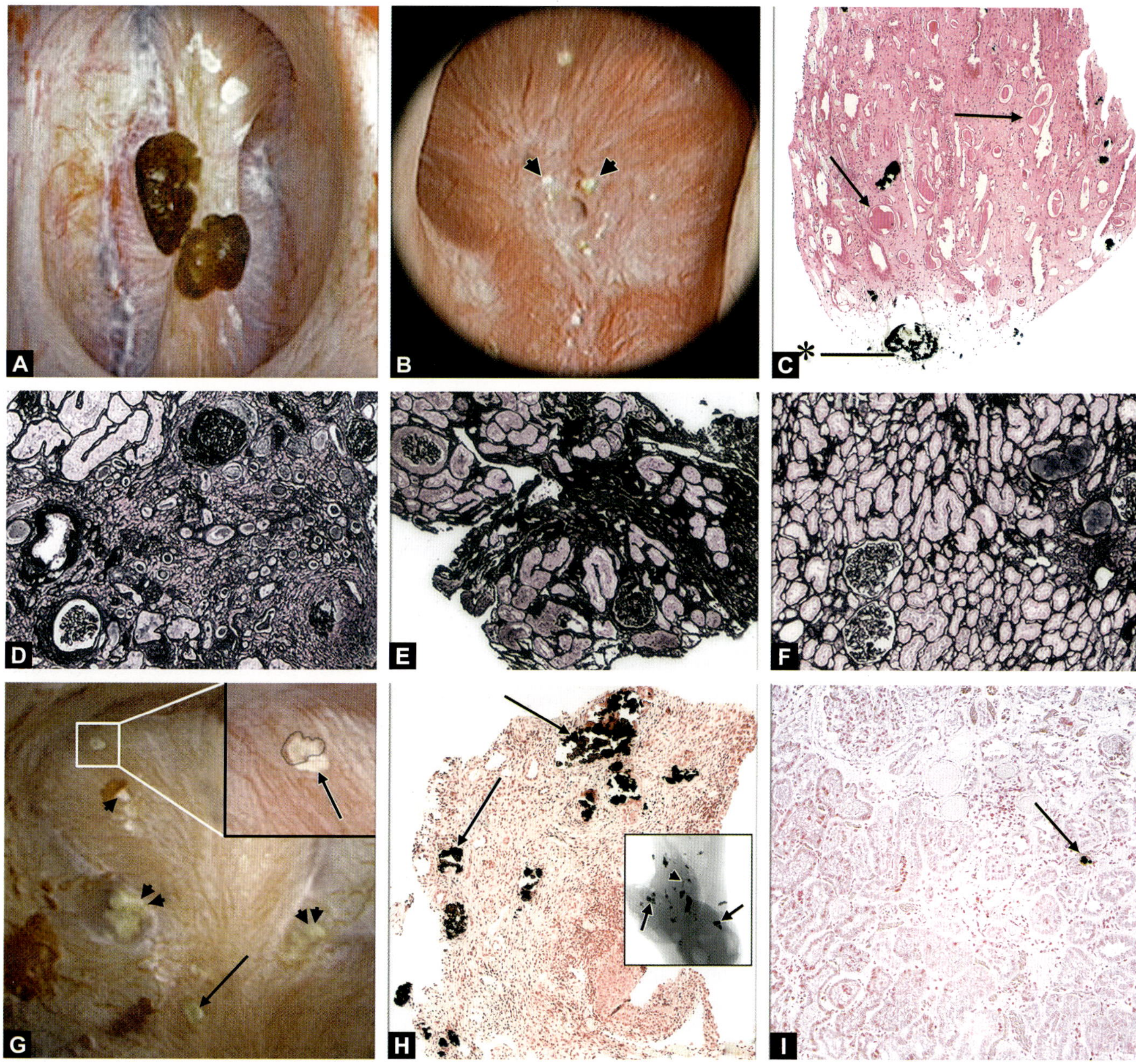

Figs. 5.27A to I: Endoscopic and histopathologic images of papillary biopsies from idiopathic calcium oxalate stone former (ICSF), bypass, brushite and primary hyperparathyroidism (PHPT) stone formers. Panel (A) shows a papilla from an ICSF stone former with idiopathic hypercalciuria (IH). Two large, brownish, 3- to 4-mm calcium oxalate (CaOx) stones are seen attached to the papillary tip region. Just above these stones are several sites of interstitial (white) plaque. Panel (B) is an example of a papilla from an intestinal bypass stone former, revealing no regions of white plaque but instead several nodular-appearing structures (arrowheads) near a dilated opening of a duct of Bellini. A light microscopic histopathologic image (C) of the same papilla shows several dilated inner medullary collecting ducts (IMCD) (arrows) with cast material and regions of fibrosis surrounding crystal filled tubules. A large intraluminal plug is seen near the opening of a duct of Bellini (BD, asterisk). Panels (D) to (F) are cortical biopsies from a brushite stone former (D) and apatite stone formers (E and F), seen by light microscopy. Extensive glomerulosclerosis and interstitial fibrosis are seen in brushite stone formers (D) while the apatite stone formers showed a more normal (F) to moderate level of change. Panels (G) to (I) are from a primary hyperparathyroid stone former. Panel (G) shows areas of yellow plaque in IMCD (double arrowheads), and white (Randall's) plaque (single arrowhead). A dilated BD has a crystalline plug (arrow) protruding from its opening. A stone attached at an area of white plaque (within the white box) is magnified in the inset; the stone is outlined within the inset by a black dotted overlay and the plaque border is indicated with an arrow. Panel (H) is a Yasue-stained section of the papilla in panel (G) showing large IMCD intraluminal deposits (arrows). The micro-CT inset reveals a number of large deposits (arrows) and sites of Randall's plaque (arrowhead). Panel (I) is also a Yasue-stained cortical biopsy from the same patients showing an intraluminal deposit in a cortical collecting duct (arrow).

deposits were found to be hydroxyapatite by micro-FTIR. As the intraluminal deposits increased in size, clear cell injury was always detected to complete cell loss as the tubular lumen was completely filled (*see* Fig. 5.21C). Plugged tubules were always surrounded by a region of interstitial fibrosis. No pathologic changes were noted in the cortical biopsies.

One of the interesting findings in these patients was the hydroxyapatite mineral deposits in the IMCD and BD. We hypothesized them to be CaOx because of the pH of the ultrafiltrate. This finding suggests that the lining cells were injured, possibly from the crystals in the urine. The injury to complete denuding of IMCD cells could result in a loss of pH control, which would allow the retention of the apatite crystals. This idea has support from hyaluronan studies on the papillary biopsies of these patients.[48] Hyaluronan positive staining was detected in plugged IMCD with injured cells as well as in nearby normal-appearing cells (Fig. 5.21E and F). Because of a lack of interstitial plaque, stone formation in intestinal bypass stone formers must be from entirely different mechanisms that we do not understand at this time.

Brushite Stone Formers

Our endoscopic and histopathologic findings on ICSF and intestinal bypass patients with stones show that these two kinds of CaOx stone formers display specific pathologies and different mechanisms for stone formation. Next, we studied a group of stone formers who form calcium phosphate stones, in particular brushite ($CaHPO_4$)-containing stones.[32] About 15% of stone formers produce predominantly (>50%) calcium phosphate.

In an earlier section of this chapter on plugs, the patterns of yellow plaque were described in detail, so the description will be brief here. In these patients, high-resolution endoscopy was used to view and video all accessible papillae in a kidney. We observed three different patterns of deposits in all brushite patients. Type 1 is suburothelial white plaque or Randall's plaque described in ICSF stone formers (Fig. 5.23A). We have seen three stones attached to sites of Randall's plaque, and all three stones were CaOx. Type 2 plaque is large yellow deposits seen filling dilated BD and also protruding from dilated openings of BD, forming an overgrowth (Figs. 5.23A and B). Largely dilated BDs were seen as depressions or pits. Randall had already described this type of mineral deposition and termed it type II plaque.[1,2] The third type (type 3) was suburothelial deposits of variable size seen on the sides of the papilla away from BD (Fig. 5.23B). Type 3 plaque was located in the lumen of IMCD and/or BD (Figs. 5.23C and D). These intraluminal deposits at times enlarged an IMCD 20× normal (*see* Fig. 5.23C) while nearby tubules appeared normal. The only other literature that had previously described this type 3 pattern was a single patient with acute lymphatic leukemia and uric acid nephropathy.[61] Many papillae in the kidney of a brushite patient possess all three plaque patterns, which gives the brushite stone former unique endoscopic characteristics that can be recognized by the urologist. In contrast, some papillae showed minimal changes determined by endoscopy and histopathology.

Tubular plugging was focal in nature and varied between patients (Figs. 5.23C and 5.24B). Some brushite patients had minor histopathologic changes in the inner medulla while others possessed extensive damage. Those IMCD and BD that had extensive plugging also showed severe cell injury to complete cell loss (*see* Fig. 5.25A to C). Although the primary mineral type in IMCD is apatite, BD plugs can have a mixture of apatite, brushite and CaOx (*see* Fig. 5.22). All severely plugged tubules were encased in fields of extensive interstitial fibrosis with an occasional giant cell (*see* Fig. 5.25C). Because some brushite stone formers receive many SWL procedures (20–30 treatments) and we know that SWL injures the renal medulla, it is possible that some of the papillary changes seen in brushite patients were induced by SWL. In addition, we have recently shown in an animal model that SWL can induce an increase urinary pH, which would support apatite deposit formation and growth.[62]

Cortical biopsies of brushite stone formers revealed severe glomerular, tubular and interstitial fibrosis in the majority of patients studied. Glomerulosclerosis had progressed to moderate or global (*see* Figs. 5.27D to F). All brushite stone formers displayed advanced tubular atrophy and interstitial fibrosis (Figs. 5.27D to F). Of great interest is that the degree of papillary change did not correlate with the level of cortical damage. In addition, the degree of cortical damage did not correlate with the level of renal function glomerular filration rate (GFR).

We discovered overgrowths on the distal ends of BD plugs first in brushite stone formers (*see* Fig. 5.26C and Table 5.2). These initially viewed overgrowths were only a few mm in size; however, we have recently found one about 4 mm, suggesting that it could present as a clinical stone. Mineral composition of these overgrowths is a mixture of apatite, CaOx and brushite, a similar composition of the BD plugs.

PHPT

Primary hyperparathyroidism with kidney stones spans a spectrum from CaOx to calcium phosphate stones. Thus, we expected our PHPT stone formers who form calcium phosphate stones to have endoscopic and histopathologic changes similar to brushite and apatite stone formers. However, surprisingly, those PHPT patients forming apatite stones possessed both IMCD plugging with associated papillary injury and interstitial fibrosis as well as abundant interstitial plaque with attached stones.[44] Our PHPT patients had a range of stone compositions from predominantly CaOx admixed with apatite, brushite with apatite and primarily apatite with brushite or CaOx.

By endoscopy, papilla varied from a normal appearance to showing extensive changes that included areas of yellow plaque on the side of the papilla as well as filling dilated BD, overgrowths on BD plugs, heavy regions of white plaque and several attached stones (*see* Fig. 5.27B). All of these changes could be seen on the same papilla or scattered between papillae. Occasionally, the papilla was flattened with numerous dilated BD.

Histopathologic examination of cortical and papillary Yasue-stained sections revealed apatite intraluminal deposits scattered along the cortical collecting ducts, outer medullary collecting ducts, IMCD and BD (Figs. 5.27H and I). All plugged tubules were surrounded by interstitial fibrosis but not as extensively as reported in brushite stone formers. The number of plugged medullary tubules varied greatly between patients, some with numerous deposits and others with only a few (Fig. 5.24C). Some plugs were very large in size, the largest of all phenotypes studied. The abundance of white plaque also varied greatly between patients, with some PHPT stone formers possessing as much white plaque as ICSF stone formers with IH. Cortical changes were minimal.

Overgrowths on the distal end of BD were seen but usually small in size, with a mineral composition primarily of apatite (Fig. 5.26E). The structure of the mineral layers of the overgrowth and BD plugs of PHPT stone formers was unique in that they had a globular organization rather than layers.

Distal Renal Tubular Acidosis

In these patients we are focusing on apatite stone formers with the syndrome of distal renal tubular acidosis (dRTA). Because dRTA is a specific form of renal dysfunction, we expected a unique pathology of its own. Prior studies on dRTA have focused on cortical biopsies while we included cortical and papillary studies for the first time as well as high-resolution endoscopy. It is important to state that all of our patients had overt nephrocalcinosis. Although the majority of the stones from these patients were 100% apatite, some had an admixture of apatite and CaOx but no brushite. If one compares a CT of a kidney for a dRTA patient before and after PNL, it is clear that these patients have a distinct nephrocalcinosis but there may be surgically removable stones during PNL, especially in patients with well-preserved renal function.

Endoscopy showed a variation in severity of the papilla. Some patients had rather normal-appearing papilla while the majority of patients had severely damaged papilla detected by flattening, retraction and a whitish appearance to the papillary surface (Fig. 5.28A). The severely damaged papilla possessed numerous BD plugs seen as yellow plaque, some with small overgrowths (Fig. 5.28A). Regions of white plaque were not obvious, and no attached stones were found.

Histopathologic examination of Yasue-stained papillary biopsies found minimal plugging and interstitial fibrosis in those papillae that appeared normal. However, the severely damaged papilla revealed numerous plugged IMDC, suggesting a diffuse pattern of plugging (Figs. 5.24F and 5.28B). Extensive cell injury was noted in the lining cells of the plugged IMCD and BD with extensive interstitial fibrosis encasing the plugged tubules. The interstitial fibrosis was noted throughout the interstitium of the inner medulla in a diffuse pattern. Many plugged IMCD and BD showed a complete loss of cells (Fig. 5.28C). The primary mineral type of the intraluminal deposits was apatite; however, a mixed CaOx/apatite deposit was identified in the patient who had a pelvic stone of the same mixture.

Cortical biopsies detected mild-to-advanced glomerular disease, mild interstitial fibrosis and atrophy. No intraluminal deposits were found in any cortical tubule. Regions of chronic inflammation were noted with lymphoid infiltration.

The pattern of nephrocalcinosis was supported by our histopathologic findings and is consistent with their non-anion gap metabolic acidosis accompanied by an alkaline urine pH. Because this syndrome affects all segments of the distal nephron, one would expect a diffuse pattern of intraluminal plugging, and this is what we found in our papillary biopsies.

Ileostomy

All of our ileostomy patients had undergone ileostomy and total colectomy.[31] By endoscopy, all patients presented

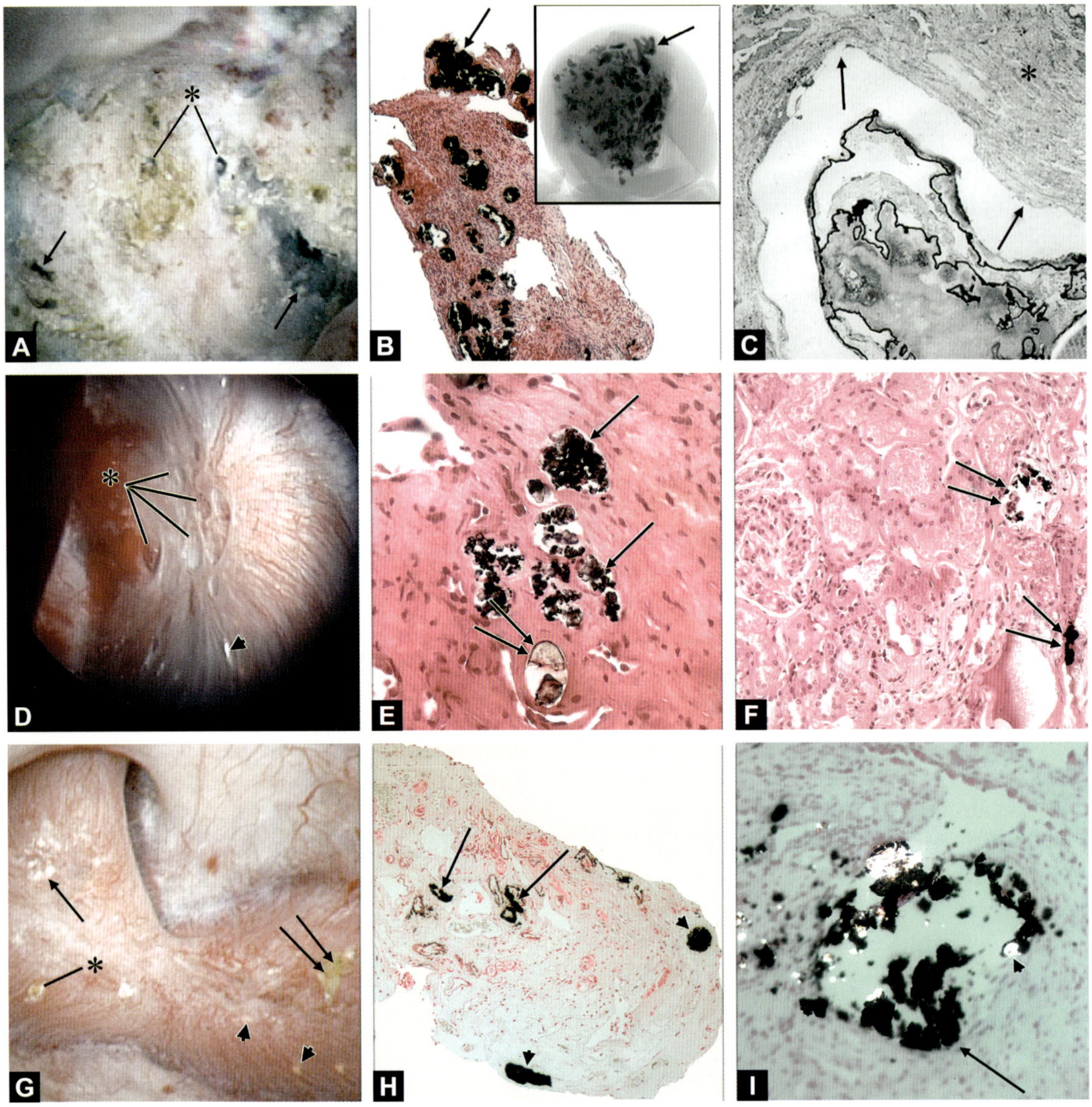

Figs. 5.28A to I: Endoscopic and histopathologic images of papillary biopsies from distal renal tubular acidosis, ileostomy and small bowel resection stone formers. Panels (A) to (C) are from renal tubular acidosis (RTA) stone formers, (D) to (F) are from ileostomy stone formers, and (G) to (I) are from small bowel resection (SBR) stone formers. The RTA stone formers show a range of papillary changes from minimal (not shown) to extremely severe (A), revealing retraction and flattening of the papilla, loss of normal architecture, multiple dilated ducts of Bellini (BD) that produce a pitted appearance (arrows), some with protruding mineral deposits (asterisk) and a whitish, thickened membrane appearance. Histopathology of Yasue-stained papillary sections shows diffuse inner medullary collecting ducts (IMCD) intraluminal plugs (arrows) with extensive fibrosis. The inset of a micro-CT image in panel (B) is of a papillary biopsy from an RTA stone former showing numerous, densely packed deposits. Panel (C) is a transmission electron microscopic image of a papillary biopsy revealing complete loss of cells (arrows) and extensive interstitial fibrosis (asterisk). Ileostomy stone patients showed a range of papillary changes from normal to flattened and retracted detected by endoscopy (D). There were also dilated opening of BD (asterisk) in normal and deformed papilla with varying amounts of yellow (arrowhead) and white (not shown) plaque. The light microscopic morphology of Yasue-stained sections (E) commonly showed numerous dilated IMCD (arrows) and BD filled with mineral. These tubules were always associated with a loss of lining cells and surrounded by interstitial fibrosis. Occasionally, sites of Randall's plaque were found (not shown). Some tubules possessed Yasue-positive (arrows) and Yasue-negative (double arrow) material. Cortical biopsies also detected Yasue-positive material in cortical collecting ducts (F, double arrows). Generally, papilla from stone patients with small bowel resection showed by endoscopy (G) areas of white (arrow) and yellow (arrowheads) plaque, attached stones to white plaque (double arrow) and BD plugs (asterisk). (H) Yasue-positive light microscopic sections revealed areas of white plaque (arrows) and plugged IMCD (arrowheads). (I) Using polarized optics, some IMCD intraluminal deposits contained nonbirefringent (arrow) and birefringent (arrowhead) material.

papilla with varying amounts of both white and yellow plaques and some dilated BD (Fig. 5.28D). Crystals were occasionally seen as overgrowths at openings of dilated BD. The percentage of abnormal papilla varied among patients from 0% to 25% with a few showing flattening and retraction. Attached stones were seen, but not in every ileostomy patient.

Histopathologic examination of Yasue-stained cortical and papillary biopsies found intraluminal deposits in a few cortical collecting ducts, thin loops of Henle, many IMCD and BD (Fig. 5.28E and F). Small-to-large crystal deposits filled IMCD tubular lumens (Figs. 5.24D and 5.28E). Injury to lining cells was detected in the completely plugged IMCD and BD. The mineral composition of most tubules was apatite except for BD plugs, which contained a mixture of apatite with sodium acid urate and ammonium acid urate (Fig. 5.28E).

Overgrowths on the distal ends of BD plugs were found and analyzed (*see* Fig. 5.26D). These overgrowths were not common. The BD plugs were a mixture of sodium acid urate and ammonium acid urate while the plug was CaOx.

These patients present unique issues for both stone formation and tubular plugging. There appears to be no reasonable explanation for the formation of plugs in these patients. This resembles our findings in intestinal bypass stone formers except that urine pH is even lower in these patients. The most reasonable assumption is that local tubular fluid pH in some ducts departs radically from that of the bulk urine pH and is high enough to make apatite a stable phase. White plaque was present as well as attached stone despite their acidic urine. These findings confirm our earlier data in that low urine volumes (known for ileostomy patients) and pH would be expected to cause plaque, and high urine SSs are present to support CaOx overgrwoth.

Small Bowel Resection

We studied 11 patients with renal stones following small bowel resection, including 10 with Crohn's disease and 1 resection in infancy for unknown causes.[33] The predominant stone was CaOx. These patients presented a risk for stone due to their hyperoxaluria, and acidic urine of reduced volume.

Endoscopy revealed large sites of white plaque with and without attached stones (Fig. 5.28G). All attached stones were composed of CaOx. In some regions, the number of attached stones to plaque was similar to that found in the ICSF stone formers. Regions of yellow plaque were also ample, suggesting IMCD plugs. Dilated BDs with and without plugs were abundant in the most severely damaged papillae. No overgrowth on BD plugs was observed.

Histopathologic examination of Yasue-stained papillary sections displayed large amount of interstitial plaque (Fig. 5.28H). Plugging was detected in both IMCD and BD. The mineral type was determined to be a mixture of apatite and CaOx. The density of plugging was less than that detected in ileostomy, but some deposits were so large that they compared to those of dRTA and brushite stone formers. Extensive cell injury and loss was common in those IMCD and BD completely plugged (Figs. 5.28H and I).

Plaque abundance is not surprising in these patients as urine pH was low and urine volume was often low. In fact, urine volumes would have been very low during episodes of diarrhea. Stone are not problematic either; in that CaOx SS was high and we found CaOx stones growing over regions of apatite plaque.

The major issue is explaining apatite plugs in IMCD and BD when urine SS would lead one to predict CaOx or uric acid deposits. This was true for the intestinal bypass and ileostomy stone formers. For ileostomy patients the effects would predictably be alkali loss and volume loss with very acid-scanty urine favoring uric acid and CaOx. For bypass and small bowel resection patients, prone to enteric hyperoxaluria, the main prediction would be extreme CaOx SS. The latter could seed IMCD or BD with initial CaOx plugs and entrain the mechanisms we have already outlined.

Cystine Stone Formers

Cystinuria is a disease arising from genetic defects of dibasic amino-acid transporters that permit excessive cystine excretion. The cystine crystallizes and forms stones. Because cystine stones are frequently large and are resistant to SWL, surgical treatments are common. Cystinuric patients are over-represented among stone formers who have lost a kidney.

Papillary morphology revealed by endoscopy varied widely from normal to extreme damage, including flattening and pallor with enlarged BD with and without plugs (Fig. 5.29A).[45] Some BD plugs revealed overgrowths of cystine (Fig. 5.29A). These plugs were not firmly attached to renal tissue, so the surgeon can easily remove the plugs at the time of PNL. Scanty regions of white plaque were noted, and no attached stones were observed. Some papillae had a billowy appearance due to the presence of free-floating tubular deposits in IMCD (Fig. 5.29B). These deposits can be deroofed, allowing the ductal stone to be released into the urine (Fig. 5.29B, inset).

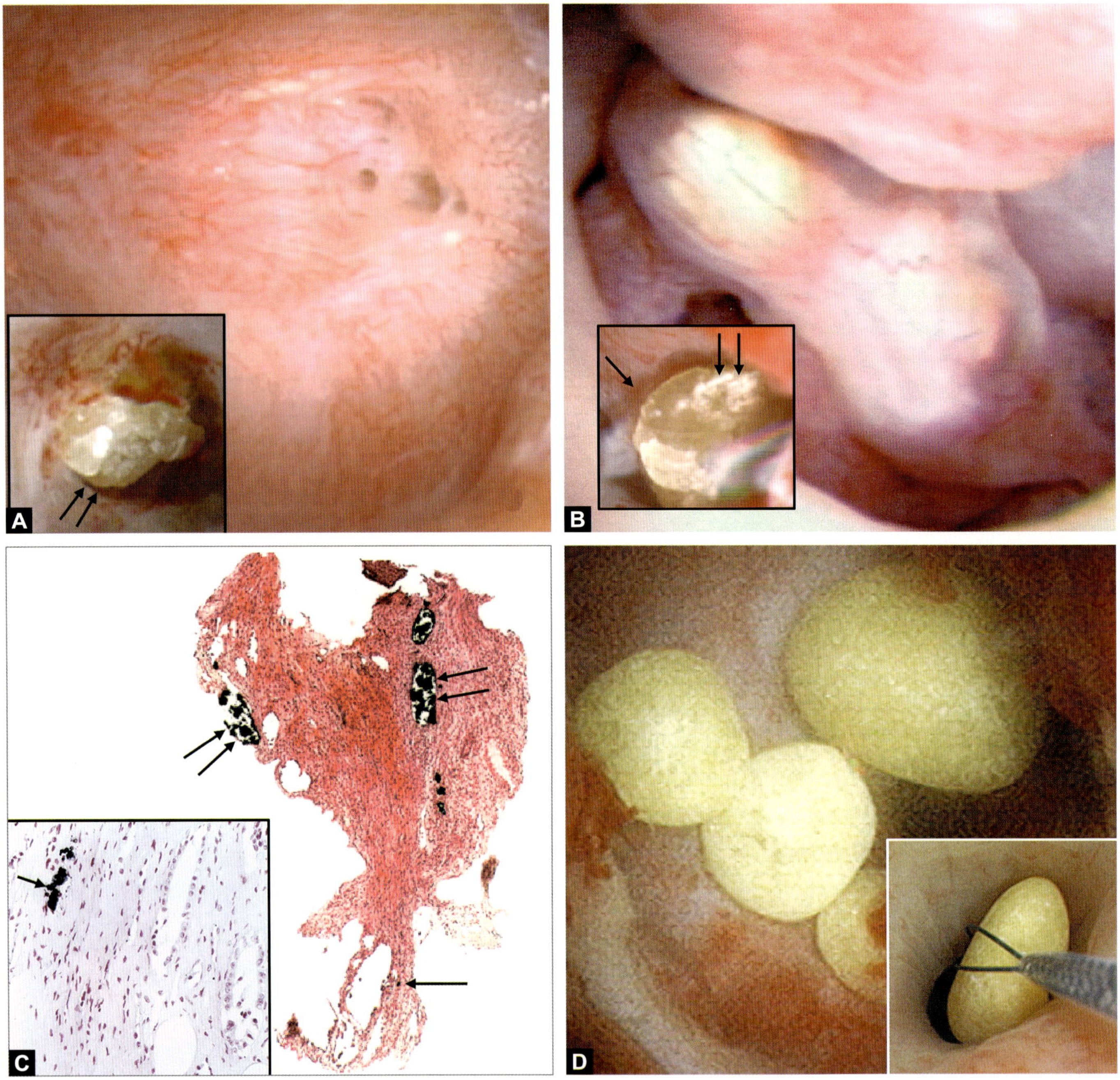

Figs. 5.29A to D: Endoscopic and histopathologic images of papillary biopsies from stone formers with cystinuria. Papillary morphology varied from normal to flattened with greatly enlarged opening of BD (A, arrows) surrounded by sites of white plaque (arrowhead). Some dilated ducts of Bellini (BD) contained overgrowths protruding into the urinary space from the distal end of plugs [inset in panel (A), double arrow]. Endoscopy also revealed sites of large mineral deposits within inner medullary collecting ducts (IMCD). These sites made the papilla look pillow like, and the mineral appeared whitish through the epithelial lining of the papilla. Using a laser, the surgeon can deroof (inset in panel (B), double arrow) the ductal stone (arrow), allowing it to be easily released into the urinary space of the minor calyx. Papillary histopathology of cystine stone formers showed numerous intraluminal plugged IMCD (double arrows) and a few thin loops of Henle (C and inset, arrows) surrounded by extensive interstitial fibrosis. Cystine stones found in the renal collection system are oval to round (D) and freely floating in the urine. They can be easily removed by a basket during PNL [inset in panel (D)].

Histopathologic examination of Yasue-stained papillary biopsies displayed plugging, dilatation and injury of IMCD (Fig. 5.29C). Plugging was also detected in numerous thin loops of Henle with a mineral composition of apatite (Fig. 5.29C, inset). The BD plugging was common. In some BDs, epithelial cells were found within the tubular lumen where they surrounded masses of crystals. These migrated BD cells appear to have altered their polarity because the cells have attached themselves to the crystal mass via their basement membrane. The mineral in these plugged BDs appears to be cystine, not apatite. Interstitial fibrosis was commonly seen at regions of plugged tubules.

Cortical biopsies varied from normal anatomy to regions of glomerular obsolescences, tubular atrophy and interstitial fibrosis. In addition, we detected Yasue-positive material in the basement membranes of the parietal layer of the glomerulus and distal convoluted tubule. The deposits had the appearance of apatite.

Cystine stones are generally seen floating in the urinary space and can easily be removed at the time of PNL (Fig. 5.29D). Whether the stones form freely in the minor calyx has not been determined. It is possible that the overgrowths with their BD plugs fall from the dilated openings of BD because they are loosely held in place. These overgrowths could progress in size to form free-floating cystine stones. To date no one has evidence for this idea.

Apatite Stone Formers

Our previous work has shown that stone formers who form calcium phosphate stones that contain any brushite have a distinctive renal histopathology and endoscopic anatomy when compared to ICSF and intestinal bypass stone formers. The phenotype that will be studied here represents a different group of idiopathic calcium phosphate stone formers: those forming stones containing primarily hydroxyapatite (>50% apatite) and no brushite. These patients are primarily female patients.

Our main finding from this study is that apatite and brushite stone formers differ greatly from each other and both differ substantially from ICSF.[44] Endoscopic examination of papilla from all apatite stone formers studied displayed tubular plugging, regions of yellow and white plaques, dilated BD with and without overgrowths and attached stones to sites of Randall's plaque (Figs. 5.30A to C). The degree of papillary change divided these patients into two groups: those with very mild change with a few pelvic stones and those with severe papillary damage with numerous pelvic stones. Only one patient had abundant white plaque and attached stones while most apatite stone formers had scanty white plaque and no attached stones. Yellow plaque was common in all papillae from all kidneys. Those patients with extensive papillary changes also presented flattening and retraction of the papilla.

Although overgrowths on distal end of BD plugs were not common, they were detected (*see* Fig. 5.26B). Their size was about 2–3 mm, with apatite as the primary composition of the BD plug. The overgrowth was mostly apatite with a thin surface layer of CaOx. This is a very different mineral pattern than that described for these structures in brushite stone formers (*see* Fig. 5.26C).

Histopathologic examination of papillary tissues stained with the Yasue method revealed two different types of interstitial plaque (Figs. 5.30D to F), intraluminal plugging of varying numbers of IMCD and BD as well as interstitial fibrosis around plugged tubules (Fig. 5.30G). The first type of interstitial plaque is the routine sites of Randall's plaque composed of numerous microspherules and organic matrix (Fig. 5.30D). The second type of interstitial plaque was termed novel interstitial plaque structures (NIPS), which appeared to replace sites of Randall's plaque (Fig. 5.30E). Novel interstitial plaque structures were plate-like-shaped deposits surrounding the lumens of capillaries and thin loops of Henle. The mineral type was biological hydroxyapatite, just like Randall's plaque. Novel interstitial plaque structures did not expand or distort the interstitial space but simply filled it. Large regions of NIPS lacked the matrix layer seen with Randall's plaque (Fig. 5.30F). By TEM, regions of NIPS were noted by its large crystals to matrix ratio (Figs. 5.30H and I).

Intraluminal plugs composited of hydroxyapatite were noted in both IMCD and BD. Those apatite stone formers with minimal papillary change displayed few plugged tubules while those with severe papillary damage have numerous intraluminal plugs. The fraction of papillary surface area covered by yellow plaque correlated significantly with the number of deposits. This suggested that in apatite stone formers the amount of yellow plaque seen at the time of surgery would be a practical gauge of determining deposit number in papillary tissue. Yellow plaque was more abundant in apatite versus brushite stone formers. The size of intraluminal deposits as determined by micro-CT was smaller in apatite versus brushite stone formers while deposit density was similar between these two groups. Deposit size correlated with deposit number in the brushites but not apatite stone formers.

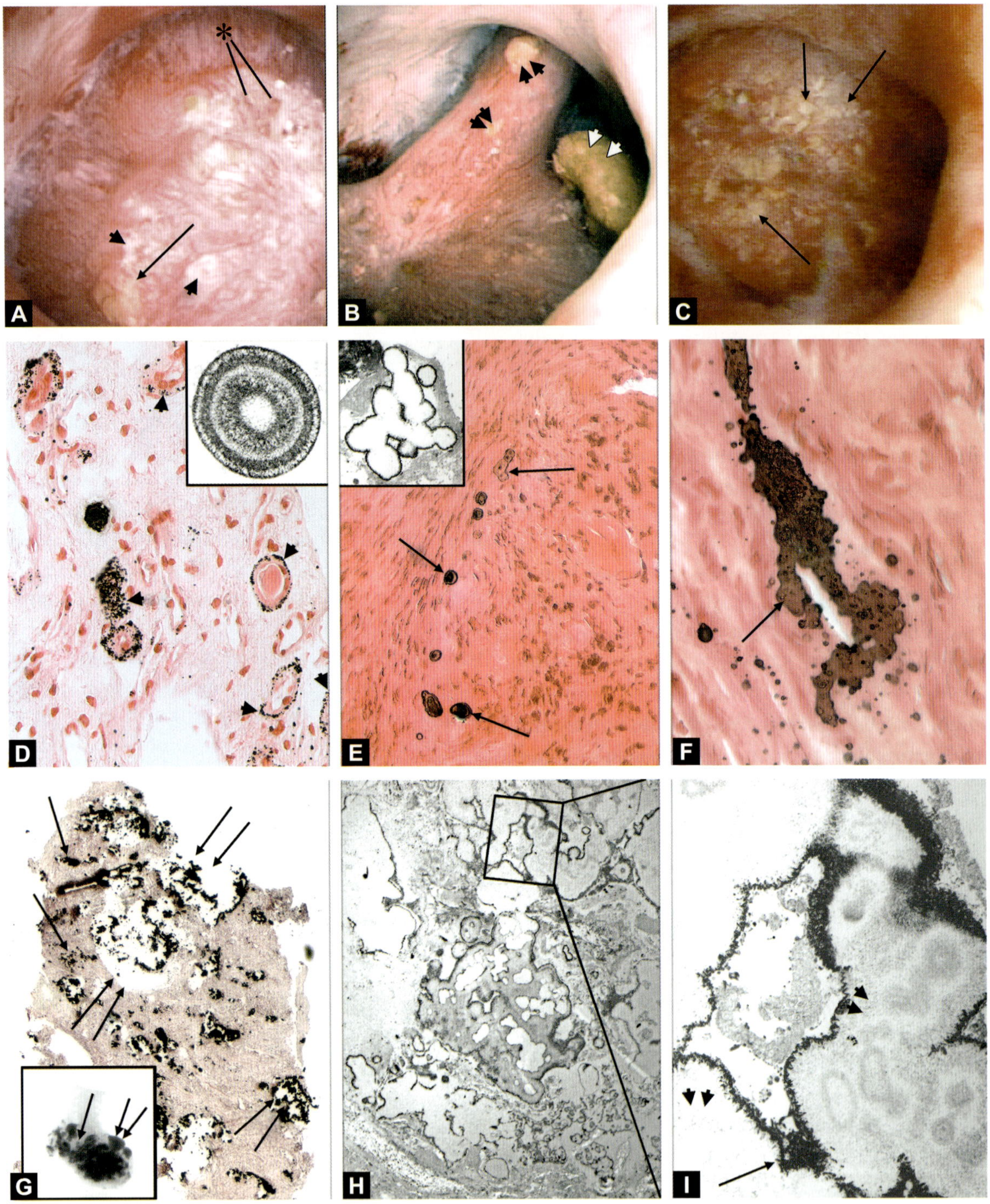

Figs. 5.30A to I: Endoscopic and histopathologic images of papillary biopsies from calcium phosphate stone formers. Endoscopy revealed a spectrum of morphological changes to the papilla of apatite stone formers (A to C), ranging from a normal conical shape (not shown) to flattened with numerous sites of white plaque (arrowheads), an occasional site of yellow plaque (A and C, arrows) and site overgrowth (asterisk) protruding from the distal end of ducts of Bellini (BD) plug. Attached stones (B, double arrowheads) to white plaque were commonly seen also. Yasue-positive light microscopic sections revealed two types of interstitial plaque: (1) sites of Randall's plaque (D, arrowheads); inset shows single plaque deposit by transmission electron microscopy (TEM) and (2) sites of novel interstitial plaque structures (NIPS) (E and F, arrows). The inset in panel (E) shows a site of NIPS by TEM. Numerous intraluminal inner medullary collecting ducts (IMCD) and BD plugs (G, double arrows) and sites of NIPS (arrows) were noted in Yasue-stained section. By TEM (H and I), the NIPS deposits were characterized by multiple regions of large crystalline material (I, arrowheads) encased in a thin electron dense matrix layer (I, arrows). The boxed area with lines seen in panel H represents the site of the enlarged region seen in panel I.

Cortical biopsies revealed rather mild-to-moderate changes in glomeruli, interstitial fibrosis levels and tubular atrophy (Figs. 5.27E and F). Perhaps of greatest clinical importance is that cortical pathology is distinctly greater in brushite than apatite stone formers.

The differing patterns of intraluminal deposits, papillary injury, white plaque abundance, production of NIPS and cortical injury suggest that brushite and apatite stone formers are not simply variations of a single disease but rather two distinct and separate diseases, and both differ from ICSF.

In trying to explain why tubular plugs are less numerous in brushite than apatite and why the mineral is apatite and not brushite, we have suggested that tissue injury related to SWL, obstruction of PNL might be the cause. These treatment procedures could impair local tubular acidification so that intratubular pH increases markedly and apatite deposits form despite inhibitors because of the extreme insolubility of apatite at high pH. The large size and focal distribution of plugs in brushite patients may reflect their formation in damaged tissue. In support of a role for injury, we have found that SWL rates in brushite exceed those of apatite stone formers.[63] Cell injury may also explain the greater cortical fibrosis and tubular atrophy in brushite stone formers.

Primary Hyperoxaluria Type 1

We studied cortical and papillary biopsies from two PH1 patients with preserved renal function and seven native kidneys removed from four PH1 patients at the time of transplant, after short-term and/or long-term dialysis.[47] Routine intraoperative endoscopy was performed on the two PH1 patients with preserved renal function while ex vivo endoscopy was used on the kidneys from PH1 patients with ESRD.

Intraoperative endoscopy of the two preserved PH1 patients revealed normal to slightly flattened papilla with a few dilated BDs with and without mineral plugs and sites of yellow plaque (Figs. 5.31A and B). Similar observations were found on the papilla from the PH1 patient with ESRD (Fig. 5.31C). In general, papilla from both groups appeared rather normal.

Histopathologic examination of Yasue-stained papillary sections from the PH1 patients with preserved renal function detected varying sized intraluminal deposits in a few IMCD and BD (Fig. 5.31C). These deposits were all composed of CaOx. Surprisingly, the entire interstitium of the papillary biopsy showed extensive interstitial fibrosis, a degree of change not seen in any other stone phenotypes (Fig. 5.31). All plugged tubules displayed extensive cell injury and loss (Figs. 5.31D and E). To determine the extent of cell injury in all IMCDs and BDs, sections were stained with hyaluronan. Hyaluronan stained all plugged tubules and a majority of nearby tubules (Fig. 5.31F). Cortical biopsies from these same patients revealed normal-appearing glomeruli and proximal tubules (Fig. 5.31G). Occasionally, however, small birefringent crystals were noted at the brush border of a few otherwise normal-appearing proximal tubules (Fig. 5.31H).

Histopathologic examination of Yasue-stained papillary sections from the PH1 patients with ESRD showed extensive tubular plugging extending from the renal capsule to the papillary tip. All deposits were composed of CaOx. Deposits were particularly dense in the S_3 segments of the proximal tubule and IMCD (Fig. 5.31I). The PH1 with short ESRD showed CaOx deposits and hyaluronan staining particularly at the corticomedullary junction in distal proximal tubules while cortical collecting ducts were spared. Longer ESRD showed widespread cortical CaOx deposits.

Medullary Sponge Kidney Disease

Medullary sponge kidney disease is associated with recurrent stone formation, but the clinical phenotype is unclear because patients with other disorders may be incorrectly labeled as MSK. Therefore, we studied all potential MSK patients using endoscopy and papillary biopsies and used the well-known triad of undifferentiated interstitial cells, abnormal multilayered IMCD epithelium and IMCD dilation as the pathognomonic traits in correctly identifying a patient with MSK.

Computed tomography imaging with contrast allows one to see the typical dense pattern of tubular deposits of MSK that extend from the renal capsule down to the corticomedullary junction (Fig. 5.32A). Without contrast, there is nothing about the radiographic pattern unique to MSK.

High-resolution endoscopy detected a unique shape of affected papilla in MSK patients. In all cases, involved papillae are generally round and enlarged with a billowy appearance we have not encountered in other types of stone formers (Fig. 5.32B). Dilated BDs are frequent (Fig. 5.32B). Despite the number of dilated BDs, only six ducts in two patients had protruding mineral plugs/overgrowths (Figs. 5.26F and 5.32C). Small sites of white and yellow plaques were commonly found, as well as a few attached

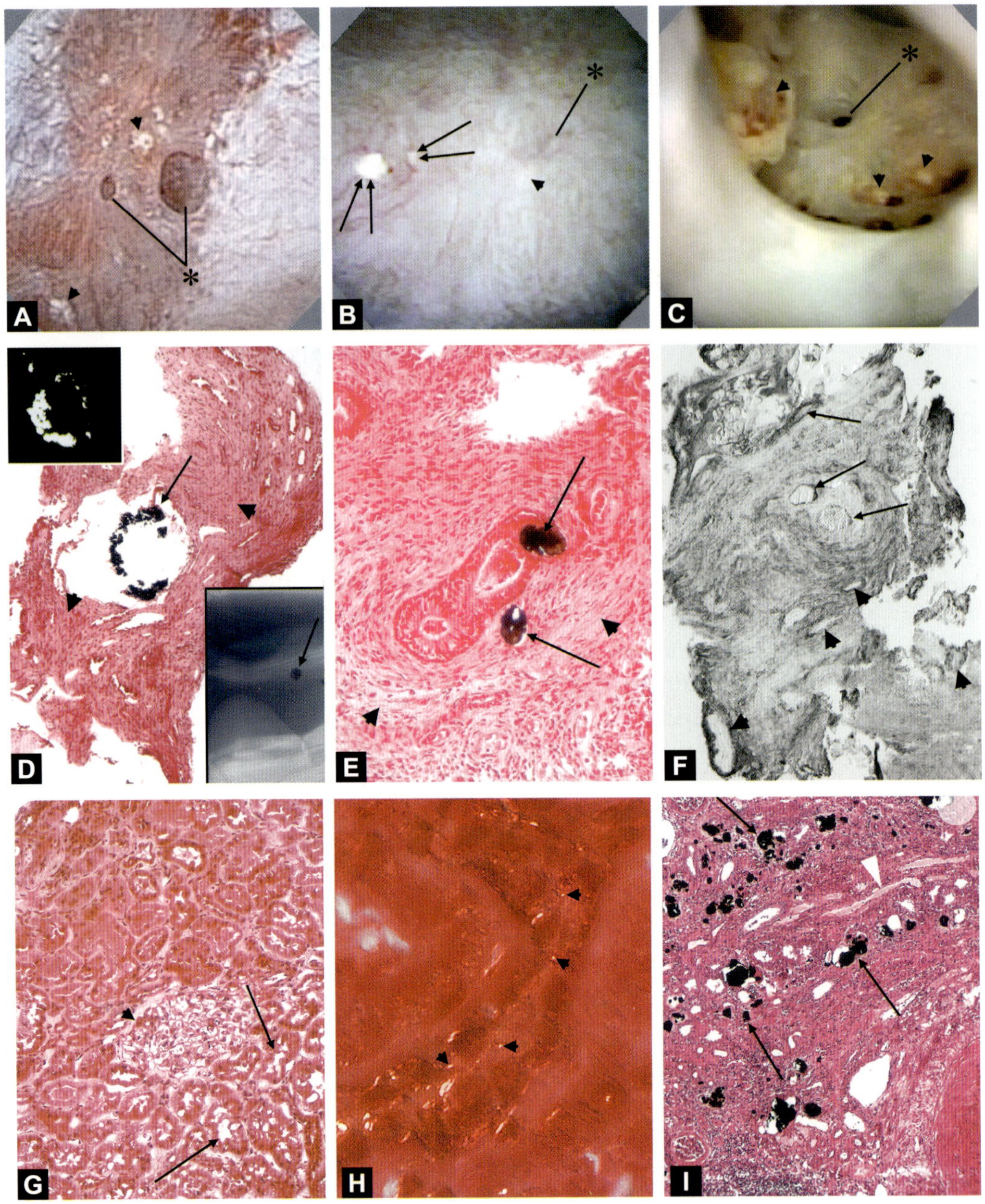

Figs. 5.31A to I: Endoscopic and histopathologic images of papillary biopsies from stone formers with primary hyperoxaluria type 1. Panels (A) and (B) show the papillary morphology of PH1 patients with normal renal function, while panel (C) shows a papilla from a primary hyperoxaluria type 1 (PH1) patient with ESRD. Papillary morphology varied from normal (B) to flattened (A) with a few dilated openings of ducts of Bellini BD (asterisk) with (B, double arrows) and without (A, asterisk) plugs. Scattered yellow plaque (arrowheads) was noted. Panel (C) shows the papilla from a PH1 patient using ex vivo ureteroscopy revealing dilated openings of BD (asterisk) and scattered yellow plaque (arrowheads) once a large calcium oxalate (CaOx) stone was removed from the minor calyx (an arrow points to remnant stone). Histopathologic examination of Yasue-stained sections of papillary biopsied from PH1 patients with normal renal function detected small to very large intraluminal deposits in a few inner medullary collecting ducts (IMCD) (D, arrow), all surrounded by dense areas of interstitial fibrosis (arrowheads). The inset in panel (D) is a micro-computed tomography (CT) image showing only a few deposits (arrow) in that papillary biopsy. Panel (E) shows at a high magnification the extensive interstitial fibrosis at (arrows) and away (arrowheads) site of tubular deposits. (F) Using hyaluronan staining, cell injury was detected in the plugged tubules (arrows) as well as nearby normal-appearing tubules (arrowheads). Cortical biopsies from PH1 stone formers with normal renal function detected normal glomeruli (G, arrowhead) and proximal tubules (arrows). However, occasional small birefringent crystals (H, arrowheads) were noted at the brush border of otherwise normal-appearing proximal tubules. Panel (**I**) shows a light micrograph of the corticomedullary junction of a PH1 patient with ESRD, revealing intraluminal deposits in most S_3 segments of the proximal tubule (arrows).

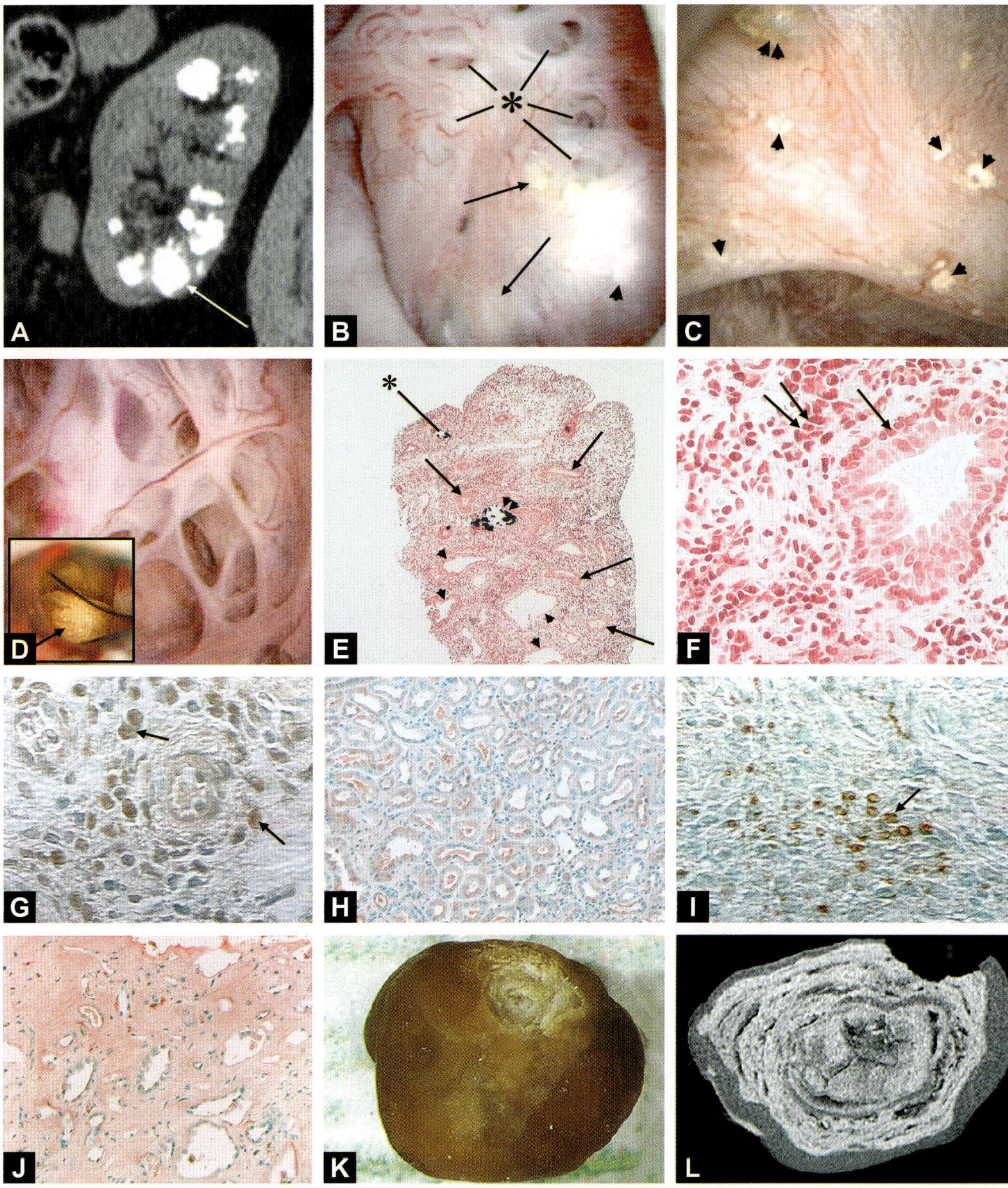

Figs. 5.32A to L: Endoscopic and histopathologic images of papillary biopsies from stone formers with medullary sponge kidney disease. Panel (A) is a computed tomography (CT) image of an medullary sponge kidney (MSK) stone former showing some deposits (arrow) in the kidney extending from the capsule to the corticomedullary junction. Medullary sponge kidneys can present affected and unaffected papilla. Unaffected papillae appear normal (not shown) but affected papillae (B and C) are characterized by a rounding of contours and enlargement, which creates a billowy appearance. As part of the general rounding of contours, the papillary tips are blunted. These papillae also show sites of white (B, arrowheads) and yellow (B, arrows) plaque and dilated opening of BD with and without plugs (B, asterisks). (C) An occasional attached stone (double arrowheads) was noted. Panel (D) shows the honeycomb appearance of a papilla when a majority of the ductal stones have been released by deroofing the dilated IMCD (the inset in panel (D); arrow points to ductal stone). The inner medulla of the MSK papilla has unique morphologic characteristics consisting of multilayered lining cells of IMCD (E and F, arrows) and a highly cellular interstitium (F, double arrows). Numerous IMCD were dilated with some containing mineral (double arrowheads) and some without mineral (arrowheads). An asterisk in panel (E) points out an IMCD that is not surrounded by interstitial fibrosis, which is the case for all plugged IMCD seen in MSK. Panel (G) shows positive immunostaining pattern for Runx2 in the interstitial cells of MSK papillary sections (arrows) and a negative staining pattern in an idiopathic calcium oxalate stone former papillary section (H). Panel (I) shows positive immunostaining pattern for Osterix in the interstitial cells of MSK papillary sections (arrow) and a negative staining pattern in an ICSF papillary section (J). Panel (K) shows a light micrograph of a ductal stone removed from an MSK patient. Panel (L) shows the same stone by micro-CT, revealing alternating layers of apatite (light layers) and calcium oxalate (CaOx) (grayish layers). Note a nick in this stone from the laser at the time of deroofing.

stones to Randall's plaque (Fig. 5.32C). A new entity was revealed in the MSK-affected papilla, ductal stones. These stones were observed in all of the MSK-involved papillae. They appeared as yellow suburothelial stones rather than as shadows as observed cystinuria. When these ducts were deroofed using a laser, numerous stones were present. Unlike plugs in BD and IMCD, which are held firmly in place, these ductal stones in dilated IMCD and BD were unattached and rolled out after deroofing like marbles on a tabletop. When a surgeon successfully removes most of these ductal stones, the papillary surface has a honeycomb appearance (Fig. 5.32D). Ductal stones were composed of a mixture of CaOx and apatite (Figs. 5.32K and L).

Histopathologic examination of Yasue-positive papillary sections revealed the triad of unique histologic characteristics of MSK papillae (Figs. 5.32E and F). Numerous dilated IMCDs were seen with and without ductal stones. Unlike other plugged IMCDs from other stone phenotypes that always show cell injury, these IMCDs had an intact multilayered epithelium. In addition, the interstitium was highly cellular (Fig. 5.32F).

Because of the unique cellular nature of the inner medulla of MSK patients, we hypothesized that stones in the MSK patients might be formed by the process of osteogenesis. Thus, we used immunohistochemistry to define the expression of two critical bone genes, Runx2 and Osterix. Both of these genes are required for osteogenesis, and both were expressed in the interstitial cells of the MSK papillary tissue but not in the similar tissue from ICSF stone formers (Figs. 5.32G to J).

Other Stone Forming Phenotypes

Two additional human stone forming phenotypes, uric acid and struvite stone formers have been examined by more modern technologies, Low and Stoller were the first to detect Randall's plaque on the papilla of uric acid stone formers using high resolution endoscopy.[6] No other abnormalities were reported. A recent study by Viers et al, noted not only Randall's plaque on the surface of papillae from all uric acid stone formers (23 patients, 100%) but tubular plugs (57% of patients) as well endoscopy.[64] These investigators obtained papillary biopsies, which confirmed the presents of intraluminal tubular plugs.

Both of these groups have also imaged the papillae of struvite stone formers.[6,23] Low and Stoller reported Randall's plaque on the papilla of only 20% of their struvite stone formers while Viers et al., found plaque on the papilla of all nine of their struvite stone formers as well as tubular plugs in 3 of their 9 patients. Little clinical data were presented on the mineral composition of these patients and potential abnomalities of the kidneys seen on X-ray.

Lastly, our group has performed preliminary analysis of papillae from stone formers who have undergone modern bariatric surgery for obesity. Initial observations of these patients suggest their surgical anatomy and histopathologic changes are similar to what we have published for intestinal bypass patients for obesity.

SUMMARY

The advent and application of modern high-resolution endoscopy, micro-computerized tomography and micro-Fourier transform infrared microspectroscopy for mineral analysis of kidney tissues of carefully phenotyped stone formers has led to the discovery of critical information on the pathogenesis of kidney stone formation. Along with the observations of Randall in the 1930's, we have presented convincing observations on idiopathic calcium oxalate stone formers showing they develop CaOx stones attached to the papillary surface at sites of interstitial (Randall's) plaque composed of calcium phosphate. Interstitial plaque is initially seen within the basement membrane of thin loops of Henle and then filling the interstitial space of the inner medulla as far down as the basal side of the urothelium covering the papilla. The interstitial plaque appears to be formed by a process of "vas washdown" aided by a defect in calcium reabsorption at the proximal tubule. If the urothelium is breached, a nidus of mineral composed of ions from the urinary space form as an overlay on a site of Randall's plaque. No other changes were noted in the tissues of the medulla or cortex of the ICSF kidneys.

This set of observations are unique to ICSF stone formers with hypercalciuria in that all of stone forming phenotypes analyzed showed a combination of intraluminal plugging of primarily IMCD and/or BD, overgrowths at the end of BD plugs, interstitial fibrosis, a few attached stones, scattered site of interstitial plaque, large pits on the papillary surface, distortion of the papillary shape, varying types of mineral deposition in tubules and an occasional ductal stone suggesting multiple mechanisms for stone formation.

We believe by carefully investigating the surgical anatomy, histopathology of the papillary tissue, patients clinical data along with a detailed study of the renal physiology of each stone formers, we will discover the precise mechanisms of stone pathogenesis of each stone forming phenotype which will lead to effective treatment protocols.

REFERENCES

1. Randall A. Papillary pathology as a precursor of primary renal calculus. J Urol. 1940;44:580-9.
2. Randall A. The origin and growth of renal calculi. Ann Surg. 1937;105:1009-27.
3. Vermooten V. Origin and development in renal papilla of Randall's calcium plaques. J Urol. 1942;48:27-37.
4. Cook SAR. The site of calcification in the human renal papilla. Brit J Surg. 1970;57:890-6.
5. Anderson WAD. Renal calcification in adults. J Urol. 1940;44:29-33.
6. Low RK, Stoller ML. Endoscopic mapping of renal papillae for Randall's plaque in patients with urinary stone disease. J Urol. 1997;158:2062-4.
7. Evan AP, Lingeman JE, Coe FL, et al. Randall's plaque of patients with nephrolithiasis begins in basement membranes of thin loops of Henle. J Clin Invest. 2003;111:607-16.
8. Khan SR, Rodriguez DE, Gower LB, et al. Association of Randall plaque with collagen fibers and membrane vesicles. J Urol. 2012;187:1094-100.
9. Evan AP, Coe FL, Rittling SR, et al. Apatite plaque particles in inner medulla of kidneys of CaOx stone formers: osteopontin localization. Kidney Int. 2005;68:145-54.
10. Evan AP, Bledsoe S, Worcester EM, et al. Renal inter-alpha-trypsin inhibitor heavy chain 3 increase in calcium oxalate stone-forming patients. Kidney Int. 2007;72:1503-11.
11. Amos FF, Olszta MJ, Khan SR, et al. Relevance of a polymer-induced liquid-precursor (PILP) mineralization process to normal and pathological biomineralization. In: Königsberger E, Königsberger L (Eds). Biomineralization-Medical Aspects of Solubility. West Sussex: Wiley; 2006. pp. 125-217.
12. Cifuentes Delatte L, Minon-Cifuentes JL, Medina JA. Papillary stones: calcified renal tubules in Randall's plaque. J Urol. 1985;133:490-4.
13. Pieras E, Costa-Bauza A, Ramis M, et al. Papillary and non-papillary calcium oxalate monohydrate renal calculi: comparative study of etiologic factors. Scientific World Journal. 2006;6:2411-9.
14. Daudon M, Traxer O, Jungers P, et al. Stone morphology suggestive of Randall's plaque. In: Evan AP, Lingeman JE, Williams JC Jr (Eds). Renal Stone Disease. Melville, NY: American Institute of Physics; 2007. pp. 26-34.
15. Cifuentes Delatte L, Minon-Cifuentes JL, Medina JA. New studies on papillary calculi. J Urol. 1987;137:1024-10.
16. Williams JC, McAteer JA, Evan AP, et al. Micro-computed tomography for analysis of urinary calculi. Urol Res. 2010;38:477-84.
17. Fernandez CM, Cifuentes Delatte L, Medina JA, et al. Nucleo con tubos renales calcificados en el interior de un pequeno calculo de Whewellita. Arch Esp Urol. 1986;39:71-3.
18. Matlaga BR, Williams C, Evan AP, et al. Calcium oxalate stones are frequently found attached to Randall's plaque. In: Evan AP, Lingeman J, Williams JC (Eds). Renal Stone Disease: Proceedings of the First International Urolithiasis Research Symposium. Melville, NY: American Institute of Physics; 2007. pp. 35-41.
19. Miller NL, Gillen DL, Williams JC, et al. A formal test of the hypothesis that idiopathic calcium oxalate stones grow on Randall's plaque. BJU Int. 2009;103:966-71.
20. Miller NL, Williams JC, Evan AP, et al. In idiopathic calcium oxalate stone formers, unattached stones show evidence of having originated as attached stones on Randall's plaque. BJU Int. 2010;105:242-5.
21. Kuo RL, Lingeman JE, Evan AP, et al. Urine calcium and volume predict coverage of renal papilla by Randall's plaque. Kidney Int. 2003;64:2150-4.
22. Kim SC, Coe FL, Tinmouth WW, et al. Stone formation is proportional to papillary surface coverage by Randall's plaque. J Urol. 2005;173:117-9.
23. Linnes MP, Krambeck AE, Cornell L, et al. Phenotypic characterization of kidney stone formers by endoscopic and histological quantitation of intrarenal calcification. Kidney Int. 2013;84:818-25.
24. Wang X, Krambeck AE, Williams JC, et al. Distinguishing characteristics of idiopathic calcium oxalate kidney stone formers with low amounts of Randall's plaque. Clin J Am Soc Nephrol. 2014;9:1757-63.
25. Ruggera L, Chiodini S, Gambaro G, et al. Does Randall's plaque represent a necessary condition in the pathogenesis of the idiopathic calcium oxalate stones? Urol Res. 2008;36:162-3.
26. Carpentier X, Daudon M, Bazin D, et al. Plaques de Randall: frequence, topographie et classification. Semin Urol Nephrol. 2009;35:86-90.
27. Evan AP, Coe L, Lingeman JE, et al. Mechanism of formation of human calcium oxalate renal stones on Randall's plaque. Anat Rec. 2007;290:1315-23.
28. Bazin D, Daudon M, Combes C, et al. Characterization and some physiochemical aspects of pathological microcalcifications. Chem Rev. 2012;112:5092-120.
29. Daudon M, Bazin D, Letavernier E. Randall's plaque as the origin of calcium oxalate kidney stones. Urolithiasis. 2015;43:S5-11.
30. Evan AP, Lingeman JE, Worcester EM, et al. Contrasting histopathology and crystal deposits in kidneys of idiopathic stone formers who produce hydroxyapatite, brushite, or calcium oxalate stones. Anat Rec. 2014;297:731-48.
31. Evan AP, Lingeman JE, Coe FL, et al. Intra-tubular deposits, urine and stone composition are divergent in patients with ileostomy. Kidney Int. 2009;67:1081-8.
32. Evan A, Lingeman JE, Coe FL, et al. Crystal associated nephropathy in patients with brushite nephrolithiasis. Kidney Int. 2005;67:576-91.
33. Evan AP, Lingeman JE, Worcester EM, et al. Renal histopathology and crystal deposits in patients with small bowel resection and calcium oxalate stone disease. Kidney Int. 2010;78:310-7.
34. Carpentier X, Bazin D, Combes C, et al. High Zn content of Randall's plaque: a micro-X-ray fluorescence investigation. J Trace Elem Electrolytes Health Dis. 2011;25:160-5.
35. Rosenow EC. Renal calculi: a study of papillary calcifications. J Urol. 1940;44:19-23.

36. Reiner AP, Kahn A, Eisner BH, et al. Kidney stones and subclinical atherosclerosis in young adults: The CARDIA study. J Urol. 2011;185:920-5.
37. Gambaro G, Abaterusso C, Fabris A, et al. The origin of nephrocalcinosis, Randall's plaque and renal stones: a cell biology viewpoint. Arch Ital Urol Androl. 2009;81:166-70.
38. Mezzabotta F, Ceol M, Torregrossa R, et al. Spontaneous calcification process in a primary culture of renal cells from a patient with MSK carrying a GDNF mutation. J Am Soc Nephrol. 2008;19:75A.
39. Kahn SR, Canales BK. Unified theory on the pathogenesis of Randall's plaque and plugs. Urolithiasis. 2015;43:S109-23.
40. Evan AP, Worcester EM, Williams JC, et al. Biopsy proven medullary sponge kidney: Clinical findings, histopathology and role of osteogenesis in stone and plaque formation. Anat Rec. 2015;298:865-77.
41. Stout HA, Akin A, Norton E. Nephrocalcinosis as a source for renal stone nuclei. J Urol. 1955;74:8.
42. Worcester EM, Gillen DL, Evan AP, et al. Evidence that postprandial reduction of renal calcium reabsorption mediates hypercalciuria of patients with calcium nephrolithiasis. Am J Physiol. 2007;292:F66-75.
43. Worcester EM, Coe FL, Evan AP, et al. Evidence for increased postprandial distal nephron calcium delivery in hypercalciuric stone-forming patients. Am J Physiol. 2008;295:F1286-94.
44. Evan AP, Lingeman JE, Coe FL, et al. Histopathology and surgical anatomy of patients with primary hyperparathyroidism and calcium phosphate stones. Kidney Int. 2008;74:223-9.
45. Evan AP, Coe FL, Lingeman JE, et al. Renal crystal deposits and histopathology of the kidney in cystinuria. Kidney Int. 2006;69:2227-35.
46. Evan AP, Lingeman J, Coe F, et al. Renal histopathology of stone-forming patients with distal renal tubular acidosis. Kidney Int. 2007;71:795-801.
47. Worcester EM, Evan AE, Coe FL, et al. A test of the hypothesis that oxalate secretion produces proximal tubule crystallization in primary hyperoxaluria Type 1. Am J Physiol. 2013;305:F1574-84.
48. Evan AP, Coe FL, Gillen D, et al. Renal intraluminal crystals and hyaluronan staining occur in stone formers with bypass surgery but not with idiopathic calcium oxalate stones. Anat Rec. 2008;291:325-34.
49. Coe FL, Evan AP, Lingeman JE, et al. Plaque and deposits in nine human stone diseases. Urol Res. 2010;38:239-47.
50. Huggins CB. Bone and calculi in the collecting tubules of the kidney. Arch Surg. 1933;27:203-15.
51. Ebisuno S, Kohjimoto Y, Tamura M, et al. Histological observations of the adhesion and endocytosis of calcium oxalate crystals MDCK cells and in rat and human kidney. Urol Int. 1997;58:227-31.
52. Khan SR, Finlayson B, Hackett RL. Renal papillary changes in patient with calcium oxalate lithiasis. Urology. 1984;23:194-9.
53. Finlayson B, Reid F. The expectation of free and fixed particles in urinary stone disease. Invest Urol. 1978;15:442-8.
54. Vervaet B. The tubular epithelium and intratubular nephrocalcinosis . Universiteit Antwerpen, CDE, Universiteitsplein 1,2610 Wilrijk, Belgium, Thesis Universiteit Antwerpten 2010.
55. Verkoelen CF, Verhulst A. Proposed mechanisms in renal tubular crystal retention. Kidney Int. 2007;72:13-8.
56. Asselman M, Verhulst A, Van Ballegooijen ES, et al. Hyaluronan is apically secreted and expressed by proliferating or regenerating renal tubular cells. Kidney Int. 2005;68:71-83.
57. Evan AP, Coe FL, Connors BA, et al. Mechanisms by which shock wave lithotripsy can promote formation of human calcium phosphate stones. Am J Physiol Renal Physiol. 2015;308:R938-49.
58. Parks JH, Worcester EM, Coe FL, et al. Clinical implications of abundant calcium phosphate in routinely analyzed kidney stones. Kidney Int. 2004;66:777-85.
59. Mulay SR, Eberhard JN, Desai J, et al. Hyperoxaluria requires TNF receptors to initiate crystal adhesion and kidney stone disease. J Am Soc Nephrol. In press.
60. Verhulst A, Asselman M, Persy VP, et al. Crystal retention capacity of cells in the human nephron: involvement of CD44 and its ligands hyaluronic acid and osteopontin in the transition of a crystal binding- into a nonadherent epithelium. J Am Soc Nephrol. 2003;14:107-15.
61. Evan AP, Worcester EM, Williams JC, et al. Biopsy proven medullary sponge kidney: clinical findings, histopathology and role of osteogenesis in stone and plaque formation. Anat Rec. 2015;298:865-77.
62. Kanwar YS, Mannaligod JR. Leukemic urate nephropathy. Arch Pathol. 1975;99:467-72.
63. Evan AP, Coe FL, Connors BA, et al. Mechanism by which shock wave lithotripsy can promote formation of human calcium phosphate stones. Am J Physiol. 2015;308:F938-49.
64. Viers BR, Lieski JC, Vrtiska TJ, et al. Urine pH in renal calcium stone formers who do and do not increase stone phosphate content with time. Nephrol Dial Transplant. 2009;24:130-6.

CHAPTER

6

Calcium Oxalate and Calcium Phosphate Crystal Interactions with Renal Cells

Benjamin A Vervaet, Patrick C D'Haese, Marc E De Broe, Anja Verhulst

Crystal retention refers to the process by which the kidney is unable to efficiently excrete urinary crystals, thereby leaving crystals behind in the tubular lumen and resulting in the histologic presentation of intratubular nephrocalcinosis (Figs. 6.1A and B). Morphologically, retained intratubular crystals can either be found occluding the tubular lumen or, when their diameters are smaller than that of the tubular lumen, adhering to the tubular epithelium. Although this difference was observed already in the late 19th and early 20th century,[1-5] mechanistic concepts explaining these observations were not developed until the second half of the 20th century. Two possible mechanisms were postulated by Vermeulen and Lyon and Finlayson and Reid: (1) a "free particle" mechanism, where crystals are retained because of their size and (2) a "fixed particle" mechanism, where smaller crystals are retained by binding to the tubular epithelium.[6-8]

Clinical observations indicate that "free particle" retention occurs and is primarily found in pathologies with acute and/or excessive forms of crystal formation, growth and/or aggregation such as acute phosphate nephropathy,[9] primary hyperoxaluria and jejunoileal bypass-induced enteric hyperoxaluria.[10-12,13] In contrast, although putative crystal adhesion has been observed in excessive forms of nephrocalcinosis as well,[4,5] it primarily is encountered in conditions presenting only moderate to even normal physiological levels of crystal formation as may occur in for example transplant patients and preterm infants.[14-20]

Mechanistically, one may reasonably assume that "free particle" retention is determined by physical parameters such as the diameter of the tubular system, the intratubular fluid flow rate and the extent of crystal formation, growth and aggregation. In contrast, "fixed particle" retention is primarily determined by the interaction between crystals and the tubular epithelium. In the current chapter, the putative mechanisms underlying crystal–cell interactions are described.

Ever since the "fixed particle" concept was postulated, several studies have focused on identifying the mechanism

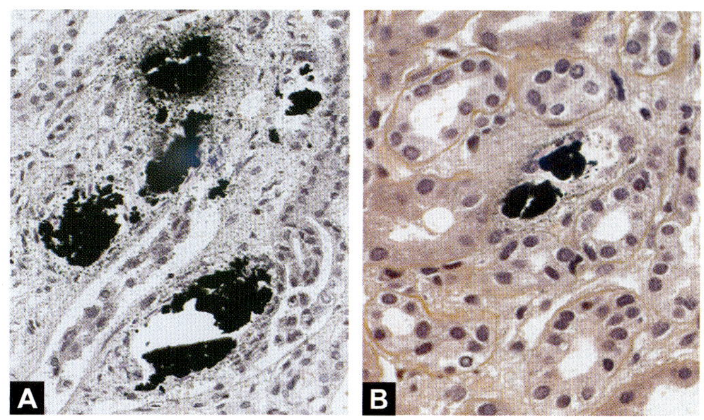

Figs. 6.1A and B: Von Kossa staining of human kidney sections from (A) preterm infant and (B) posttransplantation biopsy, clearly showing intratubular nephrocalcinosis.

by which crystals adhere to the tubular epithelium. The main questions posed in this area of research are: (1) "What is the (molecular) phenotype of crystal-binding epithelia?" and (2) "If this epithelial phenotype is aberrant from the normal situation, is its presence cause or consequence of crystal adhesion?" The following two sections aim at answering these issues.

THE (MOLECULAR) PHENOTYPE OF CRYSTAL-BINDING EPITHELIA

Several early histopathological observations in patients with nephrocalcinosis or nephrolithiasis of different etiology reported the association between intratubular crystal deposits and renal morphological alterations, which were attributed to renal injury.[2,5,21-24] These histopathological reports actually were the first indication of a link between an altered tubular epithelial phenotype and the development of intratubular calcifications. Later investigations in animal models of "nephrolithiasis," which emphasized on identifying the tubulointerstitial changes in the vicinity of intratubular crystals, provided further evidence for an association between intratubular crystal deposition and epithelial injury. These studies demonstrated that crystals can be found in contact with apoptotic and/or necrotic cells, denuded basement membranes and the surface of injured epithelial cells.[25-37] In vitro, crystals were found to preferentially adhere to either injured, depolarized, immature, migrating or proliferating tubular epithelial cells and not to fully differentiated epithelia.[38-47] Thus, an aberrant, dedifferentiated epithelial phenotype, which in general is associated with renal injury and repair processes, proofs to have the highest affinity for crystals. As mild and early forms of intratubular nephrocalcinosis generally do not display overt renal deterioration resulting in loss of tubular epithelial cells, identifying the luminal membrane characteristics and molecular composition of the luminal crystal-binding epithelia gained particular interest. In this context, the concept of crystal-binding molecules was developed.[25,33]

Crystal-binding molecules are cell-surface molecules with affinity for crystals that are expressed or produced by renal tubular epithelial cells, particularly under pathological conditions. Allegedly, these molecules are capable to anchor crystals to the luminal membrane of those cells. Thanks to the development of renal cell cultures and the relative ease by which these could be used to investigate crystal–cell interactions, the majority, if not all, currently known potential crystal-binding molecules were identified in vitro. Importantly, it is to be noted that the term "crystal-binding molecule" does not refer to urinary modulators of crystallization of which several also interact with the crystal surface and thus can be considered crystal-binding molecules as well. Nonetheless, for the remainder of this chapter, "crystal-binding molecules," as in general literature, will only refer to the membrane-bound molecules with affinity for crystals.

One of the *first* series of in vitro studies on the nature of the interaction between crystals and cells was performed by Lieske et al.[48-50] They observed that adhesion of crystals to African green monkey renal epithelial (BSC-1) cells and wild-type Madin–Darby canine kidney (MDCK) cells could be abolished either by preincubating the crystals with polyanions, i.e. negatively charged compounds, or by preincubating the epithelial monolayers with exogenous cations. These observations indicate that crystal adhesion preferentially occurs at anionic sites on the cell surface.[48-50]

In an attempt to identify the actual membrane components responsible for crystal adhesion, Lieske et al. focused on terminal sialic acid residues of the glycocalyx as these molecules considerably contribute to the overall negative charge of the cell surface.[51-55] They found that enzymatic removal of sialic acid by neuraminidase or specific blocking with lectins greatly reduces crystal binding to BSC-1 cell cultures, which allows to suggest that cell-surface glycoconjugates containing terminal sialic acid residues are potential crystal-binding molecules.[48,50] However, Verkoelen et al. showed that sialic acid might only be indirectly involved in crystal adhesion to the cell surface, as sialic acid itself has no affinity for the crystal surface.[56] Furthermore, subconfluent MDCK cell cultures, displaying proliferating and migrating cells, present markedly less sialic acid residues than confluent differentiated cell cultures, although the former are significantly more susceptible to crystal adhesion. Thus, an increase in the amount of sialic acid molecules at the cell surface associated with cellular differentiation does not lead to an increase in crystal binding. Nevertheless, the level of crystal binding could still be reduced by pretreating subconfluent cultures with neuraminidase. From these results, it was concluded that either a specific orientation of the sialic residues on the cell surface, rather than their quantity, is important in crystal binding or that sialic acid residues mediate the association of another, yet unknown crystal-binding molecule, with the cell surface.

In a *second* line of research Wiessner et al. and Bigelow et al. investigated whether certain plasma membrane phospholipids could be critical mediators of crystal attachment to epithelial cells.[47,57] Hereto these authors selectively altered the cell membrane phospholipid composition of primary and immortalized cultures of inner medullary collecting duct (IMCD) cells either by addition of exogenous phospholipid liposomes or by exposure to a membrane lipid scrambling agent, the calcium ionophore A23187. It was found that plasma membrane enrichment with the anionic phospholipid phosphatidylserine greatly increased crystal attachment to the cells. Likewise, Cao et al. found an increased level of apical membrane phosphatidylserine and crystal binding in MDCK cell cultures upon exposure to oxalate.[58] The fact that in both these approaches crystal attachment could be blocked by incubating the cells with the phosphatidylserine specific ligand annexin V supports its putative role as crystal-binding molecule. Interestingly, with respect to the overall crystal-binding phenotype, normal epithelial cells do not present phosphatidylserine in the outer leaflet of their plasma membrane's double layer, though confine it exclusively in the inner leaflet. Upon cellular injury and during apoptosis, however, this phospholipid flips to the apical leaflet,[59,60] where it potentially contributes to the overall crystal-binding capacity of injured tubular epithelial cells.

A *third* class of cell-surface molecules investigated for their potential crystal-binding capacity is membrane-bound proteins. So far, five putative mediators of crystal adhesion have been identified: collagen IV, osteopontin (OPN), annexin 2/A1 (ANX2/A1), nucleolin-related protein (NRP) and α-enolase. *First*, collagen IV is a renal tubular basement membrane multimeric protein for which Kohri et al. observed that it was specifically present on crystal-binding cell clumps of primary cultures of rat IMCD cells.[61] As collagen IV-positive mucous threads with an affinity for crystals were also present in urinary sediments of patients with kidney stones, these authors speculated that renal tubular basement membrane collagen IV is a potential crystal-binding molecule. *Second*, OPN is a glycophosphoprotein which, in the normal kidney, is abundantly secreted in the tubular fluid and only moderately expressed on the luminal membrane of distal tubules.[62,63] Upon injury/inflammation OPN is significantly upregulated throughout the nephron and is primarily thought to function as a chemokine.[62,64] Based on its (i) crystal-binding properties,[65] (ii) presence in the matrix of kidney stones,[66,67] and (iii) expression by tubular epithelial cells,[68] Yamate et al. investigated whether OPN could mediate crystal adhesion to renal epithelial MDCK cells.[69-71] These authors observed that addition of OPN to the cell cultures significantly increased crystal attachment,[69] whereas cellular incubation with either OPN antisense oligonucleotide[71] or a polyclonal OPN antibody[70] significantly reduced crystal adherence. In addition, Konya et al. observed increased crystal adhesion to immobilized OPN.[72] These results thus identified OPN as crystal-binding molecule. However, two in vivo knock out studies showed increased intratubular crystal deposition in animals lacking the OPN gene.[73,74] Therefore, despite the in vitro observations, OPN is currently considered to play an inhibitory, rather than stimulatory, role in crystal formation/retention. *Third*, Sorokina et al. identified a 110 kDa calcium-binding protein on the apical surface of IMCD cells with clear affinity for calcium crystals.[75] Amino acid sequencing revealed that this protein was highly homologous to the nucleolar protein nucleolin, a nucleus–cytoplasm shuttle protein,[76-78] and therefore was termed NRP. Further experiments by Sorokina et al. showed that proliferating/migrating IMCD cells, presenting enhanced calcium oxalate monohydrate crystal attachment, also expressed increased levels of membrane-bound NRP.[79] In addition, display vector-mediated expression of a negatively charged acidic region of NRP on the apical surface of transfected IMCD cells significantly increased crystal adhesion. Although the physiological role of NRP remains to be determined, a pathophysiological role as crystal-binding molecule could be inferred from these results. *Finally*, Kumar et al. extracted a 37 kDa protein with affinity for calcium oxalate crystals from the apical membrane of MDCK-I cells and identified it as ANX2.[80] Annexin 2 is involved in the structural organization and dynamics of endocytic and secretory pathways.[81] In normal tissue of human tumor nephrectomies ANX2 is localized at the luminal membrane, in collecting ducts, thin and (part of) the thick loop of Henle and many distal convoluted tubules.[82] Expression of ANX2, particularly cytoplasmic at corticomedullary junction, is upregulated and selectively associated with the dedifferentiation and regeneration phase following acute renal injury.[83] The observation that IMCD cells, pretreated with a monoclonal anti-ANX2 antibody, bound significantly fewer calcium oxalate crystals suggests that an increased expression of ANX2 on the surface of renal tubular cells could promote crystal retention.[80,84] Recently, identification of crystal-binding molecules was also performed via a proteomics approach: ANX2/A1 and α-enolase were found to be upregulated in MDCK cells as a result of calcium oxalate dihydrate crystal adhesion, high-calcium and high-oxalate environment respectively.[85-87] Further evidence for the crystal-binding capacity of ANX2/A1 and α-enolase was provided by using neutralizing antibodies against these proteins which significantly reduced the number of crystals adhering to the cells.

A *fourth* group of cell-surface molecules investigated in the context of crystal adhesion to epithelial cells are glycosaminoglycans (GAGs), e.g. chondroitin sulfate, dermatan sulfate, keratan sulfate, heparin, heparan sulfate and hyaluronan (HA). These long unbranched polydisaccharide chains can be present at the cell surface either freely or covalently linked (except HA) to cell-surface-associated proteins (i.e. proteoglycans).[88] Because of their negative charge and known affinity for crystals these polysaccharides have been proposed as crystal-binding molecules.[49,89] Verkoelen et al. showed that HA in particular, has to be considered a major crystal-binding molecule.[90] Previously, these authors observed that proliferating and migrating MDCK-I cells, as found in subconfluent cell cultures or in the healing wound of scrape-damaged confluent monolayers, are highly susceptible to calcium oxalate crystal binding, whereas growth-arrested differentiated cells in confluent cultures are not.[42,44] By use of a specific biotinylated HA-binding protein, HA was found to be present on the luminal surface of cells in subconfluent or healing cultures but not on cells of confluent cultures.[90] Importantly, crystal adhesion to HA-expressing proliferating/migrating MDCK-I cells decreased substantially upon treatment with *Streptomyces hyaluronidase*, an enzyme that specifically digests HA but no other GAGs or proteins.[90] Metabolic studies with [^{3}H]-labeled glucosamine, a precursor of one of the building blocks of HA, indeed confirmed that *S. hyaluronidase* cleaves HA from subconfluent cell cultures. Hyaluronan's crystal-binding capacity was further verified by the observation that plastic wells precoated with HA bind crystals, whereas uncoated wells do not. Moreover crystal binding could be abolished by *S. hyaluronidase* treatment. Importantly, in collaboration with our laboratory using primary cultures of human renal tubular cells, these workers could also confirm the specific relation between crystal adhesion and luminal expression of HA (and OPN) at the luminal cell surface of proliferating/migrating cells, but not fully differentiated cells[45] (Figs. 6.2 and 6.3). Furthermore, whereas expression of HA in the healthy kidney is primarily confined to the interstitium of the inner medulla where it plays a role in renal water handling,[91] tubular epithelial cells produce HA specifically at their apical membrane in response to mitogens, stress or mechanical injury.[92] Taken together, these results suggest a supporting role for HA in epithelial proliferation/regeneration processes and provide an explanation for the increased risk of crystal adhesion to this cellular phenotype.

Finally, although the numerous in vitro studies have provided fundamental insights in crystal–cell interactions, several important considerations have to be made when interpreting these data as conditions in culture may deviate substantially from local conditions in the kidney. Besides the type of growth substrate (i.e. solid or permeable), composition of the growth medium (either or not supplemented with serum and/or other additives), and extent and type of crystal exposure, the primary variables in this research are the segmental origin of the epithelial cells (i.e. proximal, distal, or collecting duct) on the one hand, and the differentiation/polarization status of the cells at the time of the experiment (i.e. subconfluent vs confluent) on the other hand.[38,42,44,93,94] With respect to the influence of segmental origin on crystal adhesion Verkoelen et al., Schepers et al., and Verhulst et al. showed that the level of crystal adhesion to proximal tubular cells does not depend on their differentiation status, whereas epithelial cells of distal origin acquire a noncrystal-adherent phenotype upon differentiation (Fig. 6.2).[42,45,93,95,96] As crystalluria is far more common in the human population than nephrocalcinosis/nephrolithiasis and as crystal formation in the tubular fluid particularly occurs in the distal parts of the nephron, one may reasonably assume that a default nonadherent distal epithelium plays an eminent role in renal physiology, whereas this characteristic is not required for proximal tubular cells as these only rarely encounter intratubular crystals. Furthermore, it should be noted that besides *crystal adhesion, nucleation* of crystals onto tubular epithelial cells has been observed as well which may suggest an alternative potential mechanism underlying intratubular nephrocalcinosis.[97] With this process, crystallization starts at particular sites on the epithelial surface instead of being initiated freely in the tubular fluid. Remarkably, in this process, the composition of the cell surface appears to be a critical determinant also.[56,97,98]

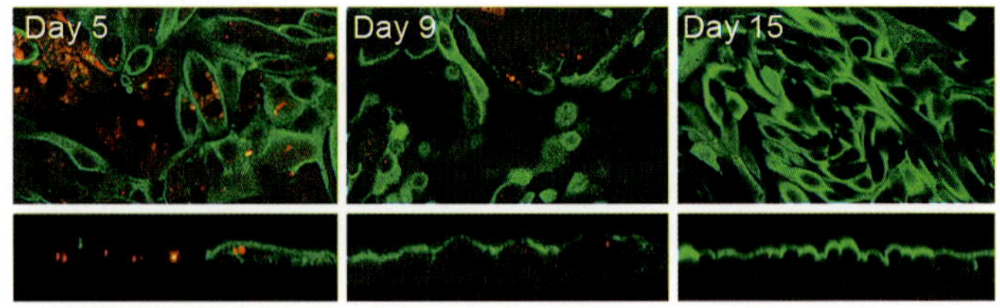

Fig. 6.2: Crystal–cell interactions analyzed by confocal microscopy. Crystals are visible by their light reflection (red). Epithelial membrane antigen (EMA) is immunofluorescently stained (green). Upper panels demonstrate overviews of the cultures at days 5, 9, and 15; lower panels demonstrate side views. Crystals interact to both distal tubular/collecting duct cells (DTC; EMA-positive) and proximal tubular cells (PTC; EMA-negative) on day 5, and selectively to PTC cells on day 9. No crystals are observed on day 15 in cultures, which almost entirely consisted of DTC. Magnification, ×630.

In conclusion, tubular epithelial cells with affinity for crystals, thus having the potential to retain crystals within the tubular lumen, have a dedifferentiated (i.e. injured, regenerating, or immature) phenotype, characterized by the expression of aberrant cell-surface molecules involved in injury, repair, maturation or pathological processes. A particular number of these membrane-bound molecules however, might be responsible for the crystal-binding capacity of this cellular phenotype and therefore are defined as crystal-binding molecules. As a fully differentiated distal epithelial phenotype has no affinity for crystals, the development of intratubular nephrocalcinosis by crystal adhesion relies on the accidental contact of crystals with aberrant epithelial cells. Increasing the expression of either one of those molecular actors considerably increases

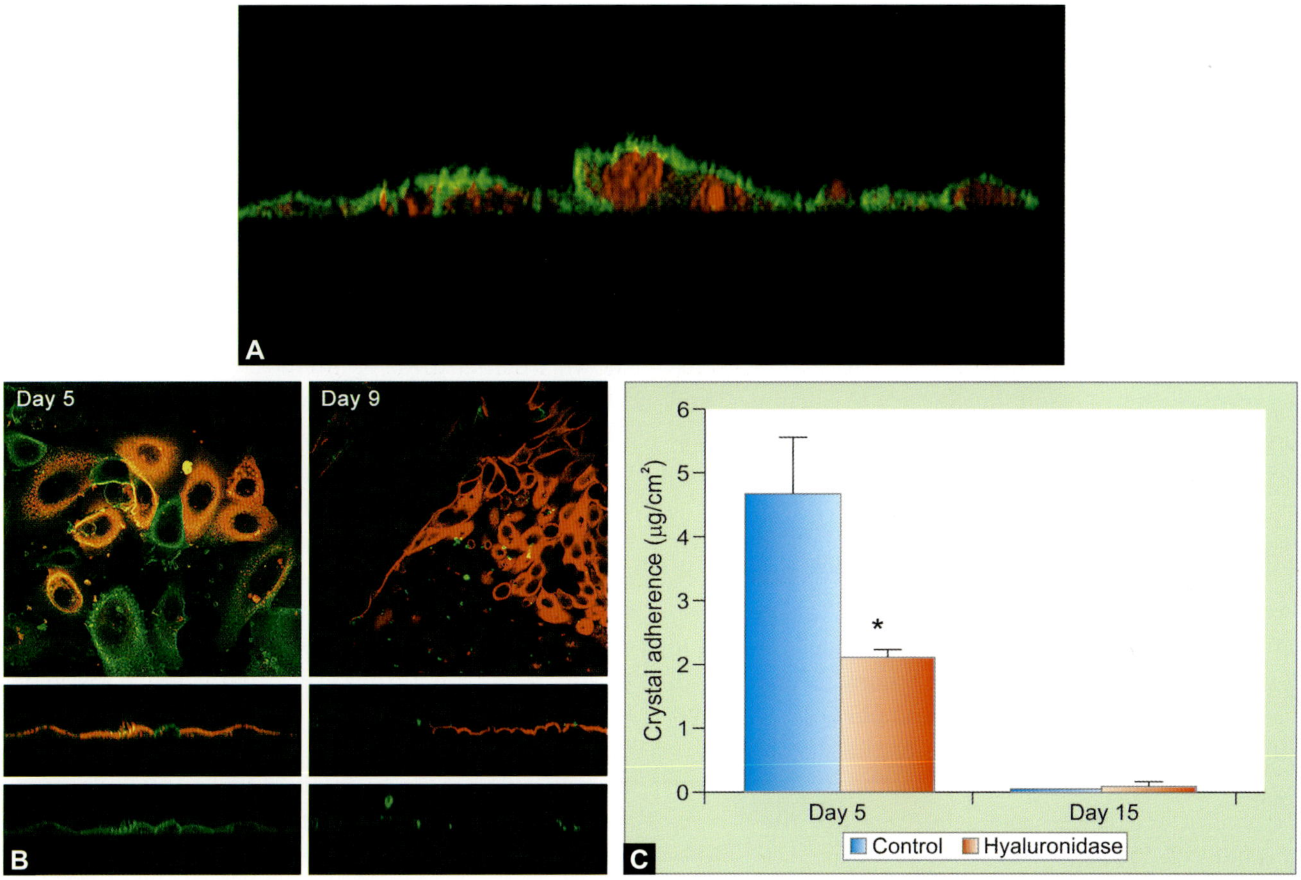

Figs. 6.3A to C: (A) Hyaluronic acid (HA; green)/propidium iodide (red) double-staining on a culture of day 5. HA is present at the apical surface of the tubular cells. (B) HA (green)/EMA (red) double-staining on cultures of days 5 and 9. Upper panels demonstrate culture overviews. Middle and lower panels represent side views (in the upper and middle panels, both EMA and HA signals are shown; in the lower panels, only the HA signal is shown). On day 5, HA is present on both EMA-positive (orange, colocalization of EMA and HA) and EMA-negative tubular cells. On day 9, HA has disappeared from tubular cells (magnification x630). (C) Crystal binding on hyaluronidase treated and control tubular cells of days 5 and 15. Hyaluronidase treatment significantly reduces crystal binding on day 5 but did not alter it on day 15. EMA, epithelial membrane antigen.

the risk for renal crystal retention. However, although it is clear from the in vitro data that phenotypical alterations of the plasma membrane cause crystal adhesion, verifying these observations in vivo and documenting their clinical relevance is of particular importance.

CRYSTAL ADHESION AS CAUSE OR CONSEQUENCE OF EPITHELIAL PHENOTYPICAL CHANGES

Whether crystal adhesion either is the consequence or the cause of the phenotypical alterations associated with epithelial injury/regeneration is a difficult question to answer as there exist two apparently conflicting observations on the interaction between crystals and cells. As described above, adhesion of crystals particularly does not occur to normal cells but at injured/regenerating epithelia, suggesting a dedifferentiated phenotype to cause crystal adhesion. On the other hand, crystals induce injury and proliferation, production of inflammatory mediators, and oxidative stress upon contact with epithelial cells in vitro, thereby suggesting that epithelial injury/dedifferentiation is the consequence rather than the cause of crystal adhesion.[99-107] There are two key aspects in this matter inferring that these confusing observations do not necessarily contradict each other.

A *first* aspect is based on the fact that crystal formation in solutions, such as original and artificial tubular fluid/urine, requires supersaturation of that solution with ions relative to the type of crystal. These ions most commonly are oxalate, phosphate and calcium. It has been hypothesized that not the crystals themselves, but rather the concomitant high concentrations of these ions might be injurious to the tubular epithelium. In particular, ionized oxalate has been considered to be the cause of oxidative stress and production of free radicals.[100,101,108] However, cell culture studies evaluating the single as well as cooperative concentration-dependent effects of both oxalate and calcium questioned the alleged toxicity of oxalate.[104,109-111] It was found that (i) free oxalate concentrations, needed to exert toxic effects, cannot be achieved in the presence of physiologic amounts of calcium,[109,110] (ii) oxalate seems to be relatively harmless in the absence of calcium,[110] and (iii) oxalate is only toxic at supraphysiological concentrations.[96,110] In addition, accumulating evidence implies that the assumed oxalate-induced cell injury most often is caused by crystals.[99,103,112-117] Nevertheless, as this issue has not been fully resolved, both passage and prolonged contact of crystals and high concentrations of oxalate, phosphate and calcium within the tubular epithelium should still be considered potential insults among the myriads of causes leading to epithelial injury and phenotypical alterations.

Second, crystal adhesion is not to be considered the only type of crystal–cell interaction. In fact, three types of crystal-cell interactions can be envisioned: (i) adhesion to cell-surface crystal-binding molecules which are expressed by injured/regenerating cells, (ii) weak, transient interactions as expected during crystalluria when crystals passing with the fluid flow shortly get in contact with the tubular wall, and (iii) a forced crystal–cell contact as expected during obstruction of the tubular lumen. As crystals do not adhere to normal epithelial cells, it is highly unlikely that crystal adhesion is the primary cause of cellular injury and phenotypical alteration. Therefore, forced contacts and transient interactions, which can occur to epithelia with a normal phenotype, are to be considered the possible initial crystal–cell interactions with injury-inducing potential. It can be suggested that obstructive crystals may harm the structural integrity of the plasma membrane primarily by denting the epithelial cells, whereas transient crystal–cell interactions might be injurious by scarring the tubular epithelium or even rip off certain membrane-bound constituents. Furthermore, prolonged nonadhesive contact between crystals and normal cells, as may occur when crystals are trapped in "dead spots" at bends in the nephron where there is little or no fluid flow, may cause injury as well. Interestingly, this situation is actually mimicked in the vast majority of in vitro studies evaluating the potential effect of crystals on cellular injury as with these experiments crystal suspensions are left on epithelial monolayers for several minutes to hours. Even so, it should be noted that in some histological studies in rat and man intratubular crystals were observed adjacent to epithelial cells which appear morphologically normal.[12,24,118] These latter observations may either suggest crystal adhesion to fully differentiated cells or alternatively may represent a "snapshot" of transient (nonadhesive) crystal–cell interactions. Although it is not known whether these epithelia actually present a normal apical membrane in terms of protein and phospholipid composition, this latter possibility cannot be excluded. Overall, although the exact mechanical and/or chemotoxical nature of crystal-induced epithelial injury remains to be determined, nonadhesive interactions may direct the normal epithelium toward a crystal-binding phenotype in such a way that a crystal may induce its own adhesion or that of a subsequently passing crystal.[119] Once adhered, crystals may then further exert their putative toxic effects, aggravating epithelial injury.

Altogether, with respect to the "cause versus consequence" issue, it can be inferred that crystal adhesion is a consequence and not an initial cause of epithelial injury. Although this concept is clear, its development is particularly based on in vitro observations. Progress in our understanding of the pathophysiological mechanisms underlying intratubular nephrocalcinosis, therefore necessitates verification of these results in animals and humans. Unfortunately, there are only little experimental studies focusing on whether this mechanism occurs in vivo as well. Therefore, as the answer to the question "Is crystal adhesion a consequence of an altered epithelial phenotype?" is clear in vitro, the next question should be "Can evidence be provided for this mechanism in vivo?." Hereto, the following paragraphs present several observations from animal studies from which the necessity of renal injury and its associated/subsequent epithelial changes in the development of crystal adhesion can be inferred.

A *first* indication is provided by experiments investigating the effect of deliberately induced epithelial injury on crystal retention. Gill et al. and Khan et al. investigated calcium oxalate crystal attachment to the normal and HCl- or Triton-X-100-pretreated urothelium of the rat bladder and observed preferential adhesion of these crystals to the chemically injured bladder urothelium, whereas control bladder samples without urothelial injury remained free of adherent crystals.[25,33] Although these studies did not involve the tubular epithelium, they provided a proof of principle that epithelial alteration can cause crystal adhesion. With respect to the renal epithelium, Kumar et al. observed that hyperoxaluric rats developed markedly more crystal deposition upon induction of renal injury by administration of gentamycin.[120] Finally, in a more relevant clinical setup, Xue et al. observed that shock wave-induced renal injury resulted in more crystal retention in the injured kidney than in the contralateral unshocked kidney upon administration of ethylene glycol (EG).[121]

A *second* line of indirect support comes from studies aiming at diminishing or abolishing crystal deposition by treating the animals with compounds that prevent renal injury. As production of reactive oxygen species has been identified as an important aspect of renal injury,[108,122-125] prevention particularly focused on restoring the normal oxidation status of the renal tissue. For example, treatment with vitamin E, a fat-soluble antioxidant, prevents EG-induced calcium oxalate crystal deposition in the kidney by attenuation of tubular injury.[126,127] Also, the cholesterol-lowering drug atorvastatin, which also has anti-inflammatory and antioxidant activities, reduces both tubular injury and crystal deposition in the EG model.[128] Likewise, Itoh et al. reported that the antioxidative effect of green tea decreased EG-induced renal calcium oxalate crystal retention in rat kidneys.[129] Furthermore, reduction of angiotensin II production via inhibition of angiotensin converting enzyme or blocking of angiotensin receptors has been shown to significantly reduce renal calcium oxalate crystal deposition as well as the development of interstitial inflammation and the level of oxidative stress in EG-treated rats.[130-132] Lastly, treatment with taurine, a naturally occurring sulfonic acid with renoprotective and antioxidant capacities, has been found to diminish crystal deposition in the rat kidney.[133-136]

Finally, a *third* approach is to verify whether the expression of known putative crystal-binding molecules is present in animal and human renal tissue and more in particular, whether it precedes or follows the onset of intratubular nephrocalcinosis. In this respect, a joint study of our laboratory with the laboratory of Experimental Urology of C. Verkoelen investigated the tubular epithelial phenotypical changes during the development of EG-induced intratubular nephrocalcinosis.[34] In this study rats were treated for 1, 4, and 8 days with 0, 0.5, and 0.75% EG, after which crystal retention and the expression of HA and OPN, and their mutual receptor CD44, was investigated. Control animals did not express HA and CD44 on renal tubular cells, whereas apical OPN expression was restricted to several distal nephron segments. This staining pattern was not altered after 1 day of treatment, and there were no visible alterations in tissue morphology. After 4 and 8 days of EG-treatment, however, the epithelial lining in the renal tubules clearly was damaged, and HA, OPN, and CD44 were expressed at the luminal surface of proliferating cell nuclear antigen (PCNA)-positive and flattened (regenerating) cells in various segments of the nephron. Although EG-induced crystalluria within 24 hours, crystals initially were not retained in the kidney. After 4 and 8 days of EG-treatment however, there was a dose- and time-dependent retention of crystals in the renal tubules. Crystals were found to be associated exclusively with regenerating renal tubular cells (Figs. 6.4A and B) expressing luminal HA, OPN, and CD44 (Figs. 6.5A to C).

In conclusion, these observations corroborated the alleged necessity of an altered epithelial phenotype in the development of intratubular nephrocalcinosis. Motivated by the lack of in vivo studies with actual emphasis on the tubular epithelial phenotype during the development of nephrocalcinosis and in extension to the work of Asselman and Verhulst,[34,45] we simultaneously investigated the temporal changes of nephrocalcinosis-associated parameters during and shortly after a 4-day EG administration period in rats. In that study, three interesting observations were made with respect to the mechanism of crystal adhesion.

First, whereas crystal formation/excretion was already present at day 1 of EG administration, crystal retention only developed gradually (Fig. 6.6), illustrating that the kidney requires a certain conditioning period toward crystal adhesion. A similar observation has been described by Marengo et al. who found that crystal retention did not develop until 2 weeks of continuous minipump-infused oxalate exposure, whereas crystalluria was already induced within 4 days.[137] The fact that their observations were seen in the presence of an average hyperoxaluria which was almost twofold of ours (4.4 mg/24 h) indicates that mere nonextreme hyperoxaluria/crystalluria might not be that effective in inducing nephrocalcinosis as compared to the EG model. Since oxalate is known to be injurious to the tubular epithelium only at supraphysiological concentrations[110] while EG, next to oxalate, also is metabolized to the nephrotoxic glycolate and glyoxylate compounds, the difference between these models in crystal retention might be explained by their distinctive effects on the tubular epithelial phenotype.

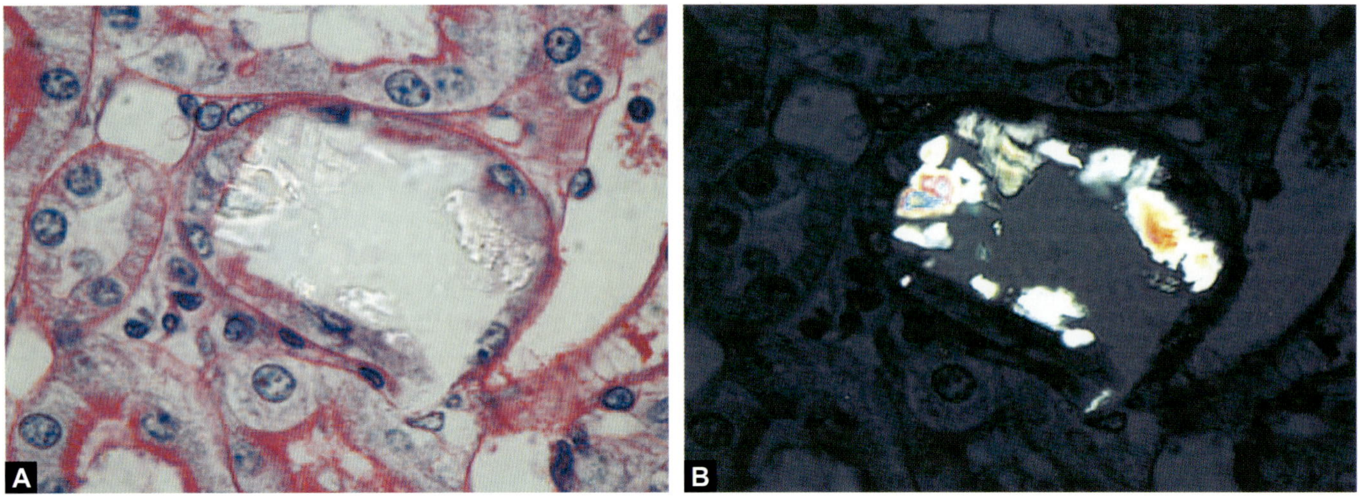

Figs. 6.4A and B: PAS stained renal tissue section of a rat treated with 0.75% EG for 4 days by optical (A) or polarized (B) light microscopy. (A) A dilated distal tubule is shown with flattened epithelial cells (score 3). (B) In the lumen of this distal tubule, crystals that are smaller than the tubular lumen are clearly visible and located at the luminal side of the injured/regenerating flattened epithelium.
(EG: Ethylene glycol; PAS: Periodic acid-Schiff).

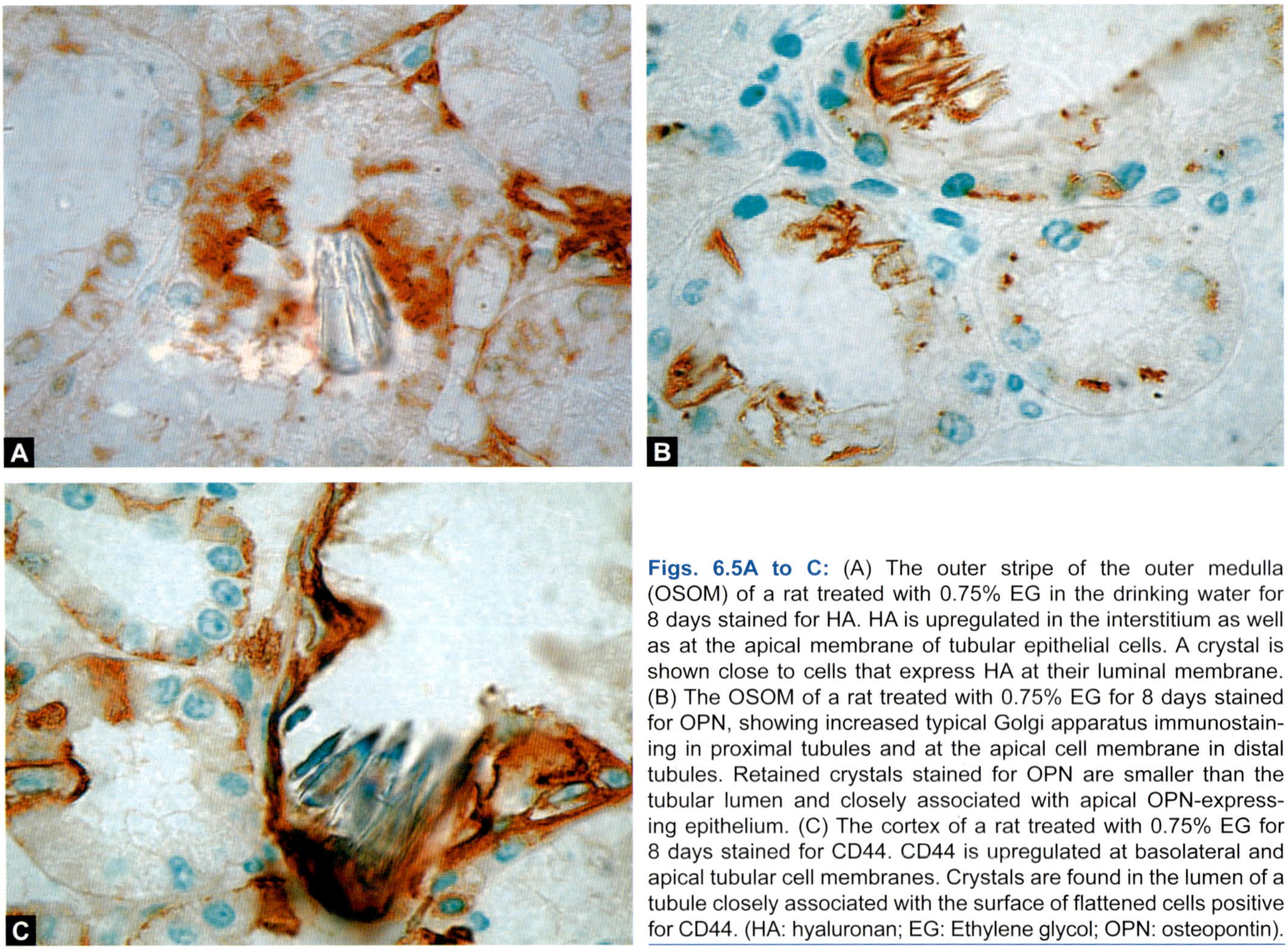

Figs. 6.5A to C: (A) The outer stripe of the outer medulla (OSOM) of a rat treated with 0.75% EG in the drinking water for 8 days stained for HA. HA is upregulated in the interstitium as well as at the apical membrane of tubular epithelial cells. A crystal is shown close to cells that express HA at their luminal membrane. (B) The OSOM of a rat treated with 0.75% EG for 8 days stained for OPN, showing increased typical Golgi apparatus immunostaining in proximal tubules and at the apical cell membrane in distal tubules. Retained crystals stained for OPN are smaller than the tubular lumen and closely associated with apical OPN-expressing epithelium. (C) The cortex of a rat treated with 0.75% EG for 8 days stained for CD44. CD44 is upregulated at basolateral and apical tubular cell membranes. Crystals are found in the lumen of a tubule closely associated with the surface of flattened cells positive for CD44. (HA: hyaluronan; EG: Ethylene glycol; OPN: osteopontin).

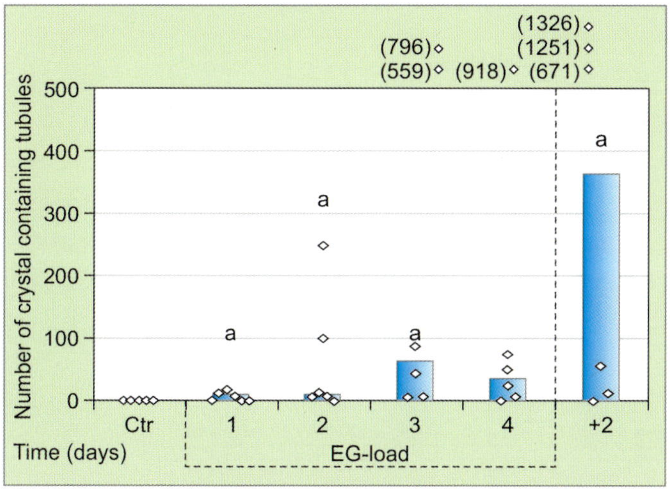

Fig. 6.6: Renal crystal content in function of time during and shortly after a 4-day EG administration period. Quantification of the amount of crystal-containing tubules on Von Kossa stained sections (n = 1/animal) shows the development of nephrocalcinosis as indicated by the gradual and dramatic increase during and following EG administration, respectively. Data are presented as individual values (diamonds) and median (bars). a, b, c, d, and e: $p < 0.05$ vs control (Ctr) and days 1, 2, 3, and 4, respectively, by Mann–Whitney U test. No significant changes were observed vs day 1, 2, 3, and 4; hence, b, c, d, and e are not displayed. Also, although cortex, OSOM, ISOM, and inner medulla were scored separately, results of these compartments were combined to avoid too complex data presentation. (EG: ethylene glycol; OSOM: Outer stripe of the outer medulla; ISOM: Inner stripe of the outer medulla).

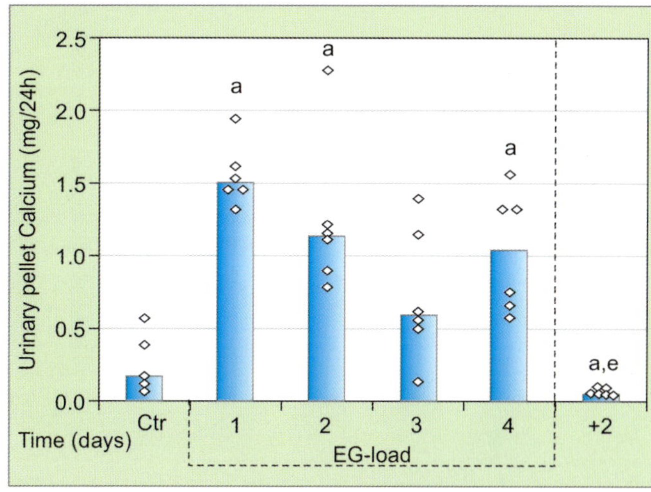

Fig. 6.7: Urinary pellet calcium analysis showing an increased calcium content in the pellet from day 1 onward. Data are presented as individual values (diamonds) and median (bars). a, b, c, d, and e: $p < 0.05$ vs control (Ctr) and days 1, 2, 3, and 4, respectively, by Mann–Whitney U test. No significant changes were observed vs day 1, 2, and 3; hence, b, c, and d are not displayed. (EG: ethylene glycol).

Second, the fact that no unequivocal temporal order of appearance between the increasing epithelial phenotypical changes and the increasing crystal adhesion could be deduced, actually supports the involvement of epithelial changes in the “fixed particle” theory, since conversion of a normal epithelium into a crystal-binding one, in an environment which is loaded with crystals, would immediately result in crystal adhesion.

Third, after arrest of EG administration, the number of crystal-containing tubules clearly increased and crystal excretion no longer occurred, whereas crystal formation was still present and comparable with (or even lower than) the level of formation during EG administration [i.e. slightly decreased hyperoxaluria and increased calcium content in urinary supernatant (urinary pellet, Fig. 6.7)]. In other words, whereas maximal hyperoxaluria (and thus maximal crystal formation) was already achieved during EG administration, tubular epithelial crystal retention further increased after arrest of EG administration. This again indicates that the development of crystal adhesion requires more than just the mere presence of crystals in the tubular fluid. Interestingly, morphological evaluation revealed an increased presence of both injured and regenerating epithelia—with known crystal-binding affinity[34]—after arrest of EG administration (Figs. 6.8A and B). As injury increased by only 50% and regeneration increased by more than 500% (Figs. 6.8A and B), the observed effects on crystal retention and excretion presumably are due to the release of the toxic EG-pressure on the kidney by which the latter could fully unfold its natural regenerating ability. In line with this, a rat study of Asselman et al., with continuous EG administration for 4 and 8 days, did not show a marked drop in crystal excretion, yet a persistent crystalluria and crystal retention,[34] indicating that withdrawal of EG apparently is necessary to induce the epithelial phenotypical shift favoring regeneration over injury as the main crystal-binding phenotype.

Preterm neonates and renal transplant patients frequently develop intratubular nephrocalcinosis. Higher mentioned experimental studies revealed that intratubular crystal retention can particularly be found in tubules presenting dedifferentiated (injured/regenerating) tubular epithelial cells expressing HA and OPN at their luminal surface. Interestingly, fetal and transplant kidneys contain either proliferating/differentiating or injured/regenerating

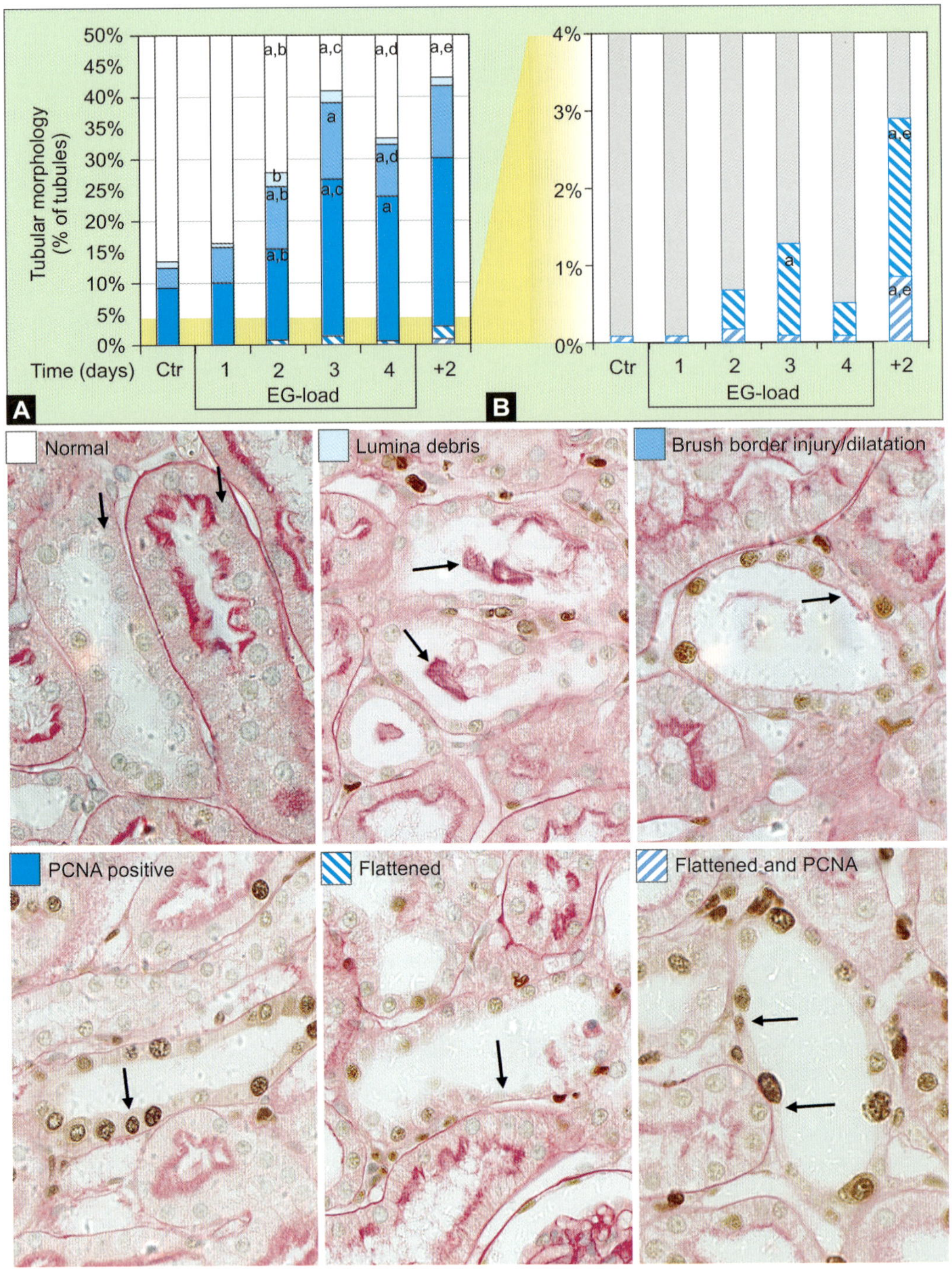

Figs. 6.8A and B: (A) General evaluation of tubular morphology. (B) Scoring results of tubules with flattened phenotype, either with or without PCNA-positive nuclei, are presented in more detail to show the relation with crystal retention in B. Data are presented as weighted mean percentages of a particular phenotype per group. a, b, c, d, and e: $p < 0.05$ vs control (Ctr) and days 1, 2, 3, and 4, respectively, by Mann–Whitney U test. Y-axis in (A) runs to 100%, but was truncated at 50%. The legend includes examples of the different phenotypical scores, with black arrows pointing toward the respective phenotypical characteristics. (EG: Ethylene glycol; PCNA: Proliferating cell nuclear antigen).

tubular epithelial cells, since nephrogenesis is not completed until 36 weeks of gestation, while ischemia and nephrotoxic immunosuppressants may lead to sustained injury and repair in renal transplants, respectively. This prompted us to investigate the luminal expression of HA and OPN on the tubular epithelium and to correlate this to

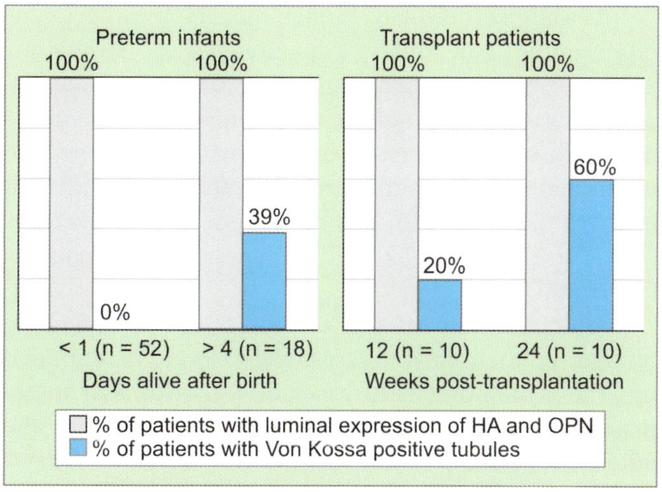

Fig. 6.9: Quantitative presentation of the fraction of tissue samples presenting luminal expression of HA and OPN on the one hand and Von Kossa positive tubules on the other hand. Whereas tubular luminal membrane expression of HA and OPN is consistently present in all investigated renal tissues, crystal retention is not, but, within the current time frame increased with time. (HA: Hyaluronan; OPN: Osteopontin).

the appearance of tubular calcifications both in fetal/preterm and transplanted kidneys.

Hyaluronan and OPN were expressed at the luminal surface of the epithelial cells lining the tubules of all fetal kidneys at birth and in all kidney graft protocol biopsies 12 and 24 weeks posttransplantation. In seven out of 18 surviving (at least 4 days) preterm neonates crystal retention developed. In renal allografts a striking increase (from 2/10 to 6/10) in tubular crystal retention between 12 and 24 weeks posttransplantation was observed. Crystals were selectively retained in renal tubules with cells expressing HA and OPN at their luminal surface.

In conclusion, the results of this study show that luminal expression of HA and OPN precedes renal tubular retention of crystals in preterm neonates and renal transplant patients, thereby providing human evidence for the putative causal role of an altered epithelial phenotype in the initiation of intratubular nephrocalcinosis (Figs. 6.9 and 6.10).

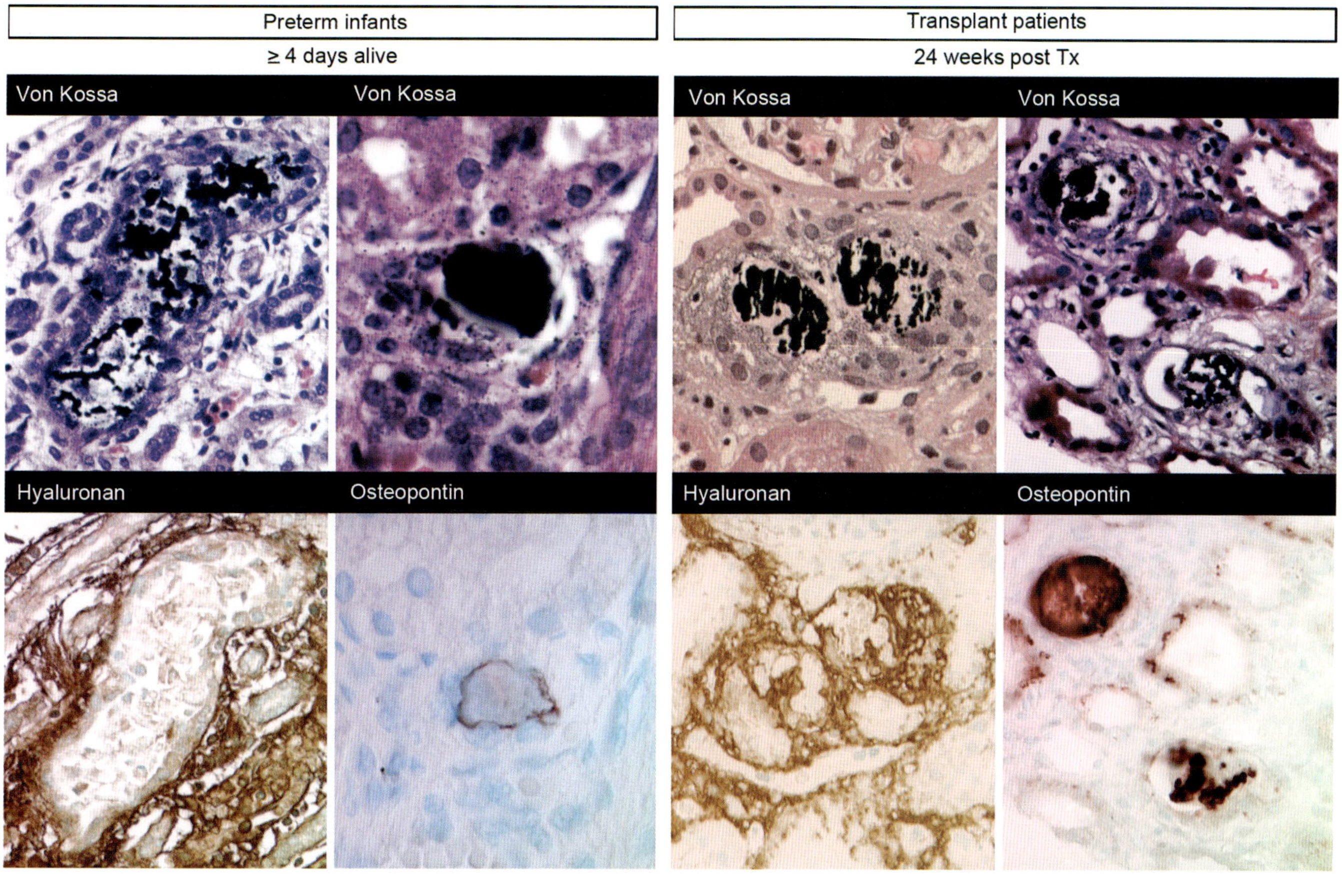

Fig. 6.10: Serial sections from preterm and transplanted kidneys stained by the Von Kossa method and either for HA or OPN. Both in preterm infants (≥4 days alive) and transplant patients (24 weeks post-Tx) intratubular crystal deposits were confined to tubulus presenting luminal expression of HA or OPN. (Tx: Transplantation; HA: Hyaluronan; OPN: Osteopontin).

POSTADHESION RENAL CRYSTAL CLEARANCE

It is obvious from human pathology and experimental studies that extensive nephrocalcinosis, as observed in acute phosphate nephropathy and primary hyperoxaluria, may lead to renal damage and functional deterioration.[15,138,139] However, the effect of less-extensive intratubular crystal adhesion on renal function is less straightforward, indicating that the kidney is functionally capable to withstand a certain degree of nephrocalcinosis and thus is able to clear crystals from the renal tissue to a certain extent.

Postadhesion renal crystal clearance was investigated in our laboratory by studying the recovery phase following EG-induced nephrocalcinosis in rats at different time points for:

1. The number of crystal-containing tubules.
2. (Semi-) quantitative morphological evaluation of tubulointerstitial changes associated with the crystal-containing tubules.
3. Morphological evaluation of the crystals.

As a clinical correlate, human renal biopsy specimens representing four different pathologies or conditions known to be associated with various degrees of nephrocalcinosis were morphologically evaluated; i.e. two disorders with extensive crystal deposition [acute phosphate nephropathy (CaP) and primary hyperoxaluria (CaOx)] and two disorders with less prominent nephrocalcinosis [preterm infants (CaOx) and kidney transplant patients (CaOx and CaP)].

After adhesion of the crystals to the regenerating tubular epithelium or, occasionally, even to denuded basement membranes in cases of severe tubular injury resulting in cell loss, the epithelial cells neighboring the adhesion site stretch and proliferate over the adhered crystals (Figs. 6.11A to F). This reaction is independent of the nature of the tubular segment, as both proximal and distal tubules show this overgrowth, and of the nature of the deposits, as CaOx (primary hyperoxaluria), CaP, cystine (cystine stone formers[140]), melamine,[141] and 2,8-dihydroxyadenine crystals are found to be overgrown by the tubu-

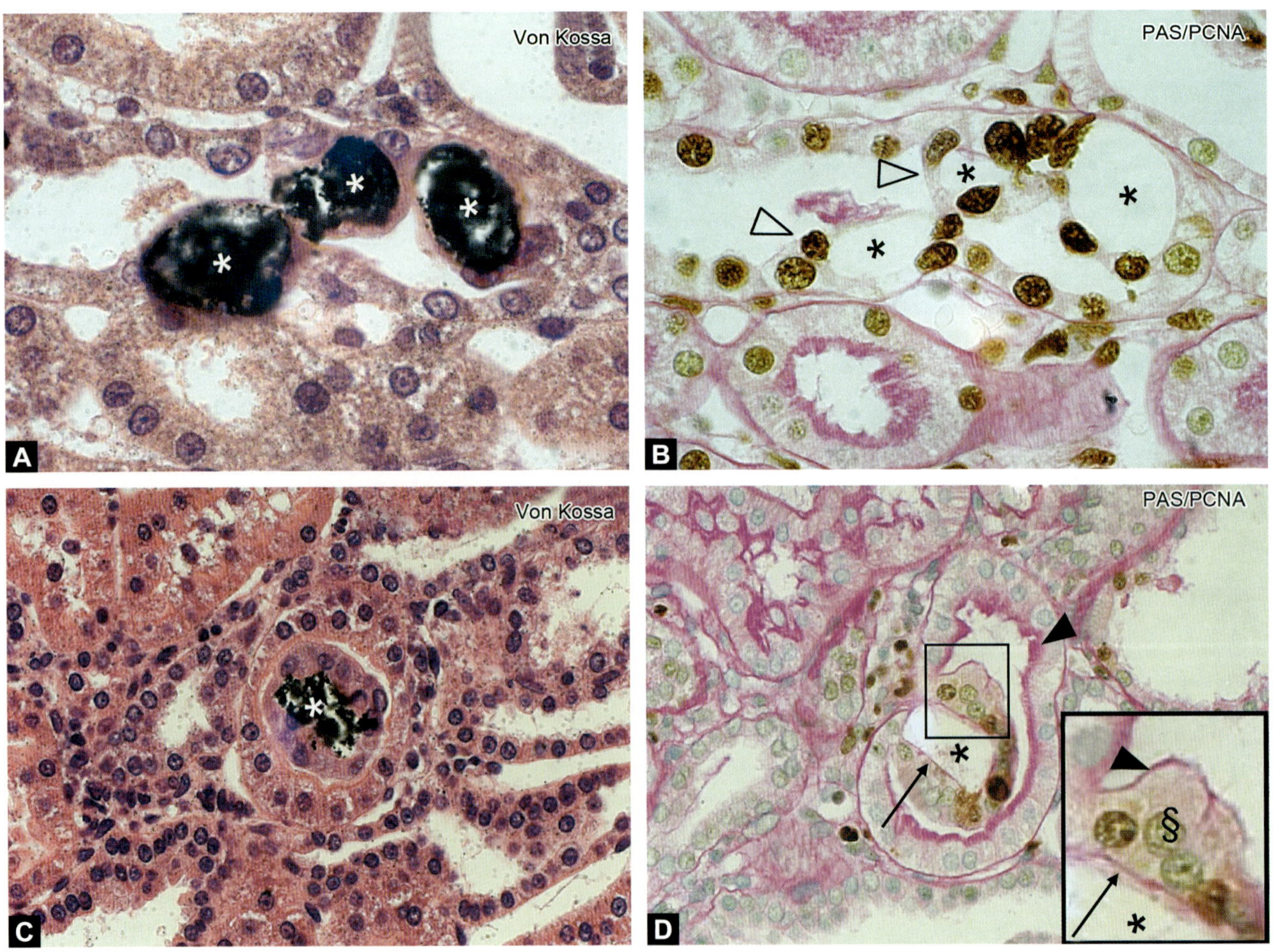

Figs. 6.11A to D

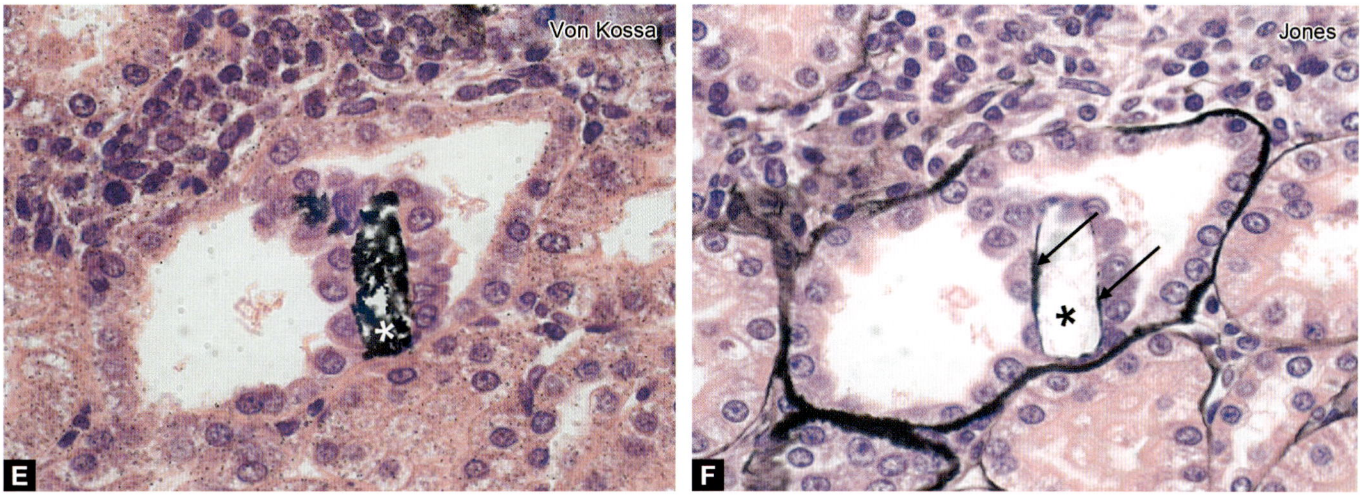

Figs. 6.11A to F: Images of serial sections showing tubules with crystals overgrown by the tubular epithelium. Serial sections are stained with Von Kossa (left) and PAS/PCNA or Jones (right). (A and B) Crystals overgrown by young flattened epithelial cells, which most likely differentiate into (C to F) where polarized epithelia cover the crystals and present basement membrane deposition (D and F) and restoration of brush border (D insert).
(Asterisk [white and black]: Location of crystals; White arrowhead: Overgrowing PCNA-positive tubular epithelial cells; Black arrowhead: Brush border; Paragraph symbol: (Re-)Differentiated tubular epithelial cells; Black arrow: Basement membrane; PAS: Periodic acid-Schiff; PCNA: Proliferating cell nuclear antigen).

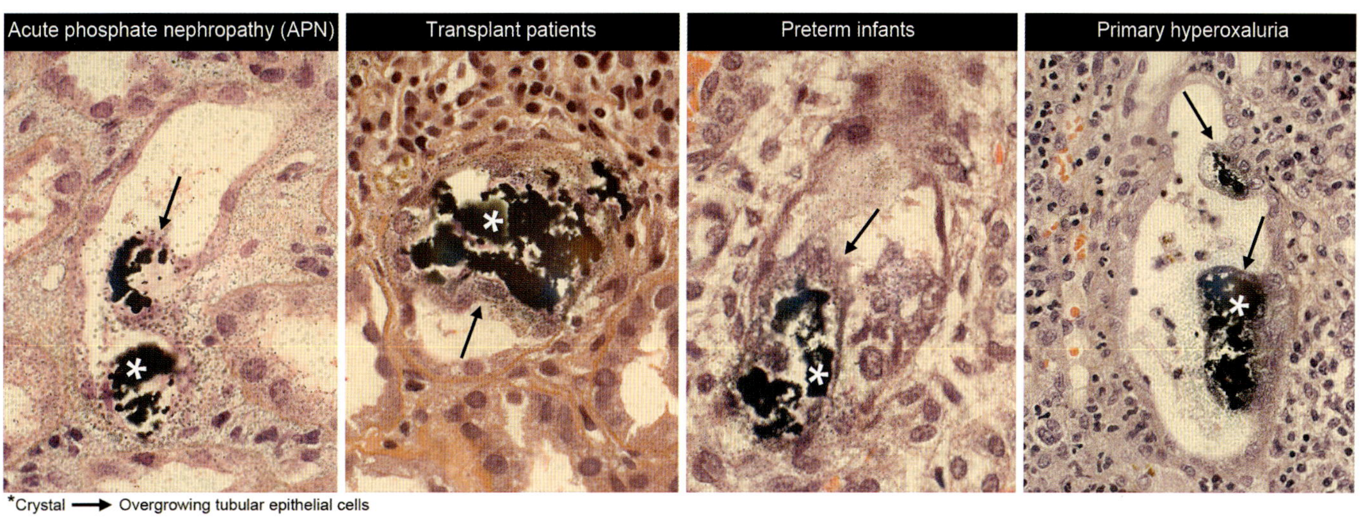

Fig. 6.12: Frequency and examples of clear overgrowth structures in human kidney biopsies with nephrocalcinosis of different etiology. Due to the extent of nephrocalcinosis and renal damage in the biopsies of primary hyperoxaluria no quantitative morphological data could be obtained.
(White asterisk: Crystals; Black arrow: Overgrowing tubular epithelial cells).

lar epithelium (Fig. 6.12). This newly formed monolayer then differentiates into a mature epithelium—with basement membranes adjacent to the crystals and restoration of brush border microvilli on the opposite luminal side (in case of proximal tubules)—thereby excluding the crystalline deposit from the tubular lumen and restoring epithelial integrity of the tubule (Figs. 6.11 and 6.13). During this overgrowth process the crystals seemingly do not undergo morphological changes, but are merely directed toward the interstitium together with the epithelial cells of the original adhesion site (Fig. 6.14). Following this translocation into the interstitium, crystal disintegration becomes morphologically apparent (Fig. 6.14). Crystals are found broken up into smaller crystallites with cellular material interspersing and surrounding the crystalline remnants, shielding them from the surrounding tissue.

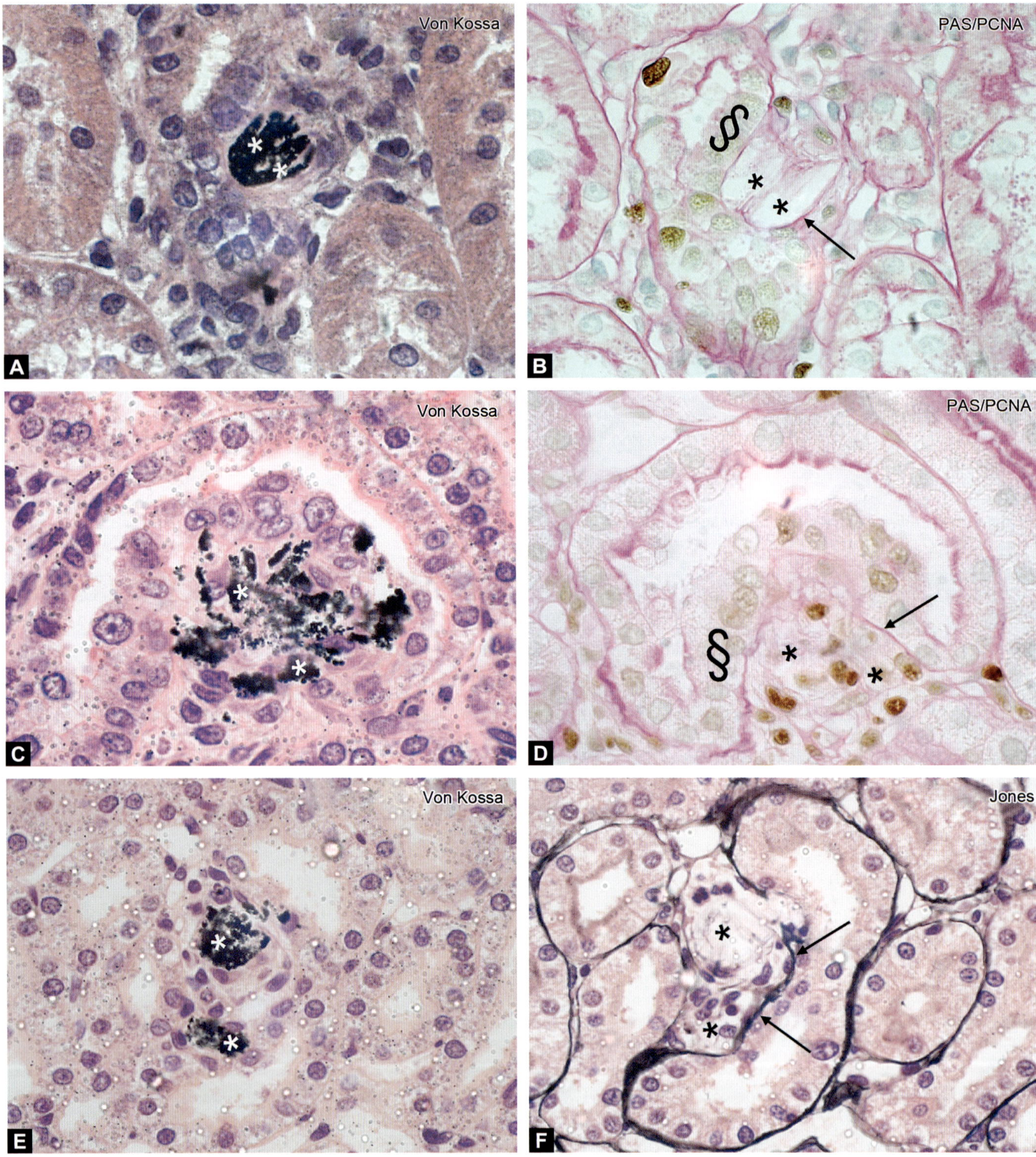

Figs. 6.13A to F: Images of serial sections showing tubules with interstitial crystals. Serial sections are stained with Von Kossa (left) and PAS/PCNA or Jones (right). Interstitial crystals either not (A and B) or already (C to F) being disintegrated in the subepithelial environment.
(PCNA: Proliferating cell nuclear antigen; PAS: Periodic acid-Schiff; Asterisk (white and black): Location of crystals; Black arrow: Basement membrane; Paragraph symbol: (Re-)Differentiated tubular epithelial cells).

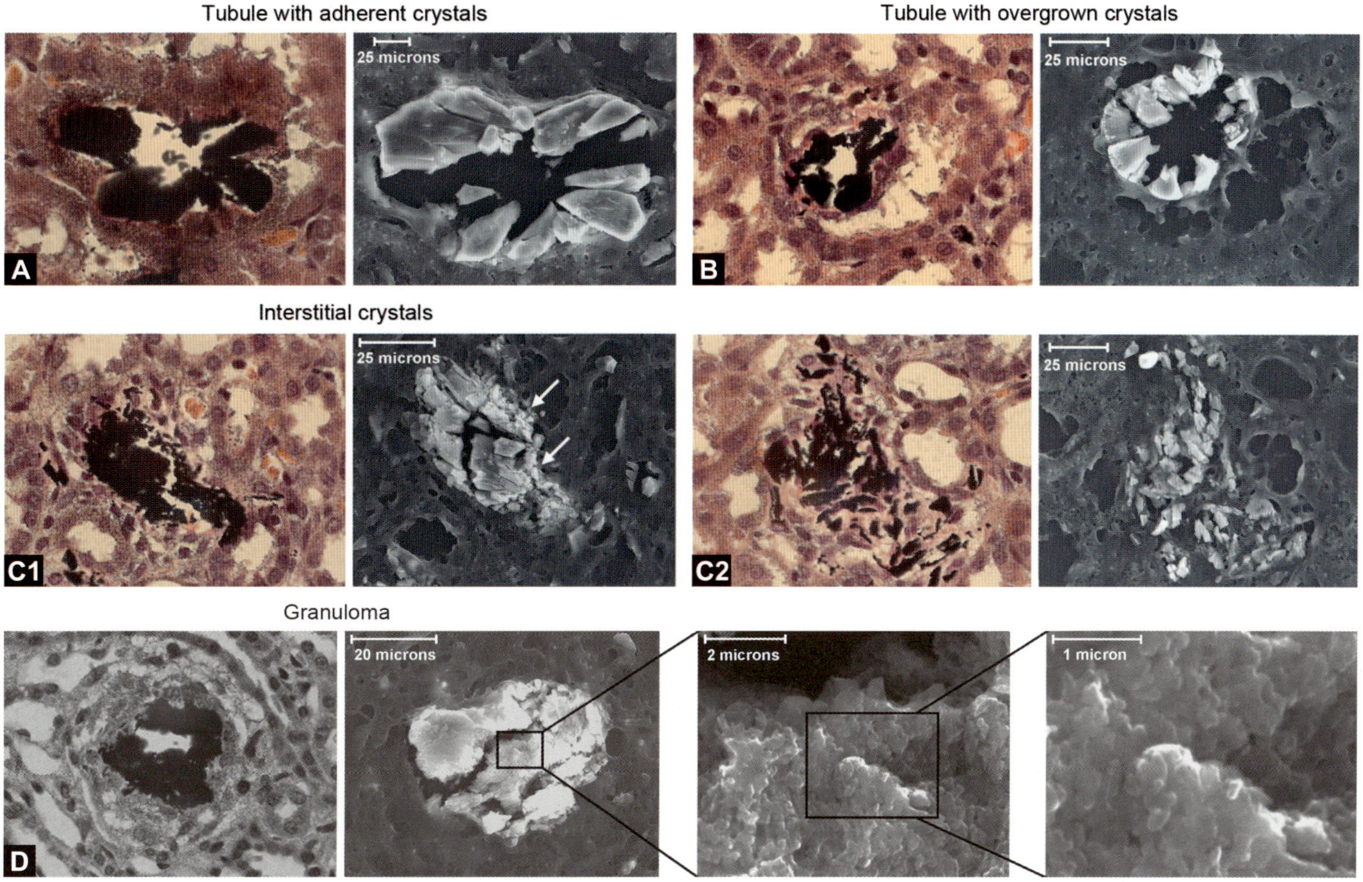

Figs. 6.14A to D: Morphology of crystals. Images of serial sections either stained with the Von Kossa method (outer left images in A, B, C, and D; crystals are black) or prepared for SEM (right-hand images). (A) Adhered crystals and (B) overgrown crystals show rather large intact crystal lattices. (C) Interstitial crystals either show smaller crystallites at their periphery (C1, white arrows) or are completely scattered and interspersed by cellular material (C2), suggesting crystal disintegration. (D) The surface of crystals in granulomatous structures has a microcrystalline appearance, as shown in the consecutive magnifications. (SEM: Scanning electron microscopy).

The biochemical mechanism by which the overgrown crystals disintegrate and eventually disappear is currently unclear. It is evident, however, that the adhered crystal deposits, ab initio, are too large to undergo endocytosis and subsequent lysosomal degradation. Therefore, following their overgrowth, an initial extracellular crystal disintegrating process must take place.

In humans, tubular epithelial overgrowth was observed, to various extents, in all four pathologies under study (*see* Fig. 6.12), corroborating the idea that the human kidney is able to actively counter progression of nephrocalcinosis and suggesting that this type of renal crystal handling is a common reaction of the tubular epithelium toward adhered crystals, unrelated to the underlying renal pathology and composition of the crystals.

In conclusion, our morphological evaluation of the fate of intratubular adhered crystals indicates the presence of an active crystal clearing mechanism in rat and man, involving epithelial crystal overgrowth, and interstitial disintegration. This mechanism seems to act independently of the underlying disorder or the nature of the crystals.

REFERENCES

1. Henle FG. Zur Anatomie der Nierre. Goettingen Nachrichten. 1863;125-35.
2. Huggins CB. Bone and calculi in the collecting tubules of the kidney. Arch Surg. 1933;27:203–15.
3. Lichtenstern R. Mikrolithiasis. Wien Klin Wchnschr. 1926;39:1156.
4. Oliver J. Nephrons and Kidneys. New York: Hoeber Medical Division, Harper & Row; 1968.

5. Morgenroth K Jr, Backmann R, Blaschke R. On the forms of calcium oxalate deposits in the human kidney in oxalosis. Beitr Pathol Anat. 1968;136: 454-63.
6. Vermeulen CW, Lyon ES, Gill WB, et al. Prevention of phosphate stones by phytate, phosphate and hexametaphosphate: experimental urolithiasis. XV. J Urol. 1959; 82:249-55.
7. Vermeulen CW, Lyon ES. Mechanisms of genesis and growth of calculi. Am J Med. 1968;45:684-92.
8. Finlayson B, Reid F. The expectation of free and fixed particles in urinary stone disease. Invest Urol. 1978;15:442-8.
9. Markowitz GS, Nasr SH, Klein P, et al. Renal failure due to acute nephrocalcinosis following oral sodium phosphate bowel cleansing. Hum Pathol. 2004;35:675-84.
10. Lieske JC, Spargo BH, Toback FG. Endocytosis of calcium oxalate crystals and proliferation of renal tubular epithelial cells in a patient with type 1 primary hyperoxaluria. J Urol. 1992;148:1517-9.
11. Worcester E, Evan A, Bledsoe S, et al. Pathophysiological correlates of two unique renal tubule lesions in rats with intestinal resection. Am J Physiol Renal Physiol. 2006;291:F1061-9.
12. Evan AP, Lingeman JE, Coe FL, et al. Randall's plaque of patients with nephrolithiasis begins in basement membranes of thin loops of Henle. J Clin Invest. 2003;111:607-16.
13. Evan AP, Lingeman JE, Coe FL, et al. Crystal-associated nephropathy in patients with brushite nephrolithiasis. Kidney Int. 2005;67:576-91.
14. Verhulst A, Asselman M, De Naeyer S, et al. Preconditioning of the distal tubular epithelium of the human kidney precedes nephrocalcinosis. Kidney Int. 2005;68:1643-7.
15. Khan SR, Shevock PN, Hackett RL. Acute hyperoxaluria, renal injury and calcium oxalate urolithiasis. J Urol. 1992;147:226-30.
16. Nankivell BJ, Borrows RJ, Fung CL, et al. The natural history of chronic allograft nephropathy. N Engl J Med. 2003;349: 2326-33.
17. Schell-Feith EA, Kist-Van Holthe JE, Conneman N, et al. Etiology of nephrocalcinosis in preterm neonates: association of nutritional intake and urinary parameters. Kidney Int. 2000;58:2102-10.
18. Vervaet BA, Verhulst A, D'Haese PC, et al. Nephrocalcinosis: new insights into mechanisms and consequences. Nephrol Dial Transplant. 2009;24:2030-5.
19. Gwinner W, Suppa S, Mengel M, et al. Early calcification of renal allografts detected by protocol biopsies: causes and clinical implications. Am J Transplant. 2005;5:1934-41.
20. Schwarz A, Mengel M, Gwinner W, et al. Risk factors for chronic allograft nephropathy after renal transplantation: a protocol biopsy study. Kidney Int. 2005;67:341-8.
21. De Albuquerque PF, De Paola D. Experiments in urolithiasis: I. Histochemical studies. J Urol. 1959;81(3):345-50.
22. Haggitt RC, Pitcock JA. Renal medullary calcifications: a light and electron microscopic study. J Urol. 1971;106:342-7.
23. King JS Jr. Etiologic factors involved in urolithiasis: a review of recent research. J Urol. 1967;97:583-91.
24. Oliver J, MacDowell M, Whang R, et al. The renal lesions of electrolyte imbalance. IV. The intranephronic calculosis of experimental magnesium depletion. J Exp Med. 1966;124:263-78.
25. Khan SR, Cockrell CA, Finlayson B, et al. Crystal retention by injured urothelium of the rat urinary bladder. J Urol. 1984;132:153-7.
26. Khan SR, Finlayson B, Hackett RL. Histologic study of the early events in oxalate induced intranephronic calculosis. Invest Urol. 1979;17:199-202.
27. Khan SR, Hackett RL, Finlayson B, et al. Light and scanning electron microscopic studies of oxamide urolithiasis in rats. Scan Electron Microsc. 1981;3:155-62.
28. Khan SR, Finlayson B, Hackett RL. Experimental calcium oxalate nephrolithiasis in the rat. Role of the renal papilla. Am J Pathol. 1982;107:59-69.
29. Khan SR, Hackett RL. The use of SEM in the study of oxalate induced experimental nephrolithiasis. Scan Electron Microsc. 1980;3:379-86.
30. Dykstra MJ, Hackett RL. Ultrastructural events in early calcium oxalate crystal formation in rats. Kidney Int. 1979;15:640-50.
31. Sarica K, Erbagci A, Yagci F, et al. Limitation of apoptotic changes in renal tubular cell injury induced by hyperoxaluria. Urol Res. 2004;32:271-7.
32. Khan SR. Calcium oxalate crystal interaction with renal tubular epithelium, mechanism of crystal adhesion and its impact on stone development. Urol Res. 1995;23:71-9.
33. GILL WB, Ruggiero K, Straus FH. Crystallization studies in a urothelial-lined living test tube (the catheterized female rat bladder). I. Calcium oxalate crystal adhesion to the chemically injured rat bladder. Invest Urol. 1979;17:257-61.
34. Asselman M, Verhulst A, De Broe ME, et al. Calcium oxalate crystal adherence to hyaluronan-, osteopontin-, and CD44-expressing injured/regenerating tubular epithelial cells in rat kidneys. J Am Soc Nephrol. 2003;14:3155-66.
35. De Bruijn WC, de Water R, Boeve ER, et al. Lectin-cytochemistry of experimental rat nephrolithiasis. Scanning Microsc. 1996;10:557-76.
36. De Bruijn WC, Ketelaars GA, Boeve ER, et al. Electron energy-loss spectroscopical and image analysis of experimentally induced rat microliths. II. J Urol. 1993;149:900-5.
37. Wiessner JH, Garrett MR, Roman RJ, et al. Dissecting the genetic basis of kidney tubule response to hyperoxaluria using chromosome substitution strains. Am J Physiol Renal Physiol. 2009;297:F301-6.
38. Bigelow MW, Wiessner JH, Kleinman JG, et al. Calcium oxalate crystal attachment to cultured kidney epithelial cell lines. J Urol. 1998;160:1528-32.
39. Riese RJ, Riese JW, Kleinman JG, et al. Specificity in calcium oxalate adherence to papillary epithelial cells in cultures. Am J Physiol. 1988;255:F1025-32.
40. Riese RJ, Mandel NS, Wiessner JH, et al. Cell polarity and calcium oxalate crystal adherence to cultured collecting duct cells. Am J Physiol. 1992;262:F177-84.
41. Wiessner JH, Kleinman JG, Blumenthal SS, et al. Calcium oxalate crystal interaction with rat renal inner papillary collecting tubule cells. J Urol. 1987;138:640-3.
42. Verkoelen CF, van der Boom BG, Kok DJ, et al. Cell type-specific acquired protection from crystal adherence by renal tubule cells in culture. Kidney Int. 1999;55:1426-33.

43. Verkoelen CF, Romijn JC, De Bruijn WC, et al. Association of calcium oxalate monohydrate crystals with MDCK cells. Kidney Int. 1995;48:129-38.
44. Verkoelen CF, van der Boom BG, Houtsmuller AB, et al. Increased calcium oxalate monohydrate crystal binding to injured renal tubular epithelial cells in culture. Am J Physiol. 1998;274:F958-65.
45. Verhulst A, Asselman M, Persy VP, et al. Crystal retention capacity of cells in the human nephron: involvement of CD44 and its ligands hyaluronic acid and osteopontin in the transition of a crystal binding into a nonadherent epithelium. J Am Soc Nephrol. 2003;14:107-15.
46. Mandel N. Crystal-membrane interaction in kidney stone disease. J Am Soc Nephrol. 1994;5:S37-45.
47. Wiessner JH, Hasegawa AT, Hung LY, et al. Mechanisms of calcium oxalate crystal attachment to injured renal collecting duct cells. Kidney Int. 2001;59:637-44.
48. Lieske JC, Leonard R, Swift H, et al. Adhesion of calcium oxalate monohydrate crystals to anionic sites on the surface of renal epithelial cells. Am J Physiol. 1996;270:F192-9.
49. Lieske JC, Leonard R, Toback FG. Adhesion of calcium oxalate monohydrate crystals to renal epithelial cells is inhibited by specific anions. Am J Physiol. 1995;268:F604-12.
50. Lieske JC, Norris R, Toback FG. Adhesion of hydroxyapatite crystals to anionic sites on the surface of renal epithelial cells. Am J Physiol. 1997;273:F224-33.
51. Glaeser RM, Mel HC. The electrophoretic behavior of osmium tetroxide-fixed and potassium permanganate-fixed rat erythrocytes. Biochim Biophys Acta. 1964;79:606-17.
52. Glaeser RM, Mel HC. Microelectrophoretic and enzymic studies concerning the carbohydrate at the surface of rat erythrocytes. Arch Biochem Biophys. 1966;113:77-82.
53. Haydon DA, Seaman GV. Electrokinetic studies on the ultrastructure of the human erythrocyte. I. Electrophoresis at high ionic strengths—the cell as a polyanion. Arch Biochem Biophys. 1967;122:126-36.
54. Sachtleben P, Ruhenstroth-Bauer G. Agglutination and the electrical surface potential of red blood cells. Nature 1961;192:982-3.
55. Eylar EH, Madoff MA, Brody OV, et al. The contribution of sialic acid to the surface charge of the erythrocyte. J Biol Chem. 1962;237:1992-2000.
56. Verkoelen CF, van der Boom BG, Kok DJ, et al. Sialic acid and crystal binding. Kidney Int. 2000;57:1072-82.
57. Bigelow MW, Wiessner JH, Kleinman JG, et al. Surface exposure of phosphatidylserine increases calcium oxalate crystal attachment to IMCD cells. Am J Physiol. 1997;272:F55-62.
58. Cao LC, Jonassen J, Honeyman TW, et al. Oxalate-induced redistribution of phosphatidylserine in renal epithelial cells: implications for kidney stone disease. Am J Nephrol. 2001;21:69-77.
59. Martin SJ, Reutelingsperger CP, McGahon AJ, et al. Early redistribution of plasma membrane phosphatidylserine is a general feature of apoptosis regardless of the initiating stimulus: inhibition by overexpression of Bcl-2 and Abl. J Exp Med. 1995;182:1545-56.
60. Buckland AG, Wilton DC. Anionic phospholipids, interfacial binding and the regulation of cell functions. Biochim Biophys Acta. 2000;1483:199-216.
61. Kohri K, Kodama M, Ishikawa Y, et al. Immunofluorescent study on the interaction between collagen and calcium oxalate crystals in the renal tubules. Eur Urol. 1991;19:249-52.
62. Xie Y, Sakatsume M, Nishi S, et al. Expression, roles, receptors, and regulation of osteopontin in the kidney. Kidney Int. 2001;60:1645-57.
63. Verhulst A, Persy VP, Van Rompay AR, et al. Osteopontin synthesis and localization along the human nephron. J Am Soc Nephrol. 2002;13:1210-8.
64. Ashkar S, Weber GF, Panoutsakopoulou V, et al. Eta-1 (osteopontin): an early component of type-1 (cell-mediated) immunity. Science. 2000;287:860-4.
65. Gorski JP. Acidic phosphoproteins from bone matrix: a structural rationalization of their role in biomineralization. Calcif Tissue Int. 1992;50:391-6.
66. Kohri K, Suzuki Y, Yoshida K, et al. Molecular cloning and sequencing of cDNA encoding urinary stone protein, which is identical to osteopontin. Biochem Biophys Res Commun. 1992;184:859-64.
67. Kohri K, Nomura S, Kitamura Y, et al. Structure and expression of the mRNA encoding urinary stone protein (osteopontin). J Biol Chem. 1993;268:15180-4.
68. Ullrich O, Mann K, Haase W, et al. Biosynthesis and secretion of an osteopontin-related 20-kDa polypeptide in the Madin–Darby canine kidney cell line. J Biol Chem. 1991;266:3518-25.
69. Yamate T, Kohri K, Umekawa T, et al. The effect of osteopontin on the adhesion of calcium oxalate crystals to Madin–Darby canine kidney cells. Eur Urol. 1996;30:388-93.
70. Yamate T, Kohri K, Umekawa T, et al. Interaction between osteopontin on Madin–Darby canine kidney cell membrane and calcium oxalate crystal. Urol Int. 1999;62:81-6.
71. Yamate T, Kohri K, Umekawa T, et al. Osteopontin antisense oligonucleotide inhibits adhesion of calcium oxalate crystals in Madin–Darby canine kidney cell. J Urol. 1998;160:1506-12.
72. Konya E, Umekawa T, Iguchi M, et al. The role of osteopontin on calcium oxalate crystal formation. Eur Urol. 2003;43:564-71.
73. Wesson JA, Johnson RJ, Mazzali M, et al. Osteopontin is a critical inhibitor of calcium oxalate crystal formation and retention in renal tubules. J Am Soc Nephrol. 2003;14:139-47.
74. Mo L, Liaw L, Evan AP, et al. Renal calcinosis and stone formation in mice lacking osteopontin, Tamm–Horsfall protein, or both. Am J Physiol Renal Physiol. 2007;293:F1935-43.
75. Sorokina EA, Kleinman JG. Cloning and preliminary characterization of a calcium-binding protein closely related to nucleolin on the apical surface of inner medullary collecting duct cells. J Biol Chem. 1999;274:27491-6.
76. Borer RA, Lehner CF, Eppenberger HM, et al. Major nucleolar proteins shuttle between nucleus and cytoplasm. Cell. 1989;56:379-90.
77. Schmidt-Zachmann MS, Dargemont C, Kuhn LC, et al. Nuclear export of proteins: the role of nuclear retention. Cell. 1993;74:493-504.

78. Nigg EA. Nucleocytoplasmic transport: signals, mechanisms and regulation. Nature. 1997;386:779-87.
79. Sorokina EA, Wesson JA, Kleinman JG. An acidic peptide sequence of nucleolin-related protein can mediate the attachment of calcium oxalate to renal tubule cells. J Am Soc Nephrol. 2004;15:2057-65.
80. Kumar V, Farell G, Deganello S, et al. Annexin II is present on renal epithelial cells and binds calcium oxalate monohydrate crystals. J Am Soc Nephrol. 2003;14:289-97.
81. Monastyrskaya K, Babiychuk EB, Hostettler A, et al. Annexins as intracellular calcium sensors. Cell Calcium. 2007;41:207-19.
82. Domoto T, Miyama Y, Suzuki H, et al. Evaluation of S100A10, annexin II and B-FABP expression as markers for renal cell carcinoma. Cancer Sci. 2007;98:77-82.
83. Cheng CW, Rifai A, Ka SM, et al. Calcium-binding proteins annexin A2 and S100A6 are sensors of tubular injury and recovery in acute renal failure. Kidney Int. 2005;68:2694-703.
84. Carr G, Simmons NL, Sayer JA. Disruption of clc-5 leads to a redistribution of annexin A2 and promotes calcium crystal agglomeration in collecting duct epithelial cells. Cell Mol Life Sci. 2006;63:367-77.
85. Chutipongtanate S, Fong-ngern K, Peerapen P, et al. High calcium enhances oxalate crystal binding capacity of renal tubular cells via increased surface annexin A1 but impairs their proliferation and healing. J Proteome Res. 2012;11:3650-63.
86. Kanlaya R, Fong-ngern K, Thongboonkerd V. Cellular adaptive response of distal renal tubular cells to high-oxalate environment highlights surface alpha-enolase as the enhancer of calcium oxalate monohydrate crystal adhesion. J Proteomics 2013;80:55-65.
87. Semangoen T, Sinchaikul S, Chen S, et al. Altered proteins in MDCK renal tubular cells in response to calcium oxalate dihydrate crystal adhesion: a proteomics approach. J Proteome Res. 2008;7:2889-96.
88. Spicer SS, Baron DA, Sato A, et al. Variability of cell surface glycoconjugates—relation to differences in cell function. J Histochem Cytochem. 1981;29:994-1002.
89. Verkoelen CF, Romijn JC, Cao LC, et al. Crystal–cell interaction inhibition by polysaccharides. J Urol. 1996;155:749-52.
90. Verkoelen CF, van der Boom BG, Romijn JC. Identification of hyaluronan as a crystal-binding molecule at the surface of migrating and proliferating MDCK cells. Kidney Int. 2000;58:1045-54.
91. Hansell P, Goransson V, Odlind C, et al. Hyaluronan content in the kidney in different states of body hydration. Kidney Int. 2000;58:2061-8.
92. Asselman M, Verhulst A, Van Ballegooijen ES, et al. Hyaluronan is apically secreted and expressed by proliferating or regenerating renal tubular cells. Kidney Int. 2005;68:71-83.
93. Schepers MS, Van Ballegooijen ES, Bangma CH, et al. Crystals cause acute necrotic cell death in renal proximal tubule cells, but not in collecting tubule cells. Kidney Int. 2005;68:1543-53.
94. Verkoelen CF. Crystal retention in renal stone disease: a crucial role for the glycosaminoglycan hyaluronan? J Am Soc Nephrol. 2006;17:1673-87.
95. Schepers MS, Duim RA, Asselman M, et al. Internalization of calcium oxalate crystals by renal tubular cells: a nephron segment-specific process? Kidney Int. 2003;64:493-500.
96. Verkoelen CF, Schepers MS, Van Ballegooijen ES, et al. Effects of luminal oxalate or calcium oxalate on renal tubular cells in culture. Urol Res. 2005;33:321-8.
97. Lieske JC, Toback FG, Deganello S. Sialic acid-containing glycoproteins on renal cells determine nucleation of calcium oxalate dihydrate crystals. Kidney Int. 2001;60:1784-91.
98. Nancollas GH, Tsortos A, Zieba A. The nucleation and growth of calcium phosphate crystals at protein and phosphatidylserine liposome surfaces. Scanning Microsc. 1996;10:499-507.
99. Thamilselvan S, Khan SR. Oxalate and calcium oxalate crystals are injurious to renal epithelial cells: results of in vivo and in vitro studies. J Nephrol. 1998;11(Suppl 1):66-9.
100. Aihara K, Byer KJ, Khan SR. Calcium phosphate-induced renal epithelial injury and stone formation: involvement of reactive oxygen species. Kidney Int. 2003;64:1283-91.
101. Thamilselvan S, Khan SR, Menon M. Oxalate and calcium oxalate mediated free radical toxicity in renal epithelial cells: effect of antioxidants. Urol Res. 2003;31:3-9.
102. Escobar C, Byer KJ, Khaskheli H, et al. Apatite induced renal epithelial injury: insight into the pathogenesis of kidney stones. J Urol. 2008;180:379-87.
103. Umekawa T, Chegini N, Khan SR. Oxalate ions and calcium oxalate crystals stimulate MCP-1 expression by renal epithelial cells. Kidney Int. 2002;61:105-12.
104. Umekawa T, Chegini N, Khan SR. Increased expression of monocyte chemoattractant protein-1 (MCP-1) by renal epithelial cells in culture on exposure to calcium oxalate, phosphate and uric acid crystals. Nephrol Dial Transplant. 2003;18:664-9.
105. Liang L, Chen J, Vittal R, et al. Expression profiling of crystal-induced injury in human kidney epithelial cells. Nephron Physiol. 2006;103:53-62.
106. Lieske JC, Walsh-Reitz MM, Toback FG. Calcium oxalate monohydrate crystals are endocytosed by renal epithelial cells and induce proliferation. Am J Physiol. 1992;262:F622-30.
107. Khan SR. Role of renal epithelial cells in the initiation of calcium oxalate stones. Nephron Exp Nephrol. 2004;98:e55-60.
108. Khan SR. Hyperoxaluria-induced oxidative stress and antioxidants for renal protection. Urol Res. 2005;33:349-57.
109. Belliveau J, Griffin H. The solubility of calcium oxalate in tissue culture media. Anal Biochem. 2001;291:69-73.
110. Schepers MS, Van Ballegooijen ES, Bangma CH, et al. Oxalate is toxic to renal tubular cells only at supraphysiologic concentrations. Kidney Int. 2005;68:1660-9.
111. Khaskhali MH, Byer KJ, Khan SR. The effect of calcium on calcium oxalate monohydrate crystal-induced renal epithelial injury. Urol Res. 2009;37:1-6.
112. Khan SR. Crystal-induced inflammation of the kidneys: results from human studies, animal models, and tissue-culture studies. Clin Exp Nephrol. 2004;8:75-88.
113. Hammes MS, Lieske JC, Pawar S, et al. Calcium oxalate monohydrate crystals stimulate gene expression in renal epithelial cells. Kidney Int. 1995;48:501-9.

114. Guo C, McMartin KE. The cytotoxicity of oxalate, metabolite of ethylene glycol, is due to calcium oxalate monohydrate formation. Toxicology. 2005;208:347-55.
115. Guo C, Cenac TA, Li Y, et al. Calcium oxalate, and not other metabolites, is responsible for the renal toxicity of ethylene glycol. Toxicol Lett. 2007;173:8-16.
116. McMartin KE, Wallace KB. Calcium oxalate monohydrate, a metabolite of ethylene glycol, is toxic for rat renal mitochondrial function. Toxicol Sci. 2005;84:195-200.
117. Tsujihata M. Mechanism of calcium oxalate renal stone formation and renal tubular cell injury. Int J Urol. 2008;15: 115-20.
118. Vervaet BA, Verhulst A, Dauwe SE, et al. An active renal crystal clearance mechanism in rat and man. Kidney Int. 2009;75:41-51.
119. Lieske JC, Norris R, Swift H, et al. Adhesion, internalization and metabolism of calcium oxalate monohydrate crystals by renal epithelial cells. Kidney Int. 1997;52:1291-301.
120. Kumar S, Sigmon D, Miller T, et al. A new model of nephrolithiasis involving tubular dysfunction/injury. J Urol. 1991;146:1384-9.
121. Xue YQ, He DL, Chen XF, et al. Shock wave induced kidney injury promotes calcium oxalate deposition. J Urol. 2009;182:762-5.
122. Baud L, Ardaillou R. Reactive oxygen species: production and role in the kidney. Am J Physiol. 1986;251:F765-76.
123. Baud L, Ardaillou R. Involvement of reactive oxygen species in kidney damage. Br Med Bull. 1993;49:621-9.
124. Andreoli SP. Reactive oxygen molecules, oxidant injury and renal disease. Pediatr Nephrol. 1991;5:733-42.
125. Abid MR, Razzaque MS, Taguchi T. Oxidant stress in renal pathophysiology. Contrib Nephrol. 2005;148:135-53.
126. Huang HS, Chen J, Chen CF, et al. Vitamin E attenuates crystal formation in rat kidneys: roles of renal tubular cell death and crystallization inhibitors. Kidney Int. 2006;70:699-710.
127. Thamilselvan S, Menon M. Vitamin E therapy prevents hyperoxaluria-induced calcium oxalate crystal deposition in the kidney by improving renal tissue antioxidant status. BJU Int. 2005;96:117-26.
128. Wassmann S, Laufs U, Muller K, et al. Cellular antioxidant effects of atorvastatin in vitro and in vivo. Arterioscler Thromb Vasc Biol. 2002;22:300-5.
129. Itoh Y, Yasui T, Okada A, et al. Preventive effects of green tea on renal stone formation and the role of oxidative stress in nephrolithiasis. J Urol. 2005;173:271-5.
130. Toblli JE, Ferder L, Stella I, et al. Effects of angiotensin II subtype 1 receptor blockade by losartan on tubulointerstitial lesions caused by hyperoxaluria. J Urol. 2002;168:1550-5.
131. Toblli JE, Ferder L, Stella I, et al. Protective role of enalapril for chronic tubulointerstitial lesions of hyperoxaluria. J Urol. 2001;166:275-80.
132. Antus B, Exton MS, Rosivall L. Angiotensin II: a regulator of inflammation during renal disease? Int J Immunopathol Pharmacol. 2001;14:25-30.
133. Li CY, Deng YL, Sun BH. Taurine protected kidney from oxidative injury through mitochondrial-linked pathway in a rat model of nephrolithiasis. Urol Res. 2009;37:211-20.
134. Erdem A, Gundogan NU, Usubutun A, et al. The protective effect of taurine against gentamicin-induced acute tubular necrosis in rats. Nephrol Dial Transplant. 2000;15:1175-82.
135. Manna P, Sinha M, Sil PC. Taurine plays a beneficial role against cadmium-induced oxidative renal dysfunction. Amino Acids. 2009;36:417-28.
136. Sener G, Sehirli O, Ipci Y, et al. Protective effects of taurine against nicotine-induced oxidative damage of rat urinary bladder and kidney. Pharmacology. 2005;74:37-44.
137. Marengo SR, Chen DH, MacLennan GT, et al. Minipump induced hyperoxaluria and crystal deposition in rats: a model for calcium oxalate urolithiasis. J Urol. 2004;171:1304-8.
138. Markowitz GS, Stokes MB, Radhakrishnan J, et al. Acute phosphate nephropathy following oral sodium phosphate bowel purgative: an underrecognized cause of chronic renal failure. J Am Soc Nephrol. 2005;16:3389-96.
139. Milliner DS, Wilson DM, Smith LH. Phenotypic expression of primary hyperoxaluria: comparative features of types I and II. Kidney Int. 2001;59:31-6.
140. Evan AP, Coe FL, Lingeman JE, et al. Renal crystal deposits and histopathology in patients with cystine stones. Kidney Int. 2006;69:2227-35.
141. Brown CA, Jeong KS, Poppenga RH, et al. Outbreaks of renal failure associated with melamine and cyanuric acid in dogs and cats in 2004 and 2007. J Vet Diagn Invest. 2007;19:525-31.

CHAPTER

7 Animal Models of Urolithiasis

Orson W Moe, David A Bushinsky

GENERAL CONSIDERATIONS

Naturally Occurring Urolithiasis in Nonhuman Species

The formation of solid inorganic crystals outside skeletal and dental tissue is pervasive throughout the animal kingdom. There are instances where the formation of these solid phase inorganic salts is clearly part of physiology, and there are examples where they definitely represent disease states. Between these extremes are conditions where it is less certain whether they represent an extreme end of physiology or pathology.

Invertebrates with Exoskeleton

The literature is replete with examples of "stones" in excretory organs of invertebrates. In the glow-worm, *Arachnocampa luminosa*,[1] crystalline concretions called "spherites" of calcium phosphate tinged with uric acid accumulate in their excretory tubules. When calcium is ingested by or injected into the hematophagous *Rhodnius prolixus*, crystalline calcium salts accumulate in tubule cells.[2] Similar mineralized substances are found ubiquitously in the common cockroach *Periplaneta americana*.[3] In the skipper butterfly, *Calpodes ethlius*, calcium phosphate accumulate in larval tubules, persists throughout metamorphosis, and decline in number in adults.[4] Mineralized concretions may serve a storage pool of calcium for later use to form the exoskeleton.

Mollusks are one of the most diverse in form and habit of all the phyla. Excretory concretions have been observed in many species of bivalves.[5] Hard, dark, and granular renal masses are extremely common in the Sunray Venus clam, *Macrocallista nimbosa*, residing off the Atlantic shoreline and Gulf of Mexico.[6] These were not considered pathologic until Tiffany and colleagues referred to them as "renal calculi."[7,8] The renal tubules of *M. nimbosa* resemble the mammalian proximal tubule. The calculi are primarily calcium phosphate with concentric laminar morphology. Tiffany and coworkers proposed that molluscan renal calculi start with intracellular "precursors" that grow by concentric deposition followed by calcification. The compression of the surrounding cells causes disruption of membrane and protrusion or extrusion of the mural stone into the lumen, where they grow by aggregation and epitaxy.[7,8] This model from the late 1970s is not very different from the paradigm for stone growth in the human kidney proposed first by Malek and Boyce[9] and later by Evan et al.[10]

Mineralized inorganic materials in invertebrate nephridia are probably as common as the ones found in insect Malpighian tubules. One should take caution in the interpretation of the examples cited above. It is unknown whether the concretions truly impact negatively on the animal's health, so one should not conclude that these are in fact disease.

Vertebrates with Endoskeletons

The aforementioned ambiguity between physiology and disease in invertebrates persists into vertebrates. Birds are uricotelic (excreting nitrogen as uric acid) organisms. Uric acid is a perfect form of nitrogenous waste as their direct discharge of urine laden with semisolid uric acid in a mucoid state into the gut lumen is advantageous for water conservation as there is minimal or no aqueous requirement for its expulsion.[11-13] While kidney stones in aquatic reptiles are extremely rare, renal calculi in desert reptiles are more common and may represent "disease."[14-16]

From here on, the examples cited are more likely to denote pathology. Reports of renal calculi in fish and aquatic amphibians are usually associated with either massive deviations from native diet changes or genitourinary infections that grossly alter urinary chemistry.[17] An example of diet-induced stone is seen in frogs.[18] Spinach-supplemented diet is used to bolster growth in tadpoles of *Rana pipiens*, and a complication of this rearing method is renal failure caused by massive calcium oxalate nephrolithiasis.[19] So even fresh water aquatic organisms can be overwhelmed by excessive loading from a dietary source. Birds, which have evolved to excrete large amounts of uric acid out of solution, can still perish from massive uric acid urolithiasis and tissue uricosis when accidentally given a large purine load.[20]

Several marine mammals succumb to urolithiasis,[21-24] but it is unclear how often this actually occurs in the wild. Bottle-nose dolphins (*Tursiops truncatus*) reared in captivity under approved managed conditions exhibit a very high prevalence of ammonium urate stones.[23,24] In contrast, it was noted that several hundred necropsies spanning two decades on wild dolphins have not disclosed urolithiasis to be a common illness.[24] By sonogram, dolphins in managed existence have a much higher incidence of ammonium urate stones[25] likely driven by high postprandial urinary ammonium and urate, conditions most likely secondary to dietary changes under managed care.[26] However, there were no demonstrable differences between the cases and controls in postprandial urinary chemistry profiles in this study, leaving one still perplexed about the propensity for stones.[26]

The prevalence of nephrolithiasis for the Asian small-clawed otter, *Aonyx cinerea*, in its natural habitat is likely very low and occurs only secondary to infection by the renal parasite *Gnathostoma vietnamicum*.[27] In sharp contrast, the exact same species reared in captivity has a 66–90% prevalence of nephrolithiasis.[28,29] The stones are primarily calcium oxalate and one study suggested hyperoxaluria as the factor, but due to lack of normal values for urinary electrolytes in otters, it is difficult to substantiate that conclusion.[29] One cannot avoid suspecting that what they are fed in the zoo is not what they forage in their natural habitats.

The high prevalence of urolithiasis in domestic animals, such as canine and feline kidney stones,[30-32] is supporting a large veterinarian health industry in the developed world. The high prevalence of urolithiasis in domestic mammals may be partially due to the processed food provided by commercial pet diets. The agricultural industry is also affected by bovine urolithiasis, which also afflicts other rumens like goats and sheep. Equine nephrolithiasis can cause obstruction and renal failure.[33-35] Compared to humans, horses have higher calcium carbonate in their calculi in addition to calcium oxalate and phosphate.[33-36] Common stone types in these domestic and agricultural species overlap with, but are also distinct from, humans (Table 7.1).[31,32] There are numerous reviews in veterinary literature, so we will not dwell on this topic further.[30,37,38]

Table 7.1: Common naturally occurring stone types in some nonhuman mammals.

Species	*Inorganic composition of stones*
Cats	Calcium oxalate Magnesium ammonium phosphate Uric acid Ammonium urate Calcium phosphate Cystine
Dogs	Magnesium ammonium phosphate Calcium oxalate Ammonium urate Cystine Sillica Calcium phosphate Xanthine
Cows	Struvite Silica Calcium carbonate Calcium oxalate
Horses	Calcium carbonate Calcium phosphate Struvite

Rare monogenic diseases do exists. The classical description of the Dalmatian as being a unique example of a uricase-positive species with hyperuricosuria[39,40] is due to inability of the hepatocyte to take up urate despite an intact ability to degrade urate.[41] This phenotype was created in a liver-specific deletion of the urate transporter GLUT9—the "Dalmatianization" of mice.[42] The chemical profile of aminoaciduria in cystinuric wolves and dogs is very similar to humans with congenital cystinuria with cystine, arginine, and lysine wasting.[43,44]

With the exception of the rare monogenic diseases, all the common urolithiasis in higher mammals can largely be attributed to some sort of exogenous factors—either infection or drastic changes in environment and diet. They represent a conflict between evolution and lifestyle, so to speak. In some ways, a lot of human urolithiasis may also represent organ dysfunction.

Model for Urolithiasis Per Se versus Pathogenic Risk Factors

It is not the objective of this chapter to summarize kidney stones in veterinarian practice for physicians, but rather to explore how one can use animals with either kidney stones or risk factors for kidney stones to enhance our understanding of human urolithiasis. At present, the large majority of animal models used to study human kidney stones are not based on naturally occurring urolithiasis despite their high prevalence. There are several reasons for this.

The pathobiology of naturally occurring stone diseases in mammals may bear some similarities to human urolithiasis, but a large number of them are quite divergent from human stone disease (e.g. canine silica stones). Even for the same type of stones with comparable pathophysiology (e.g. canine struvite stones), they may be equally complex as human urolithiasis so the advantage becomes the ability to do more invasive sampling.

The ability to manipulate the murine genome and the large battery of readily available procedures, reagents, and tools render the use of rodents highly pragmatic for biomedical research. There are formidable financial and regulatory hurdles and public opinion opposition from specific sectorsto cinduct to conducting research on larger mammals, even though they are truly valuable in some instances. As discussed below, the use of porcine models has advantages over rodents and is being pursued. In addition to discovery of disease pathways, animals are also amenable to preclinical testing and validating diagnostic and therapeutic modalities.

There are important differences between the rodent and human urinary tract, which will be discussed in more detail in a subsequent section. One major limitation of rodent models is that it is highly unusual for the organisms of the *rodentia* genus to actually develop kidney stones in nature. The commonly used Sprague-Dawley (SD) laboratory rat has a maximal urinary osmolality ($Uosm^{max}$) of 3,000 mOsm and dessert rodents can sustain $Uosm^{max}$ of over 5,000 mOsm. Yet under these most "hostile" conditions in terms of maintenance of solubility, urolithiasis is not a naturally occurring phenomenon in rodents. Crystalluria develops readily so saturation limits do get exceeded, and experimental maneuvers can successfully induce intratubular crystalline precipitations, yet true urolithiasis of the nature seen in humans is distinctly rare in rodents. One may question whether rodents are relevant to human urolithiasis research. But despite the paucity of true stones, rodents are indeed relevant.

Formation of a kidney stone is a final outcome originated from broad pathophysiologic pathways converging upon final epithelial and luminal events resulting in lithogenesis.[45] Despite the lack of this final pathology in rodents, the intermediate phenotypes that lead to stone formation are shared between humans and rodents. Within *rodentia*, there exist vast differences in pathophysiology in terms of propensity for lithogenesis.[46] The subsequent sections will illustrate how many of the biochemical risk factors for human stones were indeed successfully examined in rodents. An analogy will be a rodent model with hypertension as a complex trait (polygenic and environmental) but not prone to stroke. While such a strain may not be suitable to study the pathophysiology of a cerebrovascular event, it is still an excellent model for studying the pathogenesis of hypertension.

More than one pathogenic mechanism may exist in a given human stone former which converge and synergize to produce the final clinical picture. Despite the multiple pathogenesis, single factors—such as hypercalciuria—may carry the majority of the impact. Understanding the mechanism of intermediate phenotypes such as hypercalciuria is extremely valuable in the dissection of pathophysiology. The study of intermediate factors in isolation represents much cleaner experimental systems and will generate more precise conclusions. Again drawing on primary hypertension as an example, if impaired natriuresis due to a primary renal tubular defect is one of several pathways leading to hypertension, studying the mechanisms of this antinatriuretic propensity will beget more clear-cut and informative results than the composite pathways that cumulatively generate the complex phenotype of hypertension. In summary, the purpose of many experimental models is not directed at studying stones but rather at stone risk.

ANIMAL SPECIES CURRENTLY USED IN UROLITHIASIS RESEARCH

Rodents

Rodents still remain the mainstream model for kidney stone research. Rodents may be fed and will consume a precise quantity of food of defined composition each day for the duration of a study. Oral drugs may be mixed in with the daily food allotment and thus also completely consumed. Using metabolic cages all intake and excretion, including urine and feces, can be quantitatively collected. While similar studies can be done in humans when housed in a clinical research unit, a rodent has the research advantage that its organs, including kidney, intestine and bone, can be labeled, dissected and subjected to analysis.

There are many parallels in anatomy and physiology between rodents and humans, although rodent kidneys are anatomically distinct from human kidneys in that they have a single papilla. Ions and hormones critical to

Table 7.2: Comparison of human vs porcine kidney.

	Human	*Porcine*
Weight	110–170 g	~100–130 g
Dimesnsion Length Width Thickness	11–14 cm 6–7 cm 4–5 cm	11–12 cm 5–6 cm 3–4 cm
Papillae	Multipapillary	Multipapillary
Renal blood flow	3 ml/min/g kidney	4 ml/min/g kidney
Glomerular filtration rate	120 ml/min/70 kg BW	130 ml/min/70 kg BW
Maximal urinary osmolality	1,200 mOsm	1,100 mOsm
Maximal urine to plasma osmolality ratio	4.0	3.7

(BW: Body weight).

urolithiasis research such as calcium, phosphorus, sodium, parathyroid hormone and vitamin D, both 25(OH) and 1,25 $(OH)_2$ vitamin D are found in rodents at levels quite similar to that of humans. One distinct difference is that rodents have uricase while humans do not. While intermediate risks for uric acid stones (e.g. aciduria) can be studied, uric acid stones do not form in rodents.

Rodents, especially mice, have a genome that is quite similar to that of humans. Mouse genes may be deleted, modified or inserted, and the technology of rodent gene manipulation has become increasingly more feasible, accessible, and affordable. This is a huge advantage over large mammals. There are many examples of single gene deletions that lead to elevated stone risks. Rodents breed quickly so that genetic manipulations can be propagated and combined with other genetic alterations. Rodents are also practical with respect to housing space and costs compared to large mammals.

Pigs

There are advantages to the porcine model from both functional and structural points of view (Table 7.2).[47] The porcine kidney is anatomically highly similar to human kidney in size and anatomy. In contrast to the mouse or rat kidneys with single papilla, the pig kidney is multipyramidal with an undivided cortex. Each medullary pyramid forms a separate papilla and fusion results in the formation of some compound papillae (Figs. 7.1A to C). The prediction of single kidney glomerular filtration rate using *stereologic* methods of quantifying number or volume of glomeruli, kidney or cortical volume proved to be excellent in the Danish Landrace female pig.[48] Although rodents are clearly superior in that aspect, transgenic pigs are technically more and more feasible[49,50] and because of their anatomic likeliness to humans, they are the leading candidate species for future xenotransplantation.[51,52] Pigs are also an excellent source of pluripotent stem cells for renal application.[53]

In kidney stone research, the pig kidney has been used to evaluate imaging techniques to distinguish stone type in vivo.[54] Urologic scientists have used the pig kidney artificially implanted with stones to study efficacy and tissue damage by lithotripsy[55,56] and also ultrasonic propulsion of stones to facilitate passage.[57] These are clearly impossible ventures with rodent kidneys, but as described above and again below, rodents can be induced to have a variety of stone risk factors. However, such can also be accomplished in the pig. One is not limited to exogenously implanted stones. Diet-induced hyperoxaluria is accomplished in the pig by hydroxyproline feeding (Figs. 7.1A to C).[58-60] The full panel of urinary chemistries was not reported, but Mandel and coworkers demonstrated widespread calcium oxalate encrustations on papillary tips, and intratubular calcium oxalate crystals with evidence of tissue injury (Figs. 7.1A to C). No genuine uroliths resembling human stones were found.

One study used a presumed "acidogenic diet" on these same pigs and showed lower urine pH but unfortunately did not provide the relevant parameters of calcium, citrate, pH, ammonium, phosphate and sulfate.[58] Thus far, one cannot discern from the literature whether the major lithogenic chemical disturbances such as hypercalciuria, hypocitraturia or alterations in urine pH can be achieved with the porcine models. Overall, it appears that the pig presents an excellent model in terms of anatomy and physiology for the study of human stones, but the biochemical and local tissue defects of human lithogenesis have not been established.

Flies

At first glance, it is difficult to fathom how one can study kidney stones in organisms without kidneys (unfortunately *Malpighian* tubules do not qualify). Can one study flight physiology in a wingless bird such as the penguin? The answer is no if flight is a prerequisite of the experiment, but if the question of interest is specific aspects of thoracic

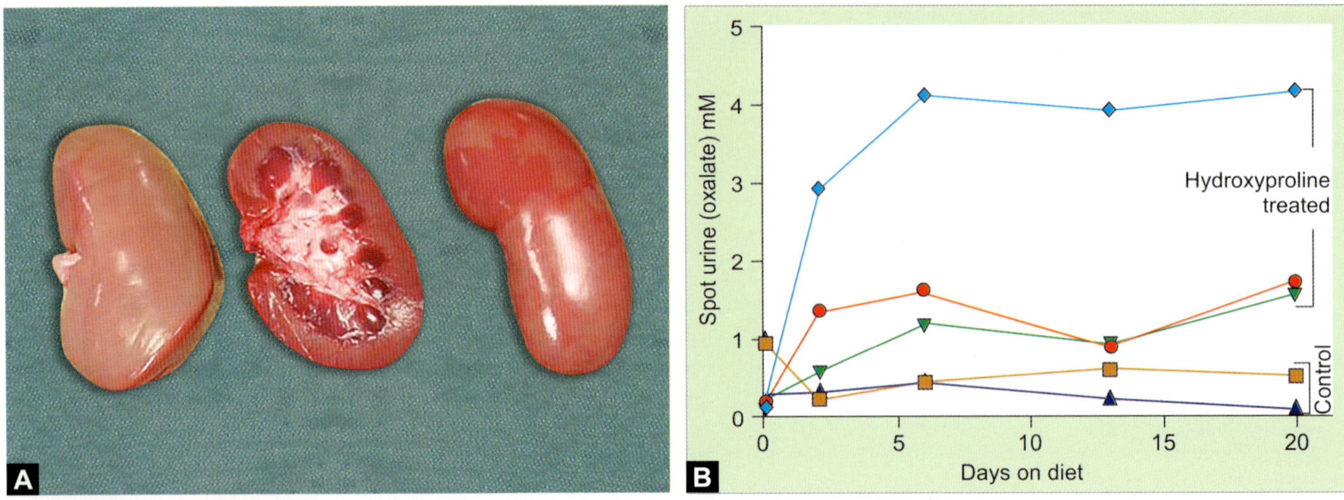

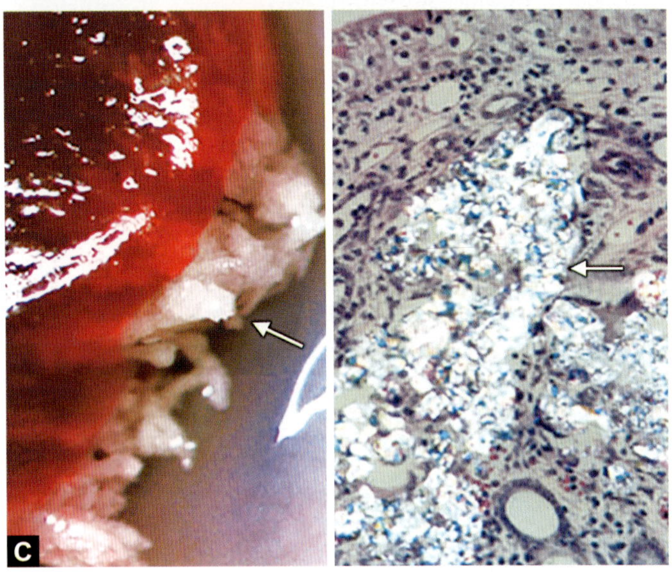

Figs. 7.1A to C: (A) Gross appearance and dimensions of porcine kidneys. (B) Hydroxyproline feeding. (C) Left: protruding calcium oxalate crystals on single papilla (arrow). Right: Pathohistology of papilla-containing birefringent calcium oxalate crystals (arrow). *Source*: (B and C) Reproduced with permission from Mandel NS, Henderson Jr JD, Hung LY, et al. A porcine model of calcium oxalate kidney stone disease. J Urol. 2004;171:1301-3.

muscle function in a homeothermic avian in cold climate, and the penguin offers clear experimental advantages, this will be an informative system.

As stated above, one does not always need to seek stone formation as a read-out. There are advantages to studying intermediate phenotypes. There is always a balance between relevance (e.g. highest in a human population with calcium oxalate stone formation as the measurement) and precision (e.g. highest in a pure preparation of the alanine: glyoxylate aminotransferase enzyme in a test tube). One sacrifices one for the other, and the choice depends on the goal of the study. The *Drosophila melanogaster* system offers more precision and investigative power than the mammalian models, which outweighs the loss in relevance due to the dearth of kidneys. This is the compromise we accept every time we obtain data from a cultured mammalian cell.

Drosophila melanogaster has two anatomically separate excretory organs—nephrocytes and Malpighian tubules. Nephrocytes are specialized cells in the thorax that filter the fly's hemolymph. In contrast, the Malpighian tubules are similar to a secretory epithelium that transports solutes from the hemolymph into the tubule lumen. There are four Malpighian tubules that coalesce into a common ureter, and each Malpighian tubule is divided into initial, transitional, and main segments.[61] The main segment is primarily responsible for urine production, which is composed of principal and stellate cells, which bear some distant organizational resemblance to principal and intercalated cells of the mammalian collecting duct. The

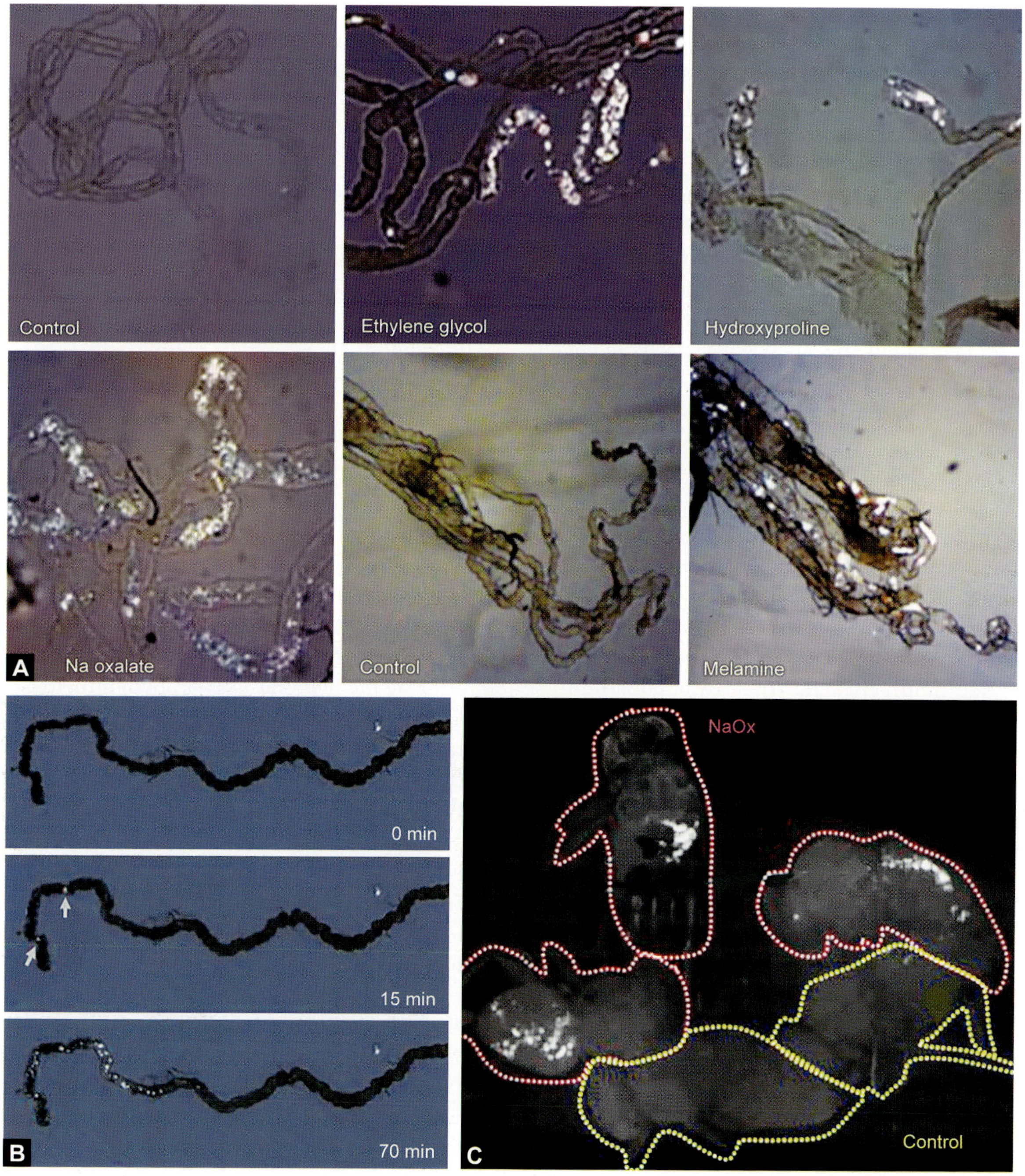

Figs. 7.2A to C: (A) Dietary models of flies fed with the indicated compounds and Malpighian tubules were isolated by dissection and CaOx crystals were identified. (B) Microdissected tubules incubated ex vivo in an oxalate-containing bath. (C) Whole-body microcomputed tomography scan with CaOx (white) inside Malpighian tubules.[63-65]

principal cells reside mostly in the main segment and contain basolateral ion cotransporters for inorganic (Na^+, K^+, and Cl^-) as well as a Na^+-dependent organic solute transporters.[62] Ion transport at the apical membrane is energized via a V-type H^+-ATPase, which extrudes H^+ into the tubule lumen providing the gradient for secondary Na^+ and K^+ excretion via cation/H^+ exchangers.

Malpighian tubules accumulate massive amounts of luminal calcium oxalate when fed ethylene glycol, hydroxyproline or sodium urate (Figs. 7.2A to C).[63] This is most likely a genuine "disease state" rather than physiologic excretion as it shortens the survival of the flies. Interestingly, melamine feeding also leads to extensive *Malpighian* crystallopathy (*see* Figs. 7.2A to C) and quite unexpectedly, the melamine stones were ameliorated by potassium citrate.[64] It has been argued that these are convenient and rapid models to study pathophysiology, which is true.[65] However, while these are all rather intriguing findings, they are more appropriately considered models of acute oxalate tubulopathy. In addition, while these studies provide proof-of-concept of the feasibility of *Drosophila* system, they have not taken full advantage of the power of genetic manipulation in fruit flies.

Human xanthinuria results from deficiency of xanthine dehydrogenase (type I) leading to increased urinary xanthine excretion and xanthine stones.[66] The rosy and maroon-like strains of *D. melanogaster* described back in 1959 suffer from whole-body accumulation of xanthine and of xanthine concretions in Malpighian tubules.[67] The cloning of the *Drosophila* maroon-like gene actually helped the identification of the human ortholog (molybdenum cofactor sulfurase gene) elucidating the genetic pathogenesis of Xanthinuria type II.[68] The rosy and maroon-like models can be manipulated with dietary restriction, and the effects can be witnessed in a much contracted time frame than rodent models.

The work of Romero, Doll and coworkers brought *Drosophila* genetic manipulation into kidney stone research. In mammals, Slc26 anion transporters are distributed in many organs and perform a variety of functions mainly via anion exchange.[69] Slc26a5/6 performs Cl^-/HCO_3^- exchange and also oxalate transport in the kidney and secretion in the small intestine (Cl^-/oxalate^{2-} exchange).[70] Gene deletion of murine Slc26a6 leads to massive hyperoxaluria and bladder calcium oxalate stones,[71] but since the same protein is responsible for intestinal oxalate secretion[72] and these animals have formidable hyperoxalemia and secondary hyperoxaluria, it is difficult to discern whether there is primary renal oxalate wasting.

The *D. melanogaster* genome contains nine homologs of the 11 human Slc26 transporters. The *Drosophila* gene CG5485 is equivalent to the human Slc26a5 and Slc26a6 transporters.[73] Malpighian tubules-specific knockdown of Slc26a5/a6 in the *D. melanogaster* was performed by Hirata and colleagues.[74] Addition of Na-oxalate to the diet of wild-type *Drosophila* larvae results formation of calcium oxalate crystals in the Malpighian tubules presumably due to a high excretory load. Adult flies fed this diet produce calcium oxalate crystals in 6–12 hours which can be quantified with birefringence microscopy of dissected tubules or at the whole organism level by *microcomputed tomography* scanning of whole flies (*see* Figs. 7.2A to C). Using *micro-dissected* Malpighian tubules bathed ex vivo in a sodium-oxalate bath, in situ formation of calcium oxalate crystals can also be observed in real time (*see* Figs. 7.2A to C). Selective knockdown of Slc26a5/a6 in the *Drosophila* Malpighian tubules results in a significant decrease in the intraluminal formation of calcium oxalate crystals proving that slc26a5/a6 are responsible for oxalate secretion in the *Malpighian* tubules.[74] The techniques described above are very useful tools of phenotyping in short time frames, which in combination with the powerful *Drosophila* genetics will prove to be a very valuable adjunct to mammalian models.

MONOGENIC MODELS OF STONE RISK

There are many rodent monogenic "disorders" that increased stone risk, although not actual stone formation (Table 7.3). These "disorders" are largely laboratory-generated by gene deletion. There are instances where a gene/protein known to regulate certain aspects of stone risk is deleted to interrogate the hypothesis as proof of principle. There are also many examples where deletion of genes of pathway not previously known to be linked to stone risk resulted in a phenotype that predisposes to stone risk. The advantage of these deletion studies is the discreet and known nature of the lesion—i.e. the inactivation of a gene. The investigative effort is devoted to connecting the lithogenic state to the function of the gene product. Although this journey can be circuitous and often has secondary and tertiary effects, the cause-and-effect relationship is certain.

There is a large number of single gene defects at the time of preparation of this chapter, and one cannot systematically go through the entire list. This is summarized in Table 7.3. We arbitrarily segregated these animal models as to whether they are related to primarily disturbances in calcium, oxalate, citrate/UpH, uric acid, or other molecules that influence stone formation.

POLYGENIC RAT MODEL OF UROLITHIASIS

The majority of humans with calcium-containing kidney stones are hypercalciuric compared to nonstone formers[113-117] and the polygenic nature of the inheritance has been discussed.[118-120] To help understand the mechanism of idiopathic hypercalciuria and stone formation in humans, an animal model of this disorder

Table 7.3: Rodent models of stone risk based on genetic deletions.

Gene/gene product	*Rodent phenotype*	*Equivalent human condition*
Hypercalciuria		
CLC5[75-78] Chloride-proton exchanger	• Hypercalciuria • Hyperphosphaturia • Proteinuria • Increased gut Ca absorption • Spinal deformities	Dent's disease[79]
NPT2a[80] Renal-specific Na-coupled phosphate cotransporter	• Hypercalciuria • Hyperphosphaturia • Renal calcifications • Retarded secondary ossification	Idiopathic infantile hypercal-cemia[81] Fanconi syndrome
NPT2c[82] Renal Na-coupled phosphate cotransporter	• Minimal abnormalities in rodents	Hereditary hypophosphatemic rickets with hypercalciuria[83]
NHERF-1[84] Na/H exchanger regulatory factor; docking protein	• Hypercalciuria • Hyperphosphaturia, hypermagnesuria • Female: reduced bone mineral density and content and fracture	Renal phosphate wasting[85]
TRPV5[86] Epithelial calcium channel	• Hypercalciuria • Hyperphosphaturia • Increased intestinal calcium absorption • Reduced trabecular and cortical thickness of bones	None to date
VDR[87,88] Vitamin D receptor	• Hypercalciuria on high-calcium and lactose diet • Rickets	Hereditary vitamin D resistant rickets[89]
CalB[90-92] Calbindin-D28k; intracellular calcium buffer	• Hypercalciuria • Normocalcemia • Normocalciuria	None to date
NKCC2[83] Na-K-Cl cotransporter	• Hypercalciuria • Polyuria, hydronephrosis • Proteinuria	Bartter's syndrome[93]
CAV1[95] Caveolin-1 scaffolding protein	• Hypercalciuria in male • Bladder stone	None to date
AKR1B1[96] Aldo keto reductase	• Hypercalciuria • Hypercalcemia • Hypermagnesemia	None to date
Hyperoxaluria		
SLC26A6[71] Oxalate-anion exchanger	• Hyperoxalemia • Hyperoxaluria • Bladder calcium oxalate stones	None to date
Agt Alanine-glyoxylate amino-transferase)[97]	• Hyperoxaluria • Calcium oxalate uroliths • Nephrocalcinosis and renal failure	Primary hyperoxaluria[98]
GRHPR Glyoxylate reductase/ hydroxypyruvate reductase[99]	• Hyperoxaluria • Calcium oxalate uroliths • Nephrocalcinosis and renal failure	Primary hyperoxaluria 2[100]
Hypocitraturia		
Atp6v1b1 *B1* Subunit of H-ATPase[101]	• Minimal disturbance at baseline • Alkaline UpH and worse metabolic acidosis after acid challenge	Distal renal tubular acidosis[102]
Atp6v0a4 *a4* Subunit of H-ATPase[103]	• Metabolic acidosis • Proximal tubular proteinuria and phosphaturia • Deafness	Distal renal tubular acidosis[104]

Contd...

Contd...

Gene/gene product	*Rodent phenotype*	*Equivalent human condition*
Hyperuricosuria		
Uricase[105]	• Hyperuricemia • Hyperuricosuria • Widespread tissue uricosis	None to date All higher primates are uricase null
UMOD *Uromodulin*[106-109]	• Deletion—changes in urinary tract immunity, papillary calcification, increased inflammation postischemia • Knock-in of human mutations—ER retention, abnormal aggregation	Cystic kidney disease type 2[110,111] Familial juvenile hyperuricemic nephropathy Glomerulocystic kidney disease
AhR *Aryl hydrocarbon receptor*[112]	• Hyperuricosuria • Uric acid bladder stones • Normouricemia	None to date

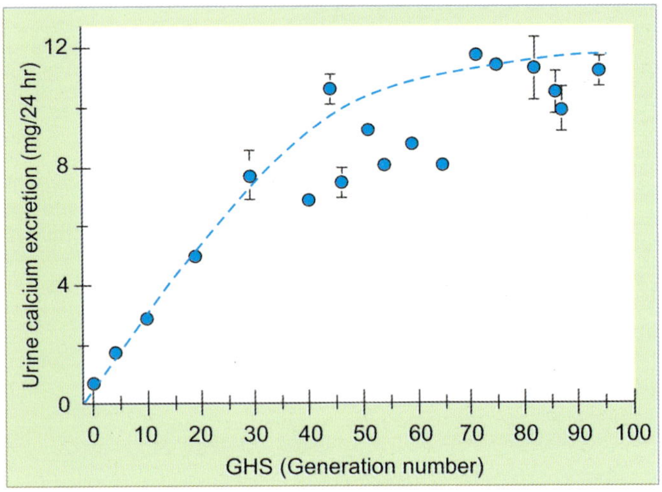

Fig. 7.3: Urine Ca excretion as a function of generation of GHS rats. Data from published studies. (GHS: Genetic hypercalciuric stone).

was developed.[121-151] Through >95 generations of successively inbreeding the most hypercalciuric progeny of the most hypercalciuric SD rats found on an initial screen, a strain of rats was established that now consistently excretes ~10 times as much urine calcium as SD controls on all diets and all feeding regimens tested (Fig. 7.3), universally forms calcium-containing kidney stones, and is termed *genetic hypercalciuric stone (GHS)-forming* rats.[121-123,125,128,130,131,133,143,146,149,150,152,153]

Genetic hypercalciuric stone rats have normal serum calcium but absorb far more dietary calcium compared to SD rats,[137,143] similar to observations in many humans with idiopathic hypercalciuria (Table 7.4).[113,115] The alterations of calcium metabolism leading to hypercalciuria are summarized in Figure 7.4. The elevated intestinal calcium absorption is due to a significant increase in the mucosal-to-serosal (absorptive) calcium fluxwith no change in the serosal-to-mucosal (secretory) flux.[139] When GHS rats are fed a diet devoid of calcium, urinary calcium excretion remains significantly elevated, indicating a defect in renal tubule calcium reabsorption, increase in bone resorption, or both,[136] again similar to observations in humans.[154,155] Cultured bone from GHS rats released more calcium than the bone of SD rats when exposed to increasing amounts of calcitriol.[132] The GHS rats, fed an ample calcium diet, have reduced *bone mineral density* (BMD) with reduced trabecular volume, mineralized volume and thickness, and their bones are more brittle and fracture prone, indicating that GHS rats have an underlying bone defect.[145] Administration of a bisphosphonate, which significantly inhibits bone resorption, to GHS rats fed a low-Ca diet significantly reduces urine calcium excretion.[128] Utilizing clearance studies, a primary defect in renal calcium reabsorption is observed.[129] Thus, compared to founder SD rats, GHS rats have a systemic abnormality in calcium homeostasis: they absorb more intestinal calcium, they resorb more bone, and they fail to adequately reabsorb filtered calcium (Fig. 7.4). The bone, kidney and intestine of our GHS rats have an increased number of vitamin D receptors (VDRs) and calcium sensing receptors (CaRs).[132,135,141,144,156] The elevation of VDR is accompanied by suppression of SNAIL gene expression.[147] SNAIL initiates epithelial to mesodermal transition in a variety of cells accompanied by a suppression of VDR and VDR-regulated genes that maintain the epithelial phenotype. In one human study, circulating monocytes from patients with idiopathic hypercalciuria were found to have an increased number of VDR.[157]

After eating standard rat chow for 18 weeks, all GHS rats form kidney stones while there is no stone formation in similarly treated SD.[133] The stones contain only calcium and phosphate without oxalate, and by X-ray diffraction are exclusively poorly crystalline apatites, a calcium phosphate

Table 7.4: Comparison of human idiopathic hypercalciuria (IH) with genetic hypercalciuric stone-forming rats.

	Hypercalciuric stone-forming (IH) humans	*Genetic hypercalciuric stone-forming (GHS) rats*
Urine Ca excretion	Increased (by definition)	Increased[116,121-135,137-140,150,153,158-160]
Intestinal Ca absorption	Increased in most patients[113,115,161-184]	Increased[121-135,137-140,158]
Renal tubular Ca reabsorption	Decreased in many patients[185-187]	Decreased[129]
Bone resorption	Increased in most patients—as evidenced by markers of bone resorption[188-194]	Increased[128,132,150,195]
Bone mineral density	Decreased in most patients [115,154,161,188,196-203]	Decreased[150,160]
Fracture propensity	Increased[204,205]	Increased[160]
Serum Ca	Normal[113,115]	Normal[137,143,149,150]
Serum PTH	Normal to reduced[172,201,206-208] or elevated[206,207]	Reduced[159]
Serum $1,25(OH)_2D_3$	Normal to elevated[164,171,172,201,209-213]	Normal to elevated[127,135,141,156,158]
Vitamin D receptor (VDR)	Increased number[157] or no change[214] Gene polymorphisms[215-228]	Increased number[127,132,135,156,229]
Biological activity of VDR	Unknown	Increased activity[149-151]
Ca receptor	Changes in number not reported Activating and inactivating mutations associated with hypercalciuria and hypocalciuria, respectively,[230,231] gene polymorphisms[232,233]	Increased number[141] Treatment with cinacalcet activates the receptor—associated with increased urine Ca in SD but not GHS rats[159]
Stone formation	Consequence of hypercalciuria[113,115,162-164,166,234-241]	Universal[121-123,128,130,131,133]

(SD: Sprague-Dawley; PTH: Parathyroid hormone).

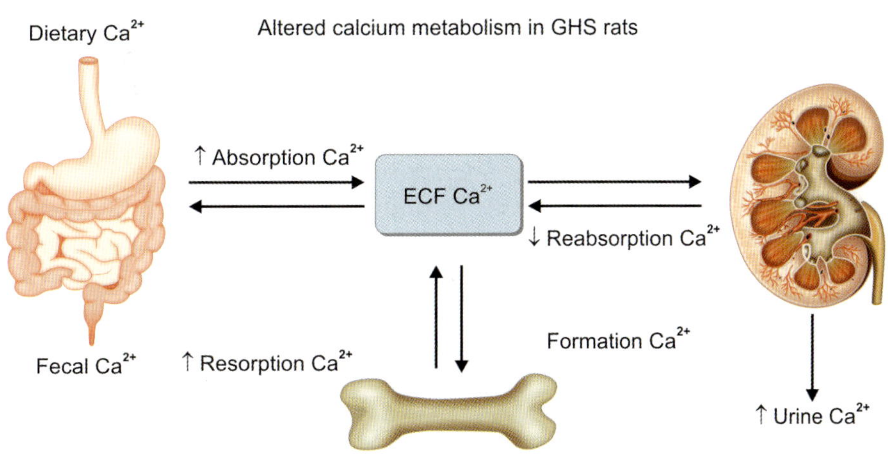

Fig. 7.4: Multiorgan abnormalities in calcium homeostasis in GHS rats. (GHS: Genetic hypercalciuric stone; ECF: Extracellular fluid).

complex.[122,123,130,133] When fed additional hydroxyproline, an amino acid which is metabolized to oxalate,[242] the GHS rats form calcium oxalate kidney stones,[121,125] the most common kidney stones in humans.[121,125]

EFFECTS OF DIET ON RODENT STONE RISK

Dietary manipulations will be discussed in the context of both the phenotypically selected GHS as well as normal rodents.

Calcium

A fundamental mechanism for hypercalciuria in genetic hypercalciuric rats appears due to a primary increase in intestinal calcium absorption. To study the effects of a reduction in dietary calcium on urine calcium excretion, GHS and SD rats were fed a normal calcium diet and then some were switched to a low-calcium diet.[158] Urine calcium excretion on a normal calcium diet was eightfold higher in GHS than in SD rats. With the low-calcium diet urine calcium excretion continued to be approximately eightfold higher in the GHS rats compared to SD. Balance studies revealed that the GHS, but not SD, rats were in negative calcium balance, that is, calcium excretion was significantly higher than that of SD. This study suggests that the provision of a low-calcium diet to hypercalciurics has the potential to have a detrimental effect of BMD.

Phosphorus

There is little direct proof that supersaturation itself regulates stone formation. Genetic hypercalciuric stone rats were used to test the hypothesis that an isolated reduction in urine supersaturation, achieved by decreasing urine phosphorus excretion, would decrease stone formation in these rats.[123] Genetic hypercalciuric stone rats received either a high- , medium-, or low-phosphorus diet for 18 weeks. The lowered dietary phosphorus would be expected to result in a decrease in urine phosphorus excretion and a decrease in urinary supersaturation with respect to the calcium phosphate solid phase. Decreasing dietary phosphorus intake led to progressive decrease in urine phosphorus excretion and increase in urine calcium excretion, the latter presumably caused by decreased intestinal calcium phosphate binding and increased calcium absorption. With decreasing dietary phosphorus intake, there was a progressive decrease in saturation with respect to the calcium phosphate solid phase. Genetic hypercalciuric stone rats fed the high-phosphorus diet had radiographic evidence of kidney stone formation, whereas rats fed either the medium- or low-phosphorus diet did not develop kidney stones. A decrease in urine phosphorus excretion not only led to a decrease in urine supersaturation with respect to the calcium phosphate solid phase but to an elimination of renal stone formation. The results of this study support the hypothesis that variation in supersaturation alone can regulate renal stone formation.

Acid

Acid is an integral component of animal protein, but the effect of protein on stone risk extends beyond acid and this will be discussed below. In humans with calcium nephrolithiasis, consumption of a diet high in acid precursors is often cited as a risk factor for the development of calcium-based kidney stones; however, the effect of this diet on urinary supersaturation with respect to the common solid phases found in kidney stones has not been determined. To determine the effect of the addition of an acid precursor on urine ion excretion, supersaturation and stone formation, GHS rats were fed a fixed amount of an ample calcium diet with three progressive, graded amounts of the acid precursor ammonium chloride (NH_4Cl) in the drinking water for 14 weeks.[122] As expected, the addition of dietary NH_4Cl led to a progressive fall in urine pH and urine citrate, while urine ammonium increased. Urine calcium and phosphorus increased, while urine oxalate fell. Increasing dietary NH_4Cl led to a fall in supersaturation with respect to brushite ($CaHPO_4$) and calcium oxalate and a rise in supersaturation with respect to uric acid. In spite of differences in supersaturation, most rats in each group formed stones that contained calcium phosphate and not calcium oxalate. Thus, while the provision of additional dietary acids alters urinary ion excretion and lowers supersaturation with respect to $CaHPO_4$ and CaO_X, it does not change the character or rate of stone formation in the GHS rats.

Protein

While the adverse effect of protein on stone risks in humans was described in epidemiologic associations[243-245] as well as intervention trials,[246] the mechanism of how protein intake leads to hypercalciuria and stone risk is still enigmatic. This was investigated in SD rats, where the acid content of a casein-based high-protein diet appeared to be responsible for the hypercalciuria and bone loss, as coadministration of the high-casein diet with alkali abrogated the hypercalciuria and bone loss.[247,248] This was in contrast with an earlier study in Wistar rats that very oddly showed that high protein decreased and sodium bicarbonate did not affect renal acid excretion.[249] Another study on Wistar rats fed a low-protein diet to pregnant females and the male offsprings seemed to have escalated renal sodium and calcium excretion suspicious of a proximal origin.[250] The experimental conditions of the above studies have sufficient variation that render a unifying interpretation difficult.

Humans on a high-protein weight-reduction diet developed hypercalciuria,[251,252] but in contrast to rodents, this hypercalciuria can only be very modestly reduced by complete neutralization of the acid,[252] suggesting that nonacid contents of the protein may be responsible for the nonacid component of hypercalciuria that is absent in casein, or there is a fundamental difference between rodents and humans. These discrepancies across species and across strains within species need to be worked out as the rodent will be an indispensable model to eventually understand the pathophysiologic mechanisms of protein-induced hypercalciuria.

Oxalate and Oxalate Precursors

Human calcium oxalate nephrolithiasis may occur if urine is supersaturated. In these patients, dietary oxalate is often restricted to reduce its absorption and subsequent excretion in an effort to lower supersaturation and to decrease stone formation. However, dietary oxalate also binds intestinal calcium, which lowers calcium absorption and excretion. The effect of increasing dietary oxalate on urinary calcium oxalate supersaturation is difficult to predict. To determine the effect of dietary oxalate intake on urinary supersaturation with respect to calcium oxalate and brushite ($CaHPO_4$) GHS rats were fed an ample calcium diet alone with the addition of graded amounts of sodium oxalate for 18 weeks.[131] Increasing dietary oxalate significantly increased urinary oxalate and decreased urinary calcium excretion, the latter presumably due to increased dietary oxalate-binding intestinal calcium. Increasing dietary oxalate actually decreased calcium oxalate supersaturation due to the decrease in urinary calcium offsetting the increase in urinary oxalate and decreased brushite supersaturation. All GHS rats formed stones. Scanning electron microscopy revealed discrete stones and not nephrocalcinosis. The stones were composed of calcium and phosphate; there were no calcium oxalate stones. Thus, increasing dietary oxalate led to a decrease in calcium oxalate and brushite supersaturation and did not alter the universal stone formation found in the GHS rats, nor the type of stones formed. These results suggest the necessity for human studies aimed at determining the role, if any, of limiting oxalate intake to prevent recurrence of calcium oxalate nephrolithiasis.

To determine if increasing urinary oxalate excretion, without the addition of dietary oxalate (which would lower dietary calcium absorption), would not only increase the calcium oxalate supersaturation, but also the ratio of calcium oxalate-to-calcium phosphate supersaturation and result in calcium oxalate stone formation in GHS rats. An oxalate precursor, hydroxyproline, was added to the diet of male GHS rats.[121] The GHS rats were fed an ample calcium diet alone or with graded amounts of hydroxyproline, which led to an increase in urinary oxalate. Small amounts of hydroxyproline did not alter urinary calcium, but a large amount led to a decrease in urine calcium, which led to an increase in urinary calcium oxalate supersaturation. Small amounts of hydroxyproline did not alter urinary supersaturation with respect to calcium hydrogen phosphate, while the addition of a large amount of hydroxyproline tended to lower this supersaturation. A large amount of hydroxyproline increased the ratio of calcium oxalate supersaturation to calcium phosphate supersaturation. Virtually, all rats formed stones. In the control and with low hydroxyproline, all of the stones were apatite; with a moderate hydroxyproline, the stones were mixed apatite and calcium oxalate; with a high hydroxyproline, all the stones were calcium oxalate. Thus, the provision of additional dietary hydroxyproline to GHS rats increases urinary oxalate excretion, calcium oxalate supersaturation and the ratio of calcium oxalate-to-calcium phosphate supersaturation, resulting in the formation of calcium oxalate stones.

Thus, with the addition of hydroxyproline, the GHS rats not only model the most common metabolic abnormality found in patients with nephrolithiasis, hypercalciuria, but also form the most common type of kidney stone, calcium oxalate.[121] Crystal deposits were found in the kidneys of all GHS rats and Yasue-stained material was detected only in the urinary space.[125] No crystal deposits were noted within the cortical or medullary segments of the nephron, and there was no evidence for tubular damage in any group. The only pathologic changes occurred in rats fed moderate and large amounts of hydroxyproline, with those fed the large amount showing the most severe changes. In these rats, which form only calcium oxalate stones, focal sites along the urothelial lining of the papilla and fornix of the urinary space demonstrated a proliferative response characterized by increased density of urothelial cells that surrounded the crystal deposits. At the fornix, some crystals were lodged within the interstitium, deep to the proliferative urothelium with increased osteopontin immunostaining in the proliferating urothelium. Thus in the GHS rat, the initial stone formation occurred solely in the urinary space. Tubular damage was not observed with either apatite or calcium oxalate stones. The apatite stones do not appear to cause any pathological change, while rats forming calcium oxalate stones have a proliferative response of the urothelium, with increased osteopontin immunostaining, around the crystal deposits in the fornix.

Sodium

While the relationship between dietary salt intake and hypertension is demonstrable in the general population, the effect of salt intake on blood pressure in individuals is extremely variable. In contrast, the linear correlative and causative relation between dietary salt intake and urinary calcium excretion is shockingly consistent in metabolic studies and population-based studies.[253] The evolutionary origin and intrarenal mechanism of this very tight relationship was speculated and discussed by Moe and Preisig.[254] The linear relationship has been used successfully as part of a larger therapeutic regimen to reduce stone recurrence.[246] In addition to hypercalciuria, a lesser-known effect of high salt is hypocitraturia and modest alkalinuria, which has been clearly shown in humans.[255] While these observations and clinical implications are unequivocal, we still do not fully understand the mechanisms of salt-induced hypercalciuria and hypocitraturia. The rodent is a good model to study this phenomenon. Rats on a normal calcium diet (0.6%) given a high NaCl diet chloride (1.8%) showed hypercalciuria and lower bone mineral content, after 4 and 12 months.[256] When the high salt was imposed on a low-calcium diet, the bone defect was further exaggerated. The effect of monovalent salt on calciuria is in the order NaCl > KCl > Controls = $NaHCO_3$ = $KHCO_3$, suggesting that the alkali may negate the effect of volume expansion.[257] This is compatible with the observation that NaCl-induced hypercalciuria but not $NaHCO_3$.

Patients with autosomal dominant pseudohypoaldosteronism type II (PHAII) caused by WNK4 mutations have low bone density and hypercalciuria.[258] It is not clear whether this is a direct effect of WNK4 mutation on distal calcium handling as these patients have hyperactive NaCl-mediated cotransport. In a murine knock-in model of a human PHAII WNK4 mutation, the source of the hypercalciuria is more compatible with a proximal tubule or thick ascending limb source secondary to the salt-induced volume expansion rather than a direct effect on DCT calcium handling.[259]

High-salt diet coupled with pharmacologic hyperaldosteronism causes hypercalciuria and secondary bone loss in rodents[260] similar to the elevated stone risk in humans with hyperaldosteronism.[261] A direct micropuncture study did not find reduced proximal tubule/thick ascending reabsorption and increased distal delivery, which argues against a volume expansion effect and rather implies aldosterone may have a direct effect on calcium handling in the mineralocorticoid-sensitive segments.[262]

EFFECTS OF MEDICATIONS ON RODENT STONE RISK

Potassium Citrate

Potassium citrate is prescribed to decrease stone recurrence in patients with calcium nephrolithiasis. Citrate binds intestinal and urine calcium and increases urine pH. $Citrate^{3-}$, when metabolized, is equivalent to generating $3HCO_3^-$ and should decrease calcium excretion by reducing bone resorption and increasing renal calcium reabsorption. However, citrate binding to intestinal calcium may increase absorption and renal excretion of both phosphate and oxalate. Thus, the effect of potassium citrate on urine calcium oxalate and calcium phosphate supersaturation and stone formation is complex and difficult to predict. To study the effects of potassium citrate on urine supersaturation and stone formation, GHS rats not given hydroxyproline were utilized; thus they form only calcium phosphate stones.[152] Rats were fed an ample calcium diet supplemented with potassium citrate or potassium chloride for 18 weeks. Urine citrate, phosphate, oxalate, and pH levels were higher and urine calcium level was lower in rats fed potassium citrate. Furthermore, calcium oxalate and calcium phosphate supersaturation were higher with potassium citrate; however, uric acid supersaturation was lower. Both groups had similar numbers of exclusively calcium phosphate stones. Thus, potassium citrate effectively raises urine citrate levels and lowers urine calcium levels; however, the increases in urine pH, oxalate, and phosphate levels lead to increased calcium oxalate and calcium phosphate supersaturation. Potassium citrate induces complex changes in urine chemistries and supersaturation, which may not be beneficial in preventing calcium phosphate stone formation. In contrast to GHS with calcium phosphate stones, the increased calcium oxalate stone risk in SD rats fed a high-casein diet can be completely neutralized by potassium citrate.[248]

Thiazide Diuretics

Hydroxyproline-supplemented GHS rats, which form only calcium oxalate stones, were used to determine if the thiazide diuretic chlorthalidone would decrease urine calcium excretion, supersaturation, and perhaps stone formation.[148] Genetic hypercalciuric stone rats were fed an ample calcium diet and hydroxyproline, so that the rats would exclusively form CaO_X stones. Compared with control, the addition of chlorthalidone led to a significant reduction of urine calcium and phosphorus excretion, whereas urine oxalate excretion increased. Supersaturation of calcium hydrogen phosphate fell, whereas supersaturation with respect to calcium oxalate was unchanged. Rats that were fed chlorthalidone had fewer stones. As calcium phosphate may be the preferred initial solid phase in patients with calcium oxalate kidney stones, the reduction in supersaturation with respect to the calcium phosphate solid phase may be the mechanism by which thiazides reduce calcium oxalate stone formation.

Thiazides also effectively decrease hypercalciuria in other rodent models such as the spontaneously hypertensive rats,[263] hyperprolactinemic hypercalciuria,[264] and vitamin-induced hypercalciuria,[265,266] which indicates that thiazides act on a very distant step that reverses the tubular mechanisms of hypercalciuria.

Thiosulfate

An uncontrolled trial reported that sodium thiosulfate reduces formation of calcium kidney stones in humans, but this has not been tested in a controlled setting in humans or animals. Genetic hypercalciuric stone rats were fed an ample calcium diet and some were given sodium thiosulfate for 18 weeks.[146] While virtually all of the untreated rats formed stones, only 25% of those given thiosulfate demonstrated stone formation. Urine calcium and phosphorus were higher and urine citrate and volume were lower in the thiosulfate-treated rats, changes that would increase calcium phosphate supersaturation. Thiosulfate treatment lowered urine pH, which would lower calcium phosphate supersaturation. Overall, there were no differences in calcium phosphate supersaturation or upper limit of metastability between thiosulfate-treated and control rats. In vitro, thiosulfate only minimally affected ionized calcium, suggesting a mechanism of action other than calcium chelation. Thus, sodium thiosulfate reduces calcium phosphate stone formation in GHS rats. Controlled trials testing the efficacy and safety of sodium thiosulfate for recurrent kidney stones in humans are needed.

Cinacalcet

Genetic hypercalciuric stone rat kidneys have an increased number of receptors for calcium (CaR) compared to SD rats. Calcimimetics, such as cinacalcet, increase the sensitivity of the CaR to calcium. The effects of cinacalcet on urine calcium are complex and difficult to predict. We determined whether cinacalcet would alter urinary calcium and supersaturation with respect to brushite and calcium oxalate.[159] Genetic hypercalciuric stone or SD rats were fed a normal calcium diet for 28 days with and cinacalcet was added to the diet of half of each group for the last 14 days. The protocol was then repeated while the rats were fed a low-calcium diet. Cinacalcet led to a marked reduction in circulating parathyroid hormone and a modest reduction in serum calcium. Cinacalcet did not alter urine calcium when the GHS rats were fed the normal calcium diet but lowered urine calcium when they were fed the low-calcium diet. However, cinacalcet did not alter urinary supersaturation with respect to either brushite or calcium oxalate on either diet. If these findings in rodents can be confirmed in man, it suggests that cinacalcet would not be an effective agent in the treatment of human idiopathic hypercalciuria and resultant stone formation.

Bisphosphonate

When GHS rats are placed on a low-calcium diet, urinary calcium excretion exceeds dietary calcium intake, suggesting that bone may contribute to the excess urine calcium excretion. Genetic hypercalciuric stone rats were utilized to determine if bone contributes to the persistent hypercalciuria on a low-calcium diet by determining if alendronate, which inhibits bone resorption, would decrease urine calcium excretion.[128] Genetic hypercalciuric stone rats and SD controls were fed a low-calcium diet and some were then injected with alendronate. On the low-calcium diet, the GHS rats excreted more calcium than they consumed and alendronate caused a significant decrease in urine calcium excretion and brought urine calcium well below intake. Alendronate also caused a marked decrease in calcium oxalate and brushite supersaturation. The alendronate-induced decrease in urine supersaturation should be beneficial in preventing stone formation in humans, if these results, observed in a short-term study using the hypercalciuric stone-forming rat, can be confirmed in longer-term human studies.

$1,25(OH)_2D_3$

Since GHS rats have normal levels of serum $1,25(OH)_2D_3$, the higher levels of VDR suggest that their VDR may be undersaturated with 1,25D. If the VDR were biologically active in GHS, then 1,25D should induce a greater increase in urine calcium in GHS compared to SD.[149] After injecting 1,25D, urine calcium in SD and GHS both increased; but the increase in GHS exceeded that of SD, indicating that the increased VDR in GHS induces a greater biological response. This increase in urine Ca must come from the intestine and/or bone.

To determine whether the origin of the excess urine calcium with 1,25D, 1,25D was administered to GHS rats fed a low-calcium diet.[267] On this low-calcium diet with 1,25D, the urine calcium in SD increased; however, urine calcium again increased significantly more in GHS. In GHS rats on low-calcium diet, with or without 1,25D, urine calcium far exceeded daily calcium intake, implying a loss of bone mineral.

To determine the role of bone resorption in the 1,25D-induced increase in GHS rat urine calcium rats were fed a low-calcium diet, coupled to inhibition of bone resorption by the bisphosphonate alendronate while receiving 1,25D.[151] Alendronate eliminated the 1,25D-induced increase in urine calcium in SD. However, in GHS alendronate decreased, but did not eliminate, the 1,25D-induced hypercalciuria, suggesting maximal alendronate cannot completely prevent the 1,25D-induced bone resorption in GHS. These results confirm the role of increased bone resorption in the hypercalciuria of GHS rats.

EFFECTS OF HYPERCALCIURIA ON RODENT BONE

Kidney stone patients tend to have a decrease in BMD and increased risk of fracture.[268] It is unclear if the reduced BMD is caused by a primary disorder of bone, the hypercalciuria itself, or both. To study the independent effects of hypercalciuria on bone, GHS and SD rats were fed a low- or high-calcium diet for 6 weeks.[160] Genetic hypercalciuric stone fed a high-calcium diet had reduced cortical (humerus) and trabecular [L(1)–L(5) vertebrae] BMD, whereas GHS rats fed a low-calcium diet had a reduction in BMD similar to SD. Genetic hypercalciuric stone rats fed a high-calcium diet had a decrease in trabecular volume and thickness, whereas a low-calcium diet led to an approximately 20-fold increase in both osteoid surface and volume. Genetic hypercalciuric stone rats fed high-calcium diet had no change in vertebral strength (failure stress), ductibility (failure strain), stiffness (modulus) or toughness, whereas in the humerus, there was reduced ductibility and toughness and an increase in modulus, indicating that the defect in mechanical properties is mainly manifested in cortical, rather than trabecular, bone. Genetic hypercalciuric stone rat cortical bone is more mineralized than trabecular bone and a low-calcium diet led to a decrease in the mineralization profile. Thus, the GHS rats, fed an ample calcium diet, have reduced BMD with reduced trabecular volume, mineralized volume and thickness, and their bones are more brittle and fracture prone, indicating that GHS rats have an intrinsic disorder of bone that is not secondary to diet.

Thiazide diuretics reduce urine calcium excretion and prevent stone formation; however, whether they benefit bone is not clear. Genetic hypercalciuric stone rats were used to test the hypothesis using chlorthalidone.[148] Genetic hypercalciuric stone rats were fed an ample calcium diet and some were given chlorthalidone. Rats treated with chlorthalidone had a marked reduction in urine calcium excretion. An increase in trabecular mineralization was observed in the axial and appendicular skeletons with chlorthalidone. Trabecular bone volume, trabecular thickness, trabecular number and connectivity were increased. Significant improvements in vertebral strength and stiffness were detected. Conversely, a slight loss of bending strength was found in the femoral diaphysis with chlorthalidone. Chlorthalidone did not alter formation parameters, suggesting that the improved vertebral bone strength was due to decreased bone resorption. Chlorthalidone can favorably influence vertebral fracture risk.

To study the effect of increased VDR on the osseous response to 1,25D, GHS, and SD rats were fed an ample Ca diet and injected with vehicle or increasing amounts of 1,25D for 16 days.[150] In GHS femoral and vertebral BMD was decreased with 1,25D and histomorphometry indicated decreased osteoclast number. In tibiae, 1,25D increased trabecular thickness, with a 12-fold increase in osteoid volume but only a threefold increase in bone volume. Bone formation rate was decreased in GHS rats receiving 1,25D, confirming the mineralization defect. The loss of BMD and the mineralization defect in GHS rats contribute to increased hypercalciuria, and if these effects persist, they would result in decreased bone strength, making these bones more fracture-prone.

REFERENCES

1. Green LF. Regional specialization in the Malpighian tubules of the New Zealand glow-worm *Arachnocampa luminosa* (Diptera: mycetophilidae). The structure and function of type I and II cells. Tissue Cell. 1979;11:673-703.
2. Maddrell SH, Whittembury G, Mooney RL, et al. The fate of calcium in the diet of *Rhodnius prolixus*: storage in concretion bodies in the Malpighian tubules. J Exp Biol. 1991;157:483-502.
3. Wall BJ, Oschman JL, Schmidt BA. Morphology and function of Malpighian tubules and associated structures in the cockroach, *Periplaneta americana*. J Morphol. 1975;146:265-306.
4. Ryerse JS. Developmental changes in Malpighian tubule cell structure. Tissue Cell. 1979;11:533-51.
5. Doyle LJ, Blake NJ, Woo CC, et al. Recent biogenic phosphorite: concretions in mollusk kidneys. Science. 1978;199:1431-3.
6. Doyle LJ, Blake NJ, Woo CC, Yevich PP. Recent Biogenuic Phosphorite: Concretions in Mollusk Kidney. Science. 1978;199:1431-3.

7. Tiffany 3rd WJ. Analysis of renal calculi from a marine mollusc (*Marcocallista nimbosa*). Implications for the study of urolithiasis. Investig Urol. 1979;17:164-5.
8. Tiffany 3rd WJ, Luer WH, Watkins MA. Intracellular and intraluminal aspects of renal calculosis in the marine mollusc *Macrocallista nimbosa*. Investig Urol. 1980;18:139-43.
9. Malek RS, Boyce WH. Observations on the ultrastructure and genesis of urinary calculi. J Urol. 1977;117:336-41.
10. Evan AP, Lingeman JE, Coe FL, et al. Randall's plaque of patients with nephrolithiasis begins in basement membranes of thin loops of Henle. J Clin Invest. 2003;111:607-16.
11. McNabb FM, McNabb RA, Ward JM Jr. The effects of dietary protein content on water requirements and ammonia excretion in pigeons, Columba livia. Comp Biochem Physiol A Comp Physiol. 1972 Sep 1;43(1):181-5.
12. McNabb RA, McNabb FA. Urate excretion by the avian kidney. Comp Biochem Physiol A: Physiol. 1975;51:253-8.
13. Shoemaker VH, Balding D, Ruibal R, et al. Uricotelism and low evaporative water loss in a South American frog. Science. 1972;175:1018-20.
14. Frye FL. Surgical removal of a cystic calculus from a desert tortoise. J Am Vet Med Assoc. 1972;161:600-2.
15. McKown RD. A cystic calculus from a wild western spiny softshell turtle (*Apalone [Trionyx] spiniferus hartwegi*). J Zoo Wildl Med. 1998;29:347.
16. Homer BL, Berry KH, Brown MB, et al. Pathology of diseases in wild desert tortoises from California. J Wildl Dis. 1998;34:508-23.
17. Walsh MT, Murru FL. Urogenital sinus calculi in a sand tiger shark (*Odontaspis taurus*). J Wildl Dis. 1987;23:428-31.
18. Smith MJ. The production and prophylaxis of calculi in *Rana pipiens*. Investig Urol. 1972;10:69-71.
19. Berns M. Mortality caused by kidney stones in spinach-fed frogs (*Rana pipiens*). BioScience 1965;15:297-8.
20. Kozhevnikov EM, Voitov LI, Efimova MN, et al. Uric acid diathesis in chickens. Veterinariia. 1978 Feb;(2):84-6.
21. Dennison S, Gulland F, Haulena M, et al. Urate nephrolithiasis in a northern elephant seal (*Mirounga angustirostris*) and a California sea lion (*Zalophus californianus*). J Zoo Wildl Med. 2007;38:114-20.
22. Stroud RK. Nephrolithiasis in a harbor seal. J Am Vet Med Assoc. 1979;175:924-5.
23. Venn-Watson S, Smith CR, Johnson S, et al. Clinical relevance of urate nephrolithiasis in bottlenose dolphins *Tursiops truncatus*. Dis Aquat Organ. 2010;89:167-77.
24. Venn-Watson SK, Townsend FI, Daniels RL, et al. Hypocitraturia in common bottlenose dolphins (*Tursiops truncatus*): assessing a potential risk factor for urate nephrolithiasis. Comp Med. 2010;60:149-53.
25. Smith CR, Venn-Watson S, Wells RS, et al. Comparison of nephrolithiasis prevalence in two bottlenose dolphin (*Tursiops truncatus*) populations. Front Endocrinol. 2013;4:145.
26. Smith CR, Poindexter JR, Meegan JM, et al. Pathophysiological and physicochemical basis of ammonium urate stone formation in dolphins. J Urol. 2014;192:260-6.
27. Daengsvang S. First report on *Gnathostoma vietnamicum* Le-Van-Hoa 1965 from urinary system of otters (*Aonyx cinerea*, Illiger) in Thailand. Southeast Asian J Trop Med Public Health. 1973;4:63-70.
28. Calle PP. Asian small-clawed otter (*Aonyx cinerea*) urolithiasis prevalence in North America. Zoo Biol. 1988;7:233-42.
29. Petrini KR, Lulich JP, Treschel L, et al. Evaluation of urinary and serum metabolites in Asian small-clawed otters (*Aonyx cinerea*) with calcium oxalate urolithiasis. J Zoo Wildl Med. 1999;30:54-63.
30. Ross SJ, Osborne CA, Lulich JP, et al. Canine and feline nephrolithiasis. Epidemiology, detection, and management. Vet Clin North Am Small Anim Pract. 1999;29:231-50, xiii-xiv.
31. Ling GV, Ruby AL, Johnson DL, et al. Renal calculi in dogs and cats: prevalence, mineral type, breed, age, and gender interrelationships (1981-1993). J Vet Intern Med. 1998;12:11-21.
32. Finco DR, Rosin E, Johnson KH. Canine urolithiasis: a review of 133 clinical and 23 necropsy cases. J Am Vet Med Assoc. 1970;157:1225-8.
33. Divers T. Chronic-renal-failure in horses. Compend Contin Educ Pract Vet. 1983;5:S310.
34. Hope W, Wilson JH, Hager D, et al. Chronic renal failure associated with bilateral nephroliths and ureteroliths in a two-year-old Thoroughbred colt. Equine Vet J. 1989;21:228-31.
35. Ehnen SJ, Divers TJ, Gillette D, et al. Obstructive nephrolithiasis and ureterolithiasis associated with chronic renal failure in horses: eight cases (1981-1987). J Am Vet Med Assoc. 1990;197:249-53.
36. Holt PE, Pearson H. Urolithiasis in the horse—a review of 13 cases. Equine Vet J. 1984;16:31-4.
37. Robinson MR, Norris RD, Sur RL, et al. Urolithiasis: not just a 2-legged animal disease. J Urol. 2008;179:46-52.
38. Lewis LD, Morris Jr ML. Diet as a causative factor of feline urolithiasis. Vet Clin North Am Small Anim Pract. 1984;14:513-27.
39. Briggs OM, Sperling O. Uric acid metabolism in the Dalmatian coach hound. J S Afr Vet Assoc. 1982;53:201-4.
40. Sorenson JL, Ling GV. Metabolic and genetic aspects of urate urolithiasis in Dalmatians. J Am Vet Med Assoc. 1993;203:857-62.
41. Simkin PA. The Dalmatian defect: a hepatic endocrinopathy of urate transport. Arthritis Rheum. 2005;52:2257-62.
42. Preitner F, Bonny O, Laverriere A, et al. Glut9 is a major regulator of urate homeostasis and its genetic inactivation induces hyperuricosuria and urate nephropathy. Proc Natl Acad Sci U S A. 2009;106:15501-6.
43. Bush M, Bovee KC. Cystinuria in a maned wolf. J Am Vet Med Assoc. 1978;173:1159-62.
44. Brand E, Cahill G. Canine cystinuria. III. J Biol Chem. 1936;114:XV.
45. Bushinsky D, Coe FC, Moe OW. Nephrolithiasis. In: Chertow G, Marsden P, Skorecki K, Yu ASL (Eds). Brenner & Rector's the Kidney, 9th edition. Philadelphia: Elsevier/Saunders; 2012.
46. Tannehill-Gregg SH, Dominick MA, Reisinger AJ, et al. Strain-related differences in urine composition of male rats of potential relevance to urolithiasis. Toxicol Pathol. 2009;37:293-305.
47. Terris J. Swine as a model in renal physiology and nephrology: an overview. In: Tumbleson M (Ed). Swine in Biomedical Research. New York: Plenum Press; 1986. pp. 1673-89.

48. Lodrup AB, Karstoft K, Dissing TH, et al. The association between renal function and structural parameters: a pig study. BMC Nephrol. 2008;9:18.
49. He J, Ye J, Li Q, et al. Construction of a transgenic pig model overexpressing polycystic kidney disease 2 (PKD2) gene. Transgenic Res. 2013;22:861-7.
50. Nagashima H, Matsunari H, Nakano K, et al. Advancing pig cloning technologies towards application in regenerative medicine. Reprod Domest Anim Zuchthygiene. 2012;47(Suppl 4):120-6.
51. Cooper DK, Satyananda V, Ekser B, et al. Progress in pig-to-non-human primate transplantation models (1998–2013): a comprehensive review of the literature. Xenotransplantation. 2014;21:397-419.
52. Sachs DH. The pig as a potential xenograft donor. Vet Immunol Immunopathol. 1994;43:185-91.
53. Kobayashi E, Hishikawa S, Teratani T, et al. The pig as a model for translational research: overview of porcine animal models at Jichi Medical University. Transplant Res. 2012;1:8.
54. Primak AN, Fletcher JG, Vrtiska TJ, et al. Noninvasive differentiation of uric acid versus non-uric acid kidney stones using dual-energy CT. Acad Radiol. 2007;14:1441-7.
55. Paterson RF, Kim SC, Kuo RL, et al. Shock wave lithotripsy of stones implanted in the proximal ureter of the pig. J Urol. 2005;173:1391-4.
56. McAteer JA, Evan AP, Williams Jr JC, et al. Treatment protocols to reduce renal injury during shock wave lithotripsy. Curr Opin Urol. 2009;19:192-5.
57. Sorensen MD, Bailey MR, Hsi RS, et al. Focused ultrasonic propulsion of kidney stones: review and update of preclinical technology. J Endourol. 2013;27:1183-6.
58. Kaplon DM, Penniston KL, Darriet C, et al. Hydroxyproline-induced hyperoxaluria using acidified and traditional diets in the porcine model. J Endourol. 2010;24:355-9.
59. Patel SR, Penniston KL, Iwicki L, et al. Dietary induction of long-term hyperoxaluria in the porcine model. J Endourol. 2012;26:433-8.
60. Mandel NS, Henderson Jr JD, Hung LY, et al. A porcine model of calcium oxalate kidney stone disease. J Urol. 2004;171:1301-3.
61. Dow JA, Maddrell SH, Gortz A, et al. The Malpighian tubules of *Drosophila melanogaster*: a novel phenotype for studies of fluid secretion and its control. J Exp Biol. 1994;197:421-8.
62. O'Donnell MJ, Ianowski JP, Linton SM, et al. Inorganic and organic anion transport by insect renal epithelia. Biochim Biophys Acta. 2003;1618:194-206.
63. Chen YH, Liu HP, Chen HY, et al. Ethylene glycol induces calcium oxalate crystal deposition in Malpighian tubules: a *Drosophila* model for nephrolithiasis/urolithiasis. Kidney Int. 2011;80:369-77.
64. Chen WC, Lin WY, Chen HY, et al. Melamine-induced urolithiasis in a *Drosophila* model. J Agric Food Chem. 2012;60:2753-7.
65. Miller J, Chi T, Kapahi P, et al. *Drosophila melanogaster* as an emerging translational model of human nephrolithiasis. J Urol. 2013;190:1648-56.
66. Pais Jr VM, Lowe G, Lallas CD, et al. Xanthine urolithiasis. Urology. 2006;67:1084 e9-11.
67. Mitchell HK, Glassman E. Hypoxanthine in rosy and maroon-like mutants of *Drosophila melanogaster*. Science. 1959;129:268.
68. Ichida K, Matsumura T, Sakuma R, et al. Mutation of human molybdenum cofactor sulfurase gene is responsible for classical xanthinuria type II. Biochem Biophys Res Commun. 2001;282:1194-200.
69. Dorwart MR, Shcheynikov N, Yang D, et al. The solute carrier 26 family of proteins in epithelial ion transport. Physiology. 2008;23:104-14.
70. Sindic A, Chang MH, Mount DB, et al. Renal physiology of SLC26 anion exchangers. Curr Opin Nephrol Hypertens. 2007;16:484-90.
71. Jiang Z, Asplin JR, Evan AP, et al. Calcium oxalate urolithiasis in mice lacking anion transporter Slc26a6. Nat Genet. 2006;38:474-8.
72. Knauf F, Ko N, Jiang Z, et al. Net intestinal transport of oxalate reflects passive absorption and SLC26A6-mediated secretion. J Am Soc Nephrol. 2011;22:2247-55.
73. Hirata T, Czapar A, Brin L, et al. Ion and solute transport by Prestin in *Drosophila* and *Anopheles*. J. Insect Physiol. 2012;58:563-9.
74. Hirata T, Cabrero P, Berkholz DS, et al. In vivo *Drosophilia* genetic model for calcium oxalate nephrolithiasis. Am J Physiol Renal Physiol. 2012;303:F1555-62.
75. Luyckx VA, Leclercq B, Dowland LK, et al. Diet-dependent hypercalciuria in transgenic mice with reduced CLC5 chloride channel expression. Proc Natl Acad Sci U S A. 1999;96:12174-9.
76. Piwon N, Gunther W, Schwake M, et al. ClC-5 Cl^--channel disruption impairs endocytosis in a mouse model for Dent's disease. Nature. 2000;408:369-73.
77. Silva IV, Cebotaru V, Wang H, et al. The ClC-5 knockout mouse model of Dent's disease has renal hypercalciuria and increased bone turnover. J Bone Miner Res. 2003;18:615-23.
78. Wang SS, Devuyst O, Courtoy PJ, et al. Mice lacking renal chloride channel, CLC-5, are a model for Dent's disease, a nephrolithiasis disorder associated with defective receptor-mediated endocytosis. Hum Mol Genet. 2000;9:2937-45.
79. Mansour-Hendili L, Blanchard A, Le Pottier N, et al. Mutation update of the CLCN5 gene responsible for dent disease 1. Hum Mutat. 2015;36:743-52.
80. Beck L, Karaplis AC, Amizuka N, et al. Targeted inactivation of Npt2 in mice leads to severe renal phosphate wasting, hypercalciuria, and skeletal abnormalities. Proc Natl Acad Sci U S A. 1998;95:5372-7.
81. Schlingmann KP, Ruminska J, Kaufmann M, et al. Autosomal-recessive mutations in SLC34A1 encoding sodium-phosphate cotransporter 2A cause idiopathic infantile hypercalcemia. J Am Soc Nephrol. 2015.
82. Segawa H, Onitsuka A, Furutani J, et al. Npt2a and Npt2c in mice play distinct and synergistic roles in inorganic phosphate metabolism and skeletal development. Am J Physiol Renal Physiol. 2009;297:F671-8.
83. Dasgupta D, Wee MJ, Reyes M, et al. Mutations in SLC34A3/NPT2c are associated with kidney stones and nephrocalcinosis. J Am Soc Nephrol. 2014;25:2366-75.

84. Shenolikar S, Voltz JW, Minkoff CM, et al. Targeted disruption of the mouse NHERF-1 gene promotes internalization of proximal tubule sodium-phosphate cotransporter type IIa and renal phosphate wasting. Proc Natl Acad Sci U S A. 2002;99:11470-5.
85. Karim Z, Gerard B, Bakouh N, et al. NHERF1 mutations and responsiveness of renal parathyroid hormone. N Engl J Med. 2008;359:1128-35.
86. Hoenderop JG, van Leeuwen JP, van der Eerden BC, et al. Renal Ca^{2+} wasting, hyperabsorption, and reduced bone thickness in mice lacking TRPV5. J Clin Invest. 2003;112:1906-14.
87. Li YC, Pirro AE, Amling M, et al. Targeted ablation of the vitamin D receptor: an animal model of vitamin D-dependent rickets type II with alopecia. Proc Natl Acad Sci U S A. 1997;94:9831-5.
88. Yoshizawa T, Handa Y, Uematsu Y, et al. Mice lacking the vitamin D receptor exhibit impaired bone formation, uterine hypoplasia and growth retardation after weaning. Nat Genet. 1997;16:391-6.
89. Hughes MR, Malloy PJ, Kieback DG, et al. Point mutations in the human vitamin D receptor gene associated with hypocalcemic rickets. Science. 1988;242:1702-5.
90. Airaksinen MS, Eilers J, Garaschuk O, et al. Ataxia and altered dendritic calcium signaling in mice carrying a targeted null mutation of the calbindin D28k gene. Proc Natl Acad Sci U S A. 1997;94:1488-93.
91. Lee CT, Huynh VM, Lai LW, et al. Cyclosporine A-induced hypercalciuria in calbindin-D28k knockout and wild-type mice. Kidney Int. 2002;62:2055-61.
92. Sooy K, Kohut J, Christakos S. The role of calbindin and 1,25dihydroxyvitamin D3 in the kidney. Curr Opin Nephrol Hypertens. 2000;9:341-7.
93. Takahashi N, Chernavvsky DR, Gomez RA, et al. Uncompensated polyuria in a mouse model of Bartter's syndrome. Proc Natl Acad Sci U S A. 2000;97:5434-9.
94. Simon DB, Karet FE, Hamdan JM, et al. Bartter's syndrome, hypokalaemic alkalosis with hypercalciuria, is caused by mutations in the Na-K-2Cl cotransporter NKCC2. Nat Genet. 1996;13:183-8.
95. Cao G, Yang G, Timme TL, et al. Disruption of the caveolin-1 gene impairs renal calcium reabsorption and leads to hypercalciuria and urolithiasis. Am J Pathol. 2003;162:1241-8.
96. Aida K, Ikegishi Y, Chen J, et al. Disruption of aldose reductase gene (Akr1b1) causes defect in urinary concentrating ability and divalent cation homeostasis. Biochem Biophys Res Commun. 2000;277:281-6.
97. Salido EC, Li XM, Lu Y, et al. Alanine-glyoxylate aminotransferase-deficient mice, a model for primary hyperoxaluria that responds to adenoviral gene transfer. Proc Natl Acad Sci U S A. 2006;103:18249-54.
98. Danpure CJ. Primary hyperoxaluria type 1: AGT mistargeting highlights the fundamental differences between the peroxisomal and mitochondrial protein import pathways. Biochim Biophys Acta. 2006;1763:1776-84.
99. Knight J, Holmes RP, Cramer SD, et al. Hydroxyproline metabolism in mouse models of primary hyperoxaluria. Am J Physiol Renal Physiol. 2012;302:F688-93.
100. Rumsby G. Primary hyperoxaluria type 2. In: Pagon RA, Adam MP, Ardinger HH, et al. (Eds). GeneReviews(R). Seattle, WA: University of Washington; 1993.
101. Finberg KE, Wagner CA, Bailey MA, et al. The B1-subunit of the H(+) ATPase is required for maximal urinary acidification. Proc Natl Acad Sci U S A. 2005;102:13616-21.
102. Karet FE, Finberg KE, Nelson RD, et al. Mutations in the gene encoding B1 subunit of H^+-ATPase cause renal tubular acidosis with sensorineural deafness. Nat Genet. 1999;21:84-90.
103. Hennings JC, Picard N, Huebner AK, et al. A mouse model for distal renal tubular acidosis reveals a previously unrecognized role of the V-ATPase a4 subunit in the proximal tubule. EMBO Mol Med. 2012;4:1057-71.
104. Stover EH, Borthwick KJ, Bavalia C, et al. Novel ATP6V1B1 and ATP6V0A4 mutations in autosomal recessive distal renal tubular acidosis with new evidence for hearing loss. J Med Genet. 2002;39:796-803.
105. Wu X, Wakamiya M, Vaishnav S, et al. Hyperuricemia and urate nephropathy in urate oxidase-deficient mice. Proc Natl Acad Sci U S A. 1994;91:742-6.
106. Liu Y, El-Achkar TM, Wu XR. Tamm-Horsfall protein regulates circulating and renal cytokines by affecting glomerular filtration rate and acting as a urinary cytokine trap. J Biol Chem. 2012;287:16365-78.
107. Mo L, Liaw L, Evan AP, et al. Renal calcinosis and stone formation in mice lacking osteopontin, Tamm-Horsfall protein, or both. Am J Physiol Renal Physiol. 2007;293:F1935-43.
108. El-Achkar TM, Wu XR, Rauchman M, et al. Tamm-Horsfall protein protects the kidney from ischemic injury by decreasing inflammation and altering TLR4 expression. Am J Physiol Renal Physiol. 2008;295:F534-44.
109. Takiue Y, Hosoyamada M, Yokoo T, et al. Progressive accumulation of intrinsic mouse uromodulin in the kidneys of transgenic mice harboring the mutant human uromodulin gene. Biol Pharm Bull. 2008;31:405-11.
110. Scolari F, Caridi G, Rampoldi L, et al. Uromodulin storage diseases: clinical aspects and mechanisms. Am J Kidney Dis. 2004;44:987-99.
111. Bollee G, Dahan K, Flamant M, et al. Phenotype and outcome in hereditary tubulointerstitial nephritis secondary to UMOD mutations. Clin J Am Soc Nephrol. 2011;6:2429-38.
112. Butler R, Inzunza J, Suzuki H, et al. Uric acid stones in the urinary bladder of aryl hydrocarbon receptor (AhR) knockout mice. Proc Natl Acad Sci U S A. 2012;109:1122-6.
113. Monk RD, Bushinsky DA. Nephrolithiasis and nephrocalcinosis. In: Frehally J, Floege J, Johnson RJ (Eds). Comprehensive Clinical Nephrology. St Louis: Elsevier; 2010. pp. 687-701.
114. Bushinsky DA, Coe FL, Moe OW. Nephrolithiasis. In: Brenner BM (Ed). The Kidney. Philadelphia: W.B. Saunders; 2012. pp. 1455-507. 9th edition.
115. Monk RD, Bushinsky DA. Kidney stones. In: Kronenberg HM, Melmed S, Polonsky KS, Larsen PR (Eds). Williams Textbook of Endocrinology. Philadelphia, PA: WB Saunders; 2011. pp. 1350-67.
116. Bushinsky DA. Calcium nephrolithiasis. In: Rosen CJ (Ed). Primer on the Metabolic Bone Diseases and Disorders of Mineral Metabolism. Washington, DC: American Society of Bone and Mineral Research; 2008. pp. 460-4.

117. Worcester EM, Coe FL. Calcium kidney stones. N Engl J Med. 2010;363:954-63.
118. Vezzoli G, Terranegra A, Arcidiacono T, et al. Genetics and calcium nephrolithiasis. Kidney Int. 2011;80:587-93.
119. Attanasio M. The genetic components of idiopathic nephrolithiasis. Pediatr Nephrol. 2011;26:337-46.
120. Devuyst O, Pirson Y. Genetics of hypercalciuric stone forming diseases. Kidney Int. 2007;72:1065-72.
121. Bushinsky DA, Asplin JR, Grynpas MD, et al. Calcium oxalate stone formation in genetic hypercalciuric stone-forming rats. Kidney Int. 2002;61:975-87.
122. Bushinsky DA, Grynpas MD, Asplin JR. Effect of acidosis on urine supersaturation and stone formation in genetic hypercalciuric stone forming rats. Kidney Int. 2001;59:1415-23.
123. Bushinsky DA, Parker WR, Asplin JR. Calcium phosphate supersaturation regulates stone formation in genetic hypercalciuric stone-forming rats. Kidney Int. 2000;57:550-60.
124. Scheinman SJ, Cox JPD, Lloyd SE, et al. Isolated hypercalciuria with mutation in CLCN5: relevance to idiopathic hypercalciuria. Kidney Int. 2000;57:232-9.
125. Evan AP, Bledsoe SB, Smith SB, et al. Calcium oxalate crystal localization and osteopontin immunostaining in genetic hypercalciuric stone-forming rats. Kidney Int. 2004;65:154-61.
126. Hoopes RR, Reid R, Sen S, et al. Quantitative trait loci for hypercalciuria in a rat model of kidney stone disease. J Am Soc Nephrol. 2003;14:1844-50.
127. Yao J, Kathpalia P, Bushinsky DA, et al. Hyperresponsiveness of vitamin D receptor gene expression to 1,25-dihydroxyvitamin D_3: a new characteristic of genetic hypercalciuric stone-forming rats. J Clin Invest. 1998;101:2223-32.
128. Bushinsky DA, Neumann KJ, Asplin J, et al. Alendronate decreases urine calcium and supersaturation in genetic hypercalciuric rats. Kidney Int. 1999;55:234-43.
129. Tsuruoka S, Bushinsky DA, Schwartz GJ. Defective renal calcium reabsorption in genetic hypercalciuric rats. Kidney Int. 1997;51:1540-7.
130. Asplin JR, Bushinsky DA, Singharetnam W, et al. Relationship between supersaturation and crystal inhibition in hypercalciuric rats. Kidney Int. 1997;51:640-5.
131. Bushinsky DA, Bashir MA, Riordon DR, et al. Increased dietary oxalate does not increase urinary calcium oxalate saturation in hypercalciuric rats. Kidney Int. 1999;55:602-12.
132. Krieger NS, Stathopoulos VM, Bushinsky DA. Increased sensitivity to 1,25(OH)2D3 in bone from genetic hypercalciuric rats. Am J Physiol. 1996 Jul;271(1 Pt 1):C130-5.
133. Bushinsky DA, Grynpas MD, Nilsson EL, et al. Stone formation in genetic hypercalciuric rats. Kidney Int. 1995;48:1705-13.
134. Bushinsky DA, Kim M, Sessler NE, et al. Increased urinary saturation and kidney calcium content in genetic hypercalciuric rats. Kidney Int. 1994;45:58-65.
135. Li XQ, Tembe V, Horwitz GM, et al. Increased intestinal vitamin D receptor in genetic hypercalciuric rats: a cause of intestinal calcium hyperabsorption. J Clin Invest. 1993;91:661-7.
136. Kim M, Sessler NE, Tembe V, et al. Response of genetic hypercalciuric rats to a low calcium diet. Kidney Int. 1993;43:189-96.
137. Bushinsky DA, Favus MJ. Mechanism of hypercalciuria in genetic hypercalciuric rats: inherited defect in intestinal calcium transport. J Clin Invest. 1988;82:1585-91.
138. Bushinsky DA. Genetic hypercalciuric stone forming rats. Semin Nephrol. 1996;16:448-57.
139. Bushinsky DA. Genetic hypercalciuric stone-forming rats. Curr Opin Nephrol Hypertens. 1999;8:479-88.
140. Bushinsky DA. Bench to bedside: lessons from the genetic hypercalciuric stone forming rat. Am J Kidney Dis. 2000;36:61-4.
141. Yao JJ, Bai S, Karnauskas AJ, et al. Regulation of renal calcium-sensing receptor gene expression in response to $1,25(OH)_2D_3$ in genetic hypercalciuric stone forming rats. J Am Soc Nephrol. 2005;16:1300-8.
142. Bushinsky DA, Asplin JR. Thiazides reduce brushite, but not calcium oxalate, supersaturation and stone formation in genetic hypercalciuric stone-forming rats. J Am Soc Nephrol. 2005;16:417-24.
143. Bushinsky DA, Frick KK, Nehrke K. Genetic hypercalciuric stone-forming rats. Curr Opin Nephrol Hypertens. 2006;15:403-18.
144. Hoopes Jr RR, Middleton FA, Sen S, et al. Isolation and confirmation of a calcium excretion quantitative trait locus on chromosome 1 in genetic hypercalciuric stone-forming congenic rats. J Am Soc Nephrol. 2006;17:1292-304.
145. Grynpas M, Waldman S, Holmyard D, et al. Genetic hypercalciuric stone-forming rats have a primary decrease in bone mineral density and strength. J Bone Miner Res. 2009;24:1420-6.
146. Asplin JR, Donahue SE, Lindeman C, et al. Thiosulfate reduces calcium phosphate nephrolithiasis. J Am Soc Nephrol. 2009;20:1246-53.
147. Bai S, Wang H, Shen J, et al. Elevated vitamin D receptor levels in genetic hypercalciuric stone-forming rats are associated with downregulation of SNAIL. J Bone Miner Res. 2010;25:830-40.
148. Bushinsky DA, Willett T, Asplin JR, et al. Chlorthalidone improves vertebral bone quality in genetic hypercalciuric stone-forming rats. J Bone Miner Res. 2011;26:1904-12.
149. Frick KK, Asplin JR, Favus MJ, et al. Increased biological response to $1,25(OH)_2D_3$ in genetic hypercalciuric stone-forming rats. Am J Physiol Renal Physiol. 2013;304:F718-26.
150. Ng AH, Frick KK, Krieger NS, et al. $1,25(OH)_2D_3$-enhanced hypercalciuria in genetic hypercalciuric stone-forming rats. Calc Tiss Int. 2014;94:531-43.
151. Frick KK, Asplin JR, Culbertson CD, et al. Persistence of $1,25(OH)_2D_3$-induced hypercalciuria in alendronate treated genetic hypercalciuric stone-forming rats fed a low calcium diet. Am J Physiol. 2014;306:F1081-7.
152. Krieger NS, Asplin JR, Frick KK, et al. Effect of potassium citrate on calcium phosphate stones in a model of hypercalciuria. J Am Soc Nephrol. 2015.
153. Frick KK, Krieger NS, Bushinsky DA. Modeling hypercalciuria in the genetic hypercalciuric stone-forming rat. Curr Opin Nephrol Hypertens. 2015;24:336-44.
154. Coe FL, Favus MJ, Crockett T, et al. Effects of low-calcium diet on urine calcium excretion, parathyroid function and serum $1,25(OH)_2D_3$ levels in patients with idiopathic hypercalciuria and in normal subjects. Am J Med. 1982;72:25-32.
155. Pak CY. Nephrolithiasis. Curr Ther Endocrinol Metab. 1997;6:572-6.

156. Karnauskas AJ1, van Leeuwen JP, van den Bemd GJ, Kathpalia PP, DeLuca HF, Bushinsky DA, Favus MJ. Mechanism and function of high vitamin D receptor levels in genetic hypercalciuric stone-forming rats. J Bone Miner Res. 2005 Mar;20(3):447-54. Epub 2004 Nov 29. Mechanism and function of high vitamin D receptor levels in genetic hypercalciuric stone-forming rats.
157. Favus MJ, Karnauskas AJ, Parks JH, et al. Peripheral blood monocyte vitamin D receptor levels are elevated in patients with idiopathic hypercalciuria. J Clin Endocrinol Metab. 2004;89:4937-43.
158. Kim M, Sessler NE, Tembe V, et al. Response of genetic hypercalciuric rats to a low calcium diet. Kidney Int. 1993;43:189-96.
159. Bushinsky DA, LaPlante K, Asplin JR. Effect of cinacalcet on urine calcium excretion and supersaturation in genetic hypercalciuric stone-forming rats. Kidney Int. 2006;69:1586-92.
160. Grynpas M, Waldman S, Holmyard D, et al. Genetic hypercalciuric stone-forming rats have a primary decrease in BMD and strength. J Bone Miner Res. 2009;24:1420-6.
161. Bushinsky DA. Recurrent hypercalciuric nephrolithiasis—does diet help? N Eng J Med 2002;346:124-5.
162. Bushinsky DA. Renal lithiasis. In: Humes HD (Ed.) Kelly's Textbook of Medicine. New York: Lippincott Williams & Wilkens; 2000. pp. 1243-8.
163. Bushinsky DA. Nephrolithiasis. J Am Soc Nephrol. 1998;9:917-24.
164. Coe FL, Favus MJ, Asplin JR. Nephrolithiasis. In: Brenner BM, Rector Jr FC (Eds). The Kidney. Philadelphia: W.B. Saunders Company; 2004. pp. 1819-66.
165. Liberman UA, Sperling O, Atsmon A, et al. Metabolic and calcium kinetic studies in idiopathic hypercalciuria. J Clin Invest. 1968;47:2580-90.
166. Coe FL, Bushinsky DA. Pathophysiology of hypercalciuria. Am J Physiol (Renal Fluid Electrolyte Physiol). 1984;247:F1-13.
167. Birge SJ, Peck WA, Berman M, et al. Study of calcium absorption in man: a kinetic analysis and physiologic model. J Clin Invest. 1969;48:1705-13.
168. Wills MR, Zisman E, Wortsman J, et al. The measurement of intestinal calcium absorption by external radioisotope counting: application to study of nephrolithiasis. Clin Sci. 1970;39:95-106.
169. Pak CYC, East DA, Sanzenbacher LJ, et al. Gastrointestinal calcium absorption in nephrolithiasis. J Clin Endocrinol Metab. 1972;35:261-70.
170. Pak CYC, Ohata M, Lawrence EC, et al. The hypercalciurias: causes, parathyroid functions, and diagnostic criteria. J Clin Invest. 1974;54:387-400.
171. Kaplan RA, Haussler MR, Deftos LJ, et al. The role of 1,25 dihydroxyvitamin D in the mediation of intestinal hyperabsorption of calcium in primary hyperparathyroidism and absorptive hypercalciuria. J Clin Invest. 1977;59:756-60.
172. Shen FH, Baylink DJ, Nielsen RL, et al. Increased serum 1,25-dihydroxyvitamin D in idiopathic hypercalciuria. J Lab Clin Med. 1977;90:955-62.
173. Frick KK, Bushinsky DA. Molecular mechanisms of primary hypercalciuria. J Am Soc Nephrol. 2003;14:1082-95.
174. Lemann Jr J. Pathogenesis of idiopathic hypercalciuria and nephrolithiasis. In: Coe FL, Favus MJ (Eds). Disorders of Bone and Mineral Metabolism. New York: Raven Press, Ltd.; 1992. pp. 685-706.
175. Henneman PH, Benedict PH, Forbes AP, et al. Idiopathic hypercalciuria. N Engl J Med. 1958;259:802.
176. Jackson WPU, Dancaster C. A consideration of the hypercalciuria in sarcoidosis, idiopathic hypercalciuria, and that produced by vitamin D. A new suggestion regarding calcium metabolism. J Clin Endocrinol Metab. 1959;19:658-81.
177. Edwards NA, Hodgkinson A. Metabolic studies in patients with idiopathic hypercalciuria. Clin Sci. 1965;29:143-57.
178. Harrison AR. Some results of metabolic investigation in cases of renal stone. Br J Urol. 1959;31:398.
179. Dent CE, Harper CM, Parfitt AM. The effect of cellulose phosphate on calcium metabolism in patients with hypercalciuria. Clin Sci. 1964;27:417.
180. Nassim JR, Higgins BA. Control of idiopathic hypercalciuria. Br Med J. 1965;1:675.
181. Caniggia A, Gennari C, Cesari L. Intestinal absorption of ^{45}Ca in stone-forming patients. Br Med J. 1965;1:427.
182. Ehrig U, Harrison JE, Wilson DR. Effect of long-term thiazide therapy on intestinal calcium absorption in patients with recurrent renal calculi. Metabolism. 1974;23:139.
183. Barilla DE, Tolentino R, Kaplan RA, et al. Selective effects of thiazide on intestinal absorption of calcium in absorptive and renal hypercalciurias. Metabolism. 1978;27:125.
184. Zerwekh JE, Pak CYC. Selective effect of thiazide therapy on serum 1, 25-dihydroxyvitamin D, and intestinal absorption in renal and absorptive hypercalciuria. Metabolism. 1980; 29:13-7.
185. Pak CYC, Kaplan R, Bone H. A simple test for the diagnosis of absorptive, resorptive and renal hypercalciurias. N Eng J Med. 1975;292:497.
186. Pak CY. Kidney stones. Lancet. 1998;351:1797-801.
187. Pak CYC, Britton F, Peterson R, et al. Ambulatory evaluation of nephrolithiasis: classification, clinical presentation and diagnostic criteria. Am J Med. 1980;69:19-30.
188. Misael da Silva AM, dos Reis LM, Pereira RC, et al. Bone involvement in idiopathic hypercalciuria. Clin Nephrol. 2002;57:183-91.
189. Heilberg IP, Weisinger JR. Bone disease in idiopathic hypercalciuria. Curr Opin Nephrol Hypertens. 2006;15:394-402.
190. Sutton RAL, Walker VR. Bone resorption and hypercalciuria in calcium stone formers. Metabolism. 1986;35:485-8.
191. Urivetzky M, Anna PS, Smith AD. Plasma osteocalcin levels in stone disease: a potential aid in the differential diagnosis of calcium nephrolithiasis. J Urol. 1988;139:12-4.
192. Pacifici R, Rothstein M, Rifas L, et al. Increased monocyte interleukin-1 activity and decreased vertebral bone density in patients with fasting idiopathic hypercalciuria. J Clin Endocrinol Metab. 1990;71:138-45.
193. Weisinger JR, Alonzo E, Bellorin-Font E, et al. Possible role of cytokines on the bone mineral loss in idiopathic hypercalciuria. Kidney Int. 1996;49:244-50.
194. Ghazali A, Fuentes V, Desaint C, et al. Low bone mineral density and peripheral blood monocyte activation profile in calcium stone formers with idiopathic hypercalciuria. J Clin Endocrinol Metab. 1997;82:32-8.
195. Krieger N, Bushinsky D. The relation between bone and stone formation. Calcif Tissue Int. 2013;93:374-81.

196. Pietschmann F, Breslau NA, Pak CYC. Reduced vertebral bone density in hypercalciuric nephrolithiasis. J Bone Miner Res. 1992;7:1383-8.
197. Jaeger P, Lippuner K, Casez JP, et al. Low bone mass in idiopathic renal stone formers: magnitude and significance. J Bone Miner Res. 1994;9:1525-32.
198. Giannini S, Nobile M, Sartori L, et al. Bone density and skeletal metabolism are altered in idiopathic hypercalciuria. Clin Nephrol. 1998;50:94-100.
199. Tasca A, Cacciola A, Ferrarese P, et al. Bone alterations in patients with idiopathic hypercalciuria and calcium nephrolithiasis. Urology. 2002;59:865-9.
200. Heilberg IP, Martini LA, Teixeira SH, et al. Effect of etidronate treatment on bone mass of male nephrolithiasis patients with idiopathic hypercalciuria and osteopenia. Nephron. 1998;79:430-7.
201. Bataille P, Achard JM, Fournier A, et al. Diet, vitamin D and vertebral mineral density in hypercalciuric calcium stone formers. Kidney Int. 1991;39:1193-205.
202. Barkin J, Wilson DR, Manuel MA, et al. Bone mineral content in idiopathic calcium nephrolithiasis. Min Electro Metab. 1985;11:19-24.
203. Alhava EM, Juuti M, Karjalainen P. Bone mineral density in patients with urolithiasis. Scan J Urol Nephrol. 1976;10:154-6.
204. Lauderdale DS, Thisted RA, Wen M, et al. Bone mineral density and fracture among prevalent kidney stone cases in the Third National Health and Nutrition Examination Survey. J Bone Miner. 2001;16:1893-8.
205. Melton III LJ, Crowson CS, Khosla S, et al. Fracture risk among patients with urolithiasis: a population based cohort study. Kidney Int. 1998;53:459-64.
206. Coe FL, Canterbury JM, Firpo JJ, et al. Evidence for secondary hyperparathyroidism in idiopathic hypercalciuria. J Clin Invest. 1973;52:134-42.
207. Bordier P, Ryckewart A, Gueris J, et al. On the pathogenesis of so-called idiopathic hypercalciuria. Am J Med. 1977;63:398.
208. Burckhardt P, Jaeger P. Secondary hyperparathyroidism in idiopathic renal hypercalciuria: fact or theory? J Clin Endocrinol Metab. 1981;55:550.
209. Monk RD, Bushinsky DA. Pathogenesis of idiopathic hypercalciuria. In: Coe F, Favus M, Pak C, Parks J, Preminger G (Eds). Kidney Stones: Medical and Surgical Management. Philadelphia: Lippincott-Raven; 1996. pp. 759-72.
210. Haussler MR, Baylink DJ, Hughes MR. The assay of 1,25-dihydroxy vitamin D_3: physiologic and pathologic modulation of circulating hormone levels. Clin Endocrinol Metab. 1976;5:151.
211. Gray RW, Wilz DR, Caldas AE, et al. The importance of phosphate in regulating plasma $1,25(OH)_2$ vitamin D levels in humans: studies in healthy subjects, in calcium stone formers and in patients with primary hyperparathyroidism. J Clin Endocrinol Metab. 1977;45:299-306.
212. Broadus AE, Insogna KL, Lang R, et al. Evidence for disordered control of 1,25-dihydroxyvitamin D production in absorptive hypercalciuria. N Engl J Med. 1984;311:73-80.
213. Insogna KL, Broadus AE, Dryer BE, et al. Elevated production rate of 1,25-dihydroxyvitamin D in patients with absorptive hypercalciuria. J Clin Endocrinol Metab. 1985;61:490-5.
214. Zerwekh JE, Reed BY, Heller HJ, et al. Normal vitamin D receptor concentration and responsiveness to 1,25-dihydroxyvitamin D_3 in skin fibroblasts from patients with absorptive hypercalciuria. Miner Electrolyte Metab. 1998;24:307-13.
215. Rendina D, Mossetti G, Viceconti R, et al. Association between vitamin D receptor gene polymorphisms and fasting idiopathic hypercalciuria in recurrent stone-forming patients. Urology. 2004;64:833-8.
216. Vezzoli G, Soldati L, Proverbio MC, et al. Polymorphism of vitamin D receptor gene start codon in patients with calcium kidney stones. J Nephrol. 2002;15:158-64.
217. Bid HK, Kumar A, Kapoor R, et al. Association of vitamin D receptor gene (Fokl) polymorphism with calcium oxalate nephrolithiasis. J Endourol. 2005;19:111-5.
218. Bid HK, Chaudhary H, Mittal RD. Association of vitamin D and calcitonin receptor gene polymorphism in paediatric nephrolithiasis. Pediatr Nephrol. 2005;20:773-6.
219. Nishijima S, Sugaya K, Naito A, et al. Association of vitamin D receptor gene polymorphism with urolithiasis. J Urol. 2002;167:2188-91.
220. Chen WC, Chen HY, Lu HF, et al. Association of the vitamin D receptor gene start codon Fok I polymorphism with calcium oxalate stone disease. BJU Int. 2001;87:168-71.
221. Valdivielso JM, Fernandez E. Vitamin D receptor polymorphisms and diseases. Clin Chim Acta. 2006;371:1-12.
222. Ozkaya O, Soylemezoglu O, Misirlioglu M, et al. Polymorphisms in the vitamin D receptor gene and the risk of calcium nephrolithiasis in children. Eur Urol. 2003;44:150-4.
223. Scott P, Ouimet D, Valiquette L, et al. Suggestive evidence for a susceptibility gene near the vitamin D receptor locus in idiopathic calcium stone formation. J Am Soc Nephrol. 1999;10:1007-13.
224. Jackman SV, Kibel AS, Ovuworie CA, et al. Familial calcium stone disease: Taql polymorphism and the vitamin D receptor. J Endourol. 1999;13:313-6.
225. Mossetti G, Vuotto P, Redina D, et al. Association between vitamin D receptor gene polymorphisms and tubular citrate handling in calcium nephrolithiasis. J Int Med. 2003;253:194-200.
226. Mossetti G, Rendina D, Viceconti R, et al. The relationship of 3'vitamin D receptor haplotypes to urinary supersaturation of calcium oxalate salts and to age at onset and familial prevalence of nephrolithiasis. Nephrol Dial Transplant. 2004;19:2259-65.
227. Ruggiero M, Pacini S, Amato M, et al. Association between vitamin D receptor gene polymorphism and nephrolithiasis. Miner Electrolyte Metab. 1999;25:185-90.
228. Uitterlinden AG, Fang Y, Van Meurs JB, et al. Genetics and biology of vitamin D receptor polymorphisms. Gene. 2004;338:143-56.
229. Favus MJ. Hypercalciuria: lessons from studies of genetic hypercalciuric rats. J Am Soc Nephrol. 1994;5:S54-8.
230. Gambaro G, Vezzoli G, Casari G, et al. Genetics of hypercalciuria and calcium nephrolithiasis: from the rare monogenic to the common polygenic forms. Am J Kidney Dis. 2004;44:963-86.
231. Chattopadhyay N, Brown EM. Role of calcium-sensing receptor in mineral ion metabolism and inherited disorders of calcium-sensing. Mol Genet Metab. 2006;89:189-202.

232. Vezzoli G, Tanini A, Ferrucci L, et al. Influence of calcium-sensing receptor gene on urinary calcium excretion in stone-forming patients. J Am Soc Nephrol. 2002;13:2517-23.
233. Scillitani A, Guarnieri V, De Geronimo S, et al. Blood ionized calcium is associated with clustered polymorphisms in the carboxyl-terminal tail of the calcium-sensing receptor. J Clin Endocrinol Metab. 2004;89:5634-8.
234. Pak CYC. Pathophysiology of calcium nephrolithiasis. In: Seldin DW, Giebisch G (Eds). The Kidney: Physiology and Pathophysiology. New York: Raven Press, Ltd; 1992. pp. 2461-80.
235. Coe FL, Parks JH, Asplin JR. The pathogenesis and treatment of kidney stones. N Engl J Med. 1992;327:1141-52.
236. Parks JH, Coe FL. Pathogenesis and treatment of calcium stones. Semin Nephrol. 1996;16:398-411.
237. Coe FL. Uric acid and calcium oxalate nephrolithiasis. Kidney Int. 1983;24:392-403.
238. Maschio G, Tessitore N, D'Angelo A, et al. Prevention of calcium nephrolithiasis with low-dose thiazide, amiloride and allopurinol. Am J Med. 1981;71:623-6.
239. Coe FL. Treated and untreated recurrent calcium nephrolithiasis in patients with idiopathic hypercalciuria, hyperuricosuria, or no metabolic disorder. Ann Int Med. 1977;87:404-10.
240. Coe FL, Parks JH, Nakagawa Y. Protein inhibitors of crystallization. Semin Nephrol. 1991;11:98-109.
241. Coe FL, Parks JH. Familial (idiopathic) hypercalciuria. In: Coe FL, Parks JH (Eds). Nephrolithiasis: Pathogenesis and Treatment. Chicago: Year Book Medical Publishers, Inc.; 1990. pp. 108-38.
242. Hagler L, Herman RH. Oxalate metabolism. I. Am J Clin Nutr. 1973;26:758-65.
243. Curhan GC. Dietary calcium, dietary protein, and kidney stone formation. Miner Electrolyte Metab. 1997;23:261-4.
244. Taylor EN, Stampfer MJ, Curhan GC. Dietary factors and the risk of incident kidney stones in men: new insights after 14 years of follow-up. J Am Soc Nephrol. 2004;15:3225-32.
245. Curhan GC, Willett WC, Knight EL, et al. Dietary factors and the risk of incident kidney stones in younger women: Nurses' Health Study II. Arch Intern Med. 2004;164:885-91.
246. Borghi L, Schianchi T, Meschi T, et al. Comparison of two diets for the prevention of recurrent stones in idiopathic hypercalciuria. N Engl J Med. 2002;346:77-84.
247. Amanzadeh J, Gitomer WL, Zerwekh JE, et al. Effect of high protein diet on stone-forming propensity and bone loss in rats. Kidney Int. 2003;64:2142-9.
248. Zerwekh JE, Zou L, Pak CY, et al. Biochemical and histological assessment of alkali therapy during high animal protein intake in the rat. Bone 2009;45:1004-9.
249. Funaba M, Yano H, Kawashima R. Effects of high protein diet and sodium bicarbonate supplementation on calcium metabolism in rats. J Nutr Sci Vitaminol. 1989;35:495-503.
250. Ashton N, Al-Wasil SH, Bond H, et al. The effect of a low-protein diet in pregnancy on offspring renal calcium handling. Am J Physiol Regul Integr Comp Physiol. 2007;293:R759-65.
251. Reddy ST, Wang CY, Sakhaee K, et al. Effect of low-carbohydrate high-protein diets on acid-base balance, stone-forming propensity, and calcium metabolism. Am J Kidney Dis. 2002;40:265-74.
252. Maalouf NM, Moe OW, Adams-Huet B, et al. Hypercalciuria associated with high dietary protein intake is not due to acid load. J Clin Endocrinol Metab. 2011;96:3733-40.
253. Ticinesi A, Nouvenne A, Maalouf NM, et al. Salt and nephrolithiasis. Nephrol Dial Transplant. 2014.
254. Moe OW, Preisig PA. Hypothesizing on the evolutionary origins of salt-induced hypercalciuria. Curr Opin Nephrol Hypertens. 2005;14:368-72.
255. Sakhaee K, Harvey JA, Padalino PK, et al. The potential role of salt abuse on the risk for kidney stone formation. J Urol. 1993;150:310-2.
256. Chan AY, Poon P, Chan EL, et al. The effect of high sodium intake on bone mineral content in rats fed a normal calcium or a low calcium diet. Osteoporos Int. 1993;3:341-4.
257. Whiting SJ. Effect of diets high in sodium and potassium on the magnitude of theophylline-induced hypercalciuria in the rat. Int J Vitam Nutr Res. 1993;63:150-5.
258. Mayan H, Vered I, Mouallem M, et al. Pseudohypoaldosteronism type II: marked sensitivity to thiazides, hypercalciuria, normomagnesemia, and low bone mineral density. J Clin Endocrinol Metab. 2002;87:3248-54.
259. Yang SS, Hsu YJ, Chiga M, et al. Mechanisms for hypercalciuria in pseudohypoaldosteronism type II-causing WNK4 knock-in mice. Endocrinology. 2010;151:1829-36.
260. Runyan AL, Chhokar VS, Sun Y, et al. Bone loss in rats with aldosteronism. Am J Med Sci. 2005;330:1-7.
261. Shey J, Cameron MA, Sakhaee K, et al. Recurrent calcium nephrolithiasis associated with primary aldosteronism. Am J Kidney Dis. 2004;44:e7-12.
262. Gehr MK, Goldberg M. Hypercalciuria of mineralocorticoid escape: clearance and micropuncture studies in the rat. Am J Physiol. 1986;251:F879-88.
263. Fanestil DD, Vaughn DA, Ma L, et al. Thiazide diuretics normalize urinary calcium in spontaneously hypertensive male rats. Kidney Int. 1997;51:1018-21.
264. Adler RA, Costanzo LS, Stauffer ME. Hypercalciuria in hyperprolactinemic rats: effects of benzthiazide. Metabolism. 1986;35:668-72.
265. Alon U, Wellons MD, Chan JC. Reversal of vitamin-D2-induced hypercalciuria by chlorothiazide. Pediatr Res. 1983;17:117-9.
266. Rizzoli R, Hugi K, Fleisch H, et al. Effect of hydrochlorothiazide on 1,25-dihydroxyvitamin D3-induced changes in calcium metabolism in experimental hypoparathyroidism in rats. Clin Sci. 1981;60:101-7.
267. Frick KK, Asplin, JR, Krieger, NS, et al. Enhanced hypercalciuria in genetic hypercalciuric stone-forming rats fed a low calcium diet. Am J Physiol Renal Physiol. 2013;305:F1132-8.
268. Sakhaee K, Maalouf NM, Kumar R, et al. Nephrolithiasis-associated bone disease: pathogenesis and treatment options. Kidney Int. 2011;79:393-403.

Section 2

Mineral Metabolism and Stone-Forming Diseases

—Elaine M Worcester

Section 2

Mineral Metabolism and Stone-Forming Diseases

—*Elaine M Worcester*

CHAPTER

8 Vitamin D, PTH and Regulation of Mineral Metabolism

Murray J Favus

INTRODUCTION

As adaptation is a coordinated physiologic attempt to preserve neutral or positive calcium (Ca) balance under a variety of developmental and pathologic conditions, and because Ca balance is negative in a considerable portion of Ca kidney stone patients with hypercalciuria, this chapter will review the adaptation process and how the multi-organ Ca homeostatic system functions in the presence of hypercalciuria.

Calcium requirements vary during the various stages of the life cycle with increases in the efficiency of intestinal Ca transport during growth, development, pregnancy, lactation, or when Ca intake is low. The supply of Ca required to meet systemic demands is determined by the efficiency of intestinal Ca absorption, and the quantities of Ca absorbed by the intestine are determined by the availability of Ca in the diet and the capacity of the intestine to absorb Ca. As major requirements for Ca occur during high rates of bone mineralization, Ca balance becomes positive and parallels increases in bone mass. The Ca homeostatic system adjusts to periods of rapid skeletal growth to meet Ca requirements through increased PTH, 1,25$(OH)_2$-vitamin D_3 production and serum levels, renal tubule Ca reabsorption and intestinal Ca absorption. Rates of bone resorption and formation adjust to maintain positive or neutral Ca balance. These coordinated physiologic adjustments in Ca metabolism that occur in intestine, kidney, bone, and parathyroids to meet changing Ca requirements are referred to in the aggregate as "adaptation." Intestinal Ca absorption was the initial component of the adaptation process to be studied in detail, and so intestinal adaptation will be examined in detail.

MINERAL DISTRIBUTION OF CALCIUM, MAGNESIUM, AND PHOSPHORUS

The distribution of minerals reflects their cellular and extracellular functions and the systemic and intracellular mineral reservoirs that can be drawn upon during periods of inadequate intake.

Calcium

Total Body

Total body content of Ca varies with the stage of skeletal development. In the fetus skeletal Ca content increases with rapid skeletal growth particularly during the third trimester.[1] Positive Ca balance (net Ca retention) continues through infancy and childhood with greater positive Ca balance during periods of accelerated skeletal growth. Mineral retention is guided by skeletal traits that are determined early in postnatal life. At 6 months of age, the measure of crown to heel length predicts body height, bone mass, size and strength in their parents and in themselves that will appear almost 20 years later.[2] Additional bone traits, including total body and regional bone mass, bone size, and radial and tibial cross-sectional area measured at 11.5 years of age, predict the bone traits at 18 years of age.

The greatest increase in Ca net retention begins with the onset of puberty and continues through the phase of rapid skeletal growth during mid-to-late adolescence with a gradual slowdown as peak adult bone mass is reached during the mid-to-late 20s.[1] While the amount of Ca retained increases throughout the formative growth years, the relative body distribution is preserved. Thus, the family resemblance of bone traits at or around peak bone mass (skeletal maturity) appears during the first year of postnatal life and influences mineral balance.

The adult body Ca content is on average 1,000 g in a 70-kg adult, of which 99% is in the crystal structure of the solid phase of bone primarily as hydroxyapatite [$Ca_{10}(PO4)_6(OH)_2$] and carbonate apatite [$Ca_{10}(PO4)_6CO_3$]. The remaining 1% of Ca is found in soft tissue, extracellular fluid, and blood. This distribution of Ca does not change with age even though the total amount of body Ca decreases with the onset of menopause in women. In men maximal total body Ca content is reached at peak adult bone density in the late 20s.[3] Stable bone density and positive or neutral Ca balance persist until about age 60 years at which time a yearly net loss of Ca and bone begins.

Quantitative differences in mineral retention in women have implications related to fracture risk. Age-related Ca loss is about 1% (one SD) and dependent upon the rate and skeletal sites of bone loss. However, the bone size difference between those at the 5th and 95th percentiles is about 50%. Therefore, differences in percentile of bone traits upon the completion of growth appear to be stronger determinants of fracture risk in women during the adult years rather than the differences in the rates of bone loss over the decades.[4]

Cellular and Subcellular

The cellular content and concentration of Ca within cells does not vary with age or Ca intake. The preservation of cell Ca concentration is required for a multitude of Ca-sensitive enzyme functions, membrane stability, and signaling between and among organelles. Intracellular Ca homeostasis begins with the limitation of total body Ca access to the intracellular space. There is a Ca gradient across the plasma membrane of 1,000:1, which is created by blood ionized Ca of 10^{-3} M and intracellular ionic Ca of 10^{-6} M. The electrical charge gradient across the plasma membrane of 50 mV (cell interior negative) also favors the inward movement of Ca. Thus, the existing electrochemical gradients favor intracellular accumulation of Ca. However, cell viability is preserved by mechanisms that limit potentially toxic Ca concentrations within the cytoplasm through binding of free Ca to intracellular membranes of the mitochondria and endoplasmic reticulum and, to a lesser extent, other intracellular organelles that have a large capacity to bind Ca. In addition, a number of Ca binding proteins with high Ca binding affinity lessen the potential for Ca toxicity. Thus, despite high extracellular Ca concentrations, the much lower cytosolic concentration of free ionic Ca in the 50- to 150-μM range is maintained through an extensive intracellular Ca buffering system. The buffering system can also mobilize Ca to maintain cytosolic Ca concentration and create receptor signaling by generating bursts of peaks of Ca levels that serve to regulate a number of biologic systems.

In addition to Ca binding to intracellular membrane sites, adenosine triphosphate (ATP)-dependent Ca pumps and Ca channels embedded in the basolateral plasma membrane extrude Ca from the cell and move it into the fluid that bathes the cells in the surrounding extracellular fluid (ECF) space. There is also a Na-Ca exchanger that moves Ca out of cells across the basolateral plasma membrane.

Blood

In adults, serum calcium concentration is an average of 2.5 mmol/L (or 5.0 mEq/L, or 10 mg/dL). Ca is found in three forms: bound to protein, ionized, and complexed. About 45% of serum Ca is bound to proteins of which 90% is bound to albumin and lesser portions to other plasma proteins including α1-, α2-, β-, and γ-globulin.[5] An additional 45% is unbound and exists in the free or ionized state. Free ionized Ca^{2+} varies inversely with blood pH with acidemia raising Ca^{2+} and alkalemia lowering Ca^{2+}. The remaining 10% of serum Ca is in the form of soluble complexes bound by electrostatic forces to small polyvalent anions primarily phosphate, citrate, bicarbonate, and sulfate. The formation of these ion pairs are subject to the concentrations of Ca^{2+}, ambient pH, and the complexing anion. Clinical laboratory assays measure both total and ionized Ca fractions. The diffusible fractions of Ca (ionized plus complexed forms) are the only portions of serum Ca that undergo filtration at the glomerulus, are capable of crossing the cellular or plasma membrane, and exert biologic actions. The hormonal maintenance of blood ionized Ca within a narrow normal range is described in Section "Calcium Homeostasis and Adaptation: Human Studies"; the biologic actions of PTH in blood Ca homeostasis and bone metabolism are detailed in Section "Parathyroid Hormone."

Phosphorus

Total Body

The average phosphorus (P) content of a 70 kg man is about 700 g of which 85% is contained in bone, 14% is in soft tissue, and 1% is intracellular and equally distributed among blood, extravascular fluid, and teeth. The P in extracellular fluid is about 600 mg, mainly in the bone matrix.

Cellular (Organelles, Storage, Signaling, and Transport): A small fraction of cytosolic P is inorganic.

Blood Levels

Unlike Ca, serum P levels fluctuate during the 24 hour cycle with a diurnal variation, rising following food intake and remaining so for hours thereafter, and then declining during fasting. Ten percent of total blood inorganic phosphorus is bound to protein and does not undergo glomerular filtration, 85% is ionized, and 5% is complexed with either Ca or Mg. The extracellular fluid pool is mainly in plasma (84%) in the inorganic form as H_2PO_4 and HPO_4. The ratio of H_2PO_4 to HPO_4 is pH dependent with a p*Ka* for phosphorus of 6.8 under conditions of plasma at 37°C. Under these conditions, the ratio of HPO_4 to H_2PO_4 is 4:1. Under acidic conditions the ratio decreases and increases with an alkaline pH.

Serum P is not tightly controlled as is Ca, but is determined by dietary intake, intestinal absorption, urinary excretion and shifts between intracellular and extracellular spaces.[6] Under stable conditions serum P concentration undergoes a diurnal variation with the lowest blood levels during the morning hours and highest levels at night. Prolonged fasting abolishes the diurnal variation.[7]

Magnesium

Total Body

Magnesium is the fourth most abundant cation in the extracellular fluid and most abundant divalent cation. Mg is primarily an intracellular ion, the second most abundant cation within cells, exceeded only by potassium. Unlike Ca, Mg concentration in the extracellular fluid is similar to that in the intracellular pool with a cytosol concentration of 5×10^{-4} M.[5] A 70 kg adult has an average Mg content of about 1.04 moles with a distribution of 66% within the skeleton, 33% within the cells, 1.0% in the blood, and the remainder in the extracellular fluid space.[8]

Cellular Location

Mg is localized to a variety of intracellular structures including microsomes, plasma membranes, and mitochondria, where 66% of intracellular Mg is found. Five to 10% of intracellular Mg is cytosolic, and intracellular Mg is modulated in part by its binding to form weak chelates with a variety of enzymes, other proteins, nucleic acids, and phospholipids. A small fraction of cytosolic Mg is free and in equilibrium with Mg bound to mitochondria and other organelles. The buffer system serves to maintain free Mg at about 1.0 mM and prevents fluctuations in total cytosolic Mg. The free cytosol Mg concentration is optimal for most intracellular Mg-dependent enzymes, including those that regulate enzymatic catalytic processes involved in the transfer, storage, and utilization of ATP.

Blood Levels

Serum Mg is partitioned with 70% either complexed or ionic and 20–30% protein-bound. Mg levels in blood are not controlled as tightly as blood Ca. Rather, serum Mg is the net result of influxes and effluxes in and out of the ECF that are driven by changes in intestinal Mg absorption, net renal Mg reabsorption, and Mg influx and efflux across bone.[6]

MINERAL HOMEOSTASIS

Hormones

Parathyroid Hormone

The evolution of animal life from the Ca-rich seawater to the Ca-deficient crust of the earth was accompanied by the appearance of parathyroid glands and their hormonal product parathyroid hormone (PTH). In healthy men and women, PTH maintains the blood ionized Ca within a narrow normal range and corrects a decrease in serum Ca by increasing Ca flux into the ECF by enhancing renal tubular Ca reabsorption, stimulating osteoclastic and osteocytic bone resorption, and increasing the efficiency and quantity of intestinal Ca absorption. Pathologic oversecretion of PTH may increase blood and urine Ca excretion and enhance the risk of Ca-containing nephrolithiasis.

PTH synthesis, secretion, and degradation: Human parathyroid glands are composed of a number of cell types, including the chief cells, which are responsible for synthesis of the nascent hormone preproPTH. In response to stimuli for PTH secretion, preproPTH is transported to the endoplasmic reticulum where the presequence is cleaved. Subsequently cleavage of the prosequence results in the biologically active 1–84 amino acid PTH molecule, which is incorporated into vesicles and secreted into the blood in response to a decrease in blood ionized Ca. Parathyroid hormone 1–84 contains all of the biological activity attributed to PTH. The pre- and propeptides are not known to contain biological activity. The PTH storage and degradation may be Ca-dependent as low ECF Ca is associated with only 10% of newly synthesized PTH degraded, whereas during high ECF Ca about 50% of newly synthesized PTH is degraded within the parathyroid tissue. Even at high ECF Ca, PTH secretion is a not completely suppressed, indicating a basal secretion level that is not subject to regulation by Ca.

The PTH is the primary hormone that maintains serum Ca within the normal range. The PTH is secreted in response to even modest decreases in blood ionized Ca. Blood ionized Ca is not solely dependent on dietary Ca intake, as serum Ca levels may be normal during low Ca intake due to elevated PTH levels that stimulate tubular Ca reabsorption (within minutes), osteoclast-mediated bone resorption (within minutes to hours), and 1,25-$(OH)_2$-vitamin D-stimulated intestinal Ca absorption (within 12–24 hours).

Measuring PTH in in vitro perfusates or in serum reveals an inverse linear relationship between extracellular Ca or Mg and PTH. Detailed analysis of the sigmoidal relationship between Ca and PTH secretion defines the set point, or the Ca concentration that produces one-half of the maximal inhibition of PTH secretion. In vitro using animal parathyroid glands, and in vivo in human subjects the shift in the set point to the right is associated with an insensitivity of PTH secretion to Ca as in patients with secondary hyperparathyroidism due to renal failure, whereas a shift to the left of the Ca-PTH set point indicates a heightened sensitivity to Ca as in newborn infants who have higher serum Ca levels than their mothers and an inappropriately normal or elevated level of PTH.

Hormone regulation of PTH secretion and function by 1,25$(OH)_2D_3$, phosphate: 1,25-Dihydroxyvitamin D_3 suppresses PTH synthesis and secretion at the level of PTH gene expression. The rise in parathyroid cell 1,25$(OH)_2D_3$ concentration increases vitamin D receptor (VDR) protein synthesis, formation of the 1,25$(OH)_2D_3$–VDR binding complex and nuclear binding of the complex to DNA sites that in turn suppress PTH gene expression and mRNA levels. The 1,25$(OH)_2D_3$ PTH-negative feedback loop is completed by PTH stimulation of the proximal renal tubule synthesis of 1,25$(OH)_2D_3$ through increased expression of the 25-hydroxy-1α hydroxylase CYP27B1 gene.

Hypocalcemia and hypophosphatemia regulate PTH gene expression post-transcriptionally by enhancing binding of proteins to the PTH mRNA 3'-UTR, which determines its stability.[9]

Estrogen stimulates phosphaturia via ERα through downregulation of NAPi-IIa and NaPi-IIc independent of PTH, FGF23, and Klotho.[10]

PTH receptor and signaling: Parathyroid hormone and the structurally related parathyroid hormone-related protein (PTHrP) share the same PTH/PTHrP receptor, referred to as the PTH/PTHrP type 1 receptor, or PTHr1. PTHr1 is a member of the G-protein-coupled receptor (GPCR) family that is expressed primarily in bone, kidney, and cartilage and to a lesser extent in the vasculature and during embryonic development of several organs.[11]

Binding of either PTH or PTHrP to PTHr1 can couple to one of several intracellular signaling pathways to generate two distinct biological functions unique to each of the two ligands.[12] PTHr1 signals primarily by coupling with the GαS–adenylyl cyclase–cAMP–protein kinase A (PKA) intracellular signaling pathway, but can also couple to the Gαq–phospholipase C (PLC) β–inositol triphosphate-cytoplasmic Ca^{2+}–protein kinase C pathway, the Gα12/13–phospholipase D–transforming protein RhoA pathway, and the β-arrestin–extracellular signal-regulated kinase 1/2 (ERK1/2) pathway.[13-16] There is overlap of specific PTH signaling in kidney and bone but with unique biologic functions generated in each target tissue. In bone, PTH binds to and activates PTHr1 in chondrocytes and osteoblasts to regulate cellular proliferation, apoptosis, and generation of signaling factors including RANKL-regulated bone resorption[17] and SOST-regulated bone formation,[18] which in turn modulate bone and cartilage metabolism.[19,20] Conversely, PTH activation of PTHr1 in renal tubule cells through cAMP-dependent and -independent mechanisms[21] modulates the expression and function of several proteins involved in transmembrane divalent mineral ion transport.[22] The biologic responses to PTH in all tissues are subject to additional modulation including control of PTH synthesis, secretion and metabolic clearance, and rates of PTHr1 internalization, endocytosis and desensitization.[23-26]

Vitamin D

Vitamin D plays a critical role in human mineral homeostasis and is essential for the homeostatic system's adaptation to changes in mineral requirements during the life cycle. Excess 1,25-$(OH)_2D_3$ production and target tissue over-responsiveness to 1,25-$(OH)_2D_3$ have been implicated in the pathogenesis of idiopathic hypercalciuria. Therefore, it is appropriate to review the physiologic functions of the vitamin D metabolic pathway, synthesis of the active vitamin D metabolite, the role of the VDR in mediating 1,25-$(OH)_2D_3$ target tissue biologic actions, and the 1,25-$(OH)_2D_3$-VDR signaling pathways.

Vitamin D Metabolic Pathway

Vitamin D_3 synthesis: The precursor to vitamin D_3 (cholecalciferol), 7-dehydrocholecalciferol (7-DHC), is synthesized in the skin and then converted to previtamin D_3 in the epidermis under conditions of UVB irradiation with optimal effects between wavelengths 290 and 310 µm. Two inactive metabolites of previtamin D_3, lumisterol and tachysterol, accumulate in the skin with continued UVB exposure but possess no biologic activity. Photolysis is the initial of two nonenzymatic steps that converts 7-dehydrocholesterol to previtamin D_3 followed by thermal-activated isomerization of previtamin D_3 to form stable cholecalciferol (vitamin D_3). The generation of previtamin D_3 is rapid and reaches maximal concentration within hours. Both the degree of pigmentation within the epidermis and the intensity of the exposure to UVB determine the time required for maximal concentration of previtamin D_3, although the maximal amount generated does not change. Melanin in the epidermis absorbs UV radiation and reduces the efficiency of sunlight to produce vitamin D_3 in the skin.[27,28] As sunlight exposure also increases melanin synthesis, the potential for excessive production of vitamin D_3 is minimized and the risk of vitamin D intoxication from sunlight is prevented. The intensity of UV irradiation is dependent on latitude with little vitamin D_3 produced in the northern latitudes and greater amounts generated closer to the equator.[29] Areas of the skin covered by clothing or sunscreen prevent or dramatically reduce vitamin D_3 production. A synthetic analog of vitamin D_3 can also be produced nonenzymatically by photolysis of the milk-derived ergosterol which forms previtamin D_2 and then thermal isomerization to form ergocalciferol, or vitamin D_2. Vitamin D_2 follows the same metabolic pathway as vitamin D_3. Recent studies suggest that active vitamin D_3 is more potent than vitamin D_2 in humans perhaps in part due to a longer retention and half-life of vitamin D_3.[30]

Following skin synthesis or ingestion and intestinal absorption, the biologically inert vitamin D_2 and vitamin D_3 circulate bound primarily to the vitamin D binding protein (DBP). The DBP is a member of the albumin family of proteins that has high capacity for binding vitamin D and its metabolites. The DBP-bound vitamin D_3 or vitamin D_2 is rapidly delivered either to storage sites in adipose tissue and muscle or to liver where the initial step in metabolism occurs.[31] The 25-hydroxylated form, 25-hydroxy-vitamin D_3, is the dominant vitamin D metabolite in the circulation and can be quantified by an enzyme-linked immunosorbent assay (ELISA) in which an antibody specific to 25-hydroxy-vitamin D is employed.[32] The distribution of serum 25-OH-D levels measured in numerous studies of healthy adults from various racial backgrounds yield contradictory results that may be resolved by using reliable assays of free 25(OH)-vitamin D.[32] The ELISA assays measure total serum 25-OH-vitamin D2 plus 25-OH-vitamin D_3, while mass spectrometry can measure individual D_2 and D_3 metabolites.[33]

25-OH-vitamin D synthesis: In the liver, vitamin D is 25-hydroxylated to 25-OHD primarily by CYP2R1, a cytochrome p450 mixed function oxidase. Several other hepatic cytochrome P450 enzymes can 25-hydroxylate vitamin D but their role in normal physiology is unclear.[34] 25-OH-vitamin D_2 and 25-OH-vitamin D_3 are the most prevalent forms of vitamin D in blood, and the 25-hydroxylated form of vitamin D is the most reliable estimate of vitamin D intake and body stores.[35]

1,25-dihydroxyvitamin D synthesis: 25-OH-vitamin D is devoid of biological activity at levels found in children and adults. In renal proximal tubules, 1α-hydroxylation is carried out by a cytochrome p450 mixed function oxidase enzyme complex located on the inner mitochondrial membrane. The complex is composed of four proteins (ferredoxin reductase, ferredoxin, ferroportin, and the cytochrome p450 CYP27B1) with specificity residing in the CYP27B1 component.[36] The bulk of 1,25-dihydroxyvitamin D [$1,25(OH)_2D$] required for physiological functions is produced in the kidney and is considered the biologically active or hormonal form of vitamin D.

While many tissues express the CYP27B1 enzyme and generate $1,25(OH)_2D$, the amounts are small, often exerting paracrine or intracellular actions. Evidence that the kidney is critical for adequate $1,25(OH)_2D$ production is supported by studies of anephric human subjects on hemodialysis in whom serum $1,25(OH)_2D$ levels are detectable, likely being generated by extrarenal CYP27B1.[37]

Regulation of CYP27B1 activity plays a critical role in integrating the effects of hormones (PTH, FGF23), mineral intake (high or low Ca, P, Mg) to meet skeletal requirements as during growth, pregnancy, lactation, and aging (see below). In proximal tubule cells 25-OH-vitamin D substrate gains access to the cell interior on the urinary luminal surface by endocytosis of filtered DBP with bound substrate. The major stimulation by PTH and inhibition by FGF23 determine 1-OHase activity by controlling the level of CYP27B1 gene expression (see PTH and FGF23 sections).

1,25(OH)2D degradation: $1,25(OH)_2D$ in proximal tubules initiates its own degradation by inducing expression of the CYP24A gene, thereby activating the mitochondrial cytochrome P450 mixed function oxidase enzyme complex.[38,39] Thus, the amount of $1,25(OH)_2D$ leaving the proximal tubule to exert its effects in multiple target tissues is determined by the net effect of synthetic action of 1α-hydroxylation on 25-OH-vitamin D by the CYP27B1 and the degradative 24-hydroxylation by CYP24A and 24-hydroxylation of the 25-hydroxyvitamin D, making less substrate available for further synthesis.[40] The product of both 1α- and 24-hydroxylation of 25-OH-vitamin D_3 creates 1,24,25-trihydroxyvitamin D_3, a molecule with markedly reduced biological activity compared to 1,25$(OH)_2D_3$ and a product likely leading to inactivation.[41]

Vitamin D receptor: The cellular biologic functions of 1,25$(OH)_2D_3$ require binding to the VDR.[42] The VDR is a member of the steroid receptor family and shares similar structural and functional characteristics with glucocorticoid, aldosterone, estrogen, progesterone, and other receptors of the family. Binding of 1,25$(OH)_2D_3$ prompts conformational changes in the receptor that facilitates RXR binding and creation of binding for nuclear coregulatory complexes to initiate transcriptional events that either activate or repress vitamin D-dependent gene transcription.[43] Genome-wide plotting of VDR binding sites reveal many VDR regulatory sites in the proximal promoter regions of target genes with additional sites located many kilobases upstream or downstream.[44,45]

The VDR-mediated transcription may be modulated by acetylation or methylation to transform nuclear histones.[46,47]

Fibroblast Growth Factor 23

Fibroblast growth factor 23 (FGF23) is a small molecular weight glycoprotein (Mol wt. 32 kD) that is a bone-derived mediator of phosphate homeostasis. The FGF23 belongs to the family of FGF ligands that signal through the FGF receptor (FGFR) tyrosine kinases primarily in a para- and/or autocrine fashion. In the presence of the cofactor αKlotho, the FGFR becomes specific for binding FGF23.[48]

FGF23 belongs to a subgroup of FGFs that function as endocrine factors.[49] Elevated serum levels of FGF-23 may be due to either increased protein production or reduced degradation. Osteocytes and osteoblasts have the highest rate of FGF23 synthesis and osteoprogenitor cells also produce FGF23 in response to increased oral phosphate.[48,50]

The FGF23 promotes phosphate retention by decreasing renal proximal tubule cell expression of two sodium-dependent phosphate transporters NPT2a and NPT2c, thereby reducing Na-dependent phosphate reabsorption.[51] Binding of FGF23 to its FGFR and simultaneous binding of the coreceptor α-Klotho are required for FGF23 to exert its physiologic actions in renal proximal tubules and parathyroid cells.[52] The FGF23 also inhibits PTH secretion in part by Klotho-induced inhibition of the PTH signaling pathway.[53] In human proximal tubule cells, in vitro addition of rhKlotho protein interacts with human PTH receptors to inhibit the binding of human PTH, suppress PTH-stimulated cAMP secretion and inositol trisphosphate generation, and in vivo reduces PTH stimulation of 1α,25-dihydroxyvitamin D_3 production through inhibition of 25-OH 1α-hydroxylation.[54] There is no evidence that FGF23 directly alters Ca metabolism; however, the suppressive effects of FGF23 on PTH secretion and 1,25(OH)2D3 synthesis have substantial impacts on renal, intestinal, and bone transport of Ca.

Gonadal Steroids

Estrogen synthesis: Both estrogens and androgens are synthesized from C19 metabolites of cholesterol. In premenopausal women, 17B-estradiol (E2) is the dominant estrogen in blood and the most potent in target tissues. A number of weaker estrogens are also produced by the ovary and adipose tissues, including estrone (E1) and estriol (E3). Circulating E2 fluctuates over a 10-fold range during the menstrual cycle depending on the stage of ovulation. In postmenopausal women, estrone is the most abundant estrogen in the circulation. E1 is synthesized in adipose tissue and other nonovarian tissues including bone.

Testosterone is the abundant sex steroid in men: Ninety-five percent of testosterone (T) is synthesized by the testes, and the remaining 5% is made in the adrenal cortex through conversion of dehydroepiandrosterone (DHEA). Enzymes 3β-hydroxysteroid dehydrogenase (HSD) and 17-β-HSD carry out the conversion of DHEA to T. The second most common circulating androgen is dihydrotestosterone (DHT), which is formed in several target tissues by the action of the enzyme 5α-reductase on T. The DHT has greater biologic potency than T, while circulating at much lower levels due to its higher affinity for the androgen receptor (AR). In women, circulating T and DHT levels are much lower than in men and arise from two sources: the conversion of C19 intermediates in the ovary to T, which in turn is then largely converted to E2 by an ovarian cytochrome P450 aromatase.

After the onset of menopause, circulating estrogens decrease to levels lower than in men of the same age. Blood levels of E2 are also present in men through aromatization of T. In men about 20% of serum E2 is synthesized in the testes by cytochrome P450 aromatase action on T. The remaining 80% of circulating E2 is made from DHEA in peripheral tissues from aromatization and then dehydrogenation to produce the weak estrogen E1. In men, serum T levels decrease modestly about 1% per year, while the level of E2 is unchanged. In elderly men, the sex hormone binding protein, which carries most of the circulating intestinal androgens and estrogens, increases substantially and decreases bioavailable T greater than E2.[55]

Cellular and subcellular mechanisms of action: Androgens and estrogens initiate their biologic functions by binding to their specific steroid receptors. There are two estrogen receptors (ERα and ERβ) and one AR.[56] The receptors function as ligand-activated transcription factors. Ligand binding induces homo- or heterodimerization with the conformational changes that result in binding of the complex to specific DNA sequences known as hormone response elements, located in the regulatory regions of target genes. Receptor-co-regulator protein complexes form and then activate or repress gene transcription. Receptors may interact with other proteins to form complexes with other nuclear transcription factors that indirectly bind to or otherwise interact with gene promoters to modify gene transcription.[57]

Nongenomic action: Estrogens and androgens may also stimulate biologic actions through nongenomic events by binding to cytoplasmic or plasma membrane ERs or ARs, and thereby activate signaling pathways to change transcription factors.[58] Through this system, ERs can control a greater number of genes that can be controlled by direct genomic actions.

Skeletal effects: Sex steroids are major determinants of the differences between the sexes in the size and shape of the skeleton. Longitudinal growth of long bones occurs at the epiphyseal growth plate through endochondral bone formation.[59] Here, chondrocytes produce cartilage, which become calcified, then resorbed by osteoclasts, and replaced by osteoblastic matrix formation. Local factors produced within the growth plate regulate longitudinal growth along with systemic hormones. At the same time, bones widen through periosteal bone formation with cortical thickening, and enlargement of the medullary cavities occurs through remodeling at the endocortical surface.

Linear growth and the growth plate: At the onset of puberty, a surge of estrogen and possibly androgen increases a linear bone growth spurt in boys and girls through stimulation of endochondral bone formation. Girls begin puberty at an earlier age, and growth rates are similar in boys and girls, but puberty lasts longer in boys. Further, boys have a greater increase in periosteal bone formation, while girls have more endochondral bone formation. These changes likely account for the differences in skeletal size and bone density between boys and girls. High levels of estrogens are responsible for epiphyseal closure and the conclusion of linear growth in both boys and girls.

The greater periosteal expansion in pubertal boys is thought to be due to higher levels of androgens. However, estrogens also appear to play a role in periosteal growth in boys, suggesting that AR and ERα are required in males for optimal periosteal growth.[60] Evidences from studies in rats suggest that estrogens may inhibit periosteal growth, but such opposite effects of androgens and estrogens observed in animal experiments are not known to occur in humans.

Aromatase: Aromatase activity is important in skeletal development, as the lack of aromatase activity results in absence of a growth spurt and the failure of epiphyseal closure in both boys and girls who are aromatase deficient. Growth can be established during estrogen administration. Aromatase gene overexpression results in accelerated growth and premature closure of the epiphyses. The importance of ERα is emphasized by lack of pubertal growth spurt when ERα receptor is nonfunctional or absent. A portion of the ERα effect is through the growth hormone (GH)–insulin-like growth factor 1 (IGF-1) signaling system.

The role of androgens and the AR in linear growth is unclear. In humans with ERα loss of function mutation or aromatase deficiency, normal serum T levels are not sufficient to support normal skeletal growth. In contrast, DHT administration stimulates longitudinal growth in boys with delayed pubertal growth. In men with AR mutations and androgen insensitivity, skeletal growth is between that of normal males and females.

At the conclusion of puberty, longitudinal skeletal growth ceases due to the decrease in the proliferative zone of the growth plate and reduced cartilage production. As a result, the growth plate closes. ERα plays a role in the closure through a direct effect of estrogen on chondrocyte proliferation. The closure is estrogen-specific, as the presence of normal T blood levels fail to stimulate the growth plate in the absence of either estrogen or ERα.

Remodeling: Bone remodeling is the periodic resorption and replacement of old bone with new bone by coordination of multicellular units. Skeletal sites designated for remodeling are targeted for remodeling by osteocytes (see the following). The specific events in identifying sites in need of repair may be driven by the ability of osteocytes to sense changes in mechanical properties of bone and initiate repair carried out by osteoclasts and osteoblasts. Estrogens and androgens can regulate the rate of bone turnover to maintain a balance between bone formation and resorption. Either estrogen or androgen deficiency increases remodeling rates with increased osteoclast and osteoblast numbers and bone cellular activities. The increase in turnover is not balanced, as osteoclastic resorption exceeds rates of bone formation. Conversely, estrogen or androgen administration reduces bone turnover rates with decreases in both osteoclast and osteoblast activities.

Cellular regulation by the sex steroids may work through either control of the birth rate of cellular differentiation from bone marrow progenitor cells or modulation of apoptotic effects on mature osteoclasts and osteoblasts.

The cellular and molecular mechanisms whereby sex steroids protect skeletal homeostasis have been investigated extensively in animal models, cell cultures, and selected knockout mice. There may be direct effects of estrogens and androgens on bone cellular function, or some functions of sex steroid actions may be indirect through production of cytokines, prostaglandins and other potential mediators. However, such studies have been inconclusive. For example, bone marrow cells from pre- and postmenopausal women suggest that estrogen deficiency increases RANKL and decreases osteoprotegrin (OPG) synthesis by osteoblast progenitor cells, and T and B cells.[61] However, estrogens do not appear to reduce RANKL gene expression, and osteoblast production of RANKL does not appear to be required for osteoclastic activity during bone remodeling.[62] In addition, serum levels of OPG are not different between pre- and postmenopausal women.[63]

Bone cellular functions: All skeletal cells including progenitor cells may contain ERα, ERβ, and the AR. In both males and females, ERα and ERβ content in bone cells are lower than in cells of the reproductive tissues, and ERβ expression is several levels of magnitude lower and may not to be required for normal bone cell functions.

- *Stromal cells*: Multipotential bone marrow primordial cells proliferate and differentiate in response to a number of hormones, receptors, and cytokines to increase cell number and functional characteristic of mature osteoclasts or osteoblasts.
- *Osteoclasts*: Recent studies using selective deletion of ERα in osteoclasts suggest that effects of estrogens mediated via the ERα can account for most of the antiresorptive properties on the female skeleton. The action may be due to the proapoptotic effects of estrogens on osteoclasts.[64]
- *Osteoblasts*: ERα deletion in osteoclasts does not alter cortical bone in females and has no effect on cortical or cancellous bone in males.[65] Several lines of evidence suggest that the effects of estrogens on proliferation and apoptosis of both osteoclasts and osteoblasts result from actions mediated by ERα.
- *Osteocytes*: While osteoblasts and osteoclasts are present only during remodeling, osteocytes have a longer lifespan and may persist in quiescent areas of bone. Osteocytes contain estrogen and ARs and respond to estrogens and androgen. Both hormones inhibit osteocyte and osteoblast apoptosis through nontranscriptional activation of Src/Shc/ERK signaling pathways and downstream transcription factors CREB and Elk-1.[66]
- *Estrogen or androgen deficiency increases osteocyte apoptosis*[67]: Osteocytes sense mechanical strain, which enhances viability and reduces apoptosis. ERα may play a role in mediating the prosurvival effect of mechanical strain on osteocytes and therefore affect bone strength.[68] Osteocytes produce molecules that control osteoclast or osteoblast formation; therefore, osteocyte apoptosis during sex steroid deficiency could adversely affect bone mass.[69]
- *Aging*: Reduction in bone mass with age had long been thought to be due to loss of ovarian function and a decline in estrogen in women and a lesser decrease in estrogen in older men. A new paradigm has emerged from recent data that shows the balance between bone formation and resorption becomes progressively negative with aging in men and women prior to and independent of significant decrease in sex steroids. Consistent with this evidence are the observations that most bone loss occurs after age 65 years at a time when most fractures occur at nonvertebral cortical sites recognized by imaging and histology as cortical porosity.[70]
- *Androgen*: The role of androgen in bone loss in elderly men remains uncertain. While androgens have a bone protective effect on the adult male skeleton, it is not clear whether it is due to the effects of T or DHT acting bound to the AR as opposed to androgens converted to estrogens and acting via estrogen binding to the ER.[71] As it is unknown whether the bone protecting action of androgen is due to direct interaction with osteoclasts and osteoblasts and how much of the low bone mass in elderly men results from sex steroid deficiency or

aging, and if a hormonal component, how much is due to decreased E2 as opposed to T or DHT. Clinical studies show a correlation between a decrease in bioavailable E2, but not T, and bone mass in elderly men.[72]

ORGANS

Bone: Structure

Composition

Bone as a tissue is composed of mineralized and unmineralized portions of cortical and trabecular bone plus the cellular elements. The bone matrix with the mineral phase contains the body's largest mass of connective tissue. Mineralization of the bone matrix is a normal function of the body that constantly regenerates during all phases of the life cycle through the process of bone turnover.

Cell types: Five cell types (see below) populate the bone and carry out both the initial building of the mineralized matrix and the adult functions related to bone turnover.

The matrix phase is protein-rich consisting predominantly (90%) of the triple helix of type I collagen (two identical $\alpha 1(I)$ chains and a genetically distinct $\alpha 2(I)$ chain). Unique to type I collagen in bone are post-translational modifications of the α chains, including covalent crosslinks between and among the three collagen chains. Small amounts of other collagens (type III, V, and fibril-associated collagens) are also found in the matrix. About 15% of matrix protein is noncollagen, including proteoglycans, glycosylated proteins, and γ-carboxylated proteins, each with specific functions including regulation of mineral phase deposition and osteoblast and osteoclast functions.

The mineral phase of bone occupies a large portion of the connective tissue matrix (osteoid) with a microcrystalline structure of hydroxylapatite $[Ca_{10}(PO4)_6(OH)_2]$ that is heavily substituted with carbonate, Mg, acid phosphate, and other elements derived from diet and the environment.

- *Stromal cells*: Bone marrow stromal cells (BMSCs) are pluripotential cells that can differentiate into bone, cartilage, muscle, and fat and so create several specific tissues. A number of cytokines stimulate BMSC differentiation through the expression of cell-specific transcription factors.

Osteocytes make up 90–95% of all bone cells in the adult skeleton, while 4–6% is osteoblasts and 1–2% is osteoclasts. The origins, factors that drive differentiation and hormones and cytokines that regulate function are reviewed in the following text.

Osteoclasts: The unique feature of osteoclast function is its ability to resorb bone. Osteoclasts arise from mononuclear macrophages within the marrow space. The phagocytic function develops in response to two essential cytokines for basal osteoclastogenesis: (1) receptor activator of nuclear factor-Kβ ligand (RANKL) and (2) the macrophage-colony stimulating factor (M-CSF). These cytokines are produced by BMSCs and their osteoblasts. Other cytokines (TGF-β, TNFα, IL-1, IL-6) and hormones (PTH, estrogens, 1,25-$(OH)_2$-vitamin D_3) are important in regulating osteoclastic bone resorptive function.

Osteoblasts: Osteoblasts and chondrocytes are thought to differentiate from a common osteochondrogenic precursor. Expression of differentiation markers can be used to track the progress of osteoblast maturation and function, including bone-specific alkaline phosphatase an early marker, and osteocalcin a marker of advanced osteoblast differentiation. Major signaling pathways are activated by cytokines that bind on their respective osteoblastic plasma membrane receptors, including bone morphogenic protein from the TGF-β superfamily; TGF-β; PTH (here as a cytokine); IGF-1; and Notch. For each pathway, signaling by cytokine binding to the receptor converges to stimulate the common Runx2 pathway, which is referred to as the indispensable "master switch" for osteoblast differentiation. There are also examples of cross-talk between and among the several pathways that modulate the extent and length of signaling.

- *Osteocytes*: These are the most common of the bone cells in the mineralized bone matrix. Osteocytes arise from bone marrow osteoprogenitor cells and then differentiate into osteoblasts on the surface of bone. Mature osteoblasts may become osteocytes as the bone matrix is produced and surrounds the osteoblasts. Osteoblasts completely embedded in the bone matrix and no longer producing matrix are called osteocytes. In addition, osteocytes are connected by cell extensions through the matrix by the creation of "tunnels" (canaliculi). Osteocytes respond to mechanical stimuli generated by bone deformation; or they may become lining cells, synthesize bone matrix and support calcification (osteoid-osteocytes); or they may undergo programmed cell death (apoptosis). Osteocytes may also resorb the walls of the bone that surrounds them.

CALCIUM HOMEOSTASIS AND ADAPTATION: HUMAN STUDIES

Intestinal Ca Absorption

The portion of dietary Ca absorbed varies by body Ca requirements, Ca intake, and age. Ca absorption increases during periods of increased Ca requirements such as skeletal growth in childhood and adolescence, pregnancy and lactation, or when diet intake is inadequate to meet body Ca requirements. Luminal Ca concentration is a function of dietary Ca intake, while Ca bioavailability for absorption is lowered when luminal Ca forms insoluble complexes with oxalate, phosphate, and other anionic molecules with high affinity for Ca. The capacity of the intestine to absorb Ca is the sum of the two pathways of transepithelial Ca transport: the saturable, energy-dependent transcellular absorption that is regulated by 1,25$(OH)_2$-vitamin D and the vitamin D-independent, nonsaturable paracellular pathway that is driven by electrochemical gradients.

Several techniques have been developed to measure intestinal Ca absorption in human studies.

External Ca Balance Technique

The external Ca balance technique requires stable Ca intake for days to weeks (10–14 days). After dietary preparation, subjects continue to ingest the same Ca intake to which a nonabsorbable marker that can be quantified in the fecal collections to verify steady state and to determine the time interval for collection. Polyethylene glycol (PEG) or small segments of radiopaque tubing can be used as markers. Samples including 24-hour urine and fecal collections are obtained during the balance period and analyzed for Ca and the nonabsorbable marker. Daily fecal Ca excretion is determined by measuring fecal Ca content corrected for the recovery of the marker. Balance data are usually collected for six consecutive 24-hour periods. Calculation of external Ca balance is intake minus excretion (urine plus fecal Ca). Neutral Ca balance is the point at which net Ca absorption (diet Ca - [fecal Ca-Ca secreted into the intestine in pancreatic and other secretions]) equals urine Ca excretion. Positive Ca balance is net Ca absorption > urine Ca; and negative Ca balance is net Ca absorption < urine Ca. Fecal Ca is composed of unabsorbed dietary Ca plus a small portion of endogenous Ca contained in intestinal, biliary and pancreatic secretions. Intestinal Ca secretion can be measured following intravenous administration of radioactive ^{45}Ca or a stable Ca isotope. Using the isotope technique, endogenous fecal Ca is usually between 100 and 200 mg per 24-hour (2.5–5.0 mmol) and is not regulated by serum Ca or hormones.

The initial experiments of intestinal Ca absorption using the external balance technique were begun in the 1930s. Adults were fed a diet of known Ca composition for 1–2 weeks to adapt to the new steady state of Ca intake before the balance collections were begun. The time for adjustment to the new Ca intake is especially important when the new intake is quite different from the habitual intake. Each phase of a balance study is usually 6 days' duration, during which time the same amount of Ca is fed and daily aliquots from duplicate diets are obtained; urine Ca excretion is measured on six daily 24-hour collections. As stool passage occurs over irregular intervals, daily fecal Ca is calculated from analysis of each of the six 24-hour fecal collections adjusted to the recovery of a continuously fed nonabsorbable marker (PEG, small pieces of radiopaque tubing) that is readily quantitated in the feces to correct fecal Ca content and determine the time interval of each collection. From the direct measurements of 24-hour Ca intake (CaI) and urine excretion (CaU) and average fecal Ca (CaF), net Ca absorption (Jnet) is calculated as the difference between CaI and fecal plus urine Ca loss (Jnet = CaI - [CaF + CaU]). The mean of the six daily 24-hour balances is expressed as mg (or mmol). Jnet Ca is in positive balance when Ca Jnet = CaI is > (CaF + CaU). Negative Ca balance predicts loss of bone and increased fracture risk.

Endogenous Ca secretion (CaE), the sum of intestinal Ca in pancreatic, bile, and intestinal secretions is relatively small (130–150 mg of Ca daily) and may not vary with CaI. CaE can be measured by fecal Ca obtained while ingesting a diet free of Ca or by intravenous administration of Ca isotope (^{45}Ca or ^{47}Ca) followed by measurement of isotope appearing in a fecal collection.

Kidney, Gastrointestinal Tract, Parathyroid Glands and Bone

The specific protein transporters of Ca, Mg and P are found imbedded in transporting surfaces of the plasma membranes of cells that participate in the quantitative delivery of the ions according to body requirements. Thus, the changes in ion delivery are reflected in the activity level of each divalent ion. A number of physiologic mechanisms have been identified that can modify transporter activities, and genetic mutations that increase or decrease transporter activity result in clinical disorders and suggest potential for targeted treatments. The transporters, their distributions in tissues and cells, physiologic actions and the molecular basis for their stimulatory and inhibitory modifications of the transporters have been presented in detail in Section 2, Chapter 2.

Intestinal Ca Absorption

Intestinal Ca absorption may also be calculated from a measured dose of ^{47}Ca administered orally followed by external counting over the forearm at a fixed time after oral dosing, or counting ^{47}Ca in serial blood samples or in the fecal collections during 4–6 days after dosing. Fractional Ca absorption (α) is that portion of the oral dose minus the ^{47}Ca isotope excreted in the fecal collection. More precise measurements of absorption can be made by simultaneous administration of intravenous ^{45}Ca and oral ^{47}Ca. The intravenous dose of ^{45}Ca permits calculation of the volume of Ca distribution, and Ca absorption can be estimated from the specific activities in serum or urine collected 4–6 hours after dosing. Dosing with stable isotopes of Ca (^{42}Ca and ^{44}Ca) measured by mass spectrometry permits studies to be conducted in children.

Intestinal Ca Absorption from an Isolated Loop of Intestine

Intestinal Ca absorption from an isolated loop of intestine is measured by intubating subjects with a triple-lumen tube positioned with the infusion aperture at the ligament of Treitz for jejunal transport and in the distal ileum for ileal absorption. Absorption is measured during constant perfusion of the 30 cm segments of jejunum or ileum. Intestinal contents are collected at two distal collecting locations 10 cm and 40 cm beyond the infusion site. Samplings taken from the collection site is started and stopped 10 minutes after the collection from the proximal site. Test solutions contain 0.5% PEG as a nonabsorbable volume marker, and the composition of the solutions is designed to minimize intestinal absorption or secretion of sodium chloride and water. A test solution containing Na and Cl of 50 meq/L and mannitol added to bring the solution to 200 mOsmol/kg has an effective osmotic solution equal to that of plasma, and causes no net water movement in the perfused jejunal segment. Ca concentration of the perfusing solutions can be varied from 0 to 20 mM with varying amounts of mannitol. Absorption or secretion rates of Ca are calculated from the perfusion rate, change in PEG concentration, and change in concentration of Ca. Unidirectional fluxes of Ca are calculated.

Evidence for Variable Intestinal Ca Absorption

Between 1918 and 1990, a large number of balance studies were conducted in healthy adult men and women over a range of CaI show that positive Jnet Ca balance with rapid increases when CaI is increased from the very lowest CaI reported of about 120 to 140 mg per 24 hour (3–4 mmol/day) and greater, although individual subjects vary widely for any given diet Ca intake. Negative Ca balance is seen when CaI is <2–4 mmol (120–140 mg/day) even though Ca Jnet is highly efficient and CaU decreased. Jnet Ca rises rapidly with CaI between 4 and 10 mmol/day and then more slowly 6–10 mmol/day CaI. CaI of 15–25 mmol/day and above may continue to increase Ca Jnet in a small number of subjects. Maintenance of neutral or positive Ca balance depends upon stabilizing Ca Jnet without increases in CaU.

Physiologic Adaptation of Intestinal Ca Absorption

The physiologic adaptation of intestinal Ca absorption to increased Ca requirements has been studied extensively using the stimulus of low Ca diet (LCD). Healthy adults can maintain neutral Ca balance during CaI as low as 2 mg/kg or about 130–150 mg/day.[73] Increased Ca requirements as during growth, pregnancy, or lactation also stimulate an increase in the efficiency of Ca absorption as detected by metabolic balance;[74] either single or double Ca isotope techniques to measure fractional Ca absorption flux from mucosa to intestinal lumen;[75] or the in situ triple lumen tube perfusion of isolated segments of duodenum, jejunum, or ileum.[76] Fractional Ca absorption may range from 20% to 40% when CaI is adequate and may increase to 60% or greater when body requirements are high or CaI is inadequate.

Vitamin D Metabolism

In rats fed a diet low in Ca for 2–3 weeks, renal proximal tubule in vitro 25-OH-vitamin D-1α-hydroxylase activity and serum 1,25-$(OH)_2$ vitamin D levels increase[77,78] through an increase in CYP 27B1 gene expression resulting in a higher rate of 1,25-$(OH)_2$ vitamin D_3 production and intestinal Ca absorption. An accompanying suppression of the 25-(OH)-24-vitamin D_3-hydroxylase and 24-hydroxylation of 25-OH-vitamin D_3 further increases serum 1,25$(OH)_2D_3$ levels.[79] A unique feature of the VDR is its upregulation during dietary Ca restriction.[80]

In healthy adults, 10 days to 2 weeks of a diet low in Ca increases in vivo conversion of ^{3}H-25-OH-vitamin D_3 to ^{3}H-1,25-$(OH)_2$-vitamin D_3 and raises serum 1,25-$(OH)_2$vitamin D_3 levels. As in animal studies, LCD raises serum PTH in healthy adults, which then stimulates mitochondrial 1-OHase activity in renal proximal tubules through generation of cAMP activation of its signaling pathways and stimulation of CYP27B1 gene expression.

Bone

Bone is involved in the adaptation to LCD. As the major site of Ca in the body, the readily mobilizable portion of bone Ca serves as the reservoir for Ca when CaI and CaA are insufficient to meet daily Ca requirements. Osteoclast-mediated bone resorption is stimulated by both PTH and 1,25D when one or both are increased during adaptation to LCD. In addition, 1,25$(OH)_2$vitamin D_3 suppresses osteoblast-mediated bone formation.[81] The net effect is reduced bone mass through both increased resorption and decreased formation with shunting of Ca from bone to the more urgent requirements of maintaining blood ionized Ca. Thus, the scarcity of Ca when Ca intake is low sets in to motion a conservation of Ca to maintain blood Ca at the expense of bone mass.

Intestinal Ca Adaptation and Aging

External balance studies have shown that the intestine adapts the rate of Ca absorption in response to the level of dietary Ca.[82-84] Using the triple lumen tube technique, 8 weeks of diet Ca restriction increased both serum 1,25$(OH)_2D_3$ and net Ca absorption across perfused segments of ileum. The ileal adaptation occurred faster and of greater magnitude than in jejunum.[85] Thus, when dietary Ca is low the fraction of dietary Ca that is absorbed is relatively high, and absorption is relatively low when Ca intake is high. However, the adaptation of jejunum absorption to low Ca diet in young adults is blunted by aging.[86]

The percentage of dietary Ca absorbed varies with the amount of Ca ingested, age, and the body requirements and may vary between 20% and 60%. Fractional Ca absorption decreases when Ca intake is high, and increases during growth, pregnancy, lactation and when dietary Ca intake is low. Net intestinal Ca absorption decreases with age in both men and women. When transport sites in all segments are stimulated, intestinal Ca absorptive capacity may increase from 20% to 45% in older men and postmenopausal women to 55–70% in children, adolescents, and young adults.

In postmenopausal women, aging and loss of estrogen decrease Ca absorption. Studies using the triple lumen tube segmental perfusion of jejunum document a rise in saturable Ca transport during low Ca intake (Ireland P, Fordtran JS). Effect of dietary calcium and age on jejunal calcium absorption in humans studied by intestinal perfusion.[86]

Ca active transport is largely located in duodenum and proximal jejunum, whereas paracellular Ca^{2+} absorption occurs throughout the entire length of the intestine.[87]

PHOSPHORUS TRANSPORT

While direct measurement of the form of P absorbed has not been done, the state of P available for absorption is that resulting from intestinal lumen pH and P ionic strength. The pK for the equilibrium between monobasic and dibasic P is 6.8 when ionic strength is that of the extracellular fluid.[88] At pH 7.4, the average valence of P is about –1.6. Therefore, the luminal pH in all but the most proximal duodenum would predict that most P is in the form of HPO_4^{2-}. Evidence supporting this species of P is derived from experiments in situ in proximal duodenum in which medium pH is increased and then decreased, with increased and decreased phosphorus absorption, respectively.[89] There is also an effect of pH on Na-P cotransport and brush border P transport where P brush border uptake increases when medium pH is reduced. At pH 7.4, brush border membrane vesicle Na-dependent P uptake is virtually independent of electrical potential gradients without requirement of accompanying cations. However, at pH 6.0 P transport has a requirement for a net negative charge.[90] The pH dependence of P transport at the brush border is related to changes in the affinity of the transporter for Na or to direct effects on the transporter.[91]

Pathways

Two pathways of transepithelial P transport are indicated from tracking in situ isotopic ^{32}P movement across intact intestinal epithelium. There is a small portion of isotope that reaches the serosal side within minutes and a large portion of isotope that equilibrates over a more prolonged period of time. The initial, smaller isotopic pool follows the paracellular pathway, and the larger, slower equilibrating pool is formed via the transcellular pathway. Both pathways are influenced to existing transepithelial electrochemical gradients. The electrical gradient is generated by the negative charge of the cell interior of –55 mV, which retards the diffusion of P across the brush border. The P concentration gradient is formed by the similar P concentrations in the extracellular fluid and cytosolic of 1–2 mM. At the brush border both gradients oppose P entry, and there is no P concentration that favors P entry across the brush border. The electrochemical gradients that oppose P entry across the brush border permit diffusional exit across the basolateral plasma membrane. The molecular mechanism(s) involved in P extrusion from the epithelial cell have not been identified.

Cellular Transport Events

The transepithelial P transport across intestinal epithelial is driven by a cellular active transport process that is dependent upon coupled sodium transport. P uptake increases linearly with luminal P and sodium concentrations.[92] Under conditions in vitro that neutralize diffusional P, transport permits the measurement of P bidirectional fluxes (Jms is mucosal to serosal; Jsm is serosal to mucosal) with net absorption (Jnet when Jms >Jsm) present in proximal (jejunum) and distal (ileum) rat small intestine, but not across colon.[93,94] The kinetics of P transport across rat jejunum is consistent with a vitamin D-dependent active transport process with a Kd for P Jms of 2.0 mM, which is within the range of concentrations found in the small intestinal lumen.[95] $1,25(OH)_2D_3$ increases intestinal Ca and Pi bidirectional transport composed of the cell-mediated absorptive flux (Jms to Jsm, mucosal-to-serosal) and paracellular diffusional flux (Jsm, serosal-to-mucosal) with Jnet positive (Jms>Jsm) indicating net absorption. The secretory flux (Jsm) increases as well and does not exceed Jms across duodenum or jejunum. The Jsm fluxes were related to tissue conductance (Gt) and short-circuit current (Isc) in duodenum and jejunum, compatible with an increase in water recycling across the paracellular tight junctions driven by a rise in sodium absorption.[96]

Sodium-Dependent P Brush Border Influx

The electrical gradient across the intestinal villus brush border is a barrier to P absorption and is overcome by a sodium-P cotransport mechanism located within the intestinal brush border plasma membrane.[92] Under conditions of low P intake, transepithelial transport of Pi in small intestine is stimulated and accompanied by an increase in the abundance of the apically localized NaPi cotransporters NaPi type IIa (NaPi-IIa). Similar events are taking place in the renal proximal tubule where NaPi type IIb (NaPi-IIb) increases in the apical brush border membrane. Studies in NaPi-IIb knockout mice confirm that this transport protein plays a significant role in intestinal phosphate absorption and is critical in the proposed feedback mechanism between the small intestine and kidney, which helps to maintain normal phosphate balance and steady-state plasma phosphate concentrations.

Low dietary P diet stimulates activity of the renal 25-hydroxyvitamin-D_3-1α-hydroxylase (1αOHase), which leads to an increase in the level of $1,25(OH)_2D_3$ and increases in VDR-$1,25(OH)_2D_3$ complexes that then stimulate upregulation by a low-Pi diet of the NaPi cotransporters NaPi-IIa and NaPi-IIb through upregulation of gene expression. There is some evidence that the regulation of NaPi cotransport in small intestine (via NaPi-IIb) by low dietary intake of P may not require vitamin D or the $1,25(OH)_2D_3$-VDR axis.[97]

Na-P(i) transport activity and NaPi-2b protein expression are differentially regulated in duodenum versus jejunum. Na-P(i) transport activity and NaPi-2b and PiT-1 proteins are mostly expressed in the in the apical membrane of enterocytes in duodenum and jejunum of rat small intestine. Their expression is negligible in the ileum. Chronic low-P(i) diet stimulates an adaptive response restricted to the jejunum, with increased brush border membrane (BBM) Na-P(i) transport activity and NaPi-2b, but not PiT-1, protein and mRNA abundance. In contrast, when dietary P is acutely switched from a low- to a high-P(i) diet, there is an acute adaptive upregulation that is restricted to the duodenum and induces an increase in serum P(i) that produces a transient postprandial hyperphosphatemia.[98]

The effect of $1,25(OH)_2D_3$ disappears when the luminal concentration of phosphate is at 2 M, suggesting that $1,25(OH)_2D_3$ stimulates active transport of phosphate but not diffusion of phosphate. Finally, unlike findings resulting from in vitro or ex vivo experiments, no evidence in vivo was obtained that phosphate absorption requires sodium or is inhibited by potassium.[99]

Diffusional Phosphorus Movement

While transcellular P transport is well characterized, there is also evidence that P can also be absorbed by diffusional pathways. From balance studies in humans, there is a linear relationship between dietary P intake and net P absorption. At high concentrations of P in rat small intestine, there is a linear increase in P absorption with no saturation observed. Triple lumen tube absorption studies in healthy humans reveal saturation at low luminal P concentrations of 1–3 mM followed by linear P absorption at higher P concentrations with no saturation observed. Paracellular P diffusional movement would be expected to be low given that the net negative charge of the paracellular space would be expected to be severely limited, especially at low luminal P concentrations. In sum, the evidence supports Na-dependent active P transport at low luminal concentrations and passive diffusional P transport at luminal P concentrations that exceed saturation.

Ca and Phosphate Cotransport

As $1,25(OH)_2D_3$ increases both intestinal Ca and P absorption, the presence of a stimulated coupled Ca-P cotransporter has been suggested. However, evidence against a Ca-P cotransporter includes intestinal brush border membrane vesicles prepared from a variety of animals in which sodium-dependent P transport is present in the absence and presence of Ca.[100-102] Also, $1,25(OH)_2D_3$ stimulates the kinetics of Ca and P active transport; however, the time course differs[103] and the distribution of Ca and P transport vary by intestinal segment with Ca Jms maximal across duodenum and P Jms maximum located in jejunum, and colon Jms increases for Ca but not P.[104] $1,25(OH)_2D_3$ stimulation increases Ca Jms and P Jms twofold for each intestinal segment, which maintains a constant Ca Jms/P Jms ratio. The data cannot distinguish a coordinated induction of separate transporters for Ca and P in response to $1,25(OH)_2D_3$ versus induction of coupled Ca-P transport.[103]

MAGNESIUM TRANSPORT

In healthy humans, net Mg absorption is 35–45% of dietary. Mg absorption is linear with intake over a range of normal Mg intake.[105] At very high Mg intake, Mg absorption is lower than predicted, suggesting a saturable mechanism at high luminal concentrations.[106] As luminal Mg absorption is dependent on lumen Mg concentration, luminal water content and water absorption may influence Mg absorption. However, Mg transport is independent of net water transport.[106]

There is limited information on the sites of intestinal Mg absorption studied using the triple lumen perfusion technique. In jejunum and ileum, Mg absorption increases linearly with increasing luminal Mg and approaches a plateau as concentrations approach 5.0 mM.[106,107] There is limited information suggesting that Mg absorption may also be absorbed by the colon. $1,25(OH)_2D_3$ administration increases net jejunal but not ileal Mg absorption in healthy human subjects.[107,108] There are conflicting results in studies of Ca and Mg and whether cotransport exists.

Ca and Mg Cotransport

Studies of simultaneous intestinal Ca and Mg absorption have yielded conflicting results, which may be due to differences between human and animal absorption or the potential formation of nonabsorbable Ca or Mg complexes created by binding with divalent ions such as oxalate or phosphate.[109] Favoring competition for a common transporter are the results conducted in humans and animals in which varied luminal Ca concentrations show a reciprocal change in Mg absorption, and vice versa.[110] Conversely, there is indirect evidence that Ca and Mg are absorbed by separate transport processes, including $1,25(OH)_2D_3$ stimulates Ca transport to a greater extent than Mg either in situ[106,111] or in vitro.[112-114] CKD impairs Ca transport to a greater extent than that of Mg[115,116] and in XLH Ca transport is decreased while Mg transport is not different from normal.[109] Further, the kinetics of Ca and Mg transport across intestine are different with greater CaV_{max}.[114] Further, Ca transport is normal in the absence of Mg, and high concentrations of Mg have little or no effect on Ca transport.

Molecular mechanisms of intestinal and renal transport in Ca homeostasis are presented in Chapters 8 and 9.

REFERENCES

1. Trotter M, Hixon B. Sequential changes in weight, density, and percentage ash weight of human skeletons from an early fetal period through old age. Anat Rec. 1974;179:1-18.
2. Wang Q, Alén M, Lyytikainen A, et al. Familial resemblance and diversity in bone mass and strength in the population are established during the first year of postnatal life. J Bone Min Res. 2010;25:1512-20.
3. Baxter-Jones ADG, Faulkner RA, Forwood MR, et al. Bone mineral accrual from 8 to 30 years of age: an estimation of peak bone mass. J Bone Miner Res. 2011;26:1729-39.
4. Hui SL, Slemenda CW, Johnston CC. The contribution of bone loss to postmenopausal osteoporosis. Osteoporosis Int. 1990;1:30-34.
5. Walser M. Ion Association: VI. Interactions between calcium, magnesium, inorganic phosphate, citrate, and protein in normal human plasma. J Clin Invest. 1961;40:723-30.
6. Lemann JJ. Calcium and phosphate metabolism: an overview in health and in stone formers, 2nd edition. New York: Lippincott Williams & Wilkins; 2002.
7. Fraser WD, Logue FC, Christie JP. Alteration of the circadian rhythm of intact parathyroid hormone following a 96-hour fast. Clin Endocrinol. 1994;40:523-8.
8. T. Günther. Concentration, compartmentation and metabolic function of intracellular free Mg2+. Magnesium Research. 2006;19:225-36.
9. Moallem E, Kilav R, Silver J, et al. RNA-Protein binding and post-transcriptional regulation of parathyroid

hormone gene expression by calcium and phosphate. J Biol Chem. 1998;273:5253-9.

10. Webster R , Sheriff S, Faroqui R, et al. Klotho/fibroblast growth factor 23- and PTH-independent estrogen receptor α mediated a direct downregulation of NaPi-IIa by estrogen in the mouse kidney. Am J Physiol Renal Physiol. 2016;311:F249-59.
11. Vilardaga JP, Romero G, Friedman PA, et al. Molecular basis of parathyroid hormone receptor signaling and trafficking: a family B GPCR paradigm. Cell Mol Life Sci. 2011;68:1-13.
12. Cheloha RW, Gellman SH, Vilardaga JP, et al. PTH receptor-1 signaling-mechanistic insights and therapeutic prospects. Nat Rev Endocrinol. 2015;11:712-24.
13. Abou-Samra AB, Jüppner H, Force T, et al. Expression cloning of a common receptor for parathyroid hormone and parathyroid hormone-related peptide from rat osteoblast-like cells: a single receptor stimulates intracellular accumulation of both cAMP and inositol trisphosphates and increases intracellular free calcium. Proc Natl Acad Sci USA. 1992;89:2732-6.
14. Singh AT, Gilchrist A, Voyno-Yasenetskaya T, et al. Gα12/Gα13 subunits of heterotrimeric G proteins mediate parathyroid hormone activation of phospholipase D in UMR-106 osteoblastic cells. Endocrinology. 2005;146:2171-5.
15. Syme CA, Friedman PA, Bisello A. Parathyroid hormone receptor trafficking contributes to the activation of extracellular signal-regulated kinases but is not required for regulation of cAMP signaling. J Biol Chem. 2005;280:11281-8.
16. Gesty-Palmer D, Chen M, Reiter E, et al. Distinct β-arrestin- and G protein-dependent pathways for parathyroid hormone receptor-stimulated ERK1/2 activation. J Biol Chem. 2006;281:10856-64.
17. Fu Q, Manolagas SC, O'Brien CA. Parathyroid hormone controls receptor activator of NF-kappa B ligand gene expression via a distant transcriptional enhancer. Mol Cell Biol. 2006;26:6453-68.
18. Keller H, Kneissel M. SOST is a target gene for PTH in bone. Bone. 2005;37:148-58.
19. Kousteni S, Bilezikin JP. The cell biology of parathyroid hormone in osteoblasts. Curr Osteoporos Rep. 2008;6:72-6.
20. Jilka RL. Molecular and cellular mechanisms of the anabolic effect of intermittent PTH. Bone. 2007;40:1434-46.
21. Pfister MF, Forgo J, Ziegler U, et al. cAMP-dependent and -independent downregulation of type II Na-Pi cotransporters by PTH. Am J Physiol. 2010;276:F720-25.
22. Blaine J, Chonchol M, Levi M. Renal control of calcium, phosphate, and magnesium homeostasis. Clin J Am Soc Nephrol. 2015;10:1257-72.
23. Habener JF, Rosenblatt M, Potts JT. Parathyroid hormone: biochemical aspects of biosynthesis, secretion, action, and metabolism. Physiol Rev. 1984;64:985-1053.
24. Brown EM. Extracellular Ca2+ sensing, regulation of parathyroid cell function, and role of Ca2+ and other ions as extracellular (first) messengers. Physiol Rev. 1991;71:371-411.
25. Lohse MJ. Molecular mechanisms of membrane-receptor desensitization. Biochim Biophys Acta. 1993;1179:171-88.
26. Tawfeek HA, Qian F, Abou-Samra AB. Phosphorylation of the receptor for PTH and PTHrP is required for internalization and regulates receptor signaling. Mol Endocrinol. 2002;16:1-13.
27. Holick MF, Richard NM, McNeill SC, et al. Isolation and identification of previtamin D3 from the skin of exposed to ultraviolet irradiation. Biochemistry. 1979;18:1003-8.
28. Holick MF, McLaughlin JA, Clark MB, et al. Factors that influence the cutaneous photosynthesis of previtamin D3. Science. 1981;211:590-93.
29. Webb AR, Kline L, Holick MF. Influence of season and latitude on the cutaneous synthesis of vitamin D_3: exposure to winter sunlight in Boston and Edmonton will not promote vitamin D3 synthesis in human skin. J Clin Endocrinol Metab. 1988;67:373-8.
30. Heaney RP, Recker RR, Grote J, et al. Vitamin D3 is more potent than vitamin D2 in humans. J Clin Endocrinol Metab. 2011;96:E447-52.
31. Heaney RP, Horst RL, Cullen DM, et al. Vitamin D3 distribution and status in body. J Am Coll Nutr. 2009;28:252-6.
32. Bouillon R. Free or total 25OHD as marker for vitamin D status? J Bone Miner Res. 2016;31:1124-7.
33. Denburg MR, Hoofnagle AN, Sayed S, et al. Leonard on behalf of the chronic renal insufficiency cohort study investigators. Comparison of two ELISA methods and mass spectrometry for measurement of vitamin D-binding protein: implications for the assessment of bioavailable vitamin D concentrations across genotypes. J Bone Miner. 2016;31:1128-36.
34. Gröschel C, Tennakoon S, Kállay E. Cytochrome P450 vitamin D hydroxylases in inflammation and cancer. Adv Pharmacol. 2015;74:413-58.
35. Holick MF. Vitamin D deficiency. N Engl J Med. 2007;357:266-81.
36. Gray RW, Omdahl JL, Ghazarian JG, et al. 25-hydroxycholecalciferol-1-hydroxylase. Subcellular location and properties. J Biol Chem. 1972;247:7528-32.
37. Jongen MJ, van der Vijgh WJ, Lips P, et al. Measurement of vitamin D metabolites in anephric subjects. Nephron. 1984;36:230-4.
38. Tanaka Y, Castillo L, DeLuca HF. 24 hydroxylation of 1,25D3-1-hydroxylase. J Biol Chem. 1977;252:1421-4.
39. Jones G, Prosser DE, Kaufmann M. 25-Hydroxyvitamin D-24-hydroxylase (CYP24A1): its important role in the degradation of vitamin D. Arch Biochem Biophys. 2012;523:9-18.
40. Shinki T, Jin CH, Nishimura A, et al. Parathyroid hormone inhibits 25-hydroxyvitamin D_3-24-hydroxylase mRNA expression stimulated by 1 alpha, 25-dihydroxyvitamin D3 in rat kidney but not in intestine. J Biol Chem. 1992;267:13757-62.
41. Castillo L, Tanaka Y, DeLuca HF, et al. On the physiological role of 1,24,25-trihydroxyvitamin D_3. Mineral Electrolyte Metab. 1978;1:198-207.
42. Christakos S, Dhawan P, Verstuyf A, et al. Vitamin D: Metabolism, molecular mechanism of action, and pleiotropic effects. Physiol Rev. 2016;96:365-408.
43. Pike JW, Meyer MB, Benkusky NA, et al. genomic determinants of vitamin D-regulated gene expression. Vitam Horm. 2016;100:21-40.
44. Lee SM, Riley EM, Meyer MB, et al. 1,25-dihydroxyvitamin D3 controls a cohort of vitamin D receptor target genes in the proximal intestine that is enriched for calcium-regulating components. J Biol Chem. 2015;290:18199-215.

45. Meyer MB, Pike JW. Corepressors (NCoR and SMRT) as well as coactivators are recruited to positively regulated 1α,25-dihydroxyvitamin D3-responsive genes. J Steroid Biochem and Mol Biol. 2013;136:120-24.
46. Kim S, Shevde N, Pike J. 1,25-Dihydroxyvitamin D3 stimulates cyclic vitamin D receptor/retinoid X receptor DNA-binding, co-activator recruitment, and histone acetylation in intact osteoblasts. J Bone Miner Res. 2005;20:305-17.
47. Ruthenburg AJ, Allis CD, Wysocka J. Methylation of lysine 4 on histone H3: Intricacy of writing and reading a single epigenetic mark. Mol Cell. 2007;25:15-30.
48. Erben RG. Update on FGF23 and Klotho signaling. Mol and Cell Endocrinol. 2016;432:56-65.
49. Lorenz-Depiereux B, Bastepe M, Benet-Pages A, et al. DMP1 mutations in autosomal recessive hypophosphatemia implicate a bone matrix protein in the regulation of phosphate homeostasis. Nat Genet. 2006;38:1248-50.
50. Riminucci M, Collins MT, Fedarko NS, et al. FGF23 in fibrous dysplasia of bone and its relationship to renal phosphate wasting. J Clin Invest. 2003;112:683-92.
51. Lanzano L, Lei T, Okamura K, et al. Differential modulation of the molecular dynamics of the type IIa and IIc sodium phosphate cotransporters by parathyroid hormone. Am J Physiol Cell Physiol. 2011;301:C850-61.
52. Kinoshita S, Kawai M. The FGF23/KLOTHO regulatory network and its roles in human disorders. Vitam Horm. 2016;101:151-74.
53. Blau JE, Collins MT. The PTH-Vitamin D-FGF23 axis. Rev Endocr Metab Dis. 2015;16:165-74.
54. Takenaka T, Inoue T, Miyazaki T, et al. Xeno klotho inhibits parathyroid hormone signaling. J Bone Miner Res. 2016;31:455-62.
55. Siiteri PK, Murai JT, Hammond GL, et al. The serum transport of steroid hormones. Recent Prog Hormone Res. 1982;38:457-510.
56. Tsai MJ, O'Malley BW. Molecular mechanisms of action of steroid/thyroid receptor superfamily members. Ann Rev Biochem. 1994;63:451-86.
57. McKenna NJ, Lanz RB, O'Malley BW. Nuclear receptor coregulators: Cellular and molecular biology. Endocr Rev. 1999;20:321-44.
58. Kousteni S, Bellido T, Plotkin LI, et al. Nongenotropic, sex-nonspecific signaling through the estrogen or androgen receptors: dissociation from transcriptional activity. Cell. 2001;104:719-30.
59. Lui JC, Nilsson O, Baron J. Recent insights into the regulation of the growth plate. J Mol Endocrinol. 2014;53:T1-9.
60. Wang Q, Nicholson PH, Suuriniemi M, et al. Relationship of sex hormones to bone geometric properties and mineral density in early pubertal girls. J Clin Endocrinol Metab. 2004;89:1698-703.
61. Eghbali-Fatourechi G, Khosla S, Sanyal A, et al. Role of RANK ligand in mediating increased bone resorption in early postmenopausal women. J Clin Invest. 2003;111:1221-30.
62. Xiong J, Onal M, Jilka RL, et al. Matrix-embedded cells control osteoclast formation. Nat Med. 2011;17:1235-41.
63. Clowes JA, Riggs BL, Khosla S. The role of the immune system in the pathophysiology of osteoporosis. Immunol Rev. 2005;208:207-27.
64. Nakamura T, Imai Y, Matsumoto T, et al. Estrogen prevents bone loss via estrogen receptor alpha and induction of Fas ligand in osteoclasts. Cell. 2007;130:811-23.
65. Martin-Millan M, Almeida M, Ambrogini E, et al. Mol Endocrinol. 2010;24:323-34.
66. Kousteni S, Bellido T, Plotkin LI, et al. Nongenotropic, sex-nonspecific signaling through the estrogen or androgen receptors: dissociation from transcriptional activity. Cell. 2001;104:719-30.
67. Tomkinson A. J Clin Endocrinol Metab. 1997;82:3128-35.
68. Lee K, Jessop H, Suswillo R, et al. Endocrinology: bone adaptation requires oestrogen receptor-α. Nature. 2003;424:389.
69. Xiong J, Onal M, Jilka RL, et al. Matrix-embedded cells control osteoclast formation. Nat Med. 2011;17:1235-41.
70. Zebaze RM, Ghasem-Zadeh A, Bohte A, et al. Intracortical remodeling and porosity in the distal radius and post-mortem femurs of women: a cross-sectional study. Lancet. 2010;375:1729-36.
71. Callewaert F, Boonen S, Vanderscheuren D. Sex steroids and the male skeleton: a tale of two hormones. Trends Endocrinol Metabol. 2010;21:89-95.
72. Cauley JA. Estrogen and bone health in men and women. Steroids. 2015;99:11-5.
73. Coe FL, Favus MJ, Asplin JR. Nephrolithiasis. In: Brenner BM (Ed). The Kidney. Philadelphia: Saunders; 2004.
74. Heaney RP, Recker RR, Saville PD. Calcium balance and calcium requirements in middle-aged women. Am J Clin Nutr. 1977; 30:1603-11.
75. Bullamore JR, Wilkinson R, Gallagher JC, et al. Effect of age on calcium absorption. Lancet. 1970; 2:535-7.
76. Ireland P, Fordtran JS. Effect of dietary calcium and age on jejunal calcium absorption in humans studied by intestinal perfusion. J Clin Invest. 1973;52:2672-81.
77. Tanaka Y, DeLuca HF. Rat renal 25-hydroxyvitamin D3 1- and 24-hydroxylases: their in vivo regulation. Am J Physiol. 1984;264:E168-73.
78. Favus MJ, Walling MW, Kimberg DV. Effects of dietary calcium restriction and chronic thyroparathyroidectomy on the metabolism of (^{3}H)25-hydroxyvitamin D_3 and the active transport of calcium by rat intestine. J Clin Invest. 1974;53:1139-48.
79. Tanaka Y, Castillo L, DeLuca HF. 24-hydroxylation of $1,25D_3$—1-hydroxylase. J Biol Chem. 1977;252:1421-4.
80. Favus MJ, Mangelsdorf DJ, Tembe V, et al. Evidence for in vivo upregulation of the intestinal vitamin D receptor during dietary calcium restriction in the rat. J Clin Invest. 1988;82:218-24.
81. Ng AH, Frick KK, Krieger NS, et al. $1,25(OH)_2D_3$ induces a mineralization defect and loss of bone mineral density in genetic hypercalciuric stone-forming rats. Calcif Tissue Int. 2014:94:531-43.
82. Leichenring JMI, Norris M, Lameson SA, et al. The effect of level of intake on calcium and phosphorus metabolism in college women. J Nutr. 1951;45:407-19.

83. Malm O. Calcium requirement and adaptation in adult man. Scand J Clin Lab Invest. 1958;10:(Suppl 36):108-99.
84. Heaney RP, Saville PD, Recker RR. Calcium absorption as a function of calcium intake. J Lab Clin Med. 1974;85:881-90.
85. Norman DA, Fordtran JS, Brinkley LJ, et al. Jejunal and ileal adaptation to alterations in dietary calcium. J Clin Invest. 1981;67:1599-603.
86. Ireland P, Fordtran JS. Effect of dietary calcium and age on jejunal calcium absorption in humans studied by intestinal perfusion. J Clin Invest. 1973;52:2672-81.
87. Brown AJ, Finch J, Slatopolsky E. Differential effects of 19-nor-1,25-dihydroxyvitamin D(2) and 1,25-dihydroxyvitamin D(3) on intestinal calcium and phosphate transport. J Lab Clin Med. 2002;139:279-84.
88. Knochel JP, Jacobson HR. Renal handling of phosphorus, clinical hypophosphatemia, and phosphorus deficiency. In: Brenner BM, Rector FC Jr (Eds). The Kidney, 3rd edition. Philadelphia: WB Saunders; 1986. pp. 619-22.
89. Danisi G, Murer H, Straub RW. Effect of pH on phosphate transport into intestinal brush-border membrane vesicles. Am J Physiol. 1984;246:G180-86.
90. Berner W, Kinne R, Murer H. Phosphate transport into brush-border membrane vesicles isolated from rat small intestine. Biochem J. 1976;160:467-74.
91. Cramer CF. Effect of Ca/P ratio and pH on calcium and phosphorus absorption from dog gut loops in vivo. Can J Physiol Pharmacol. 1968;461:171-3.
92. Danisi G, Straub RW. Unidirectional influx of phosphate across the mucosal membrane of rabbit small intestine. Pflugers Arch. 1980;385;117-22.
93. Lee DBN, Walling MW, Gafter U, et al. Calcium and inorganic phosphate transport in rat colon: dissociated response to 1,25-dihydroxyvitamin D3. J Clin Invest. 1980;65:1326-31.
94. Lee DBN, Walling MW, Levine BS, et al. Intestinal and metabolic effect of 1,25-dihydroxyvitamin D_3 in normal adult rat. Am J Physiol. 1981;240;G90-96.
95. Walling MW. Intestinal Ca and phosphate transport: differential response to vitamin D metabolites, Am J Physiol. 1977;233:E488-94.
96. Jungbluth, H. U Binswanger. Unidirectional duodenal and jejunal calcium and phosphorus transport in the rat: effects of dietary phosphorus depletion, ethane-1-hydroxy-1,1-diphosphonate and 1,25 dihydroxycholecalciferol. Res Exp Med (Berl).1989;89:439-49.
97. Capuano P, Radanovic T, Wagner CA, et al. Intestinal and renal adaptation to a low-Pi diet of type II NaPi cotransporters in vitamin D receptor- and 1alphaOHase-deficient mice. Am J Physiol Cell Physiol. 2005;288:C429-34.
98. Giral H. Renal physiology. Regulation of rat intestinal Na-dependent phosphate transporters by dietary phosphate. Am J Physiol. 2009;297:F1466-75.
99. Williams KB, HF DeLuca. Characterization of intestinal phosphate absorption using a novel in vivo method. Am J Physiol Endocrinol Metab. 2007;292:E1917-21.
100. Murer H, Hildman B. Transcellular transport of calcium and inorganic phosphate in the small intestinal epithelium. Am J Physiol. 1982;240:G409-16.
101. Berner W, Kinne R, Murer H. Phosphate transport into brush-border membrane vesicle isolated from rat small intestine. Biochem J. 1976;160(3):467-74.
102. Matsumoto T, Fontaine O, Rasmussen H. Effect of 1,25-dihydroxyvitamin D3 on phosphate uptake into chick intestinal brush border membrane vesicles. Biochem Biophys Acta. 1980;599(1):13-23.
103. Walling M. Intestinal Ca and phosphate transport: differential response to vitamin D_3 metabolites. Am J Physiol. 1977;233:E488-94.
104. Lee DBN, Walling MW, Gafter U, et al. Calcium and inorganic phosphate transport in rat colon: dissociated response to 1,25-dihydroxyvitamin D_3. J Clin Invest. 1980;65:1326-31.
105. Jones JE, Manald R, Flink EB. Magnesium requirements in adults. Am J Clin Nutr. 1967;20:632-5.
106. Brannan PG, Vergne-Marini P, Pak CYC, et al. Magnesium absorption in the human small intestine. J Clin Invest. 1976;57:1412-18.
107. Schmulen AC, Lerman M, Pak CYC, et al. Effect of $1,25(OH)_2D_3$ on jejunal absorption of Mg in patients with chronic renal disease. Am J Physiol. 1980;238:G349-52.
108. Krejs GJ, Nicar MJ, Zerwekh JE, et al. Effect of 1,25-dihydroxyvitamin D3 on calcium and Mg absorption in the healthy human jejunum and ileum. Am J Med. 1983;75:973-6.
109. Anast CS. Magnesium studies in relation to vitamin D-resistant rickets. Pediatrics. 1967;40:425-35.
110. O'Donnell JM, Smith MW. Uptake of calcium and magnesium by rat duodenal mucosa analyzed by means of competing metals. J Physiol (Lond). 1973;229:733-49.
111. Hodgkinson A, Marshall DH, Nordin BEC. Vitamin D and magnesium absorption in man. Clin Sci. 1979;57:121-3.
112. Karbach U. Cellular-mediated and diffusive magnesium transport across the descending colon of the rat. Gastroenterology. 1989;96:1282-9.
113. Karbach U, Rummel W. Cellular and paracellular magnesium transport across the terminal ileum of the rats and its interaction with the calcium transport. Gastroenterology. 1990;98:985-92.
114. Karbach U, Ewe K. Calcium and magnesium transport and influence of 1,25-dihydroxyvitamin D_3. Digestion. 1987;37:35-42.
115. Coburn JW, Brickman AS, Hartenbower DL. Effect of 1,25(OH)2D3 and 1-alpha (OH)-vitamin D3 on magnesium metabolism in man. Program Int Symp Magnesium Summ Commun. 1976;2:36.
116. Clarkson EM, McDonald SJ, de Wardener HE, et al. Magnesium metabolism in chronic renal failure. Clin Sci. 1965;28:107-15.

CHAPTER

9 Gastrointestinal and Renal Mineral Transport and Regulation

Anke L Lameris, Joost GJ Hoenderop, René JM Bindels

INTRODUCTION

Nephrolithiasis is one of the most prevalent uronephrologic disorders in the Western world as it affects up to 12% of the population, making kidney stones an important health issue as well as a major socioeconomic problem.[1,2] Kidney stones are formed when dissolved salts become supersaturated during urine concentration and precipitate. Supersaturation is approximated by the ratio between the concentration of a salt and its solubility, and in general, the composition of kidney stones reflects the supersaturation of specific ions in the urine.[3,4] The seven major minerals in the body include calcium (Ca^{2+}), phosphorus (Pi), potassium (K^+), sulfur (S), sodium (Na^+), chlorine (Cl^-), and magnesium (Mg^{2+}). Of these minerals, Ca^{2+} is the most relevant mineral in nephrolithiasis as approximately 80% of kidney stones consist of calcium oxalate (CaOx) or calcium phosphate (CaP).[5]

Nephrolithiasis is a highly heterogeneous disease due to the multiple factors involved in the precipitation of salts in the kidney.[6] Kidney stone formation depends on urinary volume, pH, and concentration of Ca^{2+}, oxalate, urate, and Na^+.[7,8] Each of these factors can be affected by the genetic background of a patient as well as by environmental influences such as diet or drug use.

Hypercalciuria is the most prevalent abnormality in patients with Ca^{2+}-containing kidney stones and is found in up to 60% of all adult nephrolithiasis patients.[3] In general, the composition of the kidney stones correlates with the supersaturation of specific ions in the patients' urine.[4] Consistent with this, hypercalciuria is the most prevalent abnormality in patients with Ca^{2+}-containing kidney stones and is found in up to 60% of all adult nephrolithiasis patients.[9] With 80% of kidney stones consisting of Ca^{2+} salts, and hypercalciuria being a major risk factor in kidney stone formation, Ca^{2+} homeostasis seems to play a central role in the etiology of nephrolithiasis. Maintenance of normal Ca^{2+} homeostasis is therefore of crucial importance to prevent kidney stone formation.

Ca^{2+} has a wide range of roles in human biology. As a major component of our bones, Ca^{2+} helps to support and protect our body. In addition, Ca^{2+} is one of the most important second messengers involved in many intracellular signaling cascades and it is required for muscle contraction, neuronal transmission, cellular motility, and fertilization.[10,11] In addition, Ca^{2+} regulates the activity of enzymes, permeability of ion channels, and activity of ion pumps.[12] Maintaining Ca^{2+} homeostasis is therefore critical for the maintenance of a normal functioning organism.

From our daily intake of 1,000 mg of Ca^{2+}, around 400 mg is absorbed along the intestinal tract.[13,14] Approximately 200 mg is excreted back into the intestine, resulting in a fecal excretion of 800 mg of Ca^{2+} per day and a net absorption of 200 mg.[15] Approximately 500 mg of all the Ca^{2+} which is stored in our bones is freely and quickly exchangeable with the extracellular fluid (ECF).[16] In the kidneys, 10,000 mg of Ca^{2+} is filtered on a daily basis; 9,800 mg is reabsorbed from the prourine, resulting in a final urinary excretion of 200 mg Ca^{2+} per day (Fig. 9.1).[17]

In normal, healthy individuals, the balance between the intestinal absorption of Ca^{2+}, its exchange with bone, and its excretion via the kidneys should be neutral, so that the total bodily content remains stable. Disturbances of Ca^{2+} homeostasis can have serious biological consequences, including an increased risk of forming kidney stones.[18] In order to maintain this balance, the transport of Ca^{2+} across the epithelial layers in various organs is tightly regulated by various transport mechanisms and hormones.[19]

EPITHELIAL TRANSPORT OF CA^{2+}

Epithelial cell layers separate compartments of different compositions such as the intestinal lumen and the interstitial space, or the lumen of the nephron and the blood compartment. Solutes, ions, and water can traverse these epithelia via either a transcellular route, passing through the apical and basolateral plasma membranes, or via a paracellular route, where the luminal compartment is

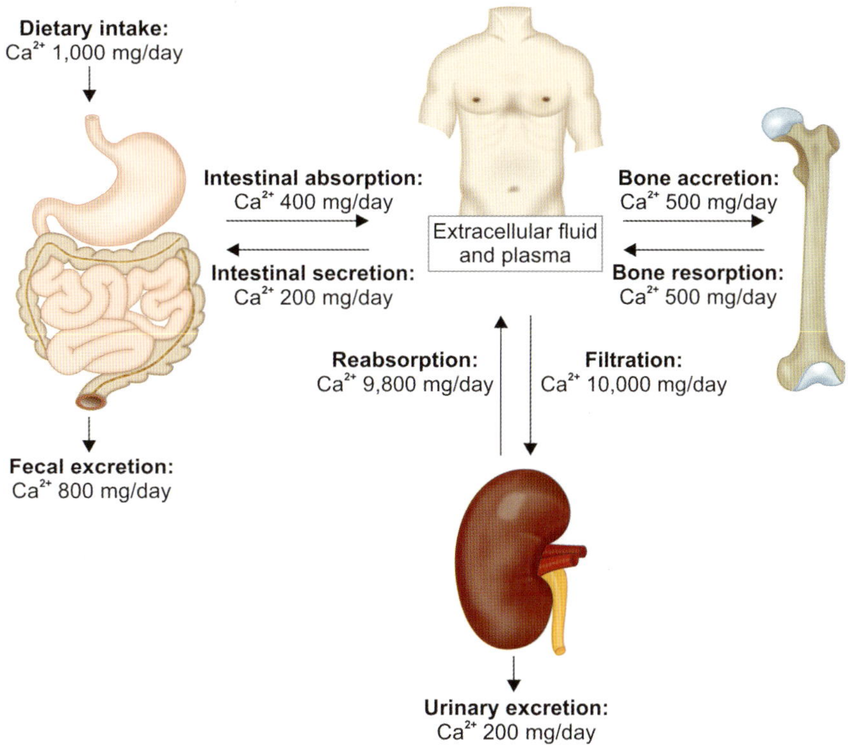

Fig. 9.1: Homeostasis of Ca^{2+} metabolism is maintained by the concerted action of the intestine, the bone, and the kidneys. Since dietary intake is the body's only source of Ca^{2+}, intestinal absorption is an essential step in Ca^{2+} homeostasis. Once absorbed into the systemic circulation Ca^{2+} can be stored in, or released from, the bone. In the kidneys Ca^{2+} is filtered from the blood and reabsorbed along the nephron to avoid excessive urinary secretion.

directly connected the interstitial space. The absorption of Ca^{2+} via the transcellular pathway is saturable, takes place via specialized transporters and can be regulated by several calciotropic hormones.[20] Transport via the paracellular pathway is nonsaturable, concentration-dependent, and mainly driven by electrochemical gradients. Together, these two routes determine the transport properties of a certain tissue.

Transcellular Transport

Transcellular transport generally requires three consecutive steps. First, ions enter the epithelial cell from the luminal compartment via specific influx proteins on the apical side of the cell. Second, ions are bound to specialized intracellular carrier proteins that facilitate the diffusion from the apical area toward the basolateral membrane. Third, the ions are extruded out of the cell and into the interstitial fluid via ion exchangers and/or pumps on the basolateral side of the epithelial cell.[21,22] Transport of Ca^{2+} across the apical membrane of epithelial cells is considered to be the rate-limiting factor in the transcellular transport pathway.[20] The discovery of the epithelial Ca^{2+} channels transient receptor potential vanilloid 5 and 6 (TRPV5 and TRPV6) in rabbit kidney and rat duodenum, respectively, gave new insights into the process of Ca^{2+} (re-) absorption.[23,24] These channels regulate the entry of Ca^{2+} across the apical membranes of the renal and intestinal epithelia.[11,20,24] The detailed characterization of these proteins reveals six membrane-spanning domains (S1–S6), a pore loop between domains S5 and S6, and intracellularly located carboxy termini and amino termini.[25] Four transient receptor potential (TRP) monomers assemble into tetramers to form a cation channel which is Ca^{2+}-selective (Figs. 9.2A and B).[20]

Once transported into the cell, Ca^{2+} is bound to calbindin proteins, which function as a buffer and facilitate diffusion of the Ca^{2+} ions toward the basolateral membrane.[26] In the intestine, calbindin-D9K is responsible for this process, whereas in the kidney calbindin-D28K is predominant.[22] By buffering intracellular Ca^{2+} levels, calbindins maintain the low intracellular free Ca^{2+} levels that facilitate the continuous inward driving force at the apical

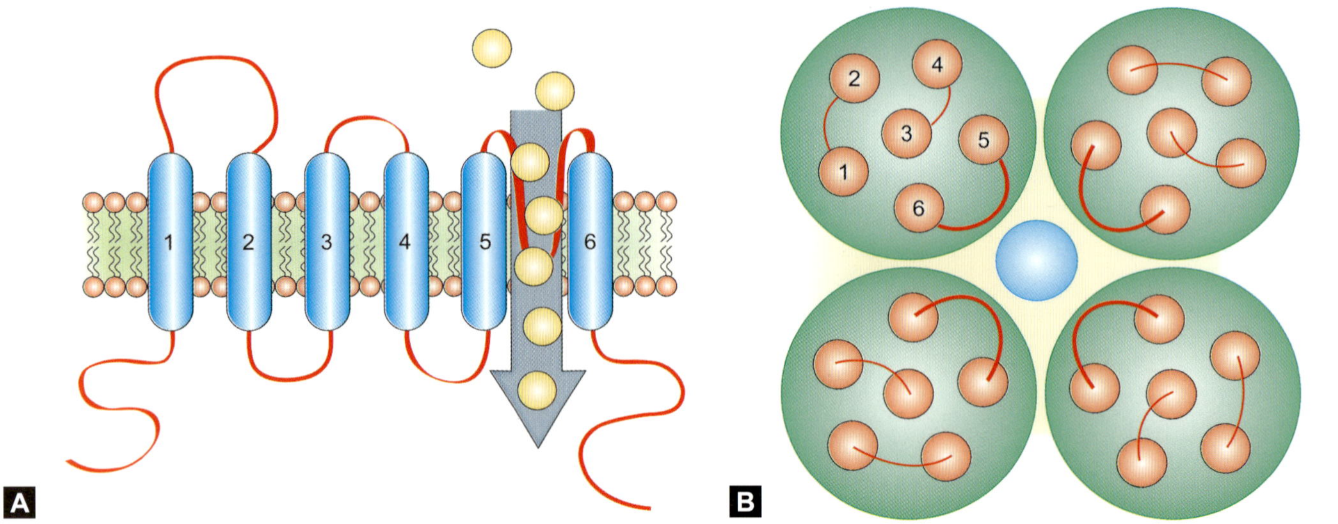

Figs. 9.2A and B: Structure of transient receptor potential (TRP) proteins: (A) A schematic representation of the six membrane-spanning domains (S1–S6) of a TRP protein, with the intracellular amino (N) and carboxy (C) termini. The pore loop, which determines size and charge selectivity of the channel is located between domain 5 and 6. (B) Four TRP monomers assemble into a tetramer forming a functional channel.

membrane.[27] At physiological intracellular Ca^{2+} concentrations, calbindins are saturated with Ca^{2+}.[28] Consequently, Ca^{2+} signaling can occur during and independently of transcellular Ca^{2+} movement.[29] At the basolateral side of the cell, efflux of Ca^{2+} takes place against a considerable electrochemical gradient. In the intestine, extrusion of Ca^{2+} across the basolateral membrane occurs via a plasma membrane Ca^{2+}-ATPase named Plasma membrane calcium pump type 1b (PMCA1b).[22] In the kidney, a Na^+/Ca^{2+} exchanger (NCX1) uses the electrochemical gradient of Na^+ at the basolateral plasma membrane to extrude Ca^{2+} from the intracellular compartment into the interstitial space.[22]

Paracellular Transport

Over the last decade, the scientific view on paracellular transport has been transformed with the identification of the various new proteins that form tight junction structures between the cells of the epithelium.[12] These tight junctions have two basic functions. First, they act as an anchor to prevent diffusion of membrane proteins from the basolateral to the apical side of the cell and vice versa, thus maintaining cell polarity.[30] Second, the tight junctions determine the permeability of the paracellular pathway to ions and water.[30] The quantity of water and small solutes exchanged passively through the paracellular junctions depends on the functional requirements of the epithelium.[31]

Tight junctions consist of several types of integral transmembrane proteins, including occludin, tricellulin, and members of the claudin family.[32] The claudin family has at least 24 members with molecular masses ranging from 20 to 28 kDa.[33] All claudins have a similar membrane topology, with four transmembrane domains and cytosolic amino termini and carboxy termini.[34] The first extracellular loop of each claudin is longer and more hydrophobic than the second extracellular loop and is believed to determine the paracellular charge selectivity.[33,35] The extracellular loops of claudin molecules make homophilic and heterophilic interactions with other claudin molecules in adjacent cells (Fig. 9.3).[34] These interactions create barriers, or pores for the passage of selected molecules.[33] The different claudin family members exhibit distinct tissue-, cell-, developmental stage-, and disease-specific expression patterns.[30,36]

The involvement of claudins in renal Ca^{2+} homeostasis has been clearly demonstrated for three isoforms: CLDN16, CLDN19, and CLDN14.[37-39] Together, CLDN16 and CLDN19 form a highly cation-specific paracellular channel, which is able to transport Ca^{2+} as well as Mg^{2+}.[40,41] CLDN14 was identified in a genome-wide association study (GWAS) in nephrolithiasis patients, and seems to have a regulatory effect on Ca^{2+} transport via CLDN16 and CLDN19.[39,42]

To date, not much is known about the role of claudins in the intestinal absorption of Ca^{2+}. In vitro studies have shown that vitamin D increases paracellular Ca^{2+} transport in Caco-2 cells.[43] In addition, in vivo studies have demonstrated that intestinal expression of claudin 2 and claudin

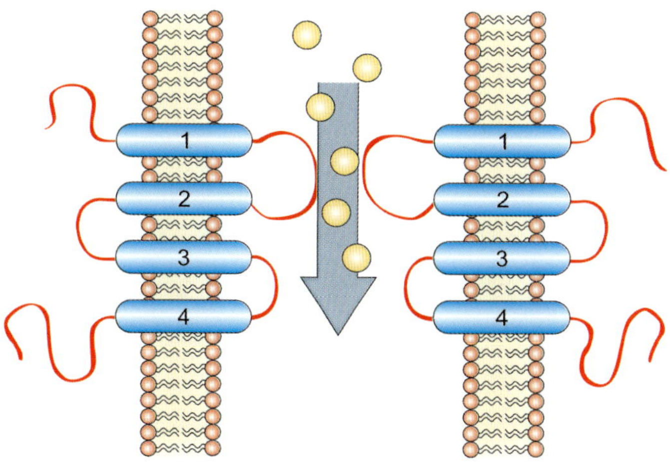

Fig. 9.3: General structure of a paracellular pore formed by claudin proteins. Claudin proteins typically consist of four transmembrane domains, with cytosolic amino termini and carboxy termini. Of the two extracellular loops, the first and larger one is considered to determine the size and charge selectivity of the paracellular pore for (cat)ions.

12 may be vitamin D-dependent.[43] Further studies are required to confirm these findings and investigate the role of these and other claudins in intestinal Ca^{2+} absorption.

CA^{2+} HOMEOSTASIS

As mentioned before, one of the major risk factors for the development of kidney stones is hypercalciuria. The pathophysiology of hypercalciuria can be classified into three categories: (1) a primary renal leak, (2) an imbalance between bone resorption and formation, and (3) intestinal hyperabsorption, which is the most common abnormality in hypercalciuric kidney stone formers.[44] These three categories represent the three major organs involved in calcium homeostasis, namely the kidneys, the bone and the intestines.

Kidney

In the kidney, the majority (50–60%) of the filtered Ca^{2+} is reabsorbed through paracellular pathways in the proximal tubule (PT), and to a lesser extent (20–25%) in the thick ascending limb (TAL) of Henle (Fig. 9.4).[22] The reabsorption of Na^+ and water in the PT creates a chemical gradient across the epithelium, increasing the luminal concentration of Ca^{2+}, which enables its paracellular reabsorption. On the apical side of the cells in the PT, Na^+ is reabsorbed from the prourine by the Na^+/H^+ exchanger 3 (NHE3), and extruded on the basolateral side via a Na^+–K^+–ATPase.[20] Water follows via aquaporin 1 (AQP1) water channels at both the apical and basolateral side of the PT cells. Although the major players in the transcellular transport processes in this segment have been identified and characterized, the identities of the proteins involved in paracellular transport in the PT are less well defined. Claudin 2 is required for paracellular Ca^{2+} reabsorption in the PT in mice; its role in human renal physiology remains to be determined.[45] In the TAL, Na^+, K^+, and Cl^- are reabsorbed from the prourine via the Na^+–K^+–$2Cl^-$ cotransporter (NKCC2). A Na^+–K^+– ATPase at the basolateral side provides the driving force for this process. The absorbed Cl^- exits via the basolateral membrane via ClC-Kb channels, whereas the renal outer medullary K^+ channel 2 (ROMK2) allows for apical recycling of K^+ to the tubular lumen. This generates a lumen-positive electrochemical gradient, which drives the reabsorption of Ca^{2+} via the paracellular pathway in this segment.[46]

In the TAL, claudin 16 and claudin 19 form a paracellular channel permeable to Ca^{2+} as well as Mg^{2+}.[41] The fine-tuning of the net urinary Ca^{2+} excretion takes place in the late distal convoluted tubule (DCT2) and in the connecting tubule (CNT), where the final 3–7% of Ca^{2+} is reabsorbed via the transcellular pathway involving TRPV5, calbindin-D_{28K}, and NCX1.[47] This process is tightly regulated by a variety of mechanisms, including hormonal regulation. In the end, only 1–2% of the Ca^{2+} that was filtered at the glomerulus is excreted via the urine.[47]

Bone

Ca^{2+} can be exchanged between ECF and bone. The maintenance of mineral stores in bone depends on the balance between bone mineralization by osteoblasts and bone resorption by osteoclasts. Various TRP channels, including TRPV4, TRPV5, and TRPV6, are involved in bone Ca^{2+} homeostasis (Fig. 9.5).[48–50] Transient receptor potential vanilloid 4 regulates intracellular Ca^{2+} concentrations both in the osteoclast and osteoblast, and plays an important role in osteoclast differentiation.[49] At the ruffled border membrane of osteoclasts, TRPV5 is involved in the removal of Ca^{2+} from the bone matrix.[48,51] Bone resorption is nearly absent osteoclasts cultured from TRPV5 knockout (KO) mice, indicating that TRPV5 deficiency impairs the osteoclasts' ability to reabsorb Ca^{2+} from bone.[51] Despite this, TRPV5 KO mice display reduced bone mineralization, probably due to excessive renal Ca^{2+} wasting.[48] Previous studies show that treatment with the bisphosphonate bone resorption inhibitor alendronate normalizes the reduced bone thickness in TRPV5 KO mice.[52] Together,

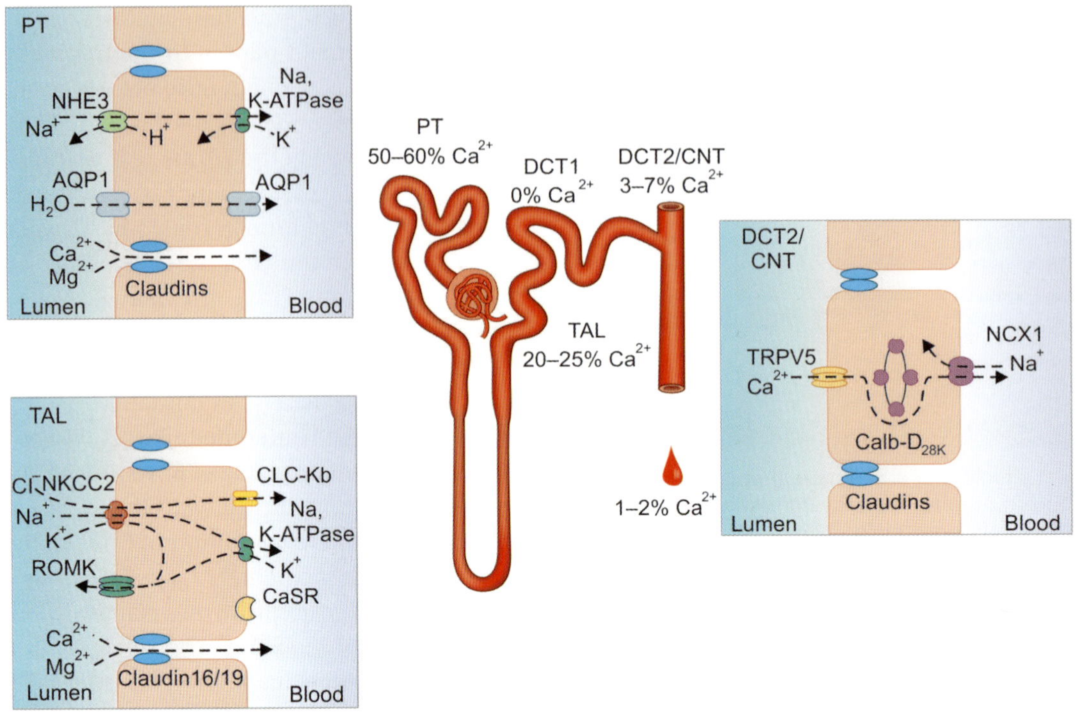

Fig. 9.4: Key players in the reabsorption of Ca^{2+} along the different segments of the nephron. In the proximal tubule (PT) and thick ascending limb (TAL) of Henle, Ca^{2+} is mainly absorbed via the paracellular pathway. Transcellular reabsorption of Ca^{2+} mainly takes place in the late distal convoluted tubule (DCT2) and connecting tubule (CNT). (NHE3, Na^+/H^+ exchanger 3; AQP1, Aquaporin 1; TRPV5, Transient receptor potential vanilloid 5; NKCC, $Na^+–K^+–2Cl^-$ cotransporter; CaSR, Ca^{2+}-sensing receptor; ROMK, Renal outer medullary K+).

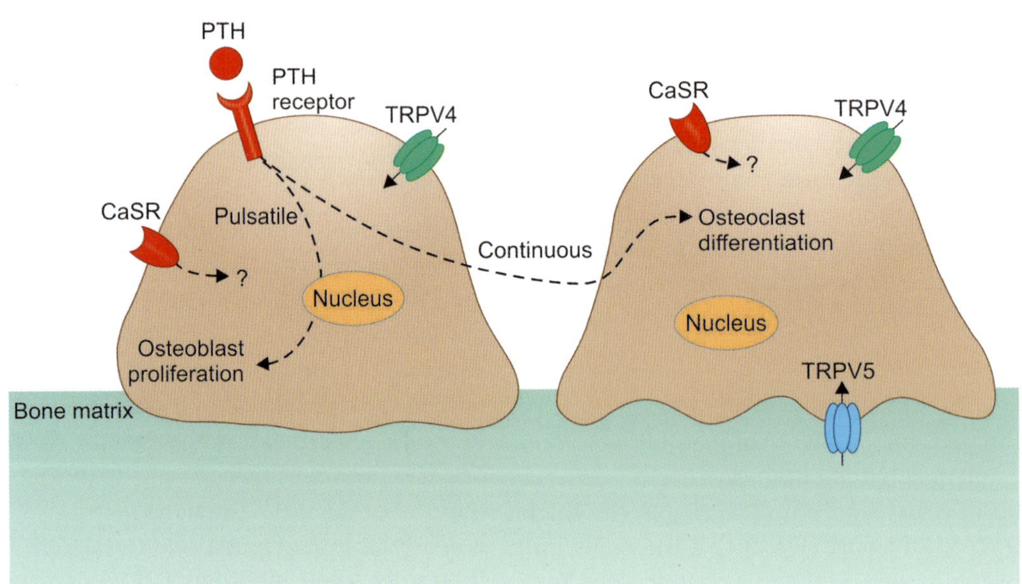

Fig. 9.5: Ca^{2+} homeostasis in osteoblasts and osteoclasts. Both osteoblasts and osteoclasts express TRPV4, which regulates intracellular Ca^{2+} concentrations. In addition, osteoclasts express TRPV5 which plays an important role in bone resorption. Osteoblasts have PTH receptors and are responsive to pulsatile PTH, which affects osteoblast proliferation. Long-term, continuous stimulation of the PTH receptor by PTH also affects osteoclast differentiation. Both osteoblasts and osteoclasts express the CaSR, the function of which in bone formation remains to be determined. (TRPV4: Transient receptor potential vanilloid 4; TRPV5: Transient receptor potential vanilloid 5; CaSR, Ca^{2+}-sensing receptor; PTH: Parathyroid hormone).

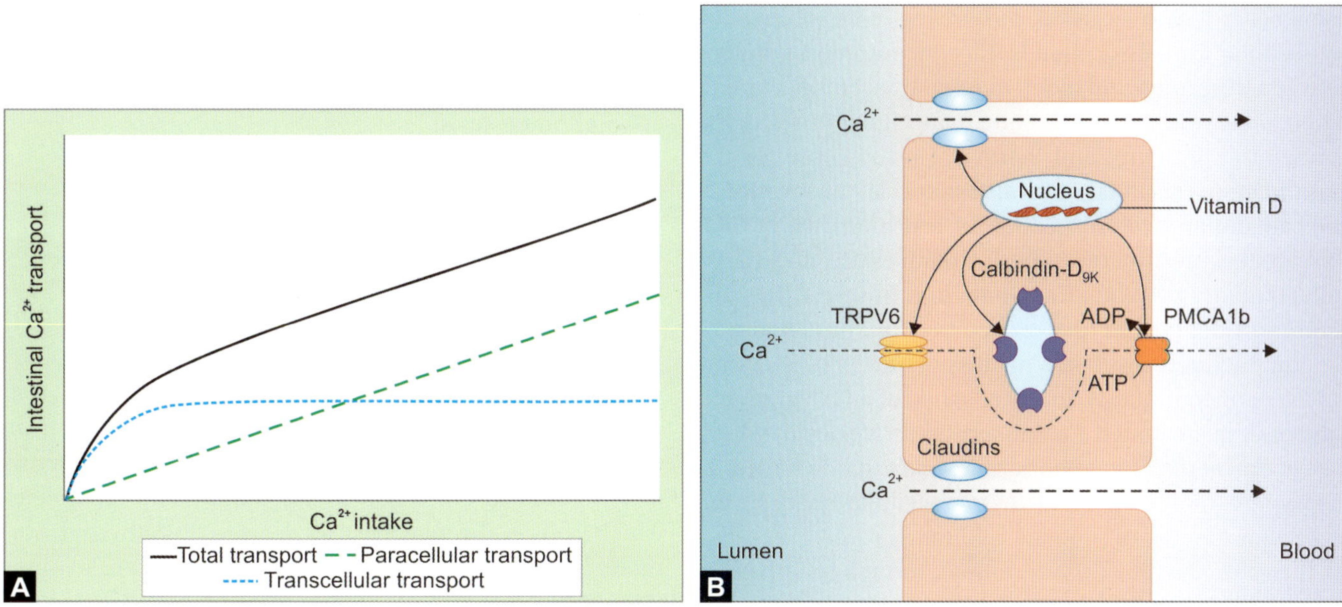

Figs. 9.6A and B: Transcellular and paracellular calcium absorption in the intestine. (A) Transport via the paracellular pathway increases linearly, depending on the luminal concentration. Transport via the transcellular pathway is saturable, and predominant when luminal concentrations are low. (B) The transcellular intestinal absorption of calcium relies on apical Ca^{2+} entry through TRPV6, intracellular calcium transport by calbindin-D9k, and basolateral Ca^{2+} extrusion via either NCX1 or PMCA1b. 1,25(OH)2-vitamin D regulates most the key players involved in this pathway on a transcriptional level. In addition, 1,25(OH)2-vitamin D regulates the permeability of tight junctions, which gate the paracellular absorption of Ca^{2+}. (TRPV6: Transient receptor potential vanilloid 6; NCX1, Na+/Ca^{2+} exchanger; ATP: Adenosine triphosphate; ADP: Adenosine diphosphate).

these findings indicate that a significant amount of resorption still occurs despite the lack of TRPV5. Apparently, alternative transport pathways exist that may compensate for the loss of TRPV5.[52] Transient receptor potential vanilloid 6 is mainly expressed at the luminal side of osteoclasts and osteoblasts; however, it does not seem crucial for bone mineralization in mice.[50]

Expression studies in bone have also reported Ca^{2+}-sensing receptor (CaSR) transcripts in osteoblasts as well as in osteoclasts.[53] In a mouse model with an osteoblast specific ablation of CaSR, mice have severe bone defects, which are independent of systemic calciotropic hormones and caused exclusively by local regulatory events involving the CaSR in bone tissue.[54] So far, it remains unknown if and how the CaSR in bone affects the expressed TRP channels.

Osteoblasts also express parathyroid hormone (PTH) receptors. Parathyroid hormone is known to exert 2 types of effects of bone, depending on the pattern of exposure: pulsatile PTH exposure exerts an anabolic effect on bone mass by stimulating osteoblast differentiation, whereas continuous PTH exposure stimulates bone resorption by osteoclasts and results in increased plasma Ca^{2+} levels.[55] The effect of PTH on TRP-channels in the bone remains to be determined.

If the balance between bone mineralization and resorption is disturbed and resorption exceeds mineralization, patients may develop resorptive hypercalciuria.[56] The most common cause of resorptive hypercalciuria is primary hyperparathyroidism.[8] Nowadays, the prevalence of this form of hypercalciuria is low (2–8%), due to early diagnosis and treatment of patients with primary hyperparathyroidism.[7] There is, however, an ongoing debate on the true origin of hypercalciuria in these patients.[57,58] Some argue that, at least in young patients with proper renal function, kidney stones are the result of intestinal hyperabsorption of Ca^{2+} due to enhanced synthesis of vitamin D.[59] Bone disease may rather occur in older patients as a result of lower vitamin D levels and consequent diminished intestinal Ca^{2+} absorption.

Intestine

Typically, the intestine absorbs between 25% and 35% of the ingested calcium; however, this fraction may vary depending on many factors, including bioavailability and bodily needs.[60] Intestinal absorption occurs through both transcellular and paracellular mechanisms (Figs. 9.6A and B).[61,62] Since the transepithelial potential difference across all intestinal segments is lumen negative, the driving force for passive paracellular Ca^{2+} absorption is the concentration gradient between the lumen and blood or interstitial compartment. When dietary Ca^{2+} levels are high, paracellular fluxes in the duodenum, jejunum, and ileum are responsible for the main fraction (80–90%) of the intestinal Ca^{2+} absorption.[63] The caecum and colon account for less than 10% of total Ca^{2+} uptake, presumably in both a paracellular and transcellular manner.[63] With a Ca^{2++}-poor diet, however, the concentration-dependent passive paracellular transport of Ca^{2+} may actually result in a net loss of Ca^{2+}.[64] At low luminal Ca^{2+} concentrations, in the absence of a Ca^{2+} gradient, solvent drag-mediated Ca^{2+} absorption may occur, where Ca^{2+} is dragged along with the water flux that is fueled by the hyperosmolar milieu in the paracellular space.[65] The molecular identity of proteins facilitating these paracellular fluxes remains to be determined, though members of the claudin family are likely candidates for the role.[66]

Intestinal Ca^{2+} transport via the transcellular pathway is well characterized. However, under normal circumstances, the contribution of the transcellular pathway to total intestinal Ca^{2+} absorption is relatively low. Ca^{2+} enters the epithelial cells via TRPV6, which is the gate-keeper for, and rate-limiting factor in, transcellular Ca^{2+} absorption. In the cell, Ca^{2+} is bound by calbindin-D9K, which keeps intracellular Ca^{2+} concentrations low and maintains the high transmembrane Ca^{2+} gradient that is essential for the absorption of Ca^{2+} via TRPV6. At the basolateral side of the cell, Ca^{2+} is extruded via PMCA1b.[22] In the intestine TRPV6 and calbindin-D9K are predominantly expressed in the duodenum.[67,68] Some expression of TRPV6 is also found in the caecum and colon.[67] The expression levels of these key players are highly sensitive to 1,25-dihydroxyvitamin D_3.[69,70] Under certain circumstances, intestinal absorption via the transcellular pathway can be increased to 50% of the total intestinal Ca^{2+} absorbed.[71] This prevents depletion of the bodily Ca^{2+} stores in case of low dietary Ca^{2+} load, or during periods in which Ca^{2+} requirements are high.

IMPORTANT REGULATORS OF CA^{2+} TRANSPORT

Ca^{2+} balance is tightly regulated by a number of hormones and receptors. The three predominant hormones in Ca^{2+} homeostasis are PTH, vitamin D and klotho.[72–74] Other hormones, such as calcitonin, adrenal corticosteroids, estrogens, thyroxine, somatotropin, and glucagon may also contribute to Ca^{2+} homeostasis.[19,22] Disturbances in PTH and vitamin D signaling often lead to nephrolithiasis, highlighting the role of these hormones in kidney stone formation.[75] Detection of local and systemic Ca^{2+} levels by the CaSR also plays an important role in the maintenance of Ca^{2+} homeostasis.

PTH

Parathyroid hormone is an 84-amino-acid polypeptide hormone, for which hypocalcemia is the primary stimulus for secretion. Once released into the circulation, PTH binds to the membrane-bound G-protein-coupled PTH receptor, which is located in bone and kidney, but can also be found in other organs.[22] The secretion of PTH from the parathyroid glands in response to hypocalcaemia is controlled by the CaSR in the parathyroid chief cells, which senses the plasma Ca^{2+} levels.[76] Parathyroid hormone helps to maintain Ca^{2+} homeostasis via three routes (Fig. 9.7).[16,77] First, PTH stimulates bone resorption, releasing Ca^{2+} and Pi from the bone into the blood. Second, it stimulates the kidney to increase the reabsorption of Ca^{2+} from the prourine. Third, it stimulates the synthesis of active vitamin D by the kidney by activating renal CYP27B1, the gene encoding the 1aOHase enzyme, which in turn leads to an increase in intestinal Ca^{2+} and Pi absorption. Once released into the circulation PTH can bind to PTH receptors that are located, among others, in the bone and kidney.[22] Parathyroid hormone also has an additional effect on the kidney, reducing the function of the Na^+-Pi-transporter NaPi2a (encoded by SLC34A1) on the apical membrane in the PT, reducing the transcellular reabsorption of filtered Pi from the prourine.[78] Although mRNA transcripts of the PTH receptor have been reported to be present in the intestine, a direct effect of PTH on intestinal Ca^{2+} handling has not been conclusively demonstrated.[79] The effect of PTH on intestinal Ca^{2+} absorption is commonly considered to be secondary to increased 1aOHase activity and the subsequent increase in circulating vitamin D levels.

The combined effects, both direct and indirect, of PTH on the intestine and kidney mean that PTH mainly affects the concentration of plasma Ca^{2+} but has very little effect on plasma Pi since the effects of PTH on Pi (re)absorption in the intestine, bone and kidney balance each other out.[74]

The effect of PTH on the major players in transcellular Ca^{2+} transport has been extensively studied. Using a rat model, Van Abel, et al. demonstrated that PTH stimulates renal Ca^{2+} reabsorption by exerting an effect on renal transcellular Ca^{2+} transport proteins.[80] They showed that

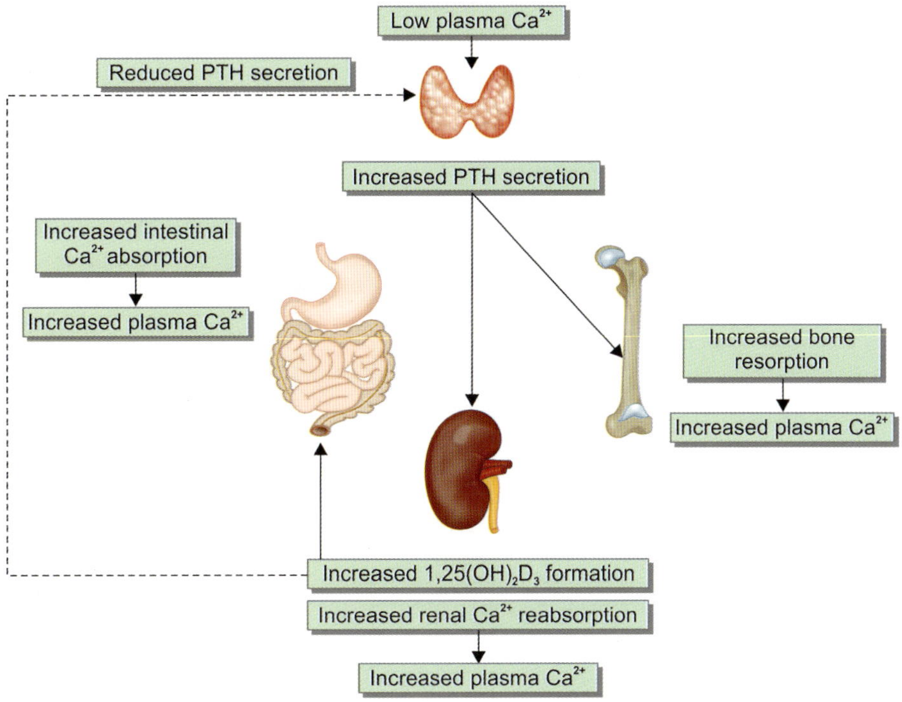

Fig. 9.7: Effects of PTH and vitamin D on Ca^{2+} homeostasis. PTH, released from the parathyroid glands, stimulates the production of active vitamin D_3 by the kidneys, which in turn stimulates intestinal Ca^{2+} absorption. It also increases bone resorption and renal Ca^{2+} reabsorption, increasing plasma Ca^{2+} levels. (PTH: Parathyroid hormone).

parathyroidectomy results in decreased serum PTH levels and hypocalcemia, most likely involving the downregulation of TRPV5, calbindin-D_{28K}, and NCX1. Transient receptor potential vanilloid 6, PMCA1b, CaSR, and vitamin D receptor (VDR) expression was unchanged. Supplementation with PTH largely restored serum Ca^{2+} concentrations as well as the abundance of the Ca^{2+} transport proteins, independent of their vitamin D status.[80] Infusion of a calcimimetic compound that activates CaSR at low serum Ca^{2+} concentrations was shown to decrease serum PTH levels and reduce renal expression of TRPV5, calbindin-D9K, calbindin-D28K, NCX1, and the CaSR.[80] Serum 1,25-dihydroxyvitamin D3 levels were unchanged as was the expression of TRPV6, PMCA1b, and VDR.[80] Together, these data indicate that PTH exerts a direct effect on renal Ca^{2+} reabsorption by influencing the expression levels of calciotropic genes, which is independent of vitamin D and CaSR.[80]

In addition to its transcriptional effects, PTH also activates the protein kinase A pathway.[81] This signaling cascade leads to PTH-dependent phosphorylation of TRPV5, which increases the open probability of TRPV5, and therefore the amount of Ca^{2+} transport.[81] Furthermore, PTH inhibits caveolae-mediated endocytosis of TRPV5, thereby increasing cell surface abundance of the channel.[82] Together, these findings demonstrate the importance of PTH in renal transcellular Ca^{2+} transport.

Vitamin D

Our body can obtain vitamin D from two sources: it can be synthesized in the skin under the influence of ultraviolet light, or it can be absorbed from our diet.[83] Few foods naturally contain vitamin D; therefore dermal synthesis is the major natural source of this vitamin. Previtamin D3 (cholecalciferol) is synthesized nonenzymatically in skin from 7-dehydrocholesterol during exposure to sunlight (Fig. 9.8). In the liver, it undergoes a hydroxylation process by an enzyme called 25-hydroxylase, turning it into 25-hydroxyvitamin D_3 (calcidiol).[16] Further hydroxylation of 25-hydroxyvitamin D_3 into the physiologically active vitamin D metabolite 1,25-dihydroxyvitamin D_3 (calcitriol) occurs in the kidney by the enzyme 1- α-hydroxylase, which is encoded by the CYP27B1 gene. The kidney also expresses CYP24A1, which codes for the enzyme 24-hydroxylase, which breaks 1,25-dihydroxyvitamin D_3 down to 24,25-dihydroxyvitamin D, which is biologically inactive. CYP24A1 is downregulated by PTH and

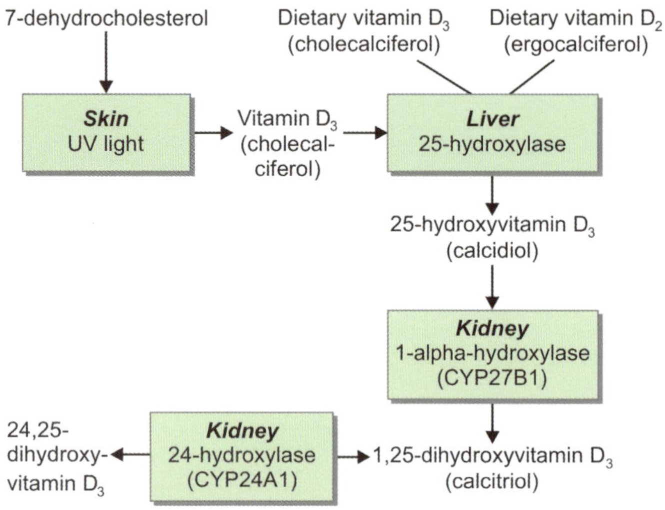

Fig. 9.8: Overview of vitamin D metabolites and enzymes involved in their synthesis. The active vitamin D metabolite, 1,25 dihydroxyvitamin D_3, is synthesized from precursors by various enzymes including 1-α-hydroxylase. The enzyme 24-hydroxylase is responsible for the breakdown of active vitamin D to 24,25-dihydroxyvitamin D_3, an inactive metabolite. (UV: Ultraviolet).

upregulated by 1,25-dihydroxyvitamin D3 in a regulatory feedback loop ensuring proper plasma 1,25-dihydroxyvitamin D_3 levels.

The renal synthesis of 1,25-dihydroxyvitamin D_3 varies according to physiologic needs. The major functions of 1,25-dihydroxyvitamin D_3 are to stimulate the absorption of Ca^{2+} in the intestine, and to inhibits the transcription of PTH in the parathyroid glands.[77] 1,25-Dihydroxyvitamin D3 can bind to the VDR, which is a transcription factor. Upon binding to 1,25-dihydroxyvitamin D3, the VDR heterodimerizes with other nuclear hormone receptors, in particular the family of retinoid X receptors.[24] This complex subsequently binds to special DNA sequences called vitamin D responsive elements in the promoters of genes.[84,85]

Recently, two groups described a new genetic defect in a large cohort of patients with infantile idiopathic hypercalcemia, and patients who were believed to exhibit symptoms of vitamin D toxicity.[86,87] These studies identified a defect in the CYP24A1 gene. Lack of functional CYP24A1 can result in elevated levels of 1,25-dihydroxyvitamin D_3 due to its reduced metabolism.[87]

A recent study in an Israeli family found that CYP24A1 mutations may also result in severe, long-standing problems with kidney stone disease in adults.[88] The patients described in this study displayed normal-high serum Ca^{2+} levels, low PTH levels, high vitamin D 25-$(OH)_2D_3$ and 1,25-dihydroxyvitamin D_3, and low levels of 24,25-$(OH)_2D_3$, resulting in severe hypercalciuric nephrolithiasis and nephrocalcinosis.[49] This study indicates that CYP24A1 mutations should be considered in the differential diagnosis of hypercalciuric nephrolithiasis.

There is ample evidence that the expression of Ca^{2+} transporters is tightly controlled by 1,25-dihydroxyvitamin D3.[89-91] Both in vivo and in vitro studies consistently show that vitamin D affects expression of calciotropic genes. The regulation of calciotropic genes by 1,25-dihydroxyvitamin D3 has been extensively studied using genetically modified mouse models in which vitamin D regulation was inactivated, such as VDR KO mice and 1aOHase KO mice.[89,91] Vitamin D receptor KO mice, displaying lower serum Ca^{2+} levels and reduced intestinal Ca^{2+} absorption, have reduced duodenal TRPV6 and calbindin-D9K mRNA expression levels, as well as reduced levels of renal TRPV5 expression.[91] 1aOHase KO mice, in which 1,25-dihydroxyvitamin D3 biosynthesis is impaired, suffer from severe hypocalcemia.[92] Renal mRNA expression of TRPV5, calbindin-D9K, calbindin-D28K, and NCX1 was decreased in these mice.[89] Administration of 1,25-dihydroxyvitamin D3 restored expression levels of calciotropic genes and normalized serum Ca^{2+} levels.[89] In line with these findings, analysis of putative promoter regions of both human and murine genes revealed potential vitamin D-response elements in genes such as TRPV5, TRPV6, calbindin-D_9k, and PMCA1b.[67,73] The effect of vitamin D on the expression of calciotropic genes is relatively fast. For example, Wood, et al. have shown that addition of 1,25-dihydroxyvitamin D3 to Caco-2 cells increases TRPV6 expression within 24 hours.[93] Time-lapse studies in mice using a single dose of 1,25-dihydroxyvitamin D3 showed that induction of duodenal TRPV6 mRNA expression occurs within 3–6 hours and precedes the functional result, i.e. the increase in intestinal Ca^{2+} absorption.[94] In line with the strong effect of Vitamin D on intestinal Ca^{2+} absorption, the expression of renal transporters involved in Ca^{2+} transport is regulated by 1,25-dihydroxyvitamin D3 to a lesser extent than the intestinal transporters.[83,95]

Klotho

A relatively new calciotropic hormone is klotho. The hormone klotho was identified in mice that displayed a phenotype similar to human ageing: a short lifespan, infertility, arteriosclerosis, skin atrophy, osteoporosis, and emphysema.[96] Klotho is a type I transmembrane protein with β-glucuronidase activity in the large extracellular domain that can be cleaved and secreted into blood, urine,

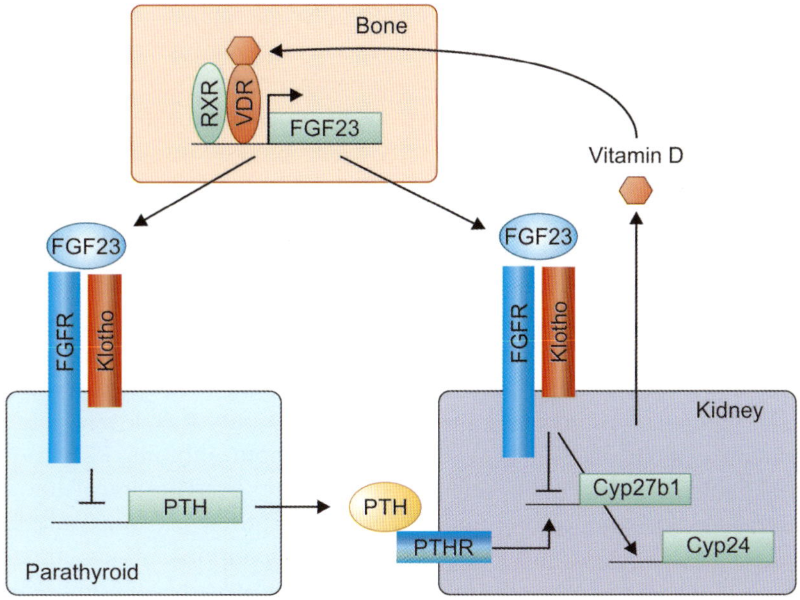

Fig. 9.9: The effect of klotho on calcium homeostasis. FGF23 released from bone acts on the FGF receptor (FGFR) complex expressed in the kidney and parathyroid gland in the presence of klotho. In the kidney, this leads to suppression of the synthesis of active vitamin D by downregulating expression of the Cyp27b1, and stimulation of vitamin D catabolism by upregulation of the Cyp24 gene. In the parathyroid gland, upon binding of the FGF receptor and klotho, FGF23 suppresses production and secretion of PTH. (PTH: Parathyroid hormone; FGF: Fibroblast growth factor).

and cerebrospinal fluid.[72,97] Klotho KO mice have elevated serum Ca^{2+} and Pi levels and display, among their other pathologies, osteopenia, and soft tissue calcifications.[96] It has been suggested that many of the abnormalities found in klotho KO mice are the result of a primary defect in Ca^{2+} and Pi homeostasis.[98,99] Klotho has been proposed to play a role in the negative feedback circuit that inhibits 1,25-dihydroxyvitamin D_3 synthesis when Ca^{2+} levels are high.[100] It is thought to transduce the signal of fibroblast growth factor 23 (FGF23) via the FGF receptor, thereby affecting PTH production as well as suppressing the conversion of 25-hydroxyvitamin D into 1,25-dihydroxyvitamin D_3 (Fig. 9.9).[101] Consequently, the absence of klotho results in increased serum levels of 1,25-dihydroxyvitamin D3 and reduced serum concentrations of PTH.[102] In addition, klotho increases cell surface expression of TRPV5 through the hydrolysis of its N-glycan, thereby exerting a direct effect on Ca^{2+} homeostasis.[72]

Extensive characterization of klotho KO mice showed that these mice display hypervitaminosis D, hypercalciuria, hyperphosphaturia, lower urinary pH, reduced urine output, and higher urine osmolarity.[103] The renal mRNA expression of TRPV5 was significantly elevated in klotho KO mice.[103] In contrast, however, the expression of both NCX1 and calbindin-D_{28K} was decreased whereas PMCA1b expression was unaltered.[103] Interestingly, the expression of calbindin-D28K and NCX1 parallels the expressions observed in the TRPV5 KO mice.[48,104] It was previously shown that the rate of Ca^{2+} influx across the apical plasma membrane into the cell determines the level of calbindin-D28K and NCX1 expression.[48,104] Consequently, the low expression levels of these proteins in klotho KO mice suggest that Ca^{2+} influx through TRPV5 is impaired. In line with this, the observed increase in TRPV5 expression in klotho KO mice is most likely functionally insignificant; due to the absence of klotho TRPV5 is likely not to be retained in the plasma membrane, leading to a failure of klotho KO mice to reabsorb Ca^{2+} in the DCT/CNT via TRPV5.[72,105]

To determine whether the renal Ca^{2+} leak observed in the klotho KO mice was primary or secondary to the increased serum Ca^{2+} and 1,25-dihydroxyvitamin D_3 levels, these parameters were normalized by feeding the animals a low Ca^{2+}, Pi, and vitamin D diet.[103] Although the diet returned serum Ca^{2+} levels back to the normal range in klotho KO animals, hypercalciuria persisted despite increased expression of TRPV5.[103] Thus, renal Ca^{2+} wasting is a primary defect in klotho KO mice.

Klotho KO mice displayed CaP precipitates throughout the renal cortex, which mainly resided in the DCT/CNT segments of the nephron.[103] This finding is consistent with the increased renal Ca^{2+} and Pi excretion observed in the klotho KO mice.[96,106] Urinary pH, unrelated to metabolic acidosis, was lower in KO mice compared to their wild-type littermates, which was not caused by metabolic acidosis.[103] In fact, the acidification of urine is a well-known protective mechanism against CaP precipitation and it is likely a response to hypercalciuria and an attempt to prevent nephrocalcinosis.[107] In fact, the acidification of urine is a well-known protective mechanism against CaP precipitation and it is likely a response to hypercalciuria and an attempt to prevent nephrocalcinosis.[108]

Another protective mechanism against nephrocalcinosis is urinary dilution. Increased delivery of Ca^{2+} to the DCT/CNT normally downregulates aquaporin-2 (AQP2) expression, diluting the urine.[109] However, klotho KO mice had more concentrated urine compared with wild-type mice, and AQP2 expression was increased in klotho KO mice compared to wild-type littermates.[103] This discrepancy is most likely due to a greater need to protect intravascular volume than to prevent stone formation. Due to their smaller size, klotho KO mice have an increased surface area to weight ratio and tend toward a reduced intravascular volume because they have increased insensible losses.[96] Therefore, they cannot afford additional fluid losses required to dilute their urine. The concentrated urine in the presence of hypercalciuria probably contributes to the formation of renal CaP precipitates in the klotho KO mice. This emphasizes that both acidification and dilution of urine are needed to prevent CaP precipitations in case of high renal Ca^{2+} excretion.

The findings in klotho KO mice support a central role for klotho in Ca^{2+} homeostasis, preventing renal Ca^{2+} loss and problems commonly associated with this loss, like nephrolithiasis and osteopenia. Interestingly, both of these clinical problems as well as hypercalciuria occur more frequently with advanced age, which coincides with decreases in circulating klotho levels, highlighting the importance of klotho in Ca^{2+} homeostasis as well as nephrolithiasis.[110] In addition, the klotho mouse model demonstrates the importance of urinary acidification and dilution in the prevention of renal stone formation of renal stones.[103]

CaSR

The Ca^{2+}-sensing receptor is a G-protein-coupled receptor that detects changes in ionized Ca^{2+} levels.[111] The Ca^{2+}-sensing receptor modulates PTH release from the parathyroid glands into the systemic circulation in response to changing Ca^{2+} levels in the blood. The Ca^{2+}-sensing receptor is expressed in other tissues as well, such as the bone and the gastrointestinal tract. Activation of the CaSR triggers adaptive responses to local variations in Ca^{2+} levels.[112] In the kidney, the CaSR is expressed at multiple sites along the nephron, and cellular localization varies in the different segments where it is expressed. The differential expression and localization of CaSR along the nephron is indicative of the variety of physiologic functions it has throughout the kidney. In the PT, the CaSR is expressed on the apical membrane of cells, where it is activated by high urinary Ca^{2+} levels.[113] Stimulation of the CaSR in this segment inhibits PTH-induced endocytosis of Pi transporters from the apical membrane, thereby increasing Pi reabsorption.[114,115] This prevents the formation of renal CaP precipitations by avoiding excess loss of Pi into a filtrate that already contains elevated Ca^{2+} concentrations. In the TAL, where 20–25% of Ca^{2+} is reabsorbed, the CaSR is expressed at the basolateral plasma membrane.[116] During hypercalcemia, activation of the basolateral CaSR inhibits ROMK and NKCC2, resulting in a loss of the driving force for paracellular transport.[117] This way, the CaSR provides a negative feedback, attenuating Ca^{2+} reabsorption to prevent hypercalcemia.[118] The expression pattern of CaSR in the DCT/CNT is diffuse, with expression on the apical as well as the basolateral side of the epithelial layer.[116] Here, the CaSR is thought to control transcellular Ca^{2+} reabsorption via modulation of apical Ca^{2+} entry through TRPV5 and/or basolateral Ca^{2+} efflux mediated by NCX1 and PMCA1B.[119,120] In the Collecting duct (CD), the CaSR is expressed at the apical membrane in principal and intercalated cells.[116] Here, the CaSR has been suggested to play an important role in the prevention of nephrolithiasis as it regulates both urinary acidification and urinary dilution.[18]

Transient receptor potential vanilloid 5 KO mice demonstrate severe hypercalciuria with hyperphosphaturia, which should increase their risk for renal CaP stone formation.[48] Interestingly, despite the fact that they display *hyperphosphaturia* and excrete 5–10 times more Ca^{2+} in their urine compared to wild-type littermates, TRPV5 KO mice do not develop kidney stones.[48] Instead, they display profound polyuria and increased urinary acidification.[48] Urinary Ca^{2+} levels in these mice correlated linearly with urinary volume as well as pH.[121] Since both urinary acidification and dilution prevent supersaturation this may explain why precipitations are not found in these mice.[48]

Urinary acidification occurs along different segments of the nephron and is essential in acid/base homeostasis.[122,123]

Together with urinary buffers, the activity of acid/base transporters in the intercalated cells of CNT and CD determines the fine-tuning of urinary pH. The multisubunit vacuolar ATP-driven proton pump (H^+-ATPase) is expressed on the apical membrane in type A intercalated cells, where it is mainly responsible for proton excretion.[124] In in vitro studies, it was shown that the exposure to high (5.0 mM) Ca^{2+} concentrations significantly enhances H^+-ATPase activity in CD cells, indicating that there might be a link between the sensing of Ca^{2+}, most likely by the CaSR, and urinary acidification via the H^+-ATPase.[121]

To address the role of the CaSR and the contribution of H^+-ATPase to the acidification of urine in response to hypercalciuria in TRPV5 KO mice, TRPV5/Atp6v1b1 double KO (DKO) mice were generated.[121] These mice are genetically ablated for both TRPV5 and the intercalated cell-specific B1 subunit of H^+-ATPase (Atp6v1b1).[125] Like TRPV5 KO mice, DKOs were hypercalciuric. The urinary pH of these mice was normalized, their urinary volume, however, was even higher compared to TRPV5 KO mice. In addition, the DKO mice showed bilateral hydronephrosis, abnormal dilation of the CD and, importantly, massive tubular CaP precipitations in the medullary CD.[121] Thus, H^+-ATPase activity is essential in the prevention of CaP stone formation during hypercalciuria.

Previous studies also provide a link between Ca^{2+} and water homeostasis, suggesting a functional role for the CaSR in final urinary concentration process in the CD.[109] The water channel AQP2, localized at the apical membrane of the CNT and CD, was significantly downregulated in TRPV5 KO mice compared with wild-type mice.[121]

In line with the increased diuresis in the DKOs, further AQP2 downregulation was detected in mice that lack both TRPV5 as well as a functional H^+-ATPase.[121] In in vitro experiments, a decreased AQP2 expression in a murine CD cell line after exposure to extracellular Ca^{2+} was shown.[121] Similar findings were done when the CaSR agonist neomycin was added to these cells.[121] Together, these findings suggest that activation of the apical CaSR reduces the water permeability of the CD when the luminal Ca^{2+} levels rise, a process which involves CaSR-mediated retrieval of AQP2 from the apical membrane into endocytic compartments. Thus, hypercalciuria activates the apical CaSR in the CD and reduces AQP2-mediated water reabsorption, permitting the disposal of excess urinary Ca^{2+}, and preventing the formation of stones. The additional decrease of AQP2 expression in the DKO mice is most likely explained by the higher sensitivity of the CaSR for Ca^{2+} at a neutral urinary pH compared to the sensitivity at a lower pH. This way, a more severe reduction in water reabsorption is induced in the absence of increased urinary acidification, in an attempt to prevent renal stone formation.

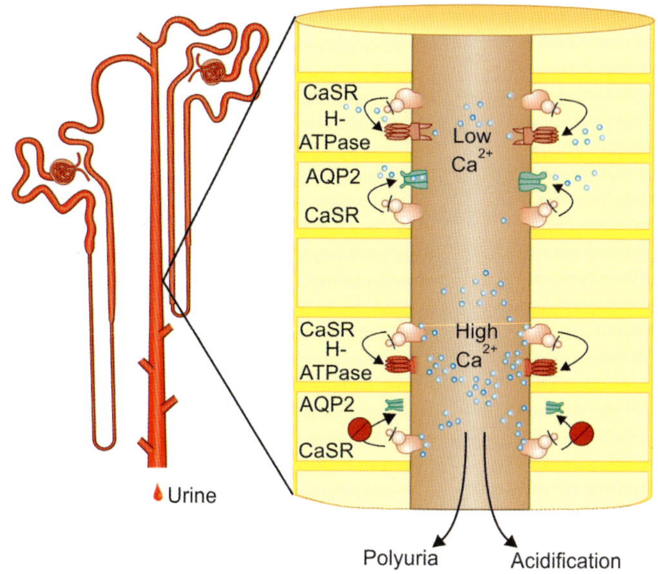

Fig. 9.10: Model of renal CaSR signaling in the collecting duct. The CaSR is located at the apical side of both principal cells and intercalated cells in the collecting duct. During hypercalciuria the CaSR is activated, leading to downregulation of the water channel AQP2, resulting in polyuria. In addition, stimulation of the CaSR increases H^+-ATPase activity, acidifying the urine. Together, polyuria and increased urinary acidification prevent renal CaP precipitation. (CaSR: Ca^{2+}-sensing receptor; AQP2: Aquaporin 2; CaP: Calcium phosphate).

Together, these observations unequivocally reveal that the naturally occurring increased urinary acidification and urinary volume through CaSR activation in the distal nephron is an essential adaptive mechanism preventing renal CaP precipitation during hypercalciuria (Fig. 9.10).

HEREDITARY DISORDERS OF MINERAL BALANCE AND NEPHROLITHIASIS

Lifestyle greatly influences the risk of nephrolithiasis but genetic factors contribute much more to the pathology of kidney stones.[126-128] Nephrolithiasis occurs more frequently in individuals whose family history is positive for renal stones and hypercalciuric nephrolithiasis is a familial phenomenon in more than 35% of patients, emphasizing the importance of genetics.[129] In addition, twin studies have shown that the proband concordance rate in monozygotic twins is significantly greater compared to dizygotic twins.[130]

Table 9.1: Known genetic defects in mineral transporters and related genes causing nephrolithiasis.

Gene	Protein	Disease	Inheritance	Pathophysiology
CLCN5	CLC5, endosomal H^+/Cl^- antiporter	Dent's disease	X-linked, recessive	PT dysfunction, proteinuria, hypercalciuria, nephrolithiasis, medullary nephrocalcinosis, and progressive renal failure
SLC34A3	NaPi-IIc, Na^+, Pi cotransporter	Hereditary hypophosphatemic rickets with hypercalciuria	Autosomal recessive	Hypercalciuria, hyperphosphaturia, hypophosphatemia, and rickets
SLC4A1	Anion exchanger 1 (AE1), Cl^- and HCO_3^- exchanger	Primary distal renal tubular acidosis	Autosomal dominant	Hyperchloremic metabolic acidosis and hypokalemia with inappropriate alkaline urine pH, nephrocalcinosis, and/or nephrolithiasis
CLDN16	Claudin 16	Familial hypomagnesemia with hypercalciuria and nephrocalcinosis	Autosomal dominant	Renal wasting of Ca^{2+} and Mg^{2+}, nephrocalcinosis, and progressive renal failure
CLDN19	Claudin 19	Familial hypomagnesemia with hypercalciuria and nephrocalcinosis with ocular impairment	Autosomal dominant	Renal wasting of Ca^{2+} and Mg^{2+}, nephrocalcinosis, and progressive renal failure
SLC12A1	NKCC2 (Na^+, K^+, $2Cl^-$ cotransporter2)	Antenatal Bartter syndrome, type I	Autosomal recessive	Salt wasting, hypokalemic metabolic acidosis, hypercalciuria, and nephrocalcinosis
KCNJ1	ROMK (renal outer medullary K^+ channel)	Antenatal Bartter syndrome, type II	Autosomal recessive	Salt wasting, hypokalemic metabolic acidosis, hypercalciuria, and nephrocalcinosis
CLCNKB	ClC-Kb, Cl^- channel	Classic Bartter syndrome, type III	Autosomal recessive	Hypokalemia, hypochloremia, variable urinary Ca^{2+} excretion

The inheritance of nephrolithiasis often is not Mendelian, and instead is consistent with a complex polygenic inheritance pattern where multiple genes exert small and additive contributions to stone susceptibility.[131,132] Genome-wide association studies to find genetic causes of nephrolithiasis often have difficulties identifying candidates that significantly correlate to kidney stone formation.[127,133] This is further evidence that stone formation often probably is not contributable to single genes but arises from the additive effects of multiple genes, the culmination of which determines whether an individual will develop nephrolithiasis or not. This greatly hampers the success of linkage analysis and GWAS approaches in the identification of the genes involved. Despite the polygenic nature of the disease, there are single genes, which contribute more to the pathology than others, which will be discussed below.

Monogenic Disturbances of Mineral Transporters in Nephrolithiasis

Over the years, linkage analysis has been successfully used to identify a number of genes encoding mineral transporters that cause monogenic forms of nephrolithiasis (Table 9.1).

CLCN5

Dent's disease (OMIM 300009) is a group of recessive, X-linked tubular disorders, including X-linked recessive nephrolithiasis with renal failure, X-linked recessive hypophosphatemic rickets and idiopathic low-molecular weight proteinuria.[134] It is characterized by PT dysfunction, and typically results in proteinuria, hypercalciuria, nephrolithiasis, medullary nephrocalcinosis, and progressive renal failure.[135] As it is linked to the X-chromosome, female patients tend to have a milder phenotype than male patients.[127]

X-linked recessive nephrolithiasis is caused by mutations in the CLCN5 gene.[134] CLCN5 encodes CLC5, which functions as an H^+/Cl^- antiporter in the subapical endosomes of kidney tubular cells.[136] It is required for the acidification of organelles involved in the endocytosis of low-molecular weight proteins.[137,138] CLC5 is expressed in the PT, the TAL, and in the α-intercalated cells of the CD.[139] The defects caused by CLCN5 mutations result in defective trafficking of several endocytic receptors, including megalin and cubilin.[140]

Currently, the exact molecular mechanisms causing hypercalciuria in Dent's disease remain unclear. In general, patients with Dent's disease display mildly elevated levels of vitamin D, which could contribute to hypercalciuria, but may also be a compensatory response to renal Ca^{2+} losses.[141,142] Some patients also present with rickets, which is normalized after pharmacologic doses of vitamin D, but physicians should be careful as this treatment could worsen the hypercalciuria.[142] Piwon, et al. suggested that the increased levels of vitamin D may be related to PTH.[143] They hypothesized that CLCN5 mutations lead to decreased PTH internalization, increasing the stimulation of luminal PTH receptors in the kidney.[143] This would stimulate the production of active vitamin D; however, the proteinuria decreases the amount of precursor $25(OH)_2D_3$ bound to vitamin D-binding protein.[143] The balance between these two processes would therefore determine the phenotype and explain the variability.[127,143]

Several groups have shown that CLC-5 plays an essential role in NHE3 endocytosis.[143,144]

Interestingly, a recent study has shown that NHE3 is essential for Ca^{2+} transport in the PT.[145] The Na^+/H^+ exchanger 3 is responsible for the majority of proximal tubular Na^+ reabsorption and, consequently, osmotically driven water reabsorption.[146,147] As a large majority of proximal tubular paracellular Ca^{2+} reabsorption is driven by active transcellular Na^+ flux, it follows that NHE3 activity drives the passive paracellular flux of Ca^{2+}.[148,149] Together, these data connect CLC-5, NHE3, and renal Ca^{2+} transport, and could explain the hypercalciuric phenotype of patients with Dents disease.

SLC34A3 and SLC34A1

Hereditary hypophosphatemic rickets with hypercalciuria (HHRH; OMIM #241530) is an autosomal recessive disorder characterized by renal Pi wasting, hypophosphatemia, and rickets.[150] As a result of hypophosphatemia, patients display a compensatory increase in 1,25(OH)2D3 levels, resulting in increased intestinal absorption of Ca^{2+} and Pi, leading to hypercalciuria.[150] The combination of hypercalciuria and *hyperphosphaturia* results in the formation of CaP kidney stones. Homozygous and compound heterozygous mutations in SLC34A3, encoding Na^+–Pi cotransporter NaPi-IIc, have been found in several families with HHRH.[151] Although SLC34A1 (encoding NaPi-IIa) is considered more important for renal phosphate transport, mutations here have not yet been conclusively linked to nephrolithiasis.[152-154]

SLC4A1

Primary distal renal tubular acidosis (dRTA) is caused by the failure of the CD to appropriately acidify the urine, resulting in hyperchloremic metabolic acidosis and hypokalemia with inappropriate alkaline urine pH.[133] It is frequently complicated by nephrocalcinosis and/or nephrolithiasis. Distal renal tubular acidosis is genetically heterogeneous in both inheritance mode and genetic defect. Among others, dRTA can be caused by mutations in SLC4A1.[155] SLC4A1 encodes anion exchanger 1 (AE1), which mediates the exchange of Cl^- and HCO_3^-.[155] It is located at the basolateral surface of the α-intercalated cells of the CD.[156] Mutations result in decreased $HCO3^-$ reabsorption at the basolateral membrane of the intercalated cells, leading to renal tubular acidosis.[156] As a result, patients develop nephrocalcinosis and nephrolithiasis.

SLC12A1 and KCNJ1

Antenatal Bartter syndrome is characterized by salt wasting, hypokalemic metabolic acidosis, hypercalciuria, and nephrocalcinosis.[157] Antenatal Bartter syndrome is caused by mutations in SLC12A1, encoding the N^+, K^+, $2Cl^-$ cotransporter NKCC2, or by mutations in KCNJ1, encoding the potassium channel ROMK1.[158,159] Na^+–K^+–$2Cl^-$ cotransporter resides in the apical membrane of the TAL where it is the major transport protein responsible for the reabsorption of Na^+. Renal outer medullary K^+ channel 1 is expressed in the apical membrane of the TAL, and recycles K^+ from the intracellular space back into the tubular lumen. It is essential for lowering intracellular K^+ levels and the maintenance of the membrane potential, which is required for NKCC2 function. Mutations in these proteins result in reduced net reabsorption of Na^+ and Cl^-, disturbing the apical membrane potential and the lumen-positive transepithelial potential.[160] The transepithelial potential is essential as it provides the driving force for the reabsorption of Ca^{2+} as well as Mg^{2+} via the paracellular pathway.[160]

CLCNKB

Classic Bartter syndrome is caused by mutations in CLCNKB, encoding ClC-Kb Cl^- channel.[161] ClC-Kb is expressed in the TAL as well as in the DCT.[162] It is localized in the basolateral membrane and mediates Cl^- efflux from the cell into the interstitium.[162] Mutations in CLC-NKB inhibit Cl^- efflux, resulting increased intracellular levels of Cl^- inhibit NKCC2 transporter activity, leading to a salt wasting phenotype similar to that of antenatal Bartter's syndrome. There is, however, a greater variability in the calciuric phenotype of the patients with classic Bartter syndrome. In contrast to the apical entry and recycling pathways, ClC-Kb appears not to be the only efflux pathway for Cl^- in the TAL; other transporters and channels may participate in the removal of intracellular Cl^- from the cell.[163,164] The level of compensation via these alternative pathways could potentially explain the clinical variability observed in patients.[164]

CDLN16 and CLDN19

Patients with mutations in *CLDN16*, the gene-encoding claudin 16, suffer from familial hypomagnesemia with hypercalciuria and nephrocalcinosis (FHHNC; OMIM 248250).[38] Patients with mutations in *CLDN19*, encoding claudin 19, have similar clinical features as patients with FHHNC, with additional ocular abnormalities (OMIM 248190).[37] In both types of patients, bilateral nephrocalcinosis is observed, ultimately leading to chronic renal failure. Expression of both claudin 16 and claudin 19 is restricted to the TAL.[38,165] Here, these two proteins form a highly cation-specific paracellular channel together, which is able to transport Mg^{2+} as well as Ca^{2+}.[40]

GWAS

Over the years, several GWAS studies have been performed to identify genes involved in nephrolithiasis. In these studies, the whole genomic DNA is mapped with polymorphic markers to identify loci associated with nephrolithiasis. By widening the scope beyond candidate genes, the involvement of genes that are not typically considered in this field can be identified. In patients with hypercalciuric nephrolithiasis, this approach has recently led to the identification of CLDN14.[39] Other studies have identified SLC34A3 (encoding NaPi-IIc) and a *bicarbonate*-sensitive adenylate cyclase gene as having a possible role in nephrolithiasis; however, these findings are still under debate and remain to be confirmed.[166,167]

CLDN14

Claudin 14, encoded by CLDN14, was initially studied due to its role in the inner ear, as mutations in this gene cause a hereditary form of deafness.[168] In the ear, claudin 14 blocks the paracellular passage of cations, including K^+.[169] The maintenance of a K^+ gradient between the different perilymph and endolymph compartments of the ear is essential for normal ear function. Interestingly, a recent GWAS identified four common synonymous variants in CLDN14 that significantly associate with kidney stones.[39] One of these Single-nucleotide polymorphism (SNPs) also correlates with increased urinary calcium excretion compared to noncarriers.[39] When coexpressed with CLDN 16, claudin 14 inhibits the permeability of the paracellular pathway for cations in the TAL.[170] Interestingly, none of the patients with CLDN14 mutations that cause deafness displayed hypercalciuria or nephrolithiasis, and CLDN14 KO mice do not display Ca^{2+} abnormalities under normal circumstances.[168,169] Like claudin 16 and 19, claudin 14 is localized in the TAL, where its expression level seems to vary depending on dietary Ca^{2+} content.[170] This suggests a regulatory role for claudin 14 in renal Ca^{2+} handling. Subsequently, it was shown that high dietary Ca^{2+} downregulates the expression level of specific microRNAs (miRs) in the TAL, miR-9 and miR-374, which in turn causes an increase in CLDN14 expression levels.[170] This process takes place under the direct regulation of the CaSR, which monitors the circulating Ca^{2+} levels and subsequently adjusts urinary excretion rates.[170] These findings correspond with previous studies, which have demonstrated that paracellular Ca^{2+} reabsorption in the TAL can be inhibited by CaSR activation during hypercalcemia.[171,172]

Candidate Screening Approach

Many studies have aimed to identify additional genes involved in nephrolithiasis in large groups of unrelated patients via candidate approaches. Candidates were mainly chosen based on their involvement in Ca^{2+} homeostasis.

TRPV5 and TRPV6

Transient receptor potential vanilloid 5 and 6 KO mice display hypercalciuria and are therefore important candidate genes in the pathogenesis of hypercalciuria and nephrolithiasis. So far, mutation analysis of TRPV5 has not revealed a primary role for this channel in idiopathic hypercalciuria.[173,174] Unusual haplotype differences can be found in the TRPV6 gene among different populations around the world; however, the functional relevance of these SNPs is under debate.[175] In in vitro studies, the SNPs did not affect the biophysical function of the channel.[176] However, the frequency of an ancestral TRPV6 haplotype consisting of three nonsynonymous polymorphisms was significantly higher in Ca^{2+} stone formers compared to nonstone-forming individuals. Nevertheless, there were no differences in plasma concentrations of 1,25-dihydroxyvitamin D3, PTH, and Ca^{2+}, or in urinary excretion Ca^{2+} between these two groups.[177]

Other Candidate Genes

Linkage disequilibrium with the loci of 1aOHase, VDR, CaSR, uromodulin, osteocalcin, and osteopontin was examined in a large cohort of French-Canadian stone formers.[178-180] Only the VDR locus (12.q12–14) showed linkage with nephrolithiasis.[180] Four of the six markers that were tested were positive for linkage with stones whereas one was positively linked with urinary Ca^{2+} excretion.[180] These findings are not yet unequivocal: they were confirmed in several Indian families, but not in a number of European families who also have a history of hypercalciuric kidney stones.[173,181]

CLDN2, CLDN10, and CLDN 15, Interesting New Candidates?

With the recent identification of three new genes in nephrolithiasis, CLDN16, CLDN19, and CLDN14, the claudin family of proteins seems to play an especially important role in Ca^{2+} homeostasis and kidney stone formation. Based on functional characteristics of other claudin family members, several other claudin isoforms could be of interest.

Claudin 2 functions as a high-conductance, cation-permeable paracellular pore, which is permeable to, and inhibited by, Ca^{2+}.[182,183] In the kidney, CLDN2 is highly expressed in the PT, where the majority of the filtered Ca^{2+} load is reabsorbed. Interestingly, CLDN2 KO mice exhibit decreased proximal reabsorption of Na^{+}, Cl^{-}, and water. In addition, CLDN2 KO mice display hypercalciuria, indicating that claudin 2 plays a role in paracellular Ca^{2+} transport in the PT.[45] In the intestine, CLDN2 expression was highest in various segments of the small intestine which are the main sites of paracellular Ca^{2+} and Mg^{2+} absorption. CLDN2 is virtually absent in the colon, where the epithelium is generally considered to be tight.[31,32] In VDR KO mice, intestinal expression of CLDN2 and CLDN12 was significantly reduced compared to wild-type mice.[43] The expression of both genes was increased by 1,25-dihydroxyvitamin D3 in an intestinal epithelial cell line, Caco-2, coinciding with an increase in paracellular Ca^{2+} transport and suggesting that tight junctions consisting of claudin 2 and/or claudin 12 form paracellular Ca^{2+} channels in intestinal as well as in renal epithelia. Importantly, they highlight a novel, vitamin D sensitive, mechanism for maintaining Ca^{2+} homeostasis.

CLDN10 KO mice develop hypermagnesemia, hypomagnesuria, and hypocalciuria, mirroring the phenotype of CLDN16 KO mice.[184] Despite the hypocalciuria, CLDN10 KO mice develop interstitial nephrocalcinosis in the outer medulla, and show paracellular hyperabsorption of Mg^{2+} and Ca^{2+} and increasing interstitial Ca^{2+} concentration.[184] The exact relevance of these observations for Ca^{2+} homeostasis and nephrolithiasis remains to be determined, and is worth investigating.

The evidence for the involvement of CLDN15 in Ca^{2+} homeostasis is incomplete, but continuously growing. Several studies suggest that CLDN15 is responsible for prolactin-stimulated paracellular intestinal Ca^{2+} absorption.[185,186] In addition, in NHE3 KO mice, which display various abnormalities in Ca^{2+} homeostasis, both CLDN2 and CLDN15 expression in the jejunum is reduced.[145] Other studies, however, showed that the overexpression of CLDN15 does not increase paracellular Ca^{2+} transport in Caco-2 cells.[43] The phenotype of the CLDN15 KO mice is in this respect informative.[187,188] Most strikingly, these mice have an enlargement of their small intestine.[187,188] Furthermore, the luminal Na^{+} concentration in their small intestine was abnormally low, and glucose absorption was impaired.[187] It has been suggested that CLDN15 could serve as a leaky Na^{+} channel.[187] At the cellular level, claudin-15 is localized in close proximity to the sodium-glucose symporter SGLT1 (sodium-glucose-linked transporter) and may contribute to the recirculation of Na^{+}.[187] The observed decrease in luminal Na^{+} directly diminishes the activity of SGLT1 in the small intestine, particularly in the jejunum, which is the major site of glucose absorption as well as paracellular Ca^{2+} transport.[187] CLDN15 is, therefore, not likely to be directly involved in paracellular Ca^{2+} transport. Instead, it probably facilitates the backleak of Na^{+}, which is important for SGLT1 and NHE3 function. The transport of Na^{+} across the apical plasma membrane, via these proteins, which potentially alters the transmembrane electrical potential, most likely plays a role in Ca^{2+} transport.

Alternatively, transcellular Na^{+} transport may contribute to the maintenance of a transepithelial electrochemical gradient facilitating paracellular Ca^{2+} transport. Since hyperabsorption of Ca^{2+} is a major cause of hypercalciuria, CLDN15 could play a relevant, if indirect, role in nephrolithiasis.

CONCLUSION

Alternations in calcium balance can play a major role in the development as well as prevention of nephrolithiasis. Maintenance of normal Ca^{2+} levels requires an intricate interplay between organs, hormones, and genes involved in maintaining Ca^{2+} homeostasis, disturbances of which may eventually lead to the formation of kidney stones. When disturbances in Ca^{2+} homeostasis lead to hypercalciuria, urinary Acidification, and dilution may help to avoid supersaturation, thereby preventing the formation of kidney stones. With the identification of new genes involved in nephrolithiasis etiology, our understanding of this multifactorial pathology continues to grow opening new opportunities for the development of new treatments.

ACKNOWLEDGMENTS

This work was supported by a Vici Grant for J. Hoenderop (NWO-ZonMw 016.130.668) and EURenOmics funding from the European Union Seventh Framework Programme (FP7/2007-2013, agreement no 305608).

REFERENCES

1. Lieske JC, Pena de la Vega LS, Slezak JM, et al. Renal stone epidemiology in Rochester, Minnesota: an update. Kidney Int. 2006;69:760-4.
2. Saigal CS, Joyce G, Timilsina AR. Direct and indirect costs of nephrolithiasis in an employed population: opportunity for disease management? Kidney Int. 2005;68:1808-14.
3. Coe FL, Favus MJ. Disorders of Bone and Mineral Metabolism. Lippincott Williams & Wilkins; 1992.
4. Parks JH, Coward M, Coe FL. Correspondence between stone composition and urine supersaturation in nephrolithiasis. Kidney Int. 1997;51:894-900.
5. Coe FL, Evan A, Worcester E. Kidney stone disease. J Clin Invest. 2005;115:2598-608.
6. Vezzoli G, Terranegra A, Arcidiacono T, et al. Genetics and calcium nephrolithiasis. Kidney Int. 2011;80:587-93.
7. Pak CY. Etiology and treatment of urolithiasis. Am J Kidney Dis. 1991;18:624-37.
8. Sakhaee K, Maalouf NM, Sinnott B. Clinical review. Kidney stones 2012: pathogenesis, diagnosis, and management. J Clin Endocrinol Metab. 2012;97:1847-60.
9. Pak CY, Britton F, Peterson R, et al. Ambulatory evaluation of nephrolithiasis. Classification, clinical presentation and diagnostic criteria. Am J Med. 1980;69:19-30.
10. de Groot T, Bindels RJ, Hoenderop JG. TRPV5: an ingeniously controlled calcium channel. Kidney Int. 2008;74:1241-6.
11. Nijenhuis T, Hoenderop JG, Bindels RJ. TRPV5 and TRPV6 in Ca(2+) (re)absorption: regulating Ca(2+) entry at the gate. Pflug Arch. 2005;451:181-92.
12. Angelow S, Ahlstrom R, Yu AS. Biology of claudins. Am J Physiol Renal Physiol. 2008;295:F867-76.
13. Bronner F, Pansu D. Nutritional aspects of calcium absorption. J Nutr. 1999;129:9-12.
14. Wasserman RH, Armbrecht HJ, Shimura F, et al. Vitamin D influences multiple phases of the intestinal calcium transport system. Prog Clin Biol Res. 1984;168:307-12.
15. Allen LH. Calcium bioavailability and absorption: a review. Am J Clin Nutr. 1982;35:783-808.
16. Favus MJ, Goltzman D. Regulation of calcium and magnesium. In: Primer on the Metabolic Bone Diseases and Disorders of Mineral Metabolism. John Wiley & Sons Inc. pp. 171-9.
17. Schrier RW. Atlas of Diseases of the Kidney. Wiley; 1999.
18. Renkema KY, Bindels RJ, Hoenderop JG. Role of the calcium-sensing receptor in reducing the risk for calcium stones. Clin J Am Soc Nephrol. 2011;6:2076-82.
19. van de Graaf SF, Bindels RJ, Hoenderop JG. Physiology of epithelial Ca^{2+} and Mg^{2+} transport. Rev Physiol Biochem Pharmacol. 2007;158:77-160.
20. Dimke H, Hoenderop JG, and Bindels RJ. Molecular basis of epithelial Ca^{2+} and Mg^{2+} transport: insights from the TRP channel family. J Physiol. 2011;589:1535-1542.
21. Hoenderop JG, Bindels RJ. Calciotropic and magnesiotropic TRP channels. Physiology (Bethesda). 2008;23:32-40.
22. Hoenderop JG, Nilius B, Bindels RJ. Calcium absorption across epithelia. Physiol Rev. 2005;85:373-422.
23. Hoenderop JG, van der Kemp AW, Hartog A, et al. Molecular identification of the apical Ca^{2+} channel in 1, 25-dihydroxyvitamin D3-responsive epithelia. J Biol Chem. 1999;274:8375-8.
24. Peng JB, Chen XZ, Berger UV, et al. Molecular cloning and characterization of a channel-like transporter mediating intestinal calcium absorption. J Biol Chem. 1999;274:22739-46.
25. Woudenberg-Vrenken TE, Bindels RJ, Hoenderop JG. The role of transient receptor potential channels in kidney disease. Nat Rev Nephrol. 2009;5:441-9.
26. Bronner F. Mechanisms and functional aspects of intestinal calcium absorption. J Exp Zool A Comp Exp Biol. 2003;300:47-52.
27. Schwaller B. The continuing disappearance of "pure" Ca^{2+} buffers. Cell Mol Life Sci. 2009;66:275-300.
28. Feher JJ. Facilitated calcium diffusion by intestinal calcium-binding protein. Am J Physiol. 1983;244:C303-7.
29. Bindels RJ. Calcium handling by the mammalian kidney. J Exp Biol. 1993;184:89-104.
30. Gunzel D, Yu AS. Claudins and the modulation of tight junction permeability. Physiol Rev. 2013;93:525-69.
31. Markov AG, Veshnyakova A, Fromm M, et al. Segmental expression of claudin proteins correlates with tight junction barrier properties in rat intestine. J Comp Physiol B. 2010;180:591-8.
32. Amasheh S, Fromm M, Gunzel D. Claudins of intestine and nephron—a correlation of molecular tight junction structure and barrier function. Acta Physiol (Oxf). 2010;201:133-40.
33. Krause G, Winkler L, Mueller SL, et al. Structure and function of claudins. Biochim Biophys Acta. 2008;1778:631-45.
34. Hou J. Lecture: New light on the role of claudins in the kidney. Organogenesis. 2012;8:1-9.
35. Suzuki H, Nishizawa T, Tani K, et al. Crystal structure of a claudin provides insight into the architecture of tight junctions. Science. 2014;344:304-7.
36. Hou J, Rajagopal M, and Yu AS. Claudins and the kidney. Annu Rev Physiol. 2013;75:479-501.

37. Konrad M, Schaller A, Seelow D, et al. Mutations in the tight-junction gene claudin 19 (CLDN19) are associated with renal magnesium wasting, renal failure, and severe ocular involvement. Am J Hum Genet. 2006;79:949-57.
38. Simon DB, Lu Y, Choate KA, et al. Paracellin-1, a renal tight junction protein required for paracellular Mg^{2+} resorption. Science. 1999;285:103-6.
39. Thorleifsson G, Holm H, Edvardsson V, et al. Sequence variants in the CLDN14 gene associate with kidney stones and bone mineral density. Nat Genet. 2009;41:926-30.
40. Hou J, Renigunta A, Gomes AS, et al. Claudin-16 and claudin-19 interaction is required for their assembly into tight junctions and for renal reabsorption of magnesium. Proc Natl Acad Sci U S A. 2009;106:15350-5.
41. Hou J, Renigunta A, Konrad M, et al. Claudin-16 and claudin-19 interact and form a cation-selective tight junction complex. J Clin Invest. 2008;118:619-28.
42. Dimke H, Desai P, Borovac J, et al. Activation of the Ca(2+)-sensing receptor increases renal claudin-14 expression and urinary Ca(2+) excretion. Am J Physiol Renal Physiol. 2013;304:F761-9.
43. Fujita H, Sugimoto K, Inatomi S, et al. Tight junction proteins claudin-2 and -12 are critical for vitamin D-dependent Ca^{2+} absorption between enterocytes. Mol Biol Cell. 2008;19: 1912-21.
44. Pak CY, Oata M, Lawrence EC, et al. The hypercalciurias. Causes, parathyroid functions, and diagnostic criteria. J Clin Invest. 1974;54:387-400.
45. Muto S, Hata M, Taniguchi J, et al. Claudin-2-deficient mice are defective in the leaky and cation-selective paracellular permeability properties of renal proximal tubules. Proc Natl Acad Sci U S A. 2010;107:8011-6.
46. Dimke H, Hoenderop JG, Bindels RJ. Hereditary tubular transport disorders: implications for renal handling of Ca^{2+} and Mg^{2+}. Clin Sci (Lond). 2009;118:1-18.
47. Boros S, Bindels RJ, Hoenderop JG. Active Ca(2+) reabsorption in the connecting tubule. Pflug Arch. 2009;458:99-109.
48. Hoenderop JG, van Leeuwen JP, van der Eerden BC, et al. Renal Ca^{2+} wasting, hyperabsorption, and reduced bone thickness in mice lacking TRPV5. J Clin Invest. 2003;112: 1906-14.
49. Masuyama R, Vriens J, Voets T, et al. TRPV4-mediated calcium influx regulates terminal differentiation of osteoclasts. Cell Metab. 2008;8:257-65.
50. van der Eerden BC, Weissgerber P, Fratzl-Zelman N, et al. The transient receptor potential channel TRPV6 is dynamically expressed in bone cells but is not crucial for bone mineralization in mice. J Cell Physiol. 2012;227:1951-9.
51. van der Eerden BC, Hoenderop JG, de Vries TJ, et al. The epithelial Ca2+ channel TRPV5 is essential for proper osteoclastic bone resorption. Proc Natl Acad Sci U S A. 2005; 102:17507-12.
52. Nijenhuis T, van der Eerden BC, Hoenderop JG, et al. Bone resorption inhibitor alendronate normalizes the reduced bone thickness of TRPV5(−/−) mice. J Bone Miner Res. 2008;23:1815-24.
53. Chang W, Tu C, Chen TH, et al. Expression and signal transduction of calcium-sensing receptors in cartilage and bone. Endocrinology. 1999;140:5883-93.
54. Chang W, Tu C, Chen TH, et al. The extracellular calcium-sensing receptor (CaSR) is a critical modulator of skeletal development. Sci Signal. 2008;1:ra1.
55. Kopic S, Geibel P. Gastric acid, calcium absorption, and their impact on bone health. Physiol Rev. 2013;93:189-268.
56. Sella S, Cattelan C, Realdi G, et al. Bone disease in primary hypercalciuria. Clin Cases Miner Bone Metab. 2008;5:118-26.
57. Pak CY, Nicar MJ, Peterson R, et al. A lack of unique pathophysiologic background for nephrolithiasis of primary hyperparathyroidism. J Clin Endocrinol Metab. 1981;53:536-42.
58. Rejnmark L, Vestergaard P, Mosekilde L. Nephrolithiasis and renal calcifications in primary hyperparathyroidism. J Clin Endocrinol Metab. 2011;96:2377-85.
59. Patron P, Gardin JP, Paillard M. Renal mass and reserve of vitamin D: determinants in primary hyperparathyroidism. Kidney Int. 1987;31:1174-80.
60. Yergey AL, Abrams SA, Vieira NE, et al. Determination of fractional absorption of dietary calcium in humans. J Nutr. 1994;124:674-82.
61. Bronner F. Mechanisms of intestinal calcium absorption. J Cell Biochem. 2003;88:387-93.
62. Hardwick LL, Jones MR, Brautbar N, et al. Magnesium absorption: mechanisms and the influence of vitamin D, calcium and phosphate. J Nutr. 1991;121:13-23.
63. Khanal RC, Nemere I. Regulation of intestinal calcium transport. Annu Rev Nutr. 2008;28:179-96.
64. Krawitt EL, Schedl HP. In vivo calcium transport by rat small intestine. Am J Physiol. 1968;214:232-6.
65. Larsen EH, Nedergaard S, Ussing HH. Role of lateral intercellular space and sodium recirculation for isotonic transport in leaky epithelia. Rev Physiol Biochem Pharmacol. 2000;141:153-212.
66. Lameris AL, Huybers S, Kaukinen K, et al. Expression profiling of claudins in the human gastrointestinal tract in health and during inflammatory bowel disease. Scand J Gastroenterol. 2013;48:58-69.
67. Nijenhuis T, Hoenderop JG, van der Kemp AW, et al. Localization and regulation of the epithelial Ca^{2+} channel TRPV6 in the kidney. J Am Soc Nephrol. 2003;14:2731-40.
68. Romagnolo B, Cluzeaud F, Lambert M, et al. Tissue-specific and hormonal regulation of calbindin-D9K fusion genes in transgenic mice. J Biol Chem. 1996;271:16820-6.
69. Christakos S, Dhawan P, Porta A, et al. Vitamin D and intestinal calcium absorption. Mol Cell Endocrinol. 2011;347:25-9.
70. Wasserman RH. Vitamin D and the dual processes of intestinal calcium absorption. J Nutr. 2004;134:3137-9.
71. Bronner F, Pansu D, Stein WD. An analysis of intestinal calcium transport across the rat intestine. Am J Physiol. 1986;250:G561-9.
72. Chang Q, Hoefs S, van der Kemp AW, et al. The beta-glucuronidase klotho hydrolyzes and activates the TRPV5 channel. Science. 2005;310:490-3.

73. Hoenderop JG, Muller D, Van Der Kemp AW, et al. Calcitriol controls the epithelial calcium channel in kidney. J Am Soc Nephrol. 2001;12:1342-9.
74. Renkema KY, Alexander RT, Bindels RJ, et al. Calcium and phosphate homeostasis: concerted interplay of new regulators. Ann Med. 2008;40:82-91.
75. D'Angelo A, Calo L, Cantaro S, et al. Calciotropic hormones and nephrolithiasis. Miner Electrolyte Metab. 1997;23:269-72.
76. Brown EM, Gamba G, Riccardi D, et al. Cloning and characterization of an extracellular Ca(2+)-sensing receptor from bovine parathyroid. Nature. 1993;366:575-80.
77. Greenberg A, Cheung AK. Primer on Kidney Diseases. Elsevier Saunders; 2005.
78. Bacic D, Lehir M, Biber J, et al. The renal Na^+/phosphate cotransporter NaPi-IIa is internalized via the receptor-mediated endocytic route in response to parathyroid hormone. Kidney Int. 2006;69:495-503.
79. Gentili C, Morelli S, de Boland AR. Characterization of PTH/PTHrP receptor in rat duodenum: effects of ageing. J Cell Biochem. 2003;88:1157-67.
80. van Abel M, Hoenderop JG, van der Kemp AW, et al. Coordinated control of renal Ca(2+) transport proteins by parathyroid hormone. Kidney Int. 2005;68:1708-21.
81. de Groot T, Lee K, Langeslag M, et al. Parathyroid hormone activates TRPV5 via PKA-dependent phosphorylation. J Am Soc Nephrol. 2009;20:1693-704.
82. Cha SK, Wu T, Huang CL. Protein kinase C inhibits caveolae-mediated endocytosis of TRPV5. Am J Physiol Renal Physiol. 2008;294:F1212-21.
83. Bouillon R, Lieben L, Mathieu C, et al. Vitamin D action: lessons from VDR and Cyp27b1 null mice. Pediatr Endocrinol Rev. 2013;10(Suppl 2):354-66.
84. Carlberg C. Mechanisms of nuclear signalling by vitamin D3. Interplay with retinoid and thyroid hormone signalling. Eur J Biochem. 1995;231:517-27.
85. Christakos S, Raval-Pandya M, Wernyj RP, et al. Genomic mechanisms involved in the pleiotropic actions of 1,25-dihydroxyvitamin D3. Biochem J. 1996;316(Pt 2):361-71.
86. Dauber A, Nguyen TT, Sochett E, et al. Genetic defect in CYP24A1, the vitamin D 24-hydroxylase gene, in a patient with severe infantile hypercalcemia. J Clin Endocrinol Metab. 2012;97:E268-74.
87. Schlingmann KP, Kaufmann M, Weber S, et al. Mutations in CYP24A1 and idiopathic infantile hypercalcemia. N Engl J Med. 2011;365:410-21.
88. Dinour D, Beckerman P, Ganon L, et al. Loss-of-function mutations of CYP24A1, the vitamin D 24-hydroxylase gene, cause long-standing hypercalciuric nephrolithiasis and nephrocalcinosis. J Urol. 2013;190:552-7.
89. Hoenderop JG, Dardenne O, Van Abel M, et al. Modulation of renal Ca^{2+} transport protein genes by dietary Ca^{2+} and 1,25-dihydroxyvitamin D3 in 25-hydroxyvitamin D3-1alpha-hydroxylase knockout mice. FASEB J. 2002;16:1398-406.
90. van Abel M, Hoenderop JG, van der Kemp AW, et al. Regulation of the epithelial Ca^{2+} channels in small intestine as studied by quantitative mRNA detection. Am J Physiol Gastrointest Liver Physiol. 2003;285:G78-85.
91. Van Cromphaut SJ, Dewerchin M, Hoenderop JG, et al. Duodenal calcium absorption in vitamin D receptor-knockout mice: functional and molecular aspects. Proc Natl Acad Sci U S A. 2001;98:13324-9.
92. Dardenne O, Prud'homme J, Arabian A, et al. Targeted inactivation of the 25-hydroxyvitamin D(3)-1(alpha)-hydroxylase gene (CYP27B1) creates an animal model of pseudovitamin D-deficiency rickets. Endocrinology. 2001;142:3135-41.
93. Wood RJ, Tchack L, Taparia S. 1,25-Dihydroxyvitamin D3 increases the expression of the CaT1 epithelial calcium channel in the Caco-2 human intestinal cell line. BMC Physiol. 2001;1:11.
94. Song Y, Peng X, Porta A, et al. Calcium transporter 1 and epithelial calcium channel messenger ribonucleic acid are differentially regulated by 1,25 dihydroxyvitamin D3 in the intestine and kidney of mice. Endocrinology. 2003;144:3885-94.
95. Cline J. Calcium and vitamin D metabolism, deficiency, and excess. Top Companion Anim Med. 2012;27:159-64.
96. Kuro-o M, Matsumura Y, Aizawa H, et al. Mutation of the mouse klotho gene leads to a syndrome resembling ageing. Nature. 1997;390:45-51
97. Imura A, Iwano A, Tohyama O, et al. Secreted Klotho protein in sera and CSF: implication for post-translational cleavage in release of Klotho protein from cell membrane. FEBS Lett. 2004;565:143-7.
98. Kuro-o M. Klotho as a regulator of fibroblast growth factor signaling and phosphate/calcium metabolism. Curr Opin Nephrol Hypertens. 2006;15:437-41.
99. Torres PU, Prie D, Molina-Bletry V, et al. Klotho: an antiaging protein involved in mineral and vitamin D metabolism. Kidney Int. 2007;71:730-7.
100. Tsujikawa H, Kurotaki Y, Fujimori T, et al. Klotho, a gene related to a syndrome resembling human premature aging, functions in a negative regulatory circuit of vitamin D endocrine system. Mol Endocrinol. 2003;17:2393-403.
101. Kuro-o M. Overview of the FGF23-Klotho axis. Pediatr Nephrol. 2010;25:583-90.
102. Yoshida T, Fujimori T, Nabeshima Y. Mediation of unusually high concentrations of 1,25-dihydroxyvitamin D in homozygous klotho mutant mice by increased expression of renal 1alpha-hydroxylase gene. Endocrinology. 2002;143:683-9.
103. Alexander RT, Woudenberg-Vrenken TE, Buurman J, et al. Klotho prevents renal calcium loss. J Am Soc Nephrol. 2009;20:2371-9.
104. Renkema KY, Nijenhuis T, van der Eerden BC, et al. Hypervitaminosis D mediates compensatory Ca^{2+} hyperabsorption in TRPV5 knockout mice. J Am Soc Nephrol. 2005;16:3188-95.
105. Cha SK, Ortega B, Kurosu H, et al. Removal of sialic acid involving Klotho causes cell-surface retention of TRPV5 channel via binding to galectin-1. Proc Natl Acad Sci U S A. 2008;105:9805-10.
106. Segawa H, Yamanaka S, Ohno Y, et al. Correlation between hyperphosphatemia and type II Na–Pi cotransporter activity in klotho mice. Am J Physiol Renal Physiol. 2007;292:F769-79.
107. Wagner CA. When proton pumps go sour: urinary acidification and kidney stones. Kidney Int. 2008;73:1103-5.

108. Wagner CA. When proton pumps go sour: urinary acidification and kidney stones. Kidney Int. 2008;73:1103-5.
109. Earm JH, Christensen BM, Frokiaer J, et al. Decreased aquaporin-2 expression and apical plasma membrane delivery in kidney collecting ducts of polyuric hypercalcemic rats. J Am Soc Nephrol. 1998;9:2181-93.
110. Xiao NM, Zhang YM, Zheng Q, et al. Klotho is a serum factor related to human aging. Chin Med J (Engl). 2004;117:742-7.
111. Nemeth EF. Regulation of cytosolic calcium by extracellular divalent cations in C-cells and parathyroid cells. Cell Calcium. 1990;11:323-7.
112. Ferre S, Hoenderop JG, Bindels RJ. Sensing mechanisms involved in Ca^{2+} and Mg^{2+} homeostasis. Kidney Int. 2012;82:1157-66.
113. Mathias RS, Brown EM. Divalent cations modulate PTH-dependent 3',5'-cyclic adenosine monophosphate production in renal proximal tubular cells. Endocrinology. 1991;128:3005-12.
114. Bajwa A, Horst RL, Beckman MJ. Gene profiling the effects of calcium deficiency versus 1,25-dihydroxyvitamin D induced hypercalcemia in rat kidney cortex. Arch Biochem Biophys. 2005;438:182-94.
115. Bland R, Walker EA, Hughes SV, et al. Constitutive expression of 25-hydroxyvitamin D3-1alpha-hydroxylase in a transformed human proximal tubule cell line: evidence for direct regulation of vitamin D metabolism by calcium. Endocrinology. 1999;140:2027-34.
116. Riccardi D, Hall AE, Chattopadhyay N, et al. Localization of the extracellular Ca^{2+}/polyvalent cation-sensing protein in rat kidney. Am J Physiol. 1998;274:F611-22.
117. Huang C, Miller RT. Novel Ca receptor signaling pathways for control of renal ion transport. Curr Opin Nephrol Hypertens. 2010;19:106-12.
118. Hebert SC, Brown EM, Harris HW. Role of the Ca(2+)-sensing receptor in divalent mineral ion homeostasis. J Exp Biol. 1997;200:295-302.
119. Hoenderop JG, Chon H, Gkika D, et al. Regulation of gene expression by dietary Ca^{2+} in kidneys of 25-hydroxyvitamin D3-1 alpha-hydroxylase knockout mice. Kidney Int. 2004;65:531-9.
120. Topala CN, Schoeber JP, Searchfield LE, et al. Activation of the Ca^{2+}-sensing receptor stimulates the activity of the epithelial Ca^{2+} channel TRPV5. Cell Calcium. 2009;45:331-9.
121. Renkema KY, Velic A, Dijkman HB, et al. The calcium-sensing receptor promotes urinary acidification to prevent nephrolithiasis. J Am Soc Nephrol. 2009;20:1705-13.
122. Kovacikova J, Winter C, Loffing-Cueni D, et al. The connecting tubule is the main site of the furosemide-induced urinary acidification by the vacuolar H+-ATPase. Kidney Int. 2006;70:1706-16.
123. Wagner CA, Kovacikova J, Stehberger PA, et al. Renal acid-base transport: old and new players. Nephron Physiol. 2006;103:p1-6.
124. Wagner CA, Finberg KE, Breton S, et al. Renal vacuolar H+-ATPase. Physiol Rev. 2004;84:1263-314.
125. Finberg KE, Wagner CA, Bailey MA, et al. The B1-subunit of the H(+) ATPase is required for maximal urinary acidification. Proc Natl Acad Sci U S A. 2005;102:13616-21.
126. Borghi L, Schianchi T, Meschi T, et al. Comparison of two diets for the prevention of recurrent stones in idiopathic hypercalciuria. N Engl J Med. 2002;346:77-84.
127. Gambaro G, Vezzoli G, Casari G, et al. Genetics of hypercalciuria and calcium nephrolithiasis: from the rare monogenic to the common polygenic forms. Am J Kidney Dis. 2004;44:963-86.
128. Goldfarb S. Dietary factors in the pathogenesis and prophylaxis of calcium nephrolithiasis. Kidney Int. 1988;34:544-55.
129. Stechman MJ, Loh NY, Thakker RV. Genetics of hypercalciuric nephrolithiasis: renal stone disease. Ann N Y Acad Sci. 2007;1116:461-84.
130. Goldfarb DS, Fischer ME, Keich Y, et al. A twin study of genetic and dietary influences on nephrolithiasis: a report from the Vietnam Era Twin (VET) Registry. Kidney Int. 2005;67:1053-61.
131. McGeown MG. Heredity in renal stone disease. Clin Sci. 1960;19:465-71.
132. Resnick M, Pridgen DB, Goodman HO. Genetic predisposition to formation of calcium oxalate renal calculi. N Engl J Med. 1968;278:1313-8.
133. Devuyst O, Pirson Y. Genetics of hypercalciuric stone forming diseases. Kidney Int. 2007;72:1065-72.
134. Lloyd SE, Pearce SH, Fisher SE, et al. A common molecular basis for three inherited kidney stone diseases. Nature. 1996;379:445-9.
135. Thakker RV. Pathogenesis of Dent's disease and related syndromes of X- linked nephrolithiasis. Kidney Int. 2000;57:787-93.
136. Gunther W, Luchow A, Cluzeaud F, et al. ClC-5, the chloride channel mutated in Dent's disease, colocalizes with the proton pump in endocytotically active kidney cells. Proc Natl Acad Sci U S A. 1998;95:8075-80.
137. Picollo A, Pusch M. Chloride/proton antiporter activity of mammalian CLC proteins ClC-4 and ClC-5. Nature. 2005;436:420-3.
138. Scheel O, Zdebik AA, Lourdel S, et al. Voltage-dependent electrogenic chloride/proton exchange by endosomal CLC proteins. Nature. 2005;436:424-7.
139. Devuyst O, Christie PT, Courtoy PJ, et al. Intra-renal and subcellular distribution of the human chloride channel, CLC-5, reveals a pathophysiological basis for Dent's disease. Hum Mol Genet. 1999;8:247-57.
140. Christensen EI, Devuyst O, Dom G, et al. Loss of chloride channel ClC-5 impairs endocytosis by defective trafficking of megalin and cubilin in kidney proximal tubules. Proc Natl Acad Sci U S A. 2003;100:8472-7.
141. Reinhart SC, Norden AG, Lapsley M, et al. Characterization of carrier females and affected males with X-linked recessive nephrolithiasis. J Am Soc Nephrol. 1995;5:1451-61.
142. Wrong OM, Norden AG, Feest TG. Dent's disease; a familial proximal renal tubular syndrome with low-molecular-weight proteinuria, hypercalciuria, nephrocalcinosis, metabolic bone disease, progressive renal failure and a marked male predominance. QJM. 1994;87:473-93.
143. Piwon N, Gunther W, Schwake M, et al. ClC-5 Cl^--channel disruption impairs endocytosis in a mouse model for Dent's disease. Nature. 2000;408:369-73.

144. Lin Z, Jin S, Duan X, et al. Chloride channel (Clc)-5 is necessary for exocytic trafficking of Na^+/H+ exchanger 3 (NHE3). J Biol Chem. 2011;286:22833-45.
145. Pan W, Borovac J, Spicer Z, et al. The epithelial sodium/proton exchanger, NHE3, is necessary for renal and intestinal calcium (re)absorption. Am J Physiol Renal Physiol. 2012;302:F943-56.
146. Lorenz JN, Schultheis PJ, Traynor T, et al. Micropuncture analysis of single-nephron function in NHE3-deficient mice. Am J Physiol 1999;277:F447-53.
147. Schultheis PJ, Clarke LL, Meneton P, et al. Targeted disruption of the murine Na^+/H+ exchanger isoform 2 gene causes reduced viability of gastric parietal cells and loss of net acid secretion. J Clin Invest. 1998;101:1243-53.
148. Suki WN. Calcium transport in the nephron. Am J Physiol. 1979;237:F1-6.
149. Sutton RA, Dirks JH. The renal excretion of calcium: a review of micropuncture data. Can J Physiol Pharmacol. 1975;53:979-88.
150. Tieder M, Modai D, Samuel R, et al. Hereditary hypophosphatemic rickets with hypercalciuria. N Engl J Med. 1985;312:611-7.
151. Bergwitz C, Roslin NM, Tieder M, et al. SLC34A3 mutations in patients with hereditary hypophosphatemic rickets with hypercalciuria predict a key role for the sodium-phosphate cotransporter NaPi-IIc in maintaining phosphate homeostasis. Am J Hum Genet. 2006;78:179-92.
152. Forster IC, Hernando N, Biber J, et al. Proximal tubular handling of phosphate: a molecular perspective. Kidney Int. 2006;70:1548-59.
153. Lapointe JY, Tessier J, Paquette Y, et al. NPT2a gene variation in calcium nephrolithiasis with renal phosphate leak. Kidney Int. 2006;69:2261-7.
154. Prie D, Huart V, Bakouh N, et al. Nephrolithiasis and osteoporosis associated with hypophosphatemia caused by mutations in the type 2a sodium-phosphate cotransporter. N Engl J Med. 2002;347:983-91.
155. Jarolim P, Shayakul C, Prabakaran D, et al.. Autosomal dominant distal renal tubular acidosis is associated in three families with heterozygosity for the R589H mutation in the AE1 (band 3) Cl^-/HCO_3^- exchanger. J Biol Chem. 1998;273:6380-8.
156. Devonald MA, Smith AN, Poon JP, et al. Non-polarized targeting of AE1 causes autosomal dominant distal renal tubular acidosis. Nat Genet. 2003;33:125-7.
157. Hou J. The role of claudin in hypercalciuric nephrolithiasis. Curr Urol Rep. 2013;14:5-12.
158. Simon DB, Karet FE, Hamdan JM, et al. Bartter's syndrome, hypokalaemic alkalosis with hypercalciuria, is caused by mutations in the Na–K–2Cl cotransporter NKCC2. Nat Genet. 1996;13:183-8.
159. Simon DB, Karet FE, Rodriguez-Soriano J, et al. Genetic heterogeneity of Bartter's syndrome revealed by mutations in the K^+ channel, ROMK. Nat Genet. 1996;14:152-6.
160. Greger R. Ion transport mechanisms in thick ascending limb of Henle's loop of mammalian nephron. Physiol Rev. 1985;65:760-797.
161. Simon DB, Bindra RS, Mansfield TA, et al. Mutations in the chloride channel gene, CLCNKB, cause Bartter's syndrome type III. Nat Genet. 1997;17:171-8.
162. Kramer BK, Bergler T, Stoelcker B, et al. Mechanisms of disease: the kidney-specific chloride channels ClCKA and ClCKB, the Barttin subunit, and their clinical relevance. Nat Clin Pract Nephrol. 2008;4:38-46.
163. Greger R, Schlatter E. Properties of the lumen membrane of the cortical thick ascending limb of Henle's loop of rabbit kidney. Pflug Arch. 1983;396:315-24.
164. Konrad M, Vollmer M, Lemmink HH, et al. Mutations in the chloride channel gene CLCNKB as a cause of classic Bartter syndrome. J Am Soc Nephrol. 2000;11:1449-59.
165. Angelow S, El-Husseini R, Kanzawa SA, et al. Renal localization and function of the tight junction protein, claudin-19. Am J Physiol Renal Physiol. 2007;293:F166-77.
166. Reed BY, Heller HJ, Gitomer WL, et al. Mapping a gene defect in absorptive hypercalciuria to chromosome 1q23.3–q24. J Clin Endocrinol Metab. 1999;84:3907-13.
167. Wolf MT, Zalewski I, Martin FC, et al. Mapping a new suggestive gene locus for autosomal dominant nephrolithiasis to chromosome 9q33.2–q34.2 by total genome search for linkage. Nephrol Dial Transplant. 2005;20:909-14.
168. Wilcox ER, Burton QL, Naz S, et al. Mutations in the gene encoding tight junction claudin-14 cause autosomal recessive deafness DFNB29. Cell. 2001;104:165-72.
169. Ben-Yosef T, Belyantseva IA, Saunders TL, et al. Claudin 14 knockout mice, a model for autosomal recessive deafness DFNB29, are deaf due to cochlear hair cell degeneration. Hum Mol Genet. 2003;12:2049-61
170. Gong Y, Renigunta V, Himmerkus N, et al. Claudin-14 regulates renal Ca(+)(+) transport in response to CaSR signalling via a novel microRNA pathway. EMBO J. 2012;31:1999-2012.
171. Desfleurs E, Wittner M, Simeone S, et al. Calcium-sensing receptor: regulation of electrolyte transport in the thick ascending limb of Henle's loop. Kidney Blood Press Res. 1998;21:401-12.
172. Motoyama HI, Friedman PA. Calcium-sensing receptor regulation of PTH-dependent calcium absorption by mouse cortical ascending limbs. Am J Physiol Renal Physiol. 2002;283:F399-406.
173. Muller D, Hoenderop JG, Vennekens R, et al. Epithelial Ca(2+) channel (ECAC1) in autosomal dominant idiopathic hypercalciuria. Nephrol Dial Transplant. 2002;17:1614-20.
174. Renkema KY, Lee K, Topala CN, et al. TRPV5 gene polymorphisms in renal hypercalciuria. Nephrol Dial Transplant. 2009;24:1919-24.
175. Akey JM, Swanson WJ, Madeoy J, et al. TRPV6 exhibits unusual patterns of polymorphism and divergence in worldwide populations. Hum Mol Genet. 2006;15:2106-13.
176. Hughes DA, Tang K, Strotmann R, et al. Parallel selection on TRPV6 in human populations. PLoS One. 2008;3:e1686.
177. Suzuki Y, Pasch A, Bonny O, et al. Gain-of-function haplotype in the epithelial calcium channel TRPV6 is a risk factor for renal calcium stone formation. Hum Mol Genet. 2008;17:1613-8.

178. Petrucci M, Scott P, Ouimet D, et al. Evaluation of the calcium-sensing receptor gene in idiopathic hypercalciuria and calcium nephrolithiasis. Kidney Int. 2000;58:38-42.
179. Scott P, Ouimet D, Proulx Y, et al. The 1 alpha-hydroxylase locus is not linked to calcium stone formation or calciuric phenotypes in French-Canadian families. J Am Soc Nephrol. 1998;9:425-32.
180. Scott P, Ouimet D, Valiquette L, et al. Suggestive evidence for a susceptibility gene near the vitamin D receptor locus in idiopathic calcium stone formation. J Am Soc Nephrol. 1999;10:1007-13.
181. Khullar M, Relan V, Singh SK. VDR gene and urinary calcium excretion in nephrolithiasis. Kidney Int. 2006;69:943.
182. Yu AS, Cheng MH, Angelow S, et al. Molecular basis for cation selectivity in claudin-2-based paracellular pores: identification of an electrostatic interaction site. J Gen Physiol. 2009;133:111-27.
183. Yu AS, Cheng MH, Coalson RD. Calcium inhibits paracellular sodium conductance through claudin-2 by competitive binding. J Biol Chem. 2010;285:37060-9.
184. Breiderhoff T, Himmerkus N, Stuiver M, et al. Deletion of claudin-10 (Cldn10) in the thick ascending limb impairs paracellular sodium permeability and leads to hypermagnesemia and nephrocalcinosis. Proc Natl Acad Sci USA. 2012;109:14241-6.
185. Charoenphandhu N, Nakkrasae LI, Kraidith K, et al. Two-step stimulation of intestinal Ca(2+) absorption during lactation by long-term prolactin exposure and suckling-induced prolactin surge. Am J Physiol Endocrinol Metab. 2009;297: E609-19.
186. Wongdee K, Teerapornpuntakit J, Siangpro C, et al. Duodenal villous hypertrophy and upregulation of claudin-15 protein expression in lactating rats. J Mol Histol. 2013;44:103-9.
187. Tamura A, Hayashi H, Imasato M, et al. Loss of claudin-15, but not claudin-2, causes Na^+ deficiency and glucose malabsorption in mouse small intestine. Gastroenterology. 2011;140:913-23.
188. Tamura A, Kitano Y, Hata M, et al. Megaintestine in claudin-15-deficient mice. Gastroenterology. 2008;134:523-34.

CHAPTER 10

Renal Citrate Metabolism and Transport: Physiology and Pathophysiology

Kathleen S Hering-Smith, Lee Hamm, Orson W Moe

INTRODUCTION

Whereas most organic anions in the urine are in micromolar quantities or less, urate and citrate are present in the urine in millimolar concentration. Urinary citrate excretion is highly regulated in humans, and reduction in urinary excretion and concentration of citrate (hypocitraturia) is a major risk factor in kidney stone formation.[1,2] Citric acid is a component of one of the best-known biochemical cycles that bears its namesake (citric acid, tricarboxylic acid, or Krebs cycle). Inside the cell, citrate serves multiple functions.[3] In the extracellular space, citrate is present in ~50–100 μM, but its physiologic role is not clearly understood. In the urinary space, citrate serves dual roles as a urinary base and a chelator of ionized calcium.[4]

Citrate is a tricarboxylic six-carbon anion (Fig. 10.1A) that exists as a polytopic acid in equilibrium with $3H^+$s to form its conjugate citric acid. The pK_a of citrate has been measured under different conditions and slightly different values have been reported.[5] The values that best approximate the urinary environment are listed in Figure 10.1A. In the plasma with an ambient pH of 7.4, citrate exists predominantly as citrate^{3-} around 100 μM. In the urine, citrate concentration is much higher in mM and is distributed between divalent and trivalent citrate. Citrate chelates a variety of cations with different stabilities. The classic functions of citrate are as a supply of reducing equivalents [i.e. adenosine triphosphate (ATP)], a source of acetyl groups, and an allosteric regulator of many enzymes.[3] The first description of the highly soluble (calcium-citrate)$^-$ complex was attributed to Sabbatini.[6] In the urine, citrate's ability to chelate calcium with high affinity and the high solubility of the complex is one of the most fundamental reasons for citrate's presence in urine in vertebrates.[4,7] The relative affinities of the different citrate species to chelate Ca^{2+} are shown in Figure 10.1A with citrate^{3-} having the highest association constant. In addition to the (calcium-citrate)$^-$ complex, there are other cationic-citrate structures of note (Fig. 10.1B).[8] The 3-calcium:2-citrate complex is a common preparation for calcium supplementation for patients.[9] The sodium and potassium complexes are structurally different from the divalent equivalent, and are prescribed by clinicians to treat hypocitraturia.

In this chapter, we will journey through some basic biology of citrate, the physiology of renal citrate handling and metabolism, pathophysiology of hypocitraturia, the clinical conditions where abnormalities of citrate are involved in urolithogenesis, and finally citrate therapy for kidney stones.

EVOLUTIONARY ORIGINS OF URINARY CITRATE

Evolution of the Tricarboxylic Acid Cycle

Of historical interest is the fact that the regulation of urinary citrate excretion (a topic of interest in this chapter) was described several years[10,11] before Hans Krebs published the components of the famous cycle.[12] One venue to understand the role of urinary citrate is to start with the tricarboxylic acid (TCA) cycle (Fig. 10.2) to appreciate the functions of a remarkable metabolic intermediate. The evolutionary origin of the TCA cycle has been a subject of much debate. The current model of the evolution of the TCA cycle favors a union of biosynthesis and bioenergetics.[13-15] Some have cited the TCA cycle with its seemingly infinite complexity as a conundrum in evolution that defies explanation by Darwinian natural selection.[16] How could natural selection construct such a complicated structure when the intermediate stages do not confer survival or reproductive fitness? In the TCA cycle, each intermediary stage is useful for different purposes, with the totality in its final, completed form being an example of opportunistic usage of existing pathways.[17]

The TCA cycle is the foundation of aerobic energy metabolism where acetyl units are converted to CO_2 and reducing equivalents, which then flow to O_2 via specialized electron and H^+ carriers embedded in mitochondrial membranes eventuating in the production of high-energy

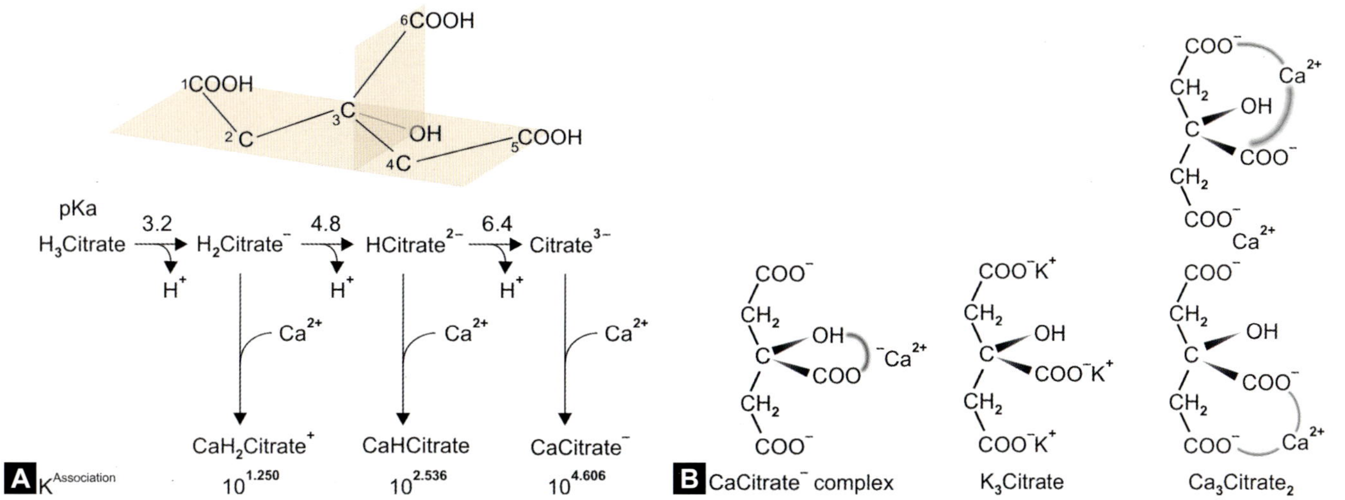

Figs. 10.1A and B: Citrate and cation metal citrate complexes. (A) Structure of citrate (top) showing the carbon skeleton (C1–C5) on a planar arrangement with the carboxyl group (C6) and hydroxyl group on C3 residing in a perpendicular plane. Citric acid dissociates (bottom) from its $3H^+$s to eventually form the trivalent citrate anion. (B) The soluble monovalent anionic calcium citrate complex in plasma and urine where the negative charge is shown to be distributed over the carboxyl and hydroxyl groups (left). The frequently prescribed tripotassium citrate salt is to treat hypocitraturia (middle). $Ca_3Citrate_2$ is prescribed as a calcium supplement (right).

ATP. Some intermediates of the TCA cycle, such as α-ketoglutarate, succinyl coenzyme A (CoA), and oxaloacetate, are also precursors of other essential molecules (glutamine, heme, aspartate, respectively) (Fig. 10.2), so certain segments of the cycle have dual bioenergetic and biosynthetic functions. One interpretation of the origin of this amalgamation is metabolic economy. In this paradigm, segments of the TCA cycle evolved in anaerobic prokaryotes as purely biosynthetic pathways.[15,16] The aerobic bioenergetic parts of the TCA cycle were the result of gradual and interrelated evolutionary improvements in both biosynthetic and bioenergetic mechanisms. Melendez-Hevia et al. performed a most interesting analysis giving consideration to different theoretical chemical solutions to the bioenergetics and biosynthetic needs of the cell, and demonstrated that the layout of the current metabolic pathway is the best chemical solution, with the least possible number of steps, and has the most ATP-generating efficiency.[14]

The concept of duality (in fact, multiplicity) of function for molecules is pervasive in biology. If the TCA cycle is ultimately optimized in cells for ATP production and amino acid synthesis, can one still assign extra roles to the TCA cycle? In the kidney, a key member of the TCA cycle, namely citrate, is called upon to fulfill yet additional functions beyond biosynthesis and bioenergetics—keeping solid-phase calcium salts from forming and maintaining acid-base balance for the whole organism. Therefore, in addition to being one of the most important intermediate metabolites for aerobic life, citrate fulfills pivotal roles in renal physiology.

Citrate as a Calcium Chelator

The existence with an apatite-based skeleton and life in terrestrial habitats mandates an obligatory amount of calcium and phosphate in the urine due to active turnover of the endoskeleton and inability to capture and recycle all the ions. Concomitant with this fact is the absolute need to conserve water and sodium on land, and hence a low urinary volume.[4] These prerequisites present a formidable conflict to the kidney and, as a result, numerous mechanisms have evolved to prevent the crystallization of calcium salts in the urine lumen. Figures 10.3A and B illustrate how the kidney utilizes two "hijack" tactics to sequester and prevent calcium and phosphate from uniting to form numerous insoluble calcium phosphate complexes. The titration of phosphate by luminal H^+ secretion (divalent:monovalent ~1:1 end proximal tubule at pH 6.8; divalent:monovalent 1:20 medullary collecting duct at pH 5.4) prevents the divalent phosphate from engaging calcium.

Citrate represents an important arm of this ensemble of mechanisms. The calcium citrate complex possesses some unique physicochemical properties. The reported

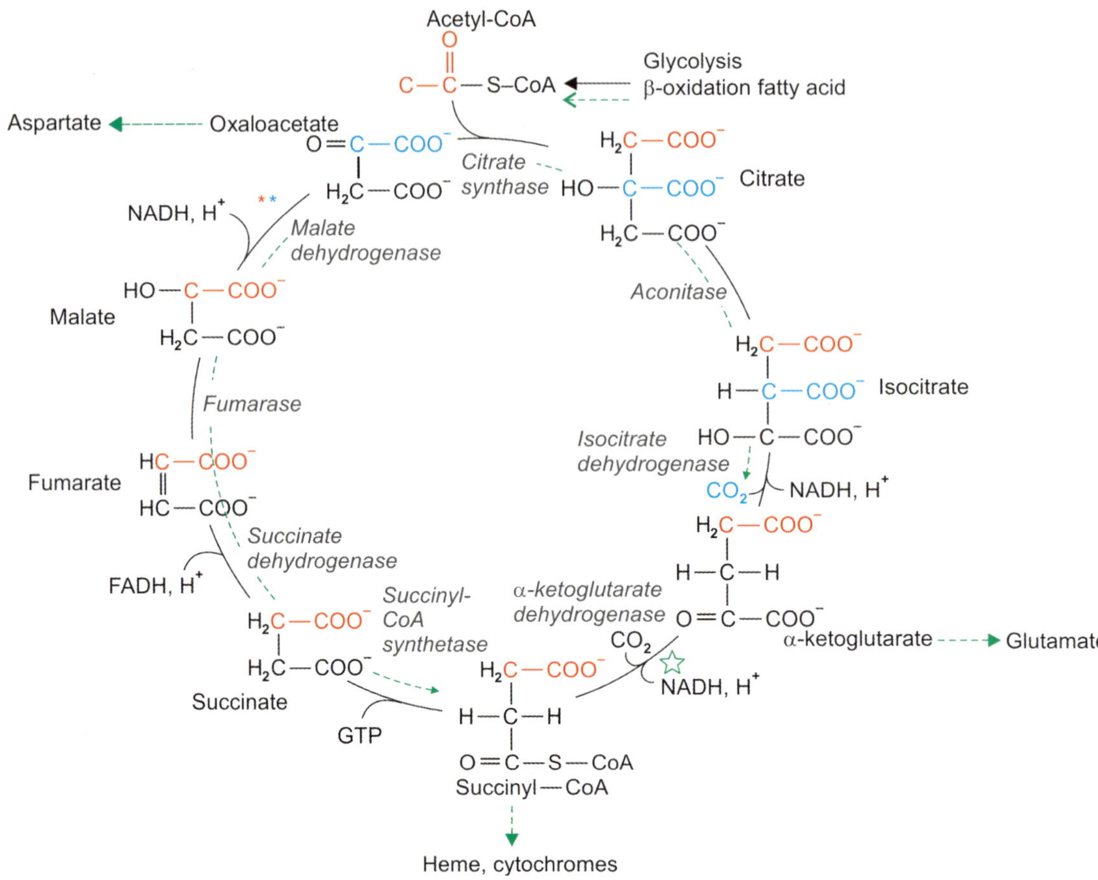

Fig. 10.2: Tricarboxylic acid (TCA, citric acid, Krebs) cycle. The modern version of the TCA cycle is shown as a bioenergetic pathway producing reducing equivalents [Nicotinamide adenine dinucleotide (reduced form) (NADH) + H^+; flavin adenine dinucleotide (reduced form) (FADH) + H^+]. The carbons that enter as acetyl-CoA are coded as red. *The color code for those same carbons is changed to blue as malate is transitioned to oxaloacetate to start a new cycle. The evolutionary origins constituting the biosynthetic segments are shown in green dotted arrows. One theory of the ancient TCA cycle is more like a "horseshoe" with the final introduction of a-ketoglutarate dehydrogenase (green star) and the oxidative direction of succinate to oxaloacetate, completing the cycle. (GTP: Guanosine triphosphate).

values of the stability constant of the (Ca^{2+} + $Citrate^{3-}$ ↔ $CaCitrate^-$) complex are in excess of 7 × 10^4 L mol^{-1} at 37°C in urinary ionic strength, which is orders of magnitude higher than values of ~ 3 × 10^2 L mol^{-1} for (Ca^{2+} + $Citrate^{2-}$ ↔ CaCitrate) and ~1.5 × 10^1 for (Ca^{2+} + $Citrate^-$ ↔ $CaCitrate^+$).[18,19] In a typical urinary pH of mid 5s, 90% of the citrate will be trivalent and most of the citrate will exist as 1:1 stoichiometric $CaCitrate^-$ complex. The solubility product (K_{sp}) of $CaCitrate^-$ is quite high. So with a typical daily excretion of calcium of 4–5 mmoles and if citrate excretion approaches that same, the ionized calcium that remains available to bind phosphate and oxalate is much diminished. In the presence of equimolar amounts of citrate and calcium in the urine, there is a vanishingly low probability of Ca^{2+} to bind phosphate or oxalate.

Citrate as a Urinary Base

Acid homeostasis is achieved by concerted efforts of extracellular and intracellular buffers and[18] multiple organs including the liver, lung, and kidneys. In terms of external nonvolatile acid-base balance, the kidney is the main interphase to the exterior. Since one virtually never ingests or produces the exact equivalent amount of acid and base in a given unit of time, the kidney is charged with the task of excreting the extra acid or base. Acid excretion is achieved by H^+ secretion into urine and carriage by buffers. Alkali excretion is primarily achieved by either bicarbonaturia or citraturia. A brief consideration of these two urinary bases is necessary.

Bicarbonaturia can be viewed as an "effortless" process. The high glomerular filtration rate required for the

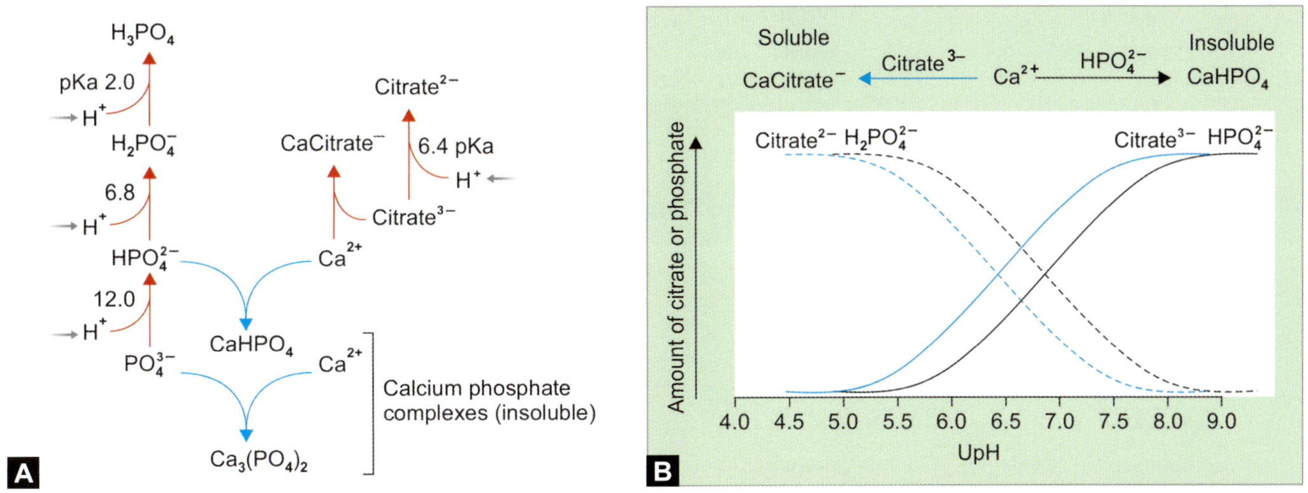

Figs. 10.3A and B: Means to prevent calcium phosphate precipitation in urine. (A) The H^+ secreted into the urine titrates phosphate to the monovalent form away from its divalent form, which binds calcium to form insoluble complexes (left). The approximate pK_a values of each acid-base pairs are shown on the left. The presence of citrate^{3-} in the urine sequesters calcium in its soluble Ca-Citrate⁻ form and prevents calcium binding with phosphate. The relative association constants (K_a; reflection of affinities) are shown. (B) Superimposition of the equilibrium of bivalent (dotted blue) versus trivalent (solid blue) citrate and monovalent phosphate (dotted black) versus bivalent (solid black) phosphate. As urine pH increases, bivalent phosphate increases, which elevates the risk of calcium phosphate precipitation. Fortunately, the rise in trivalent citrate concentration follows closely behind the rise in bivalent phosphate and partially negates the danger of calcium phosphate precipitation. Normally, urinary phosphate is much higher in concentration compared to citrate; this is offset by the much higher affinity of trivalent citrate for calcium compared to bivalent phosphate.

high metabolic rate in most mammals coupled with the high serum bicarbonate concentration mandate retrieval of the filtered bicarbonate. The fractional excretion of bicarbonate in humans is <0.1%. Much effort is devoted to the reclamation of this precious anion. When it is physiologically appropriate to excrete bicarbonate, all the tubules have to slightly reduce the large resorptive capacity, and bicarbonaturia ensues. This should be the most efficient way of ridding the body of excess base. However, bicarbonaturia carries with it an enormous price. Since urinary pCO_2, though much higher than plasma, resides in a fairly narrow range, any amount of bicarbonaturia will significantly raise the urine pH. As discussed earlier, low urine pH is required to keep calcium phosphate from precipitating. Bicarbonaturia is a powerful and efficient way of excreting base when a large amount of base needs to be excreted rapidly but infrequently. The constant use of this mode of base excretion begets serious problems of calcium phosphate precipitation; an alternative is necessary.

The need for alkali excretion without raising urine pH requires a "hydroxyl equivalent" that is in millimolar quantities in urine and does not have such a high pK_a that it binds H^+ and raises the urine pH. The concept of a base (hydroxyl or bicarbonate) equivalent is based on whether the organic anion is metabolized to neutral end products. The metabolism of glucose to CO_2 and water does not consume or generate acid or base and is therefore acid–base-neutral. The metabolism of citrate is illustrated in Figure 10.4. When trivalent citrate is completely metabolized to carbon dioxide and water, $3H^+$s are consumed. The $3H^+$s are derived from metabolic CO_2, which will leave three bicarbonates behind. Hence, trivalent citrate can be considered three hydroxyl or bicarbonate equivalents. Figure 10.4 compares the effect of addition of equivalent of bicarbonate versus citrate on urinary pH. With citraturia, significant amount of base excretion can be accommodated in the urine without an excessive rise in urine pH. While the capacity of bicarbonaturia is very high, it is not a preferred mode of sustained base excretion because of alkalinuria and the risk of calcium phosphate precipitation.

Citrate Concentration and Excretion Rates

Thus, there is duality of function of urinary citrate. On one hand, citrate chelates Ca^{2+} to prevent formation of insoluble complexes; on the other hand, it allows base excretion without a significant increase in urine pH. These are functions of equal importance, but there are scenarios where servicing one function compromises the other. "Hypoci-

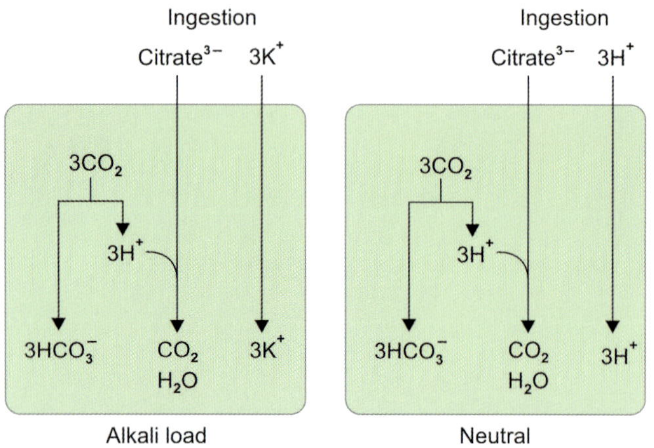

Fig. 10.4: Comparison of ingestion of K_3Citrate versus H_3Citrate (citric acid). The metabolism of citrate^{3-} to CO_2 and H_2O consumes $3H^+$s derived from metabolic CO_2 leaving $3HCO_3^-$ behind. Ingestion of K_3Citrate (left) followed by complete metabolism is equivalent to gaining $3KHCO_3$, which constitutes an alkali load. Ingestion of H_3Citrate (right) is equivalent to gain of equal amounts of HCO_3^- and H^+, which is neutral from an acid-base point of view.

traturia," as frequently referred to in common clinical parlance as a risk factor for stone risk, is actually difficult to define physiologically. Like urine calcium excretion, citraturia is not a dichotomous variable, so the question, "does the patient have hypocitraturia?" is absurd despite the fact that there is a "normal range" in clinical lab reports.

However, hypocitraturia does exist as a concept. "Low citrate" is, in fact, not necessarily an undesirable phenotype as there is no calcium crystallization and no stone formation. The duality of citrate's role mandates dual interpretation. From an acid-base point of view, urinary citrate should be expressed in milliequivalents (mEq) as that represents the number of OH^- carried into the urine. The appropriate mEq of citrate should be interpreted relative to the net acid excretion and net gastrointestinal absorption. From the calcium chelation point of view, urinary citrate should be expressed in millimoles (mmoles) as it binds calcium in a 1:1 stoichiometry, and the appropriate mmoles should be interpreted in relationship to how much calcium is in the urine and how much phosphate and oxalate are there to sequester the calcium into insoluble complexes. Under no circumstance is there any meaning in expressing urine citrate in milligrams, as it is customarily and unfortunately presented in clinical laboratory reports in the United States of America. Finally, from a mass balance viewpoint, one surveys the 24-hour excretion rate of citrate as mass/time, but from a physicochemical viewpoint it is the concentration (mass/volume) that matters.

RENAL CITRATE HANDLING

Overall renal citrate handling is summarized in Figures 10.5A and B. Species difference notwithstanding, in general, of the citrate entering the kidney, roughly 75% is returned to the body primarily as unfiltered citrate with excretion of about 5% (25% of filtered citrate; fractional excretion (FE) range from 0.1–0.3); ~20% is metabolized by the kidney.[20,21] However, it is important to note that much higher rates of metabolism have been reported, even to levels above the filtered load, indicating that the kidney consumes citrate from the filtrate as well as the plasma. All this occurs in the proximal tubule, and a cellular model is shown in Figure 10.6. Citrate transport and metabolism will be discussed separately in the following text.

Renal Citrate Transport

Apical transport of citrate representing reabsorption of filtered citrate was well characterized by membrane vesicle studies in the 1980s and 1990s. Transport was established to be via an Na-coupled dicarboxylate system that transports a variety of Krebs cycle intermediate.[22-24] Transport of citrate occurs predominantly via the divalent form, despite the fact that citrate is predominantly trivalent at physiologic pH in plasma and proximal lumen.

Basolateral uptake of citrate was suggested by studies of whole kidney demonstrating net peritubular uptake, evidenced by total uptake exceeding reabsorption of filtered citrate.[25,26] A few studies have examined basolateral membrane vesicles.[27,28] One study from rabbit renal proximal tubules found that basolateral transport of citrate was sodium-dependent but electroneutral and relatively insensitive to pH, in contrast to luminal transport.[27] The combination of the findings of insensitivity to pH and electroneutral transport suggest that citrate transport across the basolateral membrane may be coupling of one citrate^{-3} and three Na^+.[27] The mechanisms of basolateral transport have not been clearly defined, and how this may contribute to overall citrate excretion has not been determined. Thus far, there is no evidence of citrate secretion into the urine.[29] Therefore, the proximal tubule cell is a citrate uptake cell from both membranes, and the fate of citrate is either metabolism or lipid synthesis (discussed in the following text). A model that summarizes proximal tubule citrate handling is presented in Figure 10.10.

Citrate Transporters: Molecular Identities

The era of flux measurements was moved forward in 1995 when the proximal tubule apical membrane sodium-

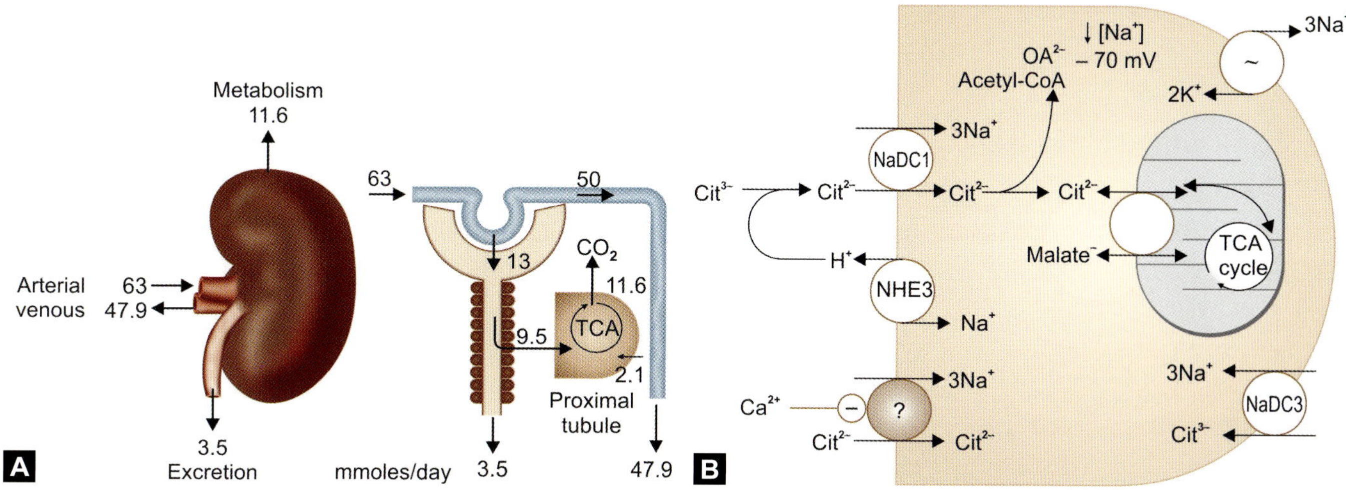

Figs. 10.5A and B: Renal handling of citrate. (A) Data extrapolated from Neith and Schollmeyer.[20,21] The numbers shown are mmoles per day in a 70 kg human. There is a negative arteriovenous content difference of ~15 mmoles in citrate indicating uptake by the kidney; only about one quarter of the 15 mmoles exits in the urine with proximal tubule metabolism to CO_2 (TCA, tricarboxylic acid cycle) accounting for three quarters of the renal uptake. About one quarter of the filtered citrate is excretion (fractional excretion ~ 25%). Citrate is taken up by the proximal tubule from both membranes and metabolized to CO_2; apical uptake exceeds basolateral by fourfold to fivefold. (B) Proximal tubule model of citrate transport and metabolism. Filtered citrate, which is mostly trivalent at early proximal tubule lumen pH, is titrated by the H^+ secreted by the Na^+/H^+ exchanger NHE3 into the bivalent form, which is transported by the Na^+–dicarboxylate cotransporter NaDC1 into the cell where it can be metabolized in the cytoplasm or mitochondria. NaDC3 is present on the basolateral membrane, which transports trivalent citrate and is responsible for citrate uptake from the blood. Another Na^+-coupled citrate transport system in the apical membrane has been functionally characterized in culture cells, is normally inhibited by luminal Ca^{2+}, and is only activated when Ca^{2+} is low.

dependent dicarboxylate cotransporter (NaDC1) was cloned by Pajor.[30,31] Unexpectedly, NaDC1 was found to be homologous to a sulfate transporter NaS-1.[32] Several sodium-dependent dicarboxylate cotransporters belonging to the solute carrier gene family SLC13A have been identified, including NaDC1; NaDC3; the sodium-dependent sulfate cotransporters, NaS-1 and SUT-1; and INDY, the transporter encoded from the gene Indy (I'm not dead yet) from *Drosophila melanogaster*. The mammalian homolog of INDY, mINDY, or sodium coupled citrate transporter (NaCT) (SLC13A5) is a sodium-coupled citrate transporter found in liver, testis and brain.[33] The transporters in the NaDC/NaSi gene family are typically composed of 590–605 aminoacids with hydropathy amino acid profiles predicting 8–13 transmembrane spanning domains.

The Na^+ to substrate stoichiometry for nearly all of the transporters of the NaDC/NaSi gene family is 3:1, with NaCT being the exception (discussed in the following text). Most of these transporters accept a broad spectrum of di- and tricarboxylates in vitro including citrate, succinate, and α-ketoglutarate. Differences in substrate affinity exist across species and between isoforms.[34]

NaDC1/SLC13A2: This is thought to be the major mechanism of proximal tubule reabsorption of citrate. NaDC1 is a low-affinity transporter with K_m values of >200 μM for the dicarboxylate succinate.[30] Antibodies directed against NaDC1 localized it to the apical membrane of the S2 segment of the proximal tubule and to the small intestine.[35] Ribonucleic acid (RNA) blots revealed that NaDC1 may also be present in lung, liver, adrenal, and epididymis, but not in heart, eye, testis, skeletal muscle, or brain.[30,36]

Chronic metabolic acidosis leads to increased citrate reabsorption by the proximal tubule, accompanied by increased expression of NaDC1 mRNA and protein levels, which is also found in potassium depletion.[35,37] Also, as mentioned above, increased acidification of the proximal tubular fluid during acidosis will in turn increase the concentration of divalent citrate. There is also increased trafficking of NaDC1 to the apical membrane with acidosis. An increase in abundance of NaDC1 and NHE3 (the major mechanism of apical H^+ excretion) was postulated to involve the Na^+/H^+ exchanger regulating factor 2, serum and glucocorticoid inducible kinase isoforms 1 and 3, and by protein kinase B.[38] Protein kinase C inhibits NaDC1;

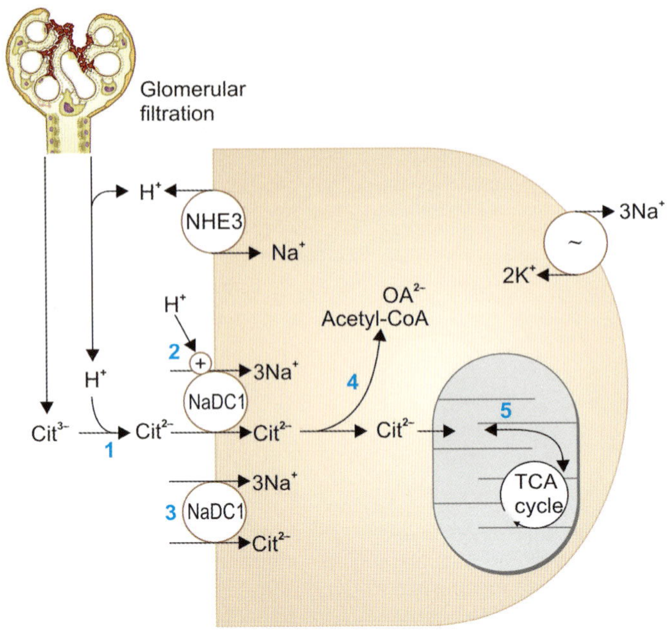

Fig. 10.6: Mechanisms of hypocitraturia in the proximal tubule during acidosis or acid-loading. Five sets of mechanisms are involved culminating in hypocitraturia. The low plasma pH in glomerular filtrate (in acidosis only) and the heightened activity of the Na^+/H^+ exchanger NHE3 titrates trivalent citrate to the preferred transported bivalent species; hence, increasing transport by increasing substrate without affecting the biology of the transporter (1). NaDC1 is directly gated by pH, so low luminal pH stimulates transport activity (2). Over longer periods of time, more transporter proteins appear in the apical membrane, thus increasing the V_{max} and J_{max} of citrate transport (3). Acidosis increases cytoplasmic ATP lyase and citrate metabolism (4). Mitochondrial citrate metabolism is stimulated by low pH and low $[HCO_3^-]$ (5). The combined end result is increased absorption of filtered citrate. (ATP: Adenosine triphosphate).

inhibition of transporter activity appears to be via a combination of endocytosis and inhibition of transporter activity.[39]

NaDC3/SLC13A3: This is a high-affinity sodium dicarboxylate cotransporter in the basolateral membrane of the renal proximal tubule, the placental brush border membrane, liver, and brain.[40] NaDC3 is 40–50% homologous with NaDC1. The location of NaDC3 at the basolateral membrane of the proximal tubule is important in the transport of Krebs cycle intermediates from the peritubular fluid, but also is important in that it maintains the driving force for the secretion of organic anions such as para-aminohippuric acid (PAH) for α-ketoglutarate via the organic anion transporter-1 (OAT1).[41] NaDC3 differs functionally from NaDC1 by its substrate affinity and specificity, and by the pH dependence of succinate transport. For NaDC3, the K_m for succinate is 2–140 μM compared to a broad range of K_ms for NaDC1 orthologs. NaDC3 may be only one mechanism of basolateral citrate transport. An unidentified electroneutral tricarboxylate transporter established in membrane vesicle studies is another possible mechanism of basolateral citrate transport.

INDY, NaCT/SLC13A5: INDY is a *Drosophila* ortholog of NaDC1; mutations in the gene resulted in nearly doubling the life span of *Drosophila*. INDY has high homology to the mammalian sodium-dicarboxylate cotransporters with ~34% identity. It is a high-affinity succinate transporter with a K_m of ~40 μM. NaCT is a mammalian carboxylate cotransporter found mainly in the liver, and also in brain. Substrates include various dicarboxylates and also the tricarboxylate form of citrate. In fact, in contrast to NaDC1, NaCT transports citrate more effectively than succinate. The stoichiometry of this sodium-dependent transport process is $4Na^+$:1 di- or tricarboxylate, even if the trivalent form of citrate is the ionic species transported. NaCT may be an important transporter linking extracellular citrate to lipid synthesis.

Mitochondrial transporters: Mitochondria have extensive transport of citrate and many other Krebs cycle intermediates using distinct transporters unrelated to the plasma membrane transporters above. The mitochondrial transporter family, SLC25, is one of the largest known family of solute carriers, comprising at least 53 members, some of which are still classified as orphan transporters such substrates as diverse as tricarboxylates, dicarboxylates, oxoglutarate, ornithine, aspartate, glutamate, phosphate, adenine nucleotides, deoxynucleotide, CoA, flavin adenine dinucleotide (FAD), FMN and adenosine monophosphate (AMP), oxiadipate, carnitine/acylcarnitine, S-adenosylmethionine, iron, folate, pyrimidine nucleotide, CoA, protons (uncoupling), and many other unidentified substrates.[42] At least three are known to transport TCA cycle intermediates as exchangers of substrates across the mitochondrial inner membrane. One mitochondrial transporter has also been reported in the plasma membrane SLC25A1 or mCiC in the prostate and may provide a K^+-dependent citrate release from normal prostate cells.[43] The role of these transporters in renal proximal tubule citrate entry and metabolism has not been uncovered.

Other transporters: Although *SLC26A6 (Pat1, CFEX)* and *SLC26A3 (DRA)* are not dicarboxylate transporters per se, they may be involved in regulation of carboxylate ion transport. These are involved in oxalate handling and are also known for chloride, sulfate, and bicarbonate exchange. Pat1 (putative anion transporter) also transports

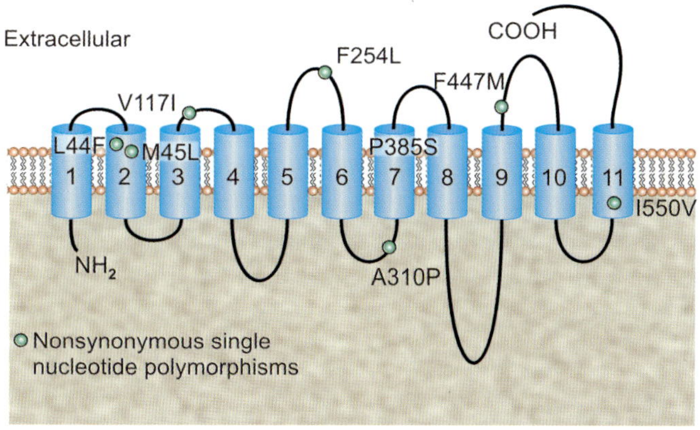

Fig. 10.7: Predicted topology model of human Na^+-dicarboxylate cotransporter (hNaDC1) showing the amino acid variants generated by nonsynonymous single nucleotide polymorphisms. The 11-putative transmembrane helices are shown as numbered cylinders. The N terminus is intracellular. The position of the variant amino acids is shown by open circles.

formate and hydroxyl ions. Although downregulated in adenoma (DRA) is present in duodenum, jejunum, ileum, and cecum, SLC26A6 is located in these same sites along with kidney, pancreas, colon, heart, muscle, and placenta. Recently, Ohana et al. determined a novel simultaneous regulation of NaDC1 and SLC26A6, both located at the apical surface of the proximal tubule. While SLC26A6 inhibits transport by NaDC1, NaDC1 simultaneously stimulates SLC26A6. This results in less citrate being taken up by the proximal tubule, which is beneficial when oxalate is being excreted at the apical side.[44]

Renal Citrate Metabolism: Cytoplasmic and Mitochondrial

Unlike metabolic solutes such as glucose, amino acids, and phosphate where the majority of the entry from the apical membrane exits the basolateral side to the peritubular capillary for the purpose of reclamation, the citrate taken up from the urine via the apical membrane and from the blood via the basolateral membrane undergoes extensive metabolism in the proximal tubule cell. Citrate was shown to provide 10–15% of the respiratory fuel of the kidney,[20,25,26] which means that if the proximal tubule is the sole site of uptake, it represents significant rates of metabolism—a fact that was confirmed in single rat proximal tubules.[45]

Since this chapter focuses on citraturia, it is important to point out that an increase in cytoplasmic citrate concentration from either decreased cellular citrate metabolism or elevated cellular citrate synthesis will decrease apical citrate uptake and lead to hypercitraturia. Conversely, increased citrate metabolism and suppressed cellular citrate synthesis will increase apical citrate uptake and hypocitraturia. One of the best pieces of supporting evidence for metabolism playing a key role in addition to transport is based on studies where tissue levels of citrate were carefully measured. Metabolic acidosis is associated with low while metabolic alkalosis is associated with renal citrate levels.[7,46-49] The carefully conducted study of Baruch et al. suggests that it is citrate metabolism and not synthetic rate that is regulated by acid-base.[50]

Citrate metabolism by the proximal tubule cell can be divided into cytoplasmic and mitochondrial. After apical (from the urine) and basolateral (from peritubular capillaries) entry, cytoplasmic citrate is metabolized by ATP citrate lyase into the 4-carbon oxaloacetate and supplies the cytoplasm with acetyl-CoA (Fig. 10.7). Acetyl-CoA is the basic building block for the endogenous synthesis of fatty acids and cholesterol, and it is involved in protein modifications such as histone acetylation.[51] The oxaloacetate thus generated can be converted to male and pyruvate via cytoplasmic enzymes (Fig. 10.7) and enters the mitochondrial matrix to enter the TCA cycle. Cytoplasmic ATP lyase is one of the enzymes increased in metabolic acidosis contributing to the hypocitraturia.[52]

Mitochondrial citrate metabolism is mediated via the TCA cycle (*see* Fig. 10.2). This is a vast topic that cannot be covered in this chapter, but selected highlights will be provided in the context of acid base. A series of important studies demonstrated the sensitivity of citrate metabolism to acid–base parameters (Fig. 10.8).[53] In these experiments in vitro where there is no perfusion and citrate oxidation rather than uptake is measured, one is examining acid-base effects on citrate metabolism. This effect is clearly renal specific and only observed in the presence of CO_2/HCO_3^- (Fig. 10.9A). The intact cell (tissue) and mitochondria appear to be differentially regulated by pH and [HCO_3^-] (Fig. 10.9B). The sensors in the cytoplasm and mitochondria are not known at present.

PHYSIOLOGIC REGULATION OF URINARY CITRATE EXCRETION

A variety of physiologic and/or clinical factors have been shown to alter urinary citrate excretion (Table 10.1). The most important of these involve some alteration in acid-base homeostasis, which will be discussed first and in some detail.

Acid-Base Parameters

Changes in acid-base homeostasis are the predominant determinant of proximal tubule reabsorption and urinary excretion of citrate. A variety of physiologic and biochemical factors likely contribute to this phenomenon. First, since citrate^{-2} is the ionic species transported by NaDC1, a lower luminal pH increases citrate^{-2} concentrations, which will increase citrate reabsorption, particularly when the luminal concentration is below the K_m.[5,54] Since the last pK_a of citric acid is 5.6, the abundance of the divalent species increases dramatically as the luminal pH falls. To illustrate the magnitude of this effect, note that the citrate^{-2} concentration increases about threefold as pH decreases from 7.4 to 6.9. A variety of *in vitro* models have shown an increase of citrate transport with acute acidosis and/or acute changes in pH.[27,54-58] Perfused tubule studies suggested that luminal pH has a more profound effect than cell pH since basolateral acidosis per se that influences cell pH did not alter luminal citrate uptake when luminal pH was buffered or was already acidic.[5,54]

A second level of regulation resides in the intrinsic properties of NaDC1. Even with the preferred substrate kept constant, low pH activates citrate transport in its native state in vesicles[58] as well as in heterologous systems.[30]

In addition, with acidosis, mRNA for NaDC1 increases and protein/transporter abundance in the apical membrane increases significantly.[35,57] This stimulation requires a functional endothelin B receptor;[59] endogenous renal endothelin 1 is known to be stimulated by acidosis.

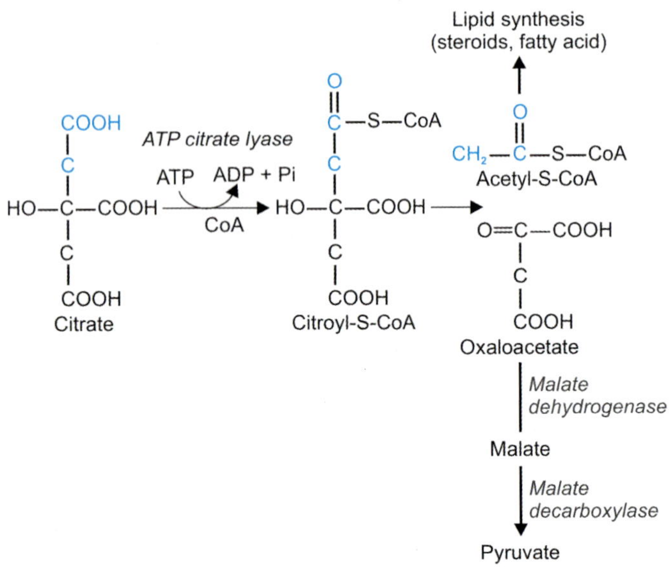

Fig. 10.8: Proximal tubule cytoplasmic citrate metabolism. After cellular uptake, citrate in the cytoplasm is metabolized by ATP citrate lyase as the main source of cytoplasmic acetyl-CoA, which supplies the carbon skeleton for lipid synthesis. The oxaloacetate and malate likely end up in the mitochondria and get metabolized there.

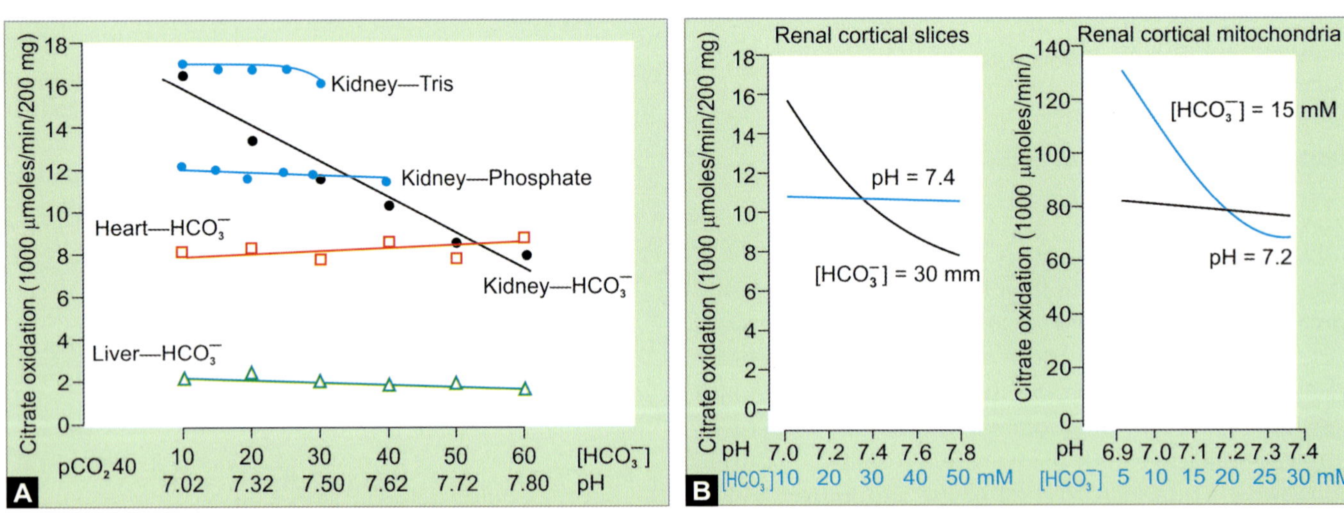

Figs. 10.9A and B: Regulation of citrate oxidation by acid-base parameters. (A) Citrate oxidation in kidney cortex is inhibited by increasing [HCO_3^-] and pH with fixed pCO_2 = 40 mm Hg in the kidney (•) but not in the heart (€) and liver (Δ). Change in pH using Tris or phosphate as buffers in the absence of HCO_3^-/CO_2 (gray lines and gray filled circles) does not affect citrate oxidation. (B) Either pH or [HCO_3^-] was varied with the other parameter kept constant. Citrate oxidation in renal cortical slices was most sensitive to changes in [HCO_3^-] (left panel) while isolated mitochondria is more sensitive to changes in [HCO_3^-] than to pH.
Source: Adapted from Simpson DP. Regulation of renal citrate metabolism by bicarbonate ion and pH: observations in tissue slices and mitochondria. J Clin Invest. 1967;46:225-38.

Table 10.1: Conditions affecting urinary citrate excretion.

Decreased urinary citrate	*Increased urinary citrate*
Metabolic acidosis (e.g. dRTA and diarrhea)	Metabolic alkalosis
Dietary and other acid loads	Increased urinary calcium
Acetazolamide	Increased urinary magnesium
Hypokalemia/potassium deficiency	Pregnancy
Thiazide diuretics	Estrogen
Intensive exercise	Advanced age
High dietary sodium	
Idiopathic	

Mitochondrial and metabolic effects also likely account for some of the changes in citrate excretion with acidosis[26] (Figs. 10.9A and B). Citrate levels in the renal cortex (which is predominantly proximal tubule) rise with alkalosis and fall with acidosis.[7,46] Acidosis stimulates citrate uptake into, and subsequent oxidation in, mitochondria.[26] Citrate entry into mitochondria is via a tricarboxylate carrier as described above, and intracellular pH alters the mitochondrial pH gradient. Also, citrate lyase activity increases in acidosis and will lower intracellular concentrations of citrate and promote reabsorption.[52] With alkali loads, urinary citrate excretion increases likely due to some reversal of the above factors. In addition, decreases in mitochondrial aconitase, the first step in mitochondrial citrate metabolism, occur.[60] The concept that citrate metabolism alters citrate reabsorption by the proximal tubule requires that intracellular citrate concentrations exert physiologic influence on citrate reabsorption via altering gradients, although there is some evidence suggesting that this is not necessarily the case.[61,62]

Estrogen

Estrogens and gender have long been thought to influence citrate excretion, based on some observations that women on average have higher urinary citrates that decline with menopause.[63,64] But direct clinical or experimental evidence of this has been minimal, and there are conflicting reports. In one population of stone formers, there were no gender differences in citrate excretion.[63] Confounding factors, such as diet, indirect effects via subtle acid base changes, or variations in calcium homeostasis which may influence urine citrate, complicate both observational studies and interventional studies. Urinary citrate is well known to vary with the menstrual cycle and to increase in pregnancy.[65,66] Lower urine citrate in postmenopausal women could result from estrogen deficiency or perhaps from a subtle imbalance between acid loads and acid excretion as part of aging or with the mild renal insufficiency that occurs with aging.[67] Studies of estrogen replacement in postmenopausal women have also been mixed, with some showing an increased citrate excretion with estrogen but others failing to show an effect.[63,68,69] Large retrospective epidemiologic studies have shown that estrogens in postmenopausal women do not decrease, and may increase, the incidence of stones);[70,71] although the mechanism(s) are not clear, an increase in urinary calcium could contribute.

Calcium

Calcium, magnesium, calcitonin, and vitamin D have all been proposed to influence urinary citrate for many years;[26] we will discuss the role of calcium briefly. Complexation of citrate by high concentrations of calcium can clearly decrease citrate movement on the proximal tubule apical transporter,[55] since total citrate concentration in the filtrate is ~ 10^{-4}–10^{-5} M while ionized calcium is in 10^{-3} M. In addition to the physicochemical chelation effect, a series of studies using the correct proximal tubule-like cell line have shown a novel calcium-sensitive dicarboxylate transport system in which citrate transport is decreased by an increase in apical calcium.[72,73,179] This transporter appears to be a high-affinity transporter (in contrast to NaDC1) for citrate, succinate, and other dicarboxylates. Multiple lines of evidence suggest that the calcium-sensitive system is distinct from NaDC1. Some studies based on human and animal have also suggested that urinary citrate increases with urinary calcium under normal conditions.[66,74–77] This may be a teleologically protective mechanism against calcium nephrolithiasis—as urinary calcium increases, increased urine citrate will bind more calcium in a soluble form, preventing crystal and stone formation. Such a calcium-sensitive process also corresponds with one epidemiologic study and a small single-center study that urinary citrate is increased in individuals with higher urinary calcium in normal patients(ref).[78] Stone-forming patients frequently have both high urinary calcium and low urinary citrate, a relationship at odds with the relationship described above, whether this is causal or just associated in stone formers is unknown. It is also challenging to extrapolate urinary calcium to proximal tubule luminal calcium given the vast modifications in calcium and water transport between the proximal tubule lumen and bladder. The calcium-sensitive system described above can conceivably be a proximal tubule-specific local mechanism to maintain calcium and citrate relationships. For the calcium concentration in the medullary collecting duct or renal pelvis to regulate proximal tubule citrate transport would require complex retrograde cross-talk, which will be fascinating to explore.

CLINICAL PATHOPHYSIOLOGY OF HYPOCITRATURIA

Hypocitraturic Nephrolithiasis

It is important to note that "hypocitraturia" may be a commonly used term in clinical practice, but as noted above, it is completely arbitrary. A cutoff of 450 mg (2.38 mmoles) per day in men or 550 mg (2.91 mmoles) per day in women is commonly used in clinical laboratories to "report" hypocitraturia, but it is crucial to once again emphasize that urinary citrate excretion is a continuous and not a dichotomous trait; strictly speaking, there is no clear cutoff between normal and abnormal.

From an acid–base balance point of view, the amount of citrate in the urine should be interpreted in the light of acid or base intake and excretion and the plasma pH and bicarbonate. For example, two subjects may both have an identical amount of 472 mg (2.5 mmoles) citrate per day. The first subject with a high acid intake and net acid excretion of 100 mEq per day will be considered to have too much citrate in the urine (hypercitraturia), while the second subject with net acid intake and excretion of –10 mEq will have too little citrate in the urine (hypocitraturia) despite the identical excretion rate.

Another parameter to consider is propensity to lithogenesis. A subject with 472 mg (2.5 mmoles) citrate per day without stones does not have hypocitraturia, but the same amount of citrate with recurrent calcium stone formation can be considered hypocitraturic as stone risk may decrease if urine citrate is raised to 660 mg (3.5 mmoles). Low urinary citrate (hypocitraturia) is a contributor to nephrolithiasis in a substantial percentage of patients (estimated as 20–60%).[64] However, hypocitraturia is seldom the sole cause of calcium or other stones. Also, low urine citrate is found accompanying significant numbers of patients in all etiologic categories of hypercalciuria.[79]

As a group, patients with calcium nephrolithiasis have lower urinary citrate excretion rates than patients without stones (reviewed in ref. 64). For instance, Parks and Coe found that urine citrate per day averaged 551 (2.91) and 516 (2.73) mg (mmoles) per 24 hours in women and men with stones, respectively, compared to 729 (8.85) and 547 (2.89) mg (mmoles) per 24 hours in women and men without stones.[80] As these numbers indicate, there is often considerable overlap in urine citrate between stone formers and nonstone formers; the urine calcium-to-citrate ratio may demonstrate more separation between groups.[64]

The low citrate undoubtedly contributes to their propensity for stone formation. Still, in many cases there is only a somewhat low urine citrate for which no clear etiology can be identified. However, in other cases there is a distinctly low urinary citrate and the etiology can be identified. Many of the causes or predispositions to hypocitraturia follow closely the physiology of citrate handling by the kidney discussed above. In particular, conditions altering acid–base balance are the most common cause of low urinary citrate.

Acidosis or Acid Load

States of chronic acidosis or acid loads are the most common and predictable of the conditions causing low urinary citrate.[5] Chronic metabolic acidosis from distal renal tubular acidosis (RTA, type I RTA, or dRTA) is a classic cause of recurrent calcium stones.[81–83] Both calcium phosphate and calcium oxalate stones occur in dRTA.[84] Calcium nephrolithiasis and nephrocalcinosis in dRTA result not only from low urinary citrate but also from acidosis-induced hypercalciuria, and from the high urine pH, which will increase calcium phosphate precipitation. The hypercalciuria from the chronic systemic acidosis of dRTA results from both dissolution of calcium from bone and decreases in distal tubule reabsorption of calcium with acidosis. The high urine pH in dRTA results from the inability of the distal nephron to acidify the urine, even in states of systemic acidosis. Low urinary citrate also occurs with incomplete dRTA where frank systemic acidosis is not present. Whether the low urine citrate despite normal systemic pH results from intermittent systemic acidosis that is not detectable in most clinical settings or from some form of intrarenal acidosis is unknown. An ammonium chloride loading test may be required to diagnose incomplete dRTA. Proximal renal tubular acidosis (pRTA) is not usually associated with calcium stones or low urine citrate,[85–87] despite a systemic acidosis. This could result from defective sodium-coupled citrate reabsorption similar to the other reabsorptive defects in the proximal tubule in pRTA[88] or in proximal tubule cell alkalinization due to defective base exit.[89] Acetazolamide via its acid-base effects can cause low urinary citrate and stones in some patients[90]; this has been reviewed in more detail previously.[5]

Other states of chronic acidosis or chronic acid loads even without frank systemic acidosis cause low urinary citrate. When a high acid load is excreted, no systemic acidosis will be detectable but part of the adaptation to restore normalcy is hypocitraturia. Alpern and Sakhaee have termed this "normobicarbonatemic acidosis," which can cause both urolithiasis and bone loss.[67] For instance, high animal protein diets that have a high acid content are particularly prone to cause low urinary citrate and stones.[91-93] How much of the predisposition to calcium stones from a high animal protein diet results from the low urinary citrate has not been defined since other factors such as hypercalciuria are also associated. Chronic diarrhea is a common cause of chronic acidosis and can cause low urinary citrate and nephrolithiasis from a variety of mechanisms, including the low urinary citrate and low urinary volumes.[94] Starvation or even fasting also decreases urinary citrate levels, perhaps related to mild systemic acidosis but perhaps from other effects on citrate reabsorption;[95] this has also been reviewed in more detail previously.[5]

Potassium Deficiency

Potassium deficiency and hypokalemia also decrease urinary citrate.[96-98] This likely occurs secondary to the known lowering of intracellular pH in potassium deficiency[99] and/or increased tubular H^+ secretion that results from potassium deficiency. An additional mechanism with potassium depletion is an increased activity of citrate transport in the proximal tubule apical membrane, probably from an increased number of transporters.[37]

Thiazide diuretics are commonly used for the prevention of recurrent calcium oxalate nephrolithiasis owing to their hypocalciuric action.[100-102] In addition to their natriuretic effects, all thiazides are also kaliuretics. Even mild degrees of potassium depletion can lead to intracellular acidosis and hypocitraturia rector.[54,103] Thiazide diuretics are known to cause a number of metabolic side effects such as hypokalemia, dyslipidemia, and insulin resistance, which raise a safety concern over lifetime use.[104,105] Thiazide diuretics can also lower urinary citrate excretion, particularly if potassium deficiency is allowed to occur;[106] in the setting of hypercalciuria treated with thiazides, the lowering of urinary citrate would offset the beneficial effect of the thiazides on potential stone formation.

Other Factors

Many factors alter urinary citrate but are not commonly a sole reason for stone disease. Potentially important is that high salt intake or volume expansion may decrease citrate excretion.[107] Chronic kidney disease, perhaps secondary to some degree of acidosis, has also been reported to reduce urinary citrate excretion.[108] Intensive exercise may also decrease urinary citrate.[109] Angiotensin converting enzyme inhibitors decrease urinary citrate, presumably via a lower intracellular pH or reduced acid secretion by the proximal tubule.[110] Other conditions reported to lower urinary citrate include environmental heat and ethacrynic acid.[26] As mentioned above, increases in urinary calcium and magnesium increase urinary citrate. During pregnancy, both urine calcium and citrate increase; the increase in citrate may protect against stone formation during the hypercalciuria.[65] These changes in urine citrate may be hormonal or possibly due to the changes in urine calcium in part. Lithium inhibits NaDC1 in many animal species, but human NaDC1 is relatively insensitive to lithium in vitro.[111] Some variants of human NaDC1 are more sensitive to lithium, but other actually have increased transport with lithium.[111] Similarly, lithium in rats causes a clear rise in urinary citrate, whereas in humans there is no clear effect of lithium on urinary citrate.[112,113] However, the effects on urinary citrate could be complex due to offsetting effects on acid-base parameters and direct effects on NaDC1 and other transporters.

Idiopathic hypocitraturia is a diagnosis by default. Some patients with low urinary citrate have no clearly identifiable cause and can be considered to be idiopathic.[114] Such patients have not been well studied in general and could have underlying dietary, metabolic, transport, or genetic factors. Decreased intestinal citrate transport or low plasma citrate has not been found to contribute to low urinary citrate in general.[115] Pajor and Sun have shown transport changes in a variety of reported single nucleotide polymorphisms, but these do not appear to account for low urinary citrate,[111] in contrast to one prior genetic linkage study.[116]

As discussed above, most studies find that urine citrate is higher in premenopausal women than in men, and that urine citrate rises with age;[64] however, this gender difference does not necessarily hold in stone formers,[63] and wide variation occurs in all ages and both genders.

Impact of Urinary Citrate on Ca Supersaturation

The role of citrate as a chelator of urinary calcium was discussed above (*see* Fig. 10.3). We will take a more in-depth look at the impact of urinary citrate on the propensity to

Table 10.2: Citrate preparations* for human and veterinary use.

Citric acid	*Sodium citrate*	*Potassium Citrate*	*Trade names (commercial preparations)*
+			Sour salt, Lemon salt
	+		Citra pH, Cystoplus, Neutramax, Tricitrasol
		+	Cymaclear, Cystopurin, Cytra-K, Effercitrate, Urocit-K, K City
+	+		Bicitra, Cytra-2, Liqui-Dual Citra, Neutracid, Oracit, Shohl's solution
	+	+	Alkasolve, Citrolith, Xitrin
+		+	Alkamax, Polycitra-K, Portrate, Pota, Uriliser, Urotrate
+	+	+	Cytra-3, Polycitra, Polycitra-LC, Tricitrates

*Citrate-containing preparations in combination with other compounds are not listed.

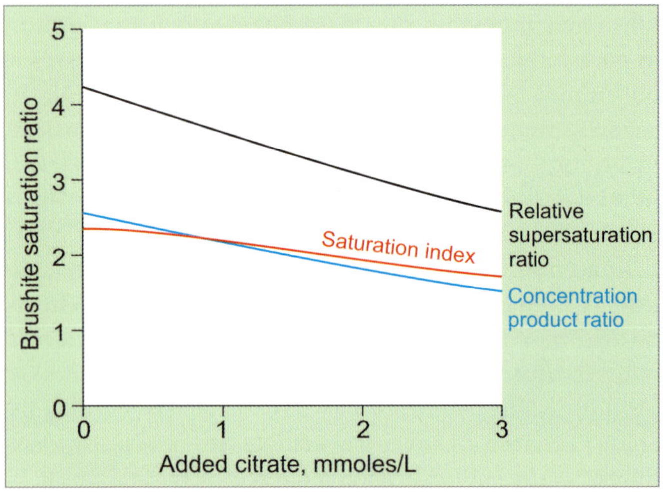

Fig. 10.10: Effect of citrate on brushite saturation. The concentration product ratio (ratio of activity or concentration of products before and after incubation with synthetic brushite) is empirically determined at the bench and provides a direct estimate of saturation from the extent of actual growth (supersaturation) or dissolution (undersaturation) of added brushite. Raising citrate within the physiologic range with all other variables kept constant lowers the saturation of brushite.

form calcium phosphate and calcium oxalate crystals. In addition to reducing urinary supersaturation of calcium salts by forming soluble complexes with calcium, citrate also inhibits the nucleation, growth, and aggregation of calcium oxalate crystals.[117,118] Citrate directly inhibits crystallization and increases the upper limit of metastability by increasing both urine citrate and pH. [119-121]

Some have proposed that citrate increases the amount and activity of some macromolecules in the urine (e.g. Tamm-Horsfall protein, THP) that inhibit calcium oxalate aggregation,[122] based on a correlation between THP excretion and citrate excretion rates[123,124] and increase in THP excretion after initiation of citrate therapy.[125] Regardless of whether citrate increases THP excretion, the inhibitory activity of THP is more active at pH 7.2 than 5.7,[126] so alkali therapy may also protect against calcium stones in this fashion.

An example of the inhibitory activity of citrate on brushite can be Demonstrated by a combination of empirical physical-chemical methods and computer-based prediction programs.[127] The concentration product ratio (CPR, ratio of activity or concentration products before and after incubation with synthetic brushite) provides a direct estimate of saturation from the extent of actual growth (supersaturation) or dissolution (undersaturation) of added brushite; thus the higher the CPR, the more the saturation.[128,129] Figures 10.9A and B show the effect of increasing citrate on lowering urine brushite saturation with all other variables kept constant (including pH) based on two prediction programs, EQUIL2[130] and JESS.[131]

CITRATE THERAPY IN NEPHROLITHIASIS

Oral citrate therapy for kidney stones was introduced >30 years ago[132] and now is a recommended therapy for calcium stones for many patients with or without low urinary citrate.[133] The oral administration of potassium or sodium citrate leads to a number of effects in urinary chemistry—decreased net acid excretion, increased citrate excretion, and increased urinary pH. There are many preparations of citrate in which the accompanying cation is either sodium, potassium, proton, or a mixture of the above (Table 10.2). It is important to note that only sodium and potassium citrate provides a base load. Citric acid is neutral from an acid-base point of view because the H^+ acquired is exactly balanced by the H^+ consumed when citrate is metabolized (*see* Fig. 10.4).

Calcium Oxalate Stones

Based on the ability of urinary citrate to complex calcium, the rationale for increasing urinary citrate in those with hypocitraturia is obvious. However, oral citrate preparations may have other benefits in addition to increasing urinary citrate. Oral citrate may decrease gut calcium absorption by binding calcium in the lumen,[134-136] although the high bioavailability of the calcium citrate complex from the intestinal lumen[115] renders the quantitative contribution of this mechanism still undefined. The main mechanism by which oral citrate decreases urinary calcium is through the systemic alkali load, which decreases calcium release from bone resorption[137]; the alkali loads also increases renal calcium reabsorption,[138,139] decreasing urinary calcium, probably predominantly via intracellular and luminal pH effects on the apical calcium channels in the distal tubule.[140,141] Citrate not only chelates calcium, rendering it unavailable to bind phosphate and oxalate, but also directly inhibits crystal nucleation and growth.[142]

Citrate is usually provided as potassium citrate or potassium-magnesium citrate.[143] Potassium citrate, rather than sodium citrate, is used since this avoids increases in urine calcium, which occur with sodium citrate (or even sodium bicarbonate), and potassium citrate has higher solubility than sodium citrate complex in the urine.[138,144] The usual amount is 40–80 mEq per day in two or three doses. Potassium-magnesium citrate has the potential additional advantage of raising urinary magnesium, which complexes oxalate and may be more efficacious than potassium citrate in reducing the supersaturation of urine.[145,146] Citrate is often used not only for hypocitraturia but also under other stone-forming conditions when thiazides are prescribed to lower urinary calcium for calcium nephrolithiasis. Citrate is well absorbed in the intestine.[115] The administered citrate is metabolized to CO_2 and water, consuming H^+ and providing an alkali load, which signals through yet unidentified pathways to induce citraturia.[147] It has been proposed that a small fraction of the administered citrate is excreted unchanged in the urine,[148] although this has never been proven. Hepatic escape past the portal circulation to reach the kidney will mandate rise in serum citrate higher than the usual 100 µM, resulting in life-threateningly low ionized calcium. The addition of fruits and vegetables may raise urinary citrate, but some of these foods will also raise urinary oxalate.[149,150] The major effect is by provision of a net dietary alkali load, in contrast to the acid load of high animal protein diets; one can elevate urinary citrate.

Clinical studies do demonstrate that citrate supplementation in general decreases the rate of calcium stone formation.[143,151-153] In a survey of the literature in 2005, Mattle and Hess identified 21 uncontrolled studies of citrate therapy with almost 1,000 patients; stone formation rate was decreased by 47–100% with citrate.[151] However, there are only a small number of prospective randomized placebo-controlled studies with reasonable numbers of patients, and not many subsets of stone formers have been studied separately. Most of the subjects were calcium oxalate stone formers with or without low urinary citrate. Two of three small randomized trials demonstrated benefit[154-156]; the study without an objective reduction in the rate of stone formation used sodium–potassium citrate compared to high fluid intake and dietary restrictions.[156] Potassium citrate has very clear benefits after shock wave lithotripsy.[157,158] Also, long-term use of citrate has been demonstrated in several nonrandomized studies to be of significant benefit.[153,159,160] The largest of the studies was a retrospective analysis of 503 patients with a mean duration of citrate therapy of 41 months. Ninety-three percent of the patients had a decrease in the stone formation rate, and 68% had no new stones.[153]

There are few safety or side effect issues with citrate therapy. Side effects are predominantly gastrointestinal in origin, with nausea, bloating, and diarrhea being the main features, although these are very variable from individual to individual. Although for many patients these are minor issues, several studies report a substantial dropout rate in individuals prone to gastrointestinal upset.[151] It is not clear why the high potassium citrate concentration in orange juice very rarely, if ever, causes gastrointestinal upset. There could possibly be other ingredients in the juice that prevent the potassium citrate from irritating the bowel. Although there have not been formal trials, many experienced clinicians have advised the ingestion of potassium citrate with orange juice.

There is also the potential risk in patients with low glomerular filtration rate (GFR) for increased aluminum absorption from the gut when citrate-containing compounds (such as calcium citrate as a phosphate binder) are taken, particularly with aluminum-containing antacids or phosphate binders.[161-163] However, other studies suggest that in patients with normal kidneys, aluminum absorption and accumulation is not an issue with oral citrate.[164,165] Therefore, this risk seems low in most stone-forming patients with preserved renal function not taking aluminum-containing compounds. One theoretical concern was alkali ingestion in the presence of salt depletion potentially resulting in metabolic alkalosis, but such complications have been shown not to occur,[166] likely due to the absence of potassium deficiency.

Uric Acid Stones and Cysteine Stones

The most common form of uric acid nephrolithiasis is not due to hyperuricosuria but is basically a disease of urine pH where the unduly low urine pH drives the protonation of urate, another abundant urinary anion, to its highly insoluble conjugate acid.[167] The rationale for using potassium or sodium citrate in treating uric acid stones is to increase urinary pH. For similar reasons, citrate is often used in cystine stones to increase solubility. The accompanying increase in urinary citrate excretion probably makes little or no contribution to the decrease in uric acid lithogenicity per se. The current model of pathogenesis of idiopathic uric acid stones espouses a two-hit hypothesis. First, there is increased net acid generation of an unknown nature.[168-170] This is an acid load presented to the kidney without overt depression of circulating plasma bicarbonate concentration, although under carefully controlled situations, a lower plasma bicarbonate concentration is detected in uric acid stone formers under metabolically controlled conditions.[171] This increased excretory load per se will not lower urine pH as long as urinary buffers carry the extra H^+. A second hit in uric acid stone formers is the inability to increase ammonia excretion.[138,172] The combination of these two factors leads to low urinary pH. From an acid-base point of view, the increased H^+ is carried by buffers other than ammonia and H^+ excretion is accomplished with these alternative buffers. Unfortunately, one of these alternative buffers is urate, and the titrated uric acid is extremely insoluble.

Potassium or sodium citrate will in fact lower the net acid load to the kidney. Urine pH will rise despite the fact that ammonia synthesis will not be improved; in fact, ammonium will fall with citrate therapy. As long as urine pH rises, the therapy will be efficacious to reduce uric acid supersaturation. Patients with uric acid nephrolithiasis (pure uric acid and mixed uric acid and calcium oxalate stones) treated with potassium citrate (30–80 mEq per day) experienced increased urinary pH and decreased new stone formation from 1.20 to 0.01 stones per year.[138,173]

Calcium Phosphate Stones

A lingering unresolved controversy in citrate therapy is calcium phosphate stones. Calcium phosphate stone formers have at least a theoretical risk with citrate administration based on the rise of calcium phosphate supersaturation with rising urine pH. Krieger et al. recently studied this in genetically hypercalciuric, stone-forming rats.[174] As predicted, oral potassium citrate raised urinary citrate and lowered slightly urine calcium; however, calcium oxalate and calcium phosphate supersaturation increased due to increases in urine pH, oxalate, and phosphate. Potassium citrate given to patient with dRTA and medullary sponge kidney with calcium phosphate stones did confer a benefit in stone recurrence.[175,176] Therefore, the effects of citrate on calcium phosphate stone formers may be complex, with some potential risks. Some clinical studies have suggested that calcium oxalate stones may transform to calcium phosphate stones over time, possibly in part due to the effects of oral citrate.[177,178] Nonetheless, citrate has been recommended for calcium phosphate stone formers.[133]

REFERENCES

1. Hamm LL, Hering-Smith KS. Pathophysiology of hypocitraturic nephrolithiasis. Endocrinol Metab Clin North Am. 2002;31:885-93, viii.
2. Moe OW. Kidney stones: pathophysiology and medical management. Lancet. 2006;367:333-44.
3. Srere PA. The molecular physiology of citrate. Nature. 1965;205:766-70.
4. Moe OW, Preisig PA. Dual role of citrate in mammalian urine. Curr Opin Nephrol Hypertens. 2006;15:419-24.
5. Hamm LL. Renal handling of citrate. Kidney Int. 1990;38:728-35.
6. Sabbatani L. Calcium et citrate trisodique dans la coagulation du sang, de la lymphe et du lait. Italian Archive of Biology Arch Ital Biol. 1901;36:1901.
7. Adler S, Anderson B, Zemotel L. Metabolic acid-base effects on tissue citrate content and metabolism in the rat. Am J Physiol. 1971;220:986-92.
8. Glusker JP. Structural aspects of citrate biochemistry. Curr Top Cell Regul. 1992;33:169-84.
9. Nicar MJ, Pak CY. Calcium bioavailability from calcium carbonate and calcium citrate. J Clin Endocrinol Metab. 1985;61:391-3.
10. Boothby WM, Adams M. The occurrence of citric acid in urine and body fluids. Am J Physiol. 1934;107:471-9.
11. Ostberg O. Studien uber die Zitronensaureausscheidung die Menschenniere in normalen und pathologischen Zustanden. Scand Arch Physiol. 1931;62:81-222.
12. Krebs HA, Johnson WA. The role of citric acid in intermediate metabolism in animal tissues. Enzymologia. 1937;4:148-56.
13. Gest H. Evolutionary roots of the citric acid cycle in prokaryotes. Biochem Soc Symp. 1987;54:3-16.
14. Melendez-Hevia E, Waddell TG, Cascante M. The puzzle of the Krebs citric acid cycle: assembling the pieces of chemically feasible reactions, and opportunism in the design of metabolic pathways during evolution. J Mol Evol. 1996;43:293-303.

15. Thauer RK. Citric-acid cycle, 50 years on. Modifications and an alternative pathway in anaerobic bacteria. Eur J Biochem. 1988;176:497-508.
16. Weitzman PDJ. Evolution of the citric acid cycle. In: Schleifer KH, Stackebrandt E (Eds). Prokaryotes, in Evolution of Prokaryotes. London: Academic Press; 1985. pp. 253-73.
17. Jacob F. Evolution and tinkering. Science. 1977;196:1161-6.
18. Muus J, Lebel H. Danske videnskabbemes selskab. In: On Complex Calcium Citrate, Kobenhavn: Levin & Munksgaard; 1936. Chap. K.
19. Singh RP, Yeboah YD, Pambid EO, et al. Stability constant of the calcium-citrate (3-) ion pair complex. J Chem Eng Data. 1991;36:52-4.
20. Nieth H, Schollmeyer P. Substrate-utilization of the human kidney. Nature. 1966;209:1244-5.
21. Nieth H, Schollmeyer P. [Citrate metabolism of the human kidney]. Verh Dtsch Ges Inn Med. 1965;71:693-9.
22. Kippen I, Hirayama B, Klinenberg JR, et al. Transport of tricarboxylic acid cycle intermediates by membrane vesicles from renal brush border. Proc Natl Acad Sci USA. 1979;76:3397-400.
23. Wright EM. Transport of carboxylic acids by renal membrane vesicles. Annu Rev Physiol. 1985;47:127-41.
24. Wright SH, Krasne S, Kippen I, et al. Na+-dependent transport of tricarboxylic acid cycle intermediates by renal brush border membranes. Effects on fluorescence of a potential-sensitive cyanine dye. Biochim Biophys Acta. 1981;640:767-78.
25. Baruch S, Burich R, Eun C, et al. Renal metabolism of citrate. Med Clin North Am. 1975;59:569-82.
26. Simpson DP. Citrate excretion: a window on renal metabolism. Am J Physiol. 1983;244:F223-34.
27. Jorgensen KE, Kragh-Hansen U, Roigaard-Petersen H, et al. Citrate uptake by basolateral and luminal membrane vesicles from rabbit kidney cortex. Am J Physiol. 1983;244:F686-95.
28. Wright SH, Wunz TM. Transport of tetraethylammonium by rabbit renal brush-border and basolateral membrane vesicles. Am J Physiol. 1987;253:F1040-50.
29. Brennan TS, Klahr S, Hamm LL. Citrate transport in rabbit nephron. Am J Physiol. 1986;251:F683-9.
30. Pajor AM. Sequence and functional characterization of a renal sodium/dicarboxylate cotransporter. J Biol Chem. 1995;270:5779-85.
31. Pajor AM. Molecular cloning and functional expression of a sodium-dicarboxylate cotransporter from human kidney. Am J Physiol 1996;270:F642-8.
32. Markovich D, Forgo J, Stange G, et al. Expression cloning of rat renal Na+/SO4(2-) cotransport. Proc Natl Acad Sci USA. 1993;90:8073-7.
33. Willmes DM, Birkenfeld AL. The Role of INDY in Metabolic Regulation. Comput Struct Biotechnol J. 2013;6:e201303020.
34. Pajor AM. Molecular properties of sodium/dicarboxylate cotransporters. Journal of Membr Biol. 2000;175:1-8.
35. Aruga S, Wehrli S, Kaissling B, et al. Chronic metabolic acidosis increases NaDC-1 mRNA and protein abundance in rat kidney. Kidney Int. 2000;58:206-15.
36. Sekine T, Cha SH, Hosoyamada M, et al. Cloning, functional characterization, and localization of a rat renal Na+-dicarboxylate transporter. Am J Physiol. 1998;275:F298-305.
37. Levi M, McDonald L, Priesig P. Chronic K depletion stimulates rat renal brush-border membrane Na-citrate cotransporter. Am J Physiol Renal Physiol. 1991;261:F767-73.
38. Boehmer C, Embark HM, Bauer A, et al. Stimulation of renal Na+ dicarboxylate cotransporter 1 by Na+/H+ exchanger regulating factor 2, serum and glucocorticoid inducible kinase isoforms, and protein kinase B. Biochem Biophys Res Commun. 2004;313:998-1003.
39. Pajor AM, Sun N. Protein kinase C-mediated regulation of the renal Na(+)/dicarboxylate cotransporter, NaDC-1. Biochim et Biophys Acta. 1999;1420:223-30.
40. Kekuda R, Wang H, Huang W, et al. Primary structure and functional characteristics of a mammalian sodium-coupled high affinity dicarboxylate transporter. J Biol Chem. 1999;274:3422-9.
41. Hagos Y, Burckhardt BC, Larsen A, et al. Regulation of sodium-dicarboxylate cotransporter-3 from winter flounder kidney by protein kinase C. Am J Physiol Renal Physiol. 2004;286:F86-93.
42. Palmieri F. The mitochondrial transporter family SLC25: identification, properties and physiopathology. Mol Aspects Med. 2013;34:465-84.
43. Mazurek MP, Prasad PD, Gopal E, et al. Molecular origin of plasma membrane citrate transporter in human prostate epithelial cells. EMBO Rep. 2010;11:431-7.
44. Ohana E, Shcheynikov N, Moe OW, et al. SLC26A6 and NaDC-1 transporters interact to regulate oxalate and citrate homeostasis. J Am Soc Nephrol. 2013;24:1617-26.
45. Klein KL, Wang MS, Torikai S, et al. Substrate oxidation by isolated single nephron segments of the rat. Kidney Int. 1981;20:29-35.
46. Crawford MA, Milne MD, Scribner BH. The effects of changes in acid-base balance on urinary citrate in the rat. J Physiol (London). 1959;149:413-23.
47. Crawford M. The effects of fluoroacetate, malonate and acid-base balance on the renal disposal of citrate. Biochem J. 1963;88:115-20.
48. Hems DA, Brosnan JT. Effects of metabolic acidosis and starvation on the content of intermediary metabolites in rat kidney. Biochem J. 1971;123:391-7.
49. Simpson DP. Tissue citrate levels and citrate utilization after sodium bicarbonate administration. Proc Soc Exp Biol Med. 1963;114:263-5.
50. Balagura-Baruch S, Burich RL, King VF. Effects of alkalosis on renal citrate metabolism in dogs infused with citrate. Am J Physiol. 1973;225:385-8.
51. Chypre M, Zaidi N, Smans K. ATP-citrate lyase: a mini-review. Biochem Biophys Res Commun. 2012;422:1-4.
52. Melnick JZ, Srere PA, Elshourbagy NA, et al. Adenosine triphosphate citrate lyase mediates hypocitraturia in rats. J Clin Invest. 1996;98:2381-7.
53. Simpson DP. Regulation of renal citrate metabolism by bicarbonate ion and pH: observations in tissue slices and mitochondria. J Clin Invest. 1967;46:225-38.

54. Brennan S, Hering-Smith K, Hamm LL. Effect of pH on citrate reabsorption in the proximal convoluted tubule. Am J Physiol. 1988;255:F301-6.
55. Barac-Nieto M. Effects of pH, calcium, and succinate on sodium citrate cotransport in renal microvilli. Am J Physiol. 1984;247:F282-90.
56. Grassl SM, Heinz E, Kinne R. Effect of K^+ and H^+ on sodium/citrate cotransport in renal brush-border vesicles. Biochim Biophys Acta. 1983;736:178-88.
57. Jenkins AD, Dousa TP, Smith LH. Transport of citrate across renal brush border membrane: effects of dietary acid and alkali loading. Am J Physiol. 1985;249:F590-5.
58. Wright SH, Kippen I, Wright EM. Effect of pH on the transport of Krebs cycle intermediates in renal brush border membranes. Biochim Biophys Acta. 1982;684:287-90.
59. Liu L, Zacchia M, Tian X, et al. Acid regulation of NaDC-1 requires a functional endothelin B receptor. Kidney Int. 2010;78:895-904.
60. Melnick JZ, Preisig PA, Moe OW, et al. Renal cortical mitochondrial aconitase is regulated in hypo- and hypercitraturia. Kidney Int. 1998;54:160-5.
61. Anaizi NH, Cohen JJ, Black AJ, et al. Renal tissue citrate: independence from citrate utilization, reabsorption, and pH. Am J Physiol. 1986;251:F547-61.
62. Gordon EE. The metabolism of citrate-C-14 in normal and in fluoroinhibitor-poisoned rats. J Clin Invest. 1961;40:1719-26.
63. Heller HJ, Sakhaee K, Moe OW, et al. Etiological role of estrogen status in renal stone formation. J Urol. 2002;168:1923-7.
64. Parks J, Ruml L, Pak C. Hypocitraturia, Chap. 40. In: Coe F, Favus M, Pak C, et al. (Eds). Kidney Stones: Medical and Surgical Management. Philadelphia, PA: Lippincott-Raven Publishers' 1996. pp. 905-20.
65. Maikranz P, Holley J, Parks J, et al. Gestational hypercalciuria causes pathological urine calcium oxalate supersaturations. Kidney Int. 1989;36:108-13.
66. Shorr E, Almy T, Sloan M, et al. The relation between the urinary excretion of citric acid and calcium; its implications for urinary calcium stone formation. Science. 1942;96:587-8.
67. Alpern RJ, Sakhaee K. The clinical spectrum of chronic metabolic acidosis: homeostatic mechanisms produce significant morbidity. Am J Kidney Dis. 1997;29:291-302.
68. Dey J, Creighton A, Lindberg JS, et al. Estrogen replacement increased the citrate and calcium excretion rates in postmenopausal women with recurrent urolithiasis. J Urol. 2002;167:169-71.
69. Hammar ML, Berg GE, Larsson L, et al. Endocrine changes and urinary citrate excretion. Scand J Urol Nephrol. 1987;21:51-3.
70. Maalouf NM, Sato AH, Welch BJ, et al. Postmenopausal hormone use and the risk of nephrolithiasis: results from the Women's Health Initiative hormone therapy trials. Arch Intern Med. 2010;170:1678-85.
71. Mattix Kramer HJ, Grodstein F, Stampfer MJ, et al. Menopause and postmenopausal hormone use and risk of incident kidney stones. J Am Soc Nephrol. 2003;14:1272-7.
72. Hering-Smith KS, Gambala CT, Hamm LL. Citrate and succinate transport in proximal tubule cells. Am J Physiol Renal Physiol 2000;278:F492-8.
73. Hering-Smith KS, Schiro FR, Pajor AM, et al. Calcium sensitivity of dicarboxylate transport in cultured proximal tubule cells. Am J Physiol Renal Physiol. 2011;300:F425-32.
74. Bushinsky DA, Kim M, Sessler NE, et al. Increased urinary saturation and kidney calcium content in genetic hypercalciuric rats. Kidney Int. 1994;45:58-65.
75. Canary J, Lynch H, Kyle L, et al. Citric acid excretion before and after calcium infusion in normal and osteoporotic subjects. J Lab Clin Med. 1961;57:230-9.
76. Crawford M, Loughridge L, Milne M, et al. Organic acid excretion after calcium gluconate infusions. J Clin Pathol. 1959;12:524-9.
77. Hodgkinson A. The relation between citric acid and calcium metabolism with particular reference to primary hyperparathyroidism and idiopathic hypercalciuria. Clin Sci. 1963;24:167-8.
78. Taylor EN, Curhan GC. Demographic, dietary, and urinary factors and 24-h urinary calcium excretion. Clin J Am Soc Nephrol. 2009;4:1980-7.
79. Nicar MJ, Skurla C, Sakhaee K, et al. Low urinary citrate excretion in nephrolithiasis. Urology. 1983;21:8-14.
80. Parks JH, Coe FL. A urinary calcium-citrate index for the evaluation of nephrolithiasis. Kidney Int. 1986;30:85-90.
81. Albright F, Consolazio W, Coombs F. Metabolic studies and therapy in a case of nephrocalcinosis with rickets and dwarfism. Bull Johns Hopkins Hosp. 1940;66:7-33.
82. Dedmon RE, Wrong O. The excretion of organic anion in renal tubular acidosis with particular reference to citrate. Clin Sci. 1962;22:19-32.
83. Morrissey JF, Ochoa MJ, Lotspeich WD, et al. Citrate excretion in renal tubular acidosis. Ann Intern Med. 1963;58:159-66.
84. Backman U, Danielson B, Johansson G, et al. Incidence and clinical importance of renal tubular defects in recurrent stone formers. Nephron. 1980;25:96.
85. Brenes L, Sanchez M, Briceno L, et al. Isolated proximal renal tubular acidosis: dissociation of cellular and systemic pH. (abstract) J Am Soc Nephrol. 1991;2:279.
86. DuBose T, Alpern R. Renal tubular acidosis, Chap. 103. In: Scriver C, Beudet A, Sly W, Valle D (Eds). The Metabolic Basis of Inherited Disease, 6th edition, New York: McGraw-Hill; 1989. pp. 2539-68.
87. Halperin ML, Kamel KS, Ethier JH, et al. What is the underlying defect in patients with isolated, proximal renal tubular acidosis? Am J Nephrol. 1989;9:265-8.
88. Moe OW, Seldin DW, Baum M. The Fanconi syndrome. In: Lifton R, Somlo S, Seldin DW, Giebisch G (Eds). Genetic Diseases of the Kidney. New York. Elsevier; 2009. pp. 171-98.
89. Kurtz I, Zhu Q. Proximal renal tubular acidosis mediated by mutations in NBCe1-A: unraveling the transporter's structure-functional properties. Front Physiol. 2013;4:350.
90. Gordon E, Sheps S. Effect of acetazolamide on citrate excretion an formation of renal calculi. Report of a case study of five normal subjects. N Engl J Med. 1957;256:1215-9.
91. Breslau NA, Brinkley L, Hill KD, et al. Relationship of animal protein-rich diet to kidney stone formation and calcium metabolism. J Clin Endocrinol Metab. 1988;66:140-6.

92. Curhan GC, Willett WC, Rimm EB, et al. A prospective study of dietary calcium and other nutrients and the risk of symptomatic kidney stones. N Engl J Med. 1993;328:833-8.
93. Mandel EI, Taylor EN, Curhan GC. Dietary and lifestyle factors and medical conditions associated with urinary citrate excretion. Clin J Am Soc Nephrol. 2013;8:901-8.
94. Pak CY, Poindexter JR, Adams-Huet B, et al. Predictive value of kidney stone composition in the detection of metabolic abnormalities. Am J Med. 2003;115:26-32.
95. Windus DW, Cohn DE, Heifets M. Effects of fasting on citrate transport by the brush-border membrane of rat kidney. Am J Physiol. 1986;251:F678-82.
96. Adler S, Zett B, Anderson B. Renal citrate in the potassium-deficient rat: role of potassium and chloride ions. J Lab Clin Med. 1974;84:307-16.
97. Evans BM, Macintyre I, Macpherson CR, et al. Alkalosis in sodium and potassium depletion; with especial reference to organic acid excretion. Clin Sci (Lond). 1957;16:53-65.
98. Fourman P, Robinson JR. Diminish urinary excretion of citrate during deficiencies of potassium in man. Lancet. 1953;2:656-7.
99. Adam WR, Koretsky AP, Weiner MW. 31P-NMR in vivo measurement of renal intracellular pH: effects of acidosis and K+ depletion in rats. Am J Physiol. 1986;251:F904-10.
100. Brickman AS, Massry SG, Coburn JW. Changes in serum and urinary calcium during treatment with hydrochlorothiazide: studies on mechanisms. J Clin Invest. 1972;51:945-54.
101. Coe FL, Parks JH, Bushinsky DA, et al. Chlorthalidone promotes mineral retention in patients with idiopathic hypercalciuria. Kidney Int. 1988;33:1140-6.
102. Ohkawa M, Tokunaga S, Nakashima T, et al. Thiazide treatment for calcium urolithiasis in patients with idiopathic hypercalciuria. Br J Urol. 1992;69:571-6.
103. Rector FC Jr, Bloomer HA, Seldin DW. Effect of potassium deficiency on the reabsorption of bicarbonate in the proximal tubule of the rat kidney. J Clin Invest. 1964;43:1976-82.
104. The Antihypertensive and Lipid-Lowering Treatment to Prevent Heart Attack Trial (ALLHAT). Major outcomes in high-risk hypertensive patients randomized to angiotensin-converting enzyme inhibitor or calcium channel blocker vs diuretic. JAMA. 2002;288:2981-997.
105. Menon DV, Arbique D, Wang Z, et al. Differential effects of chlorthalidone versus spironolactone on muscle sympathetic nerve activity in hypertensive patients. J Clin Endocrinol Metab. 2009;94:1361-1366.
106. Nicar MJ, Peterson R, Pak CY. Use of potassium citrate as potassium supplement during thiazide therapy of calcium nephrolithiasis. J Urol. 1984;131:430-3.
107. Sakhaee K, Harvey JA, Padalino PK, et al. The potential role of salt abuse on the risk for kidney stone formation. J Urol. 1993;150:310-2.
108. Marangella M, Vitale C, Manganaro M, et al. Renal handling of citrate in chronic renal insufficiency. Nephron. 1991;57:439-43.
109. Sakhaee K, Nigam S, Snell P, et al. Assessment of the pathogenetic role of physical exercise in renal stone formation. J Clin Endocrinol Metab 1987;65:974-9.
110. Melnick JZ, Preisig PA, Haynes S, et al. Converting enzyme inhibition causes hypocitraturia independent of acidosis or hypokalemia. Kidney Int. 1998;54:1670-4.
111. Pajor AM, Sun NN. Single nucleotide polymorphisms in the human Na+-dicarboxylate cotransporter affect transport activity and protein expression. Am J Physiol Renal Physiol. 2010;299:F704-11.
112. Bond PA, Jenner FA. The effect of lithium and related metal ions on the urinary excretion of 2-oxoglutarate and citrate in the rat. Br J Pharmacol. 1974;50:283-9.
113. Bond PA, Jenner FA, Lee CR, et al. The effect of lithium salts on the urinary excretion of -oxoglutarate in man. Br J Pharmacol. 1972;46:116-23.
114. Pak CY, Fuller C. Idiopathic hypocitraturic calcium-oxalate nephrolithiasis successfully treated with potassium citrate. Ann Intern Med. 1986;104:33-7.
115. Fegan J, Khan R, Poindexter J, et al. Gastrointestinal citrate absorption in nephrolithiasis. J Urol. 1992;147:1212-4.
116. Okamoto N, Aruga S, Matsuzaki S, et al. Associations between renal sodium-citrate cotransporter (hNaDC-1) gene polymorphism and urinary citrate excretion in recurrent renal calcium stone formers and normal controls. Int J Urol. 2007;14:344-9.
117. Hallson PC, Kasidas GP, Samuell CT. The inhibitory activity of some citrate analogues upon calcium crystalluria: observations using an improved urine evaporation technique. Urol Int. 1996;57:43-7.
118. Robertson WG, Scurr DS. Modifiers of calcium oxalate crystallization found in urine. I. Studies with a continuous crystallizer using an artificial urine. J Urol. 1986;135:1322-6.
119. Greischar A, Nakagawa Y, Coe FL. Influence of urine pH and citrate concentration on the upper limit of metastability for calcium phosphate. J Urol. 2003;169:867-70.
120. Nicar MJ, Hill K, Pak CY. Inhibition by citrate of spontaneous precipitation of calcium oxalate in vitro. J Bone Miner Res. 1987;2:215-20.
121. Tiselius HG, Fornander AM, Nilsson MA. The effects of citrate and urine on calcium oxalate crystal aggregation. Urol Res. 1993;21:363-6.
122. Caudarella R, Vescini F. Urinary citrate and renal stone disease: the preventive role of alkali citrate treatment. Arch Ital Urol Androl. 2009;81:182-7.
123. Ganter K, Bongartz D, Hesse A. Tamm-Horsfall protein excretion and its relation to citrate in urine of stone-forming patients. Urology. 1999;53:492-5.
124. Glauser A, Hochreiter W, Jaeger P, et al. Determinants of urinary excretion of Tamm-Horsfall protein in non-selected kidney stone formers and healthy subjects. Nephrol Dial Transplant. 2000;15:1580-7.
125. Fuselier HA, Ward DM, Lindberg JS, et al. Urinary Tamm-Horsfall protein increased after potassium citrate therapy in calcium stone formers. Urology. 1995;45:942-6.
126. Hess B, Nakagawa Y, Coe FL. Inhibition of calcium oxalate monohydrate crystal aggregation by urine proteins. Am J Physiol. 1989;257:F99-106.
127. Pak CY, Moe OW, Maalouf NM, et al. Comparison of semi-empirical and computer derived methods for estimating urinary saturation of brushite. J Urol. 2009;181:1423-8.

128. Pak CY. Physicochemical basis for formation of renal stones of calcium phosphate origin: calculation of the degree of saturation of urine with respect to brushite. J Clin Invest. 48:1914-22, 1969.
129. Pak CY, Rodgers K, Poindexter JR, et al. New methods of assessing crystal growth and saturation of brushite in whole urine: effect of pH, calcium and citrate. J Urol. 2008;180:1532-7.
130. Werness PG, Brown CM, Smith LH, et al. EQUIL2: a BASIC computer program for the calculation of urinary saturation. J Urol. 1985;134:1242-4.
131. Rodgers A, Allie-Hamdulay S, Jackson G. Therapeutic action of citrate in urolithiasis explained by chemical speciation: increase in pH is the determinant factor. Nephrol Dial Transplant. 2006;21:361-9.
132. Pak CY, Sakhaee K, Fuller CJ. Physiological and physiochemical correction and prevention of calcium stone formation by potassium citrate therapy. Trans Assoc Am Physicians. 1983;96:294-305.
133. Pearle MS, Goldfarb DS, Assimos DG, et al. Medical management of kidney stones: AUA guideline. J Urol. 2014;192:316-24.
134. Rumenapf G, Schwille PO. The influence of oral alkali citrate on intestinal calcium absorption in healthy man. Clin Sci (Lond). 1987;73:117-21.
135. Rumenapf G, Schwille PO. The influence of citrate on the duodenal absorption of calcium in the rat. Calcif Tissue Int. 1988;42:326-30.
136. Schwille PO, Rumenapf G, Kohler R, et al. Effects of acute oral sodium potassium citrate load in healthy males—outlook for treatment of patients with calcium-containing renal stones. Urol Int. 1987;42:81-8.
137. Bushinsky DA. Metabolic alkalosis decreases bone calcium efflux by suppressing osteoclasts and stimulating osteoblasts. Am J Physiol. 1996;271:F216-22.
138. Sakhaee K, Nicar M, Hill K, et al. Contrasting effects of potassium citrate and sodium citrate therapies on urinary chemistries and crystallization of stone-forming salts. Kidney Int. 1983;24:348-52.
139. Sebastian A, Harris ST, Ottaway JH, et al. Improved mineral balance and skeletal metabolism in postmenopausal women treated with potassium bicarbonate. N Engl J Med. 1994;330:1776-81.
140. Bonny O, Rubin A, Huang CL, et al. Mechanism of urinary calcium regulation by urinary magnesium and pH. J Am Soc Nephrol. 2008;19:1530-7.
141. Yeh BI, Sun TJ, Lee JZ, et al. Mechanism and molecular determinant for regulation of rabbit transient receptor potential type 5 (TRPV5) channel by extracellular pH. J Biol Chem. 2003;278:51044-52.
142. Ryall RL. Urinary inhibitors of calcium oxalate crystallization and their potential role in stone formation. World J Urol. 1997;15:155-64.
143. Moe OW, Pearle MS, Sakhaee K. Pharmacotherapy of urolithiasis: evidence from clinical trials. Kidney Int. 2011;79:385-92.
144. Lemann J Jr, Gray RW, Pleuss JA. Potassium bicarbonate, but not sodium bicarbonate, reduces urinary calcium excretion and improves calcium balance in healthy men. Kidney Int. 1989;35:688-95.
145. Pak CY, Koenig K, Khan R. et al. Physicochemical action of potassium-magnesium citrate in nephrolithiasis. J Bone Mineral Res. 1992;7:281-5.
146. Ruml LA, Pak CY. Effect of potassium magnesium citrate on thiazide-induced hypokalemia and magnesium loss. Am J Kidney Dis. 1999;34:107-13.
147. Oster JR, Stemmer CL, Perez GO, et al. Comparison of the effects of sodium bicarbonate versus sodium citrate on renal acid excretion. Miner Electrolyte Metab. 1988;14:97-102.
148. Sakhaee K, Alpern R, Poindexter J, et al. Citraturic response to oral citric acid load. J Urol. 1992;147:975-6.
149. Meschi T, Maggiore U, Fiaccadori E, et al. The effect of fruits and vegetables on urinary stone risk factors. Kidney Int. 2004;66:2402-10.
150. Prezioso D, Strazzullo P, Lotti T, et al. Dietary treatment of urinary risk factors for renal stone formation. A review of CLU Working Group. Arch Ital Urol Androl. 2015;87:105-20.
151. Mattle D, Hess B. Preventive treatment of nephrolithiasis with alkali citrate—a critical review. Urol Res. 2005;33:73-9.
152. Pearle MS, Roehrborn CG, Pak CY. Meta-analysis of randomized trials for medical prevention of calcium oxalate nephrolithiasis. J Endourol. 1999;13:679-85.
153. Robinson MR, Leitao VA, Haleblian GE, et al. Impact of long-term potassium citrate therapy on urinary profiles and recurrent stone formation. J Urol. 2009;181:1145-50.
154. Barcelo P, Wuhl O, Servitge E, et al. Randomized double-blind study of potassium citrate in idiopathic hypocitraturic calcium nephrolithiasis. J Urol. 1993;150:1761-4.
155. Ettinger B, Pak CY, Citron JT, et al. Potassium-magnesium citrate is an effective prophylaxis against recurrent calcium oxalate nephrolithiasis. J Urol. 1997;158:2069-73.
156. Hofbauer J, Hobarth K, Szabo N, et al. Alkali citrate prophylaxis in idiopathic recurrent calcium oxalate urolithiasis—a prospective randomized study. Br J Urol. 1994;73:362-5.
157. Lojanapiwat B, Tanthanuch M, Pripathanont C, et al. Alkaline citrate reduces stone recurrence and regrowth after shockwave lithotripsy and percutaneous nephrolithotomy. Int Braz J Urol. 2011;37:611-6.
158. Soygur T, Akbay A, Kupeli S. Effect of potassium citrate therapy on stone recurrence and residual fragments after shockwave lithotripsy in lower caliceal calcium oxalate urolithiasis: a randomized controlled trial. J Endourol. 2002;16:149-52.
159. Pak CY, Fuller C, Sakhaee K, et al. Long-term treatment of calcium nephrolithiasis with potassium citrate. J Urol. 1985;134:11-9.
160. Whalley NA, Meyers AM, Martins M, et al. Long-term effects of potassium citrate therapy on the formation of new stones in groups of recurrent stone formers with hypocitraturia. Br J Urol. 1996;78:10-14.
161. Coburn JW, Mischel MG, Goodman WG, et al. Calcium citrate markedly enhances aluminum absorption from aluminum hydroxide. Am J Kidney Dis. 1991;17:708-11.

162. Froment DP, Molitoris BA, Buddington B, et al. Site and mechanism of enhanced gastrointestinal absorption of aluminum by citrate. Kidney Int. 1989;36:978-84.
163. Molitoris BA, Froment DH, Mackenzie TA, et al. Citrate: a major factor in the toxicity of orally administered aluminum compounds. Kidney Int. 1989;36:949-53.
164. Sakhaee K, Ruml L, Padalino P, et al. The lack of influence of long-term potassium citrate and calcium citrate treatment in total body aluminum burden in patients with functioning kidneys. J Am Coll Nutr. 1996;15:102-6.
165. Sakhaee K, Wabner CL, Zerwekh JE, et al. Calcium citrate without aluminum antacids does not cause aluminum retention in patients with functioning kidneys. Bone Miner. 1993;20:87-97.
166. Odvina CV, Preminger GM, Lindberg JS, et al. Long-term combined treatment with thiazide and potassium citrate in nephrolithiasis does not lead to hypokalemia or hypochloremic metabolic alkalosis. Kidney Int. 2003;63:240-7.
167. Moe OW, Abate N, Sakhaee K. Pathophysiology of uric acid nephrolithiasis. Endocrinol Metab Clin North Am. 2002;31:895-914.
168. Cameron MA, Maalouf NM, Adams-Huet B, et al. Urine composition in type 2 diabetes: predisposition to uric acid nephrolithiasis. J Am Soc Nephrol. 2006;17:1422-8.
169. Maalouf NM, Cameron MA, Moe OW, et al. Low urine pH: a novel feature of the metabolic syndrome. Clin J Am Soc Nephrol. 2007;2:883-8.
170. Wiederkehr MR, Moe OW. Uric acid nephrolithiasis: a systemic metabolic disorder. Clin Rev Bone Miner Metab 9:207-217, 2011
171. Cameron M, Maalouf NM, Poindexter J, et al. The diurnal variation in urine acidification differs between normal individuals and uric acid stone formers. Kidney Int. 2012;81:1123-30.
172. Abate N, Chandalia M, Cabo-Chan AVJ, et al. The metabolic syndrome and uric acid nephrolithiasis: novel features of renal manifestation of insulin resistance. Kidney Int. 2004;65:386-92.
173. Pak CY, Sakhaee K, Fuller C. Successful management of uric acid nephrolithiasis with potassium citrate. Kidney Int. 1986;30:422-8.
174. Krieger NS, Asplin JR, Frick KK, et al. Effect of potassium citrate on calcium phosphate stones in a model of hypercalciuria. J Am Soc Nephrol. 2015;26(12):3001-8.
175. Prevention of recurrent calcium stone formation with potassium citrate therapy in patients with distal renal tubular acidosis. Preminger GM, Sakhaee K, Skurla C, Pak CY. J Urol. 1985 Jul;134(1):20-3.
176. Long-term treatment with potassium citrate and renal stones in medullary sponge kidney. Fabris A, Lupo A, Bernich P, Abaterusso C, Marchionna N, Nouvenne A, Gambaro G. Clin J Am Soc Nephrol. 2010 Sep;5(9):1663-8
177. Mandel N, Mandel I, Fryjoff K, et al. Conversion of calcium oxalate to calcium phosphate with recurrent stone episodes. J Urol. 2003;169:2026-9.
179. Parks JH, Worcester EM, Coe FL, et al. Clinical implications of abundant calcium phosphate in routinely analyzed kidney stones. Kidney Int. 2004;66:777-85.
179. Hering-Smith KS, Mao W, Schiro FR, et al. Localization of the calcium-regulated citrate transport process in proximal tubule cells. Urolithiasis. 2014;42:209-19.

CHAPTER

11

Urine pH: Relationship to Integrative Physiology of Calcium, Phosphate, and Magnesium, and Prevention of Calcium Phosphate Precipitation

Mitchell L Halperin, Orson W Moe

INTRODUCTION

The term incomplete renal tubular acidosis (iRTA) can be considered a misnomer, as there is no acidemia or acidosis. Rather, it represents a heterogeneous and incompletely defined group of disorders that have in common a high urine pH (UpH). At times, this diagnosis is incorrect because the patient actually has acidemia and thus is incompatible with the definition of the disorder. *The clinical importance of a diagnosis of iRTA is that it is associated with recurrent calcium phosphate ($CaHPO_4$) kidney stones especially in young patients and possibly nephrocalcinosis; and UpH plays a critical role in the pathogenesis.* We will present an integrative physiologic approach to enhance the understanding of a most fundamental biologic concept of prevention of calcium phosphate precipitation.

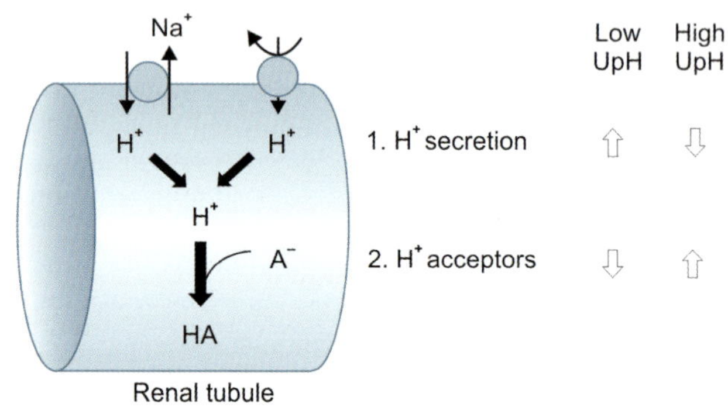

Fig. 11.1: Determinants of urine pH (UpH). Urine pH is determined by amount of H^+ secreted into the urine and the amount and propensity of H^+ acceptors to buffer the H^+ (shown as A). Low and high UpH can be caused by changes in H^+ secretion and/or H^+ acceptors.

DETERMINANTS OF UpH

In general, UpH is major a risk factor in urolithiasis.[1,2] There are separate chapters devoted to specific diseases that involve UpH, as part of the pathogenesis of stones such as calcium phosphate ($CaHPO_4$), uric acid stones, complete distal RTA (dRTA), and hypocitraturia. In this chapter, we shall focus on selected aspects of integrative physiology of calcium, inorganic phosphate, and magnesium that affect and prevent the formation of $CaHPO_4$ via modulation of UpH. We shall discuss the entity of iRTA and the importance of interorgan integrative physiology involving the gastrointestinal (GI) tract and liver, mammary gland, and the kidneys.

Normal Range of UpH

The two principal determinants of the UpH are H^+ secretion into the lumen of the nephron and the sum of all luminal ions and compounds that may bind H^+ (Fig. 11.1). For any type of H^+ acceptor, its concentration and the pH of the ambient fluid affect its ability to remove H^+. The most important physiologic closed H^+ acceptor in the urine is phosphate due to its pH and p*K* [inorganic phosphate ($H_2PO_4^-$); relevant p*K* ~6.8;[3] total excretion of 10–30 mmol/day]. In addition, there are several other closed H^+ acceptors, which include creatinine (relevant p*K* ~4.8; total excretion is 7–15 mmol/day), and urate (relevant p*K* ~5.3; total excretion is 2–3 mmol/day).[4] The other potential lithogen with Ca^{2+} is carbonate (CO_3^{2-}), but its concentration is tiny when the UpH is less than 10. Under normal conditions filtered HCO_3^- is also a major acceptor of secreted H^+, and the vast majority of conditions promote $CaHPO_4$ formation by failing to remove filtered HCO_3^- and thereby convert HPO_4^{2-} to monovalent inorganic phosphate ($H_2PO_4^-$). The only possible exception may be exaggerated secretion of HCO_3^- by the chloride Cl^-/HCO_3^- anion exchanger (AE; i.e. pendrin) if there is also poor mixing (stirring) of the luminal fluid.

For open H^+ acceptors, the buffer capacity is higher if the quantity of H^+ acceptors is increased [e.g. HCO_3^-, as described above, and ammonia (NH_3)].[5] While HCO_3^- can be a powerful H^+ acceptor, the amount of HCO_3^- in normal urine is extremely low because the usual 24-hour UpH is close to 6.0. The distribution of daily UpH in 24-hour collections in healthy subjects is shown in Figure 11.2A with a

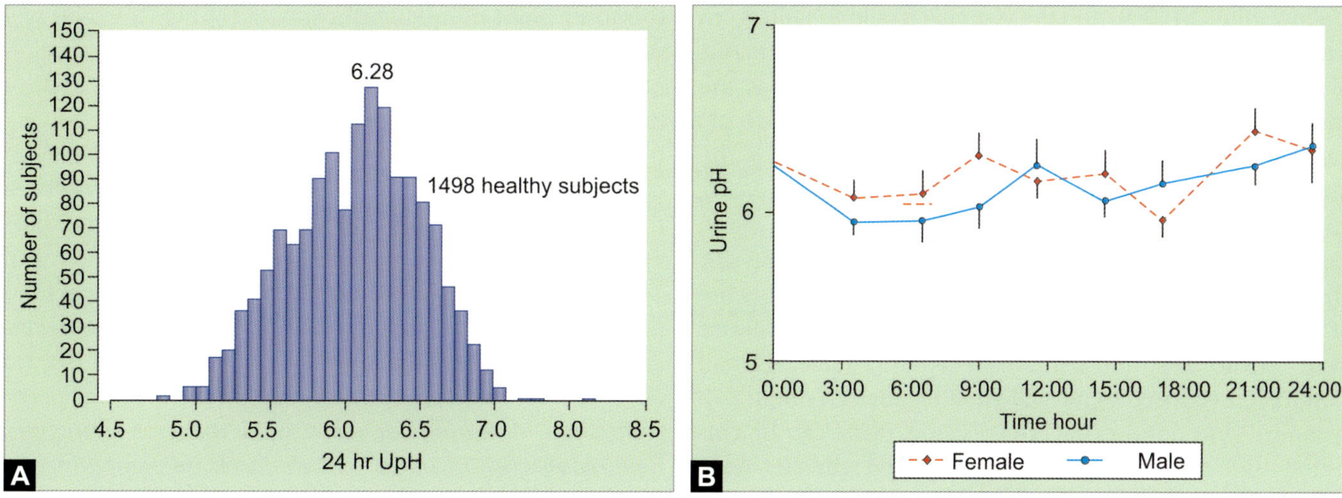

Figs. 11.2A and B: Human urine pH (UpH). (A) Distribution of 24-hour UpH in 1,498 healthy subjects on random ad lib diets (unpublished data from the Kidney Stone Registry of the Charles and Jane Pak Center of Mineral Metabolism and Clinical Research). Mean UpH 6.28 ± 0.54. (B) Urine was collected every 3 hours in 20 normal subjects (10 males and 10 females) over 24 hours (Halperin).

Table 11.1: Effect of pH on the concentrations of monovalent and divalent phosphate in an aqueous solution.

pH	$H_2PO_4^-$	HPO_4^{2-}
6.1	20	4
6.5	16	8
6.8	*12*	*12*
7.1	8	16
7.4	4	20
7.7	3	21

(We used a p*K* of $H_2PO_4^-$ of 6.8. At this pH, the concentrations of $H_2PO_4^-$ and HPO_4^{2-} are equal (bold). Moreover, the total content of $H_2PO_4^-$ plus HPO_4^{2-} is 24 mmol and the volume of this solution is one liter. Therefore, the values shown are in the mmol/L).

mean UpH on random ad lib diet around 6.28. The breakdown of this mean UpH with Q 2-hour urine collections is shown in Figure 11.2B. In fact, 80–90% of filtered HCO_3^- is reabsorbed prior to the loop of Henle (LOH) so physiologic changes in HCO_3^- in the distal nephron impart small contributions to total renal HCO_3^- reabsorption.[6]

The upper limit of UpH in higher primates is determined by physiologic needs (such as acid/base load/excretion) but constrained by solubility of uric acid in the lower range and solubility of $CaHPO_4$ in the upper range.[2] Uric acid stones are discussed elsewhere and persistently high UpH promotes $CaHPO_4$ precipitation, which is the major focus of this chapter, primarily due to high concentrations of divalent phosphate (HPO_4^{2-}) (Table 11.1).

Basis for an Increase or Decrease in Urine pH

There are limited ways to alter the UpH; it can be elevated by a decrease in the secretion of H^+, increased urinary H^+ acceptors, or both (*see* Fig. 11.1). The assumption of equivalence of UpH and acid excretion (low UpH = acid excretion) is not correct.[7] A patient with chronic kidney disease (CKD) has reduced ability to secrete H^+ but a simultaneous reduction in urinary buffering results in a low UpH in CKD.[8] An acute acid load to the organism increases net acid excretion and may lower the UpH, but when the same acid load is sustained, it may elevate ammoniagenesis and raise the UpH despite high net acid excretion.[9-12] Therefore, one should never simply equate dietary acid content with UpH.

There are multiple and highly complex systemic factors that can eventually alter H^+ secretion, H^+ acceptors abundance or both. In this chapter, we discuss a few of these factors with highlights on a challenging clinical condition, namely iRTA. We contrast that with several situations where the local concentrations of ionized calcium (Ca^{2+}) and/or HPO_4^{2-} are high, but $CaHPO_4$ does not precipitate.

Measurement of Urine pH in Clinical Practice

The usual UpH determination is by urinary dipstick on a random freshly (somewhat) voided urine. This is based on commonly used colorimetric pH indicators such methyl red (red-yellow; pH 4–6) and bromothymol blue (yellow–blue; pH 6–9) and the visualized color results from a mixture of the two dyes (orange pH 4; green pH 9). This method lacks both accuracy and precision but it is the easiest and most practical way. Accurate and precise pH determination requires a pH electrode. One issue is the relatively high pCO_2 in the normal urine of 60–80 mm Hg and can be as high as 100 in certain conditions.[13] Upon exposure to atmosphere, CO_2 escape can elevate the pH. For example, assuming a constant $[HCO_3^-]$ of 1 mm as the pCO_2 drops from 80 to 60, and 40 mm Hg, the UpH will rise from 5.72 to 5.84, and 6.02, respectively. Hence, a small sample left exposed to air will yield erroneously high pH. To retard (but not prevent) CO_2 escape, urine can be collected under mineral oil. This is often used when 24-hour urine is required. A true 24-hour urine collection removes the diurnal variations provides a representative snapshot of the mean UpH over the course of the day which is very useful for evaluation of stone risk (*see* Fig. 11.2A). Spot urines collected throughout the day are useful to examine the time profile of changes (*see* Fig. 11.2B) and will uncover extreme changes in certain times of the day.[14,15] Since, 24-hour urine collection is cumbersome, some have suggested using spot urine as a surrogate. Unfortunately, although spot UpH bears some relationship to 24-hour urine, there is insufficient correlation to justify replacing 24-hour urine with spot urine.[16]

PREVENTING FORMATION OF $CaHPO_4$ IN SITES OTHER THAN BONE

Although, these are not directly related to urolithiasis, prevention of extra-osseous $CaHPO_4$ formation is pervasive in biology and understanding how this is achieved in other organs help to understand the situation in the kidney.

Events in the GI Tract

The key elements that we consider are pH, Ca^{2+}, HPO_4^{2-}, and magnesium (Mg^{2+}) ions. The likelihood of forming precipitates varies depending formation of soluble ion complexes between two of these elements, plays a role in retarding $CaHPO_4$ precipitation in the intestinal luminal fluid.

In the Stomach and Duodenum

The low pH in the stomach (HCl secretion) has two consequences. First, alkaline calcium salts are converted to ionized Ca^{2+}, and second, since the p*K* of inorganic phosphate is ~6.8, most of the inorganic phosphate will be converted to monovalent inorganic phosphate ($H_2PO_4^-$), which will not react with Ca^{2+} to form $CaHPO_4$. Thus, the absorption of Ca^{2+} occurs early after stomach emptying into the duodenum, and it decreases when the luminal pH rises owing to alkaline pancreatic secretions, with abundant $NaHCO_3$ entering the lumen of the duodenum. Another purpose of this alkaline secretion is that it neutralizes the H^+ and prevents denaturation of the pancreatic digestive enzymes. *This is the rationale for having a significant amount of Ca^2+ absorption early in the duodenum, upstream from the pancreatic fluid addition and before conversion of $H_2PO_4^-$ to HPO_4^{2-}. This provides intestinal absorption of the Ca^{2+} needed for bone formation but not in excess thus preventing very high renal excretion of Ca^{2+} which has its inherent dangers.*

Site for Intestinal HPO_4^{2-} Formation and Absorption

Phosphate absorption must occur downstream from the duodenum after digestion of ingested organic phosphates. There is influence of Mg^{2+} on phosphate absorption because it forms a soluble ion complex with HPO_4^{2-} ($Mg{\cdot}HPO_4$) when their concentrations are high. However, this soluble complex between Mg^{2+} and HPO_4^{2-} must be lysed before or at the site for HPO_4^{2-} absorption in the jejunum. The site of absorption of Mg^{2+} must also be downstream from the site of absorption of HPO_4^{2-} otherwise the intestinal tract could not absorb dietary Mg^{2+}, and adenosine triphosphate (ATP) will not be in its biologically active form (soluble complex Mg·ATP). *Hence, the absorption of calcium, phosphate, and magnesium must occur at intestinal sites.* Moreover, more Mg^{2+} is absorbed daily than is needed in the body and the excess is excreted in the urine (~3 mmol/day) where it contributes to prevention of $CaHPO_4$ formation, as discussed below.

Events in the Kidneys

Ca^{2+} Absorption in the PCT

Much of the filtered Ca^{2+} is reclaimed in the proximal convoluted tubule (PCT) along with reabsorption of most of the filtered Na^+ and water, thereby decreasing the volume of luminal fluid, which will raise the concentration of Ca^{2+}. This will create a concentration difference favoring the passive absorption of Ca^{2+} driving its concentration to close approximate of that in plasma. Thus, there is little danger of high concentration of luminal Ca^{2+} in the early PCT because citrate is virtually all citrate^{3-}, which chelates a majority of the filtered Ca^{2+} ($Ca^{2+}{\cdot}citrate^{3-}$ = $CaCitrate^-$

complex). The large quantity of H^+ secretion in the PCT also lowers the luminal pH, converting HPO_4^{2-} to $H_2PO_4^-$.[17] Hence the concentration of HPO_4^{2-} becomes a smaller fraction of the filtered total inorganic phosphate (*see* Table 11.1). In addition, there is another defense mechanism. The amount of Mg^{2+} absorbed in the early part of the PCT is very modest resulting in the formation of a soluble ion complex ($Mg^{2+}HPO_4^{2-}$), akin to that of the soluble CaCitrate⁻ complex. Expansion of the effective arterial blood volume following a high NaCl intake will decrease reabsorption in the PCT resulting in diminished absorption of Ca^{2+} and thus a larger delivery of Ca^{2+} to the distal nephron and the urine.[18] A low intake of salt or the loss of NaCl by nonrenal routes can increase the absorption of Na^+, water, and Ca^{2+} in the PCT which is the a rationale for prescribing a low intake of NaCl in patients with calcium-containing kidney stones.[19]

Beyond the Proximal Tubule (PT)

Precipitation of Ca^{2+} and HPO_4^{2-}, as $CaHPO_4$ in the urine and in the renal medullary interstitial compartment must be avoided at all cost because these precipitates can be dangerous. *The key first step is to ensure that there will be enough citrate anions in the lumen of the nephron to prevent $CaHPO_4$ kidney stone formation. This same physiology is required in the lumen of the nephron in the bend of the LOH in the inner medulla. In addition, Mg^{2+} may play an important role by chelating HPO_4^{2-}*. Thus, both of these chelators are present in the lumen of the PCT owing to properties in cells of this nephron segment unless the proximal tubule cell is acidified (which increases proximal citrate reabsorption). In this case, the rate of excretion of citrate may be extremely low[20,21] and this contributes in a major way to the likelihood of forming calcium-containing kidney stones (*see* Chapter 10 on citrate and kidney stones) especially if there is a high concentration of HPO_4^{2-} (*i.e.* for the latter to be high, the luminal concentration of bicarbonate (HCO_3^-) must rise owing to the fact that the descending thin limbs (DtLs) of the LOH of the juxtamedullary nephrons have aquaporin-1 water channels[22] and there is an enormous osmotic force to absorb filtered water during transit through their DtL, which will raise the concentrations of Ca^{2+}, Mg^{2+}, HCO_3^-, and thereby HPO_4^{2-} will also rise in their luminal fluid in the bend of the loop. If all of this HCO_3^- were not reabsorbed in downstream nephron sites, the UpH may be high enough to have a high concentration of HPO_4^{2-} in the urine. In addition, contrary to the fact that the PCT reabsorbs virtually all of the valuable ions and compounds, this general rule does not apply for Mg^{2+}.[23] The likely rationale is that Mg^{2+} forms a soluble complex ($MgHPO_4$), which lowers the concentration of HPO_4^{2-} in the lumen of the LOH and in the urine. In this setting, $CaHPO_4$ will precipitate unless there is a high enough concentration of Mg^{2+} to lower the concentration of HPO_4^{2-} in the lumen of the juxtamedullary nephrons (JMN) deep in the inner medullary collecting duct (iMCD).

When potassium ions (K^+) are secreted through renal outer medullary potassium channel (ROMK) channels in the medullary thick ascending limbs (mTALs) of the LOH, their luminal voltage becomes positive,[24] which creates a greater driving force for the exit of divalent cations (Ca^{2+} and Mg^{2+}) in the mTAL than for the more abundant monovalent cation sodium (Na^+). The entry of Mg^{2+} into the medullary interstitial compartment could minimize **$CaHPO_4$** formation and nephrocalcinosis. There are two factors that could play an essential role in preventing this unwanted interstitial $CaHPO_4$ deposition—surprisingly low PCT reabsorption of Mg^{2+}, and the appearance of Tamm–Horsfall glycoproteins in the lumen of the mTAL. Tamm Horsfall protein (THP) is the most abundant protein in the urine of humans and has the ability to inhibit luminal Ca^{2+} precipitation.[25] *Thus, even though the concentrations of calcium and HPO_4^{2-} might seem to have exceeded their solubility constant (Ksp), precipitation of $CaHPO_4$ is not inevitable if THP-chelated Ca^{2+} and Mg^{2+} formed soluble ion complex with HPO_4^{2-} and thereby decreased the concentrations of these ions in the lumen of the mTAL.*

Events in the Mammary Gland

Mother's milk must supply the newborn with a safe, large, and timely supply of fuel and solutes to ensure that ATP regeneration is sufficient, bones become mineralized, and growth of organs occurs with synthesis of phosphate-rich essential compounds—*i.e.* to supply substances that cannot be made by the newborn which includes essential amino acids, K^+, Mg^{2+}, HPO_4^{2-}, and minor quantities of Na^+, and chloride anions (Cl^-).

Focus on Phosphate and Calcium

While both Ca^{2+} and HPO_4^{2-} are needed to form strong bones, this precipitation must not occur in other locations. Enough phosphate must be absorbed from the diet to be deposited in bones and to be converted into intracellular nucleic acids, phosphoproteins, phospholipids, and phosphoglycans. In addition, it is needed to synthesize phosphate-rich compounds essential for providing energy

Table 11.2: Examples of metabolic processes.
Oxidation of the fuel to regenerate used ATP^{4-}
Conversion of ingested fuels not needed for immediate ATP^{4-} synthesis to a storage form
Conversion of dietary protein into glucose or glycogen in liver for energy storage, or oxidation to regenerate ATP^{4-} in the brain
Conversion to a fuel of special purpose, e.g. citrate

(ATP and phosphocreatine) in the largest organ in the body (skeletal muscles).

There is a mechanism to avoid precipitation Ca^{2+} and HPO_4^{2-} in breast milk. The most abundant protein in the milk is casein which in addition to binding calcium phosphate complexes and Ca^{2+},[26] also has a large amount of covalently bound HPO_4^{2-} to it which prevents precipitation of $CaHPO_4$ despite the high concentration of Ca^{2+} in milk. This binding of HPO_4^{2-} to casein occurs because there is a kinase in mammary gland, which causes ATP to react with casein resulting in phosphorylation.

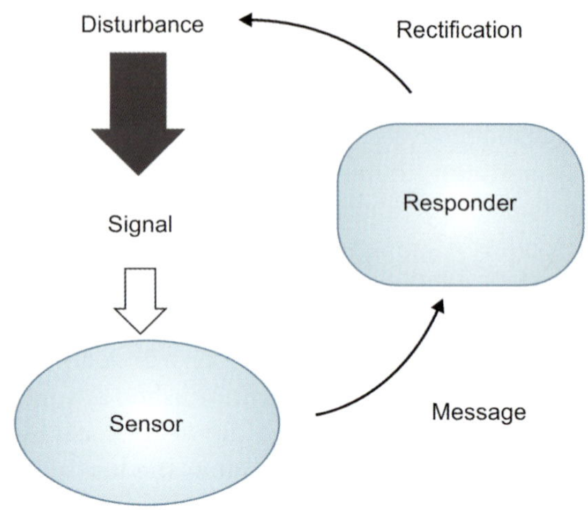

Fig. 11.3: Components of a control system. The disturbance generates a signal that is recognized by a sensor in a target organ (e.g. liver cells sensing incoming citrate from the portal system). A message is sent to response elements which may be located in other organs (e.g. the kidneys or the GI tract), which can rectify the disturbance such as removal of unwanted substances from the body without requiring very high circulating levels of these components of food.[27] (GI: Gastrointestinal).

Analysis with Emphasis on Metabolic Processes

Metabolic processes consist of a series of pathways, which may be present in the same or different organs to deal with ingested fuels to aid survival.[27] To analyze a metabolic process in acid–base terms, one must count the net valence of all of its substrates and products. If there are more anions produced than removed, there will be H^+ production to ensure electroneutrality. The best example is the complete oxidation of electroneutral sulfur-containing amino acids to $CO_2 + H_2O$, urea, and sulfate (SO_4^{2-}) plus $2H^+$. These H^+ will be removed by HCO_3^- in body water to forestall fall in pH. The decomposed HCO_3^- is replenished by metabolism of organic anions form the diet or excretion of ammonium (NH_4^+) in the urine. Some examples of metabolic processes of interest are depicted in Table 11.2. Storage forms of fuels include glycogen for carbohydrate, and triglycerides in adipose tissue for dietary fat or synthesized fatty acids. In the small intestine, more glucose is ingested and absorbed than is needed by the enterocyte to regenerate ATP^{4-} (e.g. energy expended in absorbing carbohydrates), so the extra substrate will be used for other purposes.

When viewed in the context of calcium-containing kidney stones, a fuel of special interest is citrate (Table 11.2). A separate chapter is devoted to urinary citrate handling (Chapter 10). Here, we examine the consequence oral citrate intake. Ingestion of citrate is often accompanied by K^+ in nature (e.g. in orange juice) or as a prescription for kidney stones. The components of a control system are depicted graphically in Figure 11.3. We shall illustrate one control system that deals with the challenge from dietary K^+ and more importantly with pharmacologic K^+ citrate.

Making K^+ and Citrate Ingestion Safe

K^+ and citrate are high in fruits and vegetables so omnivorous organisms have evolved ways to handle these solutes. In addition, patients with kidney stones can receive up to 60–80 mEq of K_3 citrate per day. If citrate and K^+ are not removed in a single pass by the liver, huge quantities could be added into arterial blood. The calcium-chelating effect of citrate will removed ionized calcium from blood delivered to the heart. Low ionized Ca^{2+} when coupled with the high K^+ is very detrimental to cardiac function and the subject will succumb to inadequate oxygen delivery to vital organs such as the brain. Since, all of our ancestors survived, we can anticipate that there must be control systems that are likely sensed and rectified by the liver.

Dietary sugar not completely removed a single pass in the liver increases glucose concentrations in plasma, and insulin is released into the portal vein. The release of l-lactic acid by enterocytes increases l-lactate concentration in the portal venous blood. This combination of signals form a strong stimulus for K^+ uptake into and

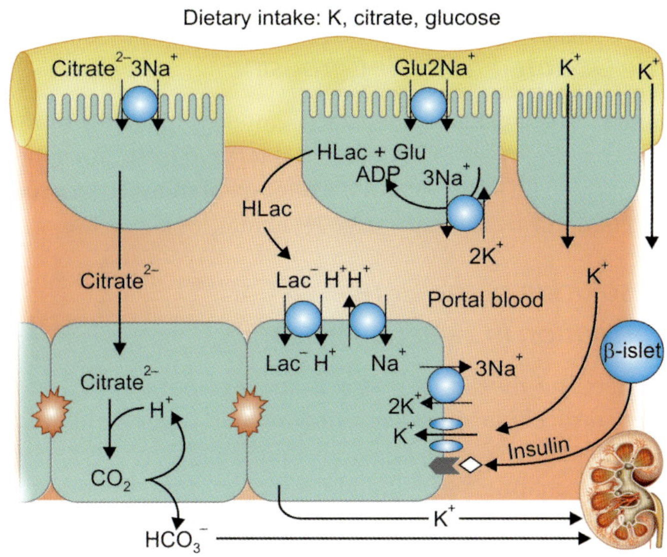

Fig. 11.4: Proposed defense mechanisms against hyperkalemia. The key is to hyperpolarization of hepatocytes as the liver is the only organ that can remove dietary K^+ and citrate before they compromise cardiac function. This model begins with the generation of l-lactic acid in enterocytes. Glucose transport uses 2 Na^+/glucose; Na exits via the basolateral Na^+–K^+-ATPase. Absorbing the normal dietary glucose mandates recruiting every Na^+ in the body to cycle 1.5 times/day in the gut which could be an enormous waste of energy unless it was a price-to-pay for survival on a K^+-rich Paleolithic diet. The ADP^{3-} generated stimulates anaerobic glycolysis in enterocytes (lack phosphocreatine^{2-}) resulting in high concentration of l-lactate in portal venous blood.[28,29] The [K^+] in portal blood is higher than the hepatic vein indicating K+ removal by the liver. Insulin stimulates Na^+–K^+-ATPase in hepatocytes[30] generating exit of a net positive charge, followed by the electroneutral entry of Na^+ on the Na^+/H^+ exchanger-1. Insulin and a low intracellular pH activate NHE-1. l-lactic acid enter hepatocytes on the monocarboxylic acid cotransporter (MCT; ref) releasing its H^+ near and activates NHE-1, providing the intracellular Na^+ for electrogenic Na^+ exit on Na–K-ATPase. Citrate is completely metabolized by the hepatocytes generating net HCO_3^- which is released from the hepatocyte and if there is a small rise in the plasma [K^+], that could provide a signal to reabsorb less $NaHCO_3$ in the PCT, and decrease activity of the H^+/K^+-ATPase in the inner medullary collecting duct.
(NHE-1: Na+/H+ exchanger-1; PCT: Proximal convoluted tubule).

temporary retention of K^+ in liver cells (Fig. 11.4), which can prevent life-threatening hyperkalemia in blood exiting the liver to reach the heart. Although, skeletal muscle is an important source of K^+ buffering, defense against dietary K^+ cannot wait until the arterial circulation because of the risk exposing the heart to hyperkalemia. Since, clinicians do not measure portal venous plasma, we never see this life-saving metabolic process in action.

A key mechanism to retain K^+ in the liver is the generation of a more negative interior voltage in hepatocytes. We alert the reader that this model is based largely hypothetical based on known properties of its key elements and evidence in experimental animals. The story is presented in detail in Figure 11.4. In summary, separate control systems deal with the need to supply vital organs with needed fuels to regenerate ATP, or to remove potentially harmful components of the diet (e.g. K^+ if ingested in amounts that exceed the immediate need for new cell formation). Accordingly, one can predict that the liver must have a signal that K^+ must not be delivered to the heart, which may be lethal. In general principle, one can predict that there must be a driving force to draw K^+ into liver cells and retain them in this location until the kidney can be sent a message to excrete this K^+ at a rapid rate without permitting a very high concentration of K^+ in plasma that will be delivered to the heart.

Events in Skeletal Muscle Cells that Prevent Formation of $CaHPO_4$

We describe the danger of $CaHPO_4$ formation in skeletal muscle and how pH is involved in its prevention. There are two phases of vigorous exercise and there is risk of $CaHPO_4$ precipitation in skeletal muscle cells. This danger becomes obvious when analyzed in quantitative and metabolic terms because the very large formation of HPO_4^{2-} in the first few seconds of a sprint when work is performed. The goal for the reader is to appreciate how the danger of forming $CaHPO_4$ is avoided in skeletal muscles in the alkaline phase of a sprint.

Alkaline Phase of a Sprint

$$\text{Work} + ATP^{4-} \rightarrow \text{adenosine diphosphate (ADP)}^{3-} + HPO_4^{2-} + H^+ \quad (1)$$

$$ADP^{3-} + \text{Phosphocreatine}^{2-} + H^+ \rightarrow \text{Creatine}^0 + ATP^{4-} \quad (2)$$

Sum of Equations (1) and (2):

$$\text{Work} + \text{Phosphocreatine}^{2-} \rightarrow HPO_4^{2-}$$

$$HPO_4^{2-} + H^+ \rightarrow H_2PO_4^- \quad (3)$$

When work is performed, ATP^{4-} is hydrolyzed and H^+ is formed [Equation (1)]. Despite this, the cell pH rises because ATP^{4-} must be regenerated rapidly to continue the essential work [Equation (2)]. ATP^{4-} is regenerated by two potential pathways. The stimulus to drive each of them is high concentration of one of the products of Equation (1)—ADP^{3-}, but one option is very rapid because it is single step and catalyzed by the enzyme, creatine phosphokinase with high abundance and activity [Equation (2)] whereas the other, which is glycolysis, has more than 10 steps with much slower kinetics. The rapid step occurs when phosphocreatine^{2-} is regenerated to maintain concentration of ATP^{4-} [Equation (2)]. The second metabolic step [Equation (2)] of the alkaline phase of a sprint removes the H$^+$ formed in Equation (1).

The sum of Equations (1) and (2) generates HPO_4^{2-}. There is one obvious way to lower the concentration of HPO_4^{2-}. Since, the quantity of phosphocreatinine^{2-} is very large (25 mmol/kg of muscle), it drives the reaction to the right, and HPO_4^{2-} accumulates, binds intracellular H$^+$, and renders the milieu alkaline. Since this new pH is higher than the p*K* for inorganic phosphate (~6.8), more than half of the total inorganic phosphate will be HPO_4^{2-} and it removes the extra H$^+$ formed in Equation (1) as well as many of the free H$^+$ in muscle cells, [Equation (3)]. When the pH rises, the H$^+$ bound to histidines in proteins and carnosine are released, making future "parking spots" for H$^+$ formed in the acid phase of the sprint *see* Equation (4) below. *In summary, one of the biochemical consequences initiated by ADP^{3-} that lead to the rapid hydrolysis of phosphocreatine^{2-} (P-Cr^{2-}) permit us to understand this alkaline phase of muscular work in which ATP^{4-} is regenerated primarily by the ADP^{3-} formed in Equation (1). Since, there are more negative charges in the substrates of Equation (2) than in its products, H$^+$ will be removed in the whole metabolic process of the alkaline phase of a sprint. In this phase of a sprint, skeletal muscle cells will be likely to produce $CaHPO_4$ because of their alkaline pH and a very large rate of concentration of HPO_4^{2-} [see sum of Equations (1) and (2)]. Thus, there must be mechanisms to prevent $CaHPO_4$ precipitation in these cells.* The reader can pause here and anticipate why $CaHPO_4$ is not formed in this stage of the sprint.

Acid Phase of a Sprint

This phase removes the alkali load described above; the sources of H$^+$ to lower the concentration of HPO_4^{2-} and to replace the H$^+$ released from nonbicarbonate buffers (e.g. H$^+$histidine in proteins and carnosine). In addition, some HCO_3^- may be exported from muscle cells (along with entry of chloride anions).

Production of H$^+$

As discussed above, accumulation of ADP^{3-} can drive anaerobic glycolysis (*i.e.* conversion of glucose to l-lactate anions, but there are no H$^+$ involved in this equation [Equation (4)]. Rather the H$^+$ are formed in Equation (1), which generates the ADP^{3-}. Thus, the first step in glycolysis is commonly overlooked.

$$\text{Glucose} + 2\,(ADP^{3-} + HPO_4^{2-}) \rightarrow 2\,(\text{l-lactate}^- + ATP^{4-}) \quad (4)$$

Removal of Surplus HPO_4^{2-} Occurs when H$^+$ are Donated from H$^+$ Carnosine

Since the cell pH is close to the p*K* for the phosphate buffer system, close to half of the HPO_4^{2-} formed from phosphocreatine^{2-} will serve to remove enough of these H$^+$ to avoid cell damage by this very large H$^+$ load.

Resolution of the Danger of $CaHPO_4$ Formation in Skeletal Muscle

Hence, the mechanism that is most important is a very low intracellular concentration of Ca^{2+}. When the voltage inside these cells becomes more negative, this causes the Ca^{2+} channels in cell membranes to close. In addition, there are proteins that will bind calcium and keep his concentration low and Ca^{2+} can be pumped into a different location using a Ca^{2+}-ATPase. Moreover maintaining a tiny initial concentration of Ca^{2+} improves the ability of having a large rise in its concentration in resting muscle cells is essential to avoid the formation of $CaHPO_4$ in skeletal muscle cells.[31]

INCOMPLETE DISTAL RTA

This diagnostic category is based primarily on the findings of a high UpH (>6.5) *and* the absence of systemic metabolic acidosis described by Wrong and Davies five and a half decades ago.[32] Notwithstanding, it includes more than one specific disease or pathophysiologic entity. It is important not to automatically equate a high UpH with dRTA. Ruling out other causes of a high UpH is necessary to improve diagnostic specificity. On the other hand, if the urine is infected with a urease-positive bacteria, there will be a simultaneous addition of NH_4^+ and HCO_3^- to the urine and the latter leads to a high UpH which is not a sign for a diagnosis of iRTA.

The label iRTA originated in an era where the lynch pin in the diagnosis of dRTA was a high UpH (>5.8) in patients with hyperchloremic metabolic acidosis (HCMA). High is defined by comparison to the 24-hour UpH in normal subjects who consume a typical Western diet. As one can see in Figure 11.2, on an outpatient ad libitum diet, normal subjects have a wide range of UpH with a mean around 6.3. Hence, it is not surprising that when patients present with recurrent stones, especially if this occurs at young age, and they have a high UpH in the absence of acidemia, a name given to this constellation of findings is iRTA because of the absence of acidemia.[33] This combination of findings, however, may be found in four circumstances; only the third one deserves the term iRTA. Therefore, of equal importance to recognizing iRTA is to identify patients with calcareous stones with features that mimic iRTA so one will not be misled.

True Distal RTA due to Low "Net" Distal Secretion of H^+

Some patients with Southeast Asian Ovalocytosis (SAO) have two mutations affecting their AE, the second mutation permits this AE to be mistargeted to the luminal membrane of α-intercalated cells[34] permitting the secretion of HCO_3^- and thereby a high UpH; the diagnostic clue for this pathophysiology was a high pCO_2 in the urine.[35] If these patients ingest potential alkali, they may not have acidemia, so it would be appropriate to call them RTA. Although patients with true dRTA usually have a low blood pH and $[HCO_3^-]$, this may not be present if they ingest a low net H^+ precursor load. For example, if their diet were to contain more alkali or potential alkali (e.g. more fruit and vegetables, and/or less precursors of H^+), acidemia may very well be absent. One option is to put the patient on a controlled metabolic diet to unmask the lesion. Alternatively, a key diagnostic step is finding a persistently low rate of ammonium (NH_4^+) excretion after chronic acidemia is induced by the administration of an acid load for several days (e.g. NH_4Cl).[32] The main point is that complete dRTA can have normal plasma parameters if the net acid load to the kidney is modest. Complete dRTA is discussed in Chapter 19.

Contamination of the Urine with a Bacterial Source of Urease

The presence of urease-containing bacteria can split urea into carbon dioxide ($[NH_2]2CO + H_2O \rightarrow CO_2 + 2NH_3$). The NH_3 combines with urinary H^+ which drives the UpH up significantly. The high UpH does not mean that the patient has impaired H^+ secretion or RTA. It is in fact a "postrenal" phenomenon. The key finding would be high UpH accompanied by an unexpected high rate of excretion of NH_4^+ (NH_4^+/SO_4^{2-} ratio >>1) and positive urine culture for organisms such as *Proteus mirabilis* and *Morganella morganii*. The stoned will also be $CaHPO_4$ and struvite ($NH_4MgPO_4{\cdot}6H_2O$).

Large Intermittent Intake of Alkali in a Normal Subject

This condition is physiologic and in fact not really a disease; it simply mimics some of the diagnostic features

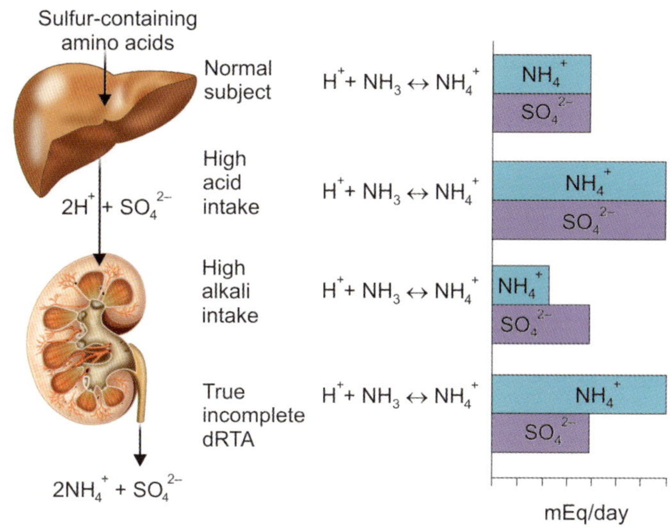

Fig. 11.5: Urinary ammonium to sulfate relationship. The amount of ammonium in the urine is approximately equal to the amount of sulfate. The ratio can often be less than 1 depending on the amount of alkali ingested and the amount of titratable acid in the urine. High acid intake raises both ammonium and sulfate while high alkali intake decreases the ratio. True incomplete RTA with intact ammoniagenesis increases the ammonium-to-sulfate ratio. (RTA: Renal tubular acidosis).

of iRTA. To exclude this subgroup of patients from those with "true" iRTA, they should be studied on a controlled metabolic diet that resembles the typical Western diet. Figure 11.5 illustrates some of the salient features of dietary changes and iRTA. Patients who have a normal plasma pH and bicarbonate (HCO_3^-) in plasma (P_{HCO_3}) along with a high UpH can have a large but episodic dietary intake of alkali (e.g. binge on fruit and berries). It is important to stress the intermittent pattern of ingestion. Additional clues to suggest that this is the basis for the high UpH are: first, the rate of excretion of NH_4^+ as compared to SO_4^{2-} in mEq terms is low; second, the calculated dietary *net* alkali intake is large (e.g. as reflected by the rate of excretion of organic anions including citrate in the urine) (Fig. 11.6). The patients in this subgroup resemble patients with dRTA due to low net H^+ secretion described above, except that they do not develop acidemia when they consume a typical Western diet, and they will be able to increase their rate of excretion of NH_4^+ appropriately when given a large and chronic acid (NH_4Cl) load.

Assessing Dietary Alkali Intake

Longer Calculation

In the absence of frank bicarbonaturia, a high rate of urinary excretion of organic anions (including citrate) is suspected when their "electrical shadow" is present in the major urinary cations exceed the major urinary anions in mEq/day terms $((U_{Na} + U_K + U_{NH4} + U_{Ca} + U_{Mg}) > (U_{Cl} + U_{HPO_4} + U_{SO_4})$ (Fig. 11.6).[36] To change concentrations into excretion rates, divide the above difference in concentration between urinary cations and urinary anions by the $U_{Creatinine}$ and multiply this ratio by the expected rate of excretion of creatinine (20 mg/kg or 0.2 μmol/kg).

Shorter Calculation

Since, the major source of Na^+ and Cl^- in the urine came from NaCl, the rate of excretion of these ions is often equal in mEq terms and they can be removed from the above calculation (*see* Fig. 11.6). By the same reasoning, in most patients under normal circumstances, HCO_3^- came from dietary organic anions in a similar quantity to urinary SO_4^{2-}, which came from sulfur-containing amino acids so NH_4^+ and SO_4^{2-} are also often equal in mEq terms, so they too can be removed from the calculation. If one makes these assumptions, the calculation breaks down to the difference of rates of excretion of K^+ and inorganic phosphate in mEq in the urine. This makes sense, as the K^+ ions from meat are largely balanced by organic monovalent plus divalent phosphate anions (the latter are derived from phosphocreatine plus ATP and ADP in muscle cells in mEq terms in the urine). Thus, the reasoning is that the remaining extra K^+ (above and beyond that associated with organic phosphates) is accompanied by potential ions that generate new HCO_3^- ions, which ultimately are excreted as organic anions in the urine.

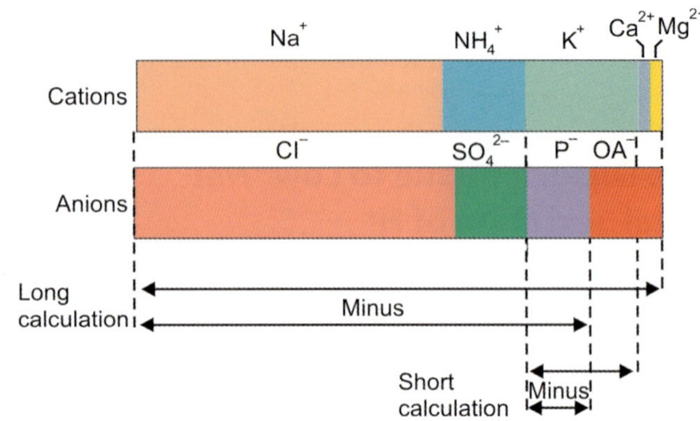

Fig. 11.6: Estimation of dietary alkali intake. The most abundant urinary cations and anions (inorganic and organic) are listed. Two calculations (long and short) are shown. Details of the rationale for these two formulae are in the text.

PATHOPHYSIOLOGY OF INCOMPLETE RTA

In contrast to the more severe presentations of congenital dRTA,[37] patients with iRTA usually come to medical attention because they have recurrent kidney stones; often as adults and less commonly in childhood. The initial diagnostic workup reveals a persistently high UpH for much of the day (>6.5 for 12 or 24 hours, an admittedly arbitrary definition).[38] A key diagnostic feature is a relatively higher rate of excretion of NH_4^+ than that of SO_4^{2-} in mEq/day terms (Fig. 11.5). In contrast, normal subjects have near-equal daily excretions of NH_4^+ and SO_4^{2-} and patients with dRTA excrete less NH_4^+ than SO_4^{2}. We envisage two subtypes of "true iRTA" from a pathophysiologic viewpoint.

Patients with an Acidified Proximal Cell pH

The lesion can begin with a higher than expected rate of production of NH_4^+ in the proximal cell due to a high concentration of H^+ in these cells. In the absence of hypokalemia, an acidified cell pH could theoretically be due to a lesion that activates the exit step for the $Na(HCO_3)_3^{2-}$ ion complex in the basolateral membrane or inactivation of apical H^+ secretion by the Na^+/H^+ exchanger-3 (NHE-3). As a result of the low intracellular pH, there would be a greater rate of production of NH_4^+, and thereby, a higher concentration of NH_3 in the renal medullary interstitial compartment. If this were to lead to a greater rate of NH_3 entry into the lumen of the iMCD, the UpH will be >6.5 and the rate of excretion of NH_4^+ will also be normal or unusually high.

As a result of the low pH in PCT cells, the rate of reabsorption and metabolism of citrate anions should rise and the excretion of citrate would be extremely low.[21] This contributes in a major way to the likelihood of forming calcium kidney stones because of the low content of this chelator in the urine (*see* Chapter 10 on citrate) and a high content of divalent phosphate (HPO_4^{2-}) (*see* Table 11.1).

There is also an interesting potential long-term issue in this diagnostic category—a high medullary NH_3 concentration may activate the complement system and thereby lead to secondary medullary interstitial damage.[39] If this were to lead to a decrease in excretion of NH_4^+, the patient would develop full dRTA later in life. These findings would now be those in the subtype of dRTA with a UpH that is ~6.0.

Patients with a Primary Increase in the Medullary NH_3 Shunt

It is also possible to have a high excretion of NH_4^+ ($U_{NH4} > U_{SO4}$ in mEq terms) and a high UpH if there were a higher rate of entry of NH_3 into the lumen of the MCD (*see* Fig. 11.5). While these findings are similar to those in subtype of patients with "true" iRTA discussed above, patients with this disorder would lack the findings directly attributable to a low pH in PCT cells. This, in effect, means that this subgroup would not have a low rate of excretion of citrate. Hence, they would form $CaHPO_4$ stones/precipitates in the mouth of the ducts of Bellini due to the high urine HPO_4^{2-} concentration, especially if they had another lesion that led to a high rate of excretion of calcium and/or a low urine flow rate (the latter may raise the concentration of Ca^{2+} and HPO_4^{2-} in the urine, which may exceed the solubility product (K_{sp}) for $CaHPO_4$). When this $CaHPO_4$ deposits at the mouth of the ducts of Bellini, the MCD can become obstructed, leading ultimately to chronic renal insufficiency.[40]

Pathophysiology-Based Analytic Approach to Incomplete RTA

The diagnostic category of "true iRTA" is a heterogeneous one even after eliminating patients with another cause for a high UpH. Hence, our recommendation is to rely on pathophysiologic parameters such as NH_4^+ excretion different subtypes depending on the rate of excretion of citrate.[38] Understanding the pathophysiology in the individual patient may have implications for therapy to prevent the recurrence of kidney stones once these separate diagnostic categories are revealed in more detail. This is particularly important because of recent findings that patients with this type of kidney stone develop progressive parenchymal damage and nephron loss due to plugging of the terminal MCD with $CaHPO_4$ crystals.[40]

We propose an analytic scheme summarized in Figure 11.7. Note that this is purely a pathophysiologic-based approach and some molecular lesions listed are in fact theoretical. The first step is to make sure that the patient with a high UpH (>7.0) does not have HCMA accompanied by a normal anion gap. True dRTA can further be analyzed by urine pCO_2 (Fig. 11.7, left). The absence of HCMA rules out most patients with dRTA; the exception to this statement includes patients who ate a diet with a low and number of precursors of H^+ [i.e. a low protein diet with low sulfur-containing amino acids (precursors of H_2SO_4), as mentioned earlier in this chapter; this diet may also contain a large quantity of potential HCO_3^- (e.g. fruit and berries, where the anion in citrus fruit might be citrate^{3-} plus 3 K^+) or malate^{2-} plus 2 K^+ in apples. Both of these anions are members of the citric acid cycle and once they are imported into the liver and metabolized into neutral end products (e.g. carbon dioxide, glucose, glycogen, or triglycerides), "potential" HCO_3^- is converted into actual HCO_3^-] and thereby decrease the net load of H^+. In this setting there is no need for a high rate of excretion of NH_4^+ and the resulting high arterial pH may contribute to the high UpH. Hence, one expects to find a high rate of excretion of K^+, high UpH, and a low rate of excretion of NH_4^+.

At this point, the subjects can be given an acid load (usually NH_4Cl)[32] and if HCMA develops without a high rate of excretion of NH_4^+, and potentially a degree of hyperkalemia if there is also a defect in the rate of excretion of K^+ (e.g. low levels of aldosterone in plasma) or have an intake of drugs that block the aldosterone receptor, suspect type IV dRTA. This patient will likely have true dRTA but masked by low acid and/or high alkali intake. Otherwise the patient is likely to have iRTA (Fig. 11.7, right).

With this latter diagnosis, the next step is to establish why this disorder may be present. There are three possible bases for this diagnosis, and one can use the urine citrate excretion rate to subdivide the first two categories (Fig. 11.7, right). Those with a low rate of excretion of citrate could have an acidified proximal tubular cell pH, as suggested by Kamel, et al..[38] These authors speculated that the acidified proximal tubular cell pH, may be due to an activating mutation of the exit step for HCO_3^- in the basolateral membrane of these cells. On the other hand, they found another patient who had a high rate of citrate in her urine and in this patient they speculated that the basis of the lesion was an activating mutation that led to the transfer of NH_3 in her urine. Since, NH_3 is an H^+ acceptor in the urine, its addition to the urine, will lead to a higher UpH, despite the secretion of H^+ by the luminal H^+/K^+-ATPase into the luminal fluid of the inner MCD. This latter H^+ pump is normally upregulated in the presence of hypokalemia and downregulated in the presence of hyperkalemia.[41] Of special interest in this patient, she developed recurrent $CaHPO_4$ kidney stones before the age of 10, which suggested that she would likely have an inborn error of metabolism. The third possible basis for a higher UpH is purely speculative at the moment, but it is an ion translocator in the β-intercalated cells, which reabsorbs Na^+ and HCO_3^- while secreting Cl^- into the lumen (Na-dependent chloride bicarbonate exchanger). In so doing, it is the concentration of HCO_3^- in the luminal fluid and may raise the UpH. Several other inborn errors of metabolism can also cause dRTA with a high UpH, include defects in intracellular carbonic anhydrase (CAII); these patients also have an alkalinized PCT pH and thereby a low rate of production of NH_4^+ so they may have high rates of excretion

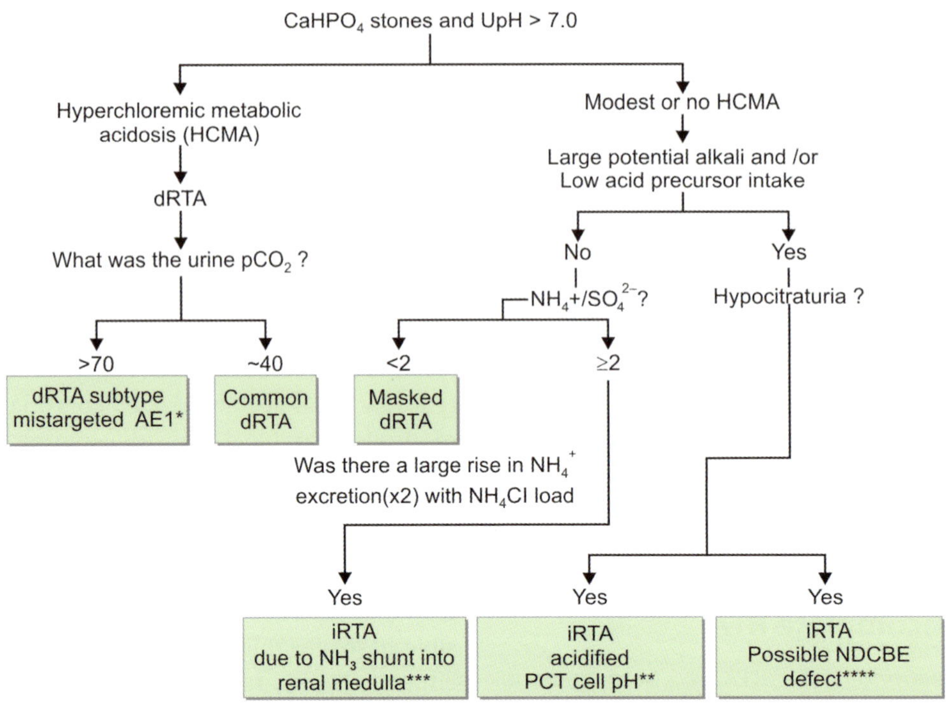

Fig. 11.7: Pathophysiology-based consideration to the patient with a high urine pH and calcium phosphate kidney stones. Patients with a low serum bicarbonate and high serum chloride (hyperchloremic metabolic acidosis, HCMA) likely has true distal renal tubular acidosis (dRTA). Patients with true dRTA usually cannot elevate their urine pCO_2 much higher than that in plasma except in those with apical mistargeting of AE1* which can theoretically mount a high urine pCO_2. A normal (or near normal) serum bicarbonate concentration justifies the diagnosis of incomplete RTA except when it is a true dRTA masked by a low net acid or high alkali load to the kidney. Without such dietary factors (see the text for calculation of alkali load), further clues can be obtained from the $NH4^+/SO_4^{2-}$ ratio. If the NH4+/SO_4^{2-} ratio is low, this can still be dRTA masked by dietary factors. Diagnostic subgroups can be distinguished by the rate of excretion of citrate excretion. Inappropriate hypocitraturia suggests an acidified proximal convoluted tubule (PCT) cell**. A large rise in NH_4^+ with NH4Cl loading can be due to NH_3 shunt from the collecting duct into renal medulla***. A hypothetical defect in the Na-dependent chloride bicarbonate exchanger (*see* the text for details) can also lead to iRTA****. (iRTA: incomplete renal tubular acidosis).

of NH_4^+ in the face of HCMA, if so, the basis for their high UpH is relatively easy to detect. The other group of patients with HCMA (dRTA) and unusually high UpH are patients with SAO with a second mutation on their AE1 that leads to abnormal migration of AE to the luminal membrane of the inner MCD. The net result is the reabsorption of Cl^- in parallel with the secretion of HCO_3^- in the luminal fluid of the inner MCD. In patients with two different mutations in their AE1, a high PCO_2 in their urine suggests that there was secretion of HCO_3^- into their inner MCD.[34] Those patients with a high U_{pH} and low concentrations of citrate in the urine are particularly likely to develop $CaHPO_4$ kidney stones.[38]

CONCLUDING REMARKS

Urine pH affects many processes in the urine, many of which are directly or indirectly relevant to prevention of precipitation of solutes. The risk of calcium phosphate precipitation is pervasive in many organs during normal physiology and multiple mechanisms are in place to prevent this from occurring. We presented examples in three organs, the GI tract, mammary gland, and skeletal muscle, to highlight how evolution has secured multiple ways to prevent such complications. The urinary environment represents a niche where prevention of calcium phosphate precipitation is of particular importance as water conservation in terrestrial vertebrates mandates low urine volume. In addition, the differential reabsorption of solutes axially down the nephron can create imbalances that promote precipitation.

Because of our evolutionary history, we have powerful hepatic defense mechanisms to allow us to binged on large amounts of potassium citrate in foraged fruits and not succumb to hyperkalemia and hypocalcemia. These same fundamental survival mechanisms today allow clinicians to prescribe large doses of potassium citrate to treat kidney stones.

Clinicians measure pH basically in bladder urine which does not provide information on UpH in the kidney and are not always cognizant of the intricacies of the physicochemical and biologic impact of UpH. Luminal pH changes significantly from one segment of the nephron to another and within each segment, there are likely microdomains of pH that serves specific purposes. For example, the apical extrusion of H^+ in the PCT helps to titrate citrate^{3-} to citrate^{2-} so it can absorbed and contemporaneously titrate HPO_4^{2-} to H_2PO^{4-} which protects against $CaHPO_4$ precipitation when citrate^{3-} is removed from the lumen. In the collecting duct where the urine volume is the lowest and risk for $CaHPO_4$ crystallization is highest, UpH also is brought down to a lowest point by the H^+-ATPase and absence of carbonic anhydrase. Failure to do so begets calcium phosphate precipitation. Because urate is unusually high in the urine in higher primates, a higher acid load coupled with inadequate ammonia excretion will drive the UpH further down to promote uric acid stones. The clinical evaluation and management of kidney stones can benefit greatly from a clinician who understands why UpH is poised where it is and what happens when it deviates outside the safety zone.

REFERENCES

1. Halperin ML, Cheema Dhadli S, Kamel KS. Physiology of acid-base balance: links with kidney stone prevention. Semin Nephrol. 2006;26(6):441-6.
2. Wagner CA, Mohebbi N. Urinary pH and stone formation. J Nephrol. 2010, 23 Suppl 16:S165-9.
3. Bank N, Schwartz WB. Influence of certain urinary solutes on acidic dissociation constant of ammonium at 37 degrees C. J Appl Physiol. 1960;15:125-7.
4. Asplin JR. Uric acid stones. Semin Nephrol. 1996;16(5): 412-24.
5. Hamm LL, Simon EE. Roles and mechanisms of urinary buffer excretion. Am J Physiol. 1987;253(4 Pt 2):F595-605.
6. Hamm LL, Alpern R, Presig PA. Cellular mechanisms of renal tubular acidification. In: Alpern RJ, Caplan M, Moe OW (Eds). Seldin and Giebisch's The Kidney: Pathophysiology. 5th ed. London, UK: Elsevier; 2013. pp. 1917-78.
7. Carlisle EJ, Donnelly SM, Halperin ML. Renal tubular acidosis (RTA): recognize the ammonium defect and pHorget the urine pH. Pediatr Nephrol. 1991;5(2):242-8.
8. Sabatini S. The acidosis of chronic renal failure. Med Clin North Am. 1983;67(4):845-58.
9. Fulgraff G, Pitts RF. Kinetics of ammonia production and excretion in the acidotic dog. Am J Physiol. 1965;209(6): 1206-12.
10. Hu MC, Shiizaki K, Kuro-o M, et al. Fibroblast growth factor 23 and Klotho: physiology and pathophysiology of an endocrine network of mineral metabolism. Annu Rev Physiol. 2013;75:503-33.
11. Lowenstam HA. Minerals formed by organisms. Science. 1981;211(4487):1126-31.
12. Pautard, FG. Calcium, phosphorus and the origin of backbones. 1961. New Scientist 12:364-6. https://books.google.co.uk/books?id=lo7r0zX_T0sC&printsec=frontcover&hl=EN#v=onepage&q&f=false
13. Pitts RF, Ayer JL, Schiess WA. The renal regulation of acid-base balance in man; the reabsorption and excretion of bicarbonate. J Clin Invest. 1949;28(1):35-44.
14. Cameron M, Maalouf NM, Poindexter J, et al. The diurnal variation in urine acidification differs between normal individuals and uric acid stone formers. Kidney Int. 2012;81(11): 1123-30.
15. Cameron MA, Baker LA, Maalouf NM, et al. Circadian variation in urine pH and uric acid nephrolithiasis risk. Nephrol Dial Transplant. 2007;22(8):2375-8.
16. Capolongo G, Sakhaee K, Pak CY, et al. Fasting versus 24-h urine pH in the evaluation of nephrolithiasis. Urol Res. 2011;39(5):367-72.
17. DuBose TD, Jr., Pucacco LR, Seldin DW, et al. Microelectrode determination of pH and PCO_2 in rat proximal tubule after benzolamide: evidence for hydrogen ion secretion. Kidney Int. 1979;15(6):624-9.
18. Rector FC, Jr., Sellman JC, Martinez-Maldonado M, et al. The mechanism of suppression of proximal tubular reabsorption by saline infusions. J Clin Invest. 1967;46(1):47-56.
19. Moe OW, Preisig PA. Hypothesizing on the evolutionary origins of salt-induced hypercalciuria. Curr Opin Nephrol Hypertens. 2005;14(4):368-72.
20. Dedmon RE, Wrong O. The excretion of organic anion in renal tubular acidosis with particular reference to citrate. Clin Sci. 1962;22:19-32.
21. Simpson DP. Citrate excretion: a window on renal metabolism. Am J Physiol. 1983;244(3):F223-34.
22. Zhai XY, Fenton RA, Andreasen A, et al. Aquaporin-1 is not expressed in descending thin limbs of short-loop nephrons. J Am Soc Nephrol. 2007;18(11):2937-44.
23. Quamme GA, Smith CM. Magnesium transport in the proximal straight tubule of the rabbit. Am J Physiol. 1984;246 (5 Pt 2):F544-50.
24. Hebert SC, Andreoli TE. Ionic conductance pathways in the mouse medullary thick ascending limb of Henle. The paracellular pathway and electrogenic Cl^- absorption. J Gen Physiol. 1986;87(4):567-90.
25. Hess B, Nakagawa Y, Coe FL. Inhibition of calcium oxalate monohydrate crystal aggregation by urine proteins. Am J Physiol. 1989;257(1 Pt 2):F99-106.
26. Holt C. Inorganic constituents of milk. III. The colloidal calcium phosphate of cow's milk. J Dairy Res. 1982;49(1):29-38.
27. Halperin ML. Metabolic Process for H^+ Production and Removal. Clinical Detective Stories: A Problem Based Approach to Energy and Acid-Base Metabolism. London, England: Portland Press; 1993.
28. Kamel KS, Schreiber M, Halperin ML. Integration of the response to a dietary potassium load: a paleolithic perspective. Nephrol Dial Transplant. 2014;29(5):982-9.

29. Cheema-Dhadli S, Chong CK, Kamel KS, et al. An acute infusion of lactic acid lowers the concentration of potassium in arterial plasma by inducing a shift of potassium into cells of the liver in fed rats. Nephron Physiol. 2012;120(2):p7-15.
30. Fehlmann M, Freychet P. Insulin and glucagon stimulation of (Na^+–K^+)-ATPase transport activity in isolated rat hepatocytes. J Biol Chem. 1981;256(14):7449-53.
31. Davids MR, Edoute Y, Jungas RL, et al. Facilitating an understanding of integrative physiology: emphasis on the composition of body fluid compartments. Can J Physiol Pharmacol. 2002;80(9):835-50.
32. Wrong O, Davies HE. The excretion of acid in renal disease. QJM. 1959;28(110):259-313.
33. Twenty-five year sentence for male sperm. New Sci. 1973;60(877):827.
34. Kaitwatcharachai C, Vasuvattakul S, Yenchitsomanus P, et al. Distal renal tubular acidosis and high urine carbon dioxide tension in a patient with southeast Asian ovalocytosis. Am J Kidney Dis. 1999;33(6):1147-52.
35. Rungroj N, Devonald MA, Cuthbert AW, et al. A novel missense mutation in AE1 causing autosomal dominant distal renal tubular acidosis retains normal transport function but is mistargeted in polarized epithelial cells. J Biol Chem. 2004;279(14):13833-8.
36. Uribarri J, Douyon H, Oh MS. A re-evaluation of the urinary parameters of acid production and excretion in patients with chronic renal acidosis. Kidney Int. 1995;47(2):624-7.
37. Batlle D, Haque SK. Genetic causes and mechanisms of distal renal tubular acidosis. Nephrol Dial Transplant. 2012;27(10):3691-704.
38. Kamel KS, Shafiee MA, Cheema-Dhadli S, et al. Studies to identify the basis for an alkaline urine pH in patients with calcium hydrogen phosphate kidney stones. Nephrol Dial Transplant. 2007;22(2):424-31.
39. Nath KA, Hostetter MK, Hostetter TH. Pathophysiology of chronic tubulo-interstitial disease in rats. Interactions of dietary acid load, ammonia, and complement component C3. J Clin Invest. 1985;76(2):667-75.
40. Gillen DL, Worcester EM, Coe FL. Decreased renal function among adults with a history of nephrolithiasis: a study of NHANES III. Kidney Int. 2005;67(2):685-90.
41. Eiam-Ong S, Kurtzman NA, Sabatini S. Regulation of collecting tubule adenosine triphosphatases by aldosterone and potassium. J Clin Invest. 1993;91(6):2385-92.

CHAPTER

12

Acid-Base Balance, Hypercalciuria, and Bone

Kevin K Frick, Nancy S Krieger, David A Bushinsky

INTRODUCTION

Adults eating a typical Western diet produce ~1 mEq of acid (H^+, protons) per day.[1,2] Much of this acid is generated from metabolism of cysteine and methionine residues in proteins to sulfate[3-5]; consequently, a diet rich in animal protein will result in greater acid production than a vegetarian diet.[1] To maintain a stable systemic pH, these protons must be buffered prior to renal excretion. Extracellular fluid bicarbonate,[6] soft tissues,[7-9] and bone[10-18] buffer these acids. Bone contains ~98% of body Ca,[19,20] which is bound to the proton buffers carbonate and phosphate and is released as these buffers neutralize the metabolic acids.[4,21-25] Diets rich in animal protein result in higher urine calcium (uCa) excretion.[26-29] The increase in uCa, from buffering of metabolic acids, would be expected to increase the risk for kidney stone formation and growth. Humans with hypercalciuria and kidney stones often have reduced bone mineral density (BMD), perhaps due to the ongoing consumption of a diet rich in acid precursors.

HYPERCALCIURIA AND BMD

Bone mineral density is correlated inversely with uCa excretion in both men[30] and women.[31] This relationship was confirmed in stone formers, but not in nonstone formers.[32] A number of studies demonstrate that patients with nephrolithiasis have a reduction in BMD compared to matched controls.[33-45] After adjusting for a large number of variables, an analysis of the 3rd National Health and Nutrition Examination Survey (NHANES III) demonstrated that men with a history of kidney stones have a lower femoral neck BMD than those with no history of stones.[46] Analysis of ~6,000 older men again demonstrated an association of kidney stones with decreased BMD.[47] Stone formers have an increased risk of fractures.[34,46] There was an increased risk of wrist and spine fractures in stone formers in NHANES III[46] and, in a retrospective analysis, stone formers had an increased incidence of vertebral fractures, but not fractures at other sites.[34]

The majority of kidney stone-forming patients with calcium-containing kidney stones are hypercalciuric as compared to nonstone formers.[42,48-51] Patients with idiopathic hypercalciuria (IH, an increase in uCa with no demonstrable metabolic cause) often excrete more calcium in their urine than they absorb from the diet, indicating a net loss of total body calcium.[41,42,48,52-59] The source of this excess uCa is almost certainly bone, as the skeleton is the largest repository of calcium in the body.[45,59,60] Idiopathic hypercalciuria has been associated with markers of increased bone turnover[32,44,61]: urinary hydroxyproline is increased in IH patients[32] and serum osteocalcin levels are elevated in stone formers who have a defect in renal tubule calcium reabsorption but not in those with exclusively excessive intestinal calcium absorption.[62] Studies with ^{47}Ca demonstrate that patients with IH have both increased bone formation and resorption, with the latter predominating.[63] Cytokines implicated in bone metabolism are altered in patients with IH.[38,64-66] In 70 children and adolescents with IH, plasma and urine levels of monocyte chemoattractant protein (MCP-1) were increased and positively correlated with BMD[67]; MCP-1 recruits monocytes to bone, resulting in an increase in osteoblast number.[68] Immunohistochemical analysis of bone samples from patients with IH showed higher expression of Receptor Activator of NFκB Ligand (RANKL).[69] Osteoprotegerin expression was also increased, possibly in an attempt to counteract the actions of RANKL.[69] Expression of transforming growth factor-β (TGFβ) was reduced, potentially contributing to delayed mineralization.[69]

EFFECTS OF ACID ON HYPERCALCIURIA *IN VIVO*

Patients with IH have normal serum Ca, normal or elevated $1,25(OH)_2D_3$, normal or elevated serum parathyroid hormone (PTH), normal or low serum phosphate, and low bone mass.[49] Idiopathic hypercalciuria exhibits a polygenic mode of inheritance.[49,70,71] As a model for IH, we have generated a novel rat strain, the genetic stone-forming hypercalciuric (GHS) rat, by inbreeding successive generations of Sprague–Dawley (SD) rats with selection for increased uCa excretion.[72-99] When fed a standard, ample Ca diet, each GHS rat now consistently excretes ~10-fold more uCa than SD controls.[72-99] Like patients with IH, GHS rats have normal serum Ca, [73] increased intestinal Ca absorption[79] and enhanced bone resorption,[78] decreased renal tubule Ca reabsorption, [80] and normal serum 1,25$(OH)_2D_3$ levels,[77,79,88,89,96] in addition to decreased BMD.[76,81] Hypercalciuria is a polygenic trait in GHS rats[86] as it is in humans.[70,71,100] When fed a standard, ample Ca diet all GHS rats develop kidney stones,[74,95,97,98] which are composed of CaP.[74,92,93,97] Addition of hydroxyproline to the diet of GHS rats results in CaOx stone formation.[72,75,90]

When GHS rats were made acidotic by including NH_4Cl in their drinking water, uCa and urine phosphorus increased while urine pH and urine citrate fell.[92] NH_4Cl led to a fall in supersaturation with respect to $CaHPO_4$ (brushite) and CaOx and a rise in supersaturation with respect to uric acid. In spite of differences in supersaturation, most rats in each group formed stones that contained calcium phosphate. To assess the role of a high protein diet in hypercalciuria, Zerwekh et al.[101] fed SD rats either a low or high casein diet, supplemented with either potassium chloride as control or potassium citrate to neutralize endogenous acid production. Compared to the low casein diet with potassium chloride, uCa excretion increased with the high casein diet. Supplementation with potassium citrate reduced the elevated uCa observed with the high casein diet, but did not alter urine phosphate or urine oxalate. Thus in both of these animal models increasing dietary acids resulted in increased urine Ca excretion whose source is almost certainly bone mineral.

EFFECTS OF METABOLIC ACID ON BONE *IN VIVO*

During acute metabolic acidosis in vivo (a primary decrease in bicarbonate concentration ($[HCO_3^-]$), there is loss of bone sodium (Na^+) and/or potassium (K^+),[102-108] loss of carbonate,[17,106,109,110] and an increase in serum Ca.[111] The loss of Na^+ and/or K^+ suggest H^+ for Na^+ or K^+ exchange, and loss of bone carbonate indicates that this buffer is being consumed by the excess H^+. This acid action on bone decreases its ability to tightly bind Ca that is consequently either recovered by renal reabsorption or excreted. Metabolic acidosis reduces renal Ca reabsorption[25,112-115]: acidosis appears to reduce abundance of the Ca transporter TRPV5 resulting in hypercalciuria.[116]

During more chronic metabolic acidosis, urinary Ca excretion is increased[59,117,118] while intestinal Ca absorption is not increased,[119,120] resulting in a negative Ca balance.[22,121] This negative Ca balance appears to reflect proton-mediated dissolution of bone mineral.[2,11,12,21,59,122] Most in vivo studies indicate that chronic metabolic acidosis decreases bone mineral content.[21,22,25,121]

During chronic kidney disease (CKD) and kidney failure, there is a marked reduction in proton excretion leading to chronic metabolic acidosis,[2,11] which adversely affects bone.[123-126] The loss of bone mineral can be reversed by bicarbonate administration.[127-129] In particular, acidic, uremic patients have decreased bone carbonate.[130-132] The cause of this decrease may be dissolution of bone carbonate stores and/or their replacement by phosphate, resulting in the incorporation of H^+ into bone mineral.[17,109,110]

The effects of acidosis on bone are not limited to mature bone: children with renal tubular acidosis (RTA) have stunted linear growth. The independent effect of acidosis to suppress bone formation has been elegantly demonstrated in children with RTA.[133-135] Alkali therapy dramatically increased the growth of children with RTA.[133] In a radiographic study, 67% of patients with proximal RTA had bone abnormalities (rickets in children, osteopenia in adults).[136] In adults with distal RTA and normal renal function, BMD was lower at most sites than normal controls.[137] Bone histomorphometry demonstrated that these patients had a significantly decreased bone formation rate and increased osteoid surface and volume when compared to normal controls. Treatment of distal RTA patients with potassium citrate for 1 year to correct their acidosis caused a normalization of bone formation rate and a significant increase in BMD at the trochanter of the femur and in the total femur.[138] When potassium bicarbonate was administered orally for 18 days to 18 postmenopausal women in negative calcium balance, their calcium balance became less negative.[139] Serum osteocalcin concentrations increased and urinary hydroxyproline excretion decreased. In a randomized, double-blind, placebo-controlled trial including 201 elderly healthy men and women, potassium citrate increased areal BMD at lumbar spine and volumetric BMD at tibia and radius and decreased fracture prediction score by fracture risk assessment tool (FRAX).[140]

POPULATION STUDIES

Given the effects of acidosis on bone and the high amounts of protein in the typical North American diet, it has been hypothesized that endogenous acid production may play a role in the etiology of metabolic bone disease of aging, such as osteoporosis.[21,141,142] While the young healthy kidney can efficiently eliminate H^+, as we age there is a decrease in overall renal function, including acid excretion.[143] As a result, with increasing age, our systems become slightly, but significantly, more acidic.[143,144] Administration of base appears to decrease the negative Ca balance induced by a high protein diet .[139,145,146] However, whether the dietary acid consumption has a significant effect on BMD is controversial.[147] While meta-analysis of 25 studies found that urine pH correlated with Ca excretion,[148] meta-analysis of five studies found no correlation between net acid excretion and change in calcium balance or N-telopeptides.[149] A second meta-analysis also found no causal relationship between dietary acid load and osteoporotic bone disease.[150] The Framingham Offspring Study data demonstrated that higher protein consumption correlates with greater bone loss at the trochanter in men but not women.[151] There was an inverse association between net excreted acid production and femoral neck BMD in older men in the Framingham Original Study.[152] Using the NHANES 2005–2008, an inverse association between dietary potential renal acid load and proximal femur BMD was detected for men with low dietary calcium (<800 mg/day), while no associations were found for men whose calcium intake was ≥800 mg/day.[153] Interpretation of these studies is difficult as they often correlate a measurement in a single point in time with the density of the skeleton that is the result of decades of bone formation and resorption. However, these data suggest that acid load may be a risk factor for bone demineralization, especially in those individuals with reduced kidney function consuming large amounts of animal protein.[154]

EFFECTS OF METABOLIC ACIDS ON BONE *IN VITRO*

In order to examine the mechanisms involving bone in the systemic response to acid-base disorders, we have established a model using cultured bone. Earlier investigators had established that a reduction in medium pH markedly increased hydroxyapatite solubility[155] and that acidic medium induced movement of labeled Ca from bone.[156] We hypothesized that cultured bone exposed to a physiologically acidic medium would release Ca into the medium and buffer the increased medium hydrogen ion concentration.[2,4,11,15-18,24,53,107,109,157-165] As bone source we utilized neonatal mouse calvariae (frontal and parietal bones of the skull) as these bones are populated by functioning osteoclasts and osteoblasts[166,167]; these cultured bones respond to hormones and synthesize DNA and proteins as does bone in vivo.[168] The calvariae are cultured in the physiologic carbon dioxide-bicarbonate buffer system[18] where medium pH is regulated precisely by independently altering bicarbonate concentration or the partial pressure of carbon dioxide, simulating either "metabolic" or "respiratory" (respectively) acid–base disorders[2-4,18,24] and avoiding the introduction of possibly confounding exogenous buffers.

ACUTE EFFECTS OF ACIDOSIS

Calcium Release

Proton-dependent net Ca efflux can be observed during both acute (3 hours) and more chronic (>24–99 hours) incubations in acidic medium.[4,5,17,18,24,103,107,109,158-160] During acute incubations, there was net Ca efflux from the calvariae when medium pH was decreased to less than the physiologic normal of 7.40 by decreasing the $[HCO^-_3]$. There is no net flux at a neutral physiologic pH and an influx of Ca into bone when pH was >7.40 (Fig. 12.1).[18,158]

To test the hypothesis that proton-mediated net Ca efflux from bone during these acute incubations was direct physicochemical (noncell-mediated) Ca release, calvariae were cultured with agents that would either stimulate (PTH, $1,25(OH)_2D_3$) or suppress (azide, freeze-thaw) bone cell activity but not directly affect bone mineral.[158] For each treatment, the pH-dependence of Ca efflux from bone was similar, indicating that acute (3 hours) proton-mediated Ca release was due to physicochemical and not cell-mediated mechanisms (Fig. 12.2).[158] Incubation of synthetic carbonated apatite disks, an accurate cell-free model of bone mineral,[169-174] in physiologically acid medium caused a net Ca efflux similar to that from cultured calvariae,[175] further supporting the hypothesis that physiologically acid medium induces physicochemical bone Ca release.

While the crystal form of mature bone is principally hydroxyapatite ($Ca_{10}(OH)_2(PO_4)_6$), poorly crystalline apatite, brushite ($CaHPO_4 \cdot 2H_2O$), and carbonated apatite can also be found.[172,174,176] To determine whether bone phosphate and carbonate were in equilibrium with the medium and thus might be subject to dissolution in an acid medium, calvariae were cultured in medium where the driving forces for crystallization with respect to the solid phases of bone mineral were varied by adjusting medium pH, [Ca], or $[PO_4]$.[17] With respect to Ca and carbonate, but not Ca and phosphate, there was bone formation in supersaturated medium, no change in the bone mineral when cultured in saturated medium, and bone dissolution

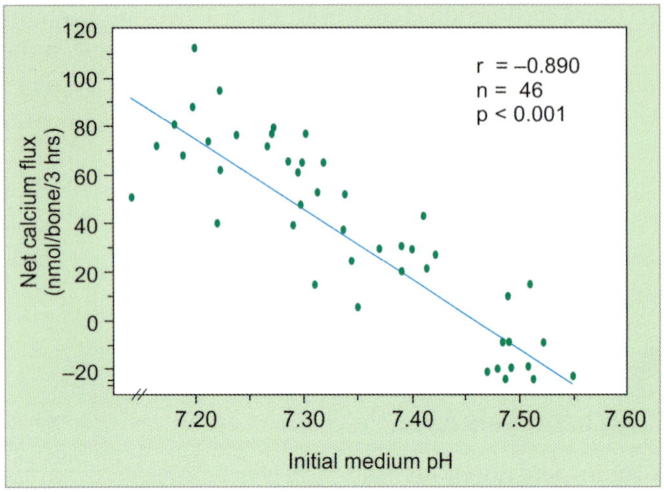

Fig. 12.1: Effect of initial medium pH on net calcium flux in neonatal mouse calvariae cultured for 3-hour. Positive flux indicates net calcium movement from the bone into the medium, a negative flux the opposite. Medium pH was adjusted with concentrated HCl or NaOH at constant partial pressure of carbon dioxide of 40 mm Hg. Calvariae were preincubated in neutral pH medium for 24 hours prior to this 3-hour incubation. $r = -0.890$, $n = 46$, $p < 0.001$.

Source: Data from Bushinsky DA, Goldring JM, Coe FL. Cellular contribution to pH-mediated calcium flux in neonatal mouse calvariae. Am J Physiol. 1985;248:F785-9.

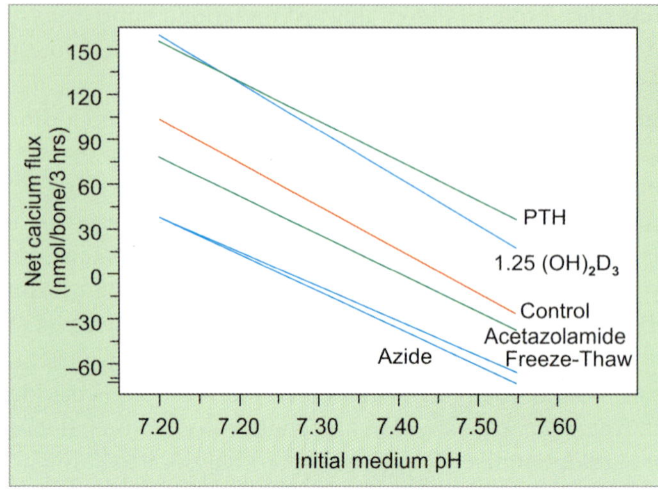

Fig. 12.2: Dependency on pH is independent of cell activity in 3-hour incubations. Comparison of regressions of initial medium pH on net calcium flux for six separate groups of calvariae. Control, calvariae incubated in control medium (pH = 7.40); PTH, calvariae incubated in control medium with parathyroid hormone (10 nM); $1,25(OH)_2D_3$, calvariae incubated in control medium with 1,25 dihydroxyvitamin D_3 (10 nM); acetazolamide, calvariae incubated in control medium with acetazolamide (0.4 mM); freeze-thaw, calvariae incubated in control medium after three successive freeze-thaw cycles to kill bone cells; azide, calvariae incubated in control medium with azide (0.1%). Calvariae were incubated for 24-hour in similar medium prior to this 3-hour incubation. Regressions are different due to a difference in intercepts of all groups except PTH and $1,25(OH)_2D_3$, which are similar and azide and freeze-thaw, which are similar. Slopes are similar in all six groups.

Source: Data from Bushinsky DA, Goldring JM, Coe FL. Cellular contribution to pH-mediated calcium flux in neonatal mouse calvariae. Am J Physiol. 1985;248:F785-9.

in undersaturated medium. A reduction in medium pH causes carbonate solubilization and Ca release. When calvariae are cultured in acidic medium, there is a progressive loss of total bone carbonate during a model of metabolic acidosis (reduced $[HCO_3]$) but not during isohydric (equivalent pH) respiratory acidosis (increased P_{CO^2}).[109] At a constant pH, whether physiologically neutral or acid, net bone Ca flux is dependent on the medium bicarbonate; the lower the bicarbonate, the greater the Ca efflux from bone.[162]

Hydrogen Ion Buffering

Incubation of calvariae in medium simulating metabolic acidosis (decreased $[HCO_3]$) results in a net influx of H^+ into the bone, decreasing the medium $[H^+]$.[16-18] Conversely, in medium with a pH above physiologically neutral, there is efflux of protons from bone (Fig. 12.3).

Exchange of Protons for Sodium and/or Potassium

Bone is relatively rich in sodium (Na^+) and potassium (K^+), which appear to freely exchange with the surrounding fluid; the bone surface has been posited to include fixed negative charges that complex with Na^+, K^+, and H^+.[20,155] By using a high resolution scanning ion microprobe to excite and release ions from the bone surface and secondary ion mass spectroscopy to identify those ions, it was determined that the calvarial bone surface is rich in Na^+ and K^+ relative to Ca.[102,103,177-180] Incubation in acidic medium causes greater loss of surface Na^+ and K^+ relative to Ca[102,103,107,108,177] in parallel with buffering of the additional H^+. These results suggest that bone can act as an ion exchange surface, where Na^+ and K^+ exchange for H^+ causing a decrease in medium acidity.[102,104,105] This exchange may be cellularly mediated: with inhibition of osteoclast function by calcitonin, physicochemical proton buffering by bone causes relatively equal loss of Ca and Na[103] and/or K.[108]

Decrease in Bone Carbonate

In addition to its role as Ca reservoir, bone also contains ~80% of the total carbon dioxide (including CO_3^{2-}, HCO_3^-,

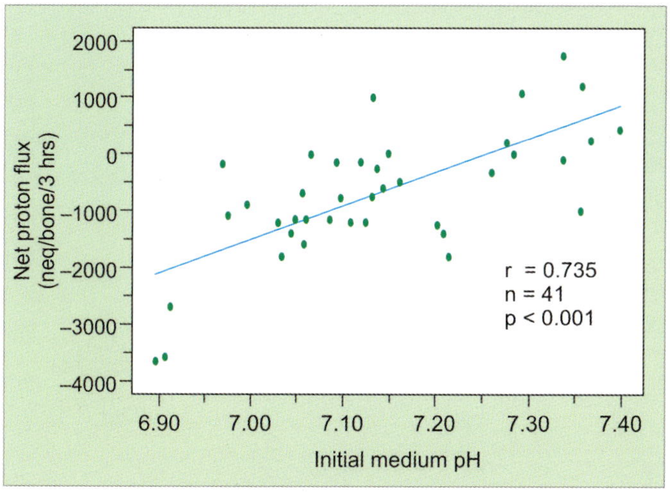

Fig. 12.3: Effect of initial medium pH on net proton flux in calvariae cultured for 3-hour. A positive flux indicates net proton movement from the bone into the medium, a negative flux the opposite. Medium pH was adjusted with concentrated HCl or NaOH at a constant partial pressure of carbon dioxide of 40 mm Hg.

Source: Data from Bushinsky DA, Krieger NS, Geisser DI, et al. Effects of pH on bone calcium and proton fluxes in vitro. Am J Physiol. 1983;245:F204-09.

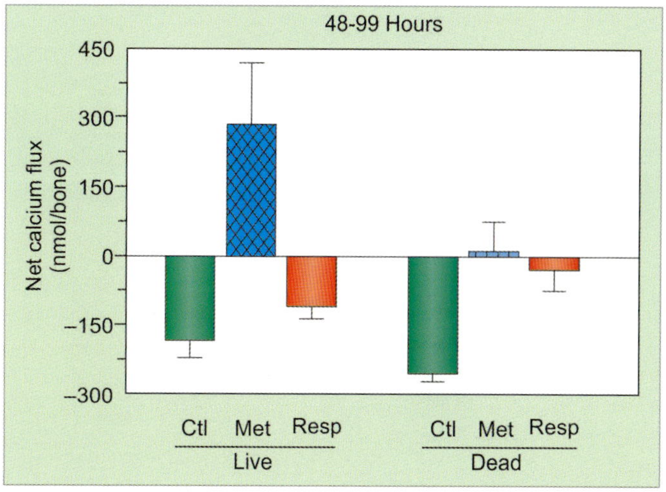

Fig. 12.4: Greater calcium efflux from living bone in response to metabolic, but not respiratory, acidosis. Net calcium flux during the final 51-hour of a 99-hour incubation for the six groups of calvariae indicated. Live, living cultured calvariae; dead, calvariae subjected to three freeze-thaw cycles to kill cells before culture; Ctl, calvariae cultured in neutral medium; Met, medium acidified by lowering the bicarbonate concentration; Resp, medium acidified by increasing the partial pressure of carbon dioxide. Values are mean + SEM.

Source: Data from Bushinsky DA. Net calcium efflux from live bone during chronic metabolic, but not respiratory, acidosis. Am J Physiol. 1989;256:F836-42.

and CO_2) in the body.[181] Most (~2/3) is in the form of carbonate (CO_3^{2-}) which complexes with cations such as H^+ (in the form of HCO_3^-), Ca, K, and Na. This carbonate is located in the lattice of the bone crystals where it is relatively inaccessible to the systemic circulation. The remaining third is readily available to the systemic circulation, in the hydration shell of hydroxyapatite.[110] *In vivo*, acute metabolic acidosis decreases bone total carbon dioxide in rats.[110] *In vitro*, acidosis induces the release of Ca and carbonate from cultured bone[17] leading to a progressive loss of bone carbonate during metabolic but not respiratory acidosis.[109]

As a whole, the *in vitro* and *in vivo* studies all provide strong evidence that bone can act as an H^+ buffer, capable of maintaining extracellular fluid pH near physiologic neutral. The response to acidosis includes Na^+ and/or K^+ for H^+ exchange and a progressive loss of carbonate.

CHRONIC EFFECTS OF ACIDOSIS

Calcium Release

As the duration of metabolic acidosis increases, the initial effects of direct physicochemical acid-induced dissolution of bone[17,18,103,158] are replaced by enhanced cell-mediated bone resorption and decreased bone formation.[159,161,163,182-184] Thyroparathyroidectomized rats made acidotic in vivo showed greater bone resorptive surface and a lower bone formation rate than thyroparathyroidectomized controls.[111,185]

After extended culture (48–99 hours) of calvarial bone, calcium release induced by metabolic acidosis is dependent on cell viability (Fig. 12.4).[159] Metabolic acidosis affects both osteoclasts and osteoblasts[161,186]; acidosis stimulates release of the osteoclastic enzyme β-glucuronidase (Fig. 12.5A) while inhibiting osteoblastic collagen synthesis (Fig. 12.5B) and alkaline phosphatase. As a result of these and other changes, there is net Ca efflux from bone (Fig. 12.5C). If [HCO_3^-] is increased, *i.e.* metabolic alkalosis, net Ca efflux from bone is decreased through increased osteoblastic bone formation and decreased osteoclastic bone resorption.[183] Primary cultures of calvarial osteoblasts cultured for 3 weeks under mineralizing conditions synthesize collagen and form nodules of apatitic bone.[187-190] Culture conditions simulating metabolic acidosis lead to fewer nodules and decreased Ca influx into those nodules (Fig. 12.6).[182] These data suggest that the hypercalciuria of chronic metabolic acidosis is a result of both augmented osteoclastic bone resorption and inhibited osteoblastic bone formation.[161,182]

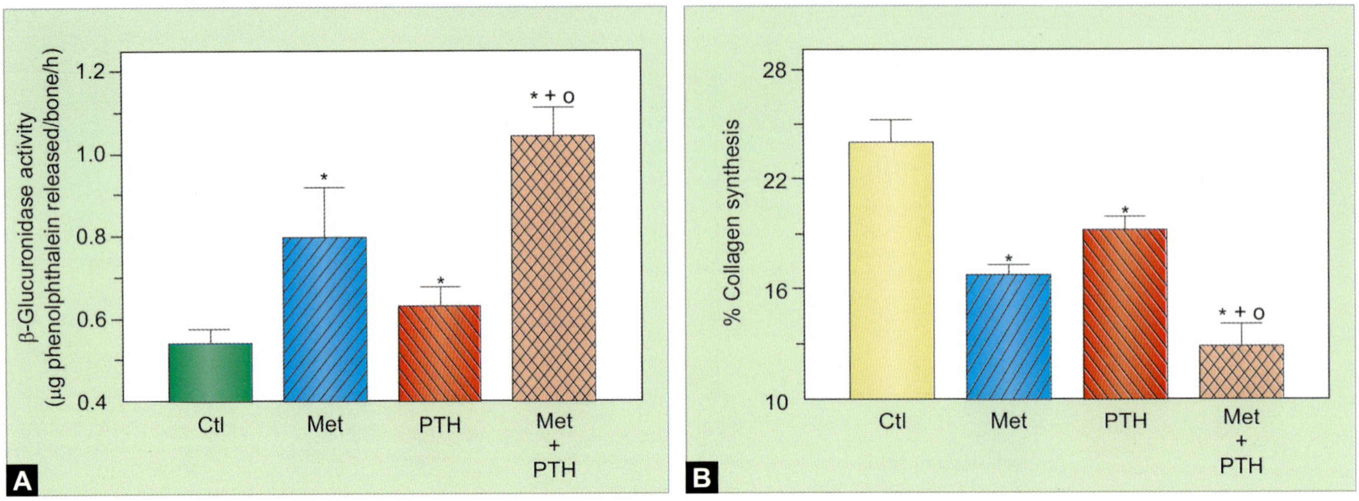

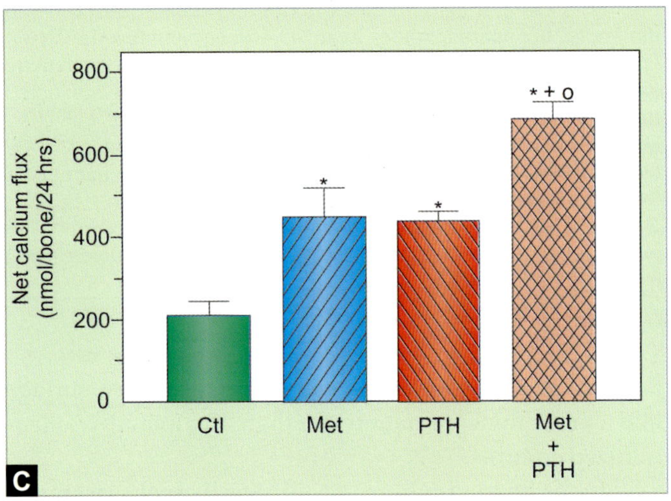

Figs. 12.5A to C: Effect of acidosis and parathyroid hormone (PTH), alone and in combination, on osteoclast and osteoblast activity. Calvariae were incubated in neutral control medium (Ctl), medium acidified to pH = 7.10 (Met); neutral medium with PTH (100 pM), or with PTH added to acidic medium (Met + PTH). Calvariae were incubated for 24-hour and then transferred to similar fresh medium for an additional 24-hour. (A) At the end of the second 24-hour incubation, aliquots of medium were removed for assay of β-glucuronidase activity. (B) Incorporation of [^{3}H]proline into collagenase-digestible protein in calvariae was measured during the final 3 hours of the second 24-hour incubation. (C) At the end of the second 24-hour incubation, aliquots of medium were removed for assay of net calcium flux. Values are mean + SEM. *, $p<0.05$ versus Ctl; +, $p<0.05$ versus Met; o, $p<0.05$ versus PTH.
Source: Data from Bushinsky DA, Nilsson EL. Additive effects of acidosis and parathyroid hormone on mouse osteoblastic and osteoclastic function. Am J Physiol. 1995; 269:C1364-70.

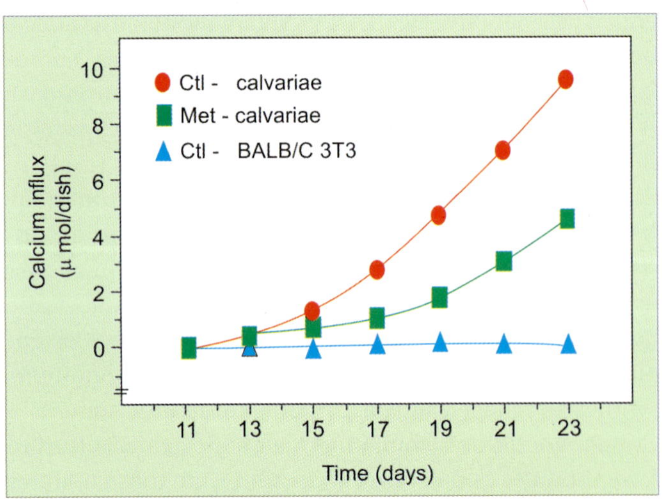

Fig. 12.6: Cumulative calcium influx as a function of incubation time for cultured neonatal mouse calvarial cells. Calvarial cells, which are predominantly osteoblasts, were incubated in neutral control medium until confluent (day 9) and then cultured for an additional 14 days in either control medium (Ctl—calvariae) or medium acidified by decreasing the medium bicarbonate concentration (Met—calvariae). As a heterologous cell type control, BALB/C 3T3 mouse fibroblasts were also incubated in control medium (Ctl—BALB/C 3T3). Changes in medium calcium concentration were calculated every 48 hours by subtracting the final calcium concentration from the initial and correcting for volume. Values are mean + SE.
Source: Data from Sprague SM, Krieger NS, Bushinsky DA. Greater inhibition of in vitro bone mineralization with metabolic than respiratory acidosis. Kidney Int. 1994;46:1199-206.

Often during renal failure, PTH is increased in addition to acidosis.[191,192] Mouse calvariae were cultured in acidic medium containing PTH to determine if acidosis and PTH have additive effects on net calcium efflux.[186] While both acidosis and PTH stimulate net calcium efflux from bone (*see* Fig. 12.5C), inhibit osteoblastic collagen synthesis (*see* Fig. 12.5B), and stimulate osteoclastic β-glucuronidase secretion (*see* Fig. 12.5A), the combination of PTH and acidosis had a greater effect on each parameter than either stimulus alone.

Changes in Gene Expression

We hypothesized that acidosis affects the pattern of gene expression in osteoblasts. To determine the early effects of acidosis on gene expression, primary neonatal mouse calvarial cells, which are principally osteoblasts,[193] were cultured in physiologically neutral pH medium until confluent, then stimulated with fresh medium at either neutral or acidic pH and RNA harvested at various times after stimulation. Expression of a group of immediate early response genes including *Egr-1, junB, c-jun, junD,* and *c-fos* was examined. Only the magnitude of *Egr-1* stimulation was dependent on medium pH.[184] At neutral pH, *Egr-1* expression is increased 10–30-fold; a progressive decrease in medium pH to 6.8 led to a parallel decrease in *Egr-1* stimulation, while conversely an increase in pH to 7.6 led to an increase in *Egr-1* stimulation.[184] Mice with a null mutation in *Egr-1* show evidence of osteopenia.[194] The major component of the bone extracellular matrix produced by osteoblasts is type 1 collagen. RNA for type I collagen was stimulated approximately threefold to fivefold by neutral medium; this stimulation was again decreased by acidosis and increased by alkalosis.[184]

Cultured primary mouse calvarial cells in mineralization medium differentiate and accumulate Ca at discrete sites of mineralization, known as bone nodules.[182,187-190] Metabolic acidosis decreases bone nodule formation and subsequent mineralization.[182] In the differentiation/mineralization process, osteoblasts express a number of matrix proteins specific to bone, including bone sialoprotein, osteocalcin, osteonectin, osteopontin, and matrix Gla protein (MGP).[195] We hypothesized that acidosis would alter the pattern of matrix gene expression in chronic cultures of bone cells, which would result in a matrix that mineralizes less extensively than that from cultures incubated at neutral pH. In neutral pH medium, there was a dramatic increase in osteopontin RNA after 3–4 weeks of incubation (Fig. 12.7A).[196,197] In contrast, in acidic cultures there was no increase in osteopontin RNA. Osteopontin plays an important role in regulating the extent of bone mineralization; OPN -/- mice have greater amounts of mineral and more mature mineral, particularly at sites of more mature bone.[198] Osteopontin contains RGD domains that may serve as an anchoring protein for macrophages and osteoclasts as well as being a chemoattractant for these cell types.[199,200] Downregulation of osteopontin expression may serve to limit recruitment of bone-resorbing cells during acidosis, perhaps a cause of low turnover renal osteodystrophy.[11,201] In neutral differentiation medium, MGP RNA expression increases by 3 weeks, reaching levels 15–20-fold greater than those before differentiation. Again, acidosis almost totally inhibits the increase in MGP RNA levels (Fig. 12.7B).[196,197] Although, MGP is expressed by other tissues in addition to bone, it comprises about 10% of the carboxyglutamic acid found in bone[202]; the Gla residue coordinates with Ca and may serve to direct calcification.[202] Deficiency in MGP leads to rapid vascular and cartilage calcification.[203] In contrast to the response of MGP to acidosis, RNA levels for the bone matrix protein osteonectin or the growth factor TGFβ1 were found not to be dependent on pH.[197] After 1 week of exposure to acidic medium, effects on osteopontin and MGP expression were fully reversible. There was only partial recovery of RNA expression for osteopontin and MGP after 3 weeks of acidosis. In the same samples, no effects of acidosis on osteonectin and glyceraldehyde 3-phosphate dehydrogenase (GAPDH) RNA expression were observed.

Intracellular Signaling Pathways in the Response to Acidosis

A variety of hormones mediate bone resorption by stimulating the production of prostaglandins, in particular prostaglandin E_2 (PGE_2).[204] The rate-limiting enzymes for prostaglandin production are cyclooxygenase 1 (COX-1, constitutive) and 2 (inducible).[205] Inhibition of both cyclooxygenases with indomethacin inhibits acid-induced calcium efflux[206] and PGE_2 secretion[164,207] after 48 hours, a time period during which acid-induced net Ca flux is predominantly cell-mediated. A specific COX-2 inhibitor, NS398, inhibited the acid-induced increase in both net Ca efflux and PGE_2 (Fig. 12.8).[208] Acidic medium also stimulated an increase in COX-2 RNA and PGE_2 levels in isolated bone cells (principally osteoblasts), which was again inhibited by NS398. In addition, calvariae from mice with a genetic deficiency in COX-2 had significantly less acid-induced Ca efflux and this Ca efflux was a function of COX-2 gene dosage.[208] These data indicate that acid-induced stimulation of cell-mediated bone resorption is mediated by osteoblastic PGE_2 synthesis.

Osteoclastogenesis and osteoclast maturation are dependent on the interaction of the osteoclastic cell-surface Receptor Activator of NFκB (RANK) with a ligand expressed on the osteoblast, RANKL.[209] The RANK/RANKL

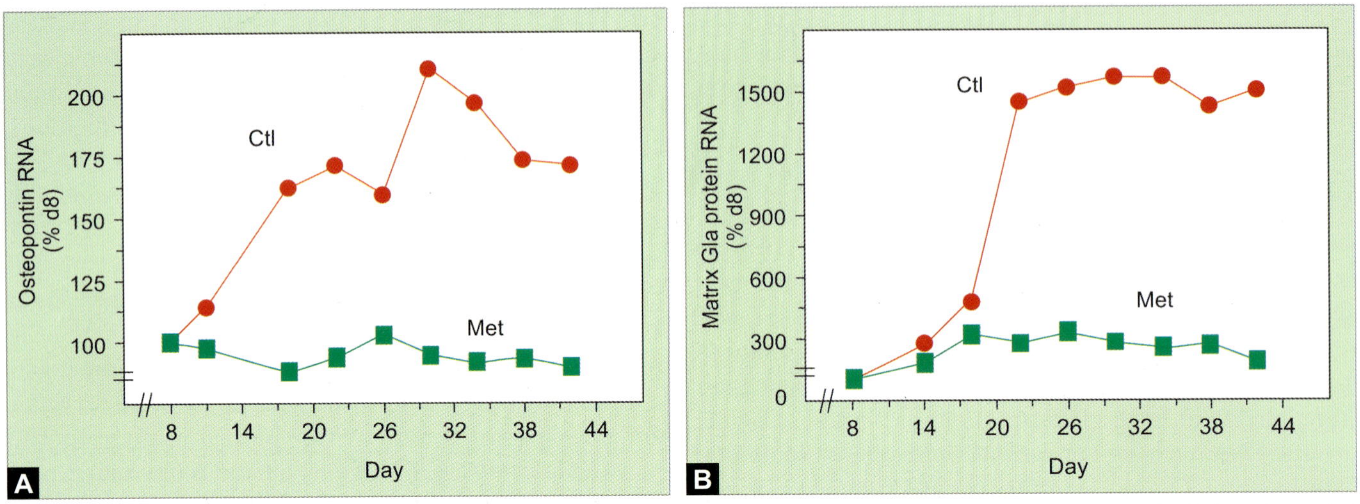

Figs. 12.7A and B: Osteopontin RNA expression is inhibited by metabolic acidosis. Calvarial cells were grown for 8 days in control medium (pH = 7.5), prior to incubation in neutral (pH = 7.5, Ctl) or acidic (pH = 7.1, Met) differentiation medium [Dulbecco's Minimal Essential Medium (DMEM) + 15% heat-inactivated horse serum + 10 mM β-glycerophosphate + 50 µg/mL ascorbic acid], and were harvested for RNA at indicated times. After Northern blotting and hybridization with an osteopontin probe, the filter was quantitated using a Molecular Dynamics PhosphorImager. To correct for variations in loading, the filter was stripped and rehybridized with GAPDH. (A) Values expressed on day 8 (d8) are the ratio of osteopontin RNA to GAPDH RNA. All values on subsequent days are expressed as the ratio of osteopontin RNA to GAPDH RNA on that day divided by the ratio on day 8 (predifferentiation). (B) Values expressed on day 8 (d8) are the ratio of matrix Gla protein RNA to GAPDH RNA. All values on subsequent days are expressed as the ratio of matrix Gla protein RNA to GAPDH RNA on that day divided by the ratio on day 8 (predifferentiation). Plots are from individual, representative experiments. *Source*: Data from Frick KK, Bushinsky DA. Chronic metabolic acidosis reversibly inhibits extracellular matrix gene expression in mouse osteoblasts. Am J Physiol. 1998;275:F840-7.

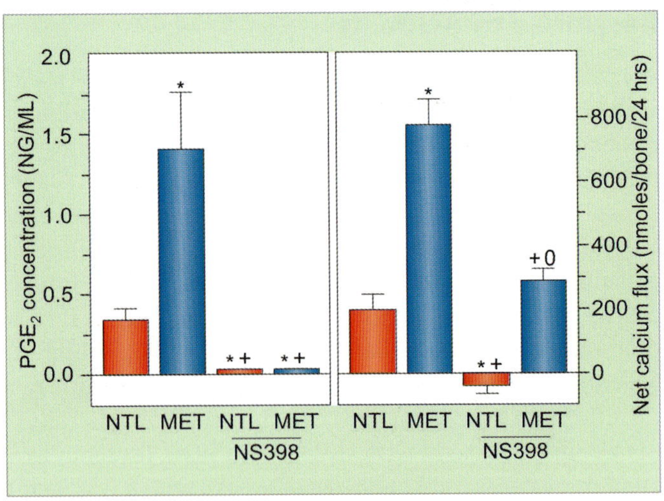

Fig. 12.8: Pharmacologic inhibition of prostaglandin E_2 production decreases acid-induced calcium efflux. Neonatal mouse calvariae were incubated in neutral (NTL) medium (pH = 7.4) or acidic (MET) medium (pH = 7.1) for 48 hours in the absence or presence of 1 µM NS398, a specific inhibitor of cyclooxygenase 1, with a medium change at 24-hour. Medium PGE2 concentration is presented in the left panel and net calcium flux is in the right panel for the 24–48 hour time period. Data are the mean + SE. *p < 0.001 versus NTL; +p<0.001 versus MET; op < 0.001 versus NTL + NS398. *Source*: Data from Krieger NS, Frick KK, LaPlante Strutz K, et al. Regulation of COX-2 mediates acid-induced bone calcium efflux in vitro. J Bone Miner Res. 2007;22:907-17.

interaction initiates a differentiation cascade that converts osteoclast precursors to bone-resorbing osteoclasts and increases the resorptive activity and survival of mature osteoclasts. To test the hypothesis that metabolic acidosis increases expression of RANKL, neonatal mouse calvariae were cultured in acidic or neutral medium, and the relative expression of RANKL RNA was significantly increased by metabolic acidosis at 24 and 48 hours compared to respective neutral controls (Fig. 12.9).[229] At 48 hours, acid-induced Ca efflux correlated directly with RANKL expression. Indomethacin, an inhibitor of prostaglandin synthesis,[210,211] prevented the acid-induced increase in RANKL RNA, indicating that prostaglandin synthesis is essential for the induction of RANKL by metabolic acidosis. Increased RANKL levels induced by acidosis would stimulate osteoclast formation, activity, and survival and help explain the acidosis-induced coupling of osteoblastic and osteoclastic activity[186] (Fig. 12.10) and increased bone Ca efflux.

Recently, we have focused on the role of the ovarian cancer G-protein coupled receptor (OGR1, also known as gpr68). Ovarian cancer G-protein coupled receptor is a member of a small family of G-protein coupled proton-sensing receptors[212] and is expressed in both osteoblasts[213] and osteoclasts.[214,215] Decreasing pH in osteoblasts

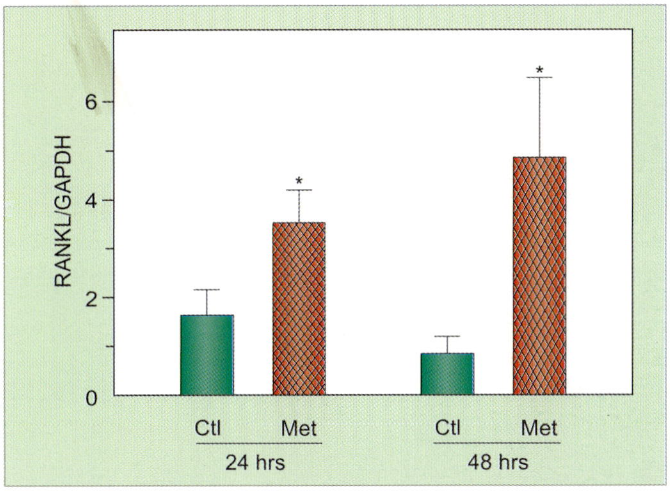

Fig. 12.9: Metabolic acidosis increases receptor activator of NFκB Ligand (RANKL) RNA expression. Neonatal mouse calvariae were incubated in neutral medium (Ctl) or in medium acidified by a primary reduction of the bicarbonate concentration, to model metabolic acidosis (Met), either for 24-hour or for 48-hour. In the 48-hour experiments, after the initial 24-hour, calvariae were moved to similar fresh preincubated medium for the final 24-hour. Calvariae from each culture dish were pooled for isolation of total RNA using a Qiagen RNeasy kit. First strand cDNA was synthesized from total RNA. Aliquots were amplified using gene-specific primers and then were electrophoresed on agarose. Filters were autoradiographed and quantitated using a densitometer and then were stripped and reprobed for GAPDH. To control for differences in RNA loading, each signal for RANKL was normalized to its respective GAPDH RNA. RANKL, receptor activator of NFκB ligand. Data are mean + SE; *, different from CTL, $p < 0.05$.
Source: Data from Frick KK, Bushinsky DA. Metabolic acidosis stimulates RANK ligand RNA expression in bone through a cyclo-oxygenase dependent mechanism. J Bone Miner Res. 2003;18: 1317-25.

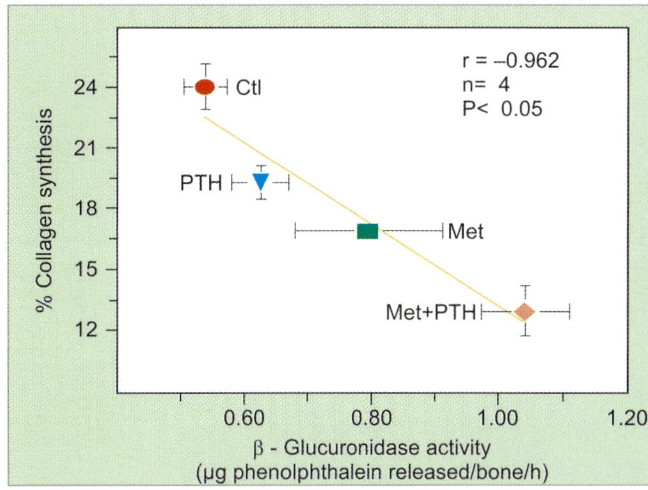

Fig. 12.10: Correlation between percent osteoblastic collagen synthesis and osteoclastic β-glucuronidase activity. Calvariae were incubated in neutral medium (Ctl), metabolic acidosis (Met), parathyroid hormone (PTH) (100 pM), or with Met + PTH. Calvariae were incubated for 24-hour and then transferred to similar fresh medium for an additional 24-hour incubation. Incorporation of [3H] proline into collagenase-digestible protein in calvariae was measured during final 3-hour of the second 24-hour incubation. At end of the second 24-hour incubation, aliquots of medium were removed for assay of βglucuronidase activity.
Source: Data from Bushinsky DA, Nilsson EL. Additive effects of acidosis and parathyroid hormone on mouse osteoblastic and osteoclastic function. Am J Physiol. 1995; 269:C1364-70.

expressing OGR1 led to accumulation of the phosphoinositide metabolites diacylglycerol and inositol triphosphate (IP_3).[213] As IP_3 leads to release of intracellular Ca (Ca_i) stores, we examined the response of primary bone cells to acidosis and found increased Ca_i.[216] Naïve Chinese hamster ovary cells (CHO), a fibroblastic cell line, show little change in Ca_i with acid stimulation. However, after transfection with mouse OGR1 cDNA, CHO cells responded to acid with a marked increase in Ca_i.[216,217] Pharmacologic inhibition of IP_3-mediated Ca signaling blocks acid-induced bone resorption in neonatal mouse calvariae as well as acid stimulation of COX-2 and RANKL in isolated osteoblasts.[218] These data are consistent with a model of metabolic acidosis action on osteoblasts in which OGR1 is activated by protons, triggering IP_3 production and Ca_i release. The increased Ca_i then acts directly or indirectly to induce COX-2, which produces PGE_2.

Regulation of Fibroblast Growth Factor 23 Expression by Acidosis

During CKD, as renal function declines there is an increase in the phosphaturic hormone, fibroblast growth factor 23 (FGF23).[219,220] Increased FGF23 results in decreased reabsorption of phosphate by renal tubules.[220,221] Fibroblast growth factor 23 also decreases renal 1α-hydroxylase and increases the catabolic 24-hydroxylase, reducing 1,25-dihydroxyvitamin D_3 levels[219,221] and subsequently decreasing intestinal phosphate absorption.[219] Fibroblast growth factor 23 directly induces left ventricular hypertrophy[222] and FGF23 levels are associated with increased mortality in patients with CKD[223] and those on dialysis.[224] Levels of phosphate, 1,25-dihydroxyvitamin D_3, and PTH have all been shown to modulate FGF23,[225-227] but it is not certain which, if any of these, is the primary regulator.

As FGF23 is produced by osteocytes and osteoblasts[221] and acidosis is often associated with CKD, we tested the hypothesis that acidosis would directly regulate FGF23 production. In both mouse calvarial cultures and cultured mouse osteoblasts, metabolic acidosis directly increases

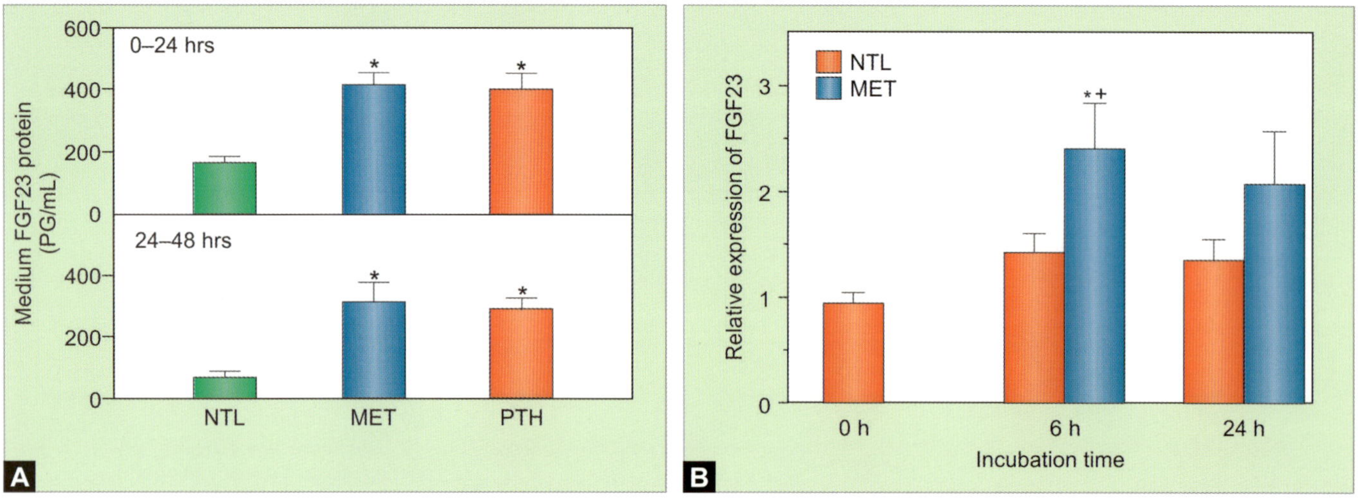

Figs. 12.11A and B: Metabolic acidosis increases expression of FGF23. Medium fibroblast growth factor 23 (FGF23) concentration after incubation of calvariae or isolated osteoblasts at neutral physiological pH (NTL) or metabolic acidosis (MET). (A) Calvariae were incubated in medium at NTL, at reduced pH simulating metabolic acidosis (MET) or with 10−8 M parathyroid hormone (PTH) in NTL for 24 hours (0–24 hours, top) or continued for an additional 24-hour in fresh pre-equilibrated medium (24–48 hours, bottom). Medium FGF23 concentration was assayed by enzyme-linked immunosorbent assay at the end of the indicated incubation time (n = 4–29 pairs of calvariae/group). (B) Primary osteoblasts were isolated from neonatal mouse calvariae. At confluence, some plates were collected for a baseline measurement of FGF23 expression (0 hour), and the remaining cells were incubated at neutral physiological pH (NTL; white bars) or at reduced pH simulating metabolic acidosis (MET; black bars) for 6 or 24-hour. At the end of the incubation period, cells were collected for RNA isolation and FGF23 expression was assayed by real-time polymerase chain reaction. Data are means ± SE for 10–20 samples/group. *$p < 0.05$ versus 0; +$p < 0.05$ versus NTL, same time period.

Source: Data from Krieger NS, Culbertson CD, Kyker-Snowman K, et al. Metabolic acidosis increases fibroblast growth factor 23 in neonatal mouse bone. Am J Physiol Renal Physiol. 2012;303:F431-6.

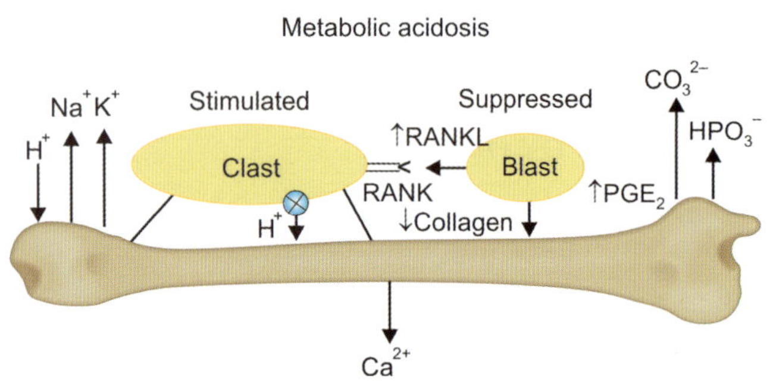

Fig. 12.12: Schematic of effects of metabolic acidosis on bone. Details as in the text. Clast, osteoclast; Blast, osteoblast.

Sources: Modified from Bushinsky DA. Acid-base imbalance and the skeleton. In: Burckhardt P, Dawson-Hughes B, Heaney RP (Eds). Nutritional Aspects of Osteoporosis. Norwell, MA: Serono Symposia USA; 1998. pp. 208-17; Bushinsky DA. Acid-base imbalance and the skeleton. Eur J Nutr. 2001;40:238-44; Lemann J, Jr, Bushinsky DA, Hamm LL. Bone buffering of acid and base in humans. Am J Physiol Renal Physiol. 2003;285:F811-32; Krieger NS, Frick KK, Bushinsky DA. Mechanism of acid-induced bone resorption. Curr Opin Nephrol Hypertens. 2004;13:423-36.

FGF23 protein (Fig. 12.11A) and RNA (Fig. 12.11B) levels.[228] These primary osteoblasts had not yet laid down a mineralized matrix, indicating the acidosis acted directly on the cells and that the FGF23 increase was not secondary to mineral phosphate release from bone. The elevated levels of FGF23 observed in CKD may result, at least in part, from metabolic acidosis directly stimulating osteoblastic production of FGF23.

HYPOTHESIS

Stone-forming patients often have reduced BMD and increased risk of fracture. There are likely multiple causes for the decreased BMD, which include the high acid load found in the typical, animal-protein-rich, Western diet. We have studied the effects of metabolic acidosis on bone and found that several mechanisms are involved in the action of acidosis on bone (Fig. 12.12). Initially, Na^+ for H^+ and K^+ for H^+ exchanges occur via physicochemical means on the mineral surface. Concurrently, there is dissolution of bone carbonate and release of Ca. Subsequently, cell-mediated processes start to predominate: osteoclastic resorption is stimulated and osteoblastic collagen deposition is inhibited. Increased bone resorption releases the buffers carbonate and phosphate as well as Ca. The decrease in bone formation in conjunction with the acidosis-induced increase in bone resorption sets the stage for a reduction in bone density increasing the risk for fracture. The Ca released from the loss of bone mineral can only exacerbate hypercalciuria and increase the risk for stone formation and growth.

REFERENCES

1. Kurtz I, Maher T, Hulter HN, et al. Effect of diet on plasma acid-base composition in normal humans. Kidney Int. 1983;24:670-80.
2. Bushinsky DA. Metabolic acidosis. In: Jacobson HR, Striker GE, Klahr S (Eds). The Principles and Practice of Nephrology. St Louis, MO: Mosby; 1995. pp. 924-32.
3. Bushinsky DA. Acid-base imbalance and the skeleton. In: Burckhardt P, Dawson-Hughes B, Heaney RP (Eds). Nutritional Aspects of Osteoporosis. Norwell, MA: Serono Symposia USA; 1998. pp. 208-17.
4. Bushinsky DA. Acid-base imbalance and the skeleton. Eur J Nutr. 2001;40:238-44.
5. Bushinsky DA. Acidosis and bone. In: Burckhardt P, Dawson-Hughes B, Weaver CM (Eds). Nutritional Influences on Bone Health, Vol 1. London: Springer-Verlag; 2010. pp. 161-7.
6. Swan RC, Pitts RF. Neutralization of infused acid by nephrectomized dogs. J Clin Invest. 1955;34:205-12.
7. Levitt MF, Turner LB, Sweet AY, et al. The response of bone, connective tissue, and muscle to acute acidosis. J Clin Invest. 1956;35:98-105.
8. Adler S, Roy A, Relman AS. Intracellular acid-base regulation. I. The response of muscle cells to changes in CO_2 tension or extra-cellular bicarbonate concentration. J Clin Invest. 1965;44:8-20.
9. Poole-Wilson PA, Cameron IR. Intracellular pH and K^+ of cardiac and skeletal muscle in acidosis and alkalosis. Am J Physiol. 1975;229:1305-10.
10. Bushinsky DA. Internal exchanges of hydrogen ions: bone. In: Seldin DW, Giebisch G (Eds). The Regulation of Acid-Base Balance. New York: Raven Press; 1989. pp. 69-88.
11. Bushinsky DA. The contribution of acidosis to renal osteodystrophy. Kidney Int. 1995;47:1816-32.
12. Bushinsky DA, Krieger NS. Regulation of bone formation and dissolution. In: Coe F, Favus M, Pak C, Parks J, Preminger G (Eds). Kidney Stones: Medical and Surgical Management. New York: Raven Press; 1996. pp. 239-58.
13. Bushinsky DA. Acidosis and bone. Miner Electrolyte Metab. 1994;20:40-52.
14. Bushinsky DA, Ori Y. Effects of metabolic and respiratory acidosis on bone. Curr Opin Nephrol Hypertens. 1993;2:588-96.
15. Bushinsky DA, Krieger NS. Role of the skeleton in calcium homeostasis. In: Seldin DW, Giebisch G (Eds). The Kidney: Physiology and Pathophysiology. New York: Raven Press; 1922. pp. 2395-430.
16. Bushinsky DA. Net proton influx into bone during metabolic, but not respiratory, acidosis. Am J Physiol. 1988;254:F306-10.
17. Bushinsky DA, Lechleider RJ. Mechanism of proton-induced bone calcium release: calcium carbonate-dissolution. Am J Physiol. 1987;253:F998-1005.
18. Bushinsky DA, Krieger NS, Geisser DI, et al. Effects of pH on bone calcium and proton fluxes in vitro. Am J Physiol. 1983;245:F204-09.
19. Widdowson EM, McCance RA, Spray CM. The chemical composition of the human body. Clin Sci. 1951;10:113-25.
20. Widdowson EM, Dickerson JWT. Chemical composition of the body. In: Comar CL, Bronner F (Eds). Mineral Metabolism. New York: Academic Press Inc; 1964. pp. 1-247.
21. Barzel US. The skeleton as an ion exchange system: implica tions for the role of acid-base imbalance in the genesis of osteoporosis. J Bone Miner Res. 1995;10:1431-6.
22. Lemann J, Jr, Litzow JR, Lennon EJ. The effects of chronic acid loads in normal man: further evidence for the participation of bone mineral in the defense against chronic metabolic acidosis. J Clin Invest. 1966;45:1608-14.
23. Lemann J, Jr, Bushinsky DA, Hamm LL. Bone buffering of acid and base in humans. Am J Physiol Renal Physiol. 2003;285:F811-32.
24. Krieger NS, Frick KK, Bushinsky DA. Mechanism of acid-induced bone resorption. Curr Opin Nephrol Hypertens. 2004;13: 423-36.
25. Lemann J, Jr, Litzow JR, Lennon EJ. Studies of the mechanism by which chronic metabolic acidosis augments urinary calcium excretion in man. J Clin Invest. 1967;46:1318-28.
26. Breslau NA, Brinkley L, Hill KD, et al. Relationship of animal protein-rich diet to kidney stone formation and calcium metabolism. J Clin Endocrinol Metab. 1988;66:140-6.
27. Robertson WG, Peacock M. The pattern of urinary stone disease in Leeds and in the United Kingdom in relation to animal protein intake during the period 1960-1980. Urol Int. 1982;37:394-9.
28. Taylor EN, Stampfer MJ, Curhan GC. Dietary factors and the risk of incident kidney stones in men: new insights after 14 years of follow-up. J Am Soc Nephrol. 2004;15:3225-32.
29. Adeva MM, Souto G. Diet-induced metabolic acidosis. Clin Nutr. 2011;30:416-21.
30. Vezzoli G, Soldati L, Arcidiacono M, et al. Urinary calcium is a determinant of bone mineral density in elderly men participating in the InCHIANTI study. Kidney Int. 2005;67:2006-14.
31. Giannini S, Nobile M, Dalle Carbonare L, et al. Hypercalciuria is a common and important finding in postmenopausal women with osteoporosis. Eur J Endocrinol. 2003;149:209-13.
32. Asplin JR, Bauer KA, Kinder J, et al. Bone mineral density and urine calcium excretion among subjects with and without nephrolithiasis. Kidney Int. 2003;63:662-9.
33. Sakhaee K, Maalouf NM, Kumar R, et al. Nephrolithiasis-associated bone disease: pathogenesis and treatment options. Kidney Int. 2011;79:393-403.
34. Melton LJ, III, Crowson CS, Khosla S, et al. Fracture risk among patients with urolithiasis: a population based cohort study. Kidney Int. 1998;53:459-64.
35. Pietschmann F, Breslau NA, Pak CY. Reduced vertebral bone density in hypercalciuric nephrolithiasis. J Bone Miner Res. 1992;7:1383-8.
36. Jaeger P, Lippuner K, Casez JP, et al. Low bone mass in idiopathic renal stone formers: magnitude and significance. J Bone Miner Res. 1994;9:1525-32.

37. Giannini S, Nobile M, Sartori L, et al. Bone density and skeletal metabolism are altered in idiopathic hypercalciuria. Clin Nephrol. 1998;50:94-100.
38. Misael da Silva AM, dos Reis LM, Pereira RC, et al. Bone involvement in idiopathic hypercalciuria. Clin Nephrol. 2002;57:183-91.
39. Tasca A, Cacciola A, Ferrarese P, et al. Bone alterations in patients with idiopathic hypercalciuria and calcium nephrolithiasis. Urology. 2002;59:865-9.
40. Heilberg IP, Martini LA, Teixeira SH, et al. Effect of etidronate treatment on bone mass of male nephrolithiasis patients with idiopathic hypercalciuria and osteopenia. Nephron. 1998;79:430-7.
41. Bushinsky DA. Recurrent hypercalciuric nephrolithiasis—does diet help? N Eng J Med. 2002;346:124-5.
42. Monk RD, Bushinsky DA. Kidney stones. In: Kronenberg HM, Melmed S, Polonsky KS, Larsen PR (Eds). Williams Textbook of Endocrinology, Vol 12. Philadelphia, PA: WB Saunders; 2011. pp. 1350-67.
43. Coe FL, Favus MJ, Crockett T, et al. Effects of low-calcium diet on urine calcium excretion, parathyroid function and serum $1,25(OH)_2D_3$ levels in patients with idiopathic hypercalciuria and in normal subjects. Am J Med. 1982;72:25-32.
44. Bataille P, Achard JM, Fournier A, et al. Diet, vitamin D and vertebral mineral density in hypercalciuric calcium stone formers. Kidney Int. 1991;39:1193-205.
45. Heilberg IP, Weisinger JR. Bone disease in idiopathic hypercalciuria. Curr Opin Nephrol Hypertens. 2006;15:394-402.
46. Lauderdale DS, Thisted RA, Wen M, et al. Bone mineral density and fracture among prevalent kidney stone cases in the Third National Health and Nutrition Examination Survey. J Bone Miner. 2001;16:1893-8.
47. Cauley JA, Fullman RL, Stone KL, et al. Factors associated with the lumbar spine and proximal femur bone mineral density in older men. Osteoporos Int. 2005;16:1525-37.
48. Monk RD, Bushinsky DA. Nephrolithiasis and nephrocalcinosis. In: Frehally J, Floege J, Johnson RJ (Eds). Comprehensive Clinical Nephrology, Vol 4. St. Louis: Elsevier; 2010. pp. 687-701.
49. Bushinsky DA, Coe FL, Moe OW. Nephrolithiasis. In: Brenner BM (Ed). The Kidney, Vol 9. Philadelphia, PA: WB Saunders; 2012. pp. 1455-507.
50. Bushinsky DA. Calcium nephrolithiasis. In: Rosen CJ (Ed). Primer on the Metabolic Bone Diseases and Disorders of Mineral Metabolism, Vol 7. Washington, DC: American Society of Bone and Mineral Research; 2008. pp. 460-4.
51. Worcester EM, Coe FL. Calcium kidney stones. N Engl J Med. 2010;363:954-63.
52. Bushinsky DA. Renal lithiasis. In: Humes HD (Ed). Kelly's Textbook of Medicine. New York: Lippincott Williams & Wilkens; 2000. pp. 1243-8.
53. Bushinsky DA, Parker WR, Alexander KM, et al. Metabolic, but not respiratory, acidosis increases bone PGE_2 levels and calcium release. Am J Physiol (Renal Fluid Electrolyte Physiol). 2001;281:F1058-66.
54. Bushinsky DA. Nephrolithiasis. J Am Soc Nephrol. 1998;9:917-24.
55. Consensus, C. Prevention and treatment of kidney stones. JAMA. 1988;260:977-81.
56. Pak CYC. Pathophysiology of calcium nephrolithiasis. In: Seldin DW, Giebisch G (Eds). The Kidney: Physiology and Pathophysiology, Vol 2. New York: Raven Press Ltd; 1992. pp. 2461-80.
57. Coe FL, Parks JH, Asplin JR. The pathogenesis and treatment of kidney stones. N Engl J Med. 1992;327:1141-52.
58. Coe FL, Favus MJ, Asplin JR. Nephrolithiasis. In: Brenner BM, Rector FC, Jr (Eds). The Kidney, Vol 7. Philadelphia, PA: WB Saunders Company; 2004. pp. 1819-66.
59. Coe FL, Bushinsky DA. Pathophysiology of hypercalciuria. Am J Physiol (Renal Fluid Electrolyte Physiol); 1984;247:F1-13.
60. Monk RD, Bushinsky DA. Pathogenesis of idiopathic hypercalciuria. In: Coe F, Favus M, Pak C, Parks J, Preminger G (Eds). Kidney Stones: Medical and Surgical Management. Philadelphia, PA: Lippincott-Raven; 1996. pp. 759-72.
61. Sutton RAL, Walker VR. Bone resorption and hypercalciuria in calcium stone formers. Metabolism. 1986;35:485-8.
62. Urivetzky M, Anna PS, Smith AD. Plasma osteocalcin levels in stone disease: a potential aid in the differential diagnosis of calcium nephrolithiasis. J Urol. 1988;139:12-14.
63. Liberman UA, Sperling O, Atsmon A, et al. Metabolic and calcium kinetic studies in idiopathic hypercalciuria. J Clin Invest. 1968;47:2580-90.
64. Pacifici R, Rothstein M, Rifas L, et al. Increased monocyte interleukin-1 activity and decreased vertebral bone density in patients with fasting idiopathic hypercalciuria. J Clin Endocrinol Metab. 1990;71:138-45.
65. Weisinger JR, Alonzo E, Bellorin-Font E, et al. Possible role of cytokines on the bone mineral loss in idiopathic hypercalciuria. Kidney Int. 1996;49:244-50.
66. Ghazali A, Fuentes V, Desaint C, et al. Low bone mineral density and peripheral blood monocyte activation profile in calcium stone formers with idiopathic hypercalciuria. J Clin Endocrinol Metab. 1997;82:32-8.
67. Santos AC, Jr, Lima EM, Penido MG, et al. Plasma and urinary levels of cytokines in patients with idiopathic hypercalciuria. Pediatr Nephrol. 2012;27:941-8.
68. Posner LJ, Miligkos T, Gilles JA, et al. Monocyte chemoattractant protein-1 induces monocyte recruitment that is associated with an increase in numbers of osteoblasts. Bone. 1997;21:321-7.
69. Gomes SA, dos Reis LM, Noronha IL, et al. RANKL is a mediator of bone resorption in idiopathic hypercalciuria. Clin J Am Soc Nephrol. 2008;3:1446-52.
70. Moe OW, Bonny O. Genetic hypercalciuria. J Am Soc Nephrol. 2005;16:729-45.
71. Stechman MJ, Loh NY, Thakker RV. Genetics of hypercalciuric nephrolithiasis: renal stone disease. Acad Sci. 2007;1116: 461-84.
72. Bushinsky DA, Asplin JR, Grynpas MD, et al. Calcium oxalate stone formation in genetic hypercalciuric stone-forming rats. Kidney Int. 2002;61:975-87.
73. Bushinsky DA, Favus MJ. Mechanism of hypercalciuria in genetic hypercalciuric rats: inherited defect in intestinal calcium transport. J Clin Invest. 1988;82:1585-91.

74. Bushinsky DA, Grynpas MD, Nilsson EL, et al. Stone formation in genetic hypercalciuric rats. Kidney Int. 1995;48: 1705-13.
75. Evan AP, Bledsoe SB, Smith SB, et al. Calcium oxalate crystal localization and osteopontin immunostaining in genetic hypercalciuric stone-forming rats. Kidney Int. 2004;65:154-61.
76. Grynpas M, Waldman S, Holmyard D, et al. Genetic hypercalciuric stone-forming rats have a primary decrease in BMD and strength. J Bone Miner Res. 2009;24:1420-6.
77. Kim M, Sessler NE, Tembe V, et al. Response of genetic hypercalciuric rats to a low calcium diet. Kidney Int. 1993;43: 189-96.
78. Krieger NS, Stathopoulos VM, Bushinsky DA. Increased sensitivity to $1,25(OH)_2D_3$ in bone from genetic hypercalciuric rats. Am J Physiol (Cell Physiol). 1996;271:C130-5.
79. Li XQ, Tembe V, Horwitz GM, et al. Increased intestinal vitamin D receptor in genetic hypercalciuric rats: a cause of intestinal calcium hyperabsorption. J Clin Invest. 1993;91:661-7.
80. Tsuruoka S, Bushinsky DA, Schwartz GJ. Defective renal calcium reabsorption in genetic hypercalciuric rats. Kidney Int. 1997;51:1540-7.
81. Bushinsky DA, Willett T, Asplin JR, et al. Chlorthalidone improves vertebral bone quality in genetic hypercalciuric stone-forming rats. J Bone Miner Res. 2011;26:1904-12.
82. Bai S, Wang H, Shen J, et al. Elevated vitamin D receptor levels in genetic hypercalciuric stone-forming rats are associated with downregulation of Snail. J Bone Miner Res. 2010;25: 830-40.
83. Asplin JR, Donahue SE, Lindeman C, et al. Thiosulfate reduces calcium phosphate nephrolithiasis. J Am Soc Nephrol. 2009;20:1246-53.
84. Solodkyy A, Shalhoub J, Chetty G, et al. A rare case of giant coronary artery aneurysm in the context of multiple arterial aneurysms. Int J Surg Case Rep. 2012;3:311-3.
85. Kelleher D, Shalhoub J, Davies AH. Venous thromboembolism in the paediatric patient. Phlebology. 2012;27(Suppl 2):81-5.
86. Hoopes RR, Jr, Middleton FA, Sen S, et al. Isolation and confirmation of a calcium excretion quantitative trait locus on chromosome 1 in genetic hypercalciuric stone-forming congenic rats. J Am Soc Nephrol. 2006;17:1292-304.
87. Bushinsky DA, LaPlante K, Asplin JR. Effect of cinacalcet on urine calcium excretion and supersaturation in genetic hypercalciuric stone-forming rats. Kidney Int. 2006;69: 1586-92.
88. Yao J, Karnauskas AJ, Bushinsky DA, et al. Regulation of renal calcium-sensing receptor gene expression in response to $1,25(OH)_2D_3$ in genetic hypercalciuric stone forming rats. J Am Soc Nephrol. 2005;16:1300-8.
89. Karnauskas AJ, van Leeuwen JP, van den Bemd GJ, et al. Mechanism and function of high vitamin D receptor levels in genetic hypercalciuric stone-forming rats. J Bone Miner Res. 2005;20:447-54.
90. Bushinsky DA, Asplin JR. Thiazides reduce brushite, but not calcium oxalate, supersaturation and stone formation in genetic hypercalciuric stone-forming rats. J Am Soc Nephrol. 2005;16:417-24.
91. Hoopes RR, Jr, Reid R, Sen S, et al. Quantitative trait loci for hypercalciuria in a rat model of kidney stone disease. J Am Soc Nephrol. 2003;14:1844-50.
92. Bushinsky DA, Grynpas MD, Asplin JR. Effect of acidosis on urine supersaturation and stone formation in genetic hypercalciuric stone forming rats. Kidney Int. 2001;59:1415-23.
93. Bushinsky DA, Parker WR, Asplin JR. Calcium phosphate supersaturation regulates stone formation in genetic hypercalciuric stone-forming rats. Kidney Int. 2000;57:550-60.
94. Bushinsky DA, Bashir MA, Riordon DR, et al. Increased dietary oxalate does not increase urinary calcium oxalate saturation in hypercalciuric rats. Kidney Int. 1999;55:602-12.
95. Bushinsky DA, Neumann KJ, Asplin J, et al. Alendronate decreases urine calcium and supersaturation in genetic hypercalciuric rats. Kidney Int. 1999;55:234-43.
96. Yao J, Kathpalia P, Bushinsky DA, et al. Hyperresponsiveness of vitamin D receptor gene expression to 1,25-dihydroxyvitamin D_3: a new characteristic of genetic hypercalciuric stone-forming rats. J Clin Invest. 1998;101:2223-32.
97. Asplin JR, Bushinsky DA, Singharetnam, et al. Relationship between supersaturation and crystal inhibition in hypercalciuric rats. Kidney Int. 1997;51:640-5.
98. Bushinsky DA, Kim M, Sessler NE, et al. Increased urinary saturation and kidney calcium content in genetic hypercalciuric rats. Kidney Int. 1994;45:58-65.
99. Shalhoub V, Shatzen EM, Ward SC, et al. FGF23 neutralization improves chronic kidney disease-associated hyperparathyroidism yet increases mortality. J Clin Invest. 2012;122:2543-53.
100. Davies KJ, Thapar A, Kasivisvanathan V, et al. Review of trans-atlantic cardiovascular best medical therapy guidelines—recommendations for asymptomatic carotid atherosclerosis. Curr Vasc Pharmacol. 2012;11:514-23.
101. Zerwekh JE, Zou L, Pak CY, et al. Biochemical and histological assessment of alkali therapy during high animal protein intake in the rat. Bone. 2009;45:1004-9.
102. Bushinsky DA, Levi-Setti R, Coe FL. Ion microprobe determination of bone surface elements: effects of reduced medium pH. Am J Physiol. 1986;250:F1090-7.
103. Bushinsky DA, Wolbach W, Sessler NE, et al. Physicochemical effects of acidosis on bone calcium flux and surface ion composition. J Bone Miner Res. 1993;8:93-102.
104. Bergstrom WH, Ruva FD. Changes in bone sodium during acute acidosis in the rat. Am J Physiol. 1960;198:1126-8.
105. Bettice JA, Gamble JL, Jr. Skeletal buffering of acute metabolic acidosis. Am J Physiol. 1975;229:1618-24.
106. Burnell JM. Changes in bone sodium and carbonate in metabolic acidosis and alkalosis in the dog. J Clin Invest. 1971;50:327-31.
107. Bushinsky DA, Gavrilov K, Stathopoulos VM, et al. Effects of osteoclastic resorption on bone surface ion composition. Am J Physiol. 1996;271:C1025-31.
108. Bushinsky DA, Gavrilov K, Chabala JM, et al. Effect of metabolic acidosis on the potassium content of bone. J Bone Min Res. 1997;12:1664-71.
109. Bushinsky DA, Lam BC, Nespeca R, et al. Decreased bone carbonate content in response to metabolic, but not respiratory, acidosis. Am J Physiol. 1993;265:F530-6.

110. Bettice JA. Skeletal carbon dioxide stores during metabolic acidosis. Am J Physiol. 1984;247:F326-30.
111. Kraut JA, Mishler DR, Kurokawa K. Effect of colchicine and calcitonin on calcemic response to metabolic acidosis. Kidney Int. 1984;25:608-12.
112. Dubb J, Goldberg M, Agus ZS. Tubular effects of acute metabolic acidosis in the rat. J Lab Clin Med. 1977;90:318-23.
113. Epstein FH. Calcium and the kidney. Am J Med. 1968;45: 700-14.
114. Stacy BD, Wilson BW. Acidosis and hypercalciuria: renal mechanism affecting calcium, magnesium, and sodium excretion in the sheep. J Physiol. 1970;210:549.
115. Beck N, Webster SK. Effects of acute metabolic acidosis on parathyroid hormone action and calcium mobilization. Am J Physiol. 1976;230:127-31.
116. Bonny O, Edwards A. Calcium reabsorption in the distal tubule: regulation by sodium, pH, and flow. Am J Physiol Renal Physiol. 2013;304:F585-600.
117. Bushinsky DA, Riera GS, Favus MJ, et al. Response of serum $1,25(OH)_2D_3$ to variation of ionized calcium during chronic acidosis. Am J Physiol. 1985;249:F361-5.
118. Lemann J, Jr, Adams ND, Gray RW. Urinary calcium excretion in human beings. N Engl J Med. 1979;301:535-41.
119. Adams ND, Gray RW, Lemann J, Jr. The calciuria of increased fixed acid production in humans: evidence against a role for parathyroid hormone and $1,25(OH)_2$-vitamin D. Calcif Tissue Int. 1979;28:233-8.
120. Weber HP, Gray RW, Dominguez JH, et al. The lack of effect of chronic metabolic acidosis on 25-OH vitamin D metabolism and serum parathyroid hormone in humans. J Clin Endocrinol Metab. 1976;43:1047-55.
121. Bushinsky DA, Favus MJ, Schneider AB, et al. Effects of metabolic acidosis on PTH and $1,25(OH)_2D_3$ response to low calcium diet. Am J Physiol. 1982;243:F570-5.
122. Green J, Kleeman CR. Role of bone in regulation of systemic acid-base balance. Kidney Int. 1991;39:9-26.
123. Goodman AD, Lemann J, Jr, Lennon EJ, et al. Production, excretion, and net balance of fixed acid in patients with renal acidosis. J Clin Invest. 1965;44:495-506.
124. Litzow JR, Lemann J, Jr, Lennon EJ. The effect of treatment of acidosis on calcium balance in patients with chronic azotemic renal disease. J Clin Invest. 1967;46:280-6.
125. Mora Palma FJ, Ellis HA, Cook DB, et al. Osteomalacia in patients with chronic renal failure before dialysis or transplantation. Q J Med. 1983;52:332-48.
126. Fletcher RF, Jones JH, Morgan DB. Bone disease in chronic renal failure. Q J Med. 1963;32:321-39.
127. Bishop MC, Ledingham JG. Alkali treatment of renal osteodystrophy. Br Med J. 1972;4: 529.
128. Cochran M, Wilkinson R. Effect of correction of metabolic acidosis on bone mineralization rates in patients with renal osteomalacia. Nephron. 1975;15:98-110.
129. Lefebvre A, de Vernejoul MC, Gueris J, et al. Optimal correction of acidosis changes progression of dialysis osteodystrophy. Kidney Int. 1989;36:1112-8.
130. Pellegrino ED, Blitz RM, Letteri JM. Inter-relationships of carbonate, phosphate, monohydrogen phosphate, calcium, magnesium, and sodium in uraemic bone: comparison of dialyzed and non-dialyzed patients. Clin Sci Mol Med. 1977;53:307-16.
131. Kaye M, Frueth AJ, Silverman M. A study of vertebral bone powder from patients with chronic renal failure. J Clin Invest. 1970;49:442-53.
132. Pellegrino ED, Blitz RM. The composition of human bone in uremia. Medicine. 1965;44:397-418.
133. McSherry E, Morris RC. Attainment and maintenance of normal stature with alkali therapy in infants and children with classic renal tubular acidosis. J Clin Invest. 1978;61:509-27.
134. McSherry E. Acidosis and growth in nonuremic renal disease. Kidney Int. 1978;14:349-54.
135. Challa A, Krieg RJ, Jr, Thabet MA, et al. Metabolic acidosis inhibits growth hormone secretion in rats: mechanism of growth retardation. Am J Physiol. 1993;265:E547-53.
136. Brenner RJ, Spring DB, Sebastian A, et al. Incidence of radiographically evident bone disease, nephrocalcinosis, and nephrolithiasis in various types of renal tubular acidosis. N Engl J Med. 1982;307:217-21.
137. Domrongkitchaiporn S, Pongskul C, Sirikulchayanonta V, et al. Bone mineral density and histology in distal renal tubular acidosis. Kidney Int. 2001;59:1086-93.
138. Domrongkitchaiporn S, Pongskul C, Sirikulchayanonta V, et al. Bone histology and bone mineral density after correction of acidosis in distal renal tubular acidosis. Kidney Int. 2002;62:2160-6.
139. Sebastian A, Harris ST, Ottaway JH, et al. Improved mineral balance and skeletal metabolism in postmenopausal women treated with potassium bicarbonate. N Engl J Med. 1994;330:1776-81.
140. Jehle S, Hulter HN, Krapf R. Effect of potassium citrate on bone density, microarchitecture, and fracture risk in healthy older adults without osteoporosis: a randomized controlled trial. J Clin Endocrinol Metab. 2013;98:207-17.
141. Lennon EJ, Lemann J, Jr, Litzow JR. The effects of diet and stool composition on the net external acid balance of normal subjects. J Clin Invest. 1966;45:1601-7.
142. Barzel US. Osteoporosis II: an overview. In: Barzel US (Ed). Osteoporosis II. New York: Grune and Stratton; 1976.
143. Frassetto LA, Morris RC, Jr, Sebastian A. Effect of age on blood acid-base composition in adult humans: role of age-related renal functional decline. Am J Physiol. 1996;271:F1114-22.
144. Frassetto L, Sebastian A. Age and systemic acid-base equilibrium: analysis of published data. J Gerontol A Biol Sci Med Sci.1996;51:B91-9.
145. Sakhaee K, Nicar M, Hill K, et al. Contrasting effects of potassium citrate and sodium citrate therapies on urinary chemistries and crystallization of stone-forming salts. Kidney Int. 1983;24:348-52.
146. Lemann J, Jr, Gray RW, Pleuss JA. Potassium bicarbonate, but not sodium bicarbonate, reduces urinary calcium excretion and improves calcium balance in healthy men. Kidney Int. 1989;35:688-95.
147. Bonjour JP. Nutritional disturbance in acid–base balance and osteoporosis: a hypothesis that disregards the essential homeostatic role of the kidney. Br J Nutr. 2013;110:1168-77.

148. Fenton TR, Eliasziw M, Lyon AW, et al. Meta-analysis of the quantity of calcium excretion associated with the net acid excretion of the modern diet under the acid-ash diet hypothesis. Am J Clin Nutr. 2008;88:1159-66.
149. Fenton TR, Lyon AW, Eliasziw M, et al. Meta-analysis of the effect of the acid-ash hypothesis of osteoporosis on calcium balance. J Bone Miner Res. 2009;24:1835-40.
150. Fenton T, Tough S, Lyon A, et al. Causal assessment of dietary acid load and bone disease: a systematic review & meta-analysis applying Hill's epidemiologic criteria for causality. Nutr J. 2011;10:41.
151. Sahni S, Broe KE, Tucker KL, et al. Association of total protein intake with bone mineral density and bone loss in men and women from the Framingham Offspring Study. Public Health Nutr. 2014;17:2570-6.
152. McLean RR, Qiao N, Broe KE, et al. Dietary acid load is not associated with lower bone mineral density except in older men. J Nutr. 2011;141:588-94.
153. Mangano KM, Walsh SJ, Kenny AM, et al. Dietary acid load is associated with lower bone mineral density in men with low intake of dietary calcium. J Bone Miner Res. 2014;29:500-6.
154. Frassetto LA, Sebastian A. Commentary to accompany the paper entitled 'Nutritional disturbance in acid–base balance and osteoporosis: a hypothesis that disregards the essential homeostatic role of the kidney,' by Jean-Philippe Bonjour. Br J Nutr. 2013;110:1935-7.
155. Neuman WF, Neuman MW. The Chemical Dynamics of Bone Mineral. Chicago: University Chicago Press; 1958.
156. Dominguez JH, Raisz LG. Effects of changing hydrogen ion, carbonic acid, and bicarbonate concentrations on bone resorption in vitro. Calcif Tissue Int. 1979;29:7-13.
157. Bushinsky DA, Frick KK. The effects of acid on bone. Curr Opin Nephrol Hypertens. 2000;9:369-79.
158. Bushinsky DA, Goldring JM, Coe FL. Cellular contribution to pH-mediated calcium flux in neonatal mouse calvariae. Am J Physiol. 1985;248:F785-9.
159. Bushinsky DA. Net calcium efflux from live bone during chronic metabolic, but not respiratory, acidosis. Am J Physiol. 1989;256:F836-42.
160. Bushinsky DA, Sessler NE, Krieger NS. Greater unidirectional calcium efflux from bone during metabolic, compared with respiratory, acidosis. Am J Physiol. 1992;262:F425-31.
161. Krieger NS, Sessler NE, Bushinsky DA. Acidosis inhibits osteoblastic and stimulates osteoclastic activity in vitro. Am J Physiol. 1992;262:F442-8.
162. Bushinsky DA, Sessler NE. Critical role of bicarbonate in calcium release from bone. Am J Physiol. 1992;263:F510-5.
163. Bushinsky DA. Stimulated osteoclastic and suppressed osteoblastic activity in metabolic but not respiratory acidosis. Am J Physiol. 1995;268:C80-8.
164. Krieger NS, Parker WR, Alexander KM, et al. Prostaglandins regulate acid-induced cell-mediated bone resorption. Am J Physiol Renal Physiol. 2000;279:F1077-82.
165. Krieger NS, Frick KK, Bushinsky DA. Cortisol inhibits acid-induced bone resorption in vitro. J Am Soc Nephrol. 2002;13:2534-9.
166. Schelling SH, Wolfe HJ, Tashjian JAH. Role of the osteoclast in prostaglandin E_2-stimulated bone resorption. A correlative morphometric and biochemical analysis. Lab Invest. 1980;42:290-5.
167. Feldman RS, Krieger NS, Tashjian JAH. Effects of parathyroid hormone and calcitonin on osteoclast formation in vitro. Endocrinology. 1980;107:1137-43.
168. Stern PH, Raisz LG. Organ culture of bone. In: Simmons DJ, Kunin AS (Eds). Skeletal Research. New York: Academic Press; 1979. pp. 21-59.
169. Ellies LG, Nelson DG, Featherstone JD. Crystallographic structure and surface morphology of sintered carbonated apatites. J Biomed Mater Res. 1988;22:541-53.
170. Ellies LG, Carter JM, Natiella JR, et al. Quantitative analysis of early in vivo tissue response to synthetic apatite implants. J Biomed Mater Res. 1988;22:137-48.
171. Nelson DG, Featherstone JD, Duncan JF, et al. Effect of carbonate and fluoride on the dissolution behavior of synthetic apatites. Caries Res. 1983;17:200-11.
172. Nelson DG, Featherstone JD. Preparation, analysis and characterization of carbonated apatites. Calcif Tissue Int. 1982;34:S69-81.
173. Nelson DG, Barry JC, Shields CP, et al. Crystal morphology, composition, and dissolution behavior of carbonated apatites prepared at controlled pH and temperature. J Colloid Interface Sci. 1989;130:467-79.
174. Boskey AL, Posner AS. Conversion of amorphous calcium phosphate to microcrystalline hydroxyapatite-pH-dependent, solution mediated, solid-solid conversion. J Phys Chem. 1973;77:2313-7.
175. Bushinsky DA, Sessler NE, Glena RE, et al. Proton-induced physicochemical calcium release from ceramic apatite disks. J Bone Miner Res. 1994;9:213-20.
176. Grynpas MD, Bonar LC, Glimcher MJ. Failure to detect an amorphous calcium-phosphate solid phase in bone mineral. A radial distribution function study. Calcif Tissue Int. 1984;36:291-301.
177. Chabala JM, Levi-Setti R, Bushinsky DA. Alteration in surface ion composition of cultured bone during metabolic, but not respiratory, acidosis. Am J Physiol. 1991;261:F76-84.
178. Bushinsky DA, Chabala JM, Levi-Setti R. Ion microprobe analysis of bone surface elements: effects of $1,25(OH)_2D_3$. Am J Physiol. 1989;257:E815-22.
179. Bushinsky DA, Chabala JM, Levi-Setti R. Ion microprobe analysis of mouse calvariae in vitro: evidence for a "bone membrane". Am J Physiol. 1989;256:E152-8.
180. Bushinsky DA, Chabala JM, Levi-Setti R. Comparison of in vitro and in vivo 44 Ca labeling of bone by scanning ion microprobe. Am J Physiol. 1990;259:E586-92.
181. Pasquale SM, Messier AA, Shea ML, et al. Bone CO_2-titration curves in acute hypercapnia obtained with a modified titration technique. J Appl Physiol. 1980;48:197-201.
182. Sprague SM, Krieger NS, Bushinsky DA. Greater inhibition of in vitro bone mineralization with metabolic than respiratory acidosis. Kidney Int. 1994;46:1199-206.
183. Bushinsky DA. Metabolic alkalosis decreases bone calcium efflux by suppressing osteoclasts and stimulating osteoblasts. Am J Physiol. 1996;271:F216-22.
184. Frick KK, Jiang L, Bushinsky DA. Acute metabolic acidosis inhibits the induction of osteoblastic egr-1 and type 1 collagen. Am J Physiol. 1997;272:C1450-6.

185. Kraut JA, Mishler DR, Singer FR, et al. The effects of metabolic acidosis on bone formation and bone resorption in the rat. Kidney Int. 1986;30:694-700.
186. Bushinsky DA, Nilsson EL. Additive effects of acidosis and parathyroid hormone on mouse osteoblastic and osteoclastic function. Am J Physiol. 1995; 269:C1364-70.
187. Bhargava U, Bar-Lev M, Bellows CG, et al. Ultrastructural analysis of bone nodules formed in vitro by isolated fetal rat calvaria cells. Bone. 1988;9:155-63.
188. Ecarot-Charrier B, Glorieux FH, van der Rest M, et al. Osteoblasts isolated from mouse calvaria initiate matrix mineralization in culture. J Cell Biol. 1983;96:639-43.
189. Sudo H, Kodama HA, Amagai Y, et al. In vitro differentiation and calcification in a new clonal osteogenic cell line derived from newborn mouse calvaria. J Cell Biol. 1983;96:191-8.
190. Sprague SM, Krieger NS, Bushinsky DA. Aluminum inhibits bone nodule formation and calcification in vitro. Am J Physiol. 1993;264:F882-90.
191. Goodman WG, Coburn JW, Slatopolsky E, et al. Renal osteodystrophy in adults and children. In: Favus MJ (Ed). Primer on the Metabolic Bone Diseases and Disorders of Mineral Metabolism, Vol 4. Philadelphia, PA: Lippincott-Raven; 1999. pp. 347-63.
192. Slatopolsky E, Delmez J. Bone disease in chronic renal failure and after renal transplantation. In: Coe F, Favus M (Eds). Disorders of Bone and Mineral Metabolism. New York, NY: Raven Press; 1992. pp. 905-34.
193. Krieger NS, Hefley TJ. Differential effects of parathyroid hormone on protein phosphorylation in two osteoblast-like cell populations isolated from neonatal mouse calvaria. Calc Tiss Int. 1989;44:192-9.
194. Reumann MK, Strachna O, Lukashova L, et al. Early growth response gene 1 regulates bone properties in mice. Calcif Tissue Int. 2011;89:1-9.
195. Stein GS, Lian JB, Stein JL, et al. Transcriptional control of osteoblast growth and differentiation. Physiol Rev. 1996;76:593-629.
196. Frick KK, Bushinsky DA. In vitro metabolic and respiratory acidosis selectively inhibit osteoblastic matrix gene expression. Am J Physiol. 1999;277:F750-5.
197. Frick KK, Bushinsky DA. Chronic metabolic acidosis reversibly inhibits extracellular matrix gene expression in mouse osteoblasts. Am J Physiol. 1998;275:F840-7.
198. Boskey A, Spevak L, Paschalis E, et al. Osteopontin deficiency increases mineral content and mineral crystallinity in mouse bone. Calc Tiss Int. 2002;71:145-54.
199. Davies JE. In vitro modeling of the bone/implant interface. Anat Rec. 1996;245:426-45.
200. Rodan GA. Osteopontin overview. Ann N Y Acad Sci. 1995; 760:1-5.
201. Shapses SA, Cifuentes M, Spevak L, et al. Osteopontin facilitates bone resorption, decreasing bone mineral crystallinity and content during calcium deficiency. Calcif Tiss Int. 2003;73:86-92.
202. Hauschka PV, Lian JB, Cole DE, et al. Osteocalcin and matrix Gla protein: vitamin K-dependent proteins in bone. Physiol Rev. 1989;69:990-1047.
203. Luo G, Ducy P, McKee MD, et al. Spontaneous calcification of arteries and cartilage in mice lacking matrix GLA protein. Nature. 1997;386:78-81.
204. Blackwell KA, Raisz LG, Pilbeam CC. Prostaglandins in bone: bad cop, good cop? Trends Endocrinol Metab. 2010;21: 294-301.
205. Smith WL. Prostanoid biosynthesis and mechanisms of action. Am J Physiol. 1992;263:F181-91.
206. Goldhaber P, Rabadjija L. H^+ stimulation of cell-mediated bone resorption in tissue culture. Am J Physiol. 1987;253:E90-8.
207. Rabadjija L, Brown EM, Swartz SL, et al. H^+-stimulated release of prostaglandin E_2 and cyclic adenosine 3', 5'-monophosphoric acid and their relationship to bone resorption in neonatal mouse calvaria cultures. Bone Miner. 1990;11:295-304.
208. Krieger NS, Frick KK, LaPlante Strutz K, et al. Regulation of COX-2 mediates acid-induced bone calcium efflux in vitro. J Bone Miner Res. 2007;22:907-17.
209. Khosla S. Minireview: the OPG/RANKL/RANK system. Endocrinology. 2001;142:5050-5.
210. Krieger NS, Stern PH. Potassium effects of bone: comparison of two model systems. Am J Physiol. 1983;245:E303-7.
211. Tashjian JAH, Hohmann EL, Antoniades HN, et al. Platelet-derived growth factor stimulates bone resorption via a prostaglandin-mediated mechanism. Endocrinology. 1982;111:118-24.
212. Seuwen K, Ludwig MG, Wolf RM. Receptors for protons or lipid messengers or both? J Recept Signal Transduct Res. 2006;26:599-610.
213. Ludwig MG, Vanek M, Guerini D, et al. Proton-sensing G-protein-coupled receptors. Nature. 2003;425:93-8.
214. Iwai K, Koike M, Ohshima S, et al. RGS18 acts as a negative regulator of osteoclastogenesis by modulating the acid-sensing OGR1/NFAT signaling pathway. J Bone Miner Res. 2007;22:1612-20.
215. Pereverzev A, Komarova SV, Korcok J, et al. Extracellular acidification enhances osteoclast survival through an NFAT-independent, protein kinase C-dependent pathway. Bone. 2008;42:150-61.
216. Frick KK, Krieger NS, Nehrke K, et al. Metabolic acidosis increases intracellular calcium in bone cells through activation of the proton receptor OGR1. J Bone Miner Res. 2009;24:305-13.
217. Frick KK, Bushinsky DA. Effect of metabolic and respiratory acidosis on intracellular calcium in osteoblasts. Am J Physiol Renal Physiol. 2010;299:418-25.
218. Krieger NS, Bushinsky DA. Pharmacologic inhibition of intracellular calcium release blocks acid-induced bone resorption. Am J Physiol Renal Physiol. 2011;300:F91-7.
219. Pande S, Ritter CS, Rothstein M, et al. FGF-23 and sFRP-4 in chronic kidney disease and post-renal transplantation. Nephron Phys. 2006;104:23-32.
220. Martin A, David V, Quarles LD. Regulation and function of the FGF23/klotho endocrine pathways. Physiol Rev. 2012;92: 131-55.
221. Razzaque MS. The FGF23-Klotho axis: endocrine regulation of phosphate homeostasis. Nat Rev Endocrinol. 2009;5:611-9.
222. Faul C, Amaral AP, Oskouei B, et al. FGF23 induces left ventricular hypertrophy. J Clin Invest. 2011;121:4393-408.

223. Kendrick J, Cheung AK, Kaufman JS, et al. FGF-23 associates with death, cardiovascular events, and initiation of chronic dialysis. J Am Soc Nephrol. 2011;22:1913-22.
224. Gutierrez OM. Fibroblast growth factor 23 and mortality among patients undergoing hemodialysis. N Engl J Med. 2008;359:584-92.
225. Liu S, Tang W, Zhou J, et al. Fibroblast growth factor 23 is a counter-regulatory phosphaturic hormone for vitamin D. J Am Soc Nephrol. 2006;17:1305-15.
226. Quarles LD. Endocrine functions of bone in mineral metabolism regulation. J Clin Invest. 2008;118:3820-8.
227. Lavi-Moshayoff V, Wasserman G, Meir T, et al. PTH increases FGF23 gene expression and mediates the high-FGF23 levels of experimental kidney failure: a bone parathyroid feedback loop. Am J Physiol Renal Physiol. 2010;299:F882-9.
228. Krieger NS, Culbertson CD, Kyker-Snowman K, et al. Metabolic acidosis increases fibroblast growth factor 23 in neonatal mouse bone. Am J Physiol Renal Physiol. 2012;303:F431-6.
229. Frick KK, Bushinsky DA. Metabolic acidosis stimulates RANK ligand RNA expression in bone through a cyclooxygenase dependent mechanism. J Bone Miner Res. 2003;18:1317-25.

CHAPTER

13 Idiopathic Hypercalciuria

Fredric L Coe, Elaine M Worcester

WHAT IS IDIOPATHIC HYPERCALCIURIA?

Idiopathic hypercalciuria (IH) is a name usually applied to a daily urine calcium excretion rate above the 90th or 95th percentile of the general population in otherwise normal people. By "otherwise normal" we mean that serum calcium is normal, no systemic disease is evident that might raise urine calcium excretion, and no excessive supplements of calcium or vitamin D are being taken.[1] Given these exclusions, the hypercalciuria is called "idiopathic" because the cause is not evident. Such high urine calcium losses may be without apparent consequences, but in some people may lead to calcium renal stones or bone disease.[2]

Because IH is simply a name for urine calcium excretion that lies in the upper percentiles of the normal range, numerical criteria for naming depend upon the normal populations used. Past common values have been above 250 and 300 mg/day for men and women, respectively,[3] but these may be low. In the two Nurses' Health Study Cohorts and the Health Professionals Follow-up Study, mean values among nonstone-forming people were 184 and 190 with standard deviations (SDs) of 95 and 91 for females, and 169 with an SD of 91 for the males.[4] This would place 1 SD limits at 279 and 281 for females and 260 for males. Corresponding 2 SD (95th percentile) values are 374 and 372 for females and 351 for males, all somewhat higher than older limits and also different because men and women have similar cut points.

Some people in these three cohorts became stone formers during the years of observation and, as blood pressure higher values are linked with risk of stroke and other cardiovascular diseases, higher values of urine calcium are linked with risk of renal stones (*see* Chapters 1 and 15). For the clinical purposes of kidney stone treatment, therefore, we advise using risk-related upper limits as described in that chapter. In both men and women, risk of stone formation begins at above 200 mg/day of calcium excretion, a value just above the median values among normal people.

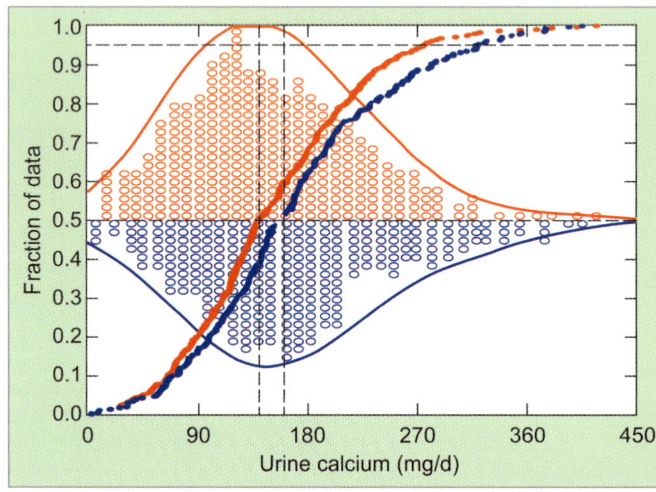

Fig. 13.1: Distribution of urine calcium excretions in normal men and women. These data have been compiled from available balance studies conducted over the past decades. In all we found 275 men (blue) and 339 women (red).

An alternative source of data that has not been extensively mined is the collection of 24-hour urines obtained in the course of the numerous metabolic balance studies performed in normal subjects over the past 100 years (Fig. 13.1). Every 6-day balance study provides a 24-hour urine calcium value, shown in red dots for females and blue dots for males. Quantile plots of the data show the locations for the medians, 161 in men and 140 in women (at the vertical dashed lines) and the 95% upper confidence interval bound (horizontal dashed line). The 2 SD upper limits, given means of 170 and 152, men and women, respectively, with SD values 83 and 72, are 336 and 296, respectively. These values are slightly below those of the three population studies, which were based on free choice diets and perhaps supplements. Even so, and despite marked differences in technique, the values are reasonably close.*

Since, the distribution of human urine calcium excretion is continuous, though left skewed with a long

*Being culled from a century of publications, and from data in a PhD thesis, it is impossible to reference the balance data within the normal confines of a chapter.

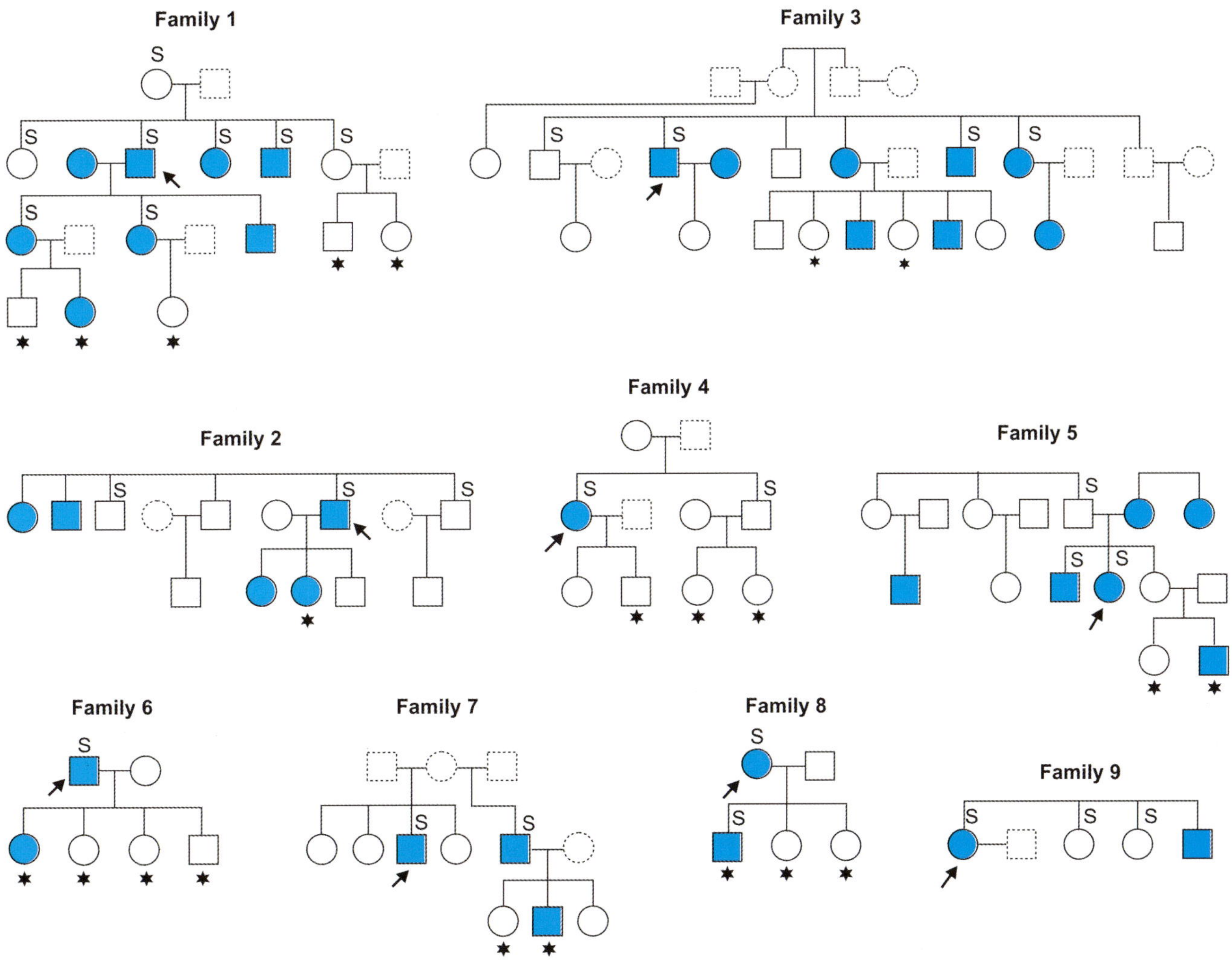

Fig. 13.2: Evidence for the familial occurrence of idiopathic hypercalciuria. S indicates stone former. Males are square, females round, filled indicates hypercalciuria. Arrows point to the probands.
Source: Redrawn from Coe FL, Parks JH, Moore ES. Familial idiopathic hypercalciuria. N Engl J Med. 1979;300:337-40.

right-high-tail (*see* Fig. 13.1), it is not that hypercalciuria marks out a category of distinct disease but rather that, like high blood pressure or even tallness, it describes people farther than usual from the center of the distribution.

For research concerning pathogenesis of hypercalciuria, the older limits—250 and 300 mg/day, women and men, respectively—are probably high enough so that one can compare people above with those below the older limits, asking in what ways the higher urine calcium arises. Perhaps for the most demanding research, for example attempts to find genes linking with hypercalciuria, the true 95% upper limits might prove more fruitful. For clinical management, 200 mg/day is a reasonable threshold of risk, which increases progressively with higher urine calcium excretion rates.

IDIOPATHIC HYPERCALCIURIA IS FAMILIAL AND CAN BE BRED FOR IN ANIMALS

Human Studies of Familial Occurrence

Among the first-degree relatives of patients with IH (Fig. 13.2), we found about half also had higher than normal urine calcium excretion.[5] A recent study shows statistical evidence that urine calcium excretion is familial[6] and reviews other studies subsequent to the one in Figure 13.2.

In a prospective study of families of calcium stone forming children, their siblings, and children from families with no history of stones,[7] we found that siblings with stones had the same high level of urine calcium as the

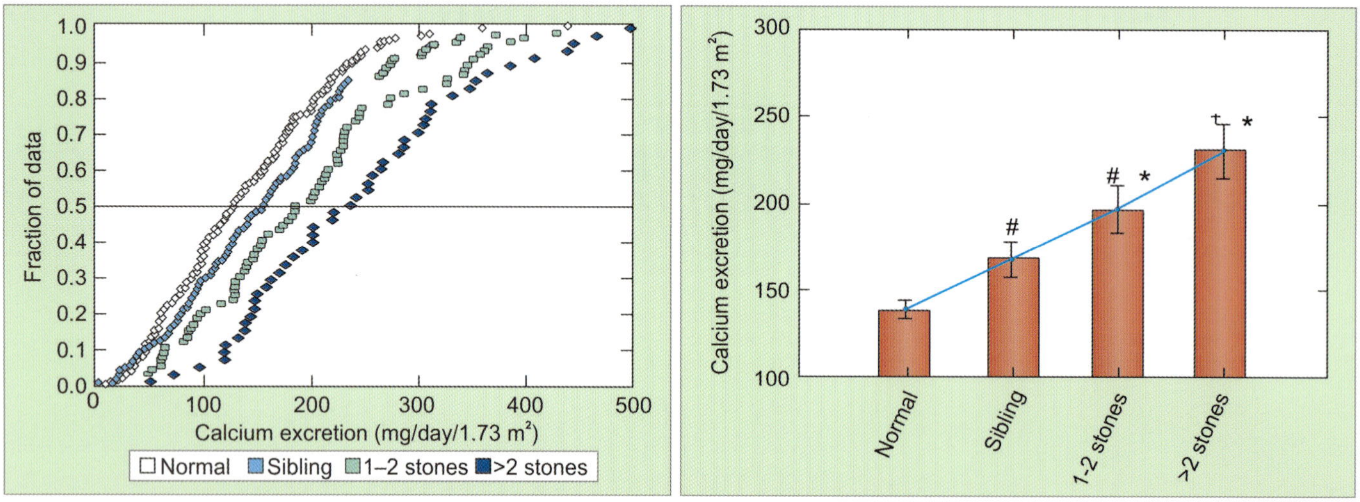

Fig. 13.3: Siblings of children with calcium kidney stones are hypercalciuric. Calcium excretion of children with calcium renal stones ('green and dark blue rectanbles', left panel) exceeded that of normal children from families without kidney stones (open rectangle). Even stone-free siblings of stone formers excreted more calcium than normal children. Urine calcium was progressively higher in siblings, children with one to two and those with more than two stones (right panel).
Source: Redrawn from Bergsland KJ, Coe FL, White MD, et al. Urine risk factors in children with calcium kidney stones and their siblings. Kidney Int. 2012;81:1140-8.

probands, whereas siblings without stones had about half that level of urine calcium excretion, and children from families with no stones even lower urine calcium excretions (Fig. 13.3). Even more, those siblings with more than two kidney stones had a higher urine calcium excretion rate than those with fewer than two kidney stones. These data support a hereditary basis for IH and also that a dose effect exists between the level of urine calcium and risk of stones, as was observed in the prospective studies of nurses and physicians mentioned above (*see* Chapters 1 and 15).

Human Monogenic Hypercalciuria

Although, the genes responsible for the common IH of calcium stone formers have not been discovered to date, numerous forms of human monogenic hypercalciuria are known and represent a priceless resource for study and thought. The best way to review this matter, in our opinion, is by reference to established compilations of genetic information, and for this purpose we have chosen OMIM (http://omim.org) as an outstanding source. In another chapter (*see* Chapter 7), Bushinsky et al. detail those animal models of hypercalciuria thus far investigated. Because this book has a strong clinical orientation and these defects are rare, we forgo their detailed presentation here. However, many recent publications are a ready entry into the literature[8-12] in addition to OMIM.

GASTROINTESTINAL AND BONE CONTRIBUTIONS TO IH

Calcium Absorption

Normal Men and Women

The same balance data we used to illustrate the distribution of urine calcium excretions demonstrate (Fig. 13.4, upper left panel) that among normal women (red) and men (blue), calcium absorption is generally a linear function of calcium intake. Each point is a single 6-day balance study from one person. The slopes differed, women higher than men, as did net absorption adjusted for intake (refer to the legend of Fig. 13.4).

The fraction of diet calcium absorbed (Fig. 13.4, upper middle panel) is generally flat above an intake of 250 mg/day; at lower intake levels, the fraction absorbed falls steeply into the negative zone, indicating net loss of bone mineral. Quantile plots of the fractional calcium absorption for men and women (Fig. 13.4, upper right panel) overlap, a fact consistent with their similar behavior concerning absorption as a function of intake. The median absorption fraction is 21%.

Idiopathic Hypercalciuria Subjects

When all 165 (eight female) available balance studies on IH subjects (Fig. 13.4, lower left panel, purple dots) are

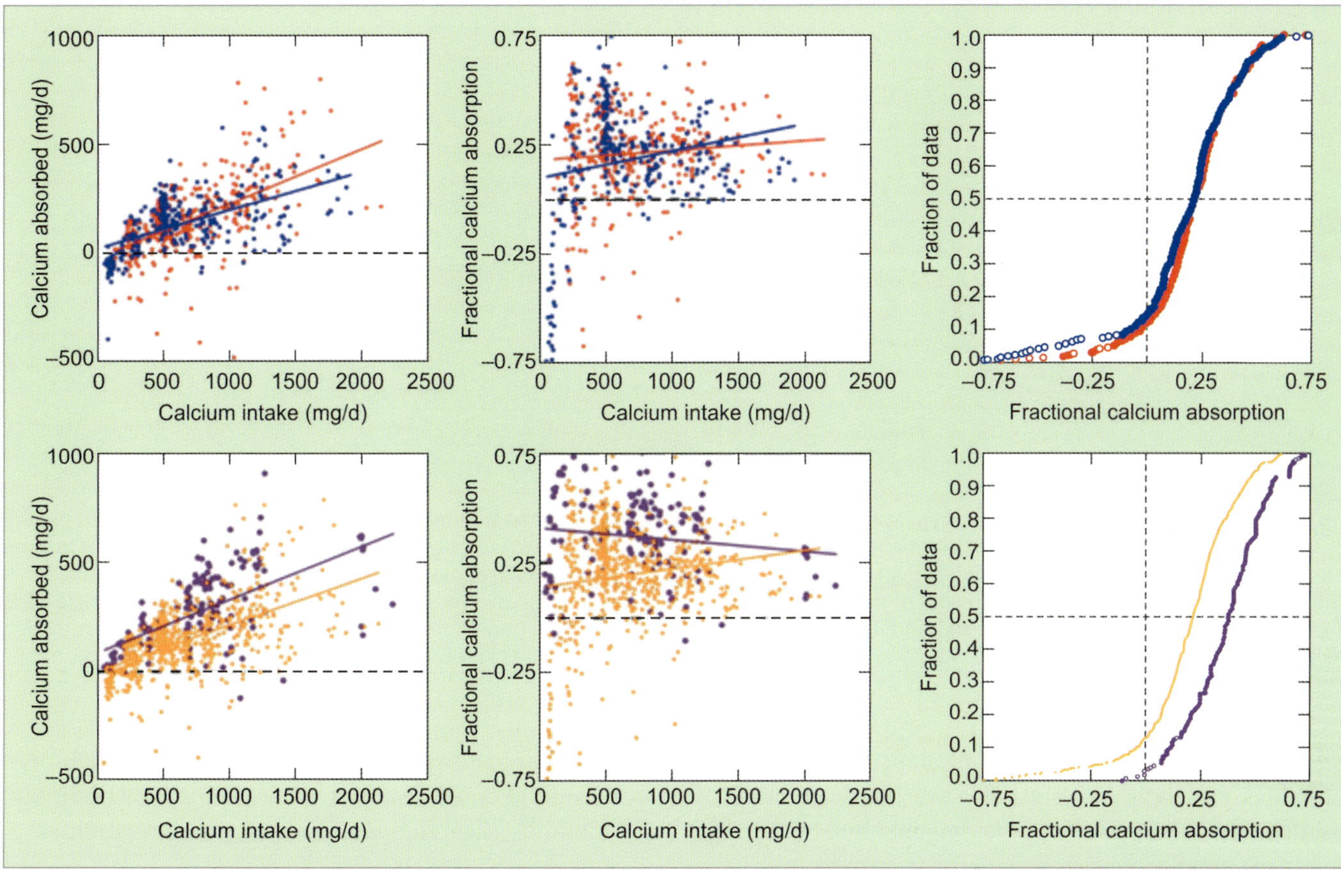

Fig. 13.4: Calcium absorption in normal people and those with idiopathic hypercalciuria (IH). Among normal men (blue) and women (red), calcium absorption (Y-axis, upper left panel) rose linearly with calcium intake (X-axis). Judged by general linear modeling, the slopes differed ($p < 0.001$), as did net absorption adjusted for intake (135 ± 8 vs 158 ± 7, $p < 0.001$, men and women, respectively). The fraction of diet calcium absorbed remains constant above an intake of 250 mg (upper middle panel) in both sexes; below that point net absorption becomes negative (stool calcium exceeds intake because of pancreatic, biliary, and intestinal calcium secretion). The distributions of fractional absorptions by women and men overlay one another (upper right panel; median 21% both sexes). Among people with IH (lower left panel, purple symbols), calcium absorption is higher than among normal men and women combined (orange symbols) at all calcium rectanbles levels (262 vs 145 mg/day adjusted for intake, $p < 0.001$), and fractional calcium intake is above normal (lower middle panel) at all but the highest calcium intakes. The entire distribution of fractional calcium absorptions is shifted upwards compared to normal (lower right panel; IH median = 37.5%).

plotted against the combined normal male and female data from the upper left panel, IH is seen to be a state of increased calcium absorption (details in the legend of the figure). Many unidirectional isotope transport studies have documented increased absorption in IH.[13,14]

As in normals, the fraction of calcium intake absorbed by IH subjects does not vary significantly with intake (Fig. 13.4, lower middle panel; regression slopes are not statistically significant). Fractional absorption by IH subjects exceeds normal throughout most of the intake range available; the few points above an intake of 2,000 mg/day appear to merge. A quantile plot of fractional calcium absorption (Fig. 13.4, lower right panel) demonstrates the markedly higher average value among IH subjects (37.5% vs 21%). Of interest is the very few negative absorption values in all three plots for IH subjects; they rarely enter negative calcium balance via an excess of gastrointestinal (GI) calcium secretion versus absorption even when calcium intake is very low.

Bone Calcium Balance

Normals

Among normal adult men and women (Fig. 13.5, left panel, blue and red dots, respectively), urine calcium excretion as measured during 6-day balance studies exceeds or lies

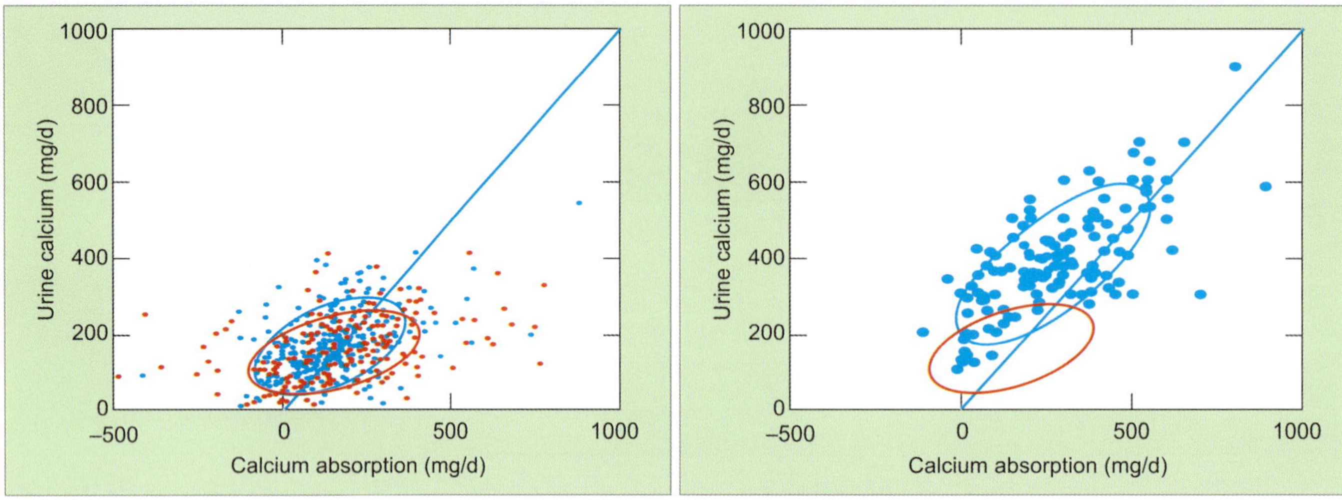

Fig. 13.5: Calcium balance in idiopathic hypercalciuria (IH) and normal people. Among normal adult men (blue) and women (left panel), urine calcium is below or above net calcium absorption about equally (points distribute above and below the line of identity). Calcium retention adjusted for absorption is slightly higher in women (−6 vs −27, $p < 0.001$). People with IH are almost always in negative calcium balance as shown by points to the left of the line of identity. Combined normal men and women are represented as a single 68% ellipse of containment. In a general linear model for normals and IH subjects (right panel), the latter have much lower calcium retention than normals (5 vs −156 mg/day, $p < 0.001$) and the slope of urine calcium on net calcium absorption is far higher in IH versus normals.

below calcium intake in the same balance periods about half the time each, as shown by the rough equality of points to the left and right of the diagonal line of identity. This is reasonably consistent with the fact that adults have finished skeletal formation and will vary in their skeletal mineral balance with their diet calcium intakes. Calcium balance is slightly higher in women than men (refer to the legend of Fig. 13.5).

Idiopathic Hypercalciuria Subjects

By contrast (Fig. 13.5, right panel), the vast majority of IH subjects excrete more calcium in their urine than they absorb; it is only at the highest calcium absorption rates that even a modest fraction enters strongly positive balance. For visual clarity, the combined normal male and female balances are shown by only their joint, empty, 68% nonparametric ellipse of containment. A few IH subjects fall into the normal zone, but most are displaced upward and to the left, meaning their hypercalciuria is a consequence or cause of negative calcium balance.

Whereas even when challenged by very low calcium intakes IH subjects can usually manage to achieve neutral or even positive net calcium absorption, they do not seem to be able to conserve calcium at a renal level, and their hypercalciuria reflects loss of bone mineral at net calcium absorption rates that overlap with those of the normal subjects. The causal mechanism for their greater loss of bone mineral could reside in bone, kidney, or both, and considerable research has concerned both possibilities.

Effects of Low-Calcium Diets

Very Low-Calcium Diet

Predictably, IH subjects should respond to a very low calcium diet by excreting in their urine more calcium than they ingest, and that is indeed the case. Nine normal subjects and 37 IH subjects ate a diet containing 2 mg/kg/day, and 24-hour urine samples were collected on days 7–9 of the diet.[15] Almost all of the IH subjects excreted more urine calcium than any of the normal, and a majority lost more calcium in their urine than they ate. This loss of calcium, which can arise only from bone mineral, confirms the predictions of the balance data and illustrates in a dramatic manner why low calcium diets are not a therapeutic option for long-term stone prevention.

Moderately Low-Calcium Diet

A large body of research[16] used a higher diet calcium intake, of 400 mg daily, in the study of IH subjects. In the absence of formal balance measurements, it would not have been an easy task to reliably identify negative bone calcium balance because the diet somewhat exceeds the amounts of

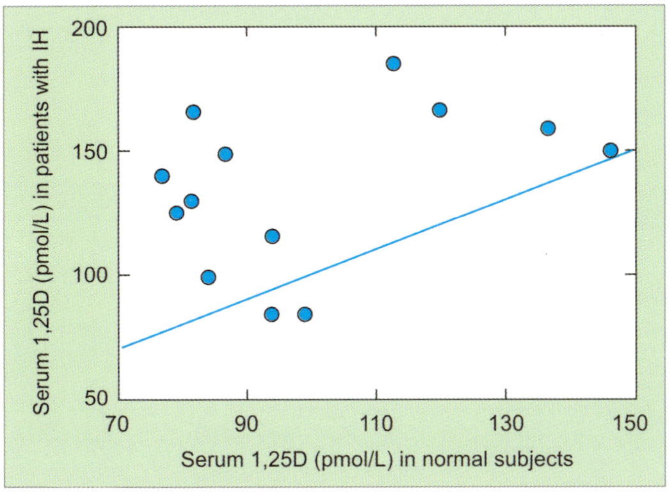

Fig. 13.6: Serum calcitriol levels in idiopathic hypercalciuria (IH) exceed normal. Each point is the mean of IH versus normal subjects within a trial. All but two trials show IH above normal—above the diagonal line of identity.[15,17-24]

urine calcium excreted by most IH subjects eating it. One way measurements of GI calcium absorption using isotopic techniques generally suggested that calcium absorption might well have balanced urine calcium losses, but calcium secretion was not measured and can easily reach values of 100 mg daily. For all these reasons, this body of work did not highlight the potential drawbacks of low calcium diets.

Vitamin D Hormone System

The increased calcium absorption in IH probably reflects activation by calcitriol (*see* Chapters 8 and 9) because in a majority of studies, serum calcitriol levels of IH subjects have exceeded those of normal people (Fig. 13.6). But serum calcitriol alone need not be the only mechanism. Increase of the vitamin D receptor (VDR) is what drives intestinal transport above normal in rats inbred for hypercalciuria (*see* Chapter 7). Serum calcitriol levels are normal in these rats, but VDR abundance and intestinal transport rates both are elevated. In one study,[25] monocyte VDR abundance was reported as higher in male IH versus normal age-matched men, but this has not thus far been tested by others.

Bone Disease

Many investigators have documented lower bone mineral densities in IH versus control subjects,[26] and increased fracture rates have also been documented. In the inbred IH rats (*see* Chapter 7), Bushinsky has shown bone abnormalities that would predispose to fracture. Mechanisms proposed are numerous, but proof in humans so far is incomplete. An extensive and recent review of this topic details results from multiple patient studies.[26]

Prospective studies of bone mineral loss in IH are not common. One in particular[27] involves no interventions but time itself (Fig. 13.7). Patients with IH were followed for 3 years after an initial bone mineral density (BMD) measurement. A second measurement was then made. The change in BMD was inversely proportional to the urine calcium excretion measured at the beginning of the observation period, especially in the femoral neck.

RENAL CALCIUM HANDLING IN IH

Because intestinal absorption is above normal, studies of renal handling require that diet intakes of IH and normal subjects be identical, a demand that can be fulfilled only in a clinical research setting. Recent studies under such conditions have clarified the role of renal calcium handling and made clear that the immediate cause of hypercalciuria in humans, as in some animal models (*see* Chapter 7), is the reduction of tubule calcium reabsorption.

A cautionary note is in order. We will be presenting published data from IH subjects who were for the most part calcium stone formers. We do not know if renal handling of calcium is the same in IH subjects who are not stone formers. Possibly stone formation is fostered precisely by the specific nephron transport abnormalities we found, and nonstone-forming IH subjects have altogether different tubule mechanisms raising urine calcium.

Overall and Segmental Tubule Reabsorptions

Overall Tubule Calcium Reabsorption

Fasting, stone formers with IH excrete more calcium in their urine than normal controls (Fig. 13.8, upper right panel), even though ultrafilterable serum calcium and filtered loads of calcium (Fig. 13.8, upper and lower left panels) are not different.[28] Fed three meals throughout the day, IH patients raise their urine calcium far above controls despite similar filtered loads, so the fraction of filtered calcium excreted (FECa) exceeds controls (Fig. 13.8, lower right panel). Tubule calcium reabsorption is reduced in IH

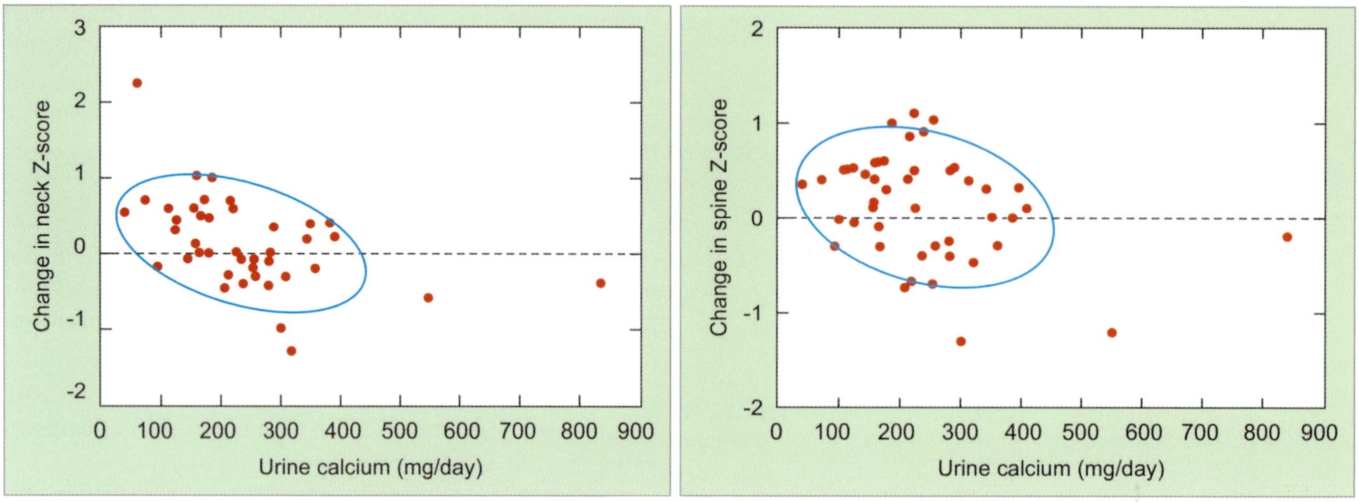

Fig. 13.7: Change in bone mineral density over time is inverse to urine calcium losses. Among stone formers with idiopathic hypercalciuria (IH), change in femoral neck (left panel) and spine (right panel) Z-score varied inversely with baseline urine calcium excretion (X-axis).

Source: Redrawn from Asplin JR, Bauer KA, Kinder J, et al. Bone mineral density and urine calcium excretion among subjects with and without nephrolithiasis. Kidney Int. 2003;63:662-9.

and it, not increased filtered load, is the immediate mechanism that raises urine calcium excretion.

Proximal Tubule Reabsorption

Using endogenous lithium clearance as a marker for proximal tubule (PT) reabsorption,[29] it is possible to calculate delivery of calcium out of PT and into the more distal nephron segments—thick ascending limbs and distal convoluted tubules. Using this technique, we[30] demonstrated that increased PT delivery is a feature of IH patients (Fig. 13.9), and that increasing delivery correlates roughly with urine calcium excretion.

Distal Nephron Reabsorption

Because we can calculate PT delivery and also measure urine calcium losses, it is possible to calculate the fraction of distal delivery reabsorbed. Using such calculations, this fraction is reduced in IH as compared to normal subjects.[31]

Integration of Proximal and Distal Nephron Reabsorptions: Calcium

Because food intake affects tubule calcium reabsorption and the final urine calcium excretion—which is what matters in terms of stone formation—is the result of distal delivery and distal fractional excretion (distal FECa) of what is delivered, the processes giving rise to IH can best be visualized from graphic presentations (Fig. 13.10).

Fast

Fasting, distal calcium delivery out of PT is higher in IH than normal subjects (N) (Fig. 13.10, upper left panel) but not significantly. Distal FECa is also higher in IH than N (Fig. 13.10, upper middle panel), although the difference is not statistically significant. The combination of the two, which is urine calcium excretion (Fig. 13.10, upper right panel), is significantly higher in IH than N.

We may have belabored the presentation of this simple point, but it is essential for understanding how IH works. The urine calcium excretion is the product of distal delivery times distal FECa, so even modest increments of both above normal, because multiplied by one another, can lead to important differences in urine calcium excretion, as demonstrated by the three top panels of the figure for fasting subjects.

Fed

Food significantly increases distal delivery for IH and N, and the difference between IH and N becomes significant. Likewise, distal FECa rises in IH and N but more in IH than N, so the difference between them becomes significant statistically: feeding increases distal delivery and FECa more in IH than in normal people. As a natural consequence of the two increases, urine calcium increases far more in IH than in N, giving rise to the hypercalciuria that increases risk of kidney stones.

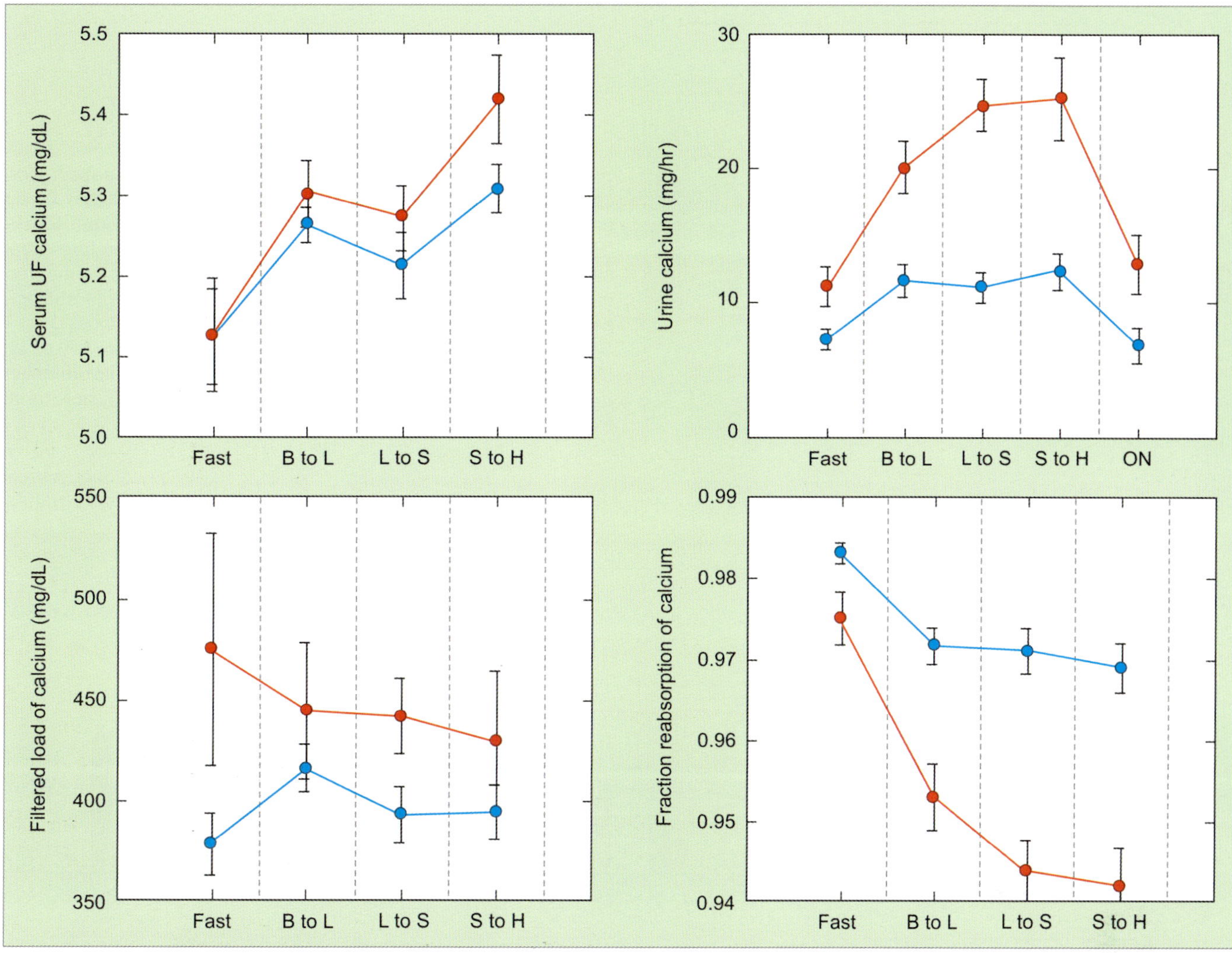

Fig. 13.8: Renal mechanisms of idiopathic hypercalciuria (IH). Urine calcium excretion by IH subjects (upper right panel, filled circles) exceeds normals fasting, and after meals: B: Breakfast; L: Lunch; S: Supper; H: Home at end of experiment; ON: Overnight. Serum ultrafilterable (UF) calcium and filtered loads of calcium (upper and lower left panels) do not differ between N and IH. Fraction of filtered calcium reabsorbed (lower right panel) by IH is far below normal, meaning that the mechanism by which excessive calcium gets into the urine is not via filtered load—as might occur from high absorption rates—but reduction of tubule calcium reabsorption.
Source: Redrawn from Worcester EM, Gillen DL, Evan AP, et al. Evidence that postprandial reduction of renal calcium reabsorption mediates hypercalciuria of patients with calcium nephrolithiasis. Am J Physiol Renal Physiol. 2007;292:F66-75.

Overnight (ON)

We have elaborated elsewhere (*see* Chapter 15) the extreme degree of urine calcium phosphate (CaP) supersaturation encountered overnight. It mainly reflects the higher urine calcium excretion of IH versus normal people during a period in which urine volumes fall remarkably and to an equal extent. Overnight, distal deliveries of IH and N become identical. But distal FECa of IH rises above even the fed period, and far above normal. The result is a marked increase of nocturnal calcium excretion in IH compared to normal subjects (*see* Fig. 13.10, upper right panel), which creates an abnormally high overnight supersaturation and therefore stone risk in people with IH.

Integration of Proximal and Distal Nephron Reabsorptions: Sodium

Fast

The higher distal delivery of calcium in IH than in N arises mainly from increased endogenous lithium clearance,

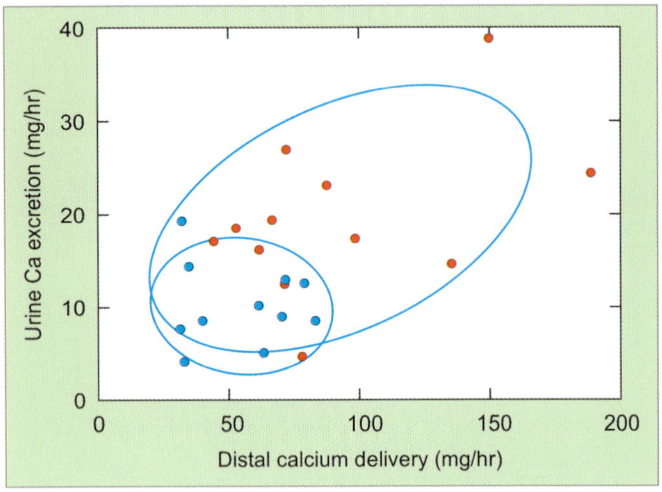

Fig. 13.9: Reduced proximal tubule calcium reabsorption contributes to hypercalciuria in idiopathic hypercalciuria (IH). Using endogenous lithium clearance as a marker for proximal tubule (PT) reabsorption, PT reabsorption is reduced and therefore distal calcium delivery (X-axis) is increased in IH (blue circles) compared to normal controls. Each point is the mean for a single subject; each subject was studied during 12 fed clearance periods.

Source: Redrawn from Worcester EM, Coe FL, Evan AP, et al. Evidence for increased postprandial distal nephron calcium delivery in hypercalciuric stone-forming patients. Am J Physiol Renal Physiol. 2008;295:F1286-94

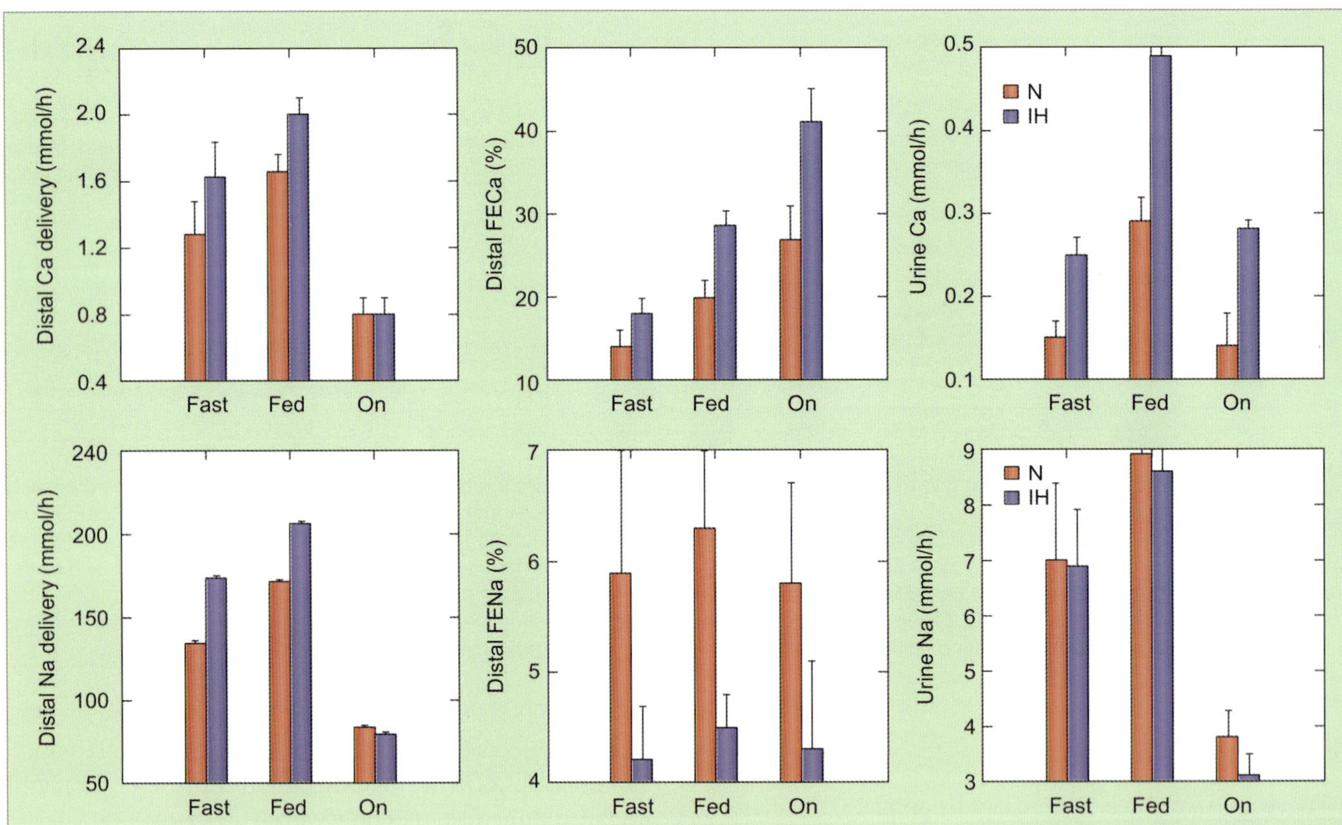

Fig. 13.10: Proximal and distal nephron calcium and sodium reabsorption in idiopathic hypercalciuria (IH) and normal subjects. Distal calcium (Ca) and sodium (Na) deliveries are higher in IH versus N fasting and fed (left panels) and fed values exceed fasting in IH and N. The fractions of distally delivered calcium excreted (upper middle panel) are higher in IH than normal fed, but not fasting. Increased delivery and distal fractional excretion combine to produce hypercalciuria (upper right panel). Urine calcium of IH exceeds N fasting, fed and overnight, and urine calcium fed exceeds fasting for both IH and N subjects. The fractions of distally delivered Na excreted are adjusted so that differing deliveries (lower middle panels) do not result in different urine Na losses.

Source: Redrawn from Ko B, Bergsland KJ, Gillen DL, et al. Gender differences in proximal and distal nephron function contribute to the mechanism of idiopathic hypercalcuria in calcium stone formers. Am J Physiol Regul Integr Comp Physiol. 2015;309:R85-92.

because filtered loads do not differ (we do not show this level of detail, which is available in the original publication).[31] Therefore, distal deliveries of calcium and sodium (*see* Fig. 13.10, lower 3 panels) must parallel each other given equal and constant levels of serum sodium and calcium. But in contrast to what happens to calcium, distal FENa of IH is far below normal, so that the final urine sodium excretions of the two groups match almost exactly.

Fed

The same is true with feeding. Distal sodium deliveries rise in IH and normals, and, to a small extent, distal FENa also rises, so urine sodium excretions rise. But they rise to an equal level, in complete contrast to the case for calcium.

Overnight

Deliveries fall remarkably, as for calcium, and distal FENa values are the same as for fasting, so urine sodium excretions fall in both IH and normals to levels far below those fasting. This contrasts with calcium excretion, which falls only to fasting levels in IH and normals, not below as for sodium. Fasting values for calcium excretion in IH are problematic overnight because urine volumes are below those fasting, as already noted.

Idiopathic Hypercalciuria is a Condition of Distal Nephron Calcium/Sodium Dissociation

It would seem a trite commonplace to point out the calcium sodium dissociation in IH, for many studies have shown that urine calcium can be high in IH in the absence of a proportional increase of urine sodium.[32] Likewise, our demonstration that the dissociation is distal to the PT is commonplace, as sodium and calcium are reabsorbed in PT together,[33] but calcium and sodium transports can be dissociated in both the thick ascending limbs and distal convoluted tubules (*see* Chapter 9).

However, our observations are rescued from the mundane because the actual situation in humans might not have been as we found it. For example, the entire mechanism of IH could have been a marked increase in distal delivery with equal distal FECa values in IH and N or even lower values of distal FECa in IH than in N but simply not low enough to offset high delivery—it could have been proximal with all the dissociation from sodium being specific to sodium itself.

In fact, the distal nephron is actively involved as distal FECa is higher in IH than normal, and rises with meals, something one might never have predicted. More so, the overnight situation is particularly odd in that distal differences in calcium handling account for all of the nocturnal hypercalciuria that is so critical to the high supersaturation one encounters.

Sex Differences in Proximal and Distal Nephron Mechanisms for IH

As if some additional bedevilment were needed in this complex physiology, it appears that men and women achieve their increases in urine calcium excretion not in the same but in somewhat different ways.[31]

Fast

Distal calcium delivery (Fig. 13.11, upper left panel) is about the same in normal women and in men and women with IH, but men with IH have far higher values. In other words, the generally higher distal delivery in IH arises from the men, not women, with IH. Distal FECa is higher in normal men than normal women and in IH than N, though none of the differences achieve significance. But once again, because of the multiplicative effects of delivery and fractional excretion, urine calcium excretion of men with IH exceeds normal men and women with IH. Essentially, men with IH have the booster effect of high delivery, which does not add to but multiplies a higher distal FECa, whereas women rely on increased distal FECa alone to achieve their hypercalciuria.

Fed

With food, these differences all become exaggerated. Distal delivery increases from fasting in women and men without IH, but especially and significantly more in men with IH. Distal FECa increases significantly in everyone compared to fasting, but it is among women that IH raises it above normal, whereas values are closer together in men with and without IH. Once again the multiplicative effects of delivery and distal FECa create a marked difference in final urine calcium excretion. Certainly, women with IH excrete more calcium than normal women, but men are more hypercalciuric because of the dual effect. Note that the obvious error—men are bigger than women, and urine is an extensive variable—has been greatly reduced by the manner of the experiment: all values are calculated to 1.73 M^2 of body surface area.

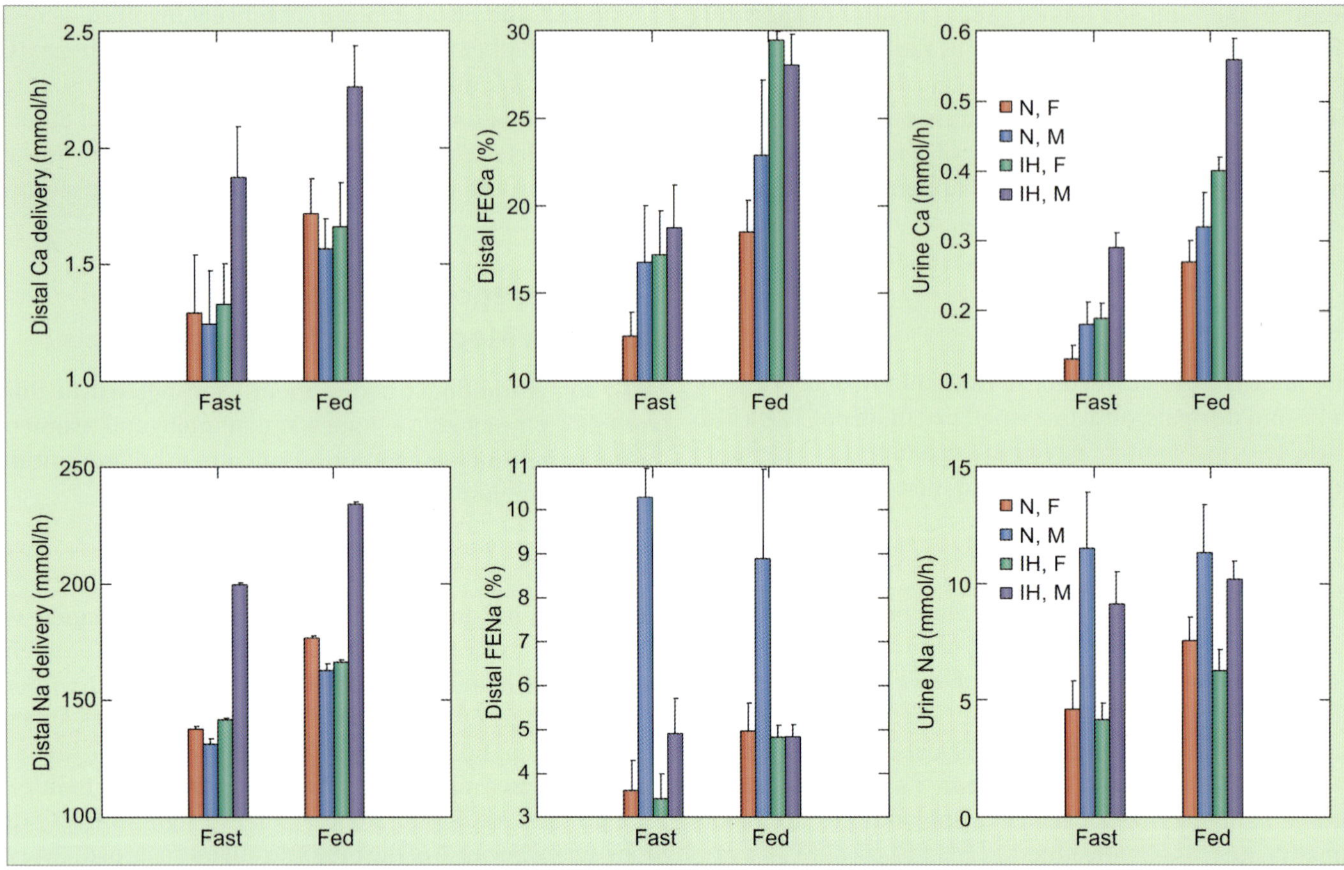

Fig. 13.11: Proximal and distal nephron calcium and sodium reabsorption in idiopathic hypercalciuria (IH) and normal subjects by sex. The high distal Ca and Na deliveries of IH subjects (left panels) arise from males not females. Fractions of distally delivered Ca excreted (upper middle panel) are higher in IH than N in both sexes and result in hypercalciuria. Both male groups ate and excreted more sodium than corresponding females and distal FENa values of IH and N males are adjusted so that urine Na excretions are not different despite the large difference in distal Na delivery.

Source: Redrawn from Ko B, Bergsland KJ, Gillen DL, et al. Gender differences in proximal and distal nephron function contribute to the mechanism of idiopathic hypercalciuria in calcium stone formers. Am J Physiol Regul Integr Comp Physiol. 2015;309:R85-92.

Sodium

The behavior of sodium reabsorption does not differ remarkably between the sexes except in the sense that higher distal delivery in men leads to higher distal sodium reabsorption and that men were in general eating more sodium—adjusted for body surface—than women. Fasting and fed, the higher delivery of sodium and calcium out of the proximal tubules of IH males is obvious.

An accident of diet offered a valuable insight into sodium physiology among the men. Both IH and normal men were less well adapted to the Clinical Research Center (CRC) diet, as noted, and the normal men lacked the high distal delivery of those with IH. In order to excrete their sodium, they greatly raised distal FENa far above what was found in men with IH, who could excrete their sodium partly through increased delivery. They, the IH men, had distal FENa values no different from normal or IH women yet excreted far more sodium.

As a result, the dissociation between sodium and calcium is perhaps most remarkable in normal men, visible by an accident of diet. Both fasting and fed and perhaps most obviously fasting, distal sodium and calcium reabsorptions diverge remarkably.

Sex Differences in Blood Pressure

In addition to differences in tubule calcium handling, men and women differ in relation to blood pressure in IH versus normal subjects.[31] Among men, those with IH had substantially lower systolic blood pressures as measured over the day of the study protocol, whereas among women the differences were less marked (120 vs 126 and 120 vs 112, IH vs N, males and females, respectively; $p < 0.01$ for the male IH vs. N comparison, p = NS for the female comparison). We could not find a link between tubule handling of calcium and blood pressure, even though other studies have suggested that higher PT reabsorption rates tend to occur in people with hypertension: older people whose blood pressures were above those of younger controls,[34] and South African Black people versus Belgian Caucasians.[35]

A General Overview of the Kidney in Hypercalciuria

One should at this point offer some kind of summary and sense of significance. Taken simply, the high calcium excretion of IH arises from variations of renal tubule reabsorption that regulate calcium excretion and presumably account for the broad spread of urine calcium excretions illustrated in Figure 13.1. Tubule reabsorption is more sensitive to food intake in hypercalciuria, so we must suppose that the regulating factors that create hypercalciuria sense nutrient intake.

But one cannot maintain a flow of water out of a bathtub simply by opening the drain. A source of renewal is essential, and that source can be only bone or diet. Ample evidence proves that high absorption rates from diet are foundational in IH, and given an adequate dietary source of calcium bone mineral loss need not, in principle, occur. Other evidence of equal quality documents that bone mineral is indeed at risk in IH, meaning that perhaps diet calcium is not commonly sufficient or, alternatively, that even high calcium diets cannot fully preserve bone. This latter seems an engaging and important direction for research.

The kidney is an executive, not a director, so one should not look to it as the prime organizer of mineral metabolism, the brains of the outfit. It almost never is in that role. Hormones, perhaps the renal nerves, possibly levels of hormone receptors, are what bring about the renal physiology of IH. Even these are simply signalers. So the real director of the program must be even further up the administrative ladder. Given that IH is heritable, that ultimate director must have been evolution, acting through regulation of the genome and its effectors. If so, it is not only enough to detail how IH may come about but why, for what reasons, evolution has seemed to favor a wide sweep of urine calcium excretions from which the hypercalciuric, and therefore stone-forming population, is commonly drawn. Here, in this chapter and at this time, we confess: such knowledge lies somewhere in the future; we hope to obtain it.

HORMONES AND RECEPTORS

Fasting Parathyroid Hormone, Calcitriol, and Fibroblast Growth Factor 23

Because these three hormones are central to modern views of mineral metabolism (*see* Chapter 8), we have sought to sort out their interactions in IH compared to normal people. In an initial stepwise analysis with serum parathyroid hormone (PTH) as dependent and serum calcium, phosphate, calcitriol, sex, and subject type as covariates, significant effects were found only for serum calcium and calcitriol. Because of limited numbers of observations, we did not use fibroblast growth factor 23 (FGF-23) as a covariate in our final models at this time.

Individual Levels

In our studies, as in others, fasting serum levels of calcitriol are higher in IH than in well-matched normal people (Fig. 13.12, upper right panel). Serum PTH levels of IH and N are not different (Fig. 13.12, upper left panel). Levels of FGF-23 are slightly higher in IH versus N, but not all subjects have this measurement, so the results are more provisional than for PTH and calcitriol. Serum phosphorus levels of IH subjects are below those of normals, a well-known finding.

Correlations between Hormones

Although, mean levels of serum PTH are not different between IH and normal, the relationships of PTH to calcitriol and serum calcium differ markedly (Fig. 13.13). Among normal subjects (red circles), serum PTH varies inversely with serum calcitriol (Fig. 13.13, upper left panel), whereas in IH subjects (blue circles and dashed ellipse), there is no relationship between them. Although, we cannot detect an inverse relationship between serum PTH and serum calcium level in fasting normal people (Fig. 13.13, upper middle panel), an inverse relationship is prominent in IH. We have published this fact in a smaller subset of subjects elsewhere[1] and ascribed the difference to a possible and as yet unproven increase in CaSR abundance or sensitivity, which might result from liganded VDR stimulation of CaSR gene expression (*see* Chapter 9). We found no relationships between FGF-23 and PTH (Fig. 13.13, upper right panel) with our rather limited set of observations.

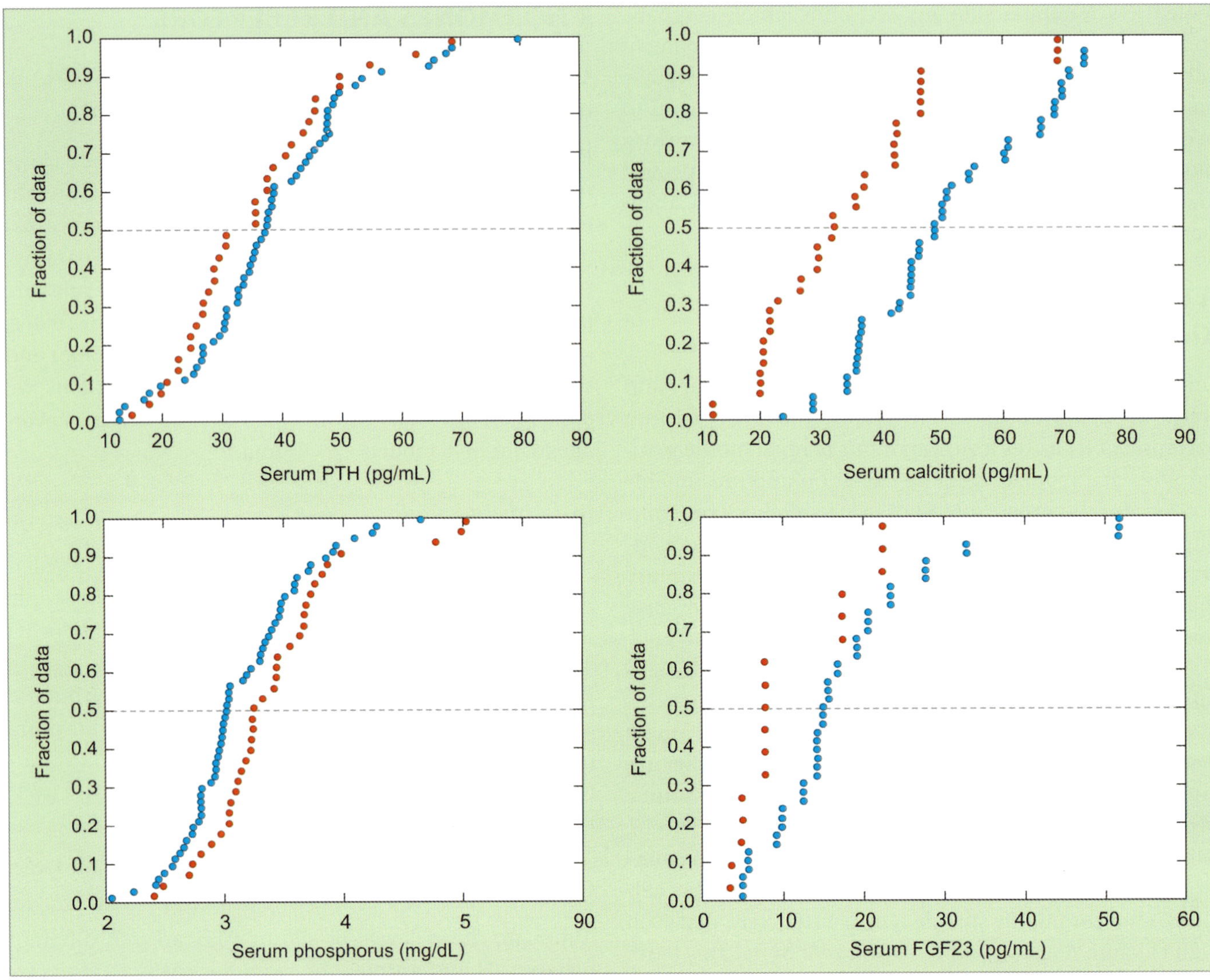

Fig. 13.12: Quantile plots of serum parathyroid hormone (PTH), calcitriol, phosphate, and fibroblast growth factor 23 (FGF-23). Serum values of calcitriol and FGF-23 idiopathic hypercalciuria (IH) differ from N ($p < 0.001$ and $p = 0.005$, respectively). Serum phosphate of IH is marginally below N ($p = 0.034$). N, red symbols; IH, blue symbols.

As expected, serum calcitriol varies inversely with serum calcium in normal people (Fig. 13.13, lower left panel) but not in IH subjects. This latter, along with the loss of any relationship between calcitriol and PTH, speaks to a disruption of normal PTH calcitriol interactions in IH that permit higher calcitriol values at overlapping serum calcium levels.

An inverse relationship is seemingly apparent between calcitriol and FGF-23 as has been suggested in more specific experimental models (*see* Chapter 8), but the scanty data set makes us unwilling to make much of this at present. Of interest, FGF-23 is strongly inverse to serum calcium in N but not IH.

An Overview

Although an increase in vitamin D-mediated calcium absorption and in serum calcitriol has been documented repeatedly by others and reproduced in part by our own work, it would be simplistic and incorrect to think about IH as simply a state of increased vitamin D activation. Such an increase would reduce serum PTH as happens when vitamin D is administered and in states of excess calcitriol production (*see* Chapter 8). Instead we find that calcitriol is increased and PTH is normal. Low calcium diet is perhaps the closest analog in that PTH and calcitriol both increase.[15] Possibly, the complex abnormalities of renal calcium handling we have shown here are a primary event

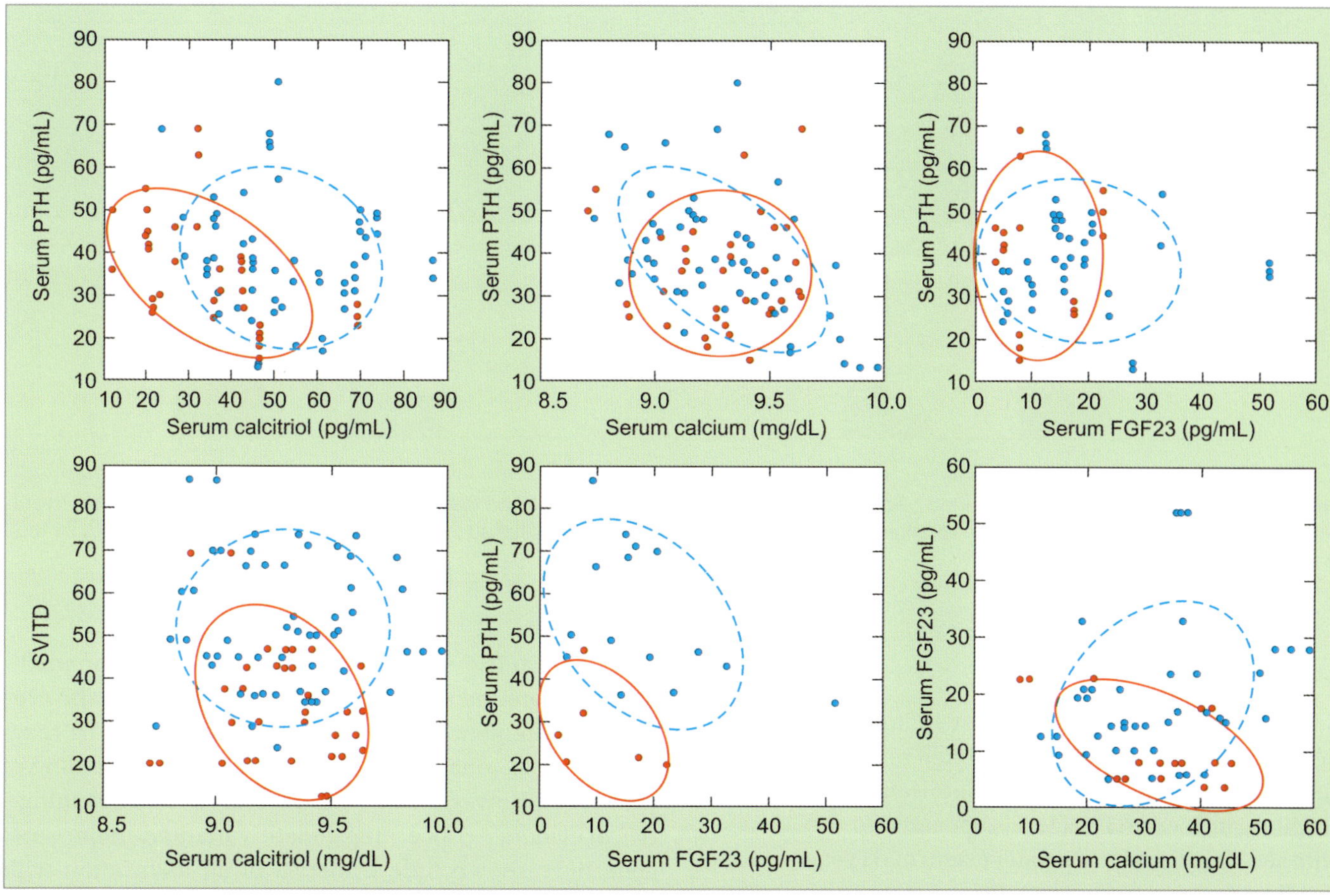

Fig. 13.13: Correlations between serum parathyroid hormone (PTH), calcitriol, calcium, and fibroblast growth factor 23 (FGF-23). Among normals (red circles) but not idiopathic hypercalciuria (IH) subjects (blue circles), serum PTH varies inversely with serum calcitriol (upper left panel). In a general linear model with PTH as dependent and serum calcitriol and calcium as covariate, the cross product of serum calcitriol and subject type was highly significant (p = 0.01). Serum PTH varies inversely with serum calcium in IH but not normal subjects (upper middle panel). The cross product of subject type by serum calcium was significant (p = 0.035).

in IH and changes in PTH and calcitriol relationships are secondary. If this were true, treatments like low sodium diet should reduce calcitriol levels, an experiment that probably should be performed.

Signalers and Renal Calcium Handling in IH

PTH

We have focused on fasting values of PTH because of an interest in the calcitriol, calcium, PTH, FGF-23 relationships, but the hypercalciuria of IH is principally manifest with meals (*see* Fig. 13.8). Parathyroid hormone stimulates calcium reabsorption mainly in the distal nephron, and if it were to fall below normal with meals could possibly contribute to reduced distal calcium reabsorption. In fact, we found the opposite: tubule reabsorption of calcium in IH was below normal at overlapping levels of serum PTH.[28] Urine calcium excretion and fractional excretion adjusted for serum PTH are both high in IH versus normal people.

Insulin

Glucose and other sugars raise urine calcium in normal people, but especially in people with IH.[36] This made insulin a prime candidate as a signaler. However, we found no evidence for higher insulin levels in our IH as opposed to our normal subjects.[1] Recent direct measurements have failed to show any effect of insulin to increase urine calcium or tubule calcium reabsorption.[37]

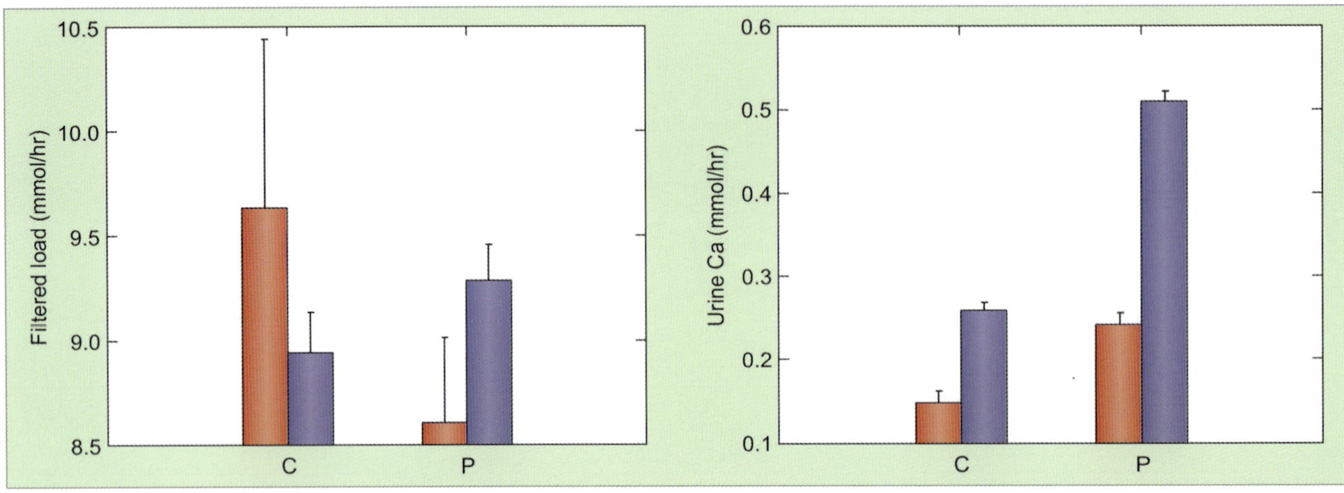

Fig. 13.14: Calcium filtered load and urine calcium excretion. Fasting (red bars) filtered load was higher in normal than idiopathic hypercalciuria (IH), whereas urine calcium excretion was higher in IH. Fed (blue bars) filtered load and urine calcium were higher in IH than in normal people.

Calcium and the CaSR

Basolateral CaSR reduces thick ascending limb reabsorption and could lead to reduced overall renal calcium reabsorption. In our experiments,[1] both renal calcium reabsorption and serum PTH levels appeared to vary inversely with serum calcium to a greater extent in IH versus normal. In a multivariate analysis, fractional excretion of calcium varied with serum calcium; serum PTH and insulin did not enter the regression. The interaction term of patient type—normal versus IH—with serum calcium was highly significant. In a second analysis, urine calcium excretion varied with calcium filtered load and with feeding, and in both cases the effects were greater in IH than in normal as judged by the interaction terms of patient type with serum calcium, filtered load, and feeding versus fasting. These findings are compatible with an enhanced CaSR responsiveness or abundance in IH. In support of this idea, PTH level itself was found to vary more with serum calcium in IH versus N. Parathyroid hormone secretion is regulated via the CaSR on PT cells (*see* Chapter 8).

Overview of Signalers

Presently, the CaSR appears to be a prime candidate as the mediator of reduced renal calcium reabsorption, perhaps by acting in the thick ascending limbs or distal convoluted tubule. Although, the effects of the slight increase of serum calcium with meals can account for only 20% of the reduction, the CaSR is known to respond to amino acids and other nutrients,[38] so the effects of meals might be mediated by more than the calcium signal. Missing is the crucial measurement of tissue CaSR in normal and IH renal tissue, which could greatly increase our understanding of the matter. However, as a cautionary note, recent summaries of evidence concerning genetic variations in the CaSR gene have shown little evidence of an association with stone disease.[12]

ABSORPTIVE HYPERCALCIURIA

A large body of data supports the idea of a nonrenal, absorptive form of IH, meaning a form of hypercalciuria in which renal calcium reabsorption is normal.[39] In the absence of reduced reabsorption, a high rate of diet calcium absorption could by itself raise urine calcium excretion only by increasing filtered load of calcium or suppressing PTH secretion via a higher level of serum ionized calcium. Our direct measurements did not correspond well with the absorptive hypothesis.

Filtered Load

Using aggregate means from all control and IH subjects studied to date (Fig. 13.14), filtered load of normals was above that of IH subjects fasting (red bars), even though urine calcium excretion was higher in IH; this is not compatible with the absorptive mechanism. Fed (blue bars) filtered load was higher in IH as was urine calcium, which is broadly compatible with an absorptive mechanism.

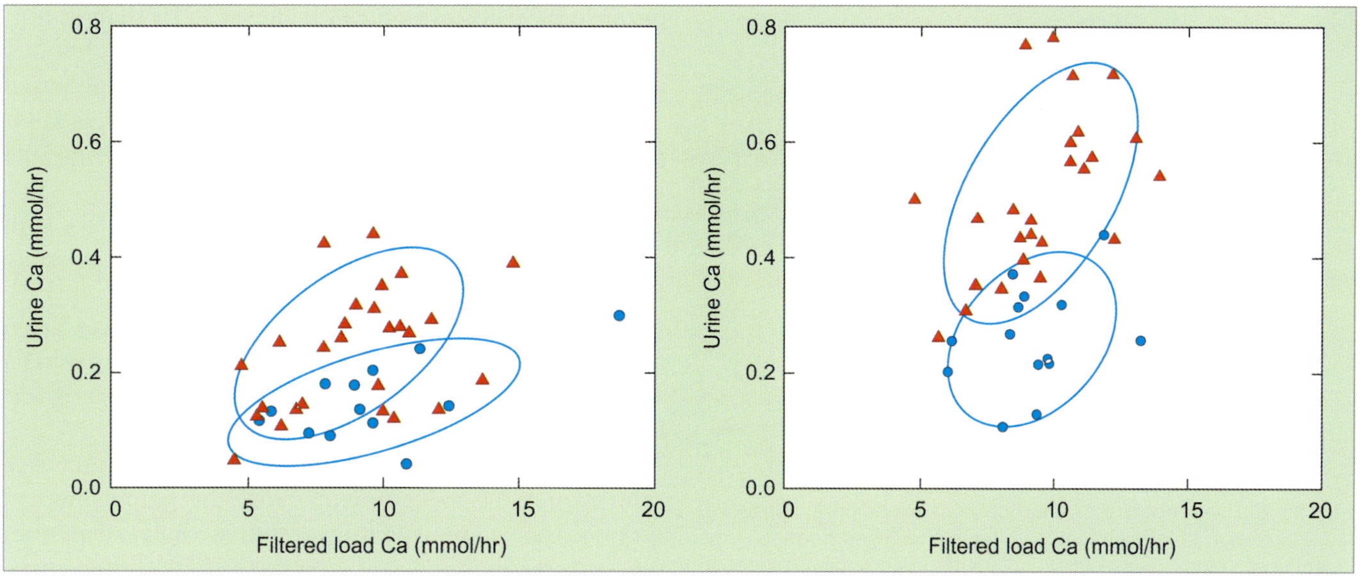

Fig. 13.15: Relationships between urine calcium excretion and calcium filtered load fasting (left panel) and fed (right panel). Fasting and fed urine calcium excretion (Y-axis) varied significantly with calcium filtered load (X-axis) in normal subjects and idiopathic hypercalciuria (IH) patients (blue circles and red triangles, respectively). The slope dependencies differed significantly between normal and IH under both conditions using general linear modeling. As is obvious from the figure, urine calcium excretion adjusted for filtered load of IH exceeded normals in both food periods.

When urine calcium excretion was plotted against filtered load (Fig. 13.15), values for IH were above normal at overlapping values of filtered loads, both fasting (left panel) and fed (right panel). If high filtered load from abnormally rapid calcium absorption were to raise urine calcium via increased filtered load, we should find significant numbers of IH points (in the figures each subject is one point) to the right of the ellipse surrounding the normal points: urine calcium is high and so is filtered load. In the fed state, where high absorption is expected to function particularly well, the IH points are dramatically above the normal points and filtered loads overlap remarkably well.

In a general linear model, urine calcium, both fasting and fed, is strongly related to filtered load, and the slope dependence is significantly different for IH and N as suggested by the tilts of the 68% nonparametric ellipses of containment on the figures. Urine calcium adjusted for filtered load is higher in IH than N under both conditions (139 vs 251 μmol/h fasting and 285 vs 503 μmol/h fed, $p < 0.001$ for both).

There is no doubt that filtered load affects urine calcium excretion, as is obvious from the graphs, but there is no evidence that filtered loads differ between N and IH. In an ANOVA with food state and subject type as categories, filtered load showed no significant differences. Instead it is fractional calcium excretion that is high in IH—urine calcium is high for the filtered load.

Parathyroid Hormone

The alternative idea, that high absorption rates lower serum PTH and thereby drive reabsorption down, is falsified by the foregoing evidence that fractional reabsorption and urine calcium excretion adjusted for PTH and filtered load both are high in IH.[28]

Overview

What all this means is that with what information we have obtained concerning renal calcium handling, we can find no apparent way for a pure absorptive model to work. On the one hand, filtered loads are not different, as one might have initially assumed from rapid calcium absorption. On the other, PTH is not suppressed and fractional calcium reabsorption is reduced in IH compared to normals at overlapping PTH values. So, reduced tubule reabsorption is the only route to the expression of hypercalciuria as a phenotype. All IH arises from reduced tubule reabsorption so far as we can tell at this time.

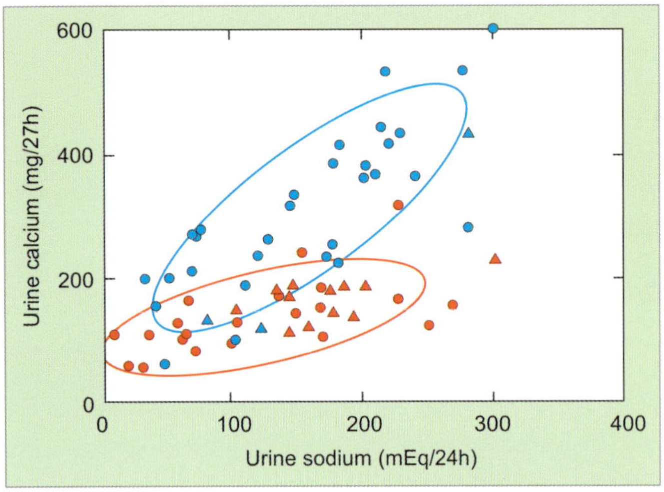

Fig. 13.16: Dependence of urine calcium excretion on urine sodium excretion in idiopathic hypercalciuria (IH) and normal. Urine calcium excretion varies significantly with urine sodium excretion in IH (blue) and non-IH subjects (red), and the slope dependencies differ significantly using general linear modeling (F = 90.9, p < 0.001). Adjusted for urine sodium, urine calcium of IH was far above normal (348 vs 154, p<0.001). Prospective trials of variation in diet sodium (filled circles) and observational studies (triangles) overlap.[32,40-53]

LESSONS ABOUT PATHOGENESIS FROM TREATMENT

Treatments may have shed more light on IH mechanisms than many observational studies, because they manipulate fundamental mechanisms of renal tubule function: changes in sodium balance and in acid loads.

Reduced Sodium Intake

Direct experimental trials and observational studies have documented a more marked effect of diet sodium intake in IH subjects than normal controls (Fig. 13.16). The slope of urine calcium excretion on urine sodium excretion in IH subjects is above that of controls, whereas the intercepts of the regressions differ only slightly.

Increasing sodium intake is known to reduce PT reabsorption in humans as well as animals, so the marked sodium effect in IH could well reflect changes in PT reabsorption.[54] Consider that urine calcium excretion is the product of PT calcium delivery times the fraction of distal delivery excreted. Since, in IH we have evidence that the fraction of distal delivery excreted is above that in normals,[30] any increase of PT delivery will give a greater increase of urine calcium than in normals. Moreover, because PT reabsorption can be lower in IH than in normals,[30] especially in men, it is possible but presently unproven that changes in PT reabsorption with increased sodium intake may be larger than in normals. This latter point is important to investigate as a clue to how the nephron of IH may differ from normal.

Even glomerular filtration rate (GFR) can vary with sodium intake,[55] and it is possible that GFR may be more responsive to salt balance in IH than in N. Presently we have no data concerning this hypothesis. However, given an abnormal balance between PT and distal nephron in IH versus normal, glomerular tubular feedback may be disordered.[56]

Clinically, reduced sodium intake stands out as a prime approach to treatment. From the graph one can estimate that at about 65 mEq of sodium daily, an amount presently recommended as ideal by the CDC (http://www.cdc.gov/Features/sodium/), urine calcium excretions of IH and normal subjects become nearly identical. As an obvious corollary, high sodium intakes pose a difficulty for treatment. Deliveries will be high, one presumes, and other measures such as thiazide diuretics and potassium alkali reduced in effectiveness.

Effects of Sodium Intake on Bone

There is little doubt that, at least in postmenopausal women, who are at particular risk for bone mineral loss, sodium intake critically determines whether bone mineral balance becomes positive (Fig. 13.17). In this study, each subject ate four diets: high and low calcium and sodium, in combination, and total mineral balance was measured.[40] On the low-calcium diets (518 mg/day), bone mineral balances were negative. On high-calcium diets (1,284 mg/day), bone balance was negative when diet sodium was high (191 mEq/day), but when it was lowered to 70 mEq/day of sodium balance became positive.

The positive balance arose from a significant fall in urine calcium loss–the expected source–and from a fall in endogenous calcium secretion into the gut lumen, which was not significant but was obviously essential numerically to achievement of positive balance. Between the low- and high-sodium diets, urine calcium changed from 153 to 112 (+ 41 mg/day retention), endogenous fecal losses from 146 to 82 (64 mg/day retention) more or less making up (41 + 64 = 105 mg/day) the net change in bone retention (–12 to 90 or 102 mg/day). The sources of endogenous calcium secretion involved were not specified and could have been pancreatic, biliary, or intestinal calcium transport. Isotope

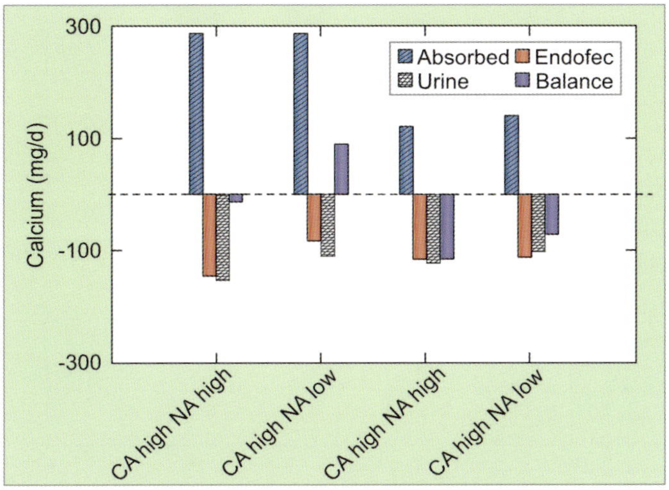

Fig. 13.17: Interaction between diet calcium and calcium in relation to bone mineral balance in menopausal women. Bone calcium balance (y axis, black bars) becomes positive only with a high calcium low sodium diet. Positive balance is achieved by increase of absorbed calcium, reduction of urine calcium, and of endogenous intestinal calcium secretion.
Source: Redrawn from Teucher B, Dainty JR, Spinks CA, et al. Sodium and bone health: impact of moderately high and low salt intakes on calcium metabolism in postmenopausal women. J Bone Miner Res. 2008;23:1477-85.

kinetics showed a change in bone off rates from 372 to 346 mg/day (+26 mg/day) and in bone on rates from 361 to 437 mg/day (76 mg/day), indicating that new bone entry was a major component of the increased balance.

This study highlights the difficulties in assessing mechanisms of calcium balance without isotope measurements. Total fecal losses of diet calcium changed from 1,110 to 1,078 mg/day (32 mg/day) as calculated from total fecal losses minus endogenous secretion. This means that it would appear that the main mechanisms driving balance in this study concerned organ calcium secretion rates as opposed to GI transepithelial transport regulation.

Thiazide Diuretics

These are well known to reduce urine calcium excretion in IH.[57] The mechanism includes changes in PT reabsorption. In four men studied before and after 6 months of chlorthalidone, a thiazide-like drug, urine calcium was reduced in the fed state, whereas urine sodium excretion (not shown) was unchanged (Fig. 13.18). As expected, blood pressure fell, and serum calcitriol also fell (65–52 pg/mL, not statistically significant).

Proximal tubule delivery of calcium and sodium were reduced.[58] The fraction of distal delivery of calcium excreted was increased by thiazide (not shown in figure) in the fed state (+8%). Thiazide causes a reduction of total body sodium stores and reduces extracellular fluid volume. This is expected to raise PT reabsorption as it is functionally identical to reduced Na intake.

Thiazide drugs have been used in three successful trials for stone prevention[57] in populations with a high, though certainly not a universal, prevalence of IH. Presumably their effectiveness arose at least in part from reduction of urine calcium excretion. The trials are summarized in Chapter 15.

Thiazide-type drugs also alter distal convoluted tubule calcium reabsorption via reduction of NaCl entry through the sodium chloride cotransporter,[59] thereby increasing transmembrane potential and facilitating calcium entry through the TRPv5 transporter.[60] However, in our study we were not able to show an increase in the distal fractional reabsorption of delivered calcium. In fact, we observed a decrease. However, since delivery of calcium and sodium was also decreased, it is difficult to sort out the precise factors influencing the DCT.

Effects on bone have been documented in many studies.[61,62] In general, thiazide appears to increase BMD. In our one balance study[63] (Fig. 13.19), 6 months of chlorthalidone led to increased net bone mineral balance. No prospective trials have tested the effects of thiazide on fracture rates, but increases in BMD have been documented.[64]

Potassium Citrate

Chronic acid loading increases urine calcium excretion.[65] The mechanisms of this phenomenon are not fully known but include PT and possibly distal nephron effects. In PT, acid load reduces overall NaCl and water reabsorption by downregulation of the SLC26a6 transporter.[66] Even though the abundance and presumed activity of NHE3, the main engine of reabsorption is increased,[67] reduction of anion exchange lowers salt and water reabsorption and increased distal delivery.

In the DCT, acid loading appears to reduce TRPv5 activity. Effects appear to include a reduction of insertion of the transporter into membranes and a direct pH sensing effect of the transporter molecule, which alters its morphology and thereby alters its transport rate.[68]

Because of long-term diet evolution, virtually everyone in First World countries today eats an acid ash diet, meaning a diet that imposes an organic acid load mainly in the form of sulfate from oxidation of sulfur on methionine and cysteine.[69] Giving alkali supplements does not so much impose an alkali load as it neutralizes the tonic acid load to which we all are accustomed. As a result, one

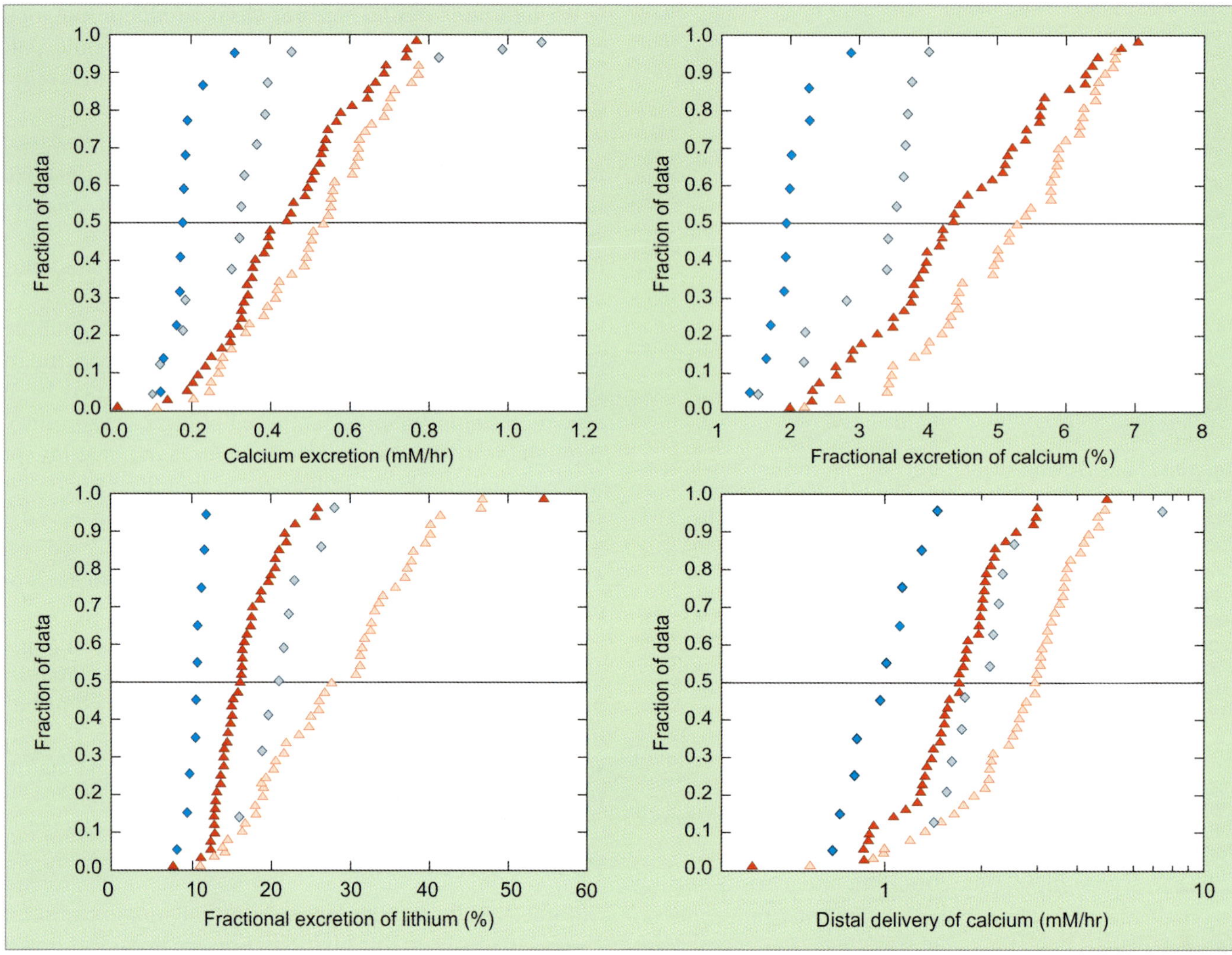

Fig. 13.18: Segmental nephron effects of thiazide on calcium reabsorption. Four men were studied in a detailed CRC protocol before (light symbols) and after 6 months of chlorthalidone (dark symbols), 25 mg daily.[58] As expected, the drug reduced urine calcium excretion (upper left panel) and fractional excretion of calcium (upper right panel) fed (triangles) and fasting (rectangle). Fractional excretion of lithium (lower left panel) and distal calcium delivery (lower right panel) also fell, denoting increased proximal tubule reabsorption.

would expect PT reabsorption to rise with alkali treatment and urine calcium to fall.

Whereas there is evidence for both PT and DCT response to acid loading, as yet no published studies have examined PT and distal nephron responses to alkali in humans. We have obtained limited and to date unpublished information on this topic using 24-hour urine samples collected from patients either untreated or receiving potassium citrate. Using lithium concentrations in each 24-hour urine sample and a single fasting blood drawn at the conclusion of the collection, we calculated distal calcium delivery. The 24-hour urine sodium excretion was used as an index of diet intake, which would condition the state of sodium balance.

Simple Comparisons

In all, we have 32 24-hour urine samples from potassium citrate treated patients and 165 from untreated patients. Urine calcium excretions and distal calcium delivery (mg/h) were lower with citrate treatment (6.5 vs 9.8, and 59 vs 76, $p < 0.003$ for both). Distal FeCa (%) was also lower (11.4 vs 14.2, $p = 0.041$). Potassium citrate appears to increase proximal and distal tubule reabsorption, and, as expected, lower urine calcium excretion.

Interactions with Sodium Intake

As expected, distal delivery rose with urine sodium excretion, our proxy for diet sodium intake (Fig. 13.20, left panel).

We presume this mirrors other data showing a response of PT reabsorption to the state of sodium balance.[70] Potassium citrate (blue circles, dashed lines) reduced distal delivery adjusted for urine sodium significantly for men and women combined (52 vs 75 mg/h, $p < 0.001$). Likewise, as expected, urine calcium varied with distal delivery, but was not significantly reduced by alkali when adjusted for distal delivery. Of note, although not significant (refer to the figure legend) given the modest numbers of observations, alkali appears to reduce the slope of distal calcium delivery on urine sodium.

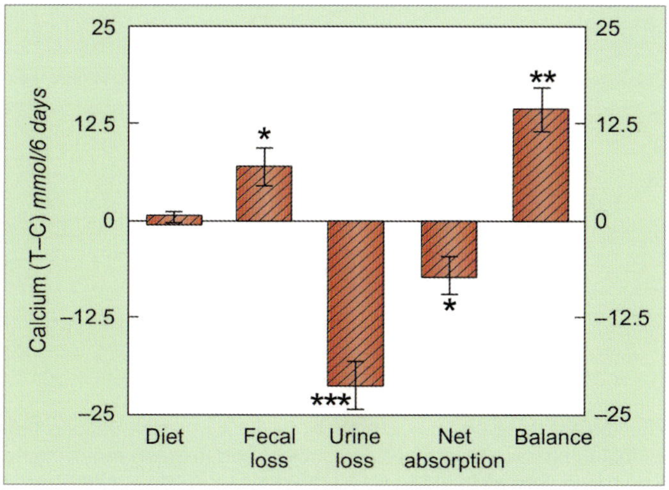

Fig. 13.19: Effects of chlorthalidone on calcium balance. Subjects with idiopathic hypercalciuria (IH) and calcium stones were studied at baseline and after 6 months of treatment with chlorthalidone, 25 mg daily. Calcium balance was determined over 6 days in a standard CRC protocol.[63] Y-axis shows the differences between treatment (T) and control (C) measurements. Fecal calcium loss increased with the drug, urine calcium fell, and balance increased. Mean differences vs. 0: *, p<0.05; ** p<0.02; ***p<0.001.

Urine calcium varied with urine sodium excretion in our studies (Fig. 13.21) and potassium citrate lowered urine calcium (236 vs 142 mg/day, $p < 0.001$) adjusted for urine sodium (left panel of figure). Among the few published studies we could find (right panel of figure), potassium citrate or bicarbonate (blue circles) lowered urine calcium excretion adjusted for urine sodium (221 vs 158, $p < 0.001$). In general, potassium citrate appeared to reduce both urine calcium, as expected, and PT fractional calcium delivery.

The interaction of alkali with sodium is instructive. From the left-hand panel, the effect seems to be on the intercept of the linear regression of urine calcium on 24-hour urine sodium. If we presume that the regression of urine calcium on urine sodium reflects mainly increase of calcium delivery distally because extracellular volume expansion reduces PT reabsorption of sodium and calcium, this would be the expected result. It is also

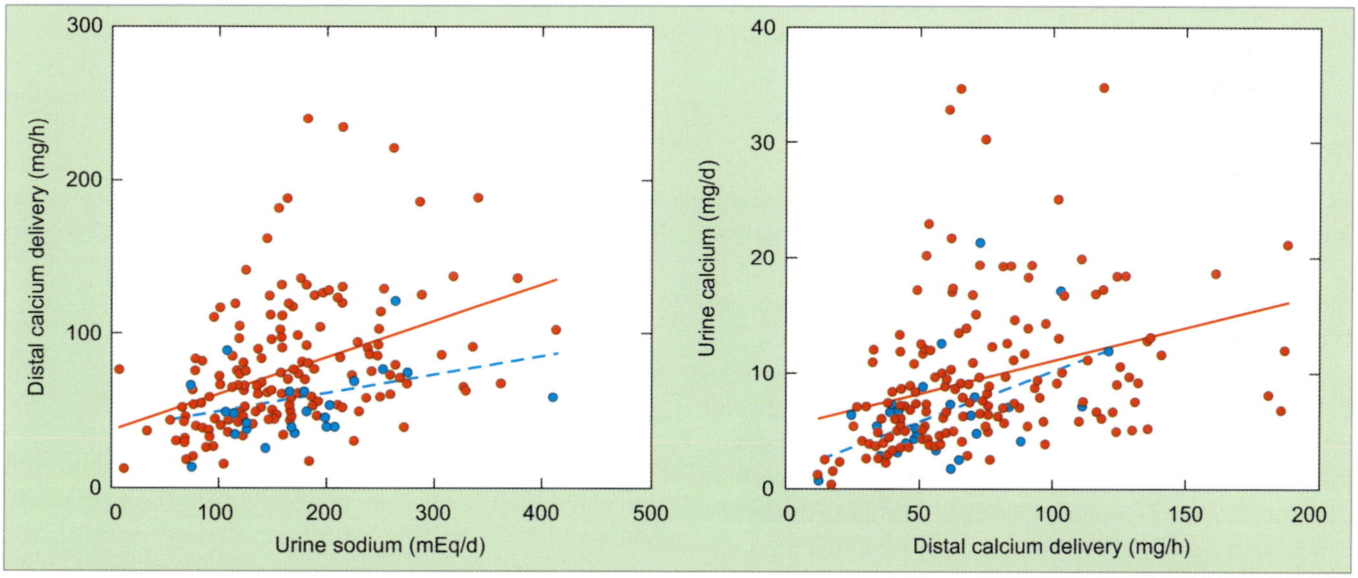

Fig. 13.20: Effects of potassium citrate on distal calcium delivery and urine calcium excretion. Distal calcium delivery (left panel, Y-axis) varied with urine sodium excretion (F = 39, p < 0.001) in 24-hour urine samples obtained from untreated calcium stone formers (red circles) and those receiving potassium citrate for treatment of stones (blue circles). Slopes appear to differ, but the difference was not significant (p = 0.252). Distal delivery adjusted for urine sodium was lower (76 vs 55 mg/h, p=0.003) in those receiving potassium citrate than in those not receiving treatment. Urine calcium excretion (right panel) varied with distal calcium delivery and was lower (7.5 vs 9.6 mg/h) in those receiving potassium citrate, but not significantly so (p = 0.058).

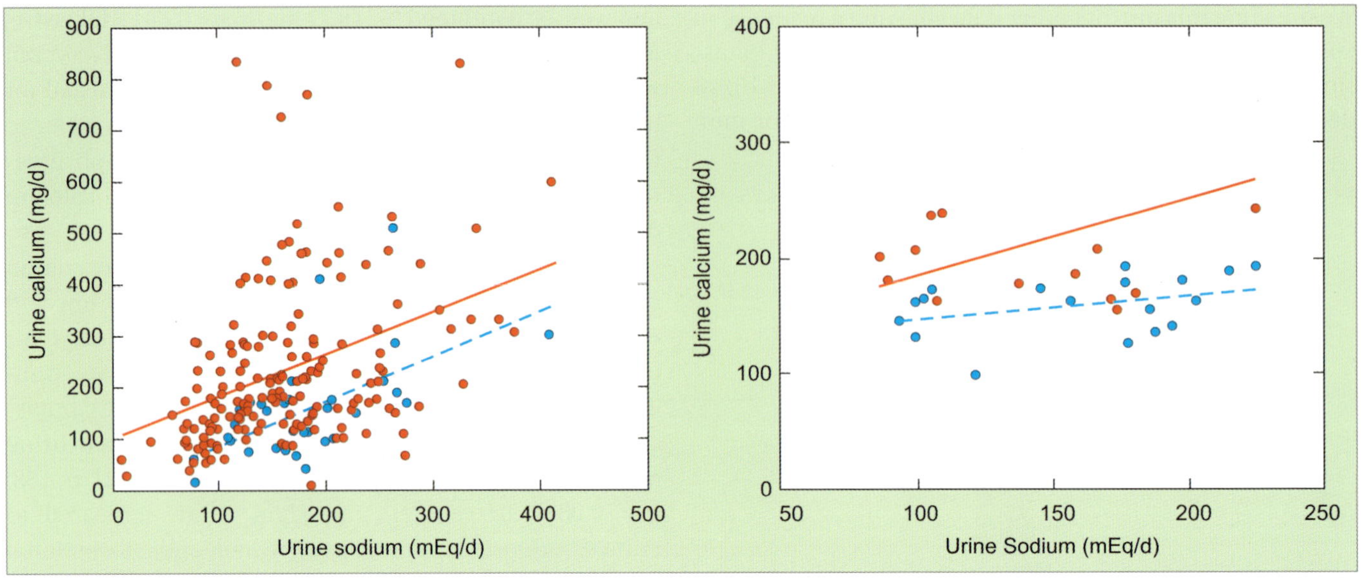

Fig. 13.21: Effects of potassium citrate on urine calcium excretion adjusted for urine sodium excretion. In our own observations (left panel), urine calcium varied with urine sodium in calcium stone formers taking potassium citrate (blue circles) and in those receiving no treatment (red circles). However, values for those being treated lie below those untreated (236 vs 142 mg/day, $p < 0.001$). In published studies,[71-85] (right panel) treated patients had lower (221 vs 158, $p < 0.001$) urine calcium excretions (blue circles) than those untreated (red circles).

compatible with the lack of a significant slope difference in Figure 13.20, left panel, between distal delivery and urine sodium. An effect mainly on distal fractional calcium reabsorption would be multiplicative, and therefore as sodium rose and calcium delivery increased, urine calcium would rise at a reduced slope. Needed are critical experiments in which sodium and alkali are altered in a controlled trial.

Interaction of Sodium and Acid Loads

At least experimentally, one can show that very low sodium intake is sufficient to prevent acid-induced hypercalciuria in normal human subjects.[15] Acid loading on a low-sodium diet (Fig. 13.22) resulted in no increase of urine calcium. When diet sodium was increased, urine calcium increased promptly. Of interest, serum PTH measured with an assay that was mainly detecting C terminal fragments showed a prompt increase despite a constant serum ionized calcium level. We presume from this experiment that low sodium diet and alkali may be synergistic in controlling the hypercalciuria of IH, but as yet no trials have demonstrated that this is the case.

Protein Intake

High protein intake raises urine calcium excretion,[86] but it does not result in negative bone calcium balance. Protein stimulates intestinal calcium absorption, so that even though urine calcium excretion rises, net intestinal calcium intake also rises, with the result that calcium balance can be maintained despite increase of urine calcium: the increased urine calcium can arise from the increased intestinal calcium absorption instead of from bone. High protein intake combined with alkali in a quantity sufficient to neutralize the acid load from the protein raises urine calcium to the same extent as without alkali, pointing to another mechanism of action than acid loading.[87] Although not an apparent cause of bone mineral loss, high protein diets raise urine calcium excretion and supersaturation, so moderation of extremely high intakes--above perhaps 1.2 g/kg/day--may be prudent.

Clinical Effects of Reduced Protein and Sodium

A single trial in men with IH has employed the combination of reduced diet protein and sodium and compared the results with reduced diet calcium over 5 years.[88] As compared with reduced calcium intake, new stone production was reduced, especially during years 3-5 of the trial. Although, bone mineral balance was not measured, nor bone density, it is likely that the reduced protein intake with reduced sodium intake would have maintained bone balance more positive—or at least less negative—than the

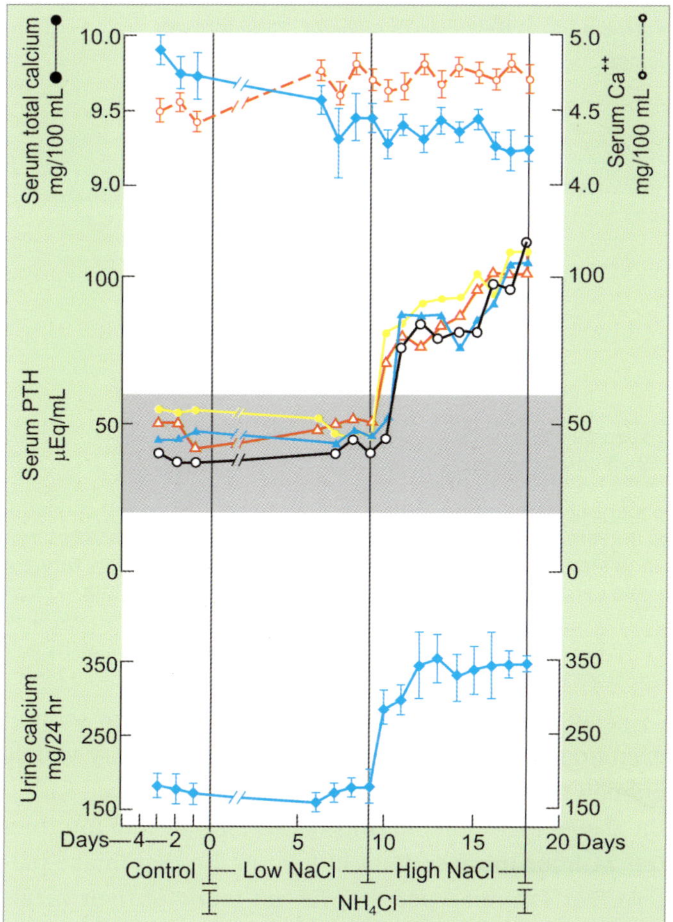

Fig. 13.22: Experimental evidence of an interaction between sodium intake and acid-induced hypercalciuria. In the control period (left panel), normal subjects ate a high-sodium diet and had normal urine calcium excretions. They were then fed a low-sodium diet and given an oral acid load of ammonium chloride. Despite the acid load, urine calcium did not increase from control (middle panel) and serum parathyroid hormone (PTH) did not increase. With high-sodium intake and acid loading (right panel), urine calcium rose far above the high-sodium control period, and serum PTH rose at a constant ionized serum calcium level.
Source: Redrawn from Coe FL, Firpo JJ, Jr, Hollandsworth DL, et al. Effect of acute and chronic metabolic acidosis on serum immunoreactive parathyroid hormone in man. Kidney Int. 1975;8:263-73.

low calcium diet without reduced sodium intake. The clinical results of this trial are reviewed in Chapter 15.

Sugar

Oral sugar loads, glucose, fructose, sucrose and their kindred all can raise urine calcium excretion briefly in normal people, but in patients with IH the response is remarkably higher and more sustained.[89] As expected, relatives of IH subjects also react with high urine calcium losses, presumably being carriers of the genes that give rise to IH (Fig. 13.23). The mediator of the sugar response was initially thought to be insulin itself. However, as has already been pointed out in this chapter, direct insulin clamping failed to increase urine calcium significantly, pointing to other possibilities.[37] Effects of sugars on bone mineral balance are not well established.

CREATION OF AN EFFECTIVE TREATMENT PLAN

Given two effective drugs that can lower urine calcium excretion, thiazides and potassium citrate, an obvious treatment approach is to use one or both long term. Since, they are inexpensive and reasonably safe, this approach would seem reasonable. However, it is a clumsy and potentially doomed way to manage patients, we think, and a far better one begins with fluids and diet.

Trials of potassium citrate and thiazide, and of water itself and reduced diet sodium and protein, are reviewed in Chapter 15. Here, we present our personal approach to management, which is naturally without proof as one cannot do a trial of a practice style in one center.

Fluids

Even when we discuss patients with an evident abnormality of urine calcium excretion, water is a premiere treatment. It undoes the work of the kidneys that creates supersaturation, and acts therefore at the very foundation of stone crystal formation. Based on the excellent available epidemiological data reviewed in Chapter 15, urine volumes of at least 2.25–2.5 L daily will greatly reduce risk of new stone onset and are therefore an ideal clinical goal. Given insensible losses, which depend on climate, work, work environment, and exercise habits, this can imply fluid intakes ranging from a low of at least 3 L to as much as 4 or 5 L in special cases.

Diet History

The main elements of diet that affect urine calcium excretion in IH are sodium, acid loads, protein intake, and sugar intake. Calcium intake does not so much affect urine calcium losses as bone mineral balance, but given the marked tendency to bone disease in IH subjects it is a crucial issue in clinical management.

Because taste, practicality, and clinical sensibility govern how physicians manage the diet history over these five

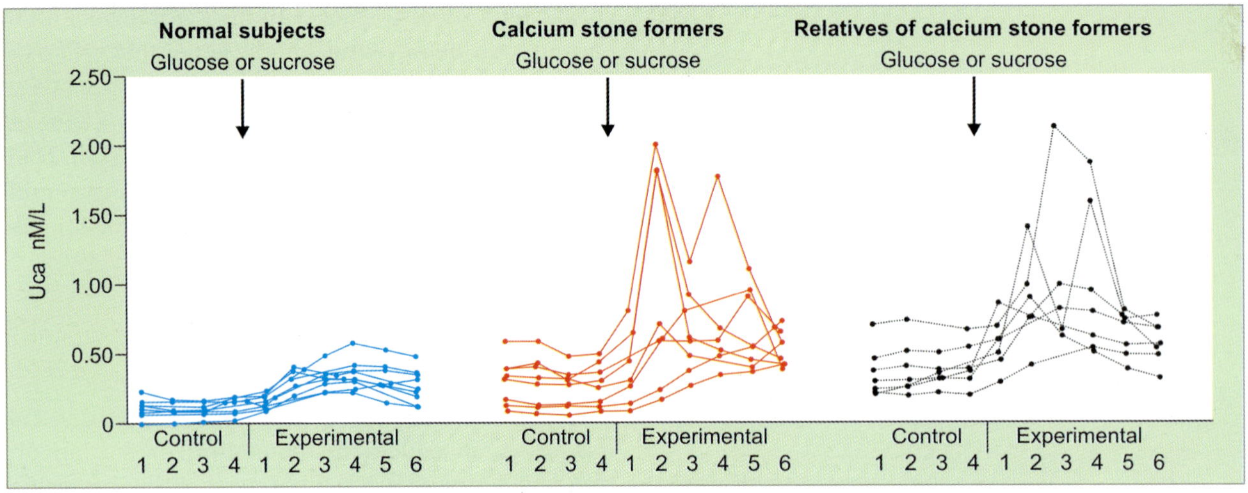

Fig. 13.23: Effects of glucose or sucrose ingestion on urine calcium concentration. In normal subjects, oral sugars (left panel) caused a slight rise in urine calcium concentration. Among calcium stone formers and their family members, the same sugars caused a very large increase of urine calcium concentration. The increase was a compound of increased calcium excretion and reduced urine flow rate. *Source*: Redrawn from Lemann J, Jr, Piering WF, Lennon EJ. Possible role of carbohydrate-induced calciuria in calcium oxalate kidney-stone formation. N Engl J Med. 1969;280:232-7.

categories, we know better than to offer more than suggestions. Our personal approach is to ask about the meals eaten each day and make coarse but robust guesses about actual intakes in each area of interest.

However, in one area we can be quite specific. It is pointless to use the results of 24-hour urine testing as a guide to diet effects without ascertaining whether the diet used during the urine collections was representative of the period in which stones occurred, of some new and presumably stable adjustments made to reduce stones, or was altogether odd in being restricted to weekends or even specially structured so as to give a "good" result.

Use of 24-Hour Urine Tests to Assess Diet Intakes

Urine Volume

The urine volume is at once the most direct measurement of the interaction between intake and need, and the least reliable index of what happens in the real life of patients. We have made this point in Chapter 15 and repeat it here for emphasis. Clinical acumen is a real skill, and essential for interpretation of this and all other elements of the 24-hour urine. Put bluntly as possible, an adequate or high urine volume commonly is an artifact not of measurement or collection but of altered habits during the collection, and only your patient can tell you which it is.

Diet sodium is very well quantified by urine sodium excretion unless day-to-day sodium intakes vary widely enough that the day's intake cannot all be excreted within the day of ingestion. For this reason, it is best to interpret the 24-hour urine sodium in light of the diet intake pattern. For example, people who eat many of their meals away from home may experience surges of diet sodium intake so that urine results lag intake.

Acid load is measured in the 24-hour collection by urine sulfate and ammonium ion excretion. Urine sulfate arises from oxidation of the sulfur on methionine and cystine to sulfuric acid whose protons are buffered by serum bicarbonate and presumably bone mineral.[90] The general physiology of acid production and renal acid excretion is reviewed in Chapters 10–12 and effects of acid loading on bone in Chapter 12.

Urinary acid excretion involves both production and excretion of ammonium ion and titration of urine phosphate by renal proton transporters. Broadly speaking, urine ammonium ion excretion accounts for about two-third of daily net acid excretion and tends to be about that fraction of daily urine sulfate excretion. For these reasons, it is reasonable to use urine sulfate and ammonium ion excretions as measures—though coarse—of net daily acid load and its disposal. Reasonable averages for these are about 40–60 mEq daily.

Protein Intake

The protein catabolic rate (PCR) can be calculated from the amount of urea nitrogen in the 24-hour urine.[91] Most vendors of 24-hour urine stone risk profiles provide this calculation, which estimates protein intake in g/kg/day. Values of less than 1.2 are reasonable as a goal of treatment.

A Strategy for Overall Diet Management

Sodium, Calcium, and Protein

One cannot do everything at once. For us, the priority is a focus on sodium and calcium. The one must be as low as one can achieve, the other as high as is reasonable. As already pointed out, recent recommendations for sodium are as low as 65 mEq daily, at which point most hypercalciuric patients will have lowered their urine calcium excretions substantially. For calcium intake, we simply recommend the current US values of 1,000–1,200 mg daily from foods. If the protein catabolic rate (PCR) is above 1.2, we try to bring it to about 1, simply by indicating that a reduction of about 20% would be valuable. But in doing this, we prioritize between sodium and protein–between the one which is most above goal, usually sodium–in hopes of achieving some changes.

Net Acid Load

The net acid load is reflected in the urine sulfate excretion, but also by the urine ammonium ion excretion. The latter reflects not only the acid from protein, but also the net alkali taken up from fruits and vegetables, which can offset acid loads from protein. In general, the urine ammonium ion excretion will be a high fraction of urine sulfate excretion—about two-third—but when food alkali is generous, this proportion can fall. When the proportion is high and sulfate and PCR are high (>1 mEq/kg/day and >1.2, respectively), we presume reduction of protein intake will reduce both the calciuric action of protein and of acid.

The key next step is to obtain another 24-hour urine sample and find out if anything has changed. Timing of follow-up can only be dictated by patients who decide they have achieved their diet goals. Otherwise, to fix some date is not productive.

A Strategy for Drug Use

Thiazide

Thiazide will not work well to lower urine calcium given high sodium loads, and will cause kaluresis[57] and hypokalemia, so its use is best reserved for after urine sodium has been reduced as much as is possible for a given patient. Chlorthalidone is our preference.[92] It has been shown to be more efficacious than hydrochlorothiazide, as well as more convenient, because the latter has a short half-life and requires twice daily dosing. Indapamide[93] shares a long half-life with chlorthalidone and should be equivalent in clinical convenience and efficacy. We have found that 25 mg of chlorthalidone daily is sufficient for most patients, and half of that dose in women and smaller men. Indapamide 2.5 mg is equivalent to chlorthalidone 25 mg daily.

If serum potassium falls, repletion can be with potassium citrate or chloride. In principle, the former is always the more desirable, but for patients who form predominantly calcium phosphate stones and have elevated urine pH values (*see* Chapter 15), the increase in urine pH may increase CaP supersaturation and stone risk. Needed is a trial of potassium citrate in such patients. Lacking a trial, we tend to use potassium chloride in these patients as a rule. Amiloride 5 mg tablets, one to three daily, can reduce potassium wasting in the event that repletion is difficult.

Potassium Citrate

Unlike thiazide, citrates will have effects at any sodium intake (Fig. 13.21) and can therefore be considered for use in parallel with diet changes. The dose we use in practice is roughly the urine ammonium ion excretion, although the trials (*see* Chapter 15) use fixed doses. One expects a rise in urine potassium and a suppression of urine ammonium ion excretion in relation to sulfate; failure to find this indicates nonuse or poor absorption. Urine pH itself is not as reliable an index of effect, nor is urine citrate excretion; both are subject to complex physiologies, whereas if ammonia does not fall alkali has not been absorbed. The standard pills are 10 mEq, and common starting doses are two pills twice daily or one pill three times daily.

Thiazide and Potassium Citrate

One can be tempted to begin both agents together, especially in someone with many stones, but we suggest this may not be clinically wise. Drugs have side effects and intolerances that discourage patients and may lead some to abandon treatment and, in the process, leave your practice. Once the diet changes have been made as best as possible, one or the other agent can be used and the urine outcomes determined. If hypercalciuria is resistant to thiazide, despite good control of protein and sodium, adding alkali may be an effective synergy. This matter has not been tested in trials to date.

REFERENCES

1. Worcester EM, Bergsland KJ, Gillen DL, et al. Evidence for increased renal tubule and parathyroid gland sensitivity to serum calcium in human idiopathic hypercalciuria. Am J Physiol Renal Physiol. 2013;305:F853-60.
2. Letavernier E, Traxer O, Daudon M, et al. Determinants of osteopenia in male renal-stone-disease patients with idiopathic hypercalciuria. Clin J Am Soc Nephrol. 2011;6: 1149-54.
3. Coe FL, Favus MJ. Idiopathic hypercalciuria. Henry Ford Hosp Med J. 1983;31:229-30.
4. Curhan GC, Taylor EN. 24-h uric acid excretion and the risk of kidney stones. Kidney Int. 2008;73:489-496.
5. Coe FL, Parks JH, Moore ES. Familial idiopathic hypercalciuria. N Engl J Med. 1979;300:337-40.
6. Lieske JC, Turner ST, Edeh SN, et al. Heritability of urinary traits that contribute to nephrolithiasis. Clin J Am Soc Nephrol. 2014;9: 943-50.
7. Bergsland KJ, Coe FL, White MD, et al. Urine risk factors in children with calcium kidney stones and their siblings. Kidney Int. 2012;81:1140-8.
8. Deeb A, Abood SA, Simon J, et al. A novel CLDN16 mutation in a large family with familial hypomagnesaemia with hypercalciuria and nephrocalcinosis. BMC Res Notes. 2013;6:527.
9. Edvardsson VO, Goldfarb DS, Lieske JC, et al. Hereditary causes of kidney stones and chronic kidney disease. Pediatr Nephrol. 2013;28:1923-42.
10. Ferre S, de Baaij JH, Ferreira P, et al. Mutations in PCBD1 cause hypomagnesemia and renal magnesium wasting. J Am Soc Nephrol. 2014;25:574-86.
11. Ichikawa S, Tuchman S, Padgett LR, et al. Intronic deletions in the SLC34A3 gene: a cautionary tale for mutation analysis of hereditary hypophosphatemic rickets with hypercalciuria. Bone. 2014;59:53-6.
12. Toka HR, Pollak MR. The role of the calcium-sensing receptor in disorders of abnormal calcium handling and cardiovascular disease. Curr Opin Nephrol Hypertens. 2014;23:494-501.
13. Pak CY. Physiological basis for absorptive and renal hypercalciurias. Am J Physiol. 1979;237:F415-23.
14. Worcester EM, Coe FL. New insights into the pathogenesis of idiopathic hypercalciuria. Semin Nephrol. 2008;28:120-32.
15. Coe FL, Favus MJ, Crockett T, et al. Effects of low-calcium diet on urine calcium excretion, parathyroid function and serum 1,25(OH)2D3 levels in patients with idiopathic hypercalciuria and in normal subjects. Am J Med. 1982;72:25-32.
16. Vezzoli G, Rubinacci A, Bianchin C, et al. Intestinal calcium absorption is associated with bone mass in stone-forming women with idiopathic hypercalciuria. Am J Kidney Dis. 2003;42:1177-83.
17. Asplin JR, Bauer KA, Kinder J, et al. Bone mineral density and urine calcium excretion among subjects with and without nephrolithiasis. Kidney Int. 2003;63:662-9.
18. Bataille P, Fardellone P, Ghazali A, et al. Pathophysiology and treatment of idiopathic hypercalciuria. Curr Opin Rheumatol. 1998;10:373-88.
19. Broadus AE, Insogna KL, Lang R. A consideration of the hormonal basis and phosphate leak hypothesis of absorptive hypercalciria. J Clin Endocrinol Metab. 1984;58:161-9.
20. Gray RW, Wilz DR, Caldas AE, et al. The importance of phosphate in regulating plasma 1,25-$(OH)_2$-vitamin D levels in humans: studies in healthy subjects in calcium-stone formers and in patients with primary hyperparathyroidism. J Clin Endocrinol Metab.1977;45:299-306.
21. Haussler MR, Baylink J, Hughes MR, et al. The assay of 1,25-dihydroxyvitamin D3: physiologic and pathologic modulation of circulating hormone levels. Clin Endocrinol Metab. 1976;5:1512-652.
22. Muller D, Hoenderop JG, Vennekens R, et al. Epithelial Ca(2+) channel (ECAC1) in autosomal dominant idiopathic hypercalciuria. Nephrol Dial Transplant. 2002;17:1614-20.
23. Rendina D, Mossetti G, Viceconti R, et al. Association between vitamin D receptor gene polymorphisms and fasting idiopathic hypercalciuria in recurrent stone-forming patients. Urology. 2004;64:833-8.
24. Shen FH, Baylink DJ, Nielsen RL, et al. Increased serum 1,25-dihydroxyvitamin D in idiopathic hypercalciuria. J Lab Clin Med. 1977;90:955-62.
25. Favus MJ, Karnauskas AJ, Parks JH, et al. Peripheral blood monocyte vitamin D receptor levels are elevated in patients with idiopathic hypercalciuria. J Clin Endocrinol Metab. 2004;89:4937-43.
26. Sakhaee K, Maalouf NM, Kumar R, et al. Nephrolithiasis-associated bone disease: pathogenesis and treatment options. Kidney Int. 2011;79:393-403.
27. Asplin JR, Donahue S, Kinder J, et al. Urine calcium excretion predicts bone loss in idiopathic hypercalciuria. Kidney Int. 2006;70:1463-7.
28. Worcester EM, Gillen DL, Evan AP, et al. Evidence that postprandial reduction of renal calcium reabsorption mediates hypercalciuria of patients with calcium nephrolithiasis. Am J Physiol Renal Physiol. 2007;292:F66-75.
29. Thomsen K, Shirley DG. The validity of lithium clearance as an index of sodium and water delivery from the proximal tubules. Nephron. 1997;77:125-38.
30. Worcester EM, Coe FL, Evan AP, et al. Evidence for increased postprandial distal nephron calcium delivery in hypercalciuric stone-forming patients. Am J Physiol Renal Physiol. 2008;295:F1286-94.
31. Ko B, Bergsland KJ, Gillen DL, et al. Gender differences in proximal and distal nephron function contribute to the mechanism of idiopathic hypercalcuria in calcium stone formers. Am J Physiol Regul Integr Comp Physiol. 2015;309:R85-92.
32. Nouvenne A, Meschi T, Prati B, et al. Effects of a low-salt diet on idiopathic hypercalciuria in calcium-oxalate stone formers: a 3-mo randomized controlled trial. Am J Clin Nutr. 2010;91:565-70.
33. Bourdeau JE. Calcium transport across the pars recta of cortical segment 2 proximal tubules. Am J Physiol. 1986;251: F718-24.

34. Fliser D, Franek E, Joest M, et al. Renal function in the elderly: impact of hypertension and cardiac function. Kidney Int. 1997;51:1196-204.
35. Bochud M, Staessen JA, Maillard M, et al. Ethnic differences in proximal and distal tubular sodium reabsorption are heritable in black and white populations. J Hypertens. 2009;27: 606-12.
36. Lennon EJ, Lemann J, Jr, Piering WF, et al. The effect of glucose on urinary cation excretion during chronic extracellular volume expansion in normal man. J Clin Invest. 1974;53: 1424-33.
37. Yoon V, Adams-Huet B, Sakhaee K, et al. Hyperinsulinemia and urinary calcium excretion in calcium stone formers with idiopathic hypercalciuria. J Clin Endocrinol Metab. 2013;98:2589-94.
38. Renkema KY, Bindels RJ, Hoenderop JG. Role of the calcium-sensing receptor in reducing the risk for calcium stones. Clin J Am Soc Nephrol. 2011;6:2076-82.
39. Heller HJ, Zerwekh JE, Gottschalk FA, et al. Reduced bone formation and relatively increased bone resorption in absorptive hypercalciuria. Kidney Int. 2007;71:808-15.
40. Teucher B, Dainty JR, Spinks CA, et al. Sodium and bone health: impact of moderately high and low salt intakes on calcium metabolism in postmenopausal women. J Bone Miner Res. 2008;23:1477-85.
41. Blackwood AM, Sagnella GA, Cook DG, et al. Urinary calcium excretion, sodium intake and blood pressure in a multi-ethnic population: results of the Wandsworth Heart and Stroke Study. J Hum Hypertens. 2001;15:229-37.
42. Breslau NA, Mcguire JL, Zerwekh JE, et al. The role of dietary sodium on renal excretion and intestinal absorption of calicum and on vitamin D metabolism. J Clin Endocrinol Metab.1982;55:369-73.
43. Burtis WJ, Gay L, Insogna KL, et al. Dietary hypercalciuria in patients with calcium oxalate kidney stones. Am J Clin Nutr. 1994;60:424-9.
44. Damasio PC, Amaro CR, Cunha NB, et al. The role of salt abuse on risk for hypercalciuria. Nutr J. 2011;10:3.
45. Frings-Meuthen P, Baecker N, Heer M. Low-grade metabolic acidosis may be the cause of sodium chloride-induced exaggerated bone resorption. J Bone Miner Res. 2008;23:517-24.
46. McCarron DA, Rankin LI, Bennett WM, et al. Urinary calcium excretion at extremes of sodium intake in normal man. Am J Nephrol. 1981;1:84-90.
47. McParland BE, Goulding A, Campbell AJ. Dietary salt affects biochemical markers of resorption and formation of bone in elderly women. BMJ. 1989;299:834-5.
48. Muldowney FP, Freaney R, Moloney MF. Importance of dietary sodium in the hypercalciuria syndrome. Kidney Int. 1982;22:292-6.
49. Nascimento L, Oliveros FH, Cunningham E. Renal handling of sodium and calcium in hypercalciuria. Clin Pharmacol Ther. 1984;35:342-7.
50. Phillips MJ, Cooke JN. Relation between urinary calcium and sodium in patients with idiopathic hypercalciuria. Lancet. 1967;1:1354-7.
51. Sakhaee K, Harvey JA, Padalino PK, et al. The potential role of salt abuse on the risk for kidney stone formation. J Urol. 1993;150:310-2.
52. Silver J, Rubinger D, Friedlaender MM, et al. Sodium-dependent idiopathic hypercalciuria in renal-stone formers. Lancet. 1983;2:484-6.
53. Taylor EN, Curhan GC. Body size and 24-hour urine composition. Am J Kidney Dis. 2006;48:905-15.
54. Roos JC, Koomans HA, Dorhout Mees EJ, et al. Renal sodium handling in normal humans subjected to low, normal, and extremely high sodium supplies. Am J Physiol. 1985;249:F941-7.
55. Bruun NE, Skott P, Damkjaer NM, et al. Normal renal tubular response to changes of sodium intake in hypertensive man. J Hypertens. 1990;8:219-27.
56. Stenvinkel P, Saggar-Malik AK, Alvestrand A. Renal haemodynamics and tubular sodium handling following volume expansion with sodium chloride (NaCl) and glucose in healthy humans. Scand J Clin Lab Invest. 1992;52:837-46.
57. Worcester EM, Coe FL. Clinical practice. Calcium kidney stones. N Engl J Med. 2010;363:954-63.
58. Bergsland KJ, Worcester EM, Coe FL. Role of proximal tubule in the hypocalciuric response to thiazide of patients with idiopathic hypercalciuria. Am J Physiol Renal Physiol. 2013;305:F592-9.
59. Dimke H. Exploring the intricate regulatory network controlling the thiazide-sensitive NaCl cotransporter (NCC). Pflugers Arch. 2011;462:767-77.
60. Leunissen EH, Nair AV, Bull C, et al. The epithelial calcium channel TRPV5 is regulated differentially by klotho and sialidase. J Biol Chem. 2013;288:29238-46.
61. Garcia-Nieto V, Monge-Zamorano M, Gonzalez-Garcia M, et al. Effect of thiazides on bone mineral density in children with idiopathic hypercalciuria. Pediatr Nephrol. 2012;27:261-8.
62. Ott SM, LaCroix AZ, Scholes D, et al. Effects of three years of low-dose thiazides on mineral metabolism in healthy elderly persons. Osteoporos Int. 2008;19:1315-22.
63. Coe FL, Parks JH, Bushinsky DA, et al. Chlorthalidone promotes mineral retention in patients with idiopathic hypercalciuria. Kidney Int. 1988;33:1140-6.
64. Moreira Guimaraes Penido MG, de Sousa TM, Campos LM, et al. Longitudinal study of bone mineral density in children with idiopathic hypercalciuria. Pediatr Nephrol. 2012;27: 123-30.
65. Lemann J, Jr, Gray RW, Maierhofer WJ, et al. The importance of renal net acid excretion as a determinant of fasting urinary calcium excretion. Kidney Int. 1986;29:743-6.
66. Wang T, Egbert AL, Jr, Aronson PS, et al. Effect of metabolic acidosis on NaCl transport in the proximal tubule. Am J Physiol. 1998;274: F1015-9.
67. Laghmani K, Preisig PA, Moe OW, et al. Endothelin-1/endothelin-B receptor-mediated increases in NHE3 activity in chronic metabolic acidosis. J Clin Invest. 2001;107:1563-9.
68. Lambers TT, Oancea E, de Groot T, et al. Extracellular pH dynamically controls cell surface delivery of functional TRPV5 channels. Mol Cell Biol. 2007;27:1486-94.

69. Mangano KM, Walsh SJ, Kenny AM, et al. Dietary acid load is associated with lower bone mineral density in men with low intake of dietary calcium. J Bone Miner Res. 2014;29:500-6.
70. Folkerd E, Singer DR, Cappuccio FP, et al. Clearance of endogenous lithium in humans: altered dietary salt intake and comparison with exogenous lithium clearance. Am J Physiol. 1995;268: F718-22.
71. Goodman JW, Asplin JR, Goldfarb DS. Effect of two sports drinks on urinary lithogenicity. Urol Res. 2009; 37:41-46.
72. Fabris A, Bernich P, Abaterusso C, et al. Bone disease in medullary sponge kidney and effect of potassium citrate treatment. Clin J Am Soc Nephrol. 2009;4:1974-9.
73. Fabris A, Lupo A, Bernich P, et al. Long-term treatment with potassium citrate and renal stones in medullary sponge kidney. Clin J Am Soc Nephrol. 2010;5:1663-8.
74. Kato Y, Yamaguchi S, Yachiku S, et al. Changes in urinary parameters after oral administration of potassium-sodium citrate and magnesium oxide to prevent urolithiasis. Urology. 2004;63:7-11.
75. Preminger GM, Sakhaee K, Skurla C, Pak CY. Prevention of recurrent calcium stone formation with potassium citrate therapy in patients with distal renal tubular acidosis. J Urol.1985; 134:20-23.
76. Marangella M, Di SM, Casalis S, et al. Effects of potassium citrate supplementation on bone metabolism. Calcif Tissue Int. 2004;74:330-5.
77. Sakhaee K, Poindexter JR, Griffith CS, Pak CY. Stone forming risk of calcium citrate supplementation in healthy postmenopausal women. J Urol. 2004: 172:958-61.
78. Moseley KF, Weaver CM, Appel L, et al. Potassium citrate supplementation results in sustained improvement in calcium balance in older men and women. J Bone Miner Res. 2013;28:497-504.
79. Pinheiro VB, Baxmann AC, Tiselius HG, et al. The effect of sodium bicarbonate upon urinary citrate excretion in calcium stone formers. Urology. 2013;82:33-7.
80. Robinson MR, Leitao VA, Haleblian GE, et al. Impact of long-term potassium citrate therapy on urinary profiles and recurrent stone formation. J Urol. 2009;181:1145-50.
81. Sebastian A, Harris ST, Ottaway JH, Todd KM, Morris RC Jr. Improved mineral balance and skeletal metabolism in postmenopausal women treated with potassium bicarbonate. N Engl J Med. 1994; 330:1776-81.
82. Sellmeyer DE, Schloetter M, Sebastian A. Potassium citrate prevents increased urine calcium excretion and bone resorption induced by a high sodium chloride diet. J Clin Endocrinol Metab. 2002;87:2008-12.
83. Spivacow FR, Negri AL, Polonsky A, et al. Long-term treatment of renal lithiasis with potassium citrate. Urology. 2010;76:1346-9.
84. Stoller ML, Chi T, Eisner BH, et al. Changes in urinary stone risk factors in hypocitraturic calcium oxalate stone formers treated with dietary sodium supplementation. J Urol. 2009;181:1140-4.
85. Whitson PA, Pietrzyk RA, Jones JA, et al. Effect of potassium citrate therapy on the risk of renal stone formation during spaceflight. J Urol. 2009;182:2490-6.
86. Fenton TR, Tough SC, Lyon AW, et al. Causal assessment of dietary acid load and bone disease: a systematic review & meta-analysis applying Hill's epidemiologic criteria for causality. Nutr J. 2011;10:41.
87. Maalouf NM, Moe OW, Adams-Huet B, et al. Hypercalciuria associated with high dietary protein intake is not due to acid load. J Clin Endocrinol Metab. 2011;96:3733-40.
88. Borghi L, Schianchi T, Meschi T, et al. Comparison of two diets for the prevention of recurrent stones in idiopathic hypercalciuria. N Engl J Med. 2002;346:77-84.
89. Lemann J, Jr, Piering WF, Lennon EJ. Possible role of carbohydrate-induced calciuria in calcium oxalate kidney-stone formation. N Engl J Med. 1969;280:232-7.
90. Lemann J, Jr, Bushinsky DA, Hamm LL. Bone buffering of acid and base in humans. Am J Physiol Renal Physiol. 2003;285:F811-32.
91. Kaysen GA, Greene T, Daugirdas JT, et al. Longitudinal and cross-sectional effects of C-reactive protein, equilibrated normalized protein catabolic rate, and serum bicarbonate on creatinine and albumin levels in dialysis patients. Am J Kidney Dis. 2003;42:1200-11.
92. Wolfgram DF, Gundu V, Astor BC, et al. Hydrochlorothiazide compared to chlorthalidone in reduction of urinary calcium in patients with kidney stones. Urolithiasis. 2013;41:315-22.
93. Alonso D, Pieras E, Piza P, et al. Effects of short and long-term indapamide treatments on urinary calcium excretion in patients with calcium oxalate dihydrate urinary stone disease: a pilot study. Scand J Urol Nephrol. 2012;46:97-101.

CHAPTER

14 Bone Histopathology and Disease in Hypercalciuria

Ita Pfeferman Heilberg, Aluizio Barbosa Carvalho

INTRODUCTION

Idiopathic hypercalciuria (IH) represents a systemic abnormality in calcium homeostasis, in which a dysregulation of calcium transport in the intestine, kidney, and bone takes place.[1-3] On a low-calcium diet, IH patients often excrete more calcium than they eat[1] and urinary calcium excretion also rises markedly after the intake of calcium-free nutrients such as simple oral glucose. In such circumstances, the only source possible is bone.

Experimental studies by Bushinsky et al.[4] reported increased urinary calcium excretion on a low-calcium diet in genetic hypercalciuric stone-forming (GHS) rats, indicating an increase in bone resorption and/or a defect in renal calcium reabsorption.[4,5] However, even when under conditions of an ample calcium diet, GHS animals exhibited reduced bone mineral density (BMD) and more brittle and fracture prone bones,[6] indicating an intrinsic disorder of bone not secondary to diet. More recently, Frick et al.[7] reported that administration of 1, 25 dihydroxyvitamin D3 (1, 25(OH)2D3) to GHS rats fed a low-calcium diet, produced a greater increase in urinary calcium than in control animals, suggesting that the additional urinary calcium might have resulted from increased bone resorption probably due to the increased number of vitamin D receptors (VDRs) in their bone cells.

The first clinical reports of reduced bone mineral content (BMC) in calcium stone-forming (CSF) patients date back to almost 40 years ago. Since then, even taking into account the heterogeneity of methods of determining BMD, decreased BMD is a homogenous finding among CSF patients, particularly in those with IH, and has been uncovered by several noninvasive techniques performed along the years in different parts of the world.[8-29] Reduced BMD has been observed in IH even in the presence of increased calcium intestinal absorption.[28] It has also been demonstrated that bone fractures are more prevalent in IH patients.[30] The nature of the defect in bone remodeling in IH patients has been explored by a small number of studies involving bone histomorphometry, which despite of nonhomogeneous results, consistently confirmed the existence of bone disease in this population.[16,24,31-36] However, the exact pathophysiological mechanism(s) of bone loss in IH remains unknown.

In this chapter we will present epidemiological, clinical, and laboratorial data supporting the evidences for an accompanying bone disease in nephrolithiasis patients, its pathogenesis, and treatment.

EPIDEMIOLOGICAL STUDIES

Increased Fracture Risk and Reduced Bone Mineral Density

In a population-based cohort study, the number of patients with a first vertebral fracture at 30 years after an initial symptomatic episode of urolithiasis were over four times the expected number on the basis of vertebral fracture incidence rates in the general population, even after adjustments for age and corticosteroids use.[30] No increases in the risk of hip, pelvis, proximal humerus or distal forearm fractures were found showing that cancellous bone was more severely affected than the cortical bone. The risk increased greatly in men who formed stones and mildly in women. A second population-based study in women failed to disclose any association between BMD and fracture and history of kidney stones,[37] but the small number of women reporting kidney stones might have accounted by for the lack of an association with BMD or fractures. A cross-sectional epidemiological study,[38] using the Third National Health and Nutrition Examination Survey, showed that men with kidney stone history (n = 477) have lower femoral neck BMD than men without kidney stones, after adjusting for age, body mass index (BMI), ethnicity, and other potential confounders, with a concomitant higher prevalence of wrist and spine fractures (odds ratio of 2.32 for spine fracture). The same was not observed among women (n = 316) who reported kidney stones.[38] Men with a history of kidney stones who reported low-milk (calcium) intake had a much lower age-adjusted BMD than men with no kidney stone history. Again, this association was not significant among women. Finally, in a large population-based sample of almost 6,000 men, 65 years of age or older, enrolled in the osteoporotic fractures in men study (MrOS), a history of kidney stones was associated with lower BMD.[39]

CLINICAL STUDIES

Bone Mineral Density

Since 1976, several studies reported decreased BMD or BMC in trabecular and cortical bone in CSF patients, in either hypercalciuric,[9,12-16,18-25] normocalciuric,[10,12,15,17,22,23] in both subgroups mixed[10,17,26] or in unselected population of stone formers,[8,11] as shown in Table 14.1. The results of BMD/BMC obtained in patients with primary hyperparathyroidism described in some of these series were not included in this table. Some of the discrepancies between these findings may be accounted for by the heterogeneity of definitions of reduced bone mass (a few studies were performed before the definition of osteoporosis and application of T-score by the World Health Organization) and the different methods of measuring BMD (neutron activation, single-photon absorptiometry, dual-energy X-ray absorptiometry, quantitative computerized tomography, and quantitative ultrasound). Accordingly, bone mineral loss was disclosed at various skeletal sites, namely vertebral spine, proximal hip, radius, tibial diaphysis and epiphysis, and distal metaphyses of the first phalanxes of the nondominant hand. Overall, as analyzed by Sakhaee et al.,[40] diminished BMD occurred at 31% at the proximal hip, 40% at the vertebral spine, and 65% at the radius. Biases in patient selection may also account for differences between results of BMD obtained by various authors. Certain investigators included postmenopausal women[26,28] or older patients, whereas others did not report the gender distribution. Even for known proportions of males and females upon inclusion, separate results from women and men have not been sorted out in some of the aforementioned studies. To avoid biases related to postmenopausal bone loss, a few studies included either only male[17,22] or a much higher proportion of males up to 79%.[10-12,21] Curiously, a handful of authors found higher prevalences of osteopenia among men[8,10,11,23] for reasons not yet completely understood. Finally, part of the studies compared BMD or BMC from stone formers with healthy subjects while others considered nonhypercalciuric stone formers as controls. Although, most studies have observed bone density below normal in all groups, hypercalciuric patients were found to have the most severe bone loss. Indeed, urinary calcium is a determinant of BMD in both postmenopausal women41 and elderly men.[42] However, among aging healthy subjects, higher calcium excretion may also be the mere consequence, not the cause of bone demineralization. But interestingly, Asplin et al.[27] have observed that spine and femoral neck BMD varied inversely with urine calcium loss in IH stone formers but not among nonstone formers.

Biochemical Markers of Bone Turnover

Bone formation markers such as serum bone alkaline phosphatase (BAP) were found to be higher in hypercalciuric than controls[21,25] or in hypercalciuric versus normocalciuric stone formers[22] while osteocalcin or GLA protein were unaltered.[12,21] As for markers of bone resorption, higher urinary total hydroxyproline (THP) in hypercalciuric versus normocalciuric patients or controls has been described by several investigators.[13,21,22,25,43] Jaeger et al.[17] found no differences in urinary fasting THP between normo- and hypercalciuric stone former but BMD at tibial diaphysis was negatively correlated with urinary collagen cross-links (pyridinoline/creatinine ratio) and skeletal score was negatively correlated with fasting THP. Finally, Asplin et al.[27] found no differences in BAP and C-terminal and N-terminal telopeptides of type I collagen in serum, and total pyridinoline/deoxypyridinoline in urine between stone formers and nonstone formers, but did not assess these markers in hypercalciuric versus nonhypercalciuric individuals.

Bone Histomorphometry

Undecalcified iliac crest bone biopsy followed by histomorphometry has been considered the gold-standard method for the diagnosis of metabolic bone disease.[44-46] It provides substantial information about bone turnover, the resultant dynamic process comprising bone formation, and resorption. This is especially true when previous tetracycline double-labeling protocol is performed, allowing the measurement of bone formation.[47] For that purpose, 18 days before the bone biopsy, patients are given oral tetracycline (20 mg/kg/day) in 2 periods of 3 days and 10 days apart. The procedure is undertaken from 3 days to 5 days after the 2nd course of tetracycline. Tetracycline uptake by active osteoblast-covered osteoid seams allows

Table 14.1: Bone mineral density (BMD) or content (BMC) in stone formers.

Authors	n	Hypercalciuric M/F AH	Hypercalciuric M/F FH	Hypercalciuric M/F RH	Normocalciuric M/F	Method	Changes in BMD or BMC
Alhava et al.[8]	59			44 / 15$^{\delta}$		Am-241 γ ray	↓ mean radius BMD of 7.7% (M) & 5.2% (F) vs HS
Lawoyin et al.[9]	161	94/23	-	28/16	-	SPA	↓ mean radius BMD of 1% in AH & 11% in RH vs mean BMD of controls
Fuss et al.[10]	119	34/19	-	7/18	35/6	SPA	↓ % of normal mean BMC in SF whole group. Trend for ↓ BMC in male RH vs AH and vs NC
Barkin et al.[11]	109			86/23		NAA	↓ BMC in 5% of SF. Low BMC in 64 M vs 21F < 50 yrs (7 vs 4%)
Pacifici et al.[12]	46	18/0	15/0	-	13/0	QCT	↓ mean spine Z-score in FH vs AH & NC
Bataille et al.[13]	42	19/7		1/0	-	QCT	↓ 9% of mean spine BMD in AH-type II (12M/6F), 29% in AH type I (7M/1F), 46% in RH & 32% in undetermined HC (9M/6F) vs HS (41M/20F)
Borghi et al.[14]	41	13/7	14/7	-	-	DPA	↓ mean spine Z-score in 13% of diet-independent HC vs diet-dependent HC
Pietschmann et al.[15]	120	42/20	24/3	-	25/6	SPA/ DEXA	↓ 10% of mean L_2L_4 BMD in AH and 12% in FH vs NC (low values in 74% of AH, 92% of FH and 48% of NC)
Heilberg et al.[16]	55	13/22	13/7	-	-	DEXA	↓ 13% of mean L_2L_4 BMD in FH vs HS (40M/144F)
Jaeger et al.[17]	110		49/0		61/0	DEXA	↓ mean BMD (spine, upper femur, tibial diaphysis and epiphysis) in all SF vs HS (234M)
Weisinger et al.[18]	29		4/13		4/8	DEXA	↓ mean L_2L_4 BMD in HC vs NC and vs HS (4M/8F)
Zanchetta et al.[19]	50	5/7	15/23	-	-	DPA	↓ 15% of mean L_1L_4 BMD in HC vs HS (20M/30F)
Ghazali et al.[20]	25		23/2		-	QCT	↓ L_1L_4 Z-score in diet-independent HC (–1.2) vs diet-dependent HC (–0.50) & vs 8M/2F HS (-0.25)
Giannini et al.[21]	49	13/5	23/8	-	-	DEXA	↓ L_2L_4 Z-score in HC (–0.92) vs 10M/3F HS (0.27)
Trinchieri et al.[22]	48		14/0		34/0	DEXA	↓ L_2L_4/femur BMD in 57% of HC and 44% of NC
Martini et al.[23]	85		29/10		18/28	DEXA	T-score < –1 in 44% of all SF patients (62% of HC and 33% of NC). Low BMD in M vs F (78 vs 37%)
Misael da Silva et al.[24]	40		11/11		8/10	DEXA	↓ L_1L_4/femur BMD and Z-scores in 45% of HC
Tasca et al.[25]	70	20/11	27/ 12	-	-	DEXA	↓ L_1L_2 BMD & Z-score (–0.93) in all HC vs 15 HS (0.28)
Caudarella et al.[26]	191			102/89		SPA/QUS	T-score < –1 in 54% of SF patients (21.7% of them HC) ↓ BMD both in pre- and postmenopausal female vs HS
Asplin et al.[27]	22		14 M/F (?)		8 M/F (?)	DEXA	Mean spine and femur Z-scores in HC did not differ from non-stone formers (14M/23F),10 of them hypercalciuric
Vezzoli et al.[28]	64		29/35		15/27	DEXA	↓ Spine Z-score in HC vs NC but only in post-menopausal HC (29F)
Tugcu et al.[29]	150		-		75/75	DEXA	T-score < –1 in 65% of NC vs 20% of HS (35M/25F)

(F: Female; M: Male; SF: Stone formers; HS: Healthy subjects; BMD: Bone mineral density; BMC: Bone mineral content; HC: Idiopathic hypercalciuria; NC: Normocalciuria; FH: Fasting hypercalciuria; AH: Absorptive hypercalciuria (type I: Calcium: independent/type II: Calcium-dependent); RH: Renal or resorptive hypercalciuria; Am-241γ ray Americium-241 gamma ray; SPA: Single Photon absorptiometry; NAA: Neutron-activation analysis; QCT: Quantitative computerized tomography; DPA: Dual photon absorptiometry; DEXA: Dual-energy X-ray absorptiometry; QUS: Quantitative ultrasound).

$^{\delta}$ First or recurrent SF (excluding patients with hyperparathyroidism or bone disease).

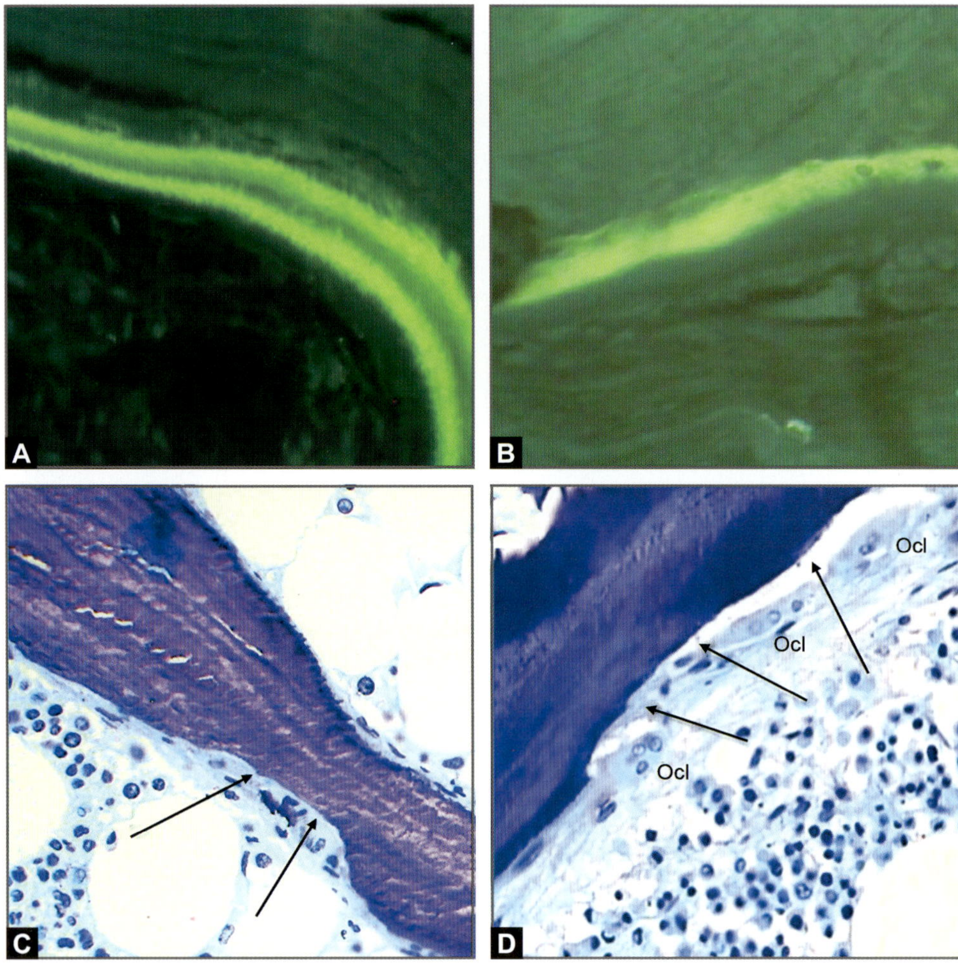

Figs. 14.1A to D: Microphotographs of undecalcified trabecular bone from iliac crest: (A) Fluorescent tetracycline double labels indicating normal bone formation. (B) Single blurred label indicating low bone formation (C) Normal eroded surface (arrows) (D) Increased extent of eroded surface (arrows), covered by multinucleated giant cells, the osteoclasts (Ocl). Toluidine blue, 200X.

the identification of two parallel fluorescent labels when bone tissue is exposed to ultraviolet (UV) light microscopy. The bone surface (BS) extension, as well as the distance between the double-labels, confers an important dynamic bone parameter, named bone formation rate (BFR/BS), as shown in Figure 14.1A. The lack of double labels, as seen in Figure 14.1B, characterizes low BFR/BS and may suggest abnormal mineralization. The mineralization lag time (MLT) determines how long the newly deposited osteoid matrix takes to be mineralized. This histomorphometric parameter derives indirectly from BFR/BS, e.g., also comes from tetracycline labeling.[46] On the other hand, there is as yet no tissue marker for bone resorption rate. Nevertheless, eroded surface (ES/BS) and osteoclast surface (Oc.S/BS) are currently used as static parameters to define bone resorption, as shown in Figures 14.1C and D. The balance between bone formation and resorption defines the bone turnover. As bone resorption and formation are a coupled process, bone formation may represent bone turnover in normal conditions, which is not true in some pathological situations.[48] The hypercalciuria-associated bone disease, as a metabolic bone disease, can be defined as an uncoupling process between bone formation and resorption that leads to a derangement of bone turnover.

The Table 14.2 summarizes the available bone histomorphometry studies involving IH patients, retrieved from eight published articles[16,24,31-34,36,49] and one abstract.[35] The parameters herein referred, were those used to define the bone turnover, mineralization, and volume (TMV) system.[50] Roughly, low-bone turnover, associated with high-bone resorption seem to be the hallmark of bone biopsies from IH patients, since all series point out to a reduced bone formation, and 66% of them shows an elevated bone resorption. However, the presented data

Table 14.2: Bone histomorphometric findings in idiopathic hypercalciuria patients

Authors	*n*	Age (years)	Gender M/F	Bone turnover: Bone formation	Bone turnover: Bone resorption	Bone mineralization	Bone volume	Tetracycline double-label protocol
Bordier et al. 1977[31]	30	38.0 ± 8.0*	38/9	Low (calcification front)	High (ES/BS)	Normal (calcification front plus OV/BV)	NA	No
Malluche et al. 1980[32]	15	41.9 ± 3.9	12/3	Low (Fmin)	Normal (ES/BS)	Abnormal (MLT)	Normal (BV/TV)	Yes
de Vernejoul et al. 1981[33]	30	46.2 ± 9.7	20/10	Low (Ob.S/BS)	Low (ES/BS)	Normal (calcification front plus OV/BV and OS/BS)	Low (BV/TV)	No
Steiniche et al. 1989[34]	33	20–68**	22/11	Low (Aj.Ar)	High (ES/BS)	Abnormal (MLT)	Normal (BV/TV)	Yes
Heilberg et al. 1994[16]	6	39.0 ± 9.6	6/0	Low (BFR/BS)	High (ES/BS)	Abnormal (MLT)	Low (BV/TV)	Yes
Bataille et al. 1995[35]	24	NA	20/4	Low (BFR/BS)	Low (ES/BS)	Normal (MLT)	Low (BV/TV)	Yes
Misael et al. 2002[24]	22	12–61	11/11	Low (BFR/BS)	High (ES/BS)	Abnormal (MLT)	Normal (BV/TV)	Yes
Heller et al. 2007[36]	9	41.0 ± 8.0	6/3	Low (BFR/BS)	High (ES/BS)	Normal (MLT)	Normal (BV/TV)	Yes
Menon et al. 2014[49]	30	32.9 ± 5.4	18/12	Low (BFR/BS)	High (ES/BS)	Abnormal (MLT)	Low (BV/TV)	Yes

* X ± SD: Mean ± SD

**: Range; histomorphometric parameter, utilized by the authors to define the presented alterations, is given between brackets. (NA: Not available; ES/BS: Eroded surface; Fmin: Fraction of mineralized osteoid seams; Ob.S/BS: Osteoblastic surface; Aj.AR: Adjusted apposition rate; BFR/BS: Bone formation rate; MLT: Mineralization lag time; OV/BV: Osteoid volume; OS/BS: Osteoid surface; BV/TV: Trabecular bone volume).

should be interpreted with caution as sample size, age, gender distribution, inclusion criteria, and diagnostic classification of hypercalciuria, disclose a remarkable heterogeneity among them. Moreover, not all the studies had performed a tetracycline double labeling protocol for their patients. In addition, the control groups of the distinct studies comprise a quite variable sample of individuals, including postmortem material obtained from subjects assumed to be healthy, albeit data regarding urinary calcium excretion are not available. Furthermore, when the bone sample is obtained after death, tetracycline labeling cannot be assessed. Thus, the dynamic parameters (bone formation and mineralization) of controls are usually the ones available in the literature, whose gender distribution, race, and diet habits may not properly match with the studied population.

When tetracycline labeling protocol was not commonly used, Bordier et al.[31] and de Vernejoul et al.[33] considered bone formation as low, either based on the calcification front or Ob.S/BS, respectively. Notwithstanding the presence of a calcification front (a single dark blue line on the osteoid surface, seen in toluidine blue staining) does indicate an active calcification process on the osteoid matrix, this parameter is not as reliable as the tetracycline labeling, in which the presence of a newly forming mineralized bone, between labels, cannot be contested. Even in the presence of normal calcification front, de Vernejoul et al.[33] reported low-bone formation in their patients, based on the diminished Ob.S/BS. The remaining studies, using tetracycline labeling, observed low-bone formation, based on either BFR/BS or related parameters, such as Fmin (fraction of mineralized osteoid seams) by Malluche et al.[32] and the adjusted apposition rate (Aj.Ar) (adjusted BFR) by Steiniche et al.[34] Of note, the study of Heilberg et al.[16] concluded that bone formation was low based on the finding that four out of six bone biopsies exhibited no tetracycline uptake. However, even without the possibility to measure bone formation in all patients, the absence of tetracycline uptake mirrored the severity of the derangement in bone formation and mineralization, allowing the authors to make that conclusion. Misael et al.[24] also detected a low BFR/BS, particularly in osteopenic patients, defined by bone densitometry. This was in accordance with their findings, as low BFR/BS could at least in part contribute to bone loss. Interestingly, although Heller et al.[36] reported that bone formation was low, based on a nonsignificant difference in BFR/BS between patients and controls, they did find a significant low Ob.S/BS, the histomorphometric parameter that gives information about the cells implicated in bone formation.

The overall results of the studies with respect to bone resorption revealed an elevated bone resorption, based on ES/BS. Even though the increase in ES/BS described by Heller et al.[36] was not significant, the Oc.S/BS was greater than controls ($p = 0.04$). Misael et al.[24] described a high ES/BS in all patients, which was even higher in osteopenic, if compared to the nonosteopenic ones. This finding, associated to the low BFR/BS, could explain the resultant osteopenia as an imbalance between bone formation and resorption.

Concerning bone mineralization, all but two studies used MLT. In fact, five out of nine studies (55.5%) found it to be abnormal. However, considering that two from the nine studies, in which bone mineralization was reported as normal, did not perform tetracycline labeling, one could assume that abnormal bone mineralization was indeed present in five out of seven studies (71%).

The last evaluated parameter was the bone volume/total volume (BV/TV), which was low in 50% of the studies (in one of them, this parameter was not available). Considering that low BFR/BS and high ES/BS are the hallmark of bone turnover in IH patients, one could expect that BV/TV would be low, in at least the majority of them. However, it is well-known that BV/TV is a parameter that varies with the technique of the bone biopsy procedure.[51] Thus, if the bone biopsy is unwittingly performed close to cortical bone, BV/TV may be mistakenly high. In summary, it seems that low bone formation, high bone resorption, abnormal mineralization, and a suspected low BV characterize the bone disorder seen in IH patients. However, further systematic trials, avoiding all biased factors that could misinterpret the real bone histologic scenario of IH patients, are still warranted.

POTENTIAL PATHOPHYSIOLOGICAL MECHANISMS FOR BONE ALTERATIONS IN HYPERCALCIURIC STONE FORMERS

Although the pathophysiology of the hypercalciuria cannot be explained by a single mechanism, and that mobilization of bone calcium by itself does not represent the only cause of hypercalciuria, bone cells involved in bone formation and resorption could play a central role in the chain of events leading to hypercalciuria.

Role of Hormones and Local Cytokines

Vitamin D

At high doses, 1, 25(OH)2D3 increases bone resorption and decreases bone collagen synthesis[52] and administration of 1, 25(OH)2D3 to healthy subjects mimics the phenotype of absorptive hypercalciuria.[53] Serum 1, 25(OH)2D3 levels in IH patients form a continuum from normal to high[1,54-59] and VDR polymorphism had been associated with elevated urinary calcium.[60] Although Zerwekh et al.,[58] found VDR concentration in fibroblasts from hypercalciuric patients to be normal, Favus et al.[59] detected a twofold increase in VDR in peripheral blood monocytes from IH patients despite normal serum 1, 25(OH)2D3, suggesting an altered tissue vitamin D response. Experimental studies have shown that GHS rats exhibit increased number of VDR coupled with normal levels of circulating 1, 25(OH)2D3 resulting in increased functional VDR-1,25(OH)2D3 complexes[61] or an increased sensitivity to its actions. Therefore, target organ action of normal circulating 1, 25(OH)2D3 in the bone, kidney, and intestine seems to be amplified by high VDR activity.[40] At a bone level, Krieger et al.[62] demonstrated increased bone resorption after calcitriol exposure in cultured calvariae from GHS rats. Increased VDR concentration and increased sensitivity of bone have been shown in this animal model.[63] Menon et al.,[49] in an immunohistochemical analysis, performed according to a technique described by their group,[64] has recently showed a strong and significant correlation between bone expression of VDR in osteoblasts with ES/BS in bone samples from IH stone formers, not evidenced in their controls.

Parathyroid Hormone

Theoretically, the negative calcium balance found among patients with renal hypercalciuria or renal leak could conceivably lead to secondary hyperparathyroidism. However, normal or low values of parathyroid hormone (PTH) despite calcium losses have been described instead.[1,65] A state of subtle primary hyperparathyroidism in patients with elevated PTH and fluctuating ionized calcium levels may be found in some IH patients, but according to Gomes et al.,[66] an oral calcium load test may be a valuable dynamic tool to identify it, avoiding numerous repeated PTH and serum calcium determinations leading to inconclusive results. Given the high-normal levels of vitamin D or higher VDR sensitivity, one can speculate about the suppression of PTH in the setting of hypercalciuria.

Interleukin-1 and Receptor Activator of Nuclear Factor Kappa-B Ligand-Osteoprotegerin System

Pioneering studies by Pacifici et al.[12] demonstrated that mononuclear cells from patients with fasting hypercalciuria had an increased spontaneous production of interleukin-1 (IL-1), which correlated negatively with lumbar spine BMD. Subsequently, Weisinger et al.[18] demonstrated that not only IL-1, but other cytokines such as IL-6, and tumor necrosis factor-α (TNF-α) were increased in peripheral monocytes of IH patients, with a significant correlation with lumbar spine BMD. Based on these findings, which were further corroborated by others,[20,24] it has been suggested that bone resorption induced by elevated cytokines could represent a primary mechanism leading to hypercalciuria.

Bone remodeling requires an interaction between osteoblasts and osteoclasts through receptor activator of nuclear factor kappa-B (RANK), the receptor activator of nuclear factor-κB (NF-κB) and its natural ligand, receptor activator of nuclear factor kappa-B ligand (RANKL), expressed by osteoblastic stromal cells and incorporated into the osteoblast membrane.[67] RANKL binding to RANK seemed to function as the primary mediator of osteoclast differentiation, activation, and survival and can be blocked by osteoprotegerin (OPG), a decoy receptor. In an immunohistochemical study, Gomes et al.[68] have shown an elevated bone expression of both RANKL and OPG in bone specimens previously obtained from 36 transiliac bone biopsies of IH stone-forming patients, when compared to controls. In addition, RANKL immunostaining was even higher in IH patients with high versus normal bone resorption, reinforcing that RANKL might be an important stimulatory local factor for bone resorption in the IH setting. Given the inhibitory osteoclastogenic effect of OPG, its unexpected higher bone expression was ascribed to an attempt to counteract the actions of RANKL. These authors also detected a trend for a higher mean value of bone immunostaining for IL-1 in bone from IH patients than in control subjects, but without statistical significance.

Transforming Growth Factor-β

The transforming growth factor-β (TGF-β is known as the most important and abundant growth factor in bone matrix, stimulating bone formation, mineralization, and inhibiting bone resorption through a proapoptotic effect on mature osteoclasts and inhibition of osteoclast differentiation.[52,69] Low levels of TGF-β were detected in immunostains of hypercalciuric stone formers by Gomes et al.,[68] in areas adjacent to osteoid surfaces. β-expression positively correlated with bone formation indices including osteoid volume, osteoblastic surface, trabecular number, and mineralization surface, and negatively correlated with bone resorption parameters such as trabecular separation. Thus, it was hypothesized that the low bone expression of TGF- could be one of the factors contributing to the delayed mineralization found in such patients.

Fibroblast Growth Factor-23

Fibroblast growth factor-23 (FGF-23) is produced in bone and acts on kidney as a systemic phosphaturic factor. Increased serum levels of FGF-23 in calcium nephrolithiasis patients with hypophosphatemia has been reported,[70] but according to Wang et al.[71] FGF-23 overexpression in cultured calvariae suppressed bone formation and matrix mineralization irrespective of the systemic effects on phosphate homeostasis. Recently, Menon et al.[49] evaluated expression of FGF-23 in bone tissue from IH patients but found no difference from controls.

Sclerostin

The signaling pathways through which sclerostin (Scl), produced in osteocytes, exerts its effects on bone metabolism are still incompletely understood. Although, Scl has emerged as a stimulator of osteoblasts apoptosis[72] and a potent inhibitor of Wnt/β-catenin signaling, hence decreasing bone formation,[73] an experimental model in which Wnt pathway was specifically inhibited in osteocytes has shown normal bone formation, but a significant increase in osteoclastic bone resorption instead.[74] It has been hypothesized that in response to catabolic stimulus, Scl expressed by mature mineral embedded or even apoptosing osteocytes may act in an autocrine manner increasing local expression of RANKL relative to OPG as well as in a paracrine manner, inducing such expression in immature osteocytes immediately below the osteoblastic lining cells.[75] Finally, a very recent randomized controlled trial (RCT) using a neutralizing antibody to Scl (romosozumab) in postmenopausal women, showed that a serum bone-resorption marker [isomer of the C-terminal telopeptide of collagen (β-CTx)] presented a significant and sustained reduction after 12 months while the increase in a bone-formation marker [procollagen type 1 N-terminal propeptide (P1NP)], was only transitory.[76] Lately, Menon et al.[49] observed that although mean bone expression of Scl in IH stone formers did not differ from healthy controls; it was significantly higher in IH patients with high versus normal bone resorption. Moreover, these investigators found a significantly positive correlation of Scl bone expression with ES/BS and with serum 1, 25(OH)2D3 in IH group, not observed in the control, raising the hypothesis that the elevated bone resorption seen in some IH patients could be mediated by an increase in vitamin D signaling stimulating Scl synthesis and leading to an imbalance in the OPG/RANKL ratio.

Role of the Diet

Calcium Intake

Large prospective observational studies showed that low-calcium intake was associated with a higher risk of kidney stones in distinct cohorts,[68-71] probably ascribed to a secondary increase in urinary oxalate, which resulted from hyperabsorption of free oxalate during low-calcium intake. In contrast, supplemental calcium was associated with a slight but significantly higher risk of incident stones in older but not younger women.[77,78] These opposing findings might have been due to different timing of ingestion of the supplements influencing calcium excretion.[79] In the general population, observational studies suggested that bone loss and fracture risk increase when calcium intake is below 700–800 mg per day,[80,81] but the risk of nephrolithiasis was modestly increased (relative risk of 1.17) with the use of calcium supplements in the Women's Health Initiative (WHI) trial.[82] Several studies have suggested a relationship between low-calcium diet and reduced BMD in IH patients.[15,17-19,22-24] Bone resorption itself may also be worsened by low-calcium intake, since even small elevations of serum 1, 25(OH)2D3 in healthy subjects or in patients with IH, seem to be sufficient to increase bone resorption when dietary calcium intake is low, indicating that 1, 25(OH)2D3 may upregulate its own receptor.[59,83] Moreover, as recently reviewed by Lieben and Carmeliet[84] when insufficient calcium is acquired from the diet and a negative calcium balance ensues, 1, 25(OH)2D3 levels increase and act directly on osteoblasts and osteocytes to enhance bone resorption and to suppress bone matrix mineralization. Therefore, to avoid the threat of bone demineralization in hypercalciuric patients, dietary calcium restriction should be avoided,[85] and a calcium intake of 800–1,200 mg (approximately 3–4 servings of dairy per day) seems to be more appropriate.[86] Calcium supplement dosing combined with dietary intake should be sufficient to approximate, but not exceed the Institute of Medicine (IOM) daily guidelines and should be taken with meals in order to avoid increasing the risk of calcium oxalate nephrolithiasis.[79] As vitamin D repletion is also useful to maintain bone health, stone formers with vitamin D deficiency and bone loss may be eligible for supplementation. According to Leaf et al.,[87] a limited course of vitamin D repletion did not augment mean urinary calcium excretion in stone formers, although a subset of individuals may have an increase. However, the amount of dietary calcium supply must be taken into account for an optimal therapeutic regimen with vitamin D as part of an antiosteoporotic therapy, in order to maximize the targeted outcome and to avoid side effects such as enhanced bone resorption.

Sodium Intake

The effect of high-sodium intake upon volume expansion and increased calcium excretion has been well documented. This has provided the physiological basis for the proposed role of increased salt intake as a risk factor for osteoporosis. In postmenopausal women, the consumption of a low-sodium diet (2 g/day) during 6 months reduced calcium excretion and the aminoterminal propeptide of type I collagen.[88] In kidney stone-forming subjects, daily urinary calcium excretion varied directly with moderate changes in dietary sodium intake.[89,90] The adverse effects of a high salt consumption upon bone loss among calcium stone formers have been evaluated by Martini et al.[23] who showed through a multiple regression analysis, that a high salt intake was the single variable predictive of risk of low bone density after adjustments for calcium and protein intakes, age, weight, BMI, urinary calcium, citrate, uric acid excretion, and duration of stone disease.

Protein Intake

Animal protein-induced hypercalciuria occurs from more bone resorption and lower tubular calcium reabsorption. The presence of nonresorbable calcium sulfate in the tubular lumen consequent to sulfate production from oxidation of excessive sulfur-containing amino acids may contribute[91] and the direct acid-mediated inhibition of renal tubule calcium reabsorption by a lower expression of transient receptor potential vanilloid-5 (TRPV5) channel in the distal tubule, also increases urine calcium excretion.[92] A high dietary animal protein intake may increase bone turnover because of the resultant subtle metabolic acidosis which suppresses osteoblastic activity and increase osteoblastic RANKL synthesis, ultimately leading to increased bone resorption to buffer the proton load.[93] In an animal model, a high-casein diet delivered a substantial acid load, which increased urinary calcium and promoted a sharp increase in bone resorption.[94] Zerwekh et al.[95,96] showed through dynamic and static bone histomorphometry, that rats fed a high-protein diet (HPD) presented a significant reduction in cancellous BV and trabecular number associated with a 2.5-fold increase in eroded and a 3.5-fold increase in osteoclastic surfaces. A near twofold increase in BFR was also disclosed. Potassium citrate (KCit) but not potassium chloride (KCl) partially or entirely prevented all changes in urine biochemistry, prevented the increase in bone resorption, but without any effect on bone formation.[96] More recently, in a short-term crossover metabolic study by Maalouf et al.,[97] although KCit neutralized the acid load delivered by a HPD given to healthy volunteers for 2 weeks, it did not prevent the hypercalciuria associated with this diet suggesting that mechanism(s) other than acid load may account for hypercalciuria induced by HPD. No significant changes in bone turnover markers were noted with the HPD in this study as well. In the general population, Feskanich et al.[98] reported an association between HPD and bone fractures. Nevertheless, the long-term effects of HPD on calcium metabolism and bone status are still controversial, since the population-based Framingham Osteoporosis Study has showed that women and men with relatively lower protein intake had increased bone loss, even after controlling for known confounders[99] and others have reported reduced BMD[100] and lower fracture risk.101 Ultimately, a recent systematic review and meta-analysis of the controversial relation between protein and bone health in healthy human adults found no definite effect of protein intake on fracture risk in the long term.[102]

Among stone formers with IH, an association of HPD with decreased BMD has been suggested by several investigators.[13,15,17,18,24] Pietschmann et al.[15] found an inverse association between vertebral BMD and 24-hour urinary sulfate and pH. Jaeger et al.[17] also showed an inverse association between these biochemical markers of increased acid load and corrected BMD at the tibia and femur. Based on the positive correlation between fasting calciuria and fasting THP, and since both correlated with urea excretion as well, Bataille et al.[13] suggested a primary bone hyperresorption as the main cause of IH and hypothesized that a higher protein intake could contribute to increase bone resorption. Although Asplin et al.[27] observed no association between femoral neck and spine Z-scores with urinary sulfate or titratable acid, they did find an inverse significant correlation of the latter with total ammonium in stone former, not evidenced among nonstone former. However, no correlations of BMD Z-score with bone markers were found. Since stone former consumed less calcium, these authors raised the hypothesis that lower calcium intake might have altered their bone responses predisposing to mineral loss. Indeed, Dawson-Hughes and Harris[103] have shown that calcium intake does influence the association of protein intake with rates of bone loss in elderly men and women.

Role of Genetics

Optimal bone mineral accretion during childhood and adolescence is critical to the attainment of a healthy adult skeleton. As in the adult population, reduced BMD has been reported in IH children as well.[104-106] Interestingly, hypercalciuria and reduced BMD were uncovered in a substantial number of their otherwise healthy asymptomatic mothers.[104] Although, growth and pubertal growth spurt have been reported to be normal in IH children and adolescents,[107,108] the diminished BMD observed in adults with IH may have started earlier, and may represent a risk factor for osteoporosis later in life. In addition, some genetically heterogeneous disorders manifested in childhood or early adulthood, are associated with hypercalciuria, nephrocalcinosis or nephrolithiasis, and rachitic bone disease, such as Dent's disease (mutations in the chloride/proton exchange transporter, CLC-5) and Lowe syndrome (mutations in phosphatidylinositol-4, 5-biphosphate-5-phosphatase, OCRL1).[109,110] Mutations in the gene encoding phosphate transporter NaPi2a, detected in two hypophosphatemic patients (one with nephrolithiasis and other with osteoporosis), which could possibly link nephrolithiasis with defective bone mineralization, have not been further supported in subsequent studies.[111,112] Whereas, hereditary monogenic kidney stone diseases are rare monogenic diseases that affect primarily the bone may also lead to hypercalciuria largely via increased calcium release into the circulating pool. As reviewed by Moe and

Bonny,[113] these conditions can be related to structural defects in bone such as osteogenesis imperfect, part of a hyperparathyroid state or rachitic-like bone lesion. Mutations or polymorphisms in the soluble adenylyl cyclase gene (ADCY10) have been linked to vertebral bone loss in stone formers with absorptive hypercalciuria[114] and a linkage to chromosome 1q23-24 was identified in three families. Although, soluble adenylyl cyclase acts as a bicarbonate sensor which mediates the inhibition of osteoclast function by bicarbonate,[115] the underlying mechanism for bone loss remains unknown and despite of the evidence of linkage and linkage disequilibrium between this gene and absorptive hypercalciuria, there is no conclusive demonstration that substitutions or mutations in ADCY10 cause absorptive hypercalciuria.[116] In a large population study from Iceland and the Netherland, Thorleifsson et al.[117] found association between sequence variants in the CLDN14 gene (which encodes for tight junction claudin-14) with kidney stones and reduced BMD at the hip. However, the mechanism of how a paracellular protein affects bone remodeling or bone cell function remains unclear and in a more recent study, conducted in other cohorts, the association of CLDN14 with urinary calcium excretion was not statistically different, hence requiring further investigation.[118]

Notwithstanding variation in urine calcium excretion does segregate in stone forming families,[119,120] and family and twin studies evidenced the importance of genes in calcium nephrolithiasis, with approximately 50% of patients showing a family history of stone disease,[121] the transmission pattern of IH does not fit into the classical Mendelian categories, but is consistent with a complex polygenic trait that may be heterogeneous in different patient groups with numerous genetic and environmental determinants.[113,122] At the same time, it is well known that BMD is under strong genetic control and as much as 75% of its variance in the normal population, has been attributed to genetic factors.[123] Single-candidate gene polymorphisms have also been explored in stone formers, and among the pursued candidate genes, the ones along the vitamin D axis were examined. The association between VDR polymorphism and BMD in the general population remains controversial since regardless of the pioneering study by Morrison et al.[124] showing that common allelic variants in the gene encoding the VDR could be used to predict differences in BMD among healthy individuals, further studies have not confirmed such an association.[125,126] Nonetheless, the potential susceptibility locus in the vicinity of the VDR gene for idiopathic stone formation[127] prompted many investigators to look for association between VDR polymorphisms and calcium excretion and/or BMD, among stone formers. Inasmuch as the *bb* genotype has been classically related to a better BMD,[124] its prevalence was expected to be lower among hypercalciuric patients, who traditionally exhibit higher rates of low BMD. However, *bb* homozygous for VDR polymorphism was shown to be overrepresented in hypercalciuric stone formers, as observed by many investigators.[60,128,129] With respect to BMD, allele distribution did not differ between osteopenic or normal BMD patients, as reported by Heilberg et al.[130] and Ferreira et al.,[60] besides a significantly lower instead of a higher mean BMD among *bb* patients, according to Rendina et al.[128] FokI VDR polymorphism also did not associate with BMD in hypercalciuric patients.[131] Such observations of an association of VDR polymorphisms with calcium excretion but not with BMD are intriguing. According to Dawson-Hughes et al.,[132] *BB* homozygous postmenopausal women, when exposed to low-calcium intake, present less efficient intestinal calcium absorption than *bb* women, despite similar levels of 1, 25(OH)2D3, pointing to VDR as functionally different between *BB* and *bb* alleles. These investigators also observed that although the altered gut VDR status in *bb* variants might have been responsible for a better ability to increase fractional calcium absorption, the patients exhibited not only slightly higher levels of urinary calcium but also somewhat lower serum PTH. The increase in calcium excretion in *bb* genotypes might have been ascribed to PTH suppression induced by increased activity of vitamin D. Another candidate gene hypothesized to be involved in the pathogenesis of hypercalciuria and bone resorption is the one encoding the G-protein coupled Ca^{++}-sensing receptor (CaSR). A single amino acid change (Arg990Gly) of the CaSR has been associated with increased urinary calcium in calcium-stone-forming patients, but BMD was not assessed in that study.[133] A gain-of-function of the CaSR with a 5.5-fold increased risk for the *G* allele to develop hypercalciuria was evidenced in a subsequent study, but the series consisted of osteoporotic women and not stone formers.[134] It is also possible to infer that in such a setting, hypercalciuria was consequent to increased bone resorption rather than being a primary mechanism leading to loss of bone mass. On the other hand, in another functional study, changes in CaSR activity in cells transfected for the *990G* allele have not been observed[135] and there was a lack of association between this and other CaSR polymorphisms with urinary calcium excretion or BMD in female twin pairs. Ferreira et al.[60] also did not find statistical differences among the various CaSR haplotype distributions in stone formers with IH when compared to normocalciurics. Finally, there were no point mutations in seven families with IH[136] and no association was found between the CaSR locus and IH.[137] A quantitative trait locus study in GHS rat showed a significant linkage to regions of chromosomes 4, 7, 10, and 14, but none of them mapped to the VDR, neither to the CaSR gene loci.[138] Mutations in the chloride channel CLCN5, responsible for Dent's disease, also do not seem to represent a common cause of IH as shown by direct sequencing in a case-control study,[139] although experimental data revealed that knockout CLCN5 mice exhibit hypercalciuria of renal and bone origin, consequent to increased bone resorption.[140] Hoenderop et al.[141] demonstrated that mice lacking TRPV5, originally called ECaC1 (epithelial Ca^{2+} channel), which facilitates Ca^{2+} influx in the kidney, small intestine, and bone,[142] display diminished active Ca^{2+} reabsorption despite enhanced vitamin D levels, severe hypercalciuria and significant disturbances in bone structure, including reduced trabecular and cortical bone thickness. However, studies performed in IH families, without available data on BMD, showed no mutations in this gene.[143]

TREATMENT OF BONE DISEASE

Although trials with thiazide diuretics and citrate have been shown to be useful in preventing stone recurrence, there have been no long-term controlled clinical studies examining the efficacy of these agents or other therapies in preventing bone loss in calcium stone formers. Among the potential pharmacological options aimed to treat nephrolithiasis-associated bone disease,[40] one can rely upon thiazides and thiazide-like agents, that reduce renal tubular calcium reabsorption and may stimulate bone formation; alkali treatment, such as citrate, which may decrease bone resorption or increase bone formation and bisphosphonates, that reduce bone resorption.

Thiazides

Thiazide diuretics, associated to a reduced sodium intake, represent the first choice of treatment in the management of IH stone formers. A meta-analysis of randomized trials revealed that in studies in which treatment lasted for more than 2 years, the reduction in stone formation recurrence rate has been significant.[144] It has been demonstrated that after adjustment for potential confounders, patients on thiazide diuretics for other medical conditions showed increased BMD and reduced forearm and hip fracture risk.[145,146] Thiazide treatment significantly diminishes the risk of hip fracture in premenopausal women, postmenopausal women, and elderly men,[147-149] but its protective effect upon reduction of fracture risk disappears within 4 months after discontinuation.[150] On the other hand, a RCT conducted in normal postmenopausal women given 50 mg hydrochlorothiazide for 4 years, showed small but sustained positive benefits on cortical bone density.[151] In 28 nephrolithiasis patients with absorptive hypercalciuria treated with thiazide or indapamide and KCit for a mean period of 3.7 years while maintained on low-calcium oxalate diet, Pak et al.[152] observed a significant increase of BMD of 7.1% at L2-L4 spine and of 4.1% at the femoral neck compared to normal age- and gender-matched patients. However, such beneficial effects could not be solely ascribed to thiazides, but might have rather resulted from the combined alkali treatment as well. Rico et al.[153] reported a decrease in 24-hour calciuria, in serum tartrate resistant acid phosphatase (TRAP) concentration and a significant increase in BMD by 3.0% in total body, 2.5% in the arms, and 3.7% in the trunk, in 14 patients with IH treated with chlorthalidone (CTD), 50 mg/day for 1 year, differing from 10 untreated patients, who lost bone mass in all three sites. A histomorphometric study performed in 27 stone formers with IH, aged 11–69 years old, both before and after thiazide treatment for 6 months (hydrochlorthiazide, 50 mg twice a day), revealed a reduction in the extent of ESs, reflecting lower bone resorption.[154] The potential favorable effect of thiazides on bone density and quality was also tested in GHS rats fed CTD for 18 weeks by means of microcomputed tomography and static histomorphometry by Bushinsky et al.,[155] who found increases in trabecular number, thickness and BV, with improvement of connectivity, vertebral strength, and stiffness. Since CTD did not alter bone formation parameters, these investigators concluded that the improved vertebral bone quality might have been due to decreased bone resorption and retention of bone structure. In IH children, the beneficial effects of thiazides on bone have been controversial. In a historical cohort of 80 pediatric patients who have been treated with both KCit and thiazides for 1 year,[156] a significant increase in BMD Z-score (z-BMD) was observed. However, in that study as well as in others undertaken in children with IH,[157,158] the positive results have not been compared with those of an untreated control group. On the other hand, a retrospective analysis by Garcia-Nieto et al.[159] involving children with IH and osteopenia followed up for 2.4 years, has shown that the z-BMD improved in 12 out of 22 (54%) patients on thiazides, but also improved spontaneously in 23 of the 32 (72%) untreated children. The spontaneous improvement was more evident when the initial BMD was not low and when the BMI had increased during the follow-up period. Nevertheless, the effects of thiazides on the bone may surpass their hypocalciuric action, for thiazides may potentially stimulate osteoblastic bone formation. In vitro, thiazides have a selective effect on human osteoblast-like cell lines, directly stimulating osteocalcin production in human osteoblasts.[160,161] They also increase the expression of thiazide-sensitive sodium chloride cotransporter (NCC) in osteoblast-like cells[162] and directly induce mineralized nodule formation by interaction with NCC and osteoblast differentiation by stimulating osteoblast differentiation markers, such as Runx2 and osteopontin.[163] The mitogenic action of thiazide has been shown in an in vitro study to be in part due to increased osteoblastic cell proliferation.[164] Therefore, thiazides do exert a direct bone-forming effect independent of their renal action. In addition, thiazides and the thiazide-related diuretic, indapamide, have been shown to decrease bone resorption both in vivo[165,166] and in vitro,[167,168] as a result of the reduction of osteoclastic cell differentiation mediated through direct inhibition of hematopoietic precursors.

Alkali Therapy and Citrate

As aforementioned, potassium alkali therapy attenuates the skeletal effect of substantial acid load provided by a HPD, reducing bone resorption[94,96] and improving bone mass because of the induced hypocalciuria[169] and stimulation of osteoblastic activity.[170,171] A RCT conducted in postmenopausal women with osteopenia by Jehle et al.[172] showed a small but significant increase of mean L2-L4 BMD by 0.89% after 1 year on KCit, compared to baseline, which contrasting with the group that received KCl, who exhibited a significant decrease of 0.98%. Conversely, another RCT by MacDonald et al.[173] showed no increased BMD in healthy postmenopausal supplemented with KCit for 2 years. Others showed that combined treatment with KCit and calcium citrate was more effective than either agent alone in inhibiting bone loss.[174] In a retrospective and uncontrolled study in 21 patients with recurrent calcium oxalate nephrolithiasis, given KCit for a mean duration of 44 months, age-dependent bone loss was averted.[175] Another study showed increases in forearm BMD in idiopathic calcium stone formers treated with KCit for 2 years.[176] No study has been undertaken specifically in population of hypercalciuric stone formers.

Bisphosphonates

An experimental study by Bushinsky et al.[177] showed that GHS rats placed on a low-calcium diet plus alendronate presented a significant decrease in urinary calcium leading to positive calcium balance, confirming the hypothesis that bone contributed to hypercalciuria. In clinical studies, Weisinger et al.[178] showed that IH patients on alendronate exhibited decreased urinary calcium starting 1 month after treatment, and increased trabecular BMD after 1 year contrasting with normocalciuric stone formers who had no significant changes in any these parameters. Similarly, Heilberg et al[179] have observed that the use of etidronate in 7 males IH stone formers, induced a significant improvement of lumbar spine BMD by 2.6% after 1 year and a non-significant increase after the 2nd year of treatment by 5.6%. In their series, histomorphometry disclosed no osteomalacia, maintenance of BV but no reduction on ESs on the second bone biopsy,[179] in agreement with other studies employing etidronate in postmenopausal osteoporosis.[180,181] In 7 children with IH, a short-term treatment with bisphosphonates normalized urine calcium excretion and significantly improved reduced BMD.[182] The combination of bisphosphonates and thiazides have also been proved useful to increase BMD in hypercalciuric stone formers with bone loss.[183]

However, considering the difficulties regarding the performance of an invasive method such as bone biopsy in the clinical practice, to evidence the presence or not of elevated bone resorption in a given patient, the benefit of the use of bisphosphonates in IH patients must be interpreted with caution, since these agents may suppress bone turnover.[184] At present, the use of bisphosphonates should be tailored based on markers of bone resorption. Of note, none of them can address if the elevated bone resorption is a primary or secondary event in hypercalciuria.

Therefore, the critical question that still remains is whether the disorder of bone metabolism is the cause or the consequence of hypercalciuria, due to the attendant negative calcium balance. New surrogate markers of bone resorption in the blood or urine are needed to better guide treatment in the future.

REFERENCES

1. Coe FL, Favus MJ, Crockett T, et al. Effects of low-calcium diet on urine calcium excretion, parathyroid function and serum 1,25(OH)2D3 levels in patients with idiopathic hypercalciuria and in normal subjects. Am J Med. 1982;72(1):25-32.
2. Worcester EM, Coe FL. Clinical practice. Calcium kidney stones. N Engl J Med. 2010;363(10):954-63.
3. Heilberg IP. Hypercalciuria. San Diego: Academic Press; 2004. pp. 530-6.
4. Bushinsky DA, Frick KK, Nehrke K. Genetic hypercalciuric stone-forming rats. Curr Opin Nephrol Hypertens. 2006;15(4):403-18.
5. Tsuruoka S, Bushinsky DA, Schwartz GJ. Defective renal calcium reabsorption in genetic hypercalciuric rats. Kidney Int. 1997;51(5):1540-7.
6. Grynpas M, Waldman S, Holmyard D, et al. Genetic hypercalciuric stone-forming rats have a primary decrease in BMD and strength. J Bone Miner Res. 2009;24(8):1420-6.
7. Frick KK, Asplin JR, Krieger NS, et al. 1,25(OH)2D3-enhanced hypercalciuria in genetic hypercalciuric stone-forming rats fed a low-calcium diet. Am J Physiol Renal Physiol. 2013;305(8):F1132-8.
8. Alhava EM, Juuti M, Karjalainen P. Bone mineral density in patients with urolithiasis. A preliminary report. Scand J Urol Nephrol. 1976;10(2):154-6.
9. Lawoyin S, Sismilich S, Browne R, et al. Bone mineral content in patients with calcium urolithiasis. Metabolism. 1979;28(12):1250-4.
10. Fuss M, Gillet C, Simon J, et al. Bone mineral content in idiopathic renal stone disease and in primary hyperparathyroidism. Eur Urol. 1983;9(1):32-4.
11. Barkin J, Wilson DR, Manuel MA, et al. Bone mineral content in idiopathic calcium nephrolithiasis. Miner Electrolyte Metab. 1985;11(1):19-24.
12. Pacifici R, Rothstein M, Rifas L, et al. Increased monocyte interleukin-1 activity and decreased vertebral bone density in patients with fasting idiopathic hypercalciuria. J Clin Endocrinol Metab. 1990;71(1):138-45.
13. Bataille P, Achard JM, Fournier A, et al. Diet, vitamin D and vertebral mineral density in hypercalciuric calcium stone formers. Kidney Int. 1991;39(6):1193-205.
14. Borghi L, Meschi T, Guerra A, et al. Vertebral mineral content in diet-dependent and diet-independent hypercalciuria. J Urol. 1991;146(5):1334-8.
15. Pietschmann F, Breslau NA, Pak CY. Reduced vertebral bone density in hypercalciuric nephrolithiasis. J Bone Miner Res. 1992;7(12):1383-8.
16. Heilberg IP, Martini LA, Szejnfeld VL, et al. Bone disease in calcium stone forming patients. Clin Nephrol. 1994;42(3):175-82.
17. Jaeger P, Lippuner K, Casez JP, et al. Low bone mass in idiopathic renal stone formers: magnitude and significance. J Bone Miner Res. 1994;9(10):1525-32.
18. Weisinger JR, Alonzo E, Bellorín-Font E, et al. Possible role of cytokines on the bone mineral loss in idiopathic hypercalciuria. Kidney Int. 1996;49(1):244-50.
19. Zanchetta JR, Rodriguez G, Negri AL, et al. Bone mineral density in patients with hypercalciuric nephrolithiasis. Nephron. 1996;73(4):557-60.
20. Ghazali A, Fuentès V, Desaint C, et al. Low bone mineral density and peripheral blood monocyte activation profile in calcium stone formers with idiopathic hypercalciuria. J Clin Endocrinol Metab. 1997;82(1):32-8.
21. Giannini S, Nobile M, Sartori L, et al. Bone density and skeletal metabolism are altered in idiopathic hypercalciuria. Clin Nephrol. 1998;50(2):94-100.
22. Trinchieri A, Nespoli R, Ostini F, et al. A study of dietary calcium and other nutrients in idiopathic renal calcium stone formers with low bone mineral content. J Urol. 1998;159(3):654-7.
23. Martini LA, Cuppari L, Colugnati FA, et al. High sodium chloride intake is associated with low bone density in calcium stone-forming patients. Clin Nephrol. 2000;54(2):85- 93.
24. Misael da Silva AM, dos Reis LM, Pereira RC, et al. Bone involvement in idiopathic hypercalciuria. Clin Nephrol. 2002;57(3):183-91.
25. Tasca A, Cacciola A, Ferrarese P, et al. Bone alterations in patients with idiopathic hypercalciuria and calcium nephrolithiasis. Urology. 2002;59(6):865-9.
26. Caudarella R, Vescini F, Buffa A, et al. Bone mass loss in calcium stone disease: focus on hypercalciuria and metabolic factors. J Nephrol. 2003;16(2):260-6.
27. Asplin JR, Bauer KA, Kinder J, et al. Bone mineral density and urine calcium excretion among subjects with and without nephrolithiasis. Kidney Int. 2003;63(2):662-9.
28. Vezzoli G, Rubinacci A, Bianchin C, et al. Intestinal calcium absorption is associated with bone mass in stone-forming women with idiopathic hypercalciuria. Am J Kidney Dis. 2003;42(6):1177-83.
29. Tugcu V, Ozbek E, Aras B, et al. Bone mineral density measurement in patients with recurrent normocalciuric calcium stone disease. Urol Res. 2007;35(1):29-34.
30. Melton LJ 3rd, Crowson CS, Khosla S, et al. Fracture risk among patients with urolithiasis: a population-based cohort study. Kidney Int. 1998;53(2):459-64.
31. Bordier P, Ryckewart A, Gueris J, et al. On the pathogenesis of so-called idiopathic hypercalciuria. Am J Med. 1977;63(3):398-409.
32. Malluche HH, Tschoepe W, Ritz E, et al. Abnormal bone histology in idiopathic hypercalciuria. J Clin Endocrinol Metab. 1980;50(4):654-8.
33. De Vernejoul MC, Hioco D, Villiaumey J, et al. Bone histomorphometric study in idiopathic hypercalciuria.. Rev Rhum Mal Osteoartic. 1981;48(5):389-95.
34. Steiniche T, Mosekilde L, Christensen MS, et al. A histomorphometric determination of iliac bone remodeling in patients with recurrent renal stone formation and idiopathic hypercalciuria. APMIS. 1989;97(4):309-16.
35. Bataille P, Hardy P, Marie A, et al. Decreased bone formation in idiopathic hypercalciuric calcium stone formers explains reduced bone density (abstract). J Bone Min Res. 1995;10 (Suppl 1):401.

36. Heller HJ, Zerwekh JE, Gottschalk FA, et al. Reduced bone formation and relatively increased bone resorption in absorptive hypercalciuria. Kidney Int. 2007;71(8):808-15.
37. Sowers MR, Jannausch M, Wood C, et al. Prevalence of renal stones in a population-based study with dietary calcium, oxalate, and medication exposures. Am J Epidemiol. 1998;147(10):914-20.
38. Lauderdale DS, Thisted RA, Wen M, et al. Bone mineral density and fracture among prevalent kidney stone cases in the Third National Health and Nutrition Examination Survey. J Bone Miner Res. 2001;16(10):1893-8.
39. Cauley JA, Fullman RL, Stone KL, et al. Factors associated with the lumbar spine and proximal femur bone mineral density in older men. Osteoporos Int. 2005;16(12):1525- 37.
40. Sakhaee K, Maalouf NM, Kumar R, et al. Nephrolithiasis-associated bone disease: pathogenesis and treatment options. Kidney Int. 2011;79(4):393-403.
41. Giannini S, Nobile M, Dalle Carbonare L, et al. Hypercalciuria is a common and important finding in postmenopausal women with osteoporosis. Eur J Endocrinol. 2003;149(3): 209-13.
42. Vezzoli G, Soldati L, Arcidiacono T, et al. Urinary calcium is a determinant of bone mineral density in elderly men participating in the InCHIANTI study. Kidney Int. 2005;67(5):2006-14.
43. Sutton RA, Walker VR. Bone resorption and hypercalciuria in calcium stoneformers. Metabolism. 1986;35(6):485–8.
44. Malluche HH, Langub MC, Monier-Faugere MC. The role of bone biopsy in clinical practice and research. Kidney Int Suppl. 1999;73:S20-5.
45. Jorgetti V. Review article: bone biopsy in chronic kidney disease: patient level end- point or just another test? Nephrology (Carlton). 2009;14(4):404-7.
46. Dempster DW, Compston JE, Drezner MK, et al. Standardized nomenclature, symbols, and units for bone histomorphometry: a 2012 update of the report of the ASBMR Histomorphometry Nomenclature Committee. J Bone Miner Res. 2013;28(1):2-17.
47. Frost HM, Villaneuva AR. Tetracycline staining of newly forming bone and mineralizing cartilage in vivo. Stain Technol. 1960;35:135-8.
48. Ott SM. Histomorphometric measurements of bone turnover, mineralization, and volume. Clin J Am Soc Nephrol. 2008;3 (Suppl 3):S151-6.
49. Menon V, Moyses R, Gomes S, et al. Expression of fibroblast growth factor 23, vitamin D receptor, and sclerostin in bone tissue from hypercalciuric stone formers. Clin J Am Soc Nephrol. 2014;9(7):1263-70.
50. Moe S, Drüeke T, Cunningham J, et al. Definition, evaluation, and classification of renal osteodystrophy: a position statement from Kidney Disease: Improving Global Outcomes (KDIGO). Kidney Int. 2006;69(11):1945-53.
51. Jorgetti V, Dos Reis LM, Ott SM. Ethnic differences in bone and mineral metabolism in healthy people and patients with CKD. Kidney Int. 2013; 85(6):1283-9.
52. Raisz LG, Kream BE, Smith MD, et al. Comparison of the effects of vitamin D metabolites on collagen synthesis and resportion of fetal rat bone in organ culture. Calcif Tissue Int. 1980;32(2):135-8.
53. Broadus AE, Erickson SB, Gertner JM, et al. An experimental human model of 1,25- dihydroxyvitamin D-mediated hypercalciuria. J Clin Endocrinol Metab. 1984;59(2):202-6.
54. Kaplan RA, Haussler MR, Deftos LJ, et al. The role of 1 alpha, 25-dihydroxyvitamin D in the mediation of intestinal hyper-absorption of calcium in primary hyperparathyroidism and absorptive hypercalciuria. J Clin Invest. 1977;59(5):756-60.
55. Broadus AE, Insogna KL, Lang R, et al. Evidence for disordered control of 1,25- dihydroxyvitamin D production in absorptive hypercalciuria. N Engl J Med. 1984;311(2):73-80.
56. Insogna KL, Broadus AE, Dreyer BE, et al. Elevated production rate of 1,25- dihydroxyvitamin D in patients with absorptive hypercalciuria. J Clin Endocrinol Metab. 1985;61(3):490-5.
57. Breslau NA, Preminger GM, Adams BV, et al. Use of ketoconazole to probe the pathogenetic importance of 1,25-dihydroxyvitamin D in absorptive hypercalciuria. J Clin Endocrinol Metab. 1992;75(6):1446-52.
58. Zerwekh JE, Reed BY, Heller HJ, et al. Normal vitamin D receptor concentration and responsiveness to 1, 25-dihydroxyvitamin D3 in skin fibroblasts from patients with absorptive hypercalciuria. Miner Electrolyte Metab. 1998;24:307-13.
59. Favus MJ, Karnauskas AJ, Parks JH, et al. Peripheral blood monocyte vitamin D receptor levels are elevated in patients with idiopathic hypercalciuria. J Clin Endocrinol Metab. 2004;89:4937-43.
60. Ferreira LG, Pereira AC, Heilberg IP. Vitamin D receptor and calcium-sensing receptor gene polymorphisms in hypercalciuric stone-forming patients. Nephron Clin Pract. 2010;114:c135-44.
61. Li XQ, Tembe V, Horwitz GM, et al. Increased intestinal vitamin D receptor in genetic hypercalciuric rats. A cause of intestinal calcium hyperabsorption. J Clin Invest. 1993;91:661-7.
62. Krieger NS, Stathopoulos VM, Bushinsky DA. Increased sensitivity to 1,25(OH)2D3 in bone from genetic hypercalciuric rats. Am J Physiol. 1996;271:C130-5.
63. Karnauskas AJ, van Leeuwen JP, van den Bemd GJ, et al. Mechanism and function of high vitamin D receptor levels in genetic hypercalciuric stone-forming rats. J Bone Miner Res. 2005;20(3):447-54.
64. Gomes SA, dos Reis LM, de Oliveira IB, et al. Usefulness of a quick decalcification of bone sections embedded in methyl methacrylate corrected.: an improved method for immunohistochemistry. J Bone Miner Metab. 2008;26:110-3.
65. Olmer M, Berland Y, Argemi B. Absence of secondary hyperparathyroidism in most patients with renal hypercalciuria. Kidney Int Suppl. 1983;16:S175-9.
66. Gomes SA, Lage A, Lazaretti-Castro M, et al. Response to an oral calcium load in nephrolithiasis patients with fluctuating parathyroid hormone and ionized calcium levels. Braz J Med Biol Res. 2004;37(9):1379-88.
67. Raisz LG. Pathogenesis of osteoporosis: concepts, conflicts, and prospects. J Clin Invest. 2005;115:3318-25.

68. Gomes SA, dos Reis LM, Noronha IL, et al. RANKL is a mediator of bone resorption in idiopathic hypercalciuria. Clin J Am Soc Nephrol. 2008;3(5):1446-52.
69. Mundy GR, Boyce B, Hughes D, et al. The effects of cytokines and growth factors on osteoblastic cells. Bone. 1995;17 (2 Suppl):71S-75S.
70. Rendina D, Mossetti G, De Filippo G, et al. Fibroblast growth factor 23 is increased in calcium nephrolithiasis with hypophosphatemia and renal phosphate leak. J Clin Endocrinol Metab. 2006;91:959-63.
71. Wang H, Yoshiko Y, Yamamoto R, et al. Overexpression of fibroblast growth factor 23 suppresses osteoblast differentiation and matrix mineralization in vitro. J Bone Miner Res. 2008;23:939-48.
72. Moester MJC, Papapoulos SE, Löwik CWGM, et al. Sclerostin: current knowledge and future perspectives. Calcif Tissue Int. 2010;87:99-107.
73. Schaffler MB, Kennedy OD. Osteocyte signaling in bone. Curr Osteoporos Rep. 2012;10:118-25.
74. Kramer I, Halleux C, Keller H, et al. Osteocyte Wnt/beta-catenin signaling is required for normal bone homeostasis. Mol Cell Biol. 2010;30:3071-85.
75. Atkins GJ, Findlay DM. Osteocyte regulation of bone mineral: a little give and take. Osteoporos Int. 2012;23(8):2067-79.
76. McClung MR, Grauer A, Boonen S, et al. Romosozumab in postmenopausal women with low bone mineral density. N Engl J Med. 2014;370:412-20.
77. Curhan GC, Willett WC, Knight EL, et al. Dietary factors and the risk of incident kidney stones in younger women: Nurses' Health Study II. Arch Intern Med. 2004;164(8):885-91.
78. Curhan GC, Willett WC, Speizer FE, et al. Comparison of dietary calcium with supplemental calcium and other nutrients as factors affecting the risk for kidney stones in women. Ann Intern Med. 1997;126:497-504.
79. Domrongkitchaiporn S, Sopassathit W, Stitchantrakul W, et al. Schedule of taking calcium supplement and the risk of nephrolithiasis. Kidney Int. 2004;65:1835-41.
80. Dawson-Hughes B. Calcium insufficiency and fracture risk. Osteoporos Int. 1996;6 Suppl 3:37-41.
81. Warensjö E, Byberg L, Melhus H, et al. Dietary calcium intake and risk of fracture and osteoporosis: prospective longitudinal cohort study. BMJ. 2011;342:d1473.
82. Wallace RB, Wactawski-Wende J, O'Sullivan MJ, et al. Urinary tract stone occurrence in the Women's Health Initiative (WHI) randomized clinical trial of calcium and vitamin D supplements. Am J Clin Nutr. 2011;94:270-7.
83. Maierhofer WJ, Gray RW, Cheung HS, et al. Bone resorption stimulated by elevated serum 1,25-(OH)2-vitamin D concentrations in healthy men. Kidney Int. 1983;24:555- 60.
84. Lieben L, Masuyama R, Torrekens S, et al. Normocalcemia is maintained in mice under conditions of calcium malabsorption by vitamin D-induced inhibition of bone mineralization. J Clin Invest. 2012;122:1803-15.
85. Martini LA, Heilberg IP. Stop dietary calcium restriction in kidney stone-forming patients. Nutr Rev. 2002;60:212-4.
86. Heilberg IP, Goldfarb DS. Optimum nutrition for kidney stone disease. Adv Chronic Kidney Dis. 2013;20:165-74.
87. Leaf DE, Korets R, Taylor EN, et al. Effect of vitamin D repletion on urinary calcium excretion among kidney stone formers. Clin J Am Soc Nephrol. 2012;7(5):829-34.
88. Carbone LD, Barrow KD, Bush AJ, et al. Effects of a low sodium diet on bone metabolism. J Bone Miner Metab. 2005;23:506-13.
89. Martini LA, Cuppari L, Cunha MA, et al. Potassium and sodium intake and excretion in calcium stone forming patients. J Ren Nutr. 1998;8(3):127-31.
90. Muldowney FP, Freaney R, Moloney MF. Importance of dietary sodium in the hypercalciuria syndrome. Kidney Int. 1982;22:292-6.
91. Reddy ST, Wang C-Y, Sakhaee K, et al. Effect of low-carbohydrate high-protein diets on acid-base balance, stone-forming propensity, and calcium metabolism. Am J Kidney Dis. 2002;40(2):265-74.
92. Bonny O, Edwards A. Calcium reabsorption in the distal tubule: regulation by sodium, pH, and flow. Am J Physiol Renal Physiol. 2013;304:F585-600.
93. Frick KK, LaPlante K, Bushinsky DA. RANK ligand and TNF-alpha mediate acid- induced bone calcium efflux in vitro. Am J Physiol Renal Physiol. 2005;289:F1005- 1011.
94. Amanzadeh J, Gitomer WL, Zerwekh JE, et al. Effect of high protein diet on stone- forming propensity and bone loss in rats. Kidney Int. 2003;64:2142-9.
95. Zerwekh JE. Bone disease and idiopathic hypercalciuria. Semin Nephrol. 2008;28:133- 42.
96. Zerwekh JE, Zou L, Pak CYC, et al. Biochemical and histological assessment of alkali therapy during high animal protein intake in the rat. Bone. 2009;45:1004-9.
97. Maalouf NM, Moe OW, Adams-Huet B, et al. Hypercalciuria associated with high dietary protein intake is not due to acid load. J Clin Endocrinol Metab. 2011;96:3733- 40.
98. Feskanich D, Willett WC, Stampfer MJ, et al. Protein consumption and bone fractures in women. Am J Epidemiol. 1996;143:472-9.
99. Hannan MT, Tucker KL, Dawson-Hughes B, et al. Effect of dietary protein on bone loss in elderly men and women: the Framingham Osteoporosis Study. J Bone Miner Res. 2000;15(12):2504-12.
100. Cooper C, Atkinson EJ, Hensrud DD, et al. Dietary protein intake and bone mass in women. Calcif Tissue Int. 1996;58:320-5.
101. Wengreen HJ, Munger RG, West NA, et al. Dietary protein intake and risk of osteoporotic hip fracture in elderly residents of Utah. J Bone Miner Res. 2004;19:537- 45.
102. Darling AL, Millward DJ, Torgerson DJ, et al. Dietary protein and bone health: a systematic review and meta-analysis. Am J Clin Nutr. 2009;90:1674-92.
103. Dawson-Hughes B, Harris SS. Calcium intake influences the association of protein intake with rates of bone loss in elderly men and women. Am J Clin Nutr. 2002;75:773- 9.
104. Freundlich M, Alonzo E, Bellorin-Font E, et al. Reduced bone mass in children with idiopathic hypercalciuria and in their asymptomatic mothers. Nephrol Dial Transplant. 2002;17(8):1396-401.

105. García-Nieto V, Navarro JF, Monge M, et al. Bone mineral density in girls and their mothers with idiopathic hypercalciuria. Nephron Clin Pract. 2003;94:c89-93.
106. Penido M-GMG, Lima EM, Souto MFO, et al. Hypocitraturia: a risk factor for reduced bone mineral density in idiopathic hypercalciuria? Pediatr Nephrol Berl Ger. 2006;21:74-8.
107. Polito C, Iolascon G, Nappi B, et al. Growth and bone mineral density in long-lasting idiopathic hypercalciuria. Pediatr Nephrol Berl Ger. 2003;18:545-7.
108. Skalova S, Palicka V, Kutilek S. Bone mineral density and urinary N-acetyl-beta-D- glucosaminidase activity in paediatric patients with idiopathic hypercalciuria. Nephrol Carlton Vic. 2005;10:99-102.
109. Lloyd SE, Pearce SH, Fisher SE, et al. A common molecular basis for three inherited kidney stone diseases. Nature. 1996;379:445-9.
110. Hoopes RR Jr, Shrimpton AE, Knohl SJ, et al. Dent Disease with mutations in OCRL1. Am J Hum Genet. 2005;76:260-7.
111. Lapointe J-Y, Tessier J, Paquette Y, et al. NPT2a gene variation in calcium nephrolithiasis with renal phosphate leak. Kidney Int. 2006;69:2261-7.
112. Virkki LV, Forster IC, Hernando N, et al. Functional characterization of two naturally occurring mutations in the human sodium-phosphate cotransporter type IIa. J Bone Miner Res. 2003;18:2135-41.
113. Moe OW, Bonny O. Genetic hypercalciuria. J Am Soc Nephrol. 2005;16:729-45.
114. Reed BY, Gitomer WL, Heller HJ, et al. Identification and characterization of a gene with base substitutions associated with the absorptive hypercalciuria phenotype and low spinal bone density. J Clin Endocrinol Metab. 2002;87:1476-85.
115. Geng W, Hill K, Zerwekh JE, et al. Inhibition of osteoclast formation and function by bicarbonate: role of soluble adenylyl cyclase. J Cell Physiol. 2009;220:332-40.
116. Econs MJ, Foroud T. The genetics of absorptive hypercalciuria—a note of caution. J Clin Endocrinol Metab. 2002;87:1473-5.
117. Thorleifsson G, Holm H, Edvardsson V, et al. Sequence variants in the CLDN14 gene associate with kidney stones and bone mineral density. Nat Genet. 2009;41:926-30.
118. Toka HR, Genovese G, Mount DB, et al. Frequency of rare allelic variation in candidate genes among individuals with low and high urinary calcium excretion. PloS One. 2013;8:e71885.
119. Goldfarb DS, Fischer ME, Keich Y, et al. A twin study of genetic and dietary influences on nephrolithiasis: a report from the Vietnam Era Twin (VET) Registry. Kidney Int. 2005;67:1053-61.
120. Loredo-Osti JC, Roslin NM, Tessier J, et al. Segregation of urine calcium excretion in families ascertained for nephrolithiasis: evidence for a major gene. Kidney Int. 2005;68:966-71.
121. Coe FL, Parks JH, Moore ES. Familial idiopathic hypercalciuria. N Engl J Med. 1979;300:337-40.
122. Gambaro G, Vezzoli G, Casari G, et al. Genetics of hypercalciuria and calcium nephrolithiasis: from the rare monogenic to the common polygenic forms. Am J Kidney Dis. 2004;44:963-86.
123. Zmuda JM, Sheu Y-T, Moffett SP. Genetic epidemiology of osteoporosis: past, present, and future. Curr Osteoporos Rep. 2005;3:111-5.
124. Morrison NA, Qi JC, Tokita A, et al. Prediction of bone density from vitamin D receptor alleles. Nature. 1994;367:284-7.
125. Macdonald HM, McGuigan FE, Stewart A, et al. Large-scale population-based study shows no evidence of association between common polymorphism of the VDR gene and BMD in British women. J Bone Miner Res. 2006;21:151-62.
126. Uitterlinden AG, Ralston SH, Brandi ML, et al. The association between common vitamin D receptor gene variations and osteoporosis: a participant-level meta-analysis. Ann Intern Med. 2006;145:255-64.
127. Scott P, Ouimet D, Valiquette L, et al. Suggestive evidence for a susceptibility gene near the vitamin D receptor locus in idiopathic calcium stone formation. J Am Soc Nephrol. 1999;10:1007-13.
128. Rendina D, Mossetti G, Viceconti R, et al. Association between vitamin D receptor gene polymorphisms and fasting idiopathic hypercalciuria in recurrent stone-forming patients. Urology. 2004;64:833-8.
129. Relan V, Khullar M, Singh SK, et al. Association of vitamin D receptor genotypes with calcium excretion in nephrolithiatic subjects in northern India. Urol Res. 2004;32:236- 40.
130. Heilberg IP, Teixeira SH, Martini LA, et al. Vitamin D receptor gene polymorphism and bone mineral density in hypercalciuric calcium-stone-forming patients. Nephron. 2002;90:51-7.
131. Vezzoli G, Soldati L, Proverbio MC, et al. Polymorphism of vitamin D receptor gene start codon in patients with calcium kidney stones. J Nephrol. 2002;15:158-64.
132. Dawson-Hughes B, Harris SS, Finneran S. Calcium absorption on high and low calcium intakes in relation to vitamin D receptor genotype. J Clin Endocrinol Metab. 1995;80:3657-61.
133. Vezzoli G, Tanini A, Ferrucci L, et al. Influence of calcium-sensing receptor gene on urinary calcium excretion in stone-forming patients. J Am Soc Nephrol. 2002;13:2517- 23.
134. Vezzoli G, Terranegra A, Arcidiacono T, et al. R990G polymorphism of calcium-sensing receptor does produce a gain-of-function and predispose to primary hypercalciuria. Kidney Int. 2007;71:1155-62.
135. Harding B, Curley AJ, Hannan FM, et al. Functional characterization of calcium sensing receptor polymorphisms and absence of association with indices of calcium homeostasis and bone mineral density. Clin Endocrinol (Oxf). 2006;65:598-605.
136. Lerolle N, Coulet F, Lantz B, et al. No evidence for point mutations of the calcium- sensing receptor in familial idiopathic hypercalciuria. Nephrol Dial Transplant. 2001;16:2317–22.
137. Petrucci M, Scott P, Ouimet D, et al. Evaluation of the calcium-sensing receptor gene in idiopathic hypercalciuria and calcium nephrolithiasis. Kidney Int. 2000;58:38-42.
138. Hoopes RR Jr, Reid R, Sen S, et al. Quantitative trait loci for hypercalciuria in a rat model of kidney stone disease. J Am Soc Nephrol. 2003;14:1844-50.

139. Scheinman SJ, Cox JP, Lloyd SE, et al. Isolated hypercalciuria with mutation in CLCN5: relevance to idiopathic hypercalciuria. Kidney Int. 2000;57:232-9.
140. Silva IV, Cebotaru V, Wang H, et al. The ClC-5 knockout mouse model of Dent's disease has renal hypercalciuria and increased bone turnover. J Bone Miner Res. 2003;18:615-23.
141. Hoenderop JGJ, van Leeuwen JPTM, van der Eerden BCJ, et al. Renal Ca^{2+} wasting, hyperabsorption, and reduced bone thickness in mice lacking TRPV5. J Clin Invest. 2003;112:1906-14.
142. Hoenderop JGJ, Bindels RJM. Epithelial Ca2+ and Mg2+ channels in health and disease. J Am Soc Nephrol. 2005;16:15-26.
143. Müller D, Hoenderop JGJ, Vennekens R, et al. Epithelial Ca(2+) channel (ECAC1) in autosomal dominant idiopathic hypercalciuria. Nephrol Dial Transplant. 2002;17:1614- 20.
144. Pearle MS, Roehrborn CG, Pak CY. Meta-analysis of randomized trials for medical prevention of calcium oxalate nephrolithiasis. J Endourol Endourol Soc. 1999;13:679- 85.
145. Lau EMC, Leung PC, Kwok T, et al. The determinants of bone mineral density in Chinese men--results from Mr. Os (Hong Kong), the first cohort study on osteoporosis in Asian men. Osteoporos Int. 2006;17:29-303.
146. Wasnich RD, Davis JW, He YF, et al. A randomized, double-masked, placebo- controlled trial of chlorthalidone and bone loss in elderly women. Osteoporos Int. 1995;5:247-51.
147. LaCroix AZ, Wienpahl J, White LR, et al. Thiazide diuretic agents and the incidence of hip fracture. N Engl J Med. 1990;322:286-90.
148. Cauley JA, Cummings SR, Seeley DG, et al. Effects of thiazide diuretic therapy on bone mass, fractures, and falls. The Study of Osteoporotic Fractures Research Group. Ann Intern Med. 1993;118:666-73.
149. Felson DT, Sloutskis D, Anderson JJ, et al. Thiazide diuretics and the risk of hip fracture. Results from the Framingham Study. J Am Med Assoc. 1991;265:370-3.
150. Schoofs MWCJ, van der Klift M, Hofman A, et al. Thiazide diuretics and the risk for hip fracture. Ann Intern Med. 2003;139:476-82.
151. Bolland MJ, Ames RW, Horne AM, et al. The effect of treatment with a thiazide diuretic for 4 years on bone density in normal postmenopausal women. Osteoporos Int. 2007;18:479-86.
152. Pak CY, Heller HJ, Pearle MS, et al. Prevention of stone formation and bone loss in absorptive hypercalciuria by combined dietary and pharmacological interventions. J Urol. 2003;169:465-9.
153. Rico H, Revilla M, Villa LF, et al. A longitudinal study of total and regional bone mineral content and biochemical markers of bone resorption in patients with idiopathic hypercalciuria on thiazide treatment. Miner Electrolyte Metab. 1993;19:337-42.
154. Steiniche T, Mosekilde L, Christensen MS, et al. Histomorphometric analysis of bone in idiopathic hypercalciuria before and after treatment with thiazide. Acta Pathol Microbiol Immunol Scand. 1989;97:302-8.
155. Bushinsky DA, Willett T, Asplin JR, et al. Chlorthalidone improves vertebral bone quality in genetic hypercalciuric stone-forming rats. J Bone Miner Res. 2011;26:1904- 12.
156. Moreira Guimarães Penido MG, de Sousa Tavares M, Campos Linhares M, et al. Longitudinal study of bone mineral density in children with idiopathic hypercalciuria. Pediatr Nephrol Berl Ger. 2012;27:123-30.
157. Voskaki I, al Qadreh A, Mengreli C, et al. Effect of hydrochlorothiazide on renal hypercalciuria. Child Nephrol Urol. 1992;12:6-9.
158. Reusz GS, Dobos M, Vásárhelyi B, et al. Sodium transport and bone mineral density in hypercalciuria with thiazide treatment. Pediatr Nephrol Berl Ger. 1998;12:30-4.
159. García-Nieto V, Monge-Zamorano M, González-García M, et al. Effect of thiazides on bone mineral density in children with idiopathic hypercalciuria. Pediatr Nephrol Berl Ger. 2012;27:261-8.
160. Aubin R, Ménard P, Lajeunesse D. Selective effect of thiazides on the human osteoblast-like cell line MG-63. Kidney Int. 1996;50:1476-82.
161. Lajeunesse D, Delalandre A, Guggino SE. Thiazide diuretics affect osteocalcin production in human osteoblasts at the transcription level without affecting vitamin D3 receptors. J Bone Miner Res. 2000;15:894-901.
162. Barry EL, Gesek FA, Kaplan MR, et al. Expression of the sodium-chloride cotransporter in osteoblast-like cells: effect of thiazide diuretics. Am J Physiol. 1997;272:C109-16.
163. Dvorak MM, De Joussineau C, Carter DH, et al. Thiazide diuretics directly induce osteoblast differentiation and mineralized nodule formation by interacting with a sodium chloride co-transporter in bone. J Am Soc Nephrol. 2007;18:2509-16.
164. Lau KH, Song XD, Ochi M, et al. Mitogenic action of hydrochlorothiazide on human osteoblasts in vitro: requirement for platelet-derived growth factor. Calcif Tissue Int. 1996;59:505-10.
165. Lalande A, Roux C, Graulet AM, et al. The diuretic indapamide increases bone mass and decreases bone resorption in spontaneously hypertensive rats supplemented with sodium. J Bone Miner Res. 1998;13:1444-50.
166. Broulik PD, Pacovský V. Hydrochlorothiazide inhibits parathormone-stimulated increase in plasma tartrate-resistant acid phosphatase in mice. Calcif Tissue Int. 1991;49:51-2.
167. Hall TJ, Schaueblin M. Hydrochlorothiazide inhibits osteoclastic bone resorption in vitro. Calcif Tissue Int. 1994;55:266-8.
168. Lalande A, Roux S, Denne MA, et al. Indapamide, a thiazide-like diuretic, decreases bone resorption in vitro. J Bone Miner Res. 2001;16:361-70.
169. Frassetto L, Morris RC Jr, Sebastian A. Long-term persistence of the urine calcium- lowering effect of potassium bicarbonate in postmenopausal women. J Clin Endocrinol Metab. 2005;90:831-4.
170. Sebastian A, Harris ST, Ottaway JH, et al. Improved mineral balance and skeletal metabolism in postmenopausal

women treated with potassium bicarbonate. N Engl J Med. 1994;330:1776-81.

171. Zhou H, Choong P, McCarthy R, et al. In situ hybridization to show sequential expression of osteoblast gene markers during bone formation in vivo. J Bone Miner Res Off. 1994;9:1489-99.
172. Jehle S, Zanetti A, Muser J, et al. Partial neutralization of the acidogenic Western diet with potassium citrate increases bone mass in postmenopausal women with osteopenia. J Am Soc Nephrol. 2006;17:3213-22.
173. Macdonald HM, Black AJ, Aucott L, et al. Effect of potassium citrate supplementation or increased fruit and vegetable intake on bone metabolism in healthy postmenopausal women: a randomized controlled trial. Am J Clin Nutr. 2008;88:465-74.
174. Sakhaee K, Maalouf NM, Abrams SA, et al. Effects of potassium alkali and calcium supplementation on bone turnover in postmenopausal women. J Clin Endocrinol Metab. 2005;90:3528-33.
175. Pak CYC, Peterson RD, Poindexter J. Prevention of spinal bone loss by potassium citrate in cases of calcium urolithiasis. J Urol. 2002;168:31-4.
176. Vescini F, Buffa A, La Manna G, et al. Long-term potassium citrate therapy and bone mineral density in idiopathic calcium stone formers. J Endocrinol Invest. 2005;28:218- 22.
177. Bushinsky DA, Neumann KJ, Asplin J, et al. Alendronate decreases urine calcium and supersaturation in genetic hypercalciuric rats. Kidney Int. 1999;55:234-43.
178. Weisinger JR, Alonzo E, Machado C, et al. Role of bones in the physiopathology of idiopathic hypercalciuria: effect of amino-bisphosphonate alendronate. Medicina (Mex). 1997;57 Suppl 1:45-8.
179. Heilberg IP, Martini LA, Teixeira SH, et al. Effect of etidronate treatment on bone mass of male nephrolithiasis patients with idiopathic hypercalciuria and osteopenia. Nephron. 1998;79:430-7.
180. Ott SM, Woodson GC, Huffer WE, et al. Bone histomorphometric changes after cyclic therapy with phosphate and etidronate disodium in women with postmenopausal osteoporosis. J Clin Endocrinol Metab. 1994;78:968-72.
181. Steiniche T, Hasling C, Charles P, et al. The effects of etidronate on trabecular bone remodeling in postmenopausal spinal osteoporosis: a randomized study comparing intermittent treatment and an ADFR regime. Bone. 1991;12:155-63.
182. Freundlich M, Alon US. Bisphosphonates in children with hypercalciuria and reduced bone mineral density. Pediatr Nephrol Berl Ger. 2008;23:2215-20.
183. Arrabal-Polo MA, Arias-Santiago S, de Haro-Muñoz T, et al. Effects of aminobisphosphonates and thiazides in patients with osteopenia/osteoporosis, hypercalciuria, and recurring renal calcium lithiasis. Urology. 2013;81:731-7.
184. Odvina CV, Zerwekh JE, Rao DS, et al. Severely suppressed bone turnover: a potential complication of alendronate therapy. J Clin Endocrinol Metab. 2005;90:1294-301.

CHAPTER

15

Idiopathic Stone Formers

Fredric L Coe, Elaine M Worcester

CALCIUM STONE FORMERS

As the most common of all stone patients, idiopathic calcium stone formers pose a common and often perplexing treatment problem for urologists, nephrologists, and primary care physicians. One might say they are what most physicians think of as stone disease itself.

Our approach is therefore to present here the lore and evidence concerning how clinicians can evaluate a stone former to winnow out those with calcium stones, those with calcium stones from one of the many systemic diseases that cause them, and finally the "idiopathic" calcium stone formers who have no systemic cause for their stones.

Because this chapter is part of a comprehensive book, we refer readers to the chapters about the systemic causes of stones in order to avoid repeating what the experts who wrote them have to say. Similarly, kidney stones themselves, mechanisms of their formation, and surgical approaches to their management are covered in other chapters.

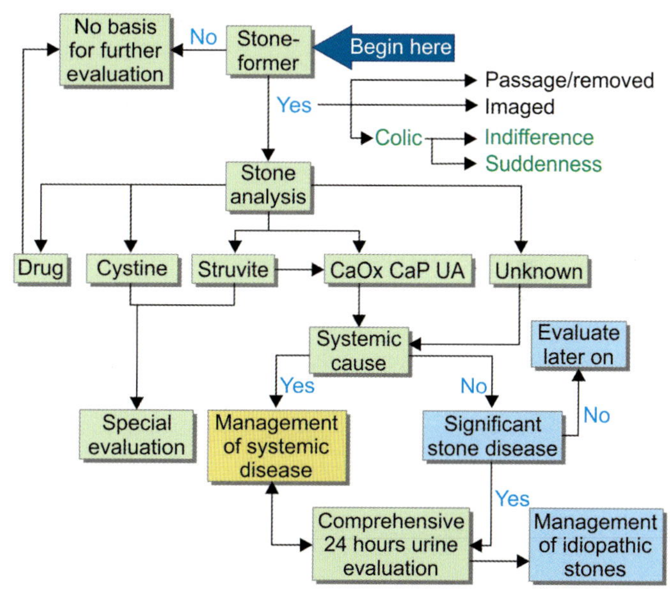

Fig. 15.1: Scheme for evaluating possible stone formers. (CaOx: Calcium oxalate; CaP: Calcium phosphate; UA: Uric acid).

CLINICAL EVALUATION OF STONE FORMATION

The first stop on any clinical roadmap is whether or not a patient really forms stones (Fig. 15.1). If not, the problem may indeed remain worthy of serious attention but not in this book. If so, the stone type comes next. Stones are hard and clinically important because of their crystals, and preventing crystallization is the key to preventing stones. Each of the crystals has its own physical chemistry and means for production, so we must know which one our patient is forming.

Is the Patient a Stone Former?

Stone Passage

Someone is surely a kidney stone former if stones are passed in a medical setting, removed, or visualized radiographically or by ultrasound. Less stringent criteria are a history of passing stones or attacks of a pain that is thought to be characteristic of stones. One might consider such stringency unnecessary, but people can confuse severe pain of other causes with that from stones. The problem is not that some rare people feign stone passage. It is that in assessing the formation of new stones we often have only reports of pain attacks, the stones being lost or even, with many episodes, passed and ignored.

Renal Colic

The best way to learn about renal colic is from the histories of patients who have experienced it during authentic episodes of stone passage. Although the story varies among people, the main outlines are clear enough. Colic pain begins suddenly, though it is often mild at the start, and tends to locate itself in one flank. Its intensity increases to a plateau over minutes to an hour or so and then remains steady. It is notoriously severe and has a burning or boring character. Most agree that the pain arises from acute obstruction of the urinary collecting system.

As stones move down the ureter, the pain also moves downward and anterolaterally across the abdomen along the path fingers make if the thumb is hooked behind at the waist and the fingers and palm spread out and pointing toward the base of the thigh and lower abdomen. When at the ureterovesical junction a stone can create urinary urgency, frequency, and burning that mimics infection.

Colic leads to, or is associated with, nausea, vomiting, sweating, and diarrhea. Nothing a patient can do changes the pain; in this sense it is indifferent to any aggravating or alleviating factors. Twisting, turning, walking, lying down, driving in a car: none of these worsen or affect the pain. In this, it differs remarkably from all musculoskeletal pains.

What is most characteristic of renal colic is not its severity, however legendary, nor its initial location, its indifference to motion, position, and jolting, nor even its migratory tendencies, although these are very useful clinical points. It is its capacity for magical disappearance. If a stone suddenly passes through the ureterovesical junction, or merely ceases to obstruct the ureter, pain can vanish in a moment. No pain we know of in all of medicine can be so severe and so suddenly gone.

Other Kinds of Pain

Sometimes, pain attacks with or without hematuria suggest stone passage but no stones pass or are visualized. Pain itself suggests stone passage when it corresponds at least in general outline to renal colic. Stone passage may cause back muscle spasms that lead to chronic back pain, often severe. Not all patients can differentiate such pain from that of stones and accordingly remain too long on pain medications or are thought to be having stone attacks. The key distinction is that all such pains are altered by position and activity, whereas renal colic is not.

Crystal Passage

Not rarely, colic attacks and hematuria arise from passage of crystals, especially calcium oxalate (CaOx) or phosphate crystals. Computed tomography (CT) and ultrasound show no stones and usually no obstruction. Sometimes patients say the urine will look white or milky. The diagnosis of these attacks requires a firm belief that colic is occurring and that at least sometimes gross or microscopic hematuria accompanies the pain.

Gravel and Sludge

Uric acid (UA) especially produces a red-orange gravel that patients easily notice. Although visually dramatic, it may not cause as much pain as that from calcium-based crystals. Occasionally, massive loads of uric acid from tumor lysis or sudden effects of a uricosuric drug will plug ureters and produce renal obstruction that may or may not cause classic colic. The renal inner medullary collecting duct (IMCD) and Bellini duct (BD) may plug, leaving the ureters normal but causing acute renal failure, which is often painless and presents with anuria.[1] Many drugs can do the same.[2]

Radiographic Patterns

From a clinical point of view, we see a few patterns that influence our behavior concerning diagnosis and prevention. Surgeons use the radiology quite differently, to determine need for procedures.

Single Stones

A patient has but one stone altogether—passed or in a kidney and come to light because of pain or bleeding, or during an X-ray done for another reason. Is it really single? Given a flat plate or ultrasound examination, there may be others, so we recommend a CT scan to be sure there is really only one. If flexible ureteroscopy is undertaken for the stone, the surgeon may see others, often tiny, meaning the patient has formed more than one. Many times the clinical setting and radiology eventuate in diagnosis of a single stone, and that has some influence on what we do.

Large Stones (>1 cm)

These mostly require surgical management. Medically, they prove that stone disease in that patient has a potential to cause serious disease, for large stones usually cannot pass through the ureters. They may obstruct at the ureteropelvic junction or block calyceal drainage, fostering infection and renal damage. Evaluation for cause and vigorous prevention are crucial. Under the heading of large stones we include both separate stones and the so-called "staghorn" stones, single stones whose body extends from the pelvis into multiple calyces.

Multiple Small Stones

When all or most papillae have stones growing on or in them, the problem may not be so much surgical as it is intriguing—why so many? Systemic and renal diseases often come to mind, such as renal tubular acidosis and medullary sponge kidney, however the radiographic picture is not diagnostic of these disorders. We are not moved especially by such "nephrocalcinosis" as it can occur in such a wide variety of disorders that it lacks specificity. However, being numerous, these stones motivate patients to obtain treatment and stay with it.

Radiolucent Stones

Long ago when simple abdominal flat plate radiographs were commonly done to evaluate stones, some stones showed faintly or not at all, unlike calcium-containing stones. If contrast was injected for intravenous pyelography, they appeared as lucencies in the contrast. Modern CT shows all stones as alike unless one has special techniques. If one happens to encounter radiolucent stones, they are usually uric acid, cystine, or rarely composed of 2,8-dihydroxyadenine or drug metabolites.

Stone Burden

As a practical matter, clinicians often summarize the mass of stones in both kidneys under this admittedly unquantitative rubric. A few big stones or many smaller stones, as an example, may both be called a moderate stone burden, the notion being intuitive. The value of the term is in the urgency of prevention treatment implied and the presumed scale of surgical stone removal if that is contemplated.

Are New Stones being Formed?

Visualization

As a definition, new stones are those passed or removed that have not been documented on prior radiographic or ultrasound image. Without a means of visualization, activity of the disease cannot be assessed. Ultrasound can give a reasonable estimate of the numbers of stones in a kidney and their approximate location but our experience is that estimates are coarse grained, dependent as they are on how well the images were obtained and which ones are available. Flat plate abdominal films are very poor for counting stones, especially small ones.

This leaves noncontrast CT (which may be low dose if body mass index permits) as both an ideal and a practical tool but one that requires significant radiation exposure. Our practice is to obtain the most recent one done by others or obtain one ourselves if that is >3 years old, and use the CT to count stones and mark their positions.

Counting New Stones

We read the CT scans ourselves and make a simple drawing of each kidney with stones we can see. A stone passage event is tallied against the change in count of stones from the side of passage or pain to distinguish new from prior stones.

New Stones versus Growth

These are very difficult to separate from each other. Growth can make visible what was a tiny deposit beyond the resolution of a CT. This is not so much a new stone as new to our eyes. Small stones of constant number that grow alarm patients and indeed should, because larger size reduces the likelihood that they will pass. So we are moved by growth to an increased effort at prevention measures.

Growth of old stones differs in its basic mechanisms from formation of new ones. De novo crystals require supersaturation (SS) exceed a threshold, the upper limit of metastability (ULM), whereas growth means merely that crystals are present in a urine that contains some degree of SS, which may be very modest. So growth is energetically easier to achieve and correspondingly harder to stop, in theory at least.

Activity of Stones

New stones occur in time; so one can speak about "stone activity" as the formation, or not, of new stones within a given time frame, which is almost inevitably enclosed in the intervals between images. The exception is a stone passage or removal from a kidney that was stone free on a prior radiograph. Growth is a different kind of activity from new stones, but growing stones pose an obvious hazard. So growth of stones is evidence of activity. Active disease in a new patient always needs treatment. Active disease during treatment indicates a need to reconsider the treatment and make changes in it to reduce activity as far as one can.

The Importance of Stone Analysis

Stones are Named for Their Crystals

The very basis of stone disease, as we know it, is the crystals, what they are, how they form, why they form in a given patient, and how one may prevent their formation. Stones are crystals embedded in a matrix of urine macromolecules, but without crystals, the matrix materials can form only soft "stones" that can, like blood clots, cause colic and obstruction. These soft stones are rare and almost never pose the surgical problems of crystal-based stones. To say all this is to say that analysis of stones for their crystal components is perhaps the central diagnostic act in clinical stone disease. How well can one prevent crystals whose composition is unknown?

Treatment is Aimed at Crystals

Almost always physicians analyze the first few stones they encounter in a patient, because these are crystals that one aims to prevent. However, subsequent analyses are just as important. For example, a patient may form stones made of CaOx for some years and then begin to form stones with higher and higher percentages of calcium phosphate (CaP). The CaP stones are a clue that renal tissue is being injured. Likewise treatment needs to focus on urine pH. The same is true for uric acid, absent at the beginning and then becoming a part of stone because urine pH has fallen. Struvite, produced by ureolytic bacteria, can appear at any time, given infection. Cystine stone formers can also form calcium stones.

Sometimes, stones are lost or discarded and all we have is what patients may have seen. Lemon-yellow stones are almost always cystine. Red or orange stones or gravel in urine are uric acid. Cystine and uric acid stones are relatively radiolucent on routine flat plate radiographs. Small black stones are usually CaOx monohydrate. Gray stones with a flaky appearance are often CaOx dihydrate.

The Value of Crystals during Urinalysis

A modest literature would argue that crystals seen at urinalysis on initial evaluation can point to the general cause of stones and especially to ongoing stone-forming propensity. One study has documented the correlation of crystals seen in first morning urine in treated patients with risk of relapse; however, the structured nature of the examination done in this study is beyond the capacity of most office settings.[3] In general, we do not place much emphasis on urinalysis in our evaluation strategy. One of us favors the search for crystals and uses the findings as part of the clinical assessment, while the other never looks.

A Clinician's Gaze at Crystal Formation

There is only one physics, so if SS is the free energy of formation of crystals, and if crystals are the absolute necessity for stones, then SS is an absolute essential in stone pathogenesis. But the matrix molecules of urine that bind crystals into stones, and that modify all aspects of their formation, determine the effectiveness of SS in achieving crystal nucleation, growth, aggregation, and cell membrane adherence. These are not available to clinicians; we cannot measure the urine matrix or assess its effects.

However, we have a kind of lemma, a way of proceeding that is of massive importance in practice. The SS we encounter in an active stone former must be too high for safety; otherwise, stones would not form. Even if a CaOx SS of 6 is common among normals, as it is, if that SS is present in an active stone former, and if we believe the measurement of 6 is a reasonable average for that patient, then 6 is too high and SS needs to be lower.

The sentence sums up much of the wisdom and power of clinical medicine. We can collect a urine and measure SS. We can know the stone crystals. But, it is an art to determine if the value we measure is pertinent. Did the patient collect under common circumstances of fluids and diet and activity? If not, do it again. The whole life of the patient needs be known in detail sufficient to answer the obvious questions.

Given what we measure is reasonable as an average: what are the limits around that average? What is the life of the patient, the diet, the work, the range? Have things changed? Have changes related to stones? Have there been events of substantial consequence related to stones? Have there been treatments, odd diet choices now gone but related to stones? In this exercise, we have the clinical art of diagnosis apart from urine measurements and finding systemic diseases. To understand stone formation, we will always need to understand the life of the patient as lived, now and in that part of the past that might have affected stone formation. To treat stones effectively, we usually need to ask that life be altered, and that is an absurd request absent a knowledge of what it is you hope to change.

CALCIUM STONES FROM SYSTEMIC DISEASES

We are at the next crossroads on our map (*see* Fig. 15.1). Patients who form drug stones may also have formed other kinds of stones, but if all the stones are made of drugs then that patient leaves the present discussion and becomes a problem in pharmacology: To find a proper substitute drug, if possible, or find some way to make the drug less of a danger. This is also true if stones are made of cystine. Even if they contain some calcium, the

Table 15.1: Screening for systemic diseases.

	Stones	Serum						Urine				Other
		Ca	PTH	CO_2	Cl	K	Cr	Ca	Ox	pH	NH_4	
PHPT	CaOx/HA	H	N/H				N	H				Hyperthyroidism, lithium
Sarcoidosis	CaOx/HA	H	L				N/H	H				Vitamin D excess, malignancy
dRTA	HA			L	H	L	N/H	H		H		CA inhibitors, Sjogren
BARTTER I-III				H	L	L		H				High urine PGE
BARTTER V		L		H	L	L		H				Low Mg
ADHH		L	N					H				
FHH		H	N					L				Not a stone disease
PH1 PH2 PH3	COM						N/H		H			Stones in childhood
Dent Disease	HA						H	H		H		Rickets; low P; Male CKD
Enteric HOX	CaOx/UA	N/L	N/H	L	H	L	N/H		H	L	H	Resection, malabsorption
Ileostomy	UA/CaOx			L	H	L	N/H			L	H	Clinically obvious
Bariatric surgery	CaOx								H			Clinically obvious
MSK/NC	CaOx/HA											Ureteroscopy; ?Radiology

(PHPT: Primary hyperparathyroidism; dRTA: Distal renal tubular acidosis; FHH: Familial hypercalcemic hypocalciuria; ADHH: Autosomal dominant hypocalcemic hypercalciuria; PH1-3: Primary hyperoxaluria types 1-3; HOX: Hyperoxaluria; MSK: Medullary sponge kidneys; NC: Nephrocalcinosis; CA: Carbonic anhydrase; CaOx: Calcium oxalate; UA: Uric acid; HA: Hydroxyapatite, PTH: Parathyroid hormone; H: High; N: Normal; L: Low; COM: Calcium oxalate monohydrate; PGE: Prostaglandin E; CKD: Chronic kidney disease).

evaluation and treatment must focus on cystinuria. Stones that contain only struvite and its invariable calcium carbonate coprecipitate arise from infection. They are infected foreign bodies in the urinary system and properly belong in the category of surgical-medical infectious disease management. Some patients form struvite stones that contain crystals that would not be produced from infection such as brushite (BR), hydroxyapatite (HA), or CaOx; they require dual evaluation. When stone composition is unknown, one can only proceed as if it was not one of these special cases, although over time that may prove false and the clinical course must be altered.

Laboratory Screening

Once in the common zone of CaP, CaOx, or UA unknown stones (*see* Fig. 15.1), the search for systemic disease begins, for any such disease requires its own special approach and usually very specific treatment. The problem is to screen intelligently because most calcium and uric acid stone formers do not have a systemic cause. So the evaluation has a dual constraint: sensitive but simple. What follows will pertain largely to calcium stones; uric acid stones are covered in a separate chapter 23.

What to Measure

A modest list of diseases causes renal stones (Table 15.1), which range from not uncommon to rare and from obvious to obscure. A few clinical, serum, and urine observations will suffice as clues, and we can gather them together to make a list of the "basic workup" for stone formers who desire, or whose physicians desire, no more than screening: Serum, calcium, creatinine, bicarbonate, chloride, potassium, phosphate, magnesium; urine calcium, pH, oxalate, creatinine, and total protein. The urine is probably best collected for 24 hours to get a daily average for which normal ranges exist. The urine and serum creatinine can give an estimate of creatinine clearance, and the creatinine, an index for completeness of collection. Cystinuria is screened for with an inexpensive qualitative urine test for cystine in all stone patients to establish that urine cystine excretion is low.

Serum Interpretation

As a practical matter, idiopathic calcium stone formers are normocalcemic and have no serum electrolyte abnormalities. Hypercalcemia is never present except from an important cause (Table 15.1). Those with overt reduction in glomerular filtration rate (GFR) are either old or have an evident clinical reason: nephrectomy, loss of renal mass from procedures or obstruction, or, e.g. a systemic disease. If decreased GFR is chronic, evaluation of the urine for protein is appropriate, which is present in some rare stone-forming conditions, such as Dent's disease. If it is of new onset, concern for silent obstruction should be addressed. Nonanion gap metabolic acidosis is expected in bowel diseases because of gastrointestinal (GI) alkali losses, but otherwise suggests some tubule disorder like distal renal tubular acidosis (RTA) or effects of a drug that reduced acidification, such as topiramate.

Hypokalemia sans GI disease is from five common causes: Diuretics that raise serum bicarbonate and are used in stone prevention or perhaps treatment of hypertension; tubule defects that cause potassium wasting that raises serum bicarbonate[4]; vomiting that raises serum bicarbonate; RTA that lowers serum bicarbonate; and laxative abuse that lowers serum bicarbonate.

Low serum hypomagnesemia is common from diuretics but can reflect an uncommon tubule defect (Table 15.1). We have seen it as a sole manifestation of malabsorption. Of course, severe Mg depletion can lead to renal potassium losses[5] and perhaps the converse, but these severe depletions are not part of the mainstream of stone disease; diuretics, GI diseases, aberrant behavior, and tubule defects are the main causes of low serum hypomagnesemia in stone formers.

In practice, expect normal serum measurement, when abnormal, look for simple causes like thiazides or bowel disease. Never neglect even slight hypercalcemia. It may be primary hyperparathyroidism (PHPT), drug effects, or even malignancy. Hypercalcemia is a cardinal finding of systemic disease.

Urine Interpretation

In all honesty, we have put on the page a sequence we never follow, because all of our stone formers collect multiple 24-hour urines before we see them. Out of respect for those who wish to stage things, however, the urine panel was chosen for safety. Positive cystine screening takes a patient to proper evaluation for that disease and ends the present discussion about screening. Far more ominous and of massive importance, a high urine oxalate can mean primary hyperoxaluria or a form of enteric hyperoxaluria. These diseases can and do cause kidney failure and require complete and detailed evaluation. Hypercalciuria is a commonplace, usually idiopathic, and also of diagnostic importance here as a way of interpreting hypercalcemia, as discussed below (see the section on primary hyperparathyroidism). Urine pH is helpful in assessing reduced serum bicarbonate: High in RTA, low in bowel diseases.

Screening History

There exist two forms of history taking, in our opinion. History can give clues to systemic diseases, the region of the chapter we presently inhabit. This is a small part of the history unless positive, whereupon it becomes a prime focus. When no clues to systemic disease arise, the history turns to factors that promote idiopathic stones, which we discuss in a later and more elaborated section.

Bowel Disease

Table 15.1 and the presumed minimal 24-hour study belie the reality of practice, which begins clinically, with history taking. Patients with almost any form of bowel disease tell you about it, and have records of past evaluations. All of them deserve a comprehensive urine study and treatment directed to the causes of their stones.

A few cannot tell you about their bowel disease because they do not know. Patients with chronic malabsorption from pancreatic insufficiency, celiac disease, otherwise silent Crohn's disease, congenital short small bowel, and more may not recognize their stools are abnormal; they may not even be perceptibly abnormal. So we must be wary of any hints. Some can tell you and will not. They use laxatives, or vomit, or both. Even stool softeners like psyllium can lower urine pH and urine volume.

Sarcoidosis that causes hypercalciuria and stones usually is, like bowel disease, clinically apparent.[6] Chest radiographs cannot be a screening test for stone formers; the yield will be too low. This is also true for angiotensin converting enzyme activity. Finding splenomegaly, hepatomegaly, enlarged nodes, or symptoms and signs of lung disease might alert one, but in all our years we have never encountered such a situation. Rather, patients with known sarcoidosis are sent for evaluation and treatment to prevent their stones.

This is also true for *drugs that cause stones*; people know they take them and can tell you. Some may not tell you because they do not know it may be important. Some drugs like lithium may be kept secret. So it is important to know all medications.

Primary hyperparathyroidism may foster hypertension, peptic ulcer, pancreatitis, bone disease, and neurological changes, but to us it is mostly diagnosed by unexplained hypercalcemia with serum parathyroid hormone (PTH) and urine calcium levels that are not low. Low PTH arises from vitamin D downregulation or the rare calcium sensing receptor (CaSR) upregulation conditions we list. Only lithium, hyperthyroidism, familial hypocalciuric hypercalcemia, and PHPT produce high serum calcium with unsuppressed PTH and high urine calcium.

Distal renal tubular acidosis (dRTA) can be inherited or acquired and is rather easy to detect. The reduced serum bicarbonate and potassium with normal anion gap and alkaline urine pH are a colorful and eye-catching combination. Family history is often positive. Even the stones, invariably HA, put one in mind of the condition. The carbonic anhydrase inhibitor drugs, like topiramate, can cause a similar picture.

Primary hyperoxaluria is the truly odd condition that is, howsoever rare, always on the mind of those who practice stone prevention. It can be missed for too long a while, and does often destroy the kidneys very rapidly. The stones are CaOx and therefore ordinary. All of the unusual traits like stones in childhood, loss of renal function, episodes of transient acute kidney injury otherwise unexplained can be absent at initial evaluation. Even the urine oxalate is sometimes deceiving, in the range of 70 or 80 mg/d which could be excused as arising from low calcium diet or diet oxalate loads. This is why even rudimentary screening should include a measurement of urine oxalate.

Uric Acid Stones without Bowel Disease

Gout, diabetes, metabolic syndrome, chronic kidney disease, and simply inheritance can lower urine pH so that uric acid crystallizes. Being a special kind of disease with its own pathophysiology, and because these stones are not common in otherwise completely healthy people, we reserve them as a form of stones in the context of systemic disease. The diagnosis is almost always by stone analysis, radiolucent stones on flat plate radiographs, or a history of red-orange gravel in the urine.

The Rarest of Rare

We mention the monogenic hypercalciuric states[7] that cause stones because, although rare, they are serious and demand proper care; however, few who read this will see one of the conditions we list in a lifetime of practice. The cases we have seen often have something odd in the history—family members with stones and renal failure, childhood stones, myriads of confused physicians, reduced renal function for no apparent reason, high salt requirements, polyuria. All have high urine calcium. None have completely normal serum screening values. This means, in a practical sense, that serum abnormalities in a hypercalciuric patient force one to look into the odd corners. Low serum phosphate is an exception. Many common idiopathic calcium stone formers have this and we have not found it has any clinical significance, although it may be of interest to those who do research on stone disease.[8]

The Special Problem of Hypercalcemia

Because PHPT is not rare among calcium stone formers[9] and because elevated serum calcium level is at once the prime hallmark of the disease and the principal means of detection, this one part of the screening evaluation has a special place in this chapter. We mean by this that most errors of omission, most missed diagnoses, occur up front, when one is looking for systemic diseases. Management of the condition, once diagnosed, belongs mainly to surgeons.

Serum Normals are Laboratory Dependent

Our experience with surgically proven primary hyperparathyroidism in calcium stone formers[9] arises from atomic absorption calcium measurements, which are very precise and accurate but impractical for commercial sale. Even so, they give an idea of how a patient can be evaluated. All of our proven PHPT cases (Fig. 15.2, upper left panel, large black squares) had serum calcium values of >10.1 on an average of the three measurements we have always chosen to make prior to treatment. Normal people (black smaller circles) and idiopathic calcium stone formers (tiny black dots) almost never had values that high. Nearly half of the PHPT patients had mean values of <10.5, so we sent these patients to surgery with "high" calciums in a range just above normal.

The general lesson from this panel of Figure 15.2 is not about our laboratory but about the very mild degree of hypercalcemia in PHPT. In practice, the laboratory that serves you will have its own range. Patients whose serum calcium is even slightly above that range probably have hypercalcemia. All you can do to make sure is measure repeatedly. Serum calcium measurements are not expensive compared to a failed or unnecessary surgery, so we recommend lavish accumulation of values when needed. In passing, serum phosphorus levels are indeed lower than normal in PHPT (Fig. 15.2, upper left panel, *y*-axis), but we, like others, have not relied on them for diagnosis.

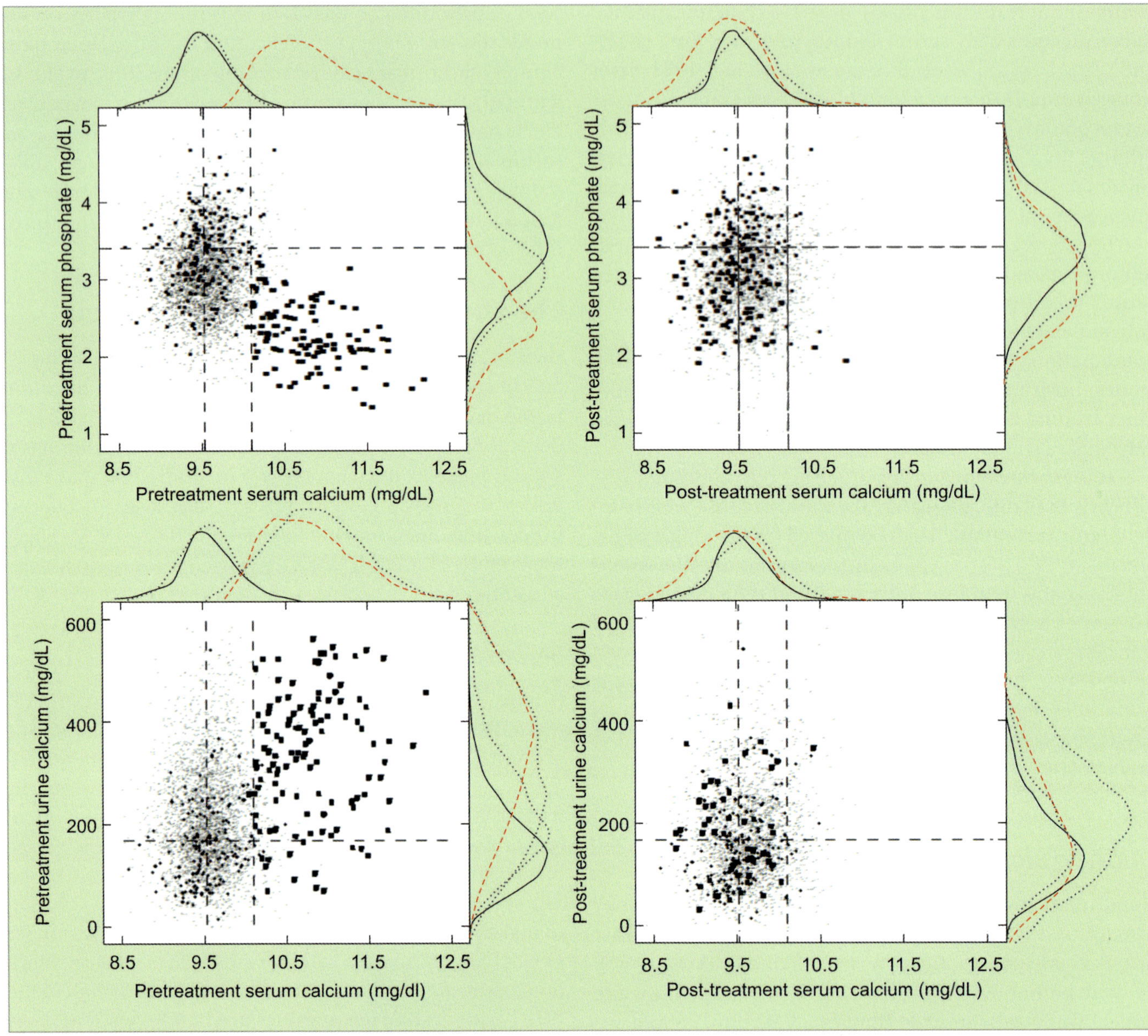

Fig. 15.2: Serum and urine chemistries in patients with primary hyperparathyroidism (PHPT) before and after parathyroidectomy. Pretreatment (left panels) serum calcium (*X*-axes of upper and lower panels) of PHPT (large black symbols) exceeds that of idiopathic stone formers (SF, cloud of small points) or normal subjects (NS, small black symbols). Serum phosphorus (*Y*-axis, upper left panel) in patients with PHPT fell as calcium rose, and urine calcium (*Y*-axis, lower left panel) rose progressively with serum calcium. Nonparametric density distributions (drawn as overlays) show the deviation of serum calcium, serum phosphorus, and urine calcium values in PHPT (dashed lines) from those in SF (dotted lines) and NS (solid lines). After treatment (right panels), values for PHPT overlap with those of SF and NS. The mean value and upper limit of normal for serum calcium, respectively, are shown as dashed vertical lines, and normal mean values for serum phosphorus (upper panels) and urine calcium (lower panels) are shown as horizontal dashed lines.
Source: With permission from Parks JH, Coe FL, Evan AP, et al. Clinical and laboratory characteristics of calcium stone-formers with and without primary hyperparathyroidism. BJU Int. 2009;103:670-8.

Urine Calcium can be Helpful

The urine calcium excretion of PHPT patients is generally, though not always, much higher than in routine calcium stone formers (Fig. 15.2, lower left panel). The points that are not as high as the other patients with PHPT arose mainly from older women and would be more impressive if scaled for their weight or urine creatinine excretion. Serum and urine calcium fall after successful surgery (Fig. 15.2, upper right and lower right panels), though the latter is often incomplete, leaving residual hypercalciuria that resembles in every way idiopathic hypercalciuria and needs to be treated to prevent more stones.[10] In other words, after cure of PHPT some patients become idiopathic calcium stone formers. Of note, hypercalcemia with low urine calcium excretion suggests familial hypocalciuric hypercalcemia, an autosomal genetic abnormality that reduces the sensitivity of the cell surface calcium receptor[11]; this is benign and not a cause of stones or any other known illness.

Serum PTH is Important but in a Special Way

The underlying physiology of PTH regulation, and of PTH regulation of urine calcium, dictate that when serum calcium is higher than normal PTH falls. Therefore, the presence of serum PTH anywhere in the normal range is compatible with PHPT in a hypercalcemic patient. Hypercalcemia in sarcoidosis, malignancy and vitamin D excess lower PTH below normal, and PTH is not suppressed in the presence of hypercalcemia; the diagnosis of PHPT should be considered.

The Diagnosis is made up Front

When referring a patient for surgery you want to be as certain as possible that PHPT is present. Furthermore, the surgeon needs to be so assured of the diagnosis as to explore the neck in whatever detail needed to find the glands. It is the surgeon who usually orders and interprets the various scans and ultrasound examinations that can sometimes identify the abnormal glands, but it is the physician who evaluates stone formers for systemic cause who generally makes the diagnosis. It is here, in the diagnosis of idiopathic calcium stone formers, that this common disease is often detected, diagnosed, and sent off to experts for cure.

An Approach to Clinical Practice

Are There Stones and What Kind?

Is the patient a stone former? If not, or if great doubt exists, we would suggest no further actions until the situation seemed to demand them. If so, stone analysis will be the immediate second level (*see* Fig. 15.1) that determines a number of outcomes. Drug stones are due to some insoluble drug or another and are managed through drug dosing or substitution. Cystine stones define an inherited amino acid transport disease with special means for evaluation and treatment. Struvite stones or struvite in stones implies an important renal infection within a foreign body. Other minerals such as CaOx and CaP may suggest that there are other stone-forming factors at work, so systemic diseases need to be sought (*see* Fig. 15.1).

Is a Systemic Disease Present that can cause Stones?

If stones are CaOx, CaP, or UA, or if they are unknown, the search for systemic causes becomes paramount because each is a disease of which stones may be only one of many consequences. Whichever is found becomes the prime focus of clinical attention. However, comprehensive stone evaluation is also reasonable because many components of the disease may be causal, and because the stone disease, arising from a systemic disease, is always clinically important.

This latter point can be lost if not repeated and emphasized. Systemic diseases produce stones through the common mechanisms of altered urine chemistry that fosters crystal formation. We treat the disease in ways that reduce its dire systemic effects and also lower urinary stone risk.

Are Idiopathic Stones Clinically Significant?

Given no reason to suspect a systemic cause, stones are presumed to be "idiopathic" by definition and the question arises as to their clinical significance. Significance is an arbitrary and personal matter. For example, a patient with one uncomplicated stone may desire all attempts at prevention, whereas another patient plagued by many stones and procedures may not feel plagued and desire nothing more than educated nostrums such as "drink more water."

When patients ask our opinion about whether to treat or not, the decision is elaborate. Are there diseases that would make a stone hazardous: clotting disorders, urinary tract anomalies, single kidney or established kidney disease, anesthesia risks? Likewise, are stones forming actively if we count them over time in the manner we have already mentioned? Is the stone burden large enough that more is very undesirable? Are stones growing? If so, comprehensive metabolic evaluation is appropriate.

If not, matters are still unfinished. Stones may grow or new ones form. We favor some form of subsequent reevaluation, but hesitate to specify overly. Perhaps an ultrasound or a CT, in a few years, is recommended, or some

Table 15.2: Serum and urine measurements for evaluation of kidney stone formers.

	Serum	*Purpose in serum*	*Normal urine range*	*Purpose in urine*
Calcium	8.9–10.2	PHPT sarcoid	<250 (F) <300 (M)	Detection of hypercalciuria
Phosphorus	2.5–4	PHPT	500–1500	Calculation of CaP SS
Creatinine	eGFR >60	Estimate renal function	15–19 (F); 20—24 (M) (mg/kg per day)	Completeness of collection, adjust excretions, calculate CCr
HCO_3	24–27	RTA	—	
Cl	98–105	RTA	—	
Sodium	138–142	Anion gap, hyponatremia	100	Diet counseling, ionic strength
Potassium	3.8–4.2	RTA; K depletion	40–80	Diet counseling; ionic strength
Uric acid	3–5	Gout	<750 <800	Hyperuricosuria in CaOx SF
Magnesium	1.8–2.2	Depletion	50–150	Detection of malabsorption
Volume	—		>1.5	Low volume as cause of stones
pH	—		5.8–6.2	UA and CaP SS
Oxalate	—		<40	Detection of HOX
Citrate	—		>500 (M) >700 (F)	Detection of hypocitraturia
NH_4	—		15—60	Renal acid excretion
SO_4	—		20–80	Metabolic acid production
PCR	—		0.8–1.2	Protein intake
SS CaOx	—		<5	
SS CaP	—		<1	
SS UA			<1	

(Units are mg/dL in serum except Na, K, Cl (mmol/d); units are mg/d in urine except Na, K, NH_4, SO_4 mmol/d; pH and SS are unit less. All urine measurements are used to calculate SS values. Purposes of serum measurements are detection of states noted. (PHPT: Primary hyperparathyroidism; RTA: Renal tubular acidosis; SS: Supersaturation; CaOx: Calcium oxalate; CaP: Calcium phosphate; UA: Uric acid; F: Female; M: Male; CCr: Creatinine clearance; SF: Stone former; HOX: Hyperoxaluria; PCR: Protein catabolic rate).

tracking of renal function in case silent obstruction has occurred. And, we always favor obvious nostrums: High fluid intake, avoidance of high-oxalate or low-calcium diets, and minimization of dehydrating conditions.

COMPREHENSIVE METABOLIC EVALUATION

The comprehensive metabolic evaluation plays different roles in stone formers with systemic diseases and in those without such diseases. For the former, treatment concerns the underlying disease process, and the metabolic panel is one of perhaps many gauges of success. For the idiopathic calcium stone formers, the metabolic evaluation is the diagnostic and therapeutic compass. Treatments are directed to the stone-forming processes it reveals.

The 24-Hour Urine Stone Risk Panel

The blood values are the same as for screening, because among the idiopathic calcium stone formers all of the stone risk factors reside in urine. As these chapters demonstrate, the crystals that make up human stones follow the laws of solution of physical chemistry concerning phase change. For CaOx stones, the main drivers of crystal formation are urine calcium and oxalate concentrations; for calcium phosphate, which begins with calcium monohydrogen phosphate crystallization, the main determinants are urine calcium, phosphate, and citrate concentrations, and urine pH. The other materials in Table 15.2 affect complex formations that remove these primary ions from mutual interactions, and the activity of the ions that are free to interact.

The Primacy of Excretion Rates

Even though concentrations of ions drive crystallization, daily excretion rates must have a powerful clinical effect. At any excretion rate the concentration of an ion will vary inversely with urine volume, so higher excretions will mean higher concentrations for a given volume. Since volume is a matter of habit, occupation, environment, mere chance, and perhaps genetics,[12] higher excretions must raise the average risk of higher concentrations.

Excretion rates, moreover, are determined to a large measure by renal function, GI transport, diet, and perhaps bone turnover, which are themselves regulated features of any one patient[13] subject to change through clinical measures. Therefore, we diagnose causes of stones in terms of excretion rates of relevant materials in urine, including urine volume, and manipulate these rates as we can so as to achieve reduced concentrations and therefore SS and crystal formation driving forces.

In doing this, we recognize that stone formation is almost certainly conditioned by the matrix molecules in urine that glue crystals together into stones, and modify crystal nucleation, growth, aggregation, and cell adhesion. These factors are presently beyond the reach of clinical practice. However, for a given SS, which is the ultimate crystallization driving force, some people will form stones while a majority of people with the same saturations will not.

Relationship of Excretion Rates to Stone Risk

Given this, one expects excretion rates to gauge the risk of being a stone former, and that expectation is supported by observational studies of female and male cohorts, some of whose subjects have become stone formers over time (Fig. 15.3).[14] The data for men are taken from the Health Professionals Follow-up Study (stone formers: 636, mean age: 63 ± 9.3 years; controls: 414, mean age: 64.6 ± 6.3 years), and data for women are taken from the Nurses' Health Study I (stone formers: 898, mean age: 66.1 ± 7.8 years; controls: 403, mean age: 65.4 ± 5.8 years) and the Nurses' Health Study II (stone formers: 703, mean age: 47.5 ± 6.1 years; controls: 296, mean age: 50.1 ± 5.2 years). Logistic regression was used to determine the relative risk of stone formation after adjusting for age and all of the 24-hour urine factors. In the figure, the two female cohorts are shown with red bars, the one male cohort with blue bars. Shown are the lower 95th percentiles for the relative risk ratio at each range of calcium and oxalate excretions (upper panels) and the upper 95th percentiles of the risk ratios for urine citrate and volume (lower panels).

Calcium

For example, at a urine calcium excretion 150–199 (*see* Fig. 15.3, upper left panel), the lower 95th percentile for relative risk (compared to a value of 1 at an excretion rate of <100 mg/d) exceeds or reaches 1 for 2 of the cohorts, meaning that it is improbable that the risk has not increased compared to <100 mg/d. Between 200 and 240 mg/d the lower bound is >1 for all three cohorts. Mean urine calcium of stone formers was greater than control in each cohort ($p < 0.001$), and was close to the risk threshold.

Oxalate

Plotted in the same manner (Fig. 15.3, upper right panel), urine oxalate poses risk [lower 95% confidence interval (CI): relative risk (RR) >1] for both sexes at 25 mg/d, substantially below the common upper limit of 40 mg/d (Table 15.2). Mean values for both normal and stone-forming women and (especially) men in these cohorts lie above the risk threshold, and mean oxalate was higher among stone formers than among controls in each cohort.

Citrate

Citrate is calcium binding and therefore lowers the concentration of calcium ion available to combine with oxalate and phosphate. Likewise, it is an inhibitor of calcium salt crystallizations. As one might, therefore, expect, rising levels of urine citrate reduce the risk of new stone onset (Fig. 15.3, lower left panel) in men and women. Mean levels of citrate were higher in controls than in stone formers in each cohort, but all lay below the risk threshold.

Urine Volume

It is traditional to take <1.5 L/d as the risk boundary (*see* Table 15.2) but stable risk reduction with the upper 95% boundary below 1 requires 1.75 L in both sexes (*see* Fig. 15.3, lower panels). Mean values for the stone formers in each cohort lie very close to the risk thresholds, whereas normal subjects had higher volumes.

Other Measurements

In women, *urine magnesium* <60 mg/d was associated with high stone risk that fell below 1 above that point without obvious progression. Among men there was no corresponding magnesium effect. Although we and others[15,16] have suggested that high urine uric acid excretion seemed to promote calcium stone risk in the women and men of this study, there was no significant effect in women and distinct risk reduction in men as one passed from <400 mg/d to >400 mg/d (not shown). The change in risk is so

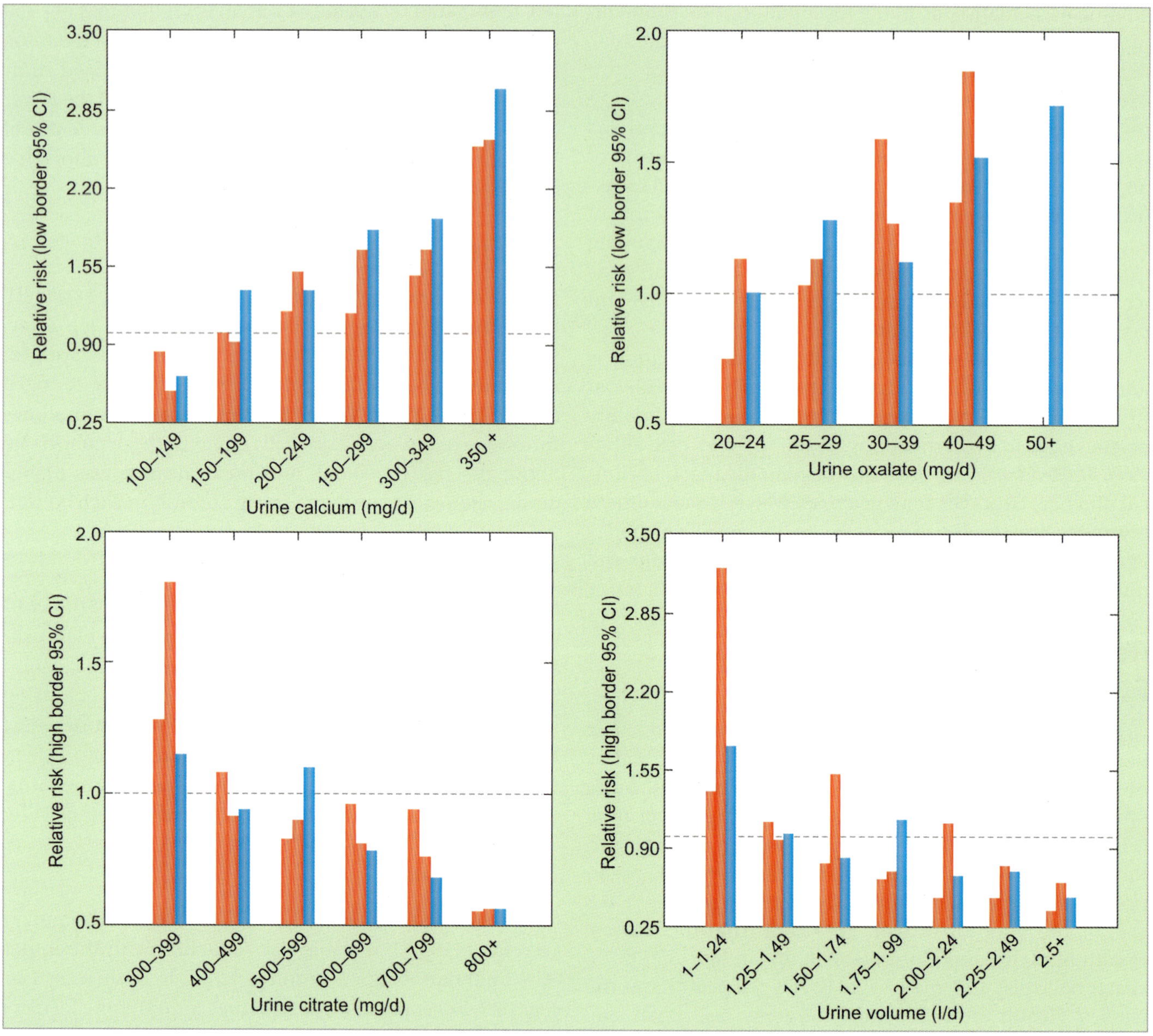

Fig. 15.3: Relative risk of kidney stone formation in three large cohorts of women (red bars) and men (blue bars) by levels of urine stone risk factors. The bars show the lower 95th percentile of the relative risk ratio at each range of calcium and oxalate excretions (upper panels) and the upper 95th percentiles of the risk ratios for urine citrate and volume (lower panels). The horizontal dashed line in each panel separates regions of decreased from increased relative risk.
Source: Redrawn from Curhan GC, Taylor EN. 24-h uric acid excretion and the risk of kidney stones. Kidney Int. 2008;73:489-96.

abrupt and the effect of increasing urine uric acid from 400 to 800 mg on risk so minimal that we suspect an artifact: Male 24-hour urine values of <400 mg/d may reflect in vitro precipitation. Those who precipitate form uric acid stones because of low urine pH and are classified as stone onset subjects. This requires further studies.

Urine pH

There was a slight increase of stone risk with pH increase above 5.5 in men but not women (not shown). However, it is not really appropriate to consider urine pH itself in relation to stones as it controls CaP and UA crystallization and has no immediate direct effects on CaOx crystallization.

Use of Deviation from Normal in Judging Urine Findings Abnormal

However rational, use of cut points from epidemiology risk studies is not the conventional approach. More common is to gauge deviation from normal, usually the upper or lower 5% or 10%, as an "abnormality" that requires treatment. For reference, we present (*see* Table 15.2) conventional limits derived from normal population.

How to Reconcile the Two Approaches

There would seem to be a schism of values implied by the differences between diagnoses based on deviation from normal and those arising from epidemiological linkages between measured values and new onset stones. However, this is not the case.

We have already mentioned that the higher the solute excretion rate for a stone-forming material, the higher the average concentration within a random bundle of urine volumes for a population and therefore an eventually higher chance of higher SS. The risk-based indices must reflect the interactions of both SS and matrix molecules as they relate excretions to stones. They are therefore preferable for practice.

On the other hand, deviations of solute excretion from normal define truly abnormal urine calcium, oxalate, citrate, and even volumes. If one believes that some or all of these arise from corresponding abnormal physiologies, then deviation from normal is appropriate for research concerning those physiologies. Hypercalciuria is surely familial, breedable in animals, and based on a complex set of abnormal physiologies. Hyperoxaluria and hypocitraturia may be similar.

Supersaturations in Clinical Practice

Practical Uses

Given this, and at the present time, evaluation of stone formers for cause of stones concerns excretion rates of key materials, urine volume, and the final result of their interactions, which are the SS. These are essentially ratios of the concentrations of the three stone-forming salts divided by their solubilities in urine at body temperature. Since uric acid and the initial CaP phases form rather readily given any SS, we view as an ideal maintaining values below 1 as much as possible. For CaOx, whose ULM is considerably >1, a reasonable choice is to lower it from wherever the patient is during active stone formation to some acceptably lower value, perhaps to one half of the initial values. As a rule, this brings most people into the range of 3–5.

The reasoning behind this idea is practical inference. There is no doubt about the physical connection between SS and crystallization in the general sense. However, urine is a complex solution that contains many modifiers of crystallization that permit metastable SS (values above 1) to persist for long periods of hours to even many days. That a person who is making stones has a particular SS means that whatever defenses may be present are not sufficient to prevent crystallization, so prevention of stones requires that SS be lowered.

Urine pH plays so special a role that we set it apart from all of the other aspects of urine chemistries. For CaP stones, calcium must initially combine with divalent phosphate. The pKa for the second proton of phosphate in urine is about 6.7, so at urine pH values as low as 5.7 very little divalent phosphate concentration is available to drive CaP SS no matter what the 24-hour urine phosphate excretion rate or urine volume. At a urine pH of 6.7, half of all the phosphate is in that form. It is for this reason that CaP stones generally form in patients with higher than normal urine pH.[9]

For uric acid, matters are the exact opposite. The N9 proton of uric acid has a pKa of about 5.35 in urine, and it is the undissociated (protonated) form of uric acid that crystallizes to make the common uric acid stone. Therefore, these stones form mainly in patients with low urine pH from diseases or perhaps heredity.

If one plots SS for CaP and uric acid against urine pH for a large number of 24-hour urine samples (Fig. 15.4, upper left panel), the powerful effects of pH are obvious. The average urine, not surprisingly, resides at the double minimum SS, a pH around 5.9–6.1. The biology that sets urine pH is not fully known, but certainly it would seem that evolution has favored a set point that minimizes both phosphate and uric acid crystallization risk.[17] By contrast, the effects of urine pH on SS for CaOx (Fig. 15.4, lower left panel) is nonexistent.

Urine Calcium and Volume

Perhaps because pH does not matter, CaOx SS is strongly dependent upon urine calcium excretion (Fig. 15.4, lower middle panel) and modestly upon urine volume (Fig. 15.4, lower right panel). Calcium phosphate SS is less influenced by urine calcium and volume (Fig. 15.4, upper middle and right panels), no doubt because pH is not a major force.

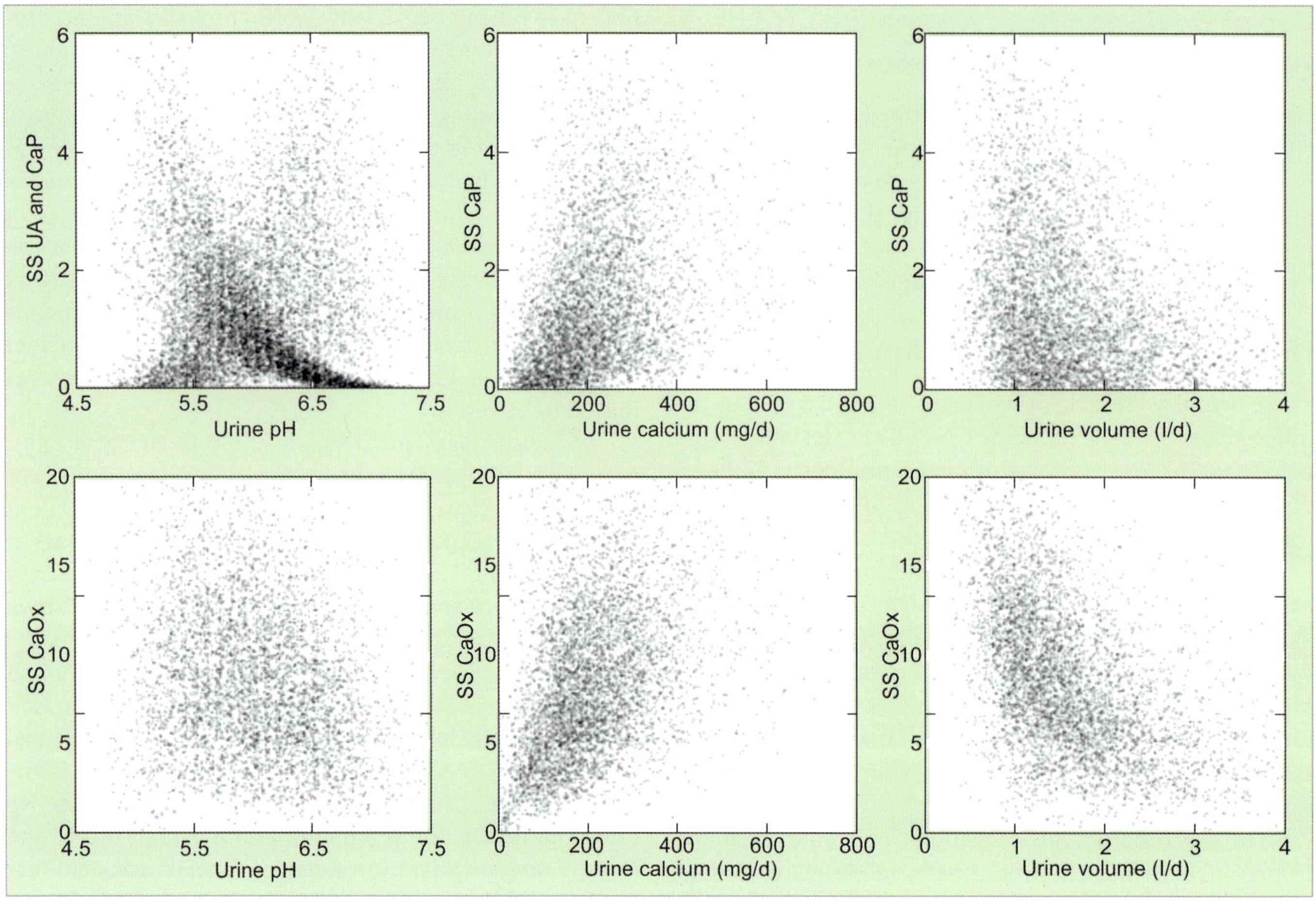

Fig. 15.4: Effects of urine pH (left panels), urine calcium excretion (middle panels), and urine volume (right panels) on levels of urinary supersaturation for uric acid (UA) and calcium phosphate (CaP) (upper panels), and calcium oxalate (CaOx) (lower panels). Each point represents a 24-hour urine. SS: Supersaturation.

We Lower SS via Changes in Excretion Rates, Urine Volume, and pH

From all the foregoing, it is obvious that treatment is to lower SS, and the only way to do this is by increasing urine volume, reducing excretions of key materials that control SS such as calcium and oxalate, reversing abnormally low or high urine pH, and raising urine citrate—the only inhibitor susceptible to change at the current time. This is true whether stones are due to systemic diseases or are idiopathic. The difference is that if systemic in origin, the means for changing excretion rates often are specific to the pathophysiology of the disease, whereas for idiopathic stones the means are universal for the class of patients depending on the urine abnormality involved.

Given the data of Figures 15.3 and 15.4, one might choose to reduce SS by working with the excretion rate(s) most deviant from the risk thresholds. For example, if volume is low, one might increase it first. If urine calcium excretion is high, one may wish to lower it. However, urine calcium can affect more than stone risk so it might warrant a special consideration.

As already mentioned, the effects of urine calcium excretion and urine volume on CaOx and CaP SS (Fig. 15.4, middle and right-hand panels) differ. The SS for CaOx is very dependent on both (Fig. 15.4, lower middle and right panels), whereas their effects on SS for CaP are more spread out and vague because urine pH is so powerful being a regulator. This means that in a patient with CaP stones and a higher than average urine pH, 6.5 for example, urine volume and calcium will need to be altered more to reduce SS than one would need for a similar change for CaOx.

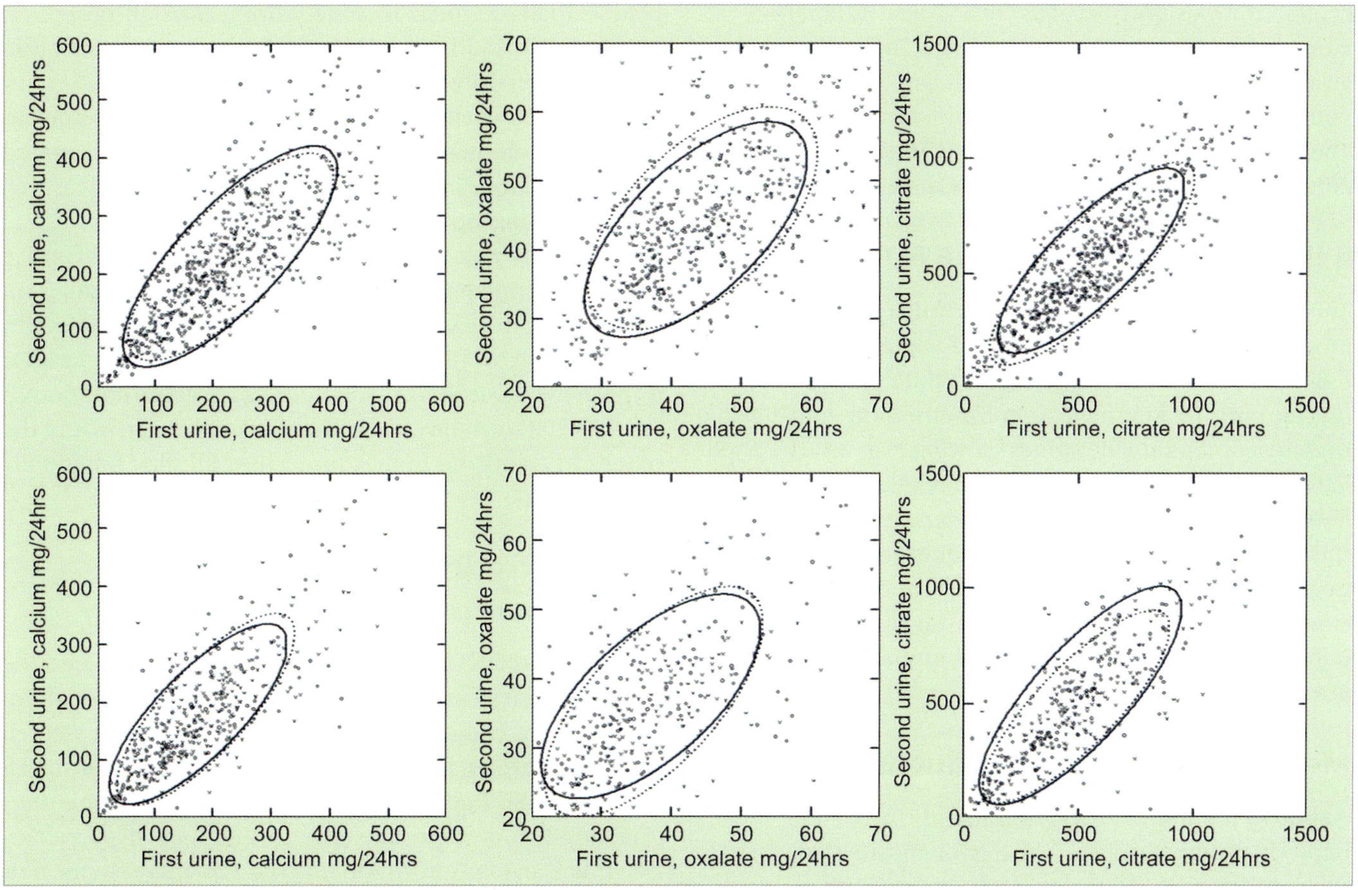

Fig. 15.5: Correspondence between daily excretions of calcium (left panels), oxalate (middle panels), and citrate (right panels) in the first and second 24-hour urine collections in male (upper panels) and female (lower panels) stone formers from two different practices. The confidence ellipses (solid, practice 1, and dotted, practice 2) contain 1 SD of the data. SD: Standard deviation.
Source: With permission from Parks JH, Goldfischer E, Asplin JR, et al. A single 24-Hour urine collection is inadequate for the medical evaluation of nephrolithiasis. J Urol. 2002;167:1607-12.

How Many 24-Hour Urines?

We and others[18-21] have pointed out that excretion rates in any two different 24-hour urines from the same person will tend to correlate rather well in the absence of treatment (Fig. 15.5). However, the range between the two urines can be large enough that if one only were obtained and used, in practice decisions and diagnoses based upon it might differ significantly from those that would arise if only the other urine were available. This is obvious from the figure. Women (lower panels) have a slightly lesser variation than men, but still the effect of chance is large enough to be clinically significant given the relationships already shown between excretion rates and stone risk.

Likewise, the variations between days offer clues to what might be accomplished in a patient with only diet and change of habits, for the variations we observe without treatment surely arise from those factors. So two collections protect the patient from errors of incomplete sampling and reveal possible ways of achieving treatment goals.

For example, an initial urine calcium excretion of 200 mg/d in a man (Fig. 15.5, upper left panel, *x*-axis) can be followed by another urine of 300 mg/d in about 30% of cases (the ellipses are nonparametric and contain about 66% of the data). Similar large variations are not uncommon for all of the other measurements.

CALCIUM STONES WITHOUT SYSTEMIC DISEASE—IDIOPATHIC

At this time, the idiopathic calcium stone formers appear to have at least two phenotypes. A large group forms CaOx stones, by which we mean stones whose crystal composition exceeds 50% CaOx [idiopathic calcium oxalate stone former (ICSF)]. The other smaller group forms stones whose crystals are >50% CaP [idiopathic calcium phosphate stone former (IPSF)].[22,23] The IPSF divide into two subtypes: Those whose stones contain BR and those whose stone CaP is entirely HA.

IDIOPATHIC CaOx STONE FORMERS

The CaOx stones form on renal papillae as overgrowths atop interstitial HA deposits called white plaque or Randall's plaque after its discoverer.[24] White plaque is visible during both percutaneous nephrolithotomy and flexible ureteroscopy, as are the stones growing over it.[25] The papillae are otherwise normal, as is the renal cortex.[26] No one knows the exact fraction of all calcium stone formers with this pure phenotype, because it requires stone analysis, a negative search for systemic diseases, and visualization of stones growing over white plaque on otherwise pristine papillae. We suspect it is not uncommon as CaOx stones are the most common type of stone.

Mechanism for Stone Production

Although the stones are predominantly CaOx, their means of production involve HA. First, HA deposits must form in the papillary interstitium to produce the white plaque the stones grow over.[27] Then, the open surface of the plaque must be covered over with an initial layer of apatite crystals.[28] Although we are speaking about work that may gradually evolve over time, it would appear that both CaOx and CaP SS are needed, and therefore clinicians need to consider both as potential risk factors in treating their patients.

Urine Matrix Molecules play a Special Role

Although we do not want to deviate too far from the clinic in this chapter, we might as well point out more of the complexity of the CaOx formation as we pass by, since it might be interesting if not particularly important for patient care. The urothelium shields plaque from the urine, so far as one can tell, so somehow it must give way over plaque deposits to begin the process. The mechanisms governing urothelial integrity and its loss are unknown.

The plaque itself, while shielded from urine by intact urothelium, is made of HA crystals covered over entirely with matrix molecules of tissue origin, which include osteopontin.[29,30] It is these tissue matrix molecules, not naked HA crystals, that are exposed to the urine. In the plaque matrix or in urine, molecules adsorb onto the plaque matrix, which include Tamm–Horsfall protein, a poorly organized form of HA nucleates.[28] This nucleation can be driven only by urine CaP SS.

Repeated cycles of new urine matrix overlay, nucleation, and more matrix deposition build up a multilayered covering ribbon.[28] Eventually, ribbon formation gives way to the heaping up of HA and matrix to form the base of the stone. By about 70–90 μm from the papillary surface CaOx first appears, and why the crystal transforms from HA to CaOx is unknown. Also unknown is why the cycles of nucleation occur to create the initial ribbon. We wonder if these cycles are hours, days, or years each, and do not know. What must be clear is that CaP and CaOx SS and the nature of the urine matrix molecules all play potentially critical roles.

Urine Excretions, Molarities, and Supersaturations throughout the Day

Since it takes CaP and CaOx SS to create CaOx stones, the levels of these SS in patients and their variation throughout the day have clinical importance. In our clinical research center setting, we have found large differences in urine SS between ICSF and normal people eating the same diets (Fig. 15.6).[31] As a group, stone formers are hypercalciuric. This is evident from the marked risk increase for new stone onset with increasing urine calcium (Fig. 15.3). Our studies focused on those in whom the hypercalciuria was clearly manifest—in other words, selected by having urinary calcium excretions far above the normal mean.

Excretions and Molarities

As we have already pointed out, higher calcium excretion must mean higher calcium molarity at any given urine flow rate, and since the urine flow rates of the three groups here (Fig. 15.6: Normals in red, CaP stone formers in blue, and CaOx stone formers in green) are more or less the same (not shown) the urine calcium molarity of patients far exceeded normals (Fig. 15.6, upper left panel). This was true fasting, all day, and most especially in the evening and overnight (B, breakfast; L, lunch; S, supper; H, home; and ON, overnight). Oxalate excretion (not shown) and molarity were also higher in patients than in normal, but the difference was much less marked than that for calcium (Fig. 15.6, upper middle panel). Urine citrate molarity was not lower in stone formers than in normals except perhaps among the CaP patients fasting; it was above normal in the CaOx patients (Fig. 15.6, upper right panel). As we have already mentioned, higher urine pH should be critical in

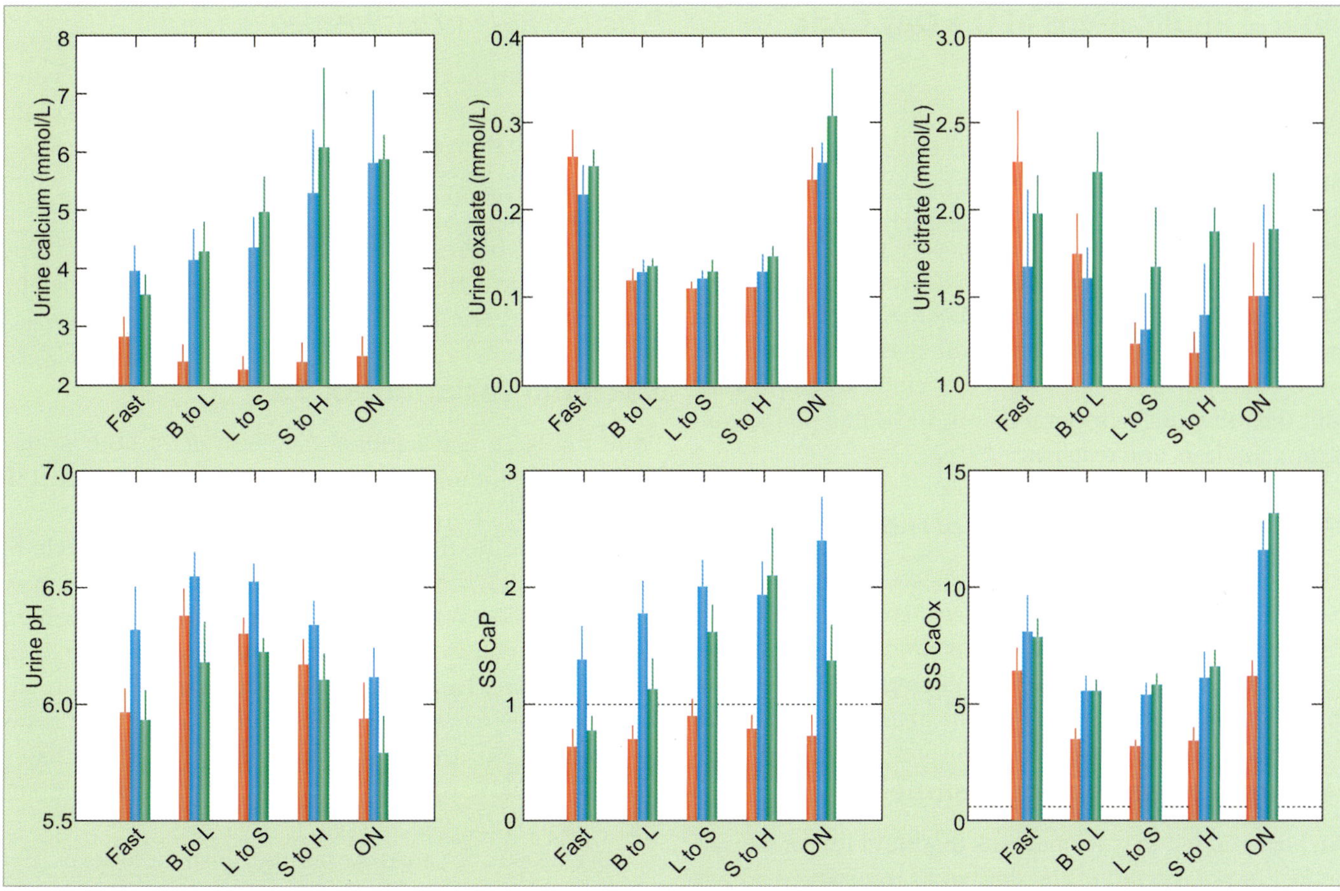

Fig. 15.6: Urinary concentrations of stone risk factors, urine pH, and urine supersaturation for CaP and CaOx (± SEM) over a 24-hour period in normal subjects (red bars), calcium phosphate (CaP) stone formers (*blue bars*), and calcium oxalate (CaOx) stone formers (*green bars*) fed the same diet. Periods of urine collection were fasting (2 hours) (FAST), between breakfast and lunch (4 hours) (B to L), between lunch and supper (5 hours) (L to S), between supper to the time the subjects went home (3 hours) (S to H), and overnight (10 hours) (ON). The horizontal dotted lines in the lower-middle and lower right panels denote the boundary between undersaturated (below 1) and supersaturated (above 1) urines. SEM: Standard error of mean.
Source: Redrawn from Bergsland KJ, Coe FL, Gillen DL, et al. A test of the hypothesis that the collecting duct calcium-sensing receptor limits rise of urine calcium molarity in hypercalciuric calcium kidney stone formers. Am J Physiol Renal Physiol. 2009;297:F1017-23.

promoting CaP crystallizations, and among the CaP stone formers it was higher than in normals or the CaOx stone formers (Fig. 15.6, lower left panel).

Supersaturations

The consequence of the hypercalciuria, higher pH, and the minimally lower urine citrate was a much higher CaP SS among CaP stone formers than in normals. Of specific importance here, however, the CaOx stone formers also generated a higher than normal CaP SS as well. In fact, our normals did not on average generate a CaP SS above 1 (Fig. 15.6, lower middle panel). It is only fasting and overnight that the CaP stone formers produced a higher urine CaP SS than did the CaOx stone formers.

It would seem that urine provides ample driving forces to create the initial HA overlay on exposed plaque, and to create the CaOx bulk of the stone body as well. It is presumably only the modest difference in CaP–CaOx SS balance that produces in one type of patient the common CaOx stone and in the others mainly CaP stones. Given that the crystallization cascade in urine is complex and may well begin with nucleation of BR, which can lead either down the CaOx or HA pathway, perhaps subtle differences in SS balance are sufficient to determine stone type. Since mixed stones with CaOx and CaP are themselves not uncommon,[32] the pattern here is reasonably consistent with the stones that have been found in large surveys.

Clinical Implications of the Day Cycle

Spot Urines are Unlikely to Support Rational Treatment

The wide variations of solute excretion during the day argue strongly against the idea that a "spot" urine can be as reliable for managing patients as one collected over the 24 hours. Since the cost of the measurements is the same, one wonders why anyone would make do with such fragmentary data. In our experience with over 50,000 24-hour urine collections, we have not been clinically impressed with the difficulties for our patients, including pilots, surgeons, children, and teachers.

The Overnight Period seems of Highest Risk

To the extent that SS controls crystallization, it would seem that fasting and overnight are the periods of highest risk for CaOx formation, and for CaP risk is progressive from fasting through the overnight period. Put together, this points to the overnight period as having the highest dual risk.

Fluid Intake needs to be Constant

We have tended to warn patients that fluid intake cannot be just in one period of the day, so as to produce a high 24-hour volume that belies periods of drought. Instead, fluids need to be constant, especially overnight. We have no trial data but would suggest that at least one nocturnal urination would be important, and that water be taken then to guard against the fasting high CaOx SS.

As a corollary, these data refute some common notions about eating. Oxalate from food is absorbed over a few hours,[33] but it is precisely during the active meal periods of the midday when urine oxalate concentration and SS are lowest. Probably breakfast and lunch are better than supper for those large bowls of berries with soy milk or that spinach salad. Here is a place for practical research we could all use. The diet in this research was, incidentally, very low in oxalate. Even so, fluids with meals seem very reasonable to recommend.

There is no time of day when CaP SS is really low in stone formers, so high fluids need to be all the time. Even if the oxalate SS is low during meals, it is far above 1, so crystals can form. Given what we know, the critical steps of HA overlay on plaque can occur at any time and the best simple defense is water.

Practical Research is Needed

Our work is artificial, being in a Clinical Research Center (CRC). However much controlled diets give insights into mechanisms, they obscure the reality of the street. Studies with open diets during normal life are needed using split urine timings, especially a division of fasting, meal periods, and overnight. We urge others to consider this kind of practical and focused research.[34] A trial of specific nocturnal hydration is also of possible value.

Seasonal Variations of SS

From the large and national database of 24-hour urines produced at Litholink, a vendor of such testing in the United States, we were able to determine the average changes in urine measurements over the yearly cycle of seasons (Fig. 15.7).[35] Urine volume of men (Fig. 15.7, upper left panel, blue dots) fell in summer, whereas women showed no such variation. Their low points were in April and December. However, urine sodium excretion, a reasonable gauge of systemic fluid volume, fell in both sexes in summer (Fig. 15.7, upper middle panel). Presumably women drank enough to maintain their urine volumes and men did not.

Because urine calcium excretion fell in both sexes (not shown), the summer increase in CaOx SS (Fig. 15.7, upper right panel) was modest in men, whereas the fall in women was large—their volume did not fall; their urine calcium did fall. Urine pH fell dramatically in men and modestly in women (Fig. 15.7, lower left panel), so CaP SS fell remarkably in both sexes (Fig. 15.7, lower middle panel). Because of their greater fall in urine volume and pH, SS UA rose far more in men than in women (Fig. 15.7, lower right panel).

We might think that summertime poses a risk for stones, and that is so for men, especially in regard to uric acid stones. For women, the highest CaOx SS are in April and December and uric acid SS never mounts significantly. It is men whom we must caution about summertime, and women, for reasons that are not evident, about April and the winter holiday season.

Upper Limits of Metastability

Something to Try at Home

You can make a metastable supersaturated solution at home. Stir table sugar into warm water until no more will

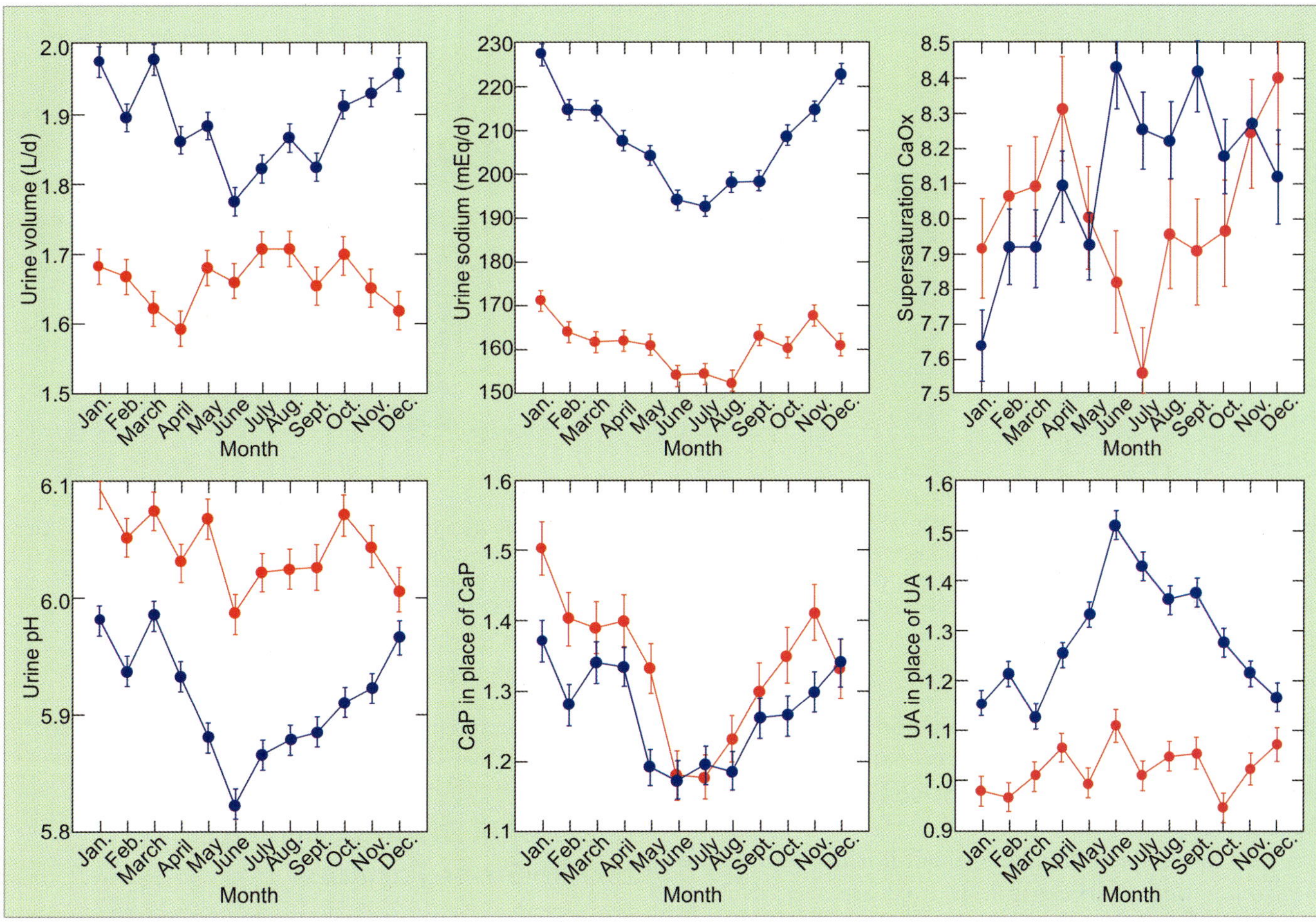

Fig. 15.7: Seasonal means (± SEM) by gender for urine volume, sodium, pH and supersaturations for CaOx, CaP, and UA among stone formers. Men—blue symbols; women—red symbols. (SEM: Standard error of mean).
Source: With permission from Parks JH, Barsky R, Coe FL. Gender differences in seasonal variation of urine stone risk factors. J Urol. 2003;170:384-8.

dissolve. Pour the solution into a jar, and let it cool. As the temperature falls, so will the solubility of the sugar, so the solution becomes supersaturated, but it will remain clear. If the glass is very clean and you are careful, you might even cool the solution in the refrigerator, although the solubility will fall a lot and the sugar or salt might crystallize. However, if you tap on the glass to create cavitation bubbles, crystals of sugar will snow down until all the SS energy is dissipated and the solution comes to solubility. The solution is called metastable because it can maintain an SS, but given some instability such as bubbles or, of course, added crystals of solid sugar, the "excess" sugar will come back out of solution.

What the Kidneys Do

Salts like CaOx and calcium phosphates form in the later nephron segments as reabsorption of water outstrips that of solutes. We have produced a map of nephron SS mainly from animal micropuncture data.[36] The urine itself may contain crystals, or may not, but urine is more stable than supersaturated sugar water. If you shake urine, or tap the side of the glass that contains urine with a spoon, crystals will not shower down. Crystals will gradually form, but over days. Urine is metastably supersaturated with respect to CaOx virtually all of the time (*see* Figs. 15.4 and 15.6) but variably for CaP and UA.

How We Measure ULM

Because it is more stable than your sugar solutions, we can let urine cool to room temperature, and it will retain most of its SS. We add one component, calcium for phosphate crystals and oxalate for CaOx crystals.[37] As you add the one component, the total salt concentration rises. You

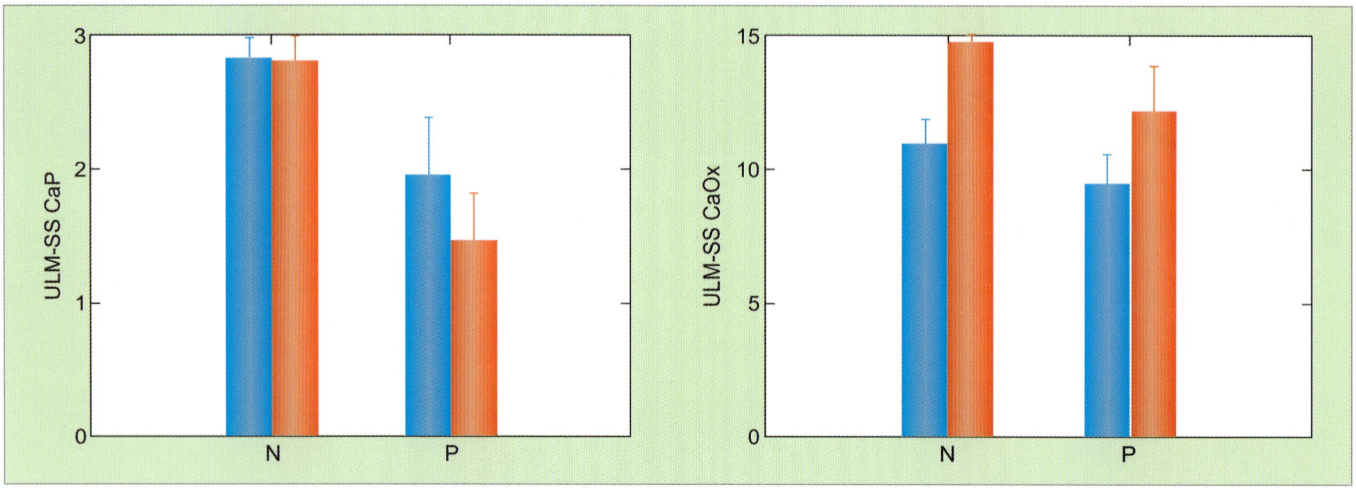

Fig. 15.8: The ULM–SS distance (± SEM) in calcium stone formers and normal subjects. The distance between the experimentally determined upper limit of metastability (ULM) and the urine supersaturation (SS) for calcium phosphate (CaP; left panel) and calcium oxalate (CaOx; right panel) is shown for men (blue bars) and women (red bars) who are either normal subjects (N) or stone formers (P). *Source*: Redrawn from Asplin JR, Parks JH, Chen MS, et al. Reduced crystallization inhibition by urine from men with nephrolithiasis. Kidney Int. 1999;56:1505-16. Asplin JR, Parks JH, Nakagawa Y, et al. Reduced crystallization inhibition by urine from women with nephrolithiasis. Kidney Int. 2002;61:1821-9.

know how much you added, so you know how much the increase is, and you can watch for crystals. The salt (CaOx or CaP) concentration at which crystals first form is called the *upper limit of metastability*.

We have not said this before, but it is the product of the concentrations of calcium and oxalate and divalent phosphate that mainly set the level of SS. The calciums interact with, as an example, the oxalates like dancers at a party ball; the more there are of, for example, men and women, the higher the likelihood they will "bump into" one another, choose to dance, and make a pairing. Salts are pairings of ligands like dancing couples are paired; the bonds are easily broken. The salt is merely the associations of calcium and oxalate ions that remain in solution.

Given that the concentration of one is less than a tenth of the other in the case of CaOx (Fig. 15.6; compare upper left and middle panels), the situation is like a party of all men with a few women, or the reverse. As we add oxalate, more and more couples form, and—though the metaphor does not hold perfectly—the higher the chance that groups of couples will get together and decide that the dance floor is too crowded and, therefore, they might want to leave.

You might say that adding one ligand of a salt is a clumsy way to do things and we would agree. We alter the balance of things. To get CaP to crystallize, we add calcium, so the ratio of calcium to phosphate changes, and it is true that the ratio of the two does affect how crystals form. For CaOx the problem is worse than for CaP because there is so much more calcium than oxalate in urine, so the ratio is very sensitive to additions of oxalate.

The SS-ULM Distance in Calcium Stone Formers

In two experiments, we compared the ULM to the SS for CaOx and CaP in men and women with and without calcium stones; the majority formed CaOx stones.[38,39] Obviously, the difference between the ULM and the SS of a urine is a critical measure as it gives the "headroom," the space between the SS and where SS has to be in order to make visible crystals.

The CaP ULM-SS Distance

Among normal men (blue) and women (red) (Fig. 15.8, left panel, "N"), the ULM–SS distance is about the same and averages about 3, meaning that you would have to raise SS by about three units on average to create crystals. Among patients (Fig. 15.8, left panel, "P"), the distance is lower than among normals for both sexes. By analysis of variance (ANOVA) the sexes do not differ; the distance between N and P is significant for women, $p = 0.02$, but not for men. The individual points for each person (Fig. 15.9, upper panels) show why the sex difference is present. Although some male patients (Fig. 15.9, upper left panel) have very low ULM-SS distances (red symbols), even negative ones

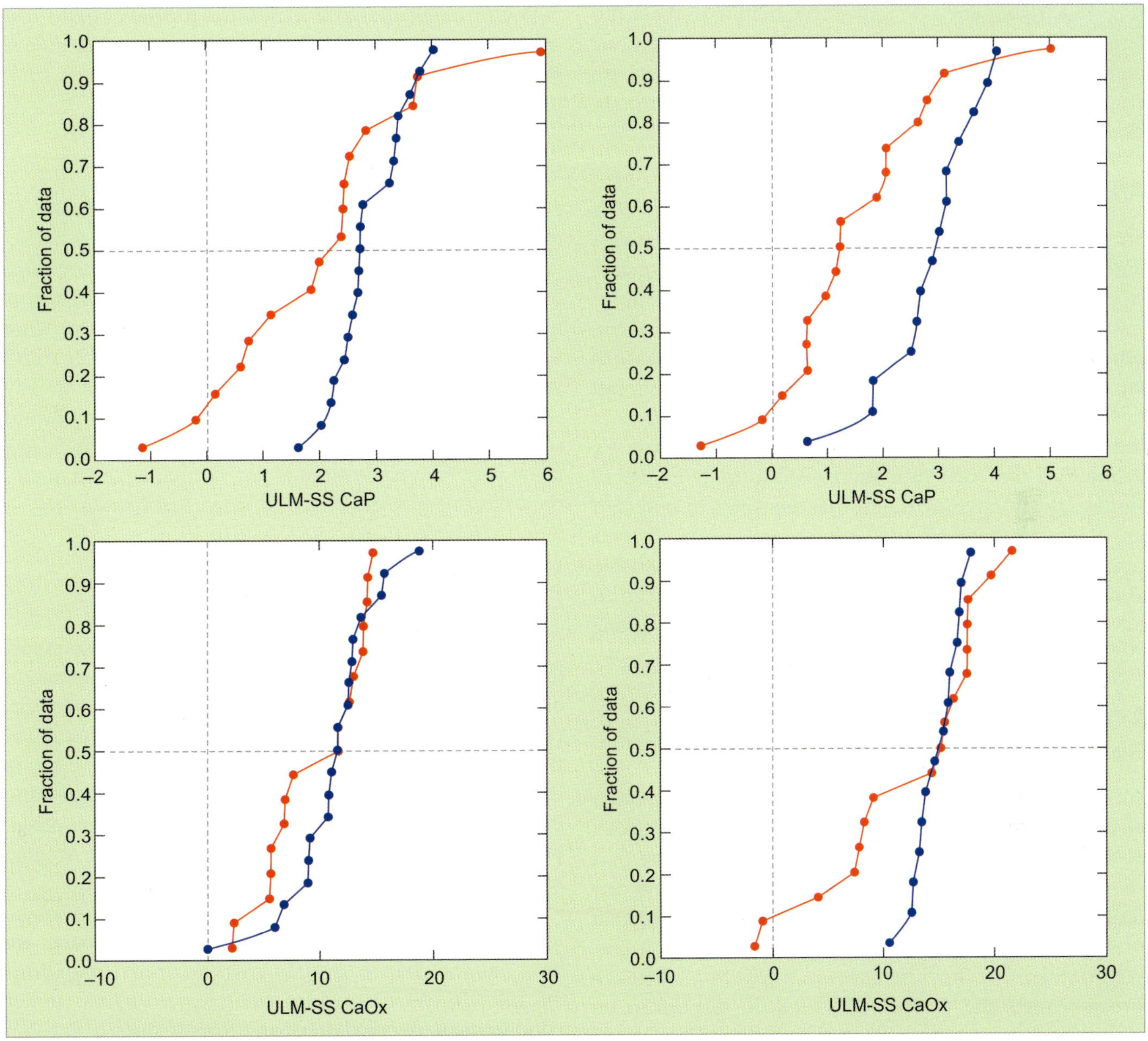

Fig. 15.9: Quantile plots of urinary ULM-SS distance in stone-formers (red symbols) and normal subjects (blue symbols) for calcium phosphate (CaP; upper panels) and calcium oxalate (CaOx; lower panels) in men (left panels) and women (right panels). The distance between the upper limit of metastability (ULM) and supersaturation (SS) represents a measure of protection against spontaneous crystallization in a given urine. Note that the distance for ULM-SS CaP is lower among stone formers than normal subjects, particularly in women.

Source: Redrawn from Asplin JR, Parks JH, Chen MS, et al. Reduced crystallization inhibition by urine from men with nephrolithiasis. Kidney Int. 1999;56:1505-16. Asplin JR, Parks JH, Nakagawa Y, et al. Reduced crystallization inhibition by urine from women with nephrolithiasis. Kidney Int. 2002;61:1821-9.

meaning that SS exceeded the ULM, others had distances close to and even overlapping with normal men (blue symbols). For women (Fig. 15.9, right upper panel) the distance between normals (blue symbols) and patients (red symbols) was far more uniform.

The CaOx ULM-SS Distance

Among normal men and women, the distance is slightly higher for women (Fig. 15.8, right panel, "N"), suggesting a greater level of protection. The same is true for stone formers

(Fig. 15.8, right panel, "P"). However, neither of these differences reaches statistical significance. The individual data show the same thing (Fig. 15.9, lower panels). In both sexes, some patients have lower distances than normals, especially among women, but the overlap is appreciable.

An Overview of the ULM-SS Distance

The distance for CaP is far more different between patients and normals than is that for CaOx, a fact very reasonable when you consider that the initial urine crystallizations over interstitial plaque are CaP. Once crystals are present, other crystals can have less trouble forming and urine is always rather saturated with CaOx. Perhaps one does not need to reach the ULM in order to grow the CaOx body over the HA starting place. Clinically, the data point strongly to the idea that CaP SS matters even in patients whose stones are entirely CaOx, and that measures to reduce it are always prudent. No trials have as yet considered this point, so we make it as a proposal that is not unreasonable and if acted on is unlikely to cause harm; a trial focused on lowering CaP SS might be highly successful in preventing CaOx stones.

Crystallization Inhibitors—Special Role of Citrate

Urine contains many molecules that slow the formation of new crystal nuclei,[40] and the growth and aggregation of those that do form.[41] No doubt many of them are part of stone matrix molecules.[42] None except citrate have any direct clinical relevance in that we cannot measure them in practice and have no means to alter their concentrations. We presume that the differences in the ULM-SS distance between men and women and between stone formers and normal people reflect, to some important extent, the activities of these many inhibitors. Unfortunately, neither the ULM nor any other measures of inhibition apart from the simple excretion of citrate are available for clinicians.

Urine Citrate Excretion

These facts have led us to emphasize urine citrate, and to treat low urine citrate as if it were a risk factor for stones. In women, new onset of stones was clearly associated with urinary citrate excretion rates below 450 mg/d (*see* Fig. 15.3) and 550 mg/d for men. These values are below the average values for female and male normals and stone formers.[14] Likewise, the risk level for women at 450 is below the conventional level of 550 as judged from the distribution of normal women (550), whereas that for men is above (550) the conventional risk level of 450 derived from normal distributions.

Urine Citrate Concentration

Presumably, lower citrate excretions will lead to lower citrate concentrations for any given urine flow, just as hypercalciuria leads to higher urine calcium concentrations. Moreover, to the extent that urine calcium excretion is higher than normal and urine citrate excretion lower than normal, their relative concentrations will change—less and less citrate for the available calcium. As we have already shown, however, at least among hypercalciuric calcium stone formers and normals, all eating the same foods, low urine citrate concentration is not a remarkable characteristic of stone formers (Fig. 15.6, upper right panel).

Urine Calcium to Citrate Concentration Differences

Relative concentrations should be among the most important factors concerning stone risk, because a main action of citrate is to bind calcium in a very soluble calcium citrate salt. That bound calcium is unavailable for crystallization with oxalate and phosphate. The epidemiologic data do not permit us to calculate the calcium-to-citrate ratio or difference and compare it to risk of new stone onset, but that could be done at some future time by the original investigators.[14]

However, our CRC-based studies give some advance idea of what might be found. As already mentioned, we have had the chance to study CaOx and CaP stone formers, albeit those selected for being hypercalciuric, under conditions of identical diets, and throughout the day and night. We have already shown (Fig. 15.6, upper left and right panels) that urine calcium molarity rises steadily throughout the day in patients, though not in normal people, and that urine citrate molarity is far less regular and generally higher in CaOx than in CaP stone formers.

If the difference between calcium and citrate molarity is calculated for every period for every subject (Fig. 15.10), the general pattern becomes clear. Among normals, the difference is rarely above 1 (horizontal dashed line). Among both forms of stone former, the difference is much higher and rises throughout the day because calcium molarity rises and citrate molarity does not do so as regularly. In fact, if one compares Figures 15.6 and 15.10,

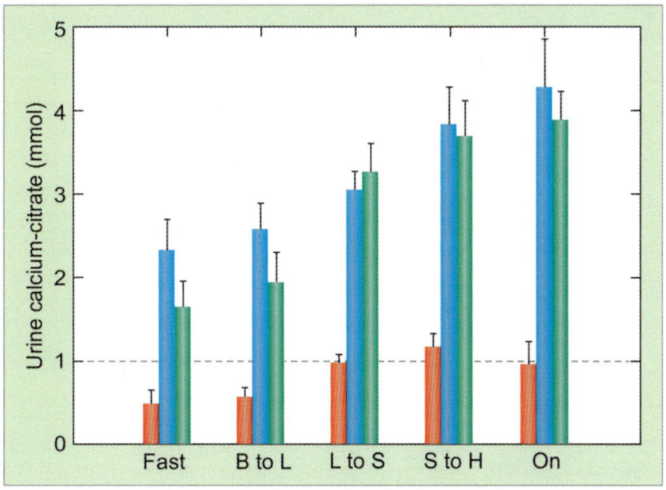

Fig. 15.10: The ratio of urinary calcium and citrate molarity (±SEM) over a 24-hour period in normal subjects (red bars), calcium phosphate (CaP) stone formers (blue bars) and calcium oxalate (CaOx) stone formers (green bars) fed the same diet. Periods of urine collection were as in Figure 15.6. The horizontal line denotes equivalent molar concentrations of calcium and citrate; bars below the line are urines in which citrate molarity exceeds calcium, and bars above the line are the reverse. (FAST: Fasting; B to L: Breakfast and lunch; L to S: Lunch and supper; S to H: Supper to the time the subjects went home; ON: Overnight.
Source: Data redrawn from Bergsland KJ, Coe FL, Gillen DL, et al. A test of the hypothesis that the collecting duct calcium-sensing receptor limits rise of urine calcium molarity in hypercalciuric calcium kidney stone-formers.
Source: Am J Physiol Renal Physiol. 2009;297:F1017-23.

the calcium–citrate difference is far more regular and uniformly abnormal in stone formers than is urine citrate molarity itself.

What this set of bars shows us is that among normal people, for every mmol/L of calcium there is about 1-2 mmol/L of citrate, so citrate can easily reduce the availability of calcium for forming oxalate and phosphate salts. Among both CaP and CaOx stone formers, for every mmol/L of urine calcium there is on average somewhere between only 0.5 mmol/L citrate (fasting) and as little as 0.25 mmol/L (late afternoon and overnight). This imbalance amplifies the effects of hypercalciuria. Not only is the ratio of urine calcium excretion high for the urine flow, which raises urine calcium molarity, but urine citrate excretion is not high enough in relation to urine flow to balance the calcium, leading to the molar imbalances on the figure.

Citrate Has More Effects than Calcium Binding

It can reduce nucleation of HA and CaOx, and slow growth of both crystals.[43] One presumes that the citrate bound to calcium will not be available for crystal surfaces where such effects are likely to occur, so the high calcium-to-citrate molarities in stone formers may well reduce the inhibition effects as it must reduce calcium binding. The latter point has not been tested rigorously and would be of possible research interest.

Calcium-Citrate Imbalance is Worst Overnight

Like the daily variations of SS we have already discussed, the overmatching of citrate by calcium during the day and night emphasizes the importance of steady fluid management which, though it cannot alter the calcium-to-citrate balance, can at least lower the SS values. It also brings to mind that whatever can maintain calcium lower in relation to citrate would be valuable. This reasoning has led to trials of potassium citrate, shown below. As well, we can point out that sodium intake affects calcium excretion[44] and is not known to reduce citrate excretion. Perhaps a low-sodium diet, especially later in the day, might be particularly important for stone prevention. Likewise, protein and sugar loads can increase urine calcium,[45,46] and perhaps the common habit of higher-protein meals at supper and liberal deserts might be less than ideal. No trials have ever been performed concerning timing of nutrient intakes, so this is mere inference, but such trials are reasonable and might be very productive.

Treatment Trials

Trials exist for high water intake,[47] reduced diet sodium and protein,[48] potassium citrate[49-51] and thiazide.[52-54] All have employed "calcium" stone formers, but not all have distinguished CaOx from CaP stone formers. Since the formers are more abundant, we present the results here with the reservation that no specific CaP stone former trials have ever been done. They should be CaP stones occur in part when urine pH is higher than in CaOx stones, so the benefits of potassium citrate, which will raise urine pH, are not certain.

Potassium Citrate

Three trials, two of them double blinded, concern this drug. The patients formed calcium stones and were "hypocitraturic" using criteria derived from normal populations. Two showed a significant reduction in new stone formation (Table 15.3).[49,50] The third used a variable dose format to keep urine pH between 7 and 7.2, and was negative.[51] It differs from the other two not in the outcome of the treated group but in that of the controls who formed very few new

Table 15.3: Treatment trials for calcium stone formers.[48-55]

Treatment	Type	Enrolled			Completed		New stones	
		%F	#C	#T	#C	#T	#C	#T
K citrate 30–60 mEq/d	RCD	56	28	27	20	18	14 (70)	**5 (28)**
K Mg citrate 60 mEq/d	RCD	21	33	31	25	16	16 (64)	**2 (13)**
K citrate (variable dose)*	RC	38	25	25	22	16	6 (27)	5 (31)
Chlorthalidone 25 mg/d	RCD	12	31	42	26	28	12 (46)	**4 (14)**
HCTZ 25 mg 2/d	RCD	24	25	25	25	23	10 (40)	**4 (17)**
Indapamide 2.5 mg/d	RCD	24	25	50	21	43	9 (43)	**6 (15)**
LCD vs reduced Na and P (diet)	RC	0	60	60	51	52	23 (45)	**12 (23)**
Allopurinol 300 mg/d	RCD	n/a	31	31	31	29	11 (35)	**5 (17)**

[K: Potassium; Mg: Magnesium; HCTZ: Hydrochlorothiazide; LCD: Low-calcium diet; P: Protein; RCD: Randomized controlled double-blind; RC: Randomized, controlled; Enrolled: Number of controls (#C) and treated (#T) subjects entering the study, and percent female (%F); Completed, number of controls (#C) and treated (#T) subjects who completed the study; new stones, number of subjects who formed stones, () percent of patients who formed one or more new stones during the trial. All studies were 3 years except for the diet study, which was 5 years. n/a: Not available; * Dose of sodium potassium citrate varied to maintain urine pH between 7 and 7.2. Bold indicates T less than C by χ^2 analysis, $p < 0.05$].

stones. Dropout was noticeable, and there is no follow-up of those who left the trial.

Certainly this should be repeated with CaP and CaOx stone formers considered separately. Given one of three negative trials, a repeat of the CaOx study would not be irrelevant. The presumed mechanism of the treatment effect would be the increase in calcium binding and crystal inhibition from urine citrate.

Thiazide

The thiazide diuretics lower urine calcium excretion by complex actions on the proximal and later nephron segments.[56,57] They also appear to increase the balance of bone mineral in a positive direction,[58] which could benefit patients with idiopathic hypercalciuria who are at risk for osteopenia and fracture.[59] Three randomized, controlled, double-blind (RCD) trials have tested thiazides and all three agree in showing a fall in the fraction of patients who form a new stone during the 3 years of trial study (Table 15.3).[52-54] In fact, as Table 15.3 makes clear, the fractions of patients who do recur are strikingly similar (14–17%) despite different investigators and cohorts and the use of three different forms of the drug. It seems unlikely that more trials will disprove the treatment efficacy of thiazide for calcium stone formers.

Unlike potassium citrate, there is little basis for believing that thiazide would be less effective for CaP stone formers than for those whose stones are CaOx, but nevertheless this matter should be tried formally at least once. Although the citrate trials concerned patients whose urine citrate excretion was low, the thiazide trials did not uniquely select for hypercalciuria. This might not be critical in light of Figurs 15.2. Even urine calcium excretions far below the conventional diagnostic cut points appear to confer stone risk, so lowering urine calcium may be indeed beneficial even in the lower ranges under 200 mg/d.

Reduced Diet Sodium and Protein versus Reduced Diet Calcium

Both sodium and protein increase urine calcium excretion.[60,61] On the other hand, reduced diet calcium might not be ideal for the purpose because idiopathic hypercalciuria has a strong renal component and a form of bone mineral instability that fosters mineral loss with low-calcium diets.[62] Yet a low-calcium diet was, for years, a mainstay of calcium stone prevention.

Here, the two were compared in hypercalciuric men eating an Italian cuisine (*see* Table 15.3).[48] The diet did not reduce stone recurrence as markedly as did thiazide, but was more like potassium citrate. Even so, it is without side effects of thiazide and ideal for people who do not want a drug unless diet proves efficacious.

High Water Intake for Patients with a Single Calcium Stone

In a single prospective observational trial, patients who had formed only one calcium stone were counseled to avoid dehydration or to maintain a urine volume above 2.5 L daily.[47] Although only 20% of those with the high urine volumes formed another stone over 5 years, 50% of the controls, who did not, in fact, increase their urine volume, formed another. Of interest, definite risk reduction seemed to occur at around 1.75 L/d in people who had no stones in that above that level the risk ratio for forming a stone was below 1 (*see* Fig. 15.3).

However, those who form new stones do so for more reasons than urine volume, and perhaps among those who make stones the threshold for risk reduction is higher. Likewise, in modern terms, not all of these patients could have been single stone formers. The CT scans were not the universal rule, and the flexible endoscopy that now regularly discloses numerous tiny stones growing on papillae over plaque, stones well below the detection threshold of even the CT scanner, had not yet become part of everyday urological practice.

Ongoing Management and Follow-Up

Only New Measurement Can Disclose Successful Changes in Urine Chemistry

We have no ways of creating trials for clinical practice, generally, so all we can offer is what we have learned to do. It seems to us thoughtless to make changes in diet, fluids, and styles of living, and to give medications as well, without measuring again in a reasonably short time to be sure what was to be changed in urine chemistries really changed. For no reason other than a guess, we chose 6 weeks as the goal, although many people choose to wait longer. When it comes to fluids and diet, at least one of us has gradually shifted to letting patients choose when to do another study—when the diet changes seemed to be not only in effect but tolerable as a long-term habit.

Diet Changes are often Paramount

Because the very physiology of the kidneys and of bone mandate close links between urine calcium excretion, net acid production, and intakes of sodium, protein, and sugar, diet change is a first step. Even more, high sodium intake, especially, reduces the effectiveness of thiazide and promotes potassium wasting.

Sodium

We use the 24-hour urine sodium excretion and protein catabolic rates to judge sodium and protein intakes, and urine sulfate for net acid production. Although we can put forward reasonable nostrums, every patient is his or her own universe. Some so much detest the idea of taking thiazide that they offer to, and in fact do, lower diet sodium so much, and raise urine volume, too, that CaOx SS falls below 4 and CaP SS below 1, goals that have no basis in trials so far but seem reasonable until such trials are done. Others have no wish to limit their culinary pleasures. Between these poles are a bulk of patients for whom a modest reduction of sodium permits a reduced dose of thiazide.

Oxalate

One can raise urine oxalate by eating high-oxalate foods or by eating a low-calcium diet,[63] and for this reason we try to achieve at least 800 mg of diet calcium for our patients and an avoidance of oxalate loads. A glance at Figure 15.2 will remind us that the risk of new stone onset increases when urine oxalate rises above 20–25 mg/d whereas even normal women, and especially normal and stone-forming men, are above that point. Smaller women have trouble getting 800 mg of calcium within their calorie envelop and ask about supplements. Lacking any trials, we assume that calcium supplements taken during a meal will be like food calcium, but this has never been tested for stone formers.

Oxalate is a special issue for another reason. Sometimes we find rather high values, even up to 60 or 70 mg/d, and believe it is from diet excess. Often this is true in that diet change eradicates the excess oxalate. Sometimes it does not, however, and there is either some failure on our part to achieve a better diet plan for our patient or the patient has a primary or secondary form of hyperoxaluria. This is always important. If the urine oxalate remains high, perhaps above 60 or so, despite what appears to be real diet change by the patients, we begin looking for a systemic disease.

Sugar and Protein

Because sugar loads cause spikes of high urine calcium,[45] we ask patients to avoid raw sugars as much as possible. Less glycemic treats like fruit can satisfy some. Others will not give up their snacks and desserts. This is also true with high protein intakes, above 1–1.2 gm/kg per day. As a rule, if possible, we try to put all available changes into play before prescribing drugs, which means follow-up urine testing may go beyond one or even two more 24-hour urine samples.

Fluids

We have already discussed the day cycle, so it is enough here to mention that we place great emphasis on even hydration throughout the day and something extra for overnight. Here, clinical history taking is paramount. Are there everyday long car drives? Long conferences? Lots of air travel? Business enough that water intake is overlooked as a rule? Teachers cannot leave their schoolrooms easily so they limit fluids. Surgeons are this way about their operations, as are pilots on local routes with tight schedules. If you do not know what your patient does all day, for work and play, you have no chance at directing hydration in a manner that will fit into his or her real life. Your efforts may well prove futile and you will seem to your patient inept and uninformed.

Prognosis

The trials are the standard gauge of what to expect, but their results need not transfer readily into real practice. What real practice means is something else altogether. How many patients will do what is advised? How many will stay in treatment or even in your practice? How well will treatment be pursued over time? For those who do persist, how well will stone prevention work? On the other hand, choice of treatment in a practice is individualized and can be adjusted over time, unlike in a trial. Patients usually require a properly chosen combination of fluid, dietary changes and medication. The chosen medication(s) and dose need to be monitored for tolerability, side effects, cost, and efficacy. Our goal with treatment has been to lower urine SS, which will decrease new stone formation—the ultimate end point.

How can one ever do a trial for these matters? It is all observation, and practices cannot, in general, support the costs of long-term observations. Even when they do, what can we learn from single clinics? They are special, their patients are not necessarily those of the common sort, their doctors are committed to stone prevention far more than is reasonable for physicians who cover more ground every day. Being a stone research center for decades, we have kept track and have presented some of our outcomes by 5-year cohorts of follow-up time.[64] We present our data in detail, because we are not aware of any other clinic experiences of this size and duration.

Few Patients Remained Long Term

Of course, all patients with initial evaluation and any follow-up at all are in the first cohort (0–5 years). Only a few hundred (Fig. 15.11) made it to over 20 years, as one might expect. Women (red bars) were the minority mainly because fewer women entered the program. The numbers of patients who entered into each of these cohorts (not shown here) were not very different, so the gradual fall represents patients leaving us. This is important. We have perhaps no less resources for maintaining follow-up than other practices, and in fact have more because grants have always supported as least some people who could help maintain patient continuity. Possibly our style of practice has been less effective in maintaining patient continuity than others might have been. This is an area of research totally relevant to clinical management and, given our results, obviously important.

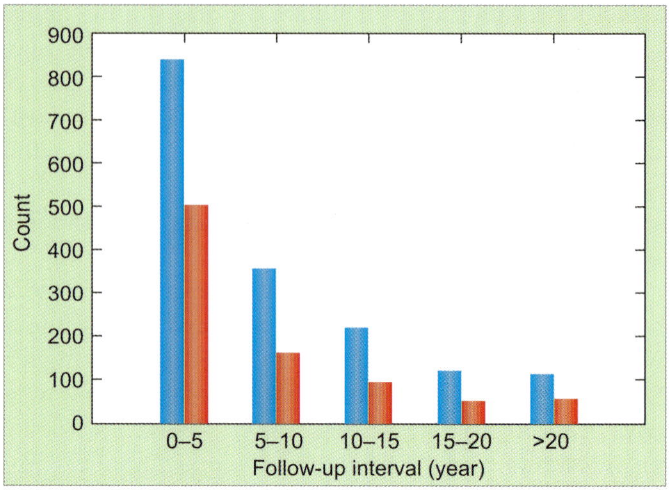

Fig. 15.11: Numbers of patients in each of five cohorts of kidney stone patients. Men (blue bars) and women (red bars) who entered the kidney stone prevention program, and had at least one laboratory follow-up after initial evaluation and treatment, by length of eventual follow-up in the program.
Source: Redrawn from Parks JH, Coe FL. Evidence for durable kidney stone prevention over several decades. BJU Int. 2009;103:1238-46.

Laboratory Stone Risk Outcomes

We chose the mean pretreatment values as a reference point and present them for men and women as the first two bars within each of the five follow-up intervals (Fig. 15.12). The means of the last follow-up are shown as the third and fourth bars, men and women respectively. Urine CaOx, CaP, and UA SS fell compared to control in both sexes (Fig. 15.12, upper panels) and in all time cohorts [compare first and third (men) and second and fourth (women) for each four-bar cluster within a time interval]. The levels of follow-up SS were quite steady, meaning control could be maintained over long periods for those who chose to stay.

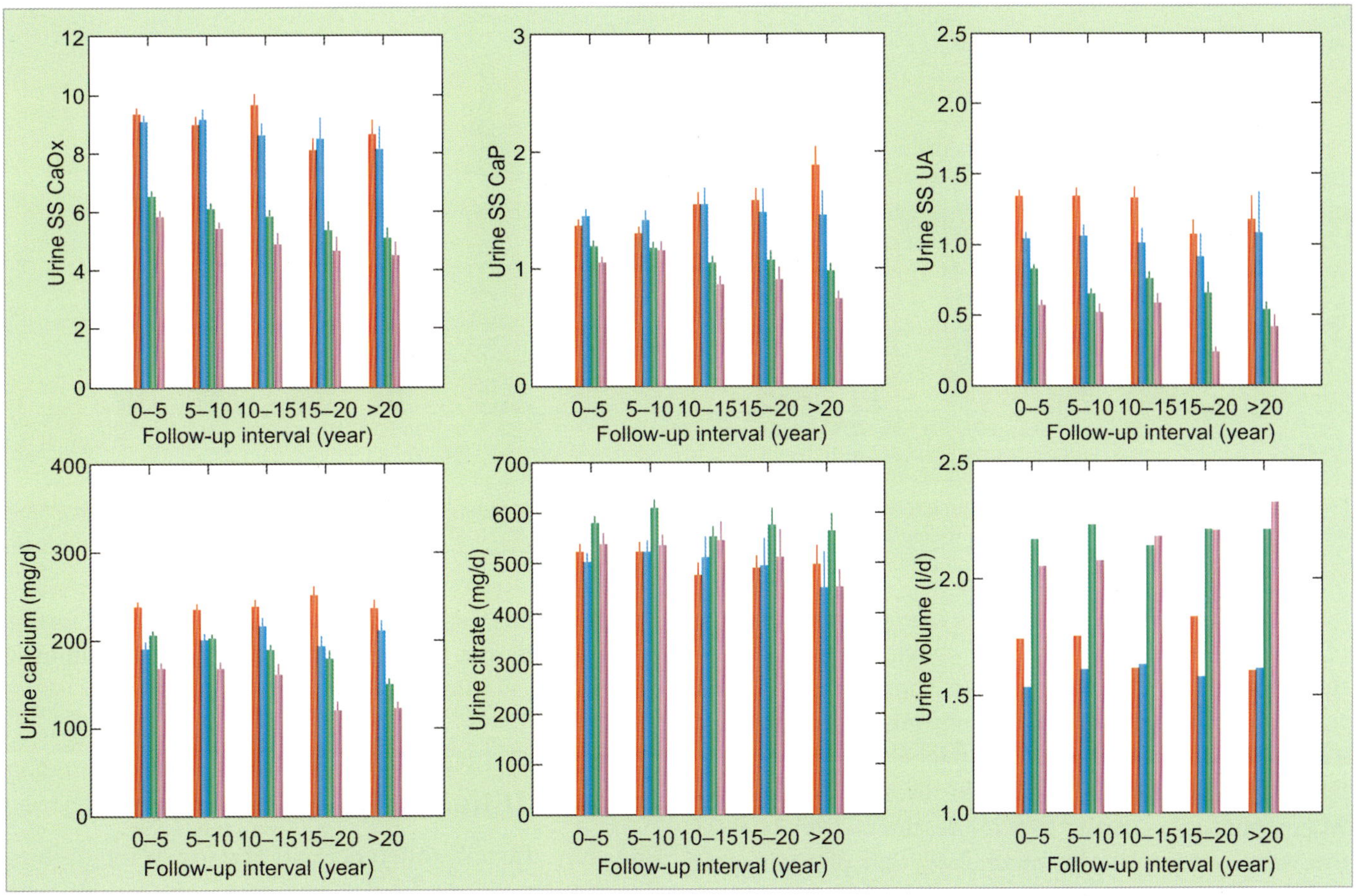

Fig. 15.12: Effects of treatment on urine supersaturation (SS; upper panels) and urine stone risk factors (lower panels) in five cohorts of kidney stone patients. Mean pretreatment values (± SEM) for men (red bars) and women (blue bars) are contrasted with mean values (± SEM) for the same measurement during the follow-up interval (men: green bars; women: pink bars). Changes in urine SS calcium oxalate (CaOx) and SS uric acid (UA), and in urine calcium and volume were significant for both sexes at each interval ($p < 0.01$). Changes in SS calcium phosphate (CaP) were significant except in men at the 5- to 10-year interval and women at the 15- to 20-year interval. Changes in citrate were significant in men ($p < 0.05$) but not in women.
Source: Redrawn from Parks JH, Coe FL. Evidence for durable kidney stone prevention over several decades. BJU Int. 2009;103:1238-46.

The fall in SS was due in part to lower urine calcium, higher citrate, and higher urine volumes (Fig. 15.12, lower panels) in both sexes. Despite what we have said about the primacy of controlling urine sodium via reduction of diet sodium intake, we were entirely unsuccessful in achieving that goal on an overall basis (Fig. 15.13, left panel). Likewise, despite the obvious risk posed by urine oxalate excretions of these patients when compared to the results in Figure 15.2, we failed utterly to achieve a reduction of urine oxalate (Fig. 15.13, right panel), and in fact there was even a slight increase in some follow-up periods, especially among women (compare second and fourth bars).

As expected, there was a marked reduction in numbers of stones and procedures documented in the original publication.[64] Even though we failed to lower urine sodium and oxalate on average, we succeeded in some, and even though we raised urine volume on average, we failed in some. Our general sense from decades of work is that with most patients SS can be lowered one way or another, through changes of volume, calcium, citrate, oxalate, even sodium, and of course by using thiazide and potassium citrate. That is the final sum of what we can say about this matter. All patients are much the same in their range of abnormalities and almost all are individual in their pattern of response to treatment.

IDIOPATHIC CALCIUM PHOSPHATE STONE FORMERS

How are They separated from CaOx Stone Formers?

Because there is often some HA in CaOx stones, the line dividing a CaOx from a CaP stone former is arbitrary. We

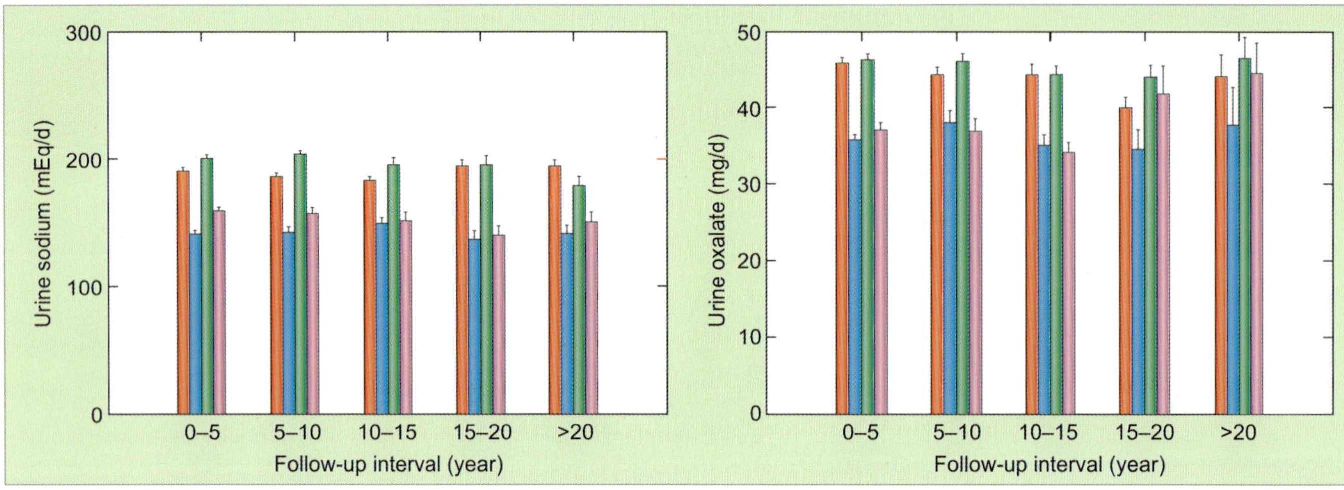

Fig. 15.13: Urine sodium (left panel) and oxalate (right panel) excretion in stone formers pretreatment and post-treatment in five follow-up intervals. Symbols are same as in Figure 15.12.

have tended to use the obvious 50% rule: when the average of all available stones is >50% HA, we name the patient for the predominant crystal. Brushite is another matter. It is a relatively soluble crystal and usually absent from stones. Any BR in stones has led us to so label the patient. Our book is as inclusive as possible of research done everywhere, but in this corner of stone research virtually all of the work relating the histopathology and physiology of patients to their clinical phenotypes has been done by us. So our work predominates for the moment until other add their contributions.

Where and How are the Stones produced?

Unlike the idiopathic CaOx stone formers whose stones often form over white plaque,[65,66] the CaP stone formers exhibit multiple possible sites and no one convincing site. First, some few stones are found over white plaque in both the BR and apatite forms of the disease.[26] Second, as we have already mentioned, the many BD plugs found in both BR and apatite CaP patients often have crystal deposits growing on them, but these overgrowths are not linked to clinical stones.[67] Because stones are usually found free in the calyces or renal pelvis, it is easiest to claim they form in free solution.

Free solution formation has its major problem in explaining why CaP crystals that form do not merely wash away unless somehow anchored. Plug overgrowths and growth on plaque derive their attractiveness precisely from this concern. If one were to identify the more perplexing open research issues in stone research, it is precisely here; we need a new testable hypothesis, or a new way of testing the hypotheses we have: growth on plugs and formation de novo in free solution.

How are Apatite and Brushite Stone Formers Different from One Another?

Clinically, the only differences are the stones themselves. Brushite stones are harder and break less readily with shock wave treatments. The sex ratio is more evenly balanced among BR patients; apatite stone formers are predominantly women.[23,32]

The main distinctions are from surgical appearance and histopathology, whose clinical significance has yet to be shown. The papillae of both forms of CaP stones show variable amounts of plugging of IMCD and terminal ducts of Bellini (BD).[26] Brushite patients exhibit extreme variability of papillae,[68] some pristine others involved with plugging; apatite patients show more consistent plugging of their papillae. The plugs in BR patients, though usually few in number, tend to be very large with extensive tubule injury and peritubular fibrosis. Those of apatite patients are more numerous but smaller.

One way, the two types of patients are alike, is in the details of stones in relation to tissue. Unlike the case of CaOx stones that grow anchored over sites of exposed plaque, many CaP stones are not found attached to papillae, but simply free in the calyces or renal pelvis. Tiny stones are not rare as overgrowths on BD plugs. In the few plug overgrowth units studied thus far, the plug itself has tended to be HA whereas the tiny overgrowths have been mixtures of HA, BR, and even CaOx. Brushite stones usually are round and unattached, giving no clue at all about a possible origin. Although the many BD plugs in HA and BR patients may have crystals growing on them, as if nascent stones, we have no evidence linking such tiny stone overgrowths to actual stones large enough to be clinically relevant.

Mechanisms Producing Phosphate Stones

CaP SS

Given our lengthy presentation about the primacy of SS, you should expect that CaP stones arise because of high urine CaP SS, and that expectation can be fulfilled (Fig. 15.14, upper left panel).[32] If our patients are categorized into octiles of stone CaP percentage (x-axes of all panels), CaP SS clearly rises with CaP% (Fig. 15.14, upper left panel). This was true in women (*red*) and men (*blue*). As small an increase as from 1% or less to 1–15% was associated with a rise in SS from 1.25 (the value at 0%) to 1.7. Thereafter, SS rose to a plateau of about 1.75 with variations in both sexes. This increase was not present for CaOx SS (Fig. 15.14, upper right panel), which showed no appreciable tendency to change among the various octiles of stone CaP.

Primacy of Urine pH

Urine volume, calcium, phosphate, citrate, and pH all affect SS CaP, but volume, phosphate, and citrate excretion rates did not vary with CaP SS and are left off this illustration, though they are detailed in the primary publication.[32] Urine calcium excretion (Fig. 15.14, lower right panel) did rise with CaP% in men and women, though it fell again in both as CaP% rose above 70%. It was urine pH (Fig. 15.14, lower left panel) that most closely tracked with both CaP SS and stone CaP%. Urine pH rose from below 5.9 to as high as 6.2 when CaP% reached 50% and to 6.3 to 6.4 at the highest stone CaP percentages. Even though urine calcium excretion in women fell rather steeply at the highest CaP percentages, SS remained high because of the high pH.

What Increases Urine pH?

Injury

Injury is a prime suspect. Stones cause obstruction; obstruction can reduce urine acidification. Obstruction needs not involve the entire urinary tract. The infundibulum of a calyx can be blocked by stones and affect acidification within only that unit, which might then produce CaP stones. Extracorporeal shock wave lithotripsy (ESWL) has become a common stone disruption modality over the past three decades, and over that same period the CaP content of stones has increased. We have observed that the number of ESWL treatments per patient, adjusted for years of stone disease and age, increases with octiles of CaP% in stones (Fig. 15.15), suggesting a strong link between damage from high-energy ultrasound and loss of acidification. In animals, a single kidney treated with ESWL produces more alkaline urine than its contralateral mate[69] for a period of some months, due apparently to a widespread loss of normal transport along the nephron.

Biology

There are reasons to think that, in part, CaP stones arise from the inherent set point of pH in an individual. An unduly alkaline urine pH in CaP stone formers always calls to mind the possibility of RTA–a group of diseases heralded by failure of normal acidification due to selective injury or mutation of proton or anion transporters.[70] Overt, or "complete" RTA, lowers serum total CO_2, but that is not present in idiopathic CaP stone formers, by definition. Some patients may have "incomplete RTA", which manifests as abnormally high urine pH, normal serum values, and normal net acid excretion but a low urine citrate. These patients have a defect in urine acidification when given an acid load with ammonium chloride;[71,72] however, most such patients appear to be able to acidify under normal conditions. The etiology of this condition is not known for most patients, but there have been descriptions of some such patients who are heterozygotes for mutations in proton transporters.[73,74]

Conversion from CaOx to CaP Stone Formers

Among our patients whose records were sufficient for the analysis, we found 243 patients who formed CaOx stones and then went on to a long enough follow-up in our clinic that we could assess conversion to CaP stones.[75] By conversion we used the criterion of a 20% or more increase of stone CaP%. Of the 243, 181 did not increase by that amount. Their change in stone CaP% (Fig. 15.16, left panel) centered on 0 (red symbols). Among the 62 who did increase their CaP%, the median increase was 60% (blue circles). When they first entered our program, before treatment had begun and their stones were CaOx, those patients who eventually increased their stone CaP% produced urine more alkaline than that of those who did not

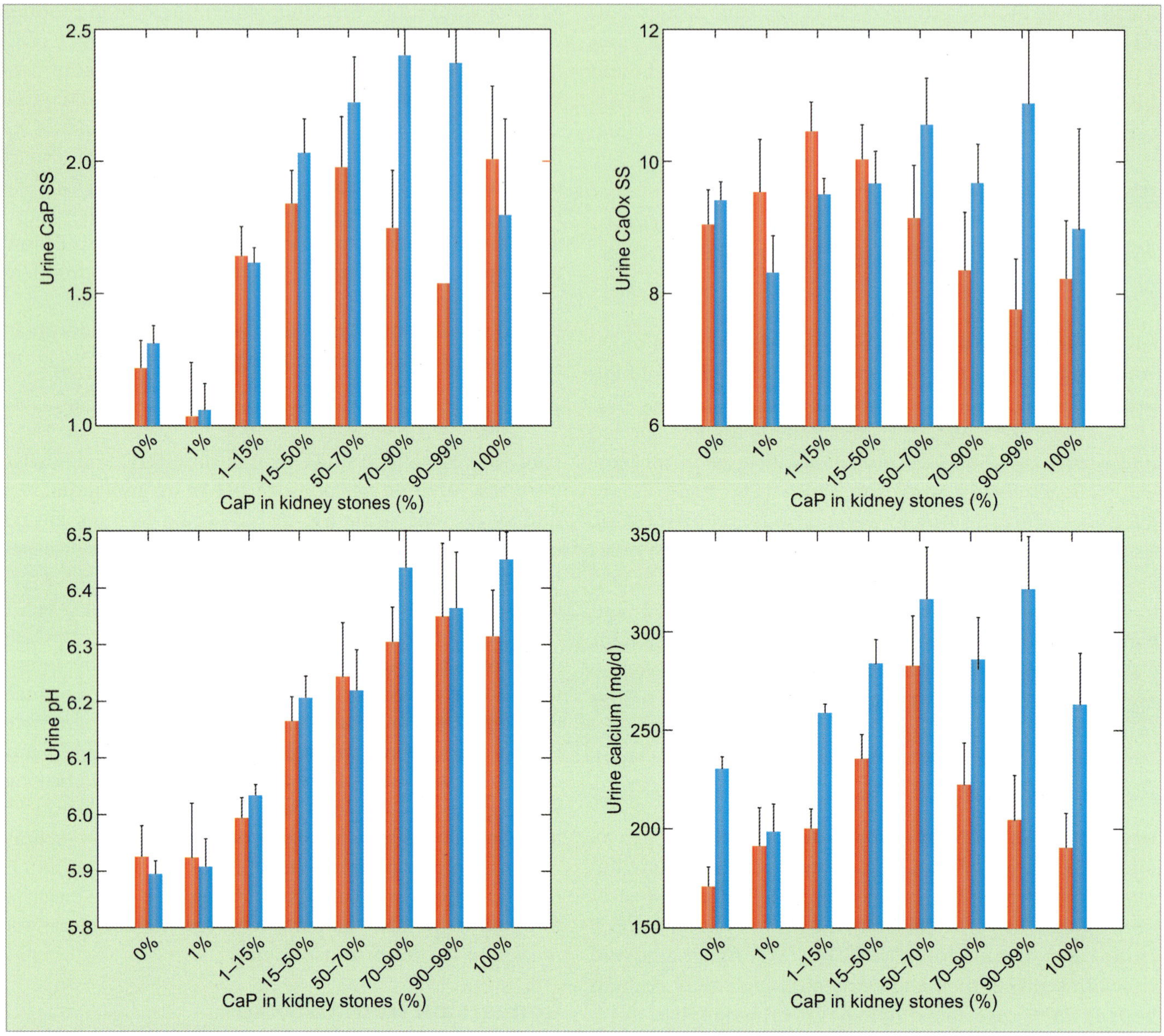

Fig. 15.14: Urine stone risk factors with increasing percentage of calcium phosphate (CaP) in stones, in men (blue bars) and women (red bars). Urine CaP supersaturation (SS) was higher in patients with more CaP in their stones (left upper panel), while calcium oxalate (CaOx) supersaturation (right upper panel) did not show a trend with stone composition. Urine pH also rose with CaP% of stones in both sexes (left lower panel). Urine calcium tended to rise with CaP% (right lower panel) but fell as CaP% rose above 70%.
Source: Redrawn from Parks JH, Worcester EM, Coe FL, et al. Clinical implications of abundant calcium phosphate in routinely analyzed kidney stones. Kidney Int. 2004;66:777-85.

increase their stone CaP%; the difference was about 0.3 units (Fig. 15.16, right panel). Urine pH not only associates with the CaP% of present stones but with the eventual stone CaP over time. Among the same subjects, those who increased stone CaP% had more ESWL treatments than those who did not (not shown).

Given conversion, one would expect some CaOx stone formers, those with higher urine pH values especially, to perhaps show some mixture of stone growth on plaque and tubule plugging with HA. In some studies of papillary pathology of stone formers based on direct operative visualization and papillary biopsy,[76,77] many CaOx stone

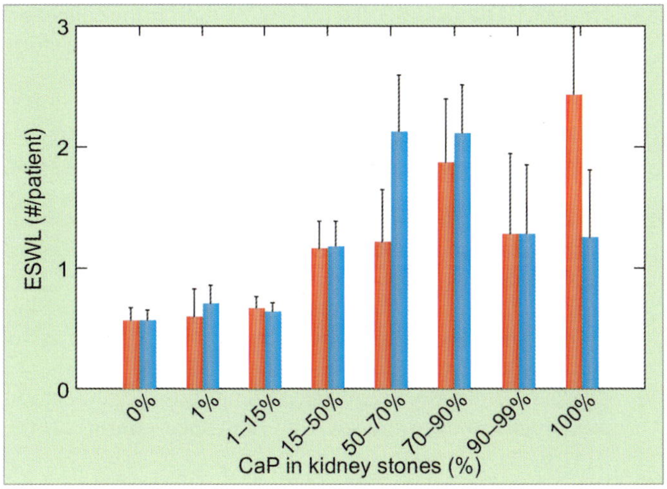

Fig. 15.15: Relationship of extracorporeal shock wave lithotripsy (ESWL) to stone composition. Calcium phosphate (CaP)% in stones rose as the number of ESWL procedures per patient (± SEM) increased, in both sexes ($p < 0.001$ for trend). SEM: Standard error of mean.

Source: Redrawn from Parks JH, Worcester EM, Coe FL, et al. Clinical implications of abundant calcium phosphate in routinely analyzed kidney stones. Kidney Int. 2004;66:777-85.

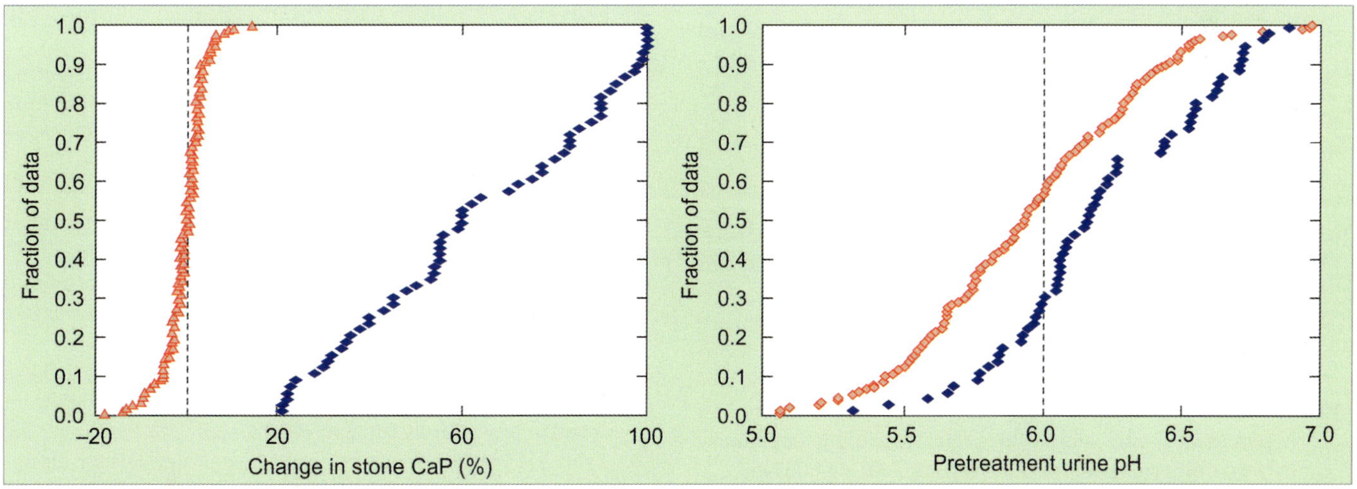

Fig. 15.16: Quantile plots of change in stone CaP% (left panel) and pretreatment urine pH (right panel) of patients who did (blue symbols) or did not (red symbols) convert from calcium oxalate (CaOx) to calcium phosphate (CaP) stone formers (defined as an increase of >20% in stone CaP content during follow-up).

Source: With permission from Parks JH, Coe FL, Evan AP, et al. Urine pH in renal calcium stone-formers who do and do not increase stone phosphate content with time. Nephrol Dial Transplant. 2009;24:130-6.

formers did in fact show plugging. However, none were described as having any CaOx stones growing on plaque, and most were not hypercalciuric. A high percentage was older women.[78]

Time and more observations are essential for us to come to a complete understanding of how stones grow and the forces that create such growths. Of immediate importance is publication of intraoperative images being obtained by numbers of surgeons during the course of stone removal from well-defined clinical phenotypes. Modern digital ureteroscopes all permit such images, and we hope we will soon be seeing them in our journals.

Treatment to Reduce Recurrences

High fluids, reduced sodium and protein diets to lower urine calcium excretion, and thiazide all seem as reasonable for CaP stones as they are for calcium stone formers in general, but because CaP stone formers will be a minority of any trial group of calcium stone formers, the available trials do not apply to them as directly as they do for CaOx stone formers, the majority of calcium stone formers.

The problem is specifically important for potassium citrates. On the one hand, increased urine citrate should reduce CaP SS via calcium binding and inhibit nucleation of BR and apatite, as well. However, these supplements will raise urine pH, which directly raises CaP SS via increase of divalent urine phosphate ion. On balance, then, the alkali salts could be beneficial or neutral or even promote more CaP stones. For this reason a trial is necessary, and in its absence it would seem prudent to use special care with dosing so as to try to increase urine citrate, when possible, without increasing urine CaP SS.

REFERENCES

1. Wilson FP, Berns JS. Tumor lysis syndrome: New challenges and recent advances. Adv Chronic Kidney Dis. 2024;21:18-26.
2. Yarlagadda SG, Perazella MA. Drug-induced crystal nephropathy: an update. Expert Opin Drug Saf. 2008;7:147-58.
3. Daudon M, Hennequin C, Boujelben G, et al. Serial crystalluria determination and the risk of recurrence in calcium stone formers. Kidney Int. 2005;67:1934-43.
4. Hamm LL, Hering-Smith KS, Nakhoul NL. Acid-base and potassium homeostasis. Semin Nephrol. 2013;33:257-64.
5. Solomon R. The relationship between disorders of K^+ and Mg^+ homeostasis. Semin Nephrol. 1987;7:253-62.
6. Gobel U, Kettritz R, Schneider W, et al. The protean face of renal sarcoidosis. J Am Soc Nephrol. 2001;12:616-23.
7. Stechman MJ, Loh NY, Thakker RV. Genetic causes of hypercalciuric nephrolithiasis. Pediatr Nephrol. 2009;24:2321-32.
8. Prie D, Beck L, Silve C, et al. Hypophosphatemia and calcium nephrolithiasis. Nephron Exp Nephrol. 2004;98:e50-4.
9. Parks JH, Coe FL, Evan AP, et al. Clinical and laboratory characteristics of calcium stone-formers with and without primary hyperparathyroidism. BJU Int. 2009;103:670-8.
10. Spivacow FR, Negri AL, del Valle EE, et al. Persistence of hypercalciuria after successful surgical treatment for primary hyperparathyroidism. Int Urol Nephrol. 2013;44:857-63.
11. Shinall MC Jr, Dahir KM, Broome JT. Differentiating familial hypocalciuric hypercalcemia from primary hyperparathyroidism. Endocr Pract. 2013;19:697-702.
12. Perinpam M, Ware EB, Smith JA, et al. Key influence of sex on urine volume and osmolality. Biol Sex Differ. 2016;7:12.
13. Lieske JC, Turner ST, Edeh SN, et al. Heritability of urinary traits that contribute to nephrolithiasis. Clin J Am Soc Nephrol. 2014;9:943-50.
14. Curhan GC, Taylor EN. 24-h uric acid excretion and the risk of kidney stones. Kidney Int. 2008;73:489-96.
15. Coe FL. Hyperuricosuric CaOx nephrolithiasis. Adv Exp Med Biol. 1980;128:439-50.
16. Pak CY, Peterson R. Successful treatment of hyperuricosuric CaOx nephrolithiasis with potassium citrate. Arch Intern Med. 1986;146:863-7.
17. Halperin ML, Cheema DS, Kamel KS. Physiology of acid-base balance: links with kidney stone prevention. Semin Nephrol. 2006;26:441-6.
18. Nayan M, Elkoushy MA, Andonian S. Variations between two 24-hour urine collections in patients presenting to a tertiary stone clinic. Can Urol Assoc J. 2012;6:30-3.
19. Healy KA, Hubosky SG, Bagley DH. 24-hour urine collection in the metabolic evaluation of stone formers: Is one study adequate? J Endourol. 2013;27:374-8.
20. Alruwaily AF, Dauw CA, Bierlein MJ, et al. How much information is lost when you only collect one 24-hour urine collection during the initial metabolic evaluation? J Urol. 2016; 196:1143-8.
21. Parks JH, Goldfischer E, Asplin JR, et al. A single 24-hour urine collection is inadequate for the medical evaluation of nephrolithiasis. J Urol. 2002;167:1607-12.
22. Singh P, Enders FT, Vaughan LE, et al. Stone composition among first-time symptomatic kidney stone formers in the community. Mayo Clin Proc. 2015;90:1356-65.
23. Lieske JC, Rule AD, Krambeck AE, et al. Stone composition as a function of age and sex. Clin J Am Soc Nephrol. 2014;9: 2141-6.
24. Randall A. The origin and growth of renal calculi. Ann Surg. 1937;105:1009-27.
25. Evan A, Lingeman J, Coe FL, et al. Randall's plaque: pathogenesis and role in CaOx nephrolithiasis. Kidney Int. 2006;69:1313-8.
26. Evan AP, Lingeman JE, Worcester EM, et al. Contrasting histopathology and crystal deposits in kidneys of idiopathic stone formers who produce hydroxyapatite, brushite, or CaOx stones. Anat Rec (Hoboken). 2014;297:731-48.
27. Evan AP, Lingeman JE, Coe FL, et al. Randall's plaque of patients with nephrolithiasis begins in basement membranes of thin loops of Henle. J Clin Invest. 2003;111:607-16.
28. Evan AP, Coe FL, Lingeman JE, et al. Mechanism of formation of human CaOx renal stones on Randall's plaque. Anat Rec (Hoboken). 2007;290:1315-23.
29. Evan AP, Coe FL, Rittling SR, et al. Apatite plaque particles in inner medulla of kidneys of CaOx stone formers: osteopontin localization. Kidney Int. 2005;68:145-54.
30. Evan AP, Bledsoe S, Worcester EM, et al. Renal inter-alpha-trypsin inhibitor heavy chain 3 increases in CaOx stone-forming patients. Kidney Int. 2007;72:1503-11.
31. Bergsland KJ, Coe FL, Gillen DL, et al. A test of the hypothesis that the collecting duct calcium-sensing receptor limits rise of urine calcium molarity in hypercalciuric calcium kidney stone formers. Am J Physiol Renal Physiol. 2009;297: F1017-23.
32. Parks JH, Worcester EM, Coe FL, et al. Clinical implications of abundant calcium phosphate in routinely analyzed kidney stones. Kidney Int. 2004;66:777-85.
33. Knight J, Jiang J, Wood KD, et al. Oxalate and sucralose absorption in idiopathic CaOx stone formers. Urology. 2011;78:475.
34. Borghi L, Guerra A, Meschi T, et al. Relationship between supersaturation and CaOx crystallization in normals and idiopathic CaOx stone formers. Kidney Int. 1999;55:1041-50.
35. Parks JH, Barsky R, Coe FL. Gender differences in seasonal variation of urine stone risk factors. J Urol. 2003;170:384-8.
36. Asplin JR, Mandel NS, Coe FL. Evidence of calcium phosphate supersaturation in the loop of Henle. Am J Physiol. 1996;270:F604-13.

37. Asplin JR, Parks JH, Coe FL. Dependence of upper limit of metastability on supersaturation in nephrolithiasis. Kidney Int. 1997;52:1602-8.
38. Asplin JR, Parks JH, Chen MS, et al. Reduced crystallization inhibition by urine from men with nephrolithiasis. Kidney Int. 1999;56:1505-16.
39. Asplin JR, Parks JH, Nakagawa Y, et al. Reduced crystallization inhibition by urine from women with nephrolithiasis. Kidney Int. 2002;61:1821-9.
40. Kumar V, Lieske JC. Protein regulation of intrarenal crystallization. Curr Opin Nephrol Hypertens. 2006;15:374-80.
41. Aggarwal KP, Narula S, Kakkar M, et al. Nephrolithiasis: molecular mechanism of renal stone formation and the critical role played by modulators. Biomed Res Int. 2013;2013: 292953.
42. Witzmann FA, Evan AP, Coe FL, et al. Label-free proteomic methodology for the analysis of human kidney stone matrix composition. Proteome Sci. 2016;14:4.
43. Qiu SR, Orme CA. Dynamics of biomineral formation at the near-molecular level. Chem Rev. 2008;108:4784-822.
44. Nouvenne A, Meschi T, Prati B, et al. Effects of a low-salt diet on idiopathic hypercalciuria in calcium-oxalate stone formers: a 3-mo randomized controlled trial. Am J Clin Nutr. 2010;91:565-70.
45. Lemann J Jr, Piering WF, Lennon EJ. Possible role of carbohydrate-induced calciuria in CaOx kidney-stone formation. N Engl J Med. 1969;280:232-7.
46. Maalouf NM, Moe OW, Adams-Huet B, et al. Hypercalciuria associated with high dietary protein intake is not due to acid load. J Clin Endocrinol Metab. 2011;96:3733-40.
47. Borghi L, Meschi T, Amato F, et al. Urinary volume, water and recurrences of idiopathic calcium nephrolithiasis: a 5-year randomized prospective study. J Urol. 1996;155:839-43.
48. Borghi L, Schianchi T, Meschi T, et al. Comparison of two diets for the prevention of recurrent stones in idiopathic hypercalciuria. N Engl J Med. 2002;346:77-84.
49. Barcelo P, Wuhl O, Servitge E, et al. Randomized double-blind study of potassium citrate in idiopathic hypocitraturic calcium nephrolithiasis. J Urol. 1993;150:1761-4.
50. Ettinger B, Pak CY, Citron JT, et al. Potassium-magnesium citrate is an effective prophylaxis against recurrent CaOx nephrolithiasis. J Urol. 1997;158(6):2069-73.
51. Hofbauer J, Hobarth K, Szabo N, et al. Alkali citrate prophylaxis in idiopathic recurrent CaOx urolithiasis—a prospective randomized study. Br J Urol. 1994;73:362-5.
52. Ettinger B, Citron JT, Livermore B, et al. Chlorthalidone reduces CaOx calculous recurrence but magnesium hydroxide does not. J Urol. 1988;139:679-84.
53. Laerum E, Larsen S. Thiazide prophylaxis of urolithiasis: a double-blind study in general practice. Acta Med Scand. 1984;215:383-9.
54. Borghi L, Meschi T, Guerra A, et al. Randomized prospective study of a nonthiazide diuretic, indapamide, in preventing calcium stone recurrences. J Cardiovasc Pharmacol. 1993;22(Suppl 6):S78-86.
55. Ettinger B, Tang A, Citron JT, et al. Randomized trial of allopurinol in the prevention of calcium oxalate calculi. New Engl J Med. 1986;315:1386-9.
56. Bergsland KJ, Worcester EM, Coe FL. Role of proximal tubule in the hypocalciuric response to thiazide of patients with idiopathic hypercalciuria. Am J Physiol Renal Physiol. 2013;305:F592-9.
57. Jang HR, Kim S, Heo NJ, et al. Effects of thiazide on the expression of TRPV5, calbindin-D28K, and sodium transporters in hypercalciuric rats. J Korean Med Sci. 2009;24(Suppl):S161-9.
58. Coe FL, Parks JH, Bushinsky DA, et al. Chlorthalidone promotes mineral retention in patients with idiopathic hypercalciuria. Kidney Int. 1988;33:1140-6.
59. Krieger NS, Bushinsky DA. The relation between bone and stone formation. Calcif Tissue Int. 2013;93:374-81.
60. Ticinesi A, Nouvenne A, Maalouf NM, et al. Salt and nephrolithiasis. Nephrol Dial Transplant. 2016;31:39-45.
61. Calvez J, Poupin N, Chesneau C, et al. Protein intake, calcium balance and health consequences. Eur J Clin Nutr. 2012;66:281-95.
62. Coe FL, Favus MJ, Crockett T, et al. Effects of low-calcium diet on urine calcium excretion, parathyroid function and serum 1,25(OH)2D3 levels in patients with idiopathic hypercalciuria and in normal subjects. Am J Med. 1982;72:25-32.
63. von Unruh GE, Voss S, Sauerbruch T, et al. Dependence of oxalate absorption on the daily calcium intake. J Am Soc Nephrol. 2004;15:1567-73.
64. Parks JH, Coe FL. Evidence for durable kidney stone prevention over several decades. BJU Int. 2009;103:1238-46.
65. Miller NL, Gillen DL, Williams JC Jr, et al. A formal test of the hypothesis that idiopathic CaOx stones grow on Randall's plaque. BJU Int. 2009;103:966-71.
66. Letavernier E, Vandermeersch S, Traxer O, et al. Demographics and characterization of 10,282 Randall plaque-related kidney stones: A new epidemic? Medicine (Baltimore). 2015;94:e566.
67. Evan AP, Worcester EM, Coe FL, et al. Mechanisms of human kidney stone formation. Urolithiasis. 2015;43(Suppl 1):19-32.
68. Evan AP, Lingeman JE, Coe FL, et al. Crystal-associated nephropathy in patients with brushite nephrolithiasis. Kidney Int. 2005;67:576-91.
69. Evan AP, Coe FL, Connors BA, et al. Mechanism by which shock wave lithotripsy can promote formation of human calcium phosphate stones. Am J Physiol Renal Physiol. 2015;308:F938-49.
70. Kurtz I. Molecular mechanisms and regulation of urinary acidification. Compr Physiol. 2014;4:1737-74.
71. Arampatzis S, Ropke-Rieben B, Lippuner K, et al. Prevalence and densitometric characteristics of incomplete distal renal tubular acidosis in men with recurrent calcium nephrolithiasis. Urol Res. 2012;40:53-9.
72. Gault MH, Chafe LL, Morgan JM et al. Comparison of patients with idiopathic calcium phosphate and CaOx stones. Medicine. 1991;70:345-58.

73. Dhayat NA, Schaller A, Albano G, et al. The vacuolar H^+-ATPase B1 subunit polymorphism p.E161K associates with impaired urinary acidification in recurrent stone formers. J Am Soc Nephrol. 2016;27:1544-54.
74. Zhang J, Fuster DG, Cameron MA, et al. Incomplete distal renal tubular acidosis from a heterozygous mutation of the V-ATPase B1 subunit. Am J Physiol Renal Physiol. 2014;307:F1063-71.
75. Parks JH, Coe FL, Evan AP, et al. Urine pH in renal calcium stone formers who do and do not increase stone phosphate content with time. Nephrol Dial Transplant. 2009;24:130-6.
76. Rivera M, Cockerill PA, Enders F, et al. Characterization of inner medullary collecting duct plug formation among idiopathic CaOx stone formers. Urology. 2016;94:47-52.
77. Linnes MP, Krambeck AE, Cornell L, et al. Phenotypic characterization of kidney stone formers by endoscopic and histological quantification of intrarenal calcification. Kidney Int. 2013;84:818-25.
78. Wang X, Krambeck AE, Williams JC Jr, et al. Distinguishing characteristics of idiopathic CaOx kidney stone formers with low amounts of Randall's plaque. Clin J Am Soc Nephrol. 2014;9:1757-63.

CHAPTER

16 Primary Hyperparathyroidism and Renal Stone Disease

Edwin L Kaplan, Megan K Applewhite, Raymon H Grogan

INTRODUCTION

Primary hyperparathyroidism (PHPT) is no longer an uncommon disease. It is diagnosed in ~100,000 people yearly in the United States with an overall prevalence of 0.2–1%.[1] The prevalence is higher in patients >65 years old (1.5%)[2] and is most common in postmenopausal women (2.1–3.4%).[3] It is the most common cause of hypercalcemia in nonhospitalized individuals. Kidney stones are a frequent complication of this disorder. Initially, patients who were diagnosed with PHPT were found to have severe bone disease; however, it was soon recognized that kidney stones were the most common manifestation of this disease. Before the advent of routine testing of serum calcium concentration, nephrolithiasis was found in >50% of patients.[4] Now, since patients are diagnosed earlier with PHPT because of routine laboratory work, they have fewer or no symptoms, and nephrolithiasis is found in <10% of those operated upon.[5] Parathyroidectomy is the only cure for PHPT and is an effective means of reducing or curing the stone disease that accompanies it. This chapter will discuss the diagnosis, location studies, and different operations that are used by surgeons as treatment for this disorder.

HISTORICAL PERSPECTIVE

In 1925, the first parathyroidectomy was performed in Vienna on "Albert," the now famous trolley car operator.[6] Albert had developed severe bone disease (Fig. 16.1), a condition that was thought by some pathologists at that time to be due to parathyroid insufficiency. Only after failure of injections of parathyroid extracts and the failure of a parathyroid transplant was surgical excision considered. In 1925, a parathyroidectomy was performed by a young surgeon, Dr Felix Mandl. One large gland was removed, and the operation resulted in dramatic symptomatic improvement of Albert's condition for about 6 years; then, his bone problems recurred.[7]

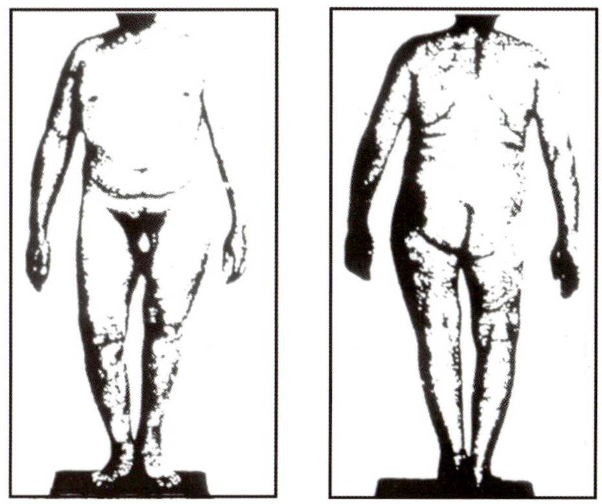

Fig. 16.1: "Albert," the now famous trolley car operator underwent the first parathyroidectomy in Vienna in 1925. His severe bone disease is pictured here.

The first patient who had an operation in the United States for PHPT was a merchant marine captain, Charles Martell (Figs. 16.2A and B).[8] Over the years, Captain Martell had developed debilitating bone disease with kyphoscoliosis and "brown tumors" that caused fractures. He was recognized to have hypercalcemia and hypophosphatemia. It was noted that these blood abnormalities were similar to changes that occurred when parathyroid extract was given to children with chronic lead poisoning to mobilize lead from their bones. They, too, developed hypercalcemia and low circulating phosphate levels. Thus, it was postulated that Martell had an overactivity of the parathyroid glands. Unaware of the successful parathyroidectomy in Vienna, doctors at Massachusetts General Hospital explored his neck in 1926.[9] Unfortunately, only normal structures were found. Five additional unsuccessful neck operations were performed over the following years. During this time he developed severe nephrolithiasis. Finally, in 1933, a large parathyroid gland was found in his mediastinum. About 90% of it was resected; the remaining part was intentionally

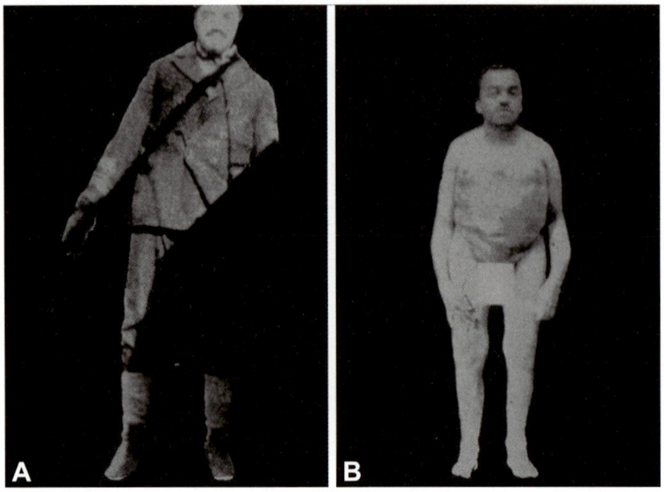

Figs. 16.2A and B: Captain Charles Martell pictured (A) as a vigorous, young merchant marine and (B) after years of a debilitating bone disease. Note his loss of stature with kyphoscoliosis.

Table 16.1: Clues to the diagnosis of hyperparathyroidism in the first 343 cases at the Massachusetts General Hospital.

Clue	*Number of cases*
Renal stones	195
Bone disease	80
Peptic ulcer	27
Fatigue	10
Pancreatitis	9
Central nervous system signs	7
Hypertension	6
Mental disturbance	3
Multiple endocrine abnormalities	3
No symptoms (routine laboratory test)	2
Lump in neck	1

left in place to try to prevent tetany. Despite this, as might be expected in a patient with very severe bone disease, postoperative tetany occurred. Six weeks later, Charles Martell died in chronic renal failure following an operation to remove a kidney stone that had blocked his ureter.

The first two patients who were operated on for PHPT had serious difficulties associated with their surgical therapies. Albert appears to have demonstrated recurrent hyperparathyroidism. Charles Martell had an ectopic parathyroid adenoma and required multiple neck operations, which resulted in removal of most, if not all, of his normal parathyroid glands before it was found in his chest. Severe hypocalcemia, which was difficult to treat, followed removal of most of his mediastinal tumor. It is interesting that now, almost 90 years after the first parathyroidectomy, the same complications still occur and remain a challenge to surgeons.

SYMPTOMS

When first described, PHPT was a disease of the bones. It soon became apparent, however, that kidney stones were more common than severe bone disease. Gradually, other symptoms and signs were added to this syndrome, largely because of the work of Oliver Cope et al. (Table 16.1).[10] Later, an increased incidence of chondrocalcinosis and pseudogout was recognized as well.[11]

As medical students, we learned that PHPT is associated with "painful bones, renal stones, abdominal groans, and psychiatric moans." Today, most individuals are discovered to have this disorder because of the recognition of hypercalcemia on multiphasic chemical blood screening tests.[12] Many of these patients are thought by their physicians to be "asymptomatic." By this designation, many physicians mean that they have none of the classic symptoms and signs that are listed in Table 16.1. However, a careful history often discloses subtle or even profound symptoms of fatigue, weakness, depression, polyuria, polydipsia, arthralgia, or constipation.[13] Further testing often shows an accelerated course of osteoporosis. Studies from Uppsala,[14] for example, have documented that alterations in neurotransmitter levels comparable to those found in endogenous depression are present in patients with PHPT. These abnormalities, they have shown, revert to normal after successful parathyroidectomy. Thus, the definition of "asymptomatic" in patients with PHPT often differs according to "the eye of the beholder."

DIAGNOSIS

To be successful, the clinician must diagnose those individuals who have PHPT and distinguish them from the many others who have hypercalcemia of other causes (Table 16.2). The diagnosis of PHPT is usually made by findings of elevated serum calcium levels or ionized calcium levels associated with elevated parathyroid hormone (PTH) concentrations. The importance of measurements of other serum and urinary values in the diagnosis of PHPT is discussed elsewhere.

Table 16.2: Differential diagnoses of hypercalcemia.
Malignancy
• Solid tumors with or without bony metastases
• Multiple myeloma
• Lymphomas and leukemias
Endocrine
• Hyperparathyroidism
• Hyper- and hypothyroidism
• Addison's disease
• VIPomas, pheochromocytoma
Granulomatous disease
• Sarcoidosis
• Tuberculosis
Increased intake
• Calcium
• Vitamin D and vitamin A intoxication
• Milk alkali syndrome
Miscellaneous
• Benign familial hypocalciuric hypercalcemia
• Paget's disease with immobilization
• Thiazides
• Lithium

Source: Adapted from Clark OH, Way LW, Hunt TK. Recurrent hyperparathyroidism. Ann Surg. 1976;184(4):391-402.

A list of the differential diagnoses of hypercalcemia is shown in Table 16.2. A detailed discussion of each disease state is beyond the scope of this chapter. It should be observed, however, that although cancer that is metastatic to bone is the most common cause of hypercalcemia in hospitalized patients, PHPT is the most common cause of hypercalcemia among outpatients who are typically otherwise healthy[13] and is the second most common cause in the hospital setting. An uncommon but difficult problem in the past has been the fact that some tumors elaborate a PTH-like peptide that is thought to be the cause of hypercalcemia. However, now PTH-related protein can be measured in the blood of such patients and can be used to differentiate them from others with PHPT.[15] Furthermore, most other diseases that produce hypercalcemia result in a suppressed serum PTH level and can be easily differentiated from PHPT. Thus, inappropriate parathyroidectomy can be avoided.

INDICATIONS FOR A PARATHYROIDECTOMY

The purpose of the parathyroidectomy in PHPT is to restore the patient to a normocalcemic, euparathyroid state, and to reverse the symptoms associated with this disease. With a correction of the hyperparathyroid state, most symptoms and signs of the disease are reversed (Table 16.3).[16,17] Bone disease and bone pain are usually benefitted. Roentgenographic evidence is seen for healing bone cysts; the "salt and pepper" osteolysis of the skull, and subperiosteal bone resorption are corrected. Patients with nephrolithiasis develop far fewer new stones. Renal function has also been shown to improve in some studies, but not in all. Symptoms of mood changes, weakness/tiredness, irritability, and thirst are often seen to improve after surgery.[18] Hypertension, seen in many patients with this disease, has only rarely been seen to improve after surgery. However, a recent study of symptomatic patients with PHPT demonstrated substantial improvement of cardiac and vascular dysfunction 6 months after parathyroidectomy.[19]

Because of the success of parathyroidectomy, most clinicians believe that if a patient is symptomatic and is not at prohibitive medical risk, a parathyroidectomy should be performed. Some differences of opinion exist about the value of parathyroidectomy for patients who are asymptomatic. Scholz and Purnell[20] at the Mayo Clinic demonstrated that about half of their asymptomatic patients with clear hyperparathyroidism who could be successfully followed for 10 years developed some problem associated with their disease. They recommended parathyroidectomy in such patients because follow-up was difficult and the operation was very successful at their institution. Other studies have demonstrated the value of parathyroidectomy in patients with PHPT and asymptomatic osteoporosis, as measured by bone densitometry.[21] Not all investigators agree, however.[17] Thus, the value of parathyroidectomy in truly asymptomatic patients is still being debated.

The most recent "Guidelines for the Management of Asymptomatic Primary Hyperparathyroidism"[22] recommend operation under the following indications:

1. All patients should be <50 years of age.
2. Serum calcium level is >1 mg/dL or above the upper limit of normal.
3. Creatinine clearance should be <60 cc/min.
4. A 24-hour urinary calcium excretion >400 mg and increased stone risk by biochemical stone risk analysis.

Table 16.3: Response of symptoms/signs to parathyroid surgery at five-year follow-up.

	Preoperative prevalence (%)		*Long-term improvement (%)*	
Symptoms and signs	*Ronni–Sivula and Sivula (n = 289)*	*Lafferty and Hubay (n = 100)*	*Ronni–Sivula and Sivula (n = 289)*	*Lafferty and Hubay (n = 68)*
Osteitis	4	6	100	100
Pancreatitis	2	3	100	100
Renal calculi	34	18	90	92
Neuropsychiatric*	61†	21	72	71
Constipation	14	15	63	70
Peptic ulcer	3	16	25	45
Hypertension	31	48	3	7
Impaired renal function	14	15	43	0
Asymptomatic	35	49	0	0

Source: Adapted from Lafferty FW, Hubay CA. Primary hyperparathyroidism. A review of the long-term surgical and nonsurgical morbidities as a basis for a rational approach to treatment. Arch Intern Med. 1989;149(4):789-96.
*It Includes fatigue, lethargy, malaise, weakness, depression, headache, irritability, and confusion.
†It combines malaise, fatigue, and weakness in 46% plus depression in 15%.

5. Presence of nephrolithiasis or nephrocalcinosis by X-ray, ultrasound, or computed tomography (CT).
6. T score < -2.5 at lumbar spine, total hip, femoral neck, or distal one-third radius.
7. Vertebral fracture by X-ray, CT, of magnetic resonance imaging (MRI).
8. Patients for whom medical surveillance is neither desired nor possible.

Over the years, the indications for operation in asymptomatic patients have broadened and more patients are now considered candidates for parathyroidectomy. It is agreed that the most important prerequisite for success is an experienced parathyroid surgeon.

PITFALLS FOR THE SURGEON

Difficulties associated with parathyroidectomy for PHPT relate to the variability in the number of parathyroid glands, the different locations of normal and pathologic glands, and problems distinguishing normal glands from others that are subtly diseased. To be successful, a parathyroid surgeon must have an excellent knowledge of the anatomy, embryology, and pathophysiology of the parathyroid glands.

Number of Parathyroid Glands

In an extensive autopsy study, Gilmour[23] found that roughly 80% of individuals had four parathyroid glands, 6% had five, and 13% had three. Two glands or six glands were present very rarely. Other anatomists and surgeons have found >6 glands to be present in some cases. This variability creates difficulties for the surgeon in several situations. First, four normal glands may be present in the neck, whereas a fifth, a supernumerary gland, which is adenomatous, may be present in the mediastinum. This situation occurred in 5 of 14 mediastinal parathyroid adenomas that were reported from the Mayo Clinic prior to 1970,[24] for example. The most common location for a supernumerary gland is in the thymus gland.

A second example in which the number of glands plays an important role is in primary parathyroid hyperplasia. Particularly in the multiple endocrine neoplasia type 1 (MEN-1), recurrent hyperparathyroidism occurs frequently, even after subtotal resection of parathyroid glands in the neck.[25,26] A thymectomy must be included as part of the standard parathyroidectomy for this condition in order to remove other parathyroid glands or parathyroid rests that might be present in this tissue.

Location of Parathyroid Glands

Embryology

The upper parathyroid glands arise embryologically from the dorsal part of the fourth branchial pouches, along with the lateral lobes of the thyroid, called the ultimobranchial bodies (Figs. 16.3A to C).[23,27] They descend only slightly

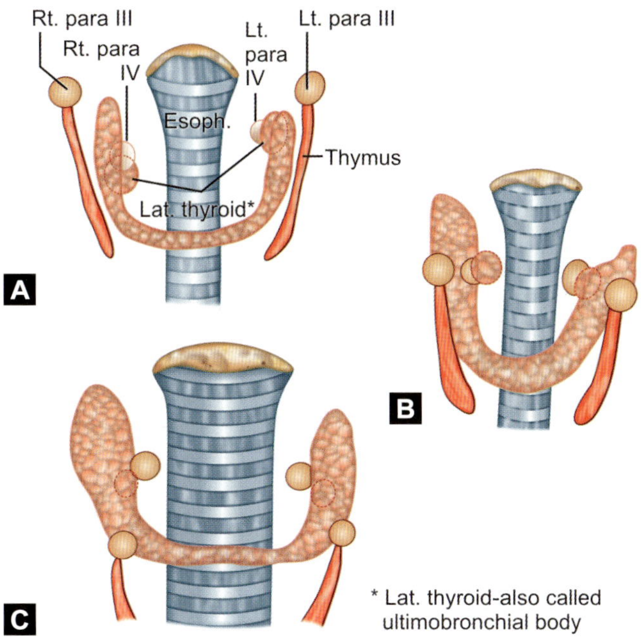

Figs. 16.3A to C: (A, B) Schematic representation of the embryologic shifts in location of the thyroid, parafollicular, and parathyroid tissues. (C) Approximation of the adult position.
Source: Redrawn with permission from Sedgwick CE, Cady B. Embryology and developmental abnormalities. Major Probl Clin Surg. 1980;15:6-18.

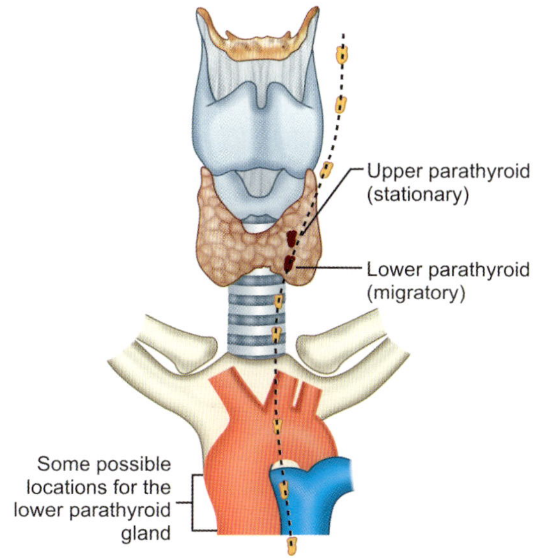

Fig. 16.4: Descent of the lower parathyroid. While the upper parathyroid occupies a relatively constant position in relation to the middle or upper third of the lateral thyroid lobe, the lower parathyroid normally migrates in embryonic life and may end up anywhere along the course of the dotted line. When this gland is in the chest, it is nearly always in the anterior mediastinum.

during embryologic life along with the thyroid and continue to remain in close association with the upper portion of the lateral thyroid lobes. Because of their relatively circumscribed migration, their position in adult life remains quite constant.

The lower parathyroids arise from the dorsal part of the third branchial pouches along with the thymus and they descend with the thymus. Because they travel so far in embryologic life, they have a very wide range of distribution in the adult. They may be found all the way from just beneath the mandible anterior to the carotid artery bifurcation, to the pericardium (Fig. 16.4). When the lower parathyroid gland descends into the mediastinum, it is almost always anterior to the recurrent laryngeal nerve and within the thymus gland.

Location of Normal Glands

The average weight of a normal parathyroid gland is between 30 and 50 mg. Some may be slightly heavier. They can be thought of as being about half the size of one's little fingernail; because they are small, they can be difficult to identify. Normal glands are usually yellow/brown in color and can look like fat, particularly to the inexperienced eye. They are also difficult to find because of their various possible locations.

In most cases, the normal upper gland may be found on the posterior portion of the middle third of the thyroid, usually toward the superior part of this area, either under a delicate fascia on the thyroid lobe or on a projecting nodule (Fig. 16.5).[23,28] It is usually found cephalad to the inferior thyroid artery and close to the recurrent laryngeal nerve as it enters the larynx.

The normal inferior parathyroid glands are more variable (Fig. 16.5).[23] In somewhat >50% of cases, the lower parathyroid is found on the lateral or posterior surface of the lower pole of the thyroid gland, not more than 0.5 cm below the lower pole. The next most common location, in 12.8% of the cases, is within 1 cm below the lower pole of the thyroid. In most of the remaining individuals, the lower parathyroid gland is found within the tongue of the thymus (called the thyrothymic ligament). The tongue of the thymus usually can be identified just below the lower pole of the thyroid gland on each side, adjacent to the inferior thyroid veins. Less frequently, normal inferior parathyroids can be located in the superior mediastinum within the thymus. Rarely, so-called "undescended" lower parathyroid glands can be found high in the neck.

Gilmour[23] found that the parathyroids, occasionally, are included within the thyroid capsule or lie beneath it.

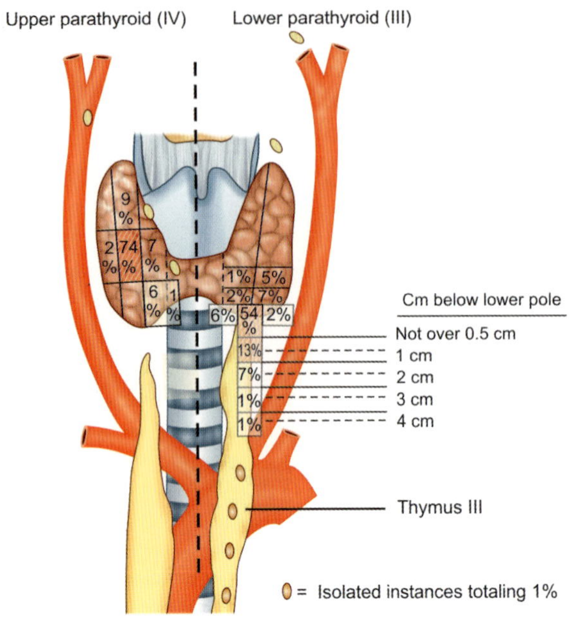

Fig. 16.5: Most frequent locations for the normal parathyroid. The locations for the upper parathyroid are shown at the left and those for the lower are shown at the right. The relative frequency with which the glands are found in the various locations is indicated on the diagram.

Source: Redrawn with permission from Gilmour J. The embryology of the parathyroid glands, the thymus and certain associated rudiments. J Pathol. 1937;45:507-22.

Sometimes a parathyroid is completely covered by the thyroid. These intrathyroidal lesions usually involve the inferior parathyroid glands. Normal lower parathyroid glands are usually anterior to the recurrent laryngeal nerves, whereas the upper parathyroid glands are usually situated more posteriorly.

Abnormal Parathyroid Glands

When parathyroid glands enlarge and become adenomatous or hyperplastic, their position can change (Figs. 16.6A and B).[29] Large upper parathyroid glands frequently fall back, posterior to the recurrent laryngeal nerve and under the inferior thyroid artery, and are found along the esophagus down into the posterior superior mediastinum. Lower parathyroid glands are displaced into the anterior superior mediastinum, either separately or along with the thymus gland. Usually, they remain anterior to the recurrent laryngeal nerves.

Although 84–94% of parathyroid adenomas are found adjacent to the thyroid gland in their normal locations, 6–16% are ectopically placed.[30] Ectopic glands can be found in the thyrothymic ligament inferior to the thyroid gland or lower in the anterior superior mediastinum either within or outside of the thymus, along the esophagus into

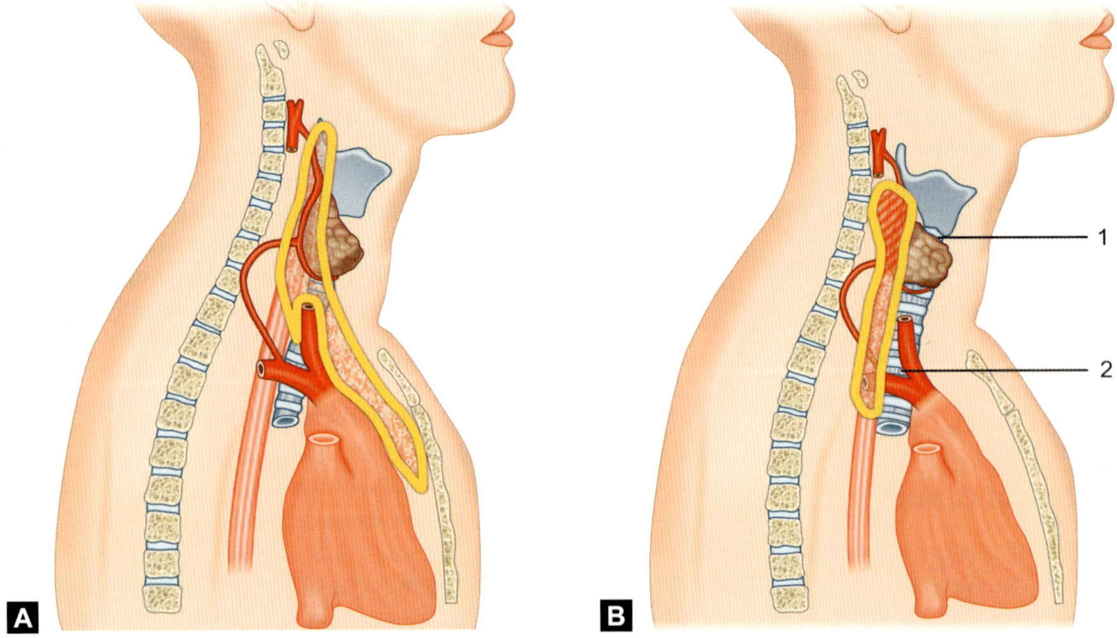

Figs. 16.6A and B: Location of adenomatous or hyperplastic parathyroid glands. (A) When a lower parathyroid gland enlarges, it frequently falls into the anterior mediastinum (highlighted area). (B) When an upper parathyroid gland enlarged, it may remain in the normal position (1), but it frequently falls into the posterior superior mediastinum (highlighted area) (2).

the posterior superior mediastinum, or very rarely in the middle mediastinum.[31] Uncommonly, they can be found within the carotid sheath or even lateral to the carotid sheath.[32] Rarely, an "undescended" lower parathyroid gland is found high up in the neck, anterior to the carotid artery bifurcation. Finally, about 5% of all parathyroid adenomas are intrathyroidal.[33] Fortunately, most of these can be felt or recognized as a mass within the thyroid lobe on ultrasound examination, but in other instances they are found only after thyroid excision or thyroidotomy. Locating and removing ectopic parathyroid glands during the initial neck operation remains one of the major pitfalls to successful parathyroid surgery. However, sestamibi and other preoperative localization scans have made this easier.

PATHOLOGY OF PRIMARY HYPERPARATHYROIDISM

One of the most difficult aspects for the surgeon is the recognition of the pathologic process that is present, for appropriate treatment is dependent on this. Primary hyperparathyroidism may be due to a single parathyroid adenoma, double adenomas, four-gland hyperplasia of the parathyroid glands, or, rarely, to a parathyroid carcinoma. The symptoms of the disease are similar regardless of the actual cause. It should also be remembered that PHPT, with parathyroid abnormalities, may result from previous low-dose radiation to the head and neck.

Today, it is generally agreed that PHPT is caused by a single adenoma in up to 85–90% of cases and that two or more enlarged parathyroid glands (called double adenomas or hyperplasia) are found in the other 10–15% of cases.[34] In MEN-1, multiple endocrine neoplasia type 2a, and the familial hyperparathyroidism syndromes, multigland hyperplasia is the rule. Parathyroid cancer is found in <1% of cases in many series, including the author's experience,[28] but makes up 3–5% of others. Perhaps it is being overdiagnosed in some institutions.

Classically, an adenoma has been defined pathologically as an enlarged gland with a rim of normal tissue. However, Roth[35] and other pathologists stated that this histologic appearance was found in cases of hyperplasia as well, and that it was not possible for the pathologist to tell the difference between a hyperplastic gland and an adenoma from looking at one gland.

In the past, when four-gland explorations were the rule and before preoperative localization tests and intraoperative PTH determinations were so commonly used, the surgeon was the diagnostician as well as the therapist. The major problem for the surgeon at the time of operation was to differentiate an adenoma from chief cell hyperplasia, or single gland disease from multigland disease of the parathyroids. Experienced surgeons evaluated the size, shape, and color of each parathyroid gland at operation and distinguished normal glands from abnormal ones. If one gland was enlarged and the others were perfectly normal, this was called an adenoma (Fig. 16.7A). If all glands were enlarged, this was called hyperplasia (or multigland disease) (Fig.16.7B). When two glands were enlarged, this was called a "double adenoma."

Most authors agree that double adenomas[26,36] occur in 5% or fewer cases; however, others believe that this represents a form of multiglandular disease. Obviously, when bilateral parathyroid explorations were the rule, the more glands the surgeon could see and evaluate, the more reliable would be the diagnosis and, hence, the treatment.

There has been a paradigm shift in the manner in which parathyroid surgery is performed in most centers. Although routine four-gland explorations are still preferred by some surgeons, most others prefer to do a minimally invasive operation when it is possible. Localization studies, usually an ultrasound examination of the neck and a sestamibi scan, are routinely performed before each parathyroidectomy. Furthermore, intraoperative PTH determinations are done before and after removal of a single large gland or glands, and this test is able to predict a cure with considerable accuracy. Thus, usually when a single gland is clearly diagnosed on preoperative localization studies, it is removed using a minimally invasive parathyroidectomy (MIP). A cure is guaranteed with 96–97% certainty when the intraoperative PTH, which was elevated, falls at least 50% and to a normal value after removal of the abnormal gland. The single gland that was removed is called an adenoma. If the intraoperative PTH does not fall appropriately, the operative approach is changed and a bilateral exploration is performed for presumed multigland disease.

LOCALIZATION PROCEDURES

Clark and Duh[13] have written an excellent summary of the advances that have been made in the preoperative localization of parathyroid tumors. With experienced radiologists and modern equipment, about 75–80% of all parathyroid adenomas can be localized using either ultrasonography, sestamibi scanning, MRI, or CT. In the best studies, using multiple techniques, as many as 80–90% of

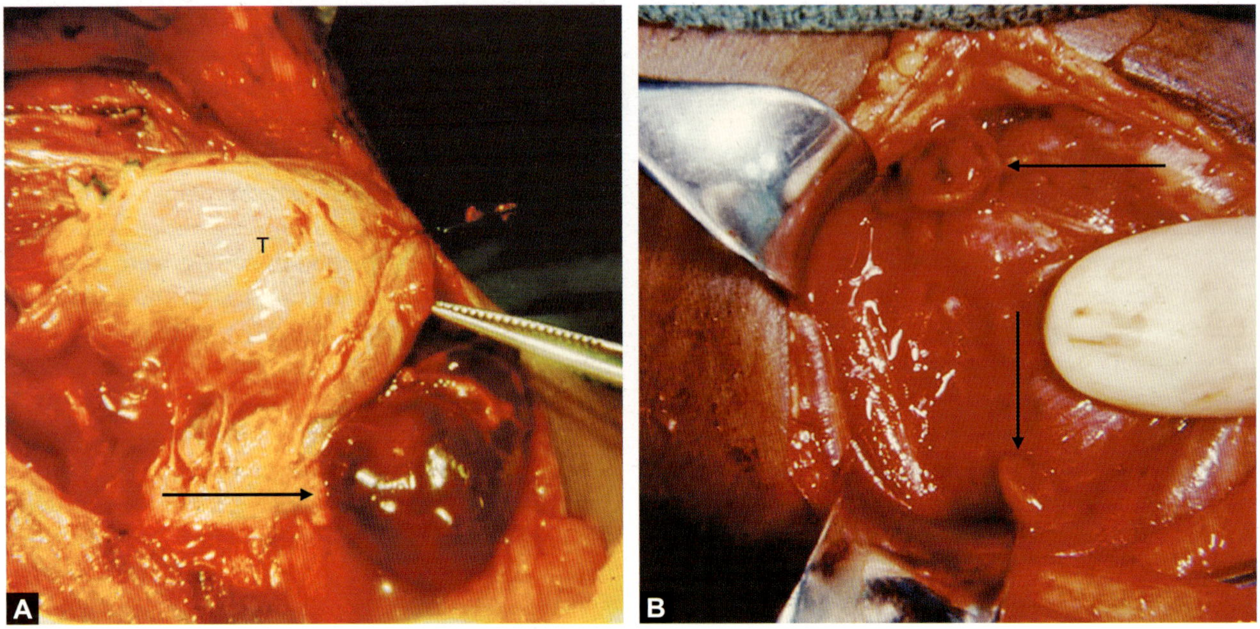

Figs. 16.7A and B: (A) On four-gland exploration, the thyroid lobe (T) was retracted medially. A large left lower parathyroid adenoma (arrow) was noted, as well as a normal left upper parathyroid gland shown at the end of the forceps. (B) In a patient with primary chief cell hyperplasia, the right thyroid lobe was retracted medially to demonstrate both an enlarged right upper (transverse arrow) and a right lower parathyroid gland (longitudinal arrow). On exploration of the left side, two similarly enlarged parathyroid glands were identified (not shown).

single parathyroid tumors have been identified. Thus, preoperative localization studies (i.e. ultrasound and sestamibi scans) are used by most parathyroid surgeons routinely.

In every series, however, both false-positive and false-negative results have been obtained. The tests are best when a single parathyroid gland enlargement is present; when this gland is >1 g in weight; and when no thyroid nodules are present. Only 20–40% of multiple gland enlargements are correctly identified in most series. Thus, localization studies of patients with parathyroid hyperplasia can be very misleading. Other problems relate to the small size of many parathyroid tumors, their position deep in the neck or chest, and the fact that thyroid nodules are frequently present especially in elderly female patients, the very individuals who have the highest prevalence of PHPT.

Ultrasonography is very operator dependent. Although experts may localize ≥80% correctly, others with less experience correctly localize far fewer.[37] This technique is good only in the neck, and is best when a 10-mHz real-time, small parts scanner is used. It often cannot identify small lesions, especially those deep in the neck or behind the esophagus. It cannot be used for lesions under the sternum. In some centers, needle aspiration of the suspected parathyroid mass is sometimes performed in difficult cases under ultrasound guidance. In such cases, measurement of the aspirate for PTH is much more accurate than cytologic evaluation and may add to the certainty of the findings. The appearance of a large parathyroid adenoma on ultrasonography is shown in Figure 16.8.

Sestamibi Scanning

Sestamibi is thought by many to be the best single test for parathyroid localization preoperatively before operating upon a patient with PHPT. Usually, it is accompanied with an ultrasound examination. In most institutions, sestamibi is given intravenously and then a scan of the neck and upper chest is obtained at about 20 minutes and again 2–3 hours after injection. At 20 minutes, the sestamibi is taken up by the thyroid gland as well as the parathyroid, and by 2 hours in a successful scan, the isotope has washed out of the thyroid and remains accumulated in the enlarged parathyroid gland (Fig. 16.9). A single-photon emission computerized tomography (SPECT) analysis with tomography may add to the accuracy of diagnosis. Furthermore, some centers utilize a SPECT–CT scan, which may be helpful in further demonstrating the anatomical location of the enlarged parathyroid gland.

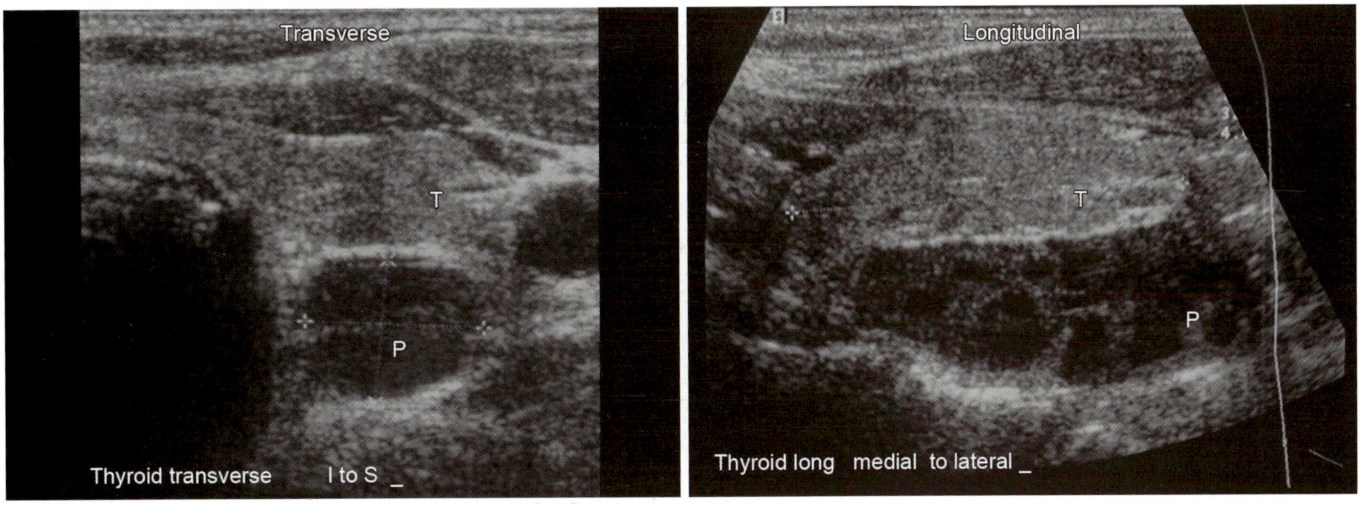

Fig. 16.8: Ultrasound examination of a large parathyroid gland (P) behind the thyroid lobe (T). Note that the parathyroid gland appears more hypoechoic than thyroid tissue.

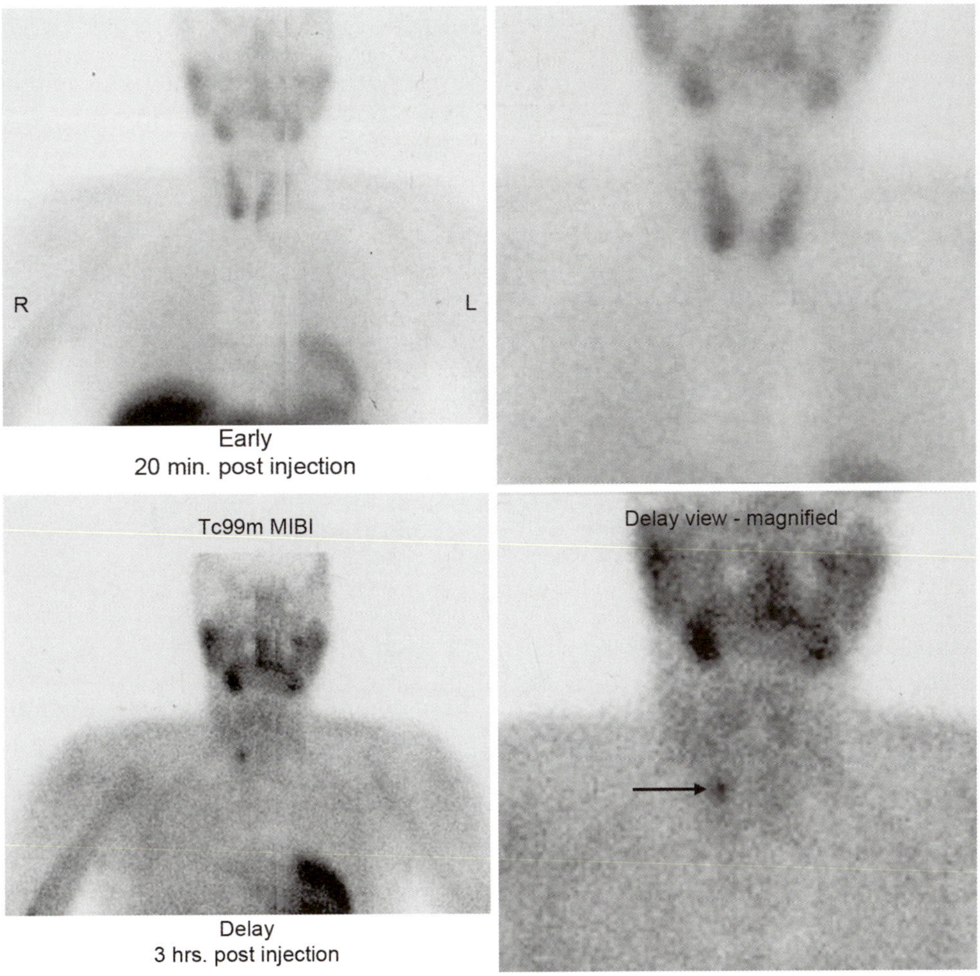

Fig. 16.9: Successful localization of a right lower parathyroid adenoma on sestamibi scan. (MIBI: Sestamibi scan).

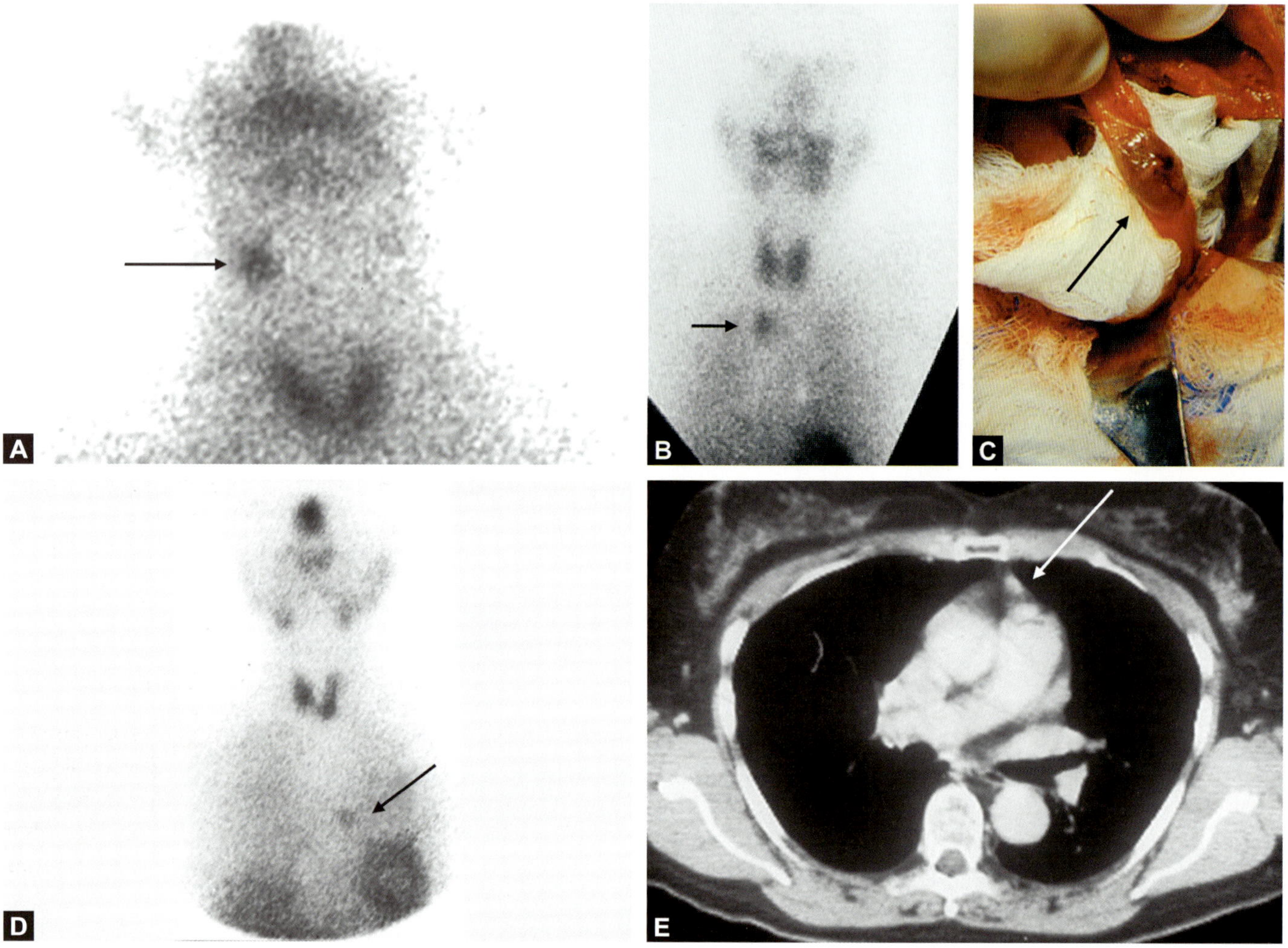

Figs. 16.10A to E: (A) Undescended right lower parathyroid adenoma (arrow) located at the carotid bifurcation. The thyroid gland is seen clearly inferior to the adenoma. (B) Intrathymic parathyroid adenoma (arrow), seen in the superior mediastinum inferior to the thyroid gland and superior to the heart. (C) Operative view through a standard neck incision. The thymus has been pulled up into the operative field from the chest. Clearly seen is the parathyroid adenoma within the thymus gland indicated by the arrow. (D and E) An elusive ectopic left inferior parathyroid was identified within the lower thymus at the level of the pulmonary artery. Shown faintly (arrow) just above the heart on sestamibi scan (D) and more definitively on CT scan (E). At the time, resection of this aberrant gland required a sternotomy; currently, however, similar glands have been removed by video-assisted thoracoscopic surgery. (CT: Computed tomography).

Sestamibi scanning is very good for identifying parathyroid adenomas in their normal locations near the thyroid, especially if the gland is larger than a gram, but these scans are very helpful for identifying ectopic parathyroid adenomas high in the neck or in the mediastinum. Successful imaging of up to 90% of adenomas has been reported; however, imaging of cases of double adenomas or hyperplasia using this technique remains much less successful. Examples of successful localization of enlarged glands in ectopic sites are illustrated in Figures 16.10A to E.

CT and MRI

These examinations can be helpful at times, especially for evaluating missing glands not imaged by ultrasound or sestamibi scanning. On MRI scans, parathyroid adenomas are recognized as bright areas on T2-weighted imaging.

4D-CT and Venous PTH Sampling

Four-dimensional computed tomography (4D-CT) is a test in which contrast is infused rapidly and a series of

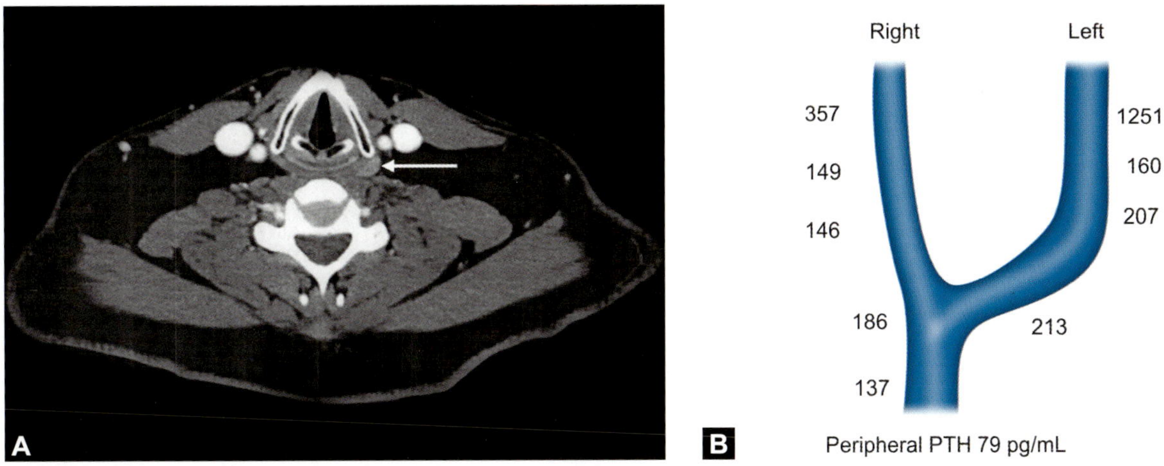

Figs. 16.11A and B: (A) A 4D-CT scan demonstrating a recurrence of parathyroid cancer (arrow) in a patient who had been previously operated upon for a large mass in this area. Neither a routine CT scan nor ultrasound and sestamibi tests were able to visualize the mass. (B) Venous sampling with measurement of parathyroid hormone in the same patient. Catheters were placed inside the right and left internal jugular veins and superior vena cava. Samples of blood were obtained from numerous locations in these vessels. The highest parathyroid hormone value correlated with the location of the recurrent focus of carcinoma in the left upper neck. (PTH: Parathyroid hormone; 4D-CT: Four-dimensional computed tomography).

three or four CT scans of the neck and upper mediastinum are obtained sequentially thereafter at timed intervals. Enlarged parathyroid glands can be recognized by their hypervascularity, but usually such glands are differentiated by a more rapid influx and efflux of contrast material than that is present in lymph nodes or thyroid tissue (Fig. 16.11A). Because of the radiation exposure, we reserve 4D-CT scanning for difficult reoperative cases of PHPT, such as when sent a patient who has failed the first operation and in whom the sestamibi and sonographic scans are negative. Usually, in such cases we combine 4D-CT scan with venous sampling with PTH determination and have found the combination of these two modalities to be the best way to locate the most difficult lesions (Fig. 16.11B). Others have used 4D-CT scanning as the primary localization test in patients who have not been operated upon and report successful localization results, which are even better than those for sestamibi scanning.

Highly selective arteriography with arterial injections of contrast material into the inferior thyroid artery has been abandoned because of the potential for severe neurologic complications.

OPERATIVE APPROACH

A number of different surgical approaches have been successfully used as treatment for PHPT. Several of these will be discussed.

Minimally Invasive Parathyroidectomy

While bilateral neck operations looking at all four parathyroid glands were done routinely by the majority of parathyroid surgeons in the past, now most prefer to do a MIP for pHPT when it is possible. By this, it is meant that when a single enlarged parathyroid gland is identified on preoperative localization studies, a small incision is made in the lower neck, either in the midline or directly over it, and the gland is removed (Fig. 16.12). To ensure a cure and to be certain that no other abnormal glands are present (double adenomas or hyperplasia), intraoperative PTH measurements are commonly used to monitor physiologic levels and guide further dissection. The half-life of PTH is about 3–5 minutes. Blood is sampled before the operation begins and before removing the enlarged gland. Then samples of blood are obtained 5, 10, and 15 minutes after removal of the adenoma (Fig. 16.13). When the pre-excision PTH concentration falls >50% and to a normal value, we consider this to be a cure and the operation is terminated (Fig. 16.14A). Others consider a 50% drop of a pre-excision PTH value alone to represent a cure. If the fall in PTH is not sufficient, then a double adenoma or hyperplasia is present and requires bilateral exploration (Fig. 16.14B).

After removing an additional gland or glands, intraoperative PTH is measured again and the process is repeated until the PTH levels fall appropriately. When a cure is obtained after removal of two enlarged glands, this

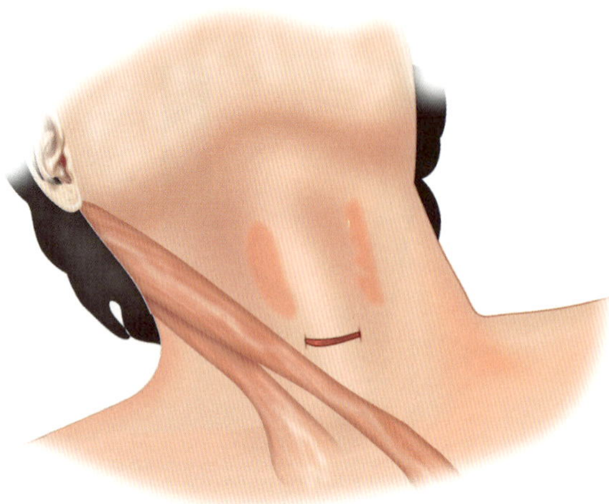

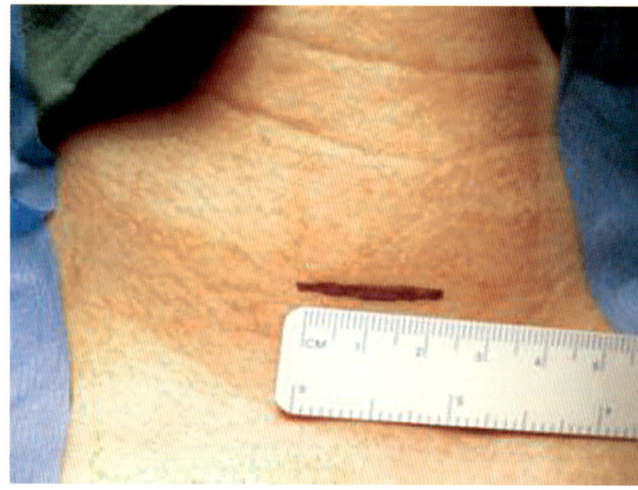

Fig. 16.12: For a minimally invasive parathyroidectomy, a small incision (~2 cm in length) is made either in the midline or over the area of the known abnormal gland.

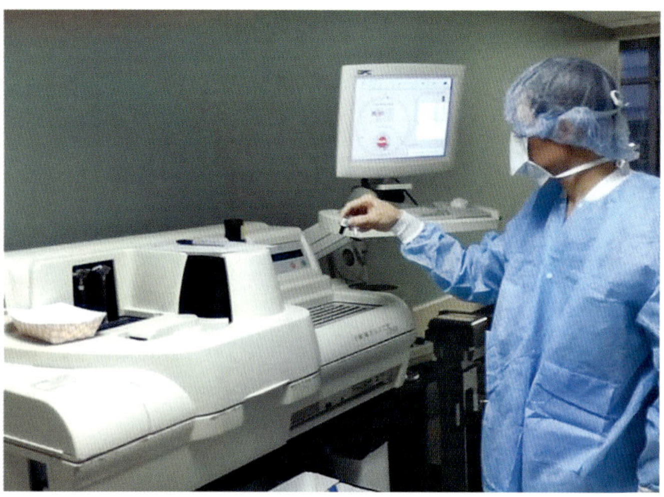

Fig. 16.13: The machine for measuring intraoperative parathyroid hormone levels is brought to the operating suite and blood samples are obtained sequentially from the patient.

is called a double adenoma. When hyperplasia is present (i.e. all four glands are abnormal), usually a subtotal parathyroidectomy is performed. Subtotal parathyroidectomy involves removal of three glands completely and partial removal of the fourth gland, making sure to leave a well-vascularized remnant. Less frequently, a total parathyroidectomy with autotransplantation of minced parathyroid tissue to small pockets made in the sternocleidomastoid muscle or in the brachioradialis of the forearm is utilized.

Another minimally invasive technique that has been described but has far less utility in the eyes of many parathyroid surgeons is the use of a nuclear probe (Fig. 16.15). Radioactive sestamibi is given preoperatively, and a nuclear probe is employed intraoperatively to detect the parathyroid gland that has the greatest amount of radioactive activity. After this gland is removed, it is placed on the probe, and a count is taken and compared with a count taken from the surface of the thyroid gland. Proponents of this technique state that if the removed gland emits ≥20% of the counts obtained from the surface of the thyroid gland, this gland is an adenoma and no other gland needs to be removed. However, we and others have reported exceptions to this rule and have not found the technique very helpful except in reoperative cases in which a great deal of scarring is present.[38,39]

Minimally invasive techniques have become popular since they employ a smaller incision than a bilateral exploration and thus may result in better cosmesis and in less pain. Furthermore, by operating on only one side of the neck, it eliminates the possibility of a bilateral recurrent laryngeal nerve injury and possibly decreases the incidence of postoperative bleeding or hematoma, uncommon events after any parathyroidectomy. Some surgeons use local infiltration of anesthesia or superficial cervical nerve block when doing an MIP, but employ general anesthesia when doing a bilateral operation. Finally, some surgeons send patients with MIP home on the same day, while those who have bilateral operations are kept in the hospital to rule out bleeding or more profound hypocalcemia.

In order to minimize or eliminate any incision in the neck, videoscopic, endoscopic, and robotic techniques of parathyroidectomy have been developed. These often use incisions in one or both axilla(e) or under the breast.

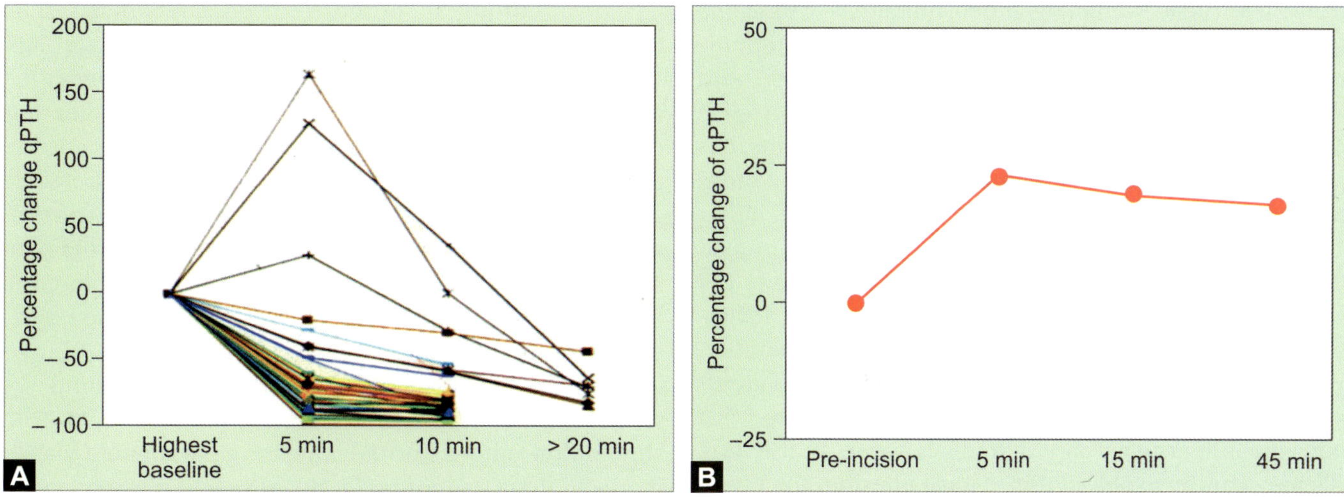

Figs. 16.14A and B: (A) Following successful removal of an adenoma, the intraoperative parathyroid hormone levels fall by 50% or greater usually within 5–10 minutes. Occasionally, as shown, manipulation of the gland can result in a transient rise in parathyroid hormone, which ultimately falls 50% or greater. (B) When intraoperative parathyroid hormone does not fall as expected, as shown in this figure, the patient is not cured of the hyperparathyroid state and further exploration is mandatory.
(qPTH: Quick parathyroid hormone).

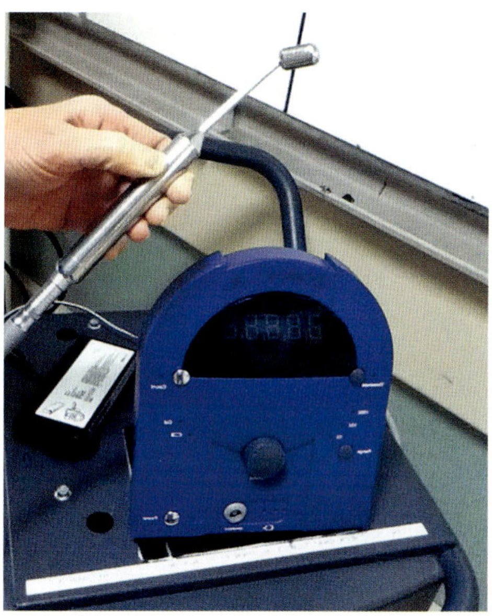

Fig. 16.15: Following injection of sestamibi, a sterile nuclear probe has been used by some surgeons to identify the parathyroid gland(s) with high radiotracer uptake.

The latest approach which shows promise is the transoral endoscopic removal of a parathyroid adenoma. An incision is made on the inside of the lower lip in the oral vestibule and access is obtained to the central neck for removal of enlarged parathyroid glands. These techniques have their own set of potential complications and their value other than cosmesis has been debated.

SUCCESS OF MINIMALLY INVASIVE PARATHYROIDECTOMY VERSUS ROUTINE FOUR-GLAND EXPLORATIONS

A minority of surgeons, including the senior author, prefer to perform bilateral explorations in most cases. This position is based on the facts that preoperative localization testing is not perfect and is less likely to identify multigland disease.[40,41] Furthermore, intraoperative PTH measurement is not perfect and has an overall accuracy of only 94%, with both false-positive and false-negative results recognized.[42]

Those who perform MIP have the greatest success in patients who have preoperative imaging that localizes the abnormal gland to one side.[43] When operated upon by an experienced parathyroid surgeon, MIP patients have been found to have indistinguishable cure rates and similar complication rates, while affording the patient shorter operating time and shorter length of hospital stay.[44] In patients with long-term follow-up after MIP, the biochemical cure rate is about 97%,[45] and is similar to that of four-gland exploration.[46] Thus, the majority of experienced parathyroid surgeons prefer to perform MIP whenever it is possible.

Multiple Endocrine Neoplasia, Type 1

Multiple endocrine neoplasia, type 1 is an autosomal dominant familial disease caused by germ line mutations of the menin gene. Numerous sites of mutations of this gene have been recognized and can be measured by appropriate blood testing preoperatively. In patients with MEN-1, parathyroid hyperplasia is the rule and recurrence after an operation is not uncommon. In such patients, it is imperative to find all parathyroid glands including those in the thymus gland. In addition to a thymectomy, either a subtotal parathyroidectomy or a total parathyroidectomy with an autotransplant of parathyroid tissue to the arm should be done. The latter technique may be advantageous because it is known that recurrent hyperparathyroidism occurs with some frequency, especially in patients with these familial, genetically induced syndromes.[25,26] If graft-dependent hyperparathyroidism occurs in the arm, this area can be explored under local anesthesia without the risk of a recurrent nerve injury, as would occur if the neck were re-explored. Wells et al.[47] recommended this approach for all cases of hyperplasia, familial, and otherwise.

Multiple Endocrine Neoplasia, Type 2a

Multiple endocrine neoplasia, type 2a is a familial disease caused by a RET oncogene point mutation. In its complete form, parathyroid hyperplasia is accompanied by medullary thyroid cancer (or C-cell hyperplasia) and bilateral pheochromocytomas (or bilateral adrenal medullary hyperplasia). The parathyroid disease is not as likely to recur as in the MEN-1 syndrome, and removal of only the enlarged parathyroid glands is favored by most surgeons at the time of total thyroidectomy, although some surgeons prefer routine subtotal parathyroidectomy.

Ectopic Parathyroid Adenomas

Although most normal or abnormal parathyroid glands are located near the thyroid, some are present in abnormal positions:

1. Within or lateral to the carotid sheath.
2. Behind the esophagus.
3. Between the trachea and esophagus.
4. Intrathyroidal parathyroid adenomas occur in about 3–5% and are usually present near the lower pole of the thyroid lobe.
5. "Undescended" lower parathyroid glands may be found near the carotid artery bifurcation.
6. Lower parathyroid glands are found in the anterior mediastinum usually but not always within the thyrothymic ligament or the thymus.
7. Upper parathyroid may fall into the posterior superior mediastinum often adjacent to the esophagus.

Most, but not all, of these ectopic adenomas can be identified by preoperative localization studies (*see* Figs. 16.10A to C). Sestamibi scanning will detect many in the upper neck or mediastinum, while ultrasound studies may demonstrate an intrathyroidal mass, usually at the lower pole. In such a case, if one is not certain, a fine-needle aspiration with measurement of a very high PTH concentration is diagnostic of an intrathyroidal parathyroid adenoma. Each of these ectopic sites should be explored at operation if the offending gland cannot be found on bilateral neck exploration.

Details of all operative techniques are beyond the scope of this chapter. However, in general, the surgeon should not remove normal appearing parathyroid glands if an adenoma cannot be found, although a careful small biopsy of each gland might be helpful.

It is imperative that the parathyroid surgeon operate in a slow, careful, meticulous fashion, keeping the operative field dry in order to succeed in curing most patients and in preventing recurrent nerve injury, injury to the external branch of the superior laryngeal nerve, hypoparathyroidism, hematoma, or hemorrhage.

Reoperation for Persistent or Recurrent Hyperparathyroidism

Before reoperating, a number of factors should be considered:[48]

1. Be certain that the patient has PHPT and not some other hypercalcemic state.
2. Be certain that the severity of the hyperparathyroid state warrants the risk of reoperative surgery.
3. Be certain that the patient does not have familial hypocalciuric hypercalcemia. If so, do not reoperate.
4. Carefully read the previous operative note and pathology report, and understand how many normal or abnormal parathyroid glands on each side were identified histologically and how many of them were removed. Review the pathologic slides of all if possible. Is this a case of a missing adenoma, incompletely treated hyperplasia, or even a recurrence of a carcinoma?
5. Use localization studies extensively in all cases preoperatively. Sonography, sestamibi scans, 4D-CT scans, and venous sampling with PTH measurement may be particularly helpful.
6. Always evaluate vocal cord function before operating.

Reoperations of the neck are more difficult because of the scarring, changes in anatomy, and loss of tissue planes

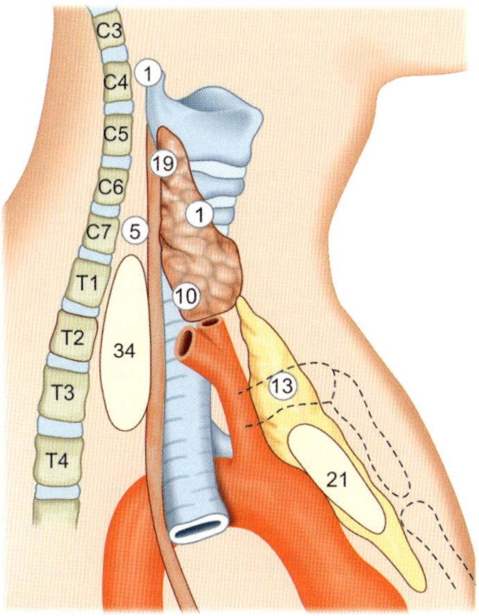

Fig. 16.16: Localization of all parathyroid adenomas found at reoperation after failure to cure hyperparathyroidism initially. Note that most of these glands could be removed through a neck incision. *Source*: Redrawn with permission from Wang CA. Parathyroid re-exploration. A clinical and pathological study of 112 cases. Ann Surg. 1977;186(2):140-5.

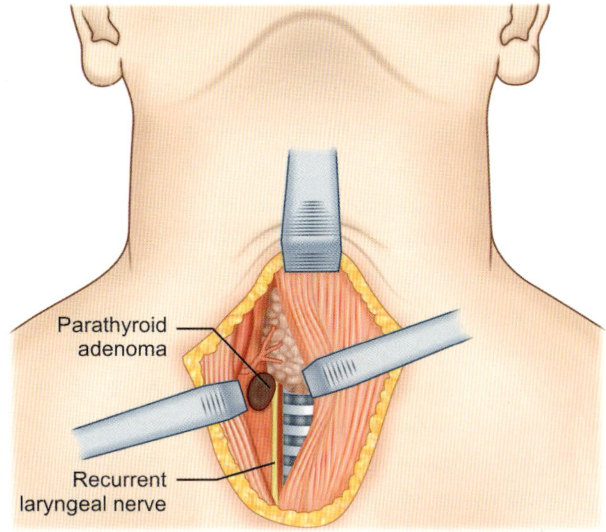

Fig. 16.17: Use of a "lateral approach" is very helpful in reoperative fields in which the strap muscles are often adherent to the anterior trachea.

that occur as a result of the first exploration, whether it was for a thyroid or a parathyroid disorder.[48-51] This is especially true if a bilateral exploration was used at the first operation. Frequently, for example, the strap muscles will be densely adherent to the anterior surface of the thyroid lobes, making entry into the usual anatomic planes more difficult. Furthermore, the recurrent laryngeal nerve is in greater jeopardy because it may be encased in scar tissue, but especially because it might lie immediately beneath the strap muscles if the thyroid lobe was previously removed. Finally, because one's knowledge of how many viable parathyroid glands remain in the neck after the first exploration is often limited, the chance of creating permanent hypoparathyroidism after removal of one or more abnormal parathyroid glands found at re-exploration is increased.

Usually, there is not a rush to reoperate, and it is better to allow some time to pass to permit the wound to heal, to re-evaluate the diagnosis, to perform localization testing, and to assess the findings of the previous operation. The location of parathyroid adenomas that were found and removed by Wang[50] at reoperation is shown in Figure 16.16.

If the gland that is causing the hyperparathyroidism is clearly localized preoperatively, the second operation is easier. However, when no localization or when only "regionalization" by venous sampling of PTH has been achieved, the operation is much more difficult and cure rates are lessened. Unless there is a rush to reoperate, one may wish to re-evaluate the situation again in the future by repeating the localization procedures. When reoperating, we almost always explore the neck again first, unless an adenoma is localized to the mediastinum or to another ectopic site preoperatively. If an experienced parathyroid surgeon did the initial operation and was "certain" that the lesion was not in the neck, it is much more likely to be found in an unusual location. On the other hand, when an inexperienced surgeon did the first operation, it is more likely to be in one of the usual locations in the neck.

In reoperative cases, because the strap muscles are often adherent to the trachea and thyroid lobes, instead of separating them in the midline, it is often easier to use a "lateral approach," as described by Fiend[52] and to dissect the plane between the sternocleidomastoid muscle and the strap muscles (Fig. 16.17). Not infrequently, this plane is totally unscarred, and by retracting the carotid sheath laterally and the thyroid gland medially, a "fresh" area containing the recurrent laryngeal nerve and parathyroid glands sometimes will be entered. If this area is scarred, the dissection should be started as low in the neck as possible, because this region has often been untouched. We use recurrent laryngeal nerve monitoring in all such cases. Once the recurrent nerve is identified, it should be treated gently. Usually, it can be safely followed in a cephalad direction. If the adenoma was not localized beforehand, a bilateral neck exploration may be necessary if it can be done safely. Be certain that the ipsilateral recurrent nerve is intact on nerve monitoring before exploring the contralateral side. In the case of positive localization, the missing gland can often be removed by a minimally invasive technique or by a unilateral conventional exploration, both of which are safer. Intraoperative PTH measurement is then performed to be certain that a cure has been obtained.

If an undescended lower parathyroid gland is recognized near the angle of the jaw, this can be removed through a small incision as one would use to approach the carotid artery bifurcation. Most substernal ectopic parathyroid glands can be removed by pulling up the thyrothymic ligament or thymus gland into the neck using a transcervical approach. If the mediastinal adenoma is too low in the mediastinum or if the enlarged gland is localized to the mid-mediastinum, a video-assisted thoracoscopic surgery technique is usually successful and eliminates the need for a sternotomy or for a formal thoracotomy.

When an adenoma is found in the neck or chest, it should be totally removed. If at least one additional normal parathyroid gland remains viable, the patient will be normocalcemic with normal postoperative parathyroid function. This fact stresses the importance of *not* removing normal parathyroid glands during an unsuccessful initial operation.

If hyperplastic glands are identified at reoperation, a subtotal parathyroidectomy can be performed. Others prefer a total parathyroidectomy, arguing that if recurrence were to occur in a remnant that is left, this would necessitate a third neck operation. If total parathyroidectomy is used, or after removal of an adenoma when one thinks that no other parathyroid tissue remains, one has the option of either immediately autotransplanting some of the abnormal parathyroid to the arm after confirming that it is not a carcinoma,[53] or else cryopreserving the tissue and waiting to see whether or not hypoparathyroidism occurs postoperatively.[54] If permanent hypoparathyroidism occurs, a subsequent autotransplant of the frozen tissue to the arm could be employed.

Either of these approaches has advantages and disadvantages. In our hands, cryopreservation has not been developed to the extent described by Wells et al.[54] and Brennan et al.[55] Furthermore, reimplantation of tissue that has been cryopreserved is not always successful. Hence, we would be more likely to use immediate autotransplantation if it were thought to be necessary, but only if we believed strongly that *all* other parathyroid tissue had been removed from the patient. Of course, patients with hypoparathyroidism and hypocalcemia require appropriate treatment with calcium and vitamin D therapy.

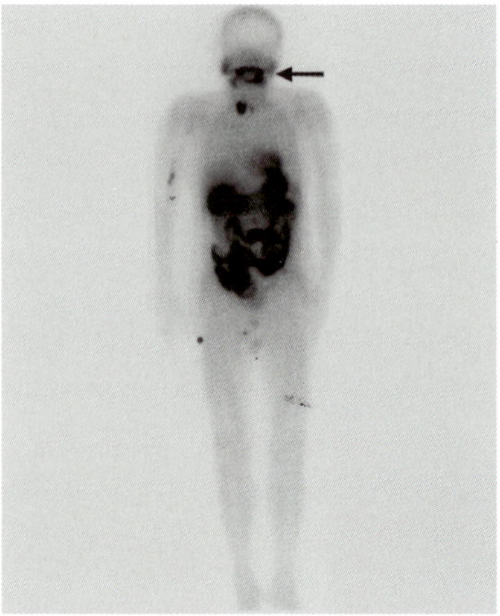

Fig. 16.18: Total body sestamibi scan showing a large parathyroid carcinoma in the right neck with a large metastasis to the occipital area (arrow). The right thigh is the site of injection.

SURGERY FOR PARATHYROID CANCER

Parathyroid cancer accounts for <1% of cases of PHPT at the University of Chicago Medical Center and elsewhere, but has been reported to occur in up to 6% of cases in other series.[56] If a carcinoma is suspected preoperatively because of a mass in the neck and severe hypercalcemia, we perform an ultrasound as well as a total-body sestamibi scan to evaluate for metastatic disease (Fig. 16.18). A carcinoma often presents as a "sticky," adherent large parathyroid gland at operation. Often a thick, dense, fibrotic, whitish capsule is present.

If recognized or suspected intraoperatively, one should not enter its capsule, for local seeding of tumor is a common occurrence. The gland should be removed widely, taking the ipsilateral thyroid lobe with it. Ipsilateral lymph nodes should be dissected in the central compartment and perhaps in the lateral neck as well, for nodal spread can occur. Distant spread occurs to the lungs, bone, brain, and elsewhere. If hypercalcemia recurs after a parathyroidectomy for parathyroid carcinoma, metastases should be aggressively localized and resected if possible,[57] because there is only limited effective therapy other than surgical excision. In general, death occurs from unrelenting hyperparathyroidism with all of the complications of this disorder, such as kidney stones and renal impairment, rather than from tumor spread by itself. Sensipar therapy, for example, has been helpful in some cases by lowering the PTH levels for a period of time. Other calcium lowering therapies may also be of benefit.

RESULTS OF PARATHYROIDECTOMY FOR PRIMARY HYPERPARATHYROIDISM

There is no question that the results of parathyroidectomy for PHPT relate to the experience of the operator. In a report from Scandinavia,[58] this was clearly shown. In centers that specialize in endocrine surgery, 90% of patients were normocalcemia, with a mean follow-up of 4.4 years after their initial parathyroidectomy, 6% were hypercalcemic, and 4% were hypocalcemic. In contrast, in a general Scandinavian survey of all hospitals done at roughly the same time and with similar follow-up, 76% of patients were normocalcemic. In hospitals where <10 operations for PHPT were done each year, only 70% were normocalcemic at follow-up, 15% had persistent or recurrent hyperparathyroidism, and 14% had permanent hypoparathyroidism.

In a number of other studies from centers that have considerable experience in parathyroid surgery, ~95% of patients or more can be rendered normocalcemic by the initial operation.[25,29,59] As practiced by surgeons in our group, patients who had four-gland explorations routinely (395 patients) had an early cure rate of 97.7%, with multiglandular disease found in 16.5%; while those who had a focused MIP exploration whenever possible (405 patients) had an early cure rate of 96.3% with multiglandular disease recognized in 11.2%. Recurrent hyperparathyroidism, defined as hyperparathyroidism recurring after 6 months of normocalcemia, occurs infrequently in nonfamilial cases[17,25] but remains a problem in familial hyperparathyroidism and in others with the MEN-1 syndrome.[25] In experienced hands, the complication rate is low in initial operations. Permanent recurrent laryngeal nerve injuries occurred in <1%.[17,58] Permanent hypoparathyroidism has been reported to be ≤2% in a number of series, but is higher in others.[17] Finally, the operative mortality rate is consistently far <1%.[17]

Reoperations for persistent or recurrent hyperparathyroidism are more difficult and have a greater potential for hypoparathyroidism, for recurrent nerve injuries, and for failure.[48] Using advanced localization studies, however, up to 90% of these tumors may be found and corrected, in the best of series.[60]

In summary, the results of parathyroid surgery for PHPT are excellent when done by experienced surgeons. As stated by Malmaeus et al.,[58] "These findings strongly advocate special training and interest in parathyroid surgery in order to ensure success."

REFERENCES

1. Adler JT, Sippel RS, Chen H. New trends in parathyroid surgery. Curr Probl Surg. 2010;47(12):958-1017.
2. Heath H 3rd, Hodgson SF, Kennedy MA. Primary hyperparathyroidism. Incidence, morbidity, and potential economic impact in a community. N Engl J Med. 1980;302(4):189-93.
3. Lundgren E, Hagström EG, Lundin J, et al. Primary hyperparathyroidism revisited in menopausal women with serum calcium in the upper normal range at population-based screening 8 years ago. World J Surg. 2002;26(8):931-6.
4. Heath H 3rd. Clinical spectrum of primary hyperparathyroidism: evolution with changes in medical practice and technology. J Bone Miner Res. 1991;6(Suppl 2):S63-70; discussion S83-4.
5. Suh JM, Cronan JJ, Monchik JM. Primary hyperparathyroidism: is there an increased prevalence of renal stone disease? AJR Am J Roentgenol. 2008;191(3):908-11.
6. Mandl F. Kliniches und Experimentelles zur Frage der lokalisierten und generalisierten Ostitis fibrosa. Arch Klin Chir. 1926;143:1-46.
7. Thompson NW. The history of hyperparathyroidism. Acta Chir Scand. 1990;156(1):5-21.
8. Bauer W, Federman DD. Hyperparathyroidism epitomized: the case of Captain Charles E. Martell. Metabolism. 1962;11:21-9.
9. Richardson EP, Aub JC, Bauer W. Parathyroidectomy in osteomalacia. Ann Surg. 1929;90:730-41.
10. Cope O. The study of hyperparathyroidism at the Massachusetts General Hospital. N Engl J Med. 1966;274(21):1174-82.
11. Pritchard MH, Jessop JD. Chondrocalcinosis in primary hyperparathyroidism. Influence of age, metabolic bone disease, and parathyroidectomy. Ann Rheum Dis. 1977;36(2):146-51.
12. Bilezikian JP, Potts JT Jr, Fuleihan GH, et al. Summary statement from a workshop on asymptomatic primary hyperparathyroidism: a perspective for the 21st century. J Clin Endocrinol Metab. 2002;87(12):5353-61.
13. Clark OH, Duh QY. Primary hyperparathyroidism. A surgical perspective. Endocrinol Metab Clin North Am. 1989;18(3):701-14.
14. Joborn C, Hetta J, Rastad J, et al. Psychiatric symptoms and cerebrospinal fluid monoamine metabolites in primary hyperparathyroidism. Biol Psychiatry. 1988;23(2):149-58.
15. Suva LJ, Winslow GA, Wettenhall RE, et al. A parathyroid hormone-related protein implicated in malignant hypercalcemia: cloning and expression. Science. 1987;237(4817):893-6.
16. Ronni-Sivula H, Sivula A. Long-term effect of surgical treatment on the symptoms of primary hyperparathyroidism. Ann Clin Res. 1985;17(4):141-7.

17. Lafferty FW, Hubay CA. Primary hyperparathyroidism. A review of the long-term surgical and nonsurgical morbidities as a basis for a rational approach to treatment. Arch Intern Med. 1989;149(4):789-96.
18. Gopinath P, Sadler GP, Mihai R. Persistent symptomatic improvement in the majority of patients undergoing parathyroidectomy for primary hyperparathyroidism. Langenbecks Arch Surg. 2010;395(7):941-6.
19. Agarwal G, Nanda G, Kapoor A, et al. Cardiovascular dysfunction in symptomatic primary hyperparathyroidism and its reversal after curative parathyroidectomy: results of a prospective case control study. Surgery. 2013;154(6):1394-403.
20. Scholz DA, Purnell DC. Asymptomatic primary hyperparathyroidism. 10-year prospective study. Mayo Clin Proc. 1981;56(8):473-8.
21. Kaplan RA, Snyder WH, Stewart A, et al. Metabolic effects of parathyroidectomy in asymptomatic primary hyperparathyroidism. J Clin Endocrinol Metab. 1976;42(3):415-26.
22. Bilezikian JP, Brandi ML, Eastell R, et al. Guidelines for the management of asymptomatic primary hyperparathyroidism: summary statement from the Fourth International Workshop. J Clin Endocrinol Metab. 2014;99(10):3561-9.
23. Gilmour J. The embryology of the parathyroid glands, the thymus and certain associated rudiments. J Pathol. 1937;45:507-22.
24. Scholz DA, Purnell DC, Woolner LB, et al. Mediastinal hyperfunctioning parathyroid tumors: review of 14 cases. Ann Surg. 1973;178(2):173-8.
25. Clark OH, Way LW, Hunt TK. Recurrent hyperparathyroidism. Ann Surg. 1976;184(4):391-402.
26. Verdonk CA, Edis AJ. Parathyroid "double adenomas": fact of fiction? Surgery. 1981;90(3):523-6.
27. Sedgwick CE, Cady B. Embryology and developmental abnormalities. Major Probl Clin Surg. 1980;15:6-18.
28. Kaplan EL. Thyroid and parathyroid. In: Schwartz S (Ed). Principles of Surgery. New York: McGraw-Hill; 1989. pp. 1613-85.
29. Bruining H. Operative strategy for primary hyperparathyroidism. In: Kaplan E (Ed). Surgery of the Thyroid and Parathyroid Glands. Edinburgh: Churchill Livingstone; 1983. pp. 158-67.
30. Roy M, Mazeh H, Chen H, et al. Incidence and localization of ectopic parathyroid adenomas in previously unexplored patients. World J Surg. 2013;37(1):102-6.
31. Curley IR, Wheeler MH, Thompson NW, et al. The challenge of the middle mediastinal parathyroid. World J Surg. 1988;12(6):818-24.
32. Udekwu AO, Kaplan EL, Wu TC, et al. Ectopic parathyroid adenoma of the lateral triangle of the neck: report of two cases. Surgery. 1987;101(1):114-8.
33. Hojaij F, Vanderlei F, Plopper C, et al. Parathyroid gland anatomical distribution and relation to anthropometric and demographic parameters: a cadaveric study. Anat Sci Int. 2011;86(4):204-12.
34. Wade TJ, Yen TW, Amin AL, et al. Surgical management of normocalcemic primary hyperparathyroidism. World J Surg. 2012;36(4):761-6.
35. Roth SI. Pathology of the parathyroids in hyperparathyroidism. Discussion of recent advances in the anatomy and pathology of the parathyroid glands. Arch Pathol. 1962;73:495-510.
36. Brothers TE, Thompson NW. Surgical treatment of primary hyperparathyroidism in elderly patients. Acta Chir Scand. 1987;153(3):175-8.
37. Lucas RJ, Welsh RJ, Glover JL. Unilateral neck exploration for primary hyperparathyroidism. Arch Surg. 1990;125(8):982-4; discussion 984-5.
38. Jaskowiak NT, Sugg SL, Helke J, et al. Pitfalls of intraoperative quick parathyroid hormone monitoring and gamma probe localization in surgery for primary hyperparathyroidism. Arch Surg. 2002;137(6):659-68; discussion 668-9.
39. Bonjer HJ, Bruining HA, Pols HA, et al. Intraoperative nuclear guidance in benign hyperparathyroidism and parathyroid cancer. Eur J Nucl Med. 1997;24(3):246-51.
40. Palestro CJ, Tomas MB, Tronco GG. Radionuclide imaging of the parathyroid glands. Semin Nucl Med. 2005;35(4):266-76.
41. Shen W, Sabanci U, Morita ET, et al. Sestamibi scanning is inadequate for directing unilateral neck exploration for first-time parathyroidectomy. Arch Surg. 1997;132(9):969-74; discussion 974-6.
42. Cho E, Chang JM, Yoon SY, et al. Preoperative localization and intraoperative parathyroid hormone assay in Korean patients with primary hyperparathyroidism. Endocrinol Metab (Seoul). 2014;29(4):464-9.
43. Reeve TS, Babidge WJ, Parkyn RF, et al. Minimally invasive surgery for primary hyperparathyroidism: a systematic review. Aust N Z J Surg. 2000;70(4):244-50.
44. Udelsman R, Donovan PI. Open minimally invasive parathyroid surgery. World J Surg. 2004;28(12):1224-6.
45. Venkat R, Kouniavsky G, Tufano RP, et al. Long-term outcome in patients with primary hyperparathyroidism who underwent minimally invasive parathyroidectomy. World J Surg. 2012;36(1):55-60.
46. Westerdahl J, Bergenfelz A. Unilateral versus bilateral neck exploration for primary hyperparathyroidism: five-year follow-up of a randomized controlled trial. Ann Surg. 2007;246(6):976-80; discussion 980-1.
47. Wells SA Jr, Ellis GJ, Gunnells JC, et al. Parathyroid autotransplantation in primary parathyroid hyperplasia. N Engl J Med. 1976;295(2):57-62.
48. Brennan MF. Reoperation for suspected hyperparathyroidism. In: Kaplan EL (Ed). Surgery of the Thyroid and Parathyroid Glands. Edinburgh: Churchill Livingstone; 1983. pp. 168-76.
49. Kadowaki MH, Fulton N, Schark C, et al. Difficulties of parathyroidectomy after previous thyroidectomy. Surgery. 1989;106(6):1018-23, discussion 1023-4.
50. Wang CA. Parathyroid re-exploration. A clinical and pathological study of 112 cases. Ann Surg. 1977;186(2):140-5.
51. Edis AJ. Surgical anatomy and technique of neck exploration for primary hyperparathyroidism. Surg Clin North Am. 1977;57(3):495-504.
52. Feind CR. Re-exploration for parathyroid adenoma. Am J Surg. 1964;108:543-6.

53. Edis AJ, Linos DA, Kao PC. Parathyroid autotransplantation at the time of reoperation for persistent hyperparathyroidism. Surgery. 1980;88(4):588-93.
54. Wells SA Jr, Gunnells JC, Gutman RA, et al. The successful transplantation of frozen parathyroid tissue in man. Surgery. 1977;81(1):86-90.
55. Brennan MF, Brown EM, Spiegel AM, et al. Autotransplantation of cryopreserved parathyroid tissue in man. Ann Surg. 1979;189(2):139-42.
56. Schantz A, Castleman B. Parathyroid carcinoma. A study of 70 cases. Cancer. 1973;31(3):600-5.
57. Flye MW, Brennan MF. Surgical resection of metastatic parathyroid carcinoma. Ann Surg. 1981;193(4):425-35.
58. Malmaeus J, Granberg PO, Halvorsen J, et al. Parathyroid surgery in Scandinavia. Acta Chir Scand. 1988;154(7-8):409-13.
59. van Heerden JA, Grant CS. Surgical treatment of primary hyperparathyroidism: an institutional perspective. World J Surg. 1991;15(6):688-92.
60. Levin KE, Clark OH. The reasons for failure in parathyroid operations. Arch Surg. 1989;124(8):911-4; discussion 914-5.

CHAPTER

17 Bowel Disease and Urolithiasis

John R Asplin

INTRODUCTION

The kidneys maintain homeostasis of the body fluids by filtering large amounts of plasma and then modifying the filtrate by the selective reabsorption or secretion of compounds to maintain optimal health. The activity of the intestinal tract is the other half of this equation, as the amount of nutrients absorbed provides the metabolic load which the kidney must excrete to maintain balance. In the setting of intestinal disease, abnormal absorption of nutrients, electrolytes and fluids leads to alterations of urine composition that puts the patient at risk of forming urolithiasis. Depending on the severity of disease and the regions of the gastrointestinal (GI) tract that are involved, characteristic changes in urine chemistry can occur leading to the formation of calcium oxalate, uric acid, or less commonly, ammonium acid urate (AmU) stones.

GASTROINTESTINAL ANATOMY AND PHYSIOLOGY

A brief review of the anatomy and functional segmentation of the gut is essential when considering how disease and surgical resection can increase the risk of stone disease. The small intestine absorbs nutrients and has large bidirectional traffic of water and electrolytes, though there is net absorption of water and electrolytes in the absence of disease. The large intestine has almost no role in nutrient absorption. The cecum, ascending, and transverse colon absorb water and electrolytes. The descending colon is mainly a storage area for waste. The total length of the small intestine varies considerably, from ~400 to 800 cm in adults.[1] The duodenum is ~25–30 cm, the jejunum 200–300 cm, and the ileum 200–400 cm in length. The colon ranges in length from 100 to 200 cm.

Water

On average, daily water intake is in the range of 2–3 L. In addition to the ingested fluids, the gut and other organs of digestion (salivary glands, gallbladder, pancreas, and the small intestine itself) deliver an additional 5–6 L of fluid into the lumen of the small intestine. Water reabsorption is coupled to solute reabsorption, mostly driven by active sodium uptake with cotransport of amino acids and sugars. The small intestine absorbs ~6 or 7 L of fluid so that ~1.5–2 L of fluid is delivered to the colon. The colon absorbs most of the fluid delivered so that stool losses of water are in the range of 100–200 mL/d. If disease reduces small intestinal water absorption, the colon has the capacity to increase absorption, but once delivery to the colon exceeds 4–5 L/d, the absorptive capacity of the colon is surpassed, resulting in diarrhea with potential dehydration and volume depletion.

Acid–Base

The intestine traffics large amounts of protons and bicarbonate, so any disturbance in their secretion or reabsorption can lead to an acid–base disturbance. Both bile and pancreatic juices are alkaline and provide large amounts of bicarbonate to the intestinal lumen. Approximately 1.5–2 L of bicarbonate-rich fluid reaches the terminal ileum to be processed by the colon. In normal health, only 150 mL of stool water is excreted and the bulk of alkali entering the cecum is reabsorbed. Bicarbonate is either reabsorbed via sodium–hydrogen exchange or is titrated by the protons from organic acids produced by colonic bacteria. The organic anions are absorbed and metabolized by colonic epithelia resulting in the production of bicarbonate, leading to a net bicarbonate absorption. Total loss of alkali in the stool is about 5 mEq of bicarbonate and 10 mEq of organic anions per day. In diarrheal states, the loss of alkali and alkali equivalents increases significantly, sufficient to produce metabolic acidosis.[2]

Minerals

Calcium is absorbed via both active transport and paracellular diffusion. Approximately 15–25% of dietary calcium is absorbed. Kidney stone patients with hypercalciuria tend to absorb a larger fraction of their calcium intake than normal subjects. In the duodenum, there is active transcellular absorption, which is stimulated by calcitriol.[3] The bulk of calcium absorption occurs in the jejunum and ileum by passive paracellular uptake.[4] There is also active absorption in the cecum, though it does not appear to be as dependent on vitamin D as that in the duodenum. The cecum probably contributes no more than 10% of total calcium absorption in health, but this fraction may increase when the small bowel is compromised. When calcium intake is adequate, transcellular absorption in the jejunum and ileum is the major absorptive pathway. When calcium intake is limited, active absorption becomes the predominate mechanism for calcium absorption.

Magnesium is absorbed in the jejunum and ileum. Most magnesium absorption is via a passive paracellular process driven by the luminal electrochemical gradient. There is also an active transcellular process in the ileum. Vitamin D is not a significant regulator of magnesium uptake. Net intestinal absorption of Mg is ~30–50%.[5] Because the distal small intestine and proximal colon play a significant role in magnesium absorption, magnesium deficiency is common in patients with ileal resection.

Phosphorus, in the form of inorganic phosphate, is absorbed along the entire length of the small intestine, with most being absorbed in the jejunum.[6] Approximately 60–80% of dietary phosphorous is absorbed, via both paracellular and active transcellular pathways. Vitamin D is not as critical in maintaining phosphorus balance as it is for calcium, such that even in vitamin D deficiency, phosphorus stores remain adequate if dietary intake is sufficient.[7]

In humans, vitamin D is either produced by fibroblasts in the skin via conversion of 7-dehydrocholesterol to cholecalciferol under the influence of ultraviolet B light, or it is absorbed from supplements and foods enriched with vitamin D (cholecalciferol or ergocalciferol). In theory, humans do not require dietary sources of vitamin D as epidermal production should be adequate given sunlight of sufficient intensity and exposure. However, in industrialized cultures, sun exposure has decreased as fewer people work outside, air-conditioned climates are preferred by many people, and sun screen is routinely used when outside. Lack of sun exposure is even more severe in northern climates and the winter season. In such situations, people are more dependent on orally ingested vitamin D to maintain adequate stores. Vitamin D is a fat-soluble vitamin that requires micelle formation in the gut lumen for adequate absorption. It is absorbed in the jejunum and ileum. Normally, about 75% of ingested vitamin D is absorbed. Any disease that leads to bile acid deficiency or loss of intestinal surface area puts the patient at risk for vitamin D deficiency and bone disease.[8] Vitamin D deficiency limits active calcium and phosphate absorption in the intestine, which in concert with reduced surface area can lead to negative calcium and phosphate balance.

Magnesium deficiency may be a direct risk factor for stone disease as low urine magnesium levels will lead to higher free oxalate levels in urine. Hypophosphaturia, hypocalciuria, and vitamin D deficiency are not risk factors for stone formation, but they can be clinical clues to help clinicians recognize the presence and severity of bowel disease that may not be obvious from the medical history.

Oxalate

Oxalate is an end-product of metabolism in humans, arising from a variety of precursors. The major route of excretion is through the kidney. Because calcium oxalate (CaOx) is highly insoluble, any increase in oxalate production or intestinal absorption increases urinary excretion of oxalate and the risk of kidney stone formation.[9] Approximately 40–50% of urine oxalate derives from intestinal absorption of dietary oxalate, the rest is from endogenous production.[10] Dietary oxalate can contribute an even larger fraction of daily oxalate excretion when intestinal absorption increases due to consumption of high oxalate diets or when fractional absorption of ingested oxalate increases. The latter is the case in enteric hyperoxaluria (EH). The normal Western diet provides about 100–200 mg of oxalate per day, though the range of intake is quite large as intake of high oxalate foods can lead to an oxalate load of over 500 mg/d. Typically, fractional absorption of oxalate is low, usually in the range of 5–15% of dietary intake. Absorption of diet oxalate depends not only on the presence of oxalate in the diet but also on the bioavailability. Oxalate that is ingested as CaOx, or ingested as part of a multicomponent meal that contains significant calcium or magnesium, is much less bioavailable than oxalate provided as sodium or potassium salts.[11-13] There is also considerable intraindividual variation of oxalate absorption as has been shown in studies using an oxalate loading test using a radiolabeled oxalate.[14]

Oxalate absorption has been demonstrated through the entire GI tract, but the relative contribution of the different segments in humans is not well quantified. The stomach has been shown to absorb oxalate, likely promoted by the low intraluminal pH that would lead to a protonated oxalate able to cross the gastric epithelia passively.[15,16] It is unclear what fraction of dietary oxalate the stomach absorbs. Nonetheless, an intact stomach may be important in downstream oxalate absorption by solubilizing oxalate salts in the acidic stomach lumen. Whether lack of stomach acidification alters oxalate excretion in humans has not been adequately studied.

The small intestine is clearly a major site of oxalate absorption. In oxalate loading studies, the peak of oxalate absorption occurs within 2–5 hours of ingestion of the oxalate load. Small intestinal transit time (from mouth to cecum) in healthy people is about 5–7 hours.[17] Unfortunately, which intestinal segment is the major site of absorption in humans is not known. Oxalate absorption occurs by both active transport via the transcellular route and passive down an electrochemical gradient via paracellular routes. The colon has clearly been shown to absorb oxalate in the setting of EH associated with fat malabsorption. How much the colon contributes to oxalate absorption in people with a healthy GI tract is uncertain. In a healthy colon, as water is extracted from colonic contents, the formation of solid fecal matter leads to reduced exposure to the intestinal surface for absorption.

Effect of Intestinal Disease/Resection

Conditions for optimal absorption of water, nutrients, and electrolytes include adequate surface area of the small intestine, a high concentration of nutrients and electrolytes in the gut lumen (i.e. adequate dietary intake), and a moderate transit time to maximize contact between the intestinal fluid and the epithelia. Any disease or procedure that reduces intestinal surface area or shortens intestinal transit time, limits intestinal absorption.

After bowel resection, there is adaptation to improve nutrient and fluid absorption in the remnant segments. Resection of the proximal intestine is more easily managed than that of the ileum as the ileum has a greater capacity for adaptation than the duodenum or jejunum.[18] Because of the specialized role the ileum plays in bile salt absorption, ileal resection can lead to steatorrhea and deficiencies in fat soluble vitamins, a role that cannot be assumed by the jejunum. Leaving the colon in continuity also improves adaptation as the colon can significantly increase daily fluid reabsorption and can contribute to caloric needs via absorption of short-chain fatty acids produced by bacteria from carbohydrates that reach the colon. Peptide YY, produced by the distal ileum and colon, reduces intestinal motility, increasing contact of nutrients and fluid with the small intestinal mucosa.[18] In patients with ileal-cecal resection or a colon no longer in continuity, loss of peptide YY contributes to malabsorption and diarrhea. When surgical resection or bypass is performed, the length of the bowel segments left intact will determine the severity of GI dysfunction. Since intestinal length varies among individuals by twofold, and women tend to have shorter small bowel than men, the remaining functional surface cannot be adequately judged by how much is resected.[1] However, the amount resected is usually the data that are available, and the clinician must use the region and length of resection as a rough guide as to the metabolic consequences of surgery.

Epidemiology

An increased prevalence of urolithiasis in patients with bowel disease has been reported by multiple investigators. The prevalence rates of urolithiasis in patients with bowel disease should not be compared to the lifetime prevalence of the general population but to an age and gender matched cohort. Patients with bowel disease will have an earlier age of onset of stone disease than the overall population. Most of our knowledge of stone rates from bowel disease comes from the study of patients with inflammatory bowel disease (IBD). Other causes of bowel disease/intestinal resection such as trauma, infections, or congenital anomalies are not sufficiently common to provide reliable data on stone prevalence specific to each disease. There is data on the prevalence of stones in patients undergoing bariatric surgery, which will be explored separately in the section on bariatric surgery below.

In 1938, Bargen et al. at Mayo Clinic were the first to report an association of urolithiasis with IBD, reporting stones in 8 of 871 patients with ulcerative colitis (UC).[19] In a follow-up study, they noted the relationship between ileostomy and stone formation, reporting urolithiasis in 6 of 182 patients who had undergone colectomy.[20] Deren et al. published one of the first reports focused specifically on the prevalence of urolithiasis in IBD.[21] They performed a retrospective review of 583 patients with IBD treated at a single institution from 1950 to 1960. Urolithiasis occurred in 3.2% of patients with UC, 6.3% of those with Crohn's disease and 16.6% of those with ileocolitis. Based on stone analysis and radiographic findings, they reported 46% of patients had uric acid stones, 32% had calcium stones, and the rest of the stones could not be classified. They

Table 17.1: Prevalence of urolithiasis in inflammatory bowel disease.

	Disease	*Medical therapy*	*Ileostomy*	*Other surgery*	*Total*
Deren et al.[21]	IBD	5/241 (2.1)	12/163 (7.4)	11/179 (6.1)	28/583 (4.8)
Maratka and Nedbal[22]	UC	1/438 (0.2)	9/74 (12.2)	NA	10/512 (2.0)
Grossman and Nugent[23]	IBD	4/273 (1.5)	16/544 (2.9)	15/283 (5.3)	35/1100 (3.2)
Gelzayd et al.[24]	IBD	35/706 (5.0)	14/79 (18)	15/100 (15.0)	64/885 (7.2)
Bennett and Hughes[29]	UC	5/125 (4.0)	28/333 (8.4)	NA	41/458 (8.9)
Shield et al.[26]	IBD	4/85 (4.7)	11/85 (12.9)	5/63 (7.9)	20/233 (8.6)
Fukushima et al.[30]	UC	5/97 (5.1)	3/15 (20)	NA	8/112 (7.1)

(UC: Ulcerative colitis only; IBD: Includes ulcerative colitis, Crohn's disease and unspecified inflammatory bowel disease. Data are presented as the number of patients with stones/total number of patients in the category; number in parentheses is the percent of patients with stones; NA: Not applicable).

noted higher rates of stones with patients who had surgical removal of a portion of the intestine compared to those with intact GI tracts (Table 17.1).

After Deren's initial report, a number of other studies reporting rates of urolithiasis in IBD quickly followed. Maratka and Nebdal found urolithiasis in 12% of patients with UC who had an ileostomy, much higher than the rate of 0.2% in those without surgery.[22] A study from the Lahey clinic reported a stone formation rate of 3.2% in 1,100 patients with IBD, with the highest stone rate in patients with ileocolitis.[23] The University of Chicago reported a significantly higher rate of urolithiasis in IBD than previous studies.[24] Of 885 IBD patients, 7.2% had urolithiasis. Stones were more frequent in those with granulomatous bowel disease (regional enteritis or ileocolitis), compared to those with UC (10.1% vs 6.4%, respectively). Calcium stones were four times more common than uric acid stones in both ulcerative and granulomatous colitis. In the subset of patients who had an ileostomy, 18% developed urolithiasis, with uric acid stones as common as calcium stones. Greenstein et al. reported rates of urolithiasis in patients with IBD followed from 1964 to 1973.[25] Of 700 patients, 5.3% of those with colitis and 8.9% of those with small bowel disease formed stones. Shield et al. reviewed 233 patients with IBD treated from 1958 to 1973.[26] Overall, 8.6% developed urolithiasis. Only 4.7% of patients without surgery developed stones, compared to 12.9% of patients who had ileostomies.

In a paper from Denmark reviewing 228 patients with IBD cared for from 1964 to 1975, 35 (15%) developed urolithiasis.[27] The prevalence of urolithiasis was the same for Crohn's disease and UC. The study only included patients who had undergone pyelography, so it likely overestimates the rate of stone disease in this patient population. A study from Leeds surveyed 426 patients who had undergone intestinal resection, 40 (9.4%) patients reported a history of symptomatic urolithiasis.[28] They separated the patients into three groups: (1) those with a colectomy and ileostomy with <10 cm of small bowel removed, (2) colectomy and ileostomy with 20–300 cm of small bowel removed, and (3) 50–300 cm of small bowel removed but colon left intact. Those with combined colectomy and small bowel resection had the highest rate of stone disease (14.8%) those with only small bowel resection and an intact colon had the lowest rate of stones (6.7%). Bennett and Hughes performed a mail survey of patients with UC; 458 patients participated. Of those treated medically, 4% developed urolithiasis after the onset of colitis symptoms. Of the patients who had an ileostomy, 8.4% developed urolithiasis.[29] In a study from Japan of 112 patients with UC, 7.1% developed urolithiasis, with higher stone rates seen in those who had ileostomies.[30] In studies where long-term follow-up was available, there was an average delay of 10 years from the onset of bowel disease to the diagnosis of urolithiasis.[21,23,24,26] Table 17.1 summarizes the studies that reported stone rates for patients who received only medical therapy compared to those who also had surgical intervention. All report higher rates with surgical resection of small or large intestine.

A more recent study from South Korea reported the incidence of urolithiasis in patients with Crohn's disease followed from 2011 to 2013.[31] Of the 387 patients evaluated, 4.7% developed new onset stone disease after the onset of their Crohn's symptoms with a mean time to stone formation of 3.9 years. The annual incidence of urolithiasis in this study was more than twice as high as the general population in Korea. Cury et al. did a cross-sectional study, performing renal ultrasounds on 168 patients with IBD in

Brazil, 93 diagnosed with Crohn's disease and 75 with UC.[32] The incidence of stones was 38% for both Crohn's and UC, all stones were asymptomatic. Only 1.2% of patients had undergone intestinal surgery. Of note, another report from Brazil reported a series of 29 patients with Crohn's disease evaluated by renal ultrasound. They found renal stones in 45% of the subjects.[33] The markedly elevated stone rate compared to other studies could be due to imaging all patients to screen for stones, or may be due to environment/diet unique to the patient population. Whether routine screening for stones in IBD would document such a high stone rate in other populations is not known.

Multiple factors may contribute to the wide variation in stone rates that have been reported. Methods of classifying patients as having urolithiasis vary from study to study. Some studies were done by chart review that included only stones requiring medical intervention. Others include any stone event as reported by patient survey, while some include asymptomatic stones that are incidental findings on radiologic studies. Because patients with GI disease are more likely to have imaging studies of the abdomen, asymptomatic stones are more likely to be discovered than in the general population. Also, as stones became a recognized complication, they were more likely to be noted by gastroenterologists caring for IBD patients, so an apparent increase in rate over time may be secondary to better recognition of the disease association as well as improved radiologic techniques. Despite variations from study to study, almost all show higher than the expected stone rate in the general population, and consistently find a higher rate of stone disease in those who have had surgical resection.

Improvements in treatment of IBD should reduce the prevalence of urolithiasis. Frolkis et al. performed a systematic literature review to document rates of surgery for IBD patients over time.[34] They reported the risk of intestinal surgery in the 10 years after diagnosis was 47% for patients with Crohn's disease and 16% for UC. Over the course of six decades, there were significant declines in the rates of surgery for both Crohn's and UC. Presumably, the improvement in medical therapy, particularly the use of biologic agents such as adalimumab and infliximab, reduce the need for surgical intervention.[35] Because surgical resection increases the risk of urolithiasis, any change in surgical rates should be reflected in fewer patients developing stones. In addition, there is a general trend to more bowel-conserving procedures, which should minimize the pathologic changes in intestinal fluid and electrolyte handling related to surgery.

Not only do patients with bowel disease have an increased rate of stone formation, they also have more complications associated with symptomatic urolithiasis. In a study using a national emergency department database from the United States, Varda et al. identified all patients presenting with urolithiasis from 2006 to 2009.[36] They then compared those patients who carried a diagnosis of IBD to those who did not. Patients with IBD had significantly higher rates of urinary infection, sepsis, organ failure, and hospital admission.

DISEASE OF THE COLON AND COLECTOMY

The following discussion separates patients with disease isolated to the colon from disease the affects the small intestine. The distinct physiologic functions of the small and large intestine lead to characteristic changes in urine chemistries when disease or surgical resection occurs. Some patients will have disease that encompasses both the small and large intestine. In such cases, prevalence of stone disease is usually greater than those with disease isolated to one intestinal segment[21,23] and the alterations in urine chemistries will depend on the extent of disease in each bowel segment.

Most of the data related to colectomy comes from series describing outcomes of patients with UC and Crohn's colitis. However, colectomy for any cause, such as familial polyposis, cancer, or trauma, places the patient at increased risk for urolithiasis. Multiple reports have shown a higher rate of stone formation in patients with colectomy compared to those with UC who had successful medical management. Surgical procedures for colectomy include proctocolectomy with or without continent pouch, ileorectal anastomosis or ileal pouch anal anastomosis (IPAA). In early series of surgical treatment of UC, proctocolectomy with terminal ileostomy was the usual procedure. Over time, ileostomy has been increasingly replaced with surgical techniques that leave the intestine in continuity, such as IPAA.[37] Many studies do not specify the type of surgery performed with colectomy or whether an ileostomy was continent or not, making it difficult to distinguish the effects of the individual surgical techniques. Epidemiologic studies specifically comparing stone rates in patients with permanent ileostomy compared to patients with continent ileostomies or IPAA are lacking. In the following discussion, specific surgical techniques will be identified when possible.

The physiologic derangements from colonic disease/resection increase risk of both uric acid and CaOx stones. Though both types of stones have been well documented, the relative incidence of uric acid vs CaOx is difficult to assess. However, it is clear that uric acid stones are more common in patients with colonic disease than those with disease of the small bowel.[24,38] Many studies documenting urolithiasis related to bowel disease have included only a smattering of stone analyses or have relied upon radiopacity of the stone to define the type of stone. In addition, many stones contain both CaOx and uric acid, and how they might be categorized varies from study to study. The following discussion approaches uric acid and calcium oxalate stones separately, but in reality, conditions amenable to formation of both types of stones often coexist.

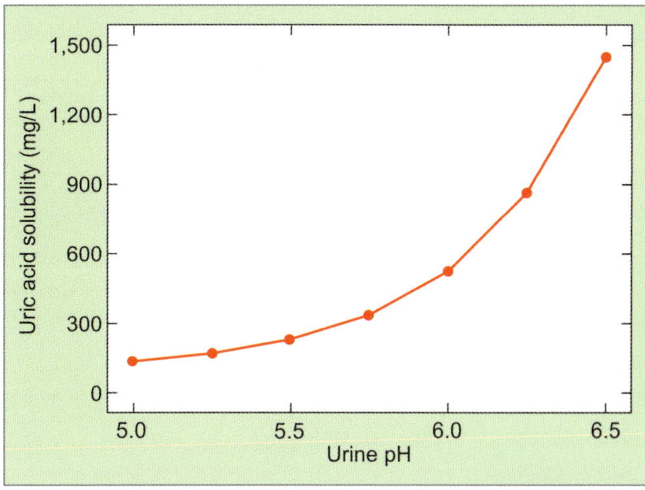

Fig. 17.1: Effect of urine pH on uric acid solubility. Total uric acid solubility is calculated assuming a solubility of deprotonated uric acid of 90 mg/L in urine.

Uric Acid Stones

An increased risk of uric acid stone formation by patients with colectomy has been well documented.[38-40] The key determinants of uric acid stone formation are urine pH, urine flow rate, and uric acid excretion. The fully protonated form of uric acid is poorly soluble with an estimated solubility in human urine of ~90 mg/L.[41] Uric acid is a weak acid with an effective pK_a of 5.35 in urine.[41,42] As urine pH falls to levels <5.5, a larger fraction of uric acid becomes protonated, such that even at normal urine flow and uric acid excretion rates, urine can become markedly supersaturated (Fig. 17.1). Patients with significant colonic disease and particularly those who have had colectomy and ileostomy typically produce an acidic urine. As noted above, ~1.5–2 L of bicarbonate-rich fluid is delivered to the colon each day. When colonic absorptive capacity is compromised, alkali, in the form of bicarbonate and organic anions, will be lost from the GI tract. The renal response will be to increase net acid excretion, by increasing ammonium and titratable acid excretion. The renal response can be quite vigorous, such that the majority of patients with colectomy do not develop overt metabolic acidosis.[43,44] But they do so by maintaining a high net acid excretion and potentially a very low urine pH. Pertinent studies of urine chemistries in relation to uric acid stone risk from patients with colectomy are summarized in Table 17.2.[28,45-48] Each of the studies provides a comparison to a healthy control group. Urine was significantly more acidic in colectomy patients in four of the five studies. Even in the study by Stern et al., a similar degree of urine acidity was found, but did not reach statistical significance due to the small number of subjects in the study (Table 17.2).[46]

Table 17.2: Colectomy and risk of uric acid stones.

	N		*Volume (mL/d)*		*pH*		*Uric acid (mg/d)*		*Mean uric acid SS*	
	Ctrl	Col	Ctrl	Col	Ctrl	Col	Ctrl	Col	Ctrl	Col
Clarke and McKenzie[45]	15	14	1342 ± 374	1082 ± 407*	6.0 ± 0.6	5.1 ± 0.5*	518 ± 234	640 ± 240	0.8	4.2
Stern et al.[46]	9	9	1221 ± 350	1095 ± 445*	5.9 ± 0.5	5.4 ± 0.6	818 ± 240	701 ± 297	1.6	3.7
Bambach et al.[28]	85	27	1700 ± 645	990 ± 363*	6.1 ± 0.5	5.2 ± 0.5*	606 ± 138	575 ± 295	0.6	3.8
Kennedy et al.[47]	39	39	1440 ± 560	1340 ± 400	5.9 ± 0.5	5.3 ± 1.0*	454 ± 185	504 ± 185	0.8	2.2
Caudarella et al.[48]	51	28	1454 ± 576	821 ± 331*	5.8 ± 0.3	5.2 ± 0.3*	514 ± 147	403 ± 223	1.0	3.2

Data are presented as mean ± SD. Uric acid SS estimated as the diprotonated uric acid concentration calculated using pK_a 5.35, divided by the diprotonated uric acid solubility of 90 mg/L.
Values marked (*) differ significantly from control group, $p < 0.05$.
(Ctrl: Control subjects; Col: Patients with colectomy; SS: Supersaturation).

Table 17.3: Effect of Ileostomy versus ileal pouch anal anastomosis on fluid and electrolyte balance.

		Urine			*Fecal output*		
	N	*Volume (mL/d)*	*Na (mmol/d)*	*K (mmol/d)*	*Weight (g/d)*	*Na (mmol/d)*	*K (mmol/d)*
Singer et al.[43]							
Ileostomy	20	623 ± 288	99 ± 70	69 ± 20	NR	NR	NR
IPAA	20	971 ± 549	114 ± 46	63 ± 27	NR	NR	NR
Christie et al.[59]							
Ileostomy	14	1171 ± 486	NR	NR	548 ± 150	74 ± 37	14 ± 19
IPAA	20	1139 ± 425	NR	NR	507 ± 40	58 ± 44	8 ± 4
Santavirta et al.[60]							
Ileostomy	10	1250 ± 543	79 ± 49	84 ± 24	688 ± 276	57 ± 25	5 ± 3
IPAA	30	1166 ± 522	73 ± 34	72 ± 24	547 ± 252	51 ± 23	7 ± 3*
Okamoto et al.[52]							
Ileostomy	24	802 ± 303	68 ± 39	47 ± 20	589 ± 205	69 ± 20	7 ± 5
IPAA	24	852 ± 201	126 ± 68	53 ± 39	410 ± 137	43 ± 10	5 ± 20

Data presented as mean ± SD. NR, not reported.
(IPAA: Ileal pouch anal anastomosis).
*$p < 0.05$ ileostomy compared to IPAA.

The colon is the final site of water and sodium reabsorption. Normal stool water is ~150 mL/d. In patients with colectomies, ileostomy fluid output is in the range of 300–1,000 mL/d (Table 17.3). As would be expected, this excess water loss leads to increased thirst and higher intake of water than healthy people.[49] However, the increased fluid intake is not sufficient to fully compensate for the GI losses, resulting in urine flow rates lower than healthy subjects, as shown in four of the five studies in Table 17.2. Accompanying the GI fluid loss is an increased loss of sodium, in the range of 25–100 mmol/d, much greater than the 5–10 mmol/d found in healthy subjects (Table 17.3).

The physiologic impact of the intestinal salt and water losses has been confirmed using isotopic methods. Measurement of total body water showed deficits of 11% in two separate studies of stable ileostomy patients at least 3 months postsurgery.[50,51] Clarke et al. showed a 7% deficit in total body sodium in 21 patients with ileostomy compared to a healthy control group.[50] Hill et al. measured total body sodium in 10 patients before and after ileostomy.[51] There was no improvement in total body sodium from the preoperative state when the patients were ill, compared to 6 months after surgery when the patients were stable. In a separate study, Kennedy et al. measured plasma renin and aldosterone in 39 patients with ileostomy for UC.[44] All were at least 1 year postsurgery and otherwise healthy. Both renin and aldosterone were significantly higher than that of the control group. Okamoto et al. measured plasma renin and aldosterone in 26 patients with UC before and after ileostomy.[52] Renin and aldosterone were higher after ileostomy, but the differences were not statistically significant, which might be due to some level of volume depletion from active colonic disease preoperatively. No comparison was made to a healthy control group in this study. Volume depletion promotes sodium retention, which maximizes bicarbonate reabsorption via Na-proton exchange in the tubule, contributing to the low urine pH. In response to the chronic volume depletion, renal sodium excretion is reduced compared to healthy people.[44,50] The chronic water and sodium deficits increase vasopressin release from the pituitary, resulting in production of a highly concentrated urine.

Uric acid excretion is dependent on purine consumption. The colon is not involved in nutrient absorption, so colonic disease does not affect purine absorption from the diet. Only a limited number of studies have included uric acid excretion data from patients with ileal disease. As shown in Table 17.2, there is not a difference in uric acid excretion between healthy subjects and patients with colectomy. In order to estimate overall uric acid stone risk, uric acid supersaturation (SS) was calculated from the mean data presented in each study in Table 17.2. The uric acid saturation was approximately three times higher in the colectomy groups compared to controls.

Of note, patients in these studies (*see* Table 17.2) were not selected for stone formation. In the Clarke study none of the subjects had urolithiasis, in the other studies ~10% of subjects had formed stones. In comparison, Parks et al. published their findings in 58 patients with urolithiasis secondary to ileostomy.[38] They found a urine pH of 5.40 ± 0.05 (mean ± SEM) and urine flow rate of 1.22 ± 0.07 L/d similar to that presented in Table 17.2, showing that those who form stones are not significantly different than those without stones. Therefore, most colectomy patients are at risk for uric acid stone formation. Whether an acute or intermittent worsening of disease and urine chemistries, not detected in routine urine testing, contributes to stone formation is not known. At times, dehydration and urine acidification can become so severe that urate nephropathy can develop leading to acute kidney injury. In any patient with colectomy and unexplained loss of kidney function is diagnosed, the possibility of acute urate nephropathy needs to be evaluated.[53]

Calcium Oxalate Stones

The major determinants of CaOx SS are urine flow rate, and the excretion of calcium, oxalate, magnesium, and citrate. As noted above, colectomy is characterized by production of small amounts of concentrated urine, a risk factor for forming any type of stone. Dietary oxalate can be absorbed from the colon, though in the absence of fat malabsorption, this is probably a minor contribution to total daily oxalate excretion. Colectomy is not associated with hyperoxaluria,[38] though a patient who has a very high dietary oxalate intake may still develop hyperoxaluria because small intestinal oxalate absorption remains intact. Urine calcium excretion tends to be normal to low in patients with colectomy.[38] Chronic volume depletion will lead to increased renal reabsorption and lower urine Ca excretion. In addition, the cecum and ascending colon do absorb 5–10% of dietary calcium, so surgical resection contributes to lower calcium absorption. If the patient has reduced intake due to lack of appetite from persistent GI disease, they may have frankly low urine calcium.

Citrate prevents crystallization of calcium oxalate by complexing calcium and by direct inhibition of calcium oxalate crystal growth.[54] Hypocitraturia is a well-documented risk factor for calcium stones. Citrate is filtered by the glomerulus and final renal excretion is determined by the extent of proximal tubule reabsorption. Metabolic acidosis and hypokalemia are the main factors that increase tubular reabsorption, lowering citrate excretion.[55] As described above, GI bicarbonate loss commonly leads to low urine citrate in patients with colectomy. Gastrointestinal potassium losses in colectomy patients are not excessive (*see* Table 17.3) and urine potassium excretion is not low, suggesting potassium depletion is not a common contributing factor of hypocitraturia in colonic disease. Multiple studies have documented hypocitraturia is common in patients with colectomy, in both patients with and without a history of urolithiasis.[38,48,56,57] Magnesium complexes oxalate in urine, thus acting as an inhibitor of CaOx crystallization. Renal magnesium excretion is lower in patients with colectomy than healthy subjects or patients with bowel disease without colonic resection.[38,47,48,56] Overt magnesium depletion as defined by hypomagnesemia seems to be rare in colectomy patients, unless small intestinal disease coexists.[47,56]

In theory, any disease that interferes with colonic function/integrity should increase the risk of stone formation. However, most studies have focused specifically on patients with ileostomy/colectomy. Stelzner et al. studied 12 patients with UC immediately before and 4 months after colectomy with ileostomy.[57] Urine citrate and sodium excretion were both low even before ileostomy. McConnell and colleagues studied 15 patients with UC, only one of whom had colon surgery and a minority had active bowel disease.[56] Urine volume and citrate excretion did not differ from controls. Caudarella et al. measured urine chemistries in 10 patients with UC prior to surgery, and 28 patients after having an IPAA.[48] Both groups had lower urine pH and citrate than healthy subjects, but only those with IPAA had lower urine volume. The differences found in these studies are likely due to differences in disease activity at the time of urine collections. It is probable that stone disease is more common in those with colonic resection as patients with uncontrollable inflammatory disease will be those who require colectomies. Patients whose UC can successfully be managed medically would be expected to have less severe derangements in urine chemistries.

Much of the data regarding colectomy and stone risk were collected from patients who had a permanent ileostomy, but surgical techniques have changed over time. The effects of the continent ileostomy and the ileoanal anastomosis on fluid and electrolyte balance have been compared to that of standard ileostomy with proctocolectomy. Stern et al. studied nine patients with conventional ileostomy to nine patients with a continent ileostomy (Kock pouch).[46] Urine volume was lower (733 ± 307 vs 1095 ± 445 mL/d) and urine pH higher (5.63 ± 0.54 vs 5.38 ± 0.62) in the patients with a Kock pouch, though neither difference reached statistical significance. At the present time, the ileoanal anastomosis is the preferred procedure for most patients requiring colectomy.[58] A number of studies have reported fluid and electrolyte balance in patients with ileoanal anastomosis compared to those with IPAA.[43,52,59,60] The results are summarized in Table 17.3. Three of the studies reported stool output and noted no significant differences in stool weight or electrolyte losses. Because GI losses did not differ, urine flow and electrolyte excretion did not differ between the two groups either. All in all, patient satisfaction is enhanced by the procedures that maintain fecal continence, but it appears that the risk of stone formation is not reduced with the continent procedures.

Renal Pathology

Historically, renal histology related to stone disease was limited to the unusual cases where kidney dysfunction necessitated a renal biopsy or in cases where stone burden was large and advanced renal parenchymal scarring was present, in which case a nephrectomy might be performed. However, these scenarios provided only glimpses of the most severe renal outcomes and did not apply to more common disease. Recently, technologic advances in minimally invasive surgery for urolithiasis have permitted groundbreaking research on the anatomy and histology of stone formation in the renal pelvis; allowing correlation of histology with medical phenotypes defined by medical history, urine chemistries and crystallographic stone analysis. Evan et al. reported renal histology in seven patients who had developed kidney stones after undergoing total colectomy with ileostomy.[61] Five of the patients had UC, one had Crohn's disease and one had colon cancer. The patients were evaluated and biopsied while undergoing percutaneous nephrolithotomy. Three patients had pure uric acid stones, three pure CaOx stones and one had mixed uric acid/CaOx stones. All patients had interstitial white plaque, which is apatite deposition in the papillary interstitium. White plaque is a frequent lesion in idiopathic calcium oxalate stone formers that appears to be a preferred growth site for CaOx stones.[62] All patients also had yellow intratubular plaque that was composed of mixed crystals, apatite as well as AmU and sodium acid urate. Papillary scarring was common and the extent of the papillary damage correlated with reduced eGFR (*see* Chapter 1.5). In idiopathic CaOx stone formers, increased levels of white plaque is related to low urine flow and low urine pH. Patients with colectomy share these traits, which explain the finding of white plaque in this group. The finding of urate salts is understandable in a group of patients that are at increased risk of uric acid stone formation. The presence of apatite in the collecting ducts of patients with persistently acidic urine is unexpected. Apatite tends to form in urine above pH 6.0. The consistent finding of apatite in tubules despite acid urine has led the investigators to hypothesize that local acidification defects occur in some papillae after obstruction, leading to apatite formation. However, this hypothesis remains to be proven.

Treatment of Stones in Patients with Colectomy

Whether the patient has uric acid or calcium oxalate stone, the focal point for therapy is to increase urine flow. The patient needs to ingest sufficient fluids to compensate for their intestinal losses. Adequate fluid intake will suppress vasopressin release and lead to formation of a dilute urine. Unfortunately, altered GI function may prevent the patient from drinking as much as directed. As fluid intake increases, ileostomy output or delivery of liquid stool to the ileoanal pouch increases as well.[49,63] Patients may find the extra GI output impacts their quality of life. Their fluid intake will be a balance of their desire to prevent additional stone formation versus the need to live as normal a life as possible. This will be even more problematic if the patient has any small bowel involvement with their disease. Consuming beverages along with solute such as sugars or electrolytes may improve water reabsorption in proximal intestinal segments, reducing delivery to the terminal ileum and total GI output. In idiopathic stone formers, it is frequently recommended that they urinate at least 2.5 L/d.[64] In patients with colectomy, their baseline urine flow rate may be well below 1 L/d; in such cases raising urine volume to 1.5–2 L/d may be sufficient to reduce stone formation. However, as in all stone patients, the greater the urine volume the better.

Alkali therapy is of benefit for both uric acid and calcium oxalate stone formers, though the goal of alkali therapy is different depending on the type of stone. In uric acid stone formers, the goal is to raise urine pH into the range of 6.0–6.5, which correlates to a uric acid solubility of ~500–1500 mg/L in urine (*see* Fig. 17.1). There is seldom reason to raise 24-hour urine pH >6.5, and doing so may put the patient at risk for calcium phosphate stone formation. Response to therapy can be monitored by 24-hour urine collections using the time averaged pH to assess risk. Alternatively, the patient can use urine dipsticks and measure urine pH multiple times during the day to see if urine pH is above 6 the majority of time. For CaOx stones, the goal of alkali therapy is not the increase in pH, but an increase in urine citrate, as CaOx stone risk is fairly independent of urine pH. Twenty-four-hour urine collections are required to assess if citrate excretion has normalized with therapy. Using urine pH as a marker of alkali effect is not adequate to insure there has been an improvement in urine citrate excretion. An alkali load sufficient to compensate for the daily GI loss of alkali is the minimum required dose. Generally, a dose of 40–60 mEq/d of alkali divided into two to three doses is a reasonable starting dose. If renal acid excretion is very high, then it may be wise to start with an even higher dose. Renal acid excretion can be estimated by how much higher urine ammonium excretion is compared to urine sulfate excretion (both measured in mEq/d) in patients with a urine pH < 6.5. Urine sulfate is a convenient marker of diet acid load. The amount of ammonium excreted in excess of sulfate is an estimate of the amount of alkali lost in diarrhea. A daily alkali dose in excess of the ammonium to sulfate difference will likely be needed to raise urine pH. It has been suggested that uric acid stone formers can be treated with a single dose of alkali per day, though there have not been prospective trials comparing multiple doses to single-dose therapy.[65] In patients with the extreme alkali loss caused by colectomy, it seems prudent to use a more standard dosing schedule.

The alkali anion is usually provided as citrate or bicarbonate salts. A key question is whether to use potassium or sodium as the accompanying cation. In most patients with kidney stones, potassium is preferred over sodium, as sodium loading may increase urine calcium excretion. In patients with bowel disease, there is often accompanying volume depletion,[44,52] in which case sodium alkali may be preferred. If a patient has potassium depletion, potassium alkali is indicated. The patients' urine sodium and potassium excretion can guide which alkali to use; in some patients, a mix of both potassium and sodium salts may be the best choice. Since the electrolytes are predominantly absorbed in the small intestine, absorption of alkali salts should not be a problem. Potassium salts tend to cause more intestinal problems, including bloating, diarrhea and GI irritation. The symptoms may be minimized by taking the potassium salts with meals. Potassium alkali may be provided as liquid or pill form. Because potassium salts have an unpleasant taste, many patients prefer to take pills. The pills are provided as a delayed release formulation that should reduce the amount of gastric irritation, though drug intolerance is still a problem. Potassium citrate is provided in a wax matrix tablet, which is not digestible. Patients will pass the pill matrix in their stool, which can lead to concerns that the medication is not being absorbed. Monitoring urine potassium excretion, which should rise significantly above baseline during therapy, will confirm if the potassium citrate is being absorbed.

If a patient with uric acid stones is unable to take sufficient alkali to raise urine pH and/or sufficient fluids to increase urine flow rate, then an alternative therapy would be to lower uric acid excretion. Reducing dietary purine intake will lower uric acid excretion. The most common high purine foods are high protein foods. One can get a reasonable assessment of protein intake from urine urea nitrogen and urine sulfate excretion, and monitor the success of dietary intervention by follow-up measurements of these diet protein markers. Lowering dietary protein intake will also lower metabolic acid production, helping to raise urine pH. However, restriction of diet protein must be done with care so as not to risk inadequate nutrition. In recalcitrant cases of uric acid stones due to bowel disease, treatment with xanthine oxidase inhibitors such as allopurinol or febuxostat can be considered. Xanthine oxidase inhibitors lower urine uric acid by 40–50%. Though lowering uric acid excretion will reduce stone risk, the five- to eightfold increase in uric acid solubility that can be obtained by increasing urine pH makes alkali therapy the optimal therapy (*see* Fig. 17.1).

The net benefit of treatment (fluids, diet, alkali, and even xanthine oxidase inhibitors) can be judged by calculations of uric acid SS. The goal of therapy should be to make urine undersaturated with respect to uric acid (a SS value of <1). If this value goal is achieved and maintained, it is highly unlikely uric acid stones will recur. In fact, urine persistently undersaturated with respect to uric acid can lead to dissolution of uric acid stones present in the renal pelvis. It is unlikely that medical therapy will lead to dissolution of calcium oxalate stones, so the goal is prevention of new stones forming and reducing the growth rate of pre existing stones.

Not all stones associated with bowel disease are composed of CaOx and/or uric acid. Aminosalicylates are part of the standard therapy for IBD. Sulfasalazine, which is metabolized by intestinal bacteria into 5-aminosalicylate and sulfapyridine, is one of the common forms of aminosalicylate in use. In acidic, concentrated urine, as might be found in patients with IBD, the risk of crystallization of the drug within the urinary tract increases. Cases have been reported of acute kidney injury due to bilateral ureteral stone formation. Maintaining high fluid intake should be emphasized during treatment with sulfasalazine.[66,67]

ENTERIC HYPEROXALURIA

Small Intestinal Disease and Resection

Enteric hyperoxaluria is the pathologic hyperabsorption of dietary oxalate that leads to increased renal excretion of the excess oxalate. Enteric hyperoxaluria is caused by reduced functional surface area of the small intestine, most commonly due to surgical bypass or resection. Paradoxically, it is intestinal malabsorption, specifically of lipids and bile salts, which leads to the increased absorption of oxalate.

Enteric hyperoxaluria was first described in the early 1970s, with the recognition of an association of small bowel resection and subsequent stone disease and hyperoxaluria.[68,69] Most commonly it was described as a consequence of intestinal resection for Crohn's disease, but EH can occur in any disease that caused malabsorption of fat and bile salts (Table 17.4). Numerous studies have shown that the excess oxalate is of dietary origin. Chadwick et al. performed oxalate loading tests in seven patients with EH due to ileal resection and found ^{14}C oxalate absorption of 52 ± 3% versus 28 ± 3% in healthy subjects.[70] In addition, they placed patients on a diet devoid of oxalate, leading to the resolution of hyperoxaluria. Earnest et al. compared ^{14}C oxalate absorption in patients with minimal (<50 cm) ileal resection to those with extensive ileal resection (>100 cm) and found oxalate absorption significantly higher in those with more extensive resection (20% vs 44%, $p < 0.001$).[71] Froeder et al. showed significantly higher urine oxalate excretion rates after an oral oxalate load in 61 patients who had undergone either Roux-en-Y gastric bypass (RYGB) or biliopancreatic diversion (BPD) compared to morbidly obese subjects who had not undergone bariatric surgery.[72] Stauffer et al. reported normalization of urine oxalate with institution of an oxalate-free diet in two patients with EH due to ileal resection.[73] Normal urinary excretion of glycolate confirmed abnormal endogenous oxalate production did not contribute to hyperoxaluria in patients with bowel resection.[71,74]

The site of excess oxalate absorption in EH proved to be the colon. Dobbins and Binder reported a urine oxalate of 84 ± 12 mg/d in 11 patients with steatorrhea and intact colons, but in 5 patients with steatorrhea and colectomy, none had hyperoxaluria.[75] A ^{14}C oxalate load test revealed absorption of >35% in all patients with steatorrhea and an intact colon, but <10% in those with an ileostomy. Andersson and associates compared 12 patients with Crohn's disease who had an ileal resection to 11 who had ileal resection with a colectomy.[76] On a high-oxalate diet, those with only ileal resection had a urine oxalate of 122 ± 24 mg/d versus 49 ± 6 mg/d in the colectomy group. Hylander et al. found significantly higher urine oxalate excretion in 36 Crohn's disease patients with steatorrhea and partial colectomy than in 20 Crohn's patients who had steatorrhea and a total colectomy.[77] Modigliani et al. reported normal urine oxalate (22 ± 4 mg/d) in 5 patients with ileal resection and colectomy compared to urine oxalate excretion of 90 ± 12 mg/d in 13 patients with ileal resection and an intact colon.[78] Though most diet oxalate is absorbed in the small intestine in healthy people, small bowel malabsorption alters colonic function to induce a remarkable increase in oxalate absorption.

Table 17.4: Causes of enteric hyperoxaluria in adults.
Bariatric surgery
• Roux-en-Y gastric bypass
• Biliopancreatic diversion
• Jejunoileal bypass
Intestinal resection for bowel disease
• Crohn's disease
• Radiation enteritis
• Mesenteric ischemia
• Trauma
Celiac disease
Pancreatic insufficiency
Intestinal lipase inhibitors

The final components in the genesis of EH are fat and bile salt malabsorption. Absorption of dietary fatty acids requires micelle formation with bile acids to insure delivery of the hydrophobic fats to the intestinal epithelia. Lipids are absorbed throughout the small intestine, but the ileum plays the most important role. Not only does the ileum provide surface area for fat absorption but it is the site of enterohepatic recirculation of bile salts. The loss of bile salts in the stool is usually compensated by increased production of bile salts in the liver, but if bile salt losses become overwhelming, a bile salt deficiency can result and further compromise intestinal fat absorption. Considering the unique role of the ileum in fat and bile acid metabolism, it is not surprising that patients with ileal resection are at such high risk of developing EH.

Fat malabsorption promotes colonic oxalate absorption in two ways. Excess free fatty acids in the intestinal lumen complex calcium, lowering the free calcium concentration. With depletion of ionized calcium, a larger percentage of dietary oxalate remains as free ion in solution, and thus is more readily absorbed by the gut. In vitro studies have shown that addition of the fatty acid oleate to an aqueous solution of calcium and oxalate increases the solubility of oxalate, presumably by lowering ionized calcium levels.[79] The critical role of calcium in regulating oxalate absorption was shown in colonic perfusion studies performed in patients with EH. In a study of three subjects with steatorrhea from ileal resection, a perfusion tube was placed at the ileocecal junction and 48 mmol of Ca in a saline solution was administered directly into the colon each day while the patients consumed a high oxalate diet. Colonic perfusion resulted in a 57% reduction in urine oxalate excretion and returned to baseline when perfusion was done with a calcium free solution.[78] This study confirms the contribution of the colon in excess oxalate absorption in EH. A study using ^{14}C oxalate load in two patients with steatorrhea from pancreatitis showed administration of 1,500 mg of Ca reduced intestinal oxalate absorption from 54% to 4%.[80] Hylander showed reductions of ^{14}C oxalate absorption (from 28% to 9%) during calcium supplementation in eight patients with jejunoileal bypass (JIB).[81] Additional studies of the effectiveness of oral calcium loading on oxalate excretion are described below in the section on treatment of EH. The second means by which steatorrhea promotes oxalate absorption is by a direct effect on the colon. Animal experiments have shown that fatty acids increase the permeability of the colonic epithelia to oxalate, allowing increased absorption down its concentration gradient.[82,83]

Bile acid malabsorption is frequently present in patients with EH and plays an important role in oxalate absorption. Multiple studies showed bile acids increased permeability of colonic epithelia to oxalate.[75,82,84] Fairclough et al. proved a link between bile acid malabsorption and oxalate absorption by the colon.[85] In two patients who had colon exclusion surgery for hepatic encephalopathy, they perfused the colon with an oxalate solution spiked with ^{14}C oxalate, with or without the bile acid chenodeoxycholate. Uptake of radiolabeled oxalate from the perfusate was much greater in the presence of the bile acid, as was the urinary excretion of oxalate after the perfusion containing bile acids. Most early studies of EH focused on patients with ileal resection or bypass, in which case bile acid malabsorption was invariably present. The recent description of EH in patients with RYGB for obesity, where the ileum is not bypassed and bile acid malabsorption is not usually present,[86] suggests bile acid malabsorption is not an absolute requirement for the development of EH.

In summary, disease or resection of the small intestine leads to the loss of jejunal and ileal surface area that will reduce fluid and electrolyte absorption, increasing delivery of fluid to the colon. Lipids are absorbed throughout the small intestine, so loss of surface area reduces fat absorption. In addition, the loss of the ileum will increase delivery of bile salts to the colon and lead to possible bile acid deficiency, further worsening steatorrhea. Nutrients delivered to the colon will produce an osmotic diarrhea, because the colon has limited capacity for nutrient absorption. Bile acids cause secretion of water and solute from the colonic epithelium, worsening diarrhea. The delivery of excess bile salts and fatty acids to the colon increases colonic permeability to oxalate and excess fatty acids prevent calcium from binding oxalate, increasing the free oxalate concentration in the colon lumen. The extra fluid in the colon lumen helps disperse oxalate across the intestinal surface, further promoting oxalate absorption, resulting in hyperoxaluria.

In addition to the aforementioned overabsorption of dietary oxalate, the stone risk associated with EH is often exacerbated by derangements in other intestinal functions. The most basic is the loss of excess water in the stool, leading to chronic dehydration. As noted previously, the small intestine traffics large amounts of fluid each day and delivers 1.5–2 L of fluid to the colon daily. If disease reduces small intestinal water absorption, the colon has the capacity to increase absorption but once delivery to the colon exceeds 4–5 L/d, the absorptive capacity of the colon is exceeded and diarrhea occurs. Of course, if a disease involves both colon and small intestine, as might be seen in Crohn's disease, then clinically significant diarrhea is even more likely. The renal response to chronic dehydration will be the excretion of small amounts of highly concentrated urine, increasing the risk of stone formation.[38,68,87]

The loss of GI alkali equivalents from chronic diarrhea leads to metabolic acidosis. Both pancreatic juice and bile are alkaline and provide large amounts of bicarbonate to the intestinal lumen. Much of the secreted bicarbonate is absorbed via sodium-hydrogen exchange in the lumen of the small intestine. In addition, organic anions, which generate bicarbonate when metabolized, are absorbed in

Table 17.5: Urinary excretions in patients with urolithiasis from small bowel disease compared to patients with idiopathic urolithiasis.

	Jejunoileal bypass	*Small bowel surgery*	*Small bowel and colon surgery*	*Idiopathic stone formers*
N	27	36	29	2,048
Volume (L/d)	1.88 ± 0.12	1.41 ± 0.11	1.41 ± 0.18	1.65 ± 0.02
pH	5.59 ± 0.06	5.78 ± 0.08	5.55 ± 0.06	6.01 ± 0.01*
Calcium (mg/d)	120 ± 19	150 ± 15	144 ± 11	221 ± 2*
Oxalate (mg/d)	104 ± 11*	57 ± 5†	47 ± 3	39 ± 0.3
Citrate (mg/d)	254 ± 60	342 ± 62	175 ± 32	521 ± 6*
Uric acid (mg/d)	608 ± 58	561 ± 21	551 ± 32	641 ± 4
Magnesium mg/d	61 ± 7	59 ± 5	48 ± 6	103 ± 1*
Sodium (mmol/d)	242 ± 20*	149 ± 11	122 ± 15	170 ± 1*
Potassium (mmol/d)	55 ± 4	48 ± 2†	54 ± 6	59 ± 1

Source: Adapted from Parks et al.[38]
Data presented as mean ± SEM.
*Differs from all other groups, $p < 0.05$.
†Differs from idiopathic stone formers, $p < 0.05$.

the small intestine. Loss of bicarbonate and organic anions is the equivalent to a metabolic acid load. When severe it can lead to an overt metabolic acidosis with low blood bicarbonate levels. Potassium deficiency is common in short bowel syndrome, due to excess loss of potassium in the stool. Both the increased metabolic acid load and potassium deficiency increase proximal tubule reabsorption of citrate, reducing urine citrate excretion (Table 17.5).[38,88-91] Low urine flow rate and hypocitraturia are well-recognized risk factors for calcium oxalate stone formation, adding these problems to hyperoxaluria creates a urine milieu that strongly favors stone formation.

Bariatric Surgery

Jejunoileal Bypass

Bariatric surgery was introduced as a treatment for morbid obesity in the early 1960s, long before the obesity epidemic began in the United States. The JIB was initially reported by Payne et al. in 1963 and was the first bariatric procedure to gain wide spread acceptance.[92] In the JIB, the terminal 10–25 cm of the ileum is connected to 30 cm of proximal jejunum, bypassing the bulk of the jejunum and ileum, greatly reducing the available absorptive surface of the intestinal tract (Fig. 17.2A). The procedure induced weight loss by a combination of reduced caloric intake and reduced absorption of ingested nutrients. Caloric intake was not limited by restricting gastric capacity but rather by the discomfort and inconvenience of malabsorption induced diarrhea, as well as a hormonally mediated decrease in appetite. Condon et al. showed caloric intake fell by 20% 6 months postsurgery compared to preoperative intake.[93] Weight loss was significant with good patient satisfaction, as dietary intake was not greatly restricted.

The first reports of kidney stones ascribed to JIB did not appear for a decade after the procedure was introduced.[94-96] The delay in recognition of the association was likely due to the delay of stone formation after the JIB procedure and the high prevalence of kidney stone disease in the general population. There is little concern when a patient passes a kidney stone that it may represent a new syndrome. Urolithiasis in patients with IBD had been recognized and many risk factors such as low urine flow, hypocitraturia, and acidic urine had been reported. An additional factor that delayed the recognition of JIB as a cause of stones and oxalate nephropathy was urine oxalate measurements were not commonly available for clinical care until the 1980s. However, the description of EH in patients with extensive small bowel disease and/or intestinal resection led investigators to consider whether a similar problem might exist in patients with JIB.[68] In most series, urolithiasis begin to appear in the first 2 years after JIB surgery, but the mean time to stone formation for a surgical cohort is dependent on the duration of follow-up of the study. The longer patients are followed, the larger the fraction of the cohort that develops stones, as would

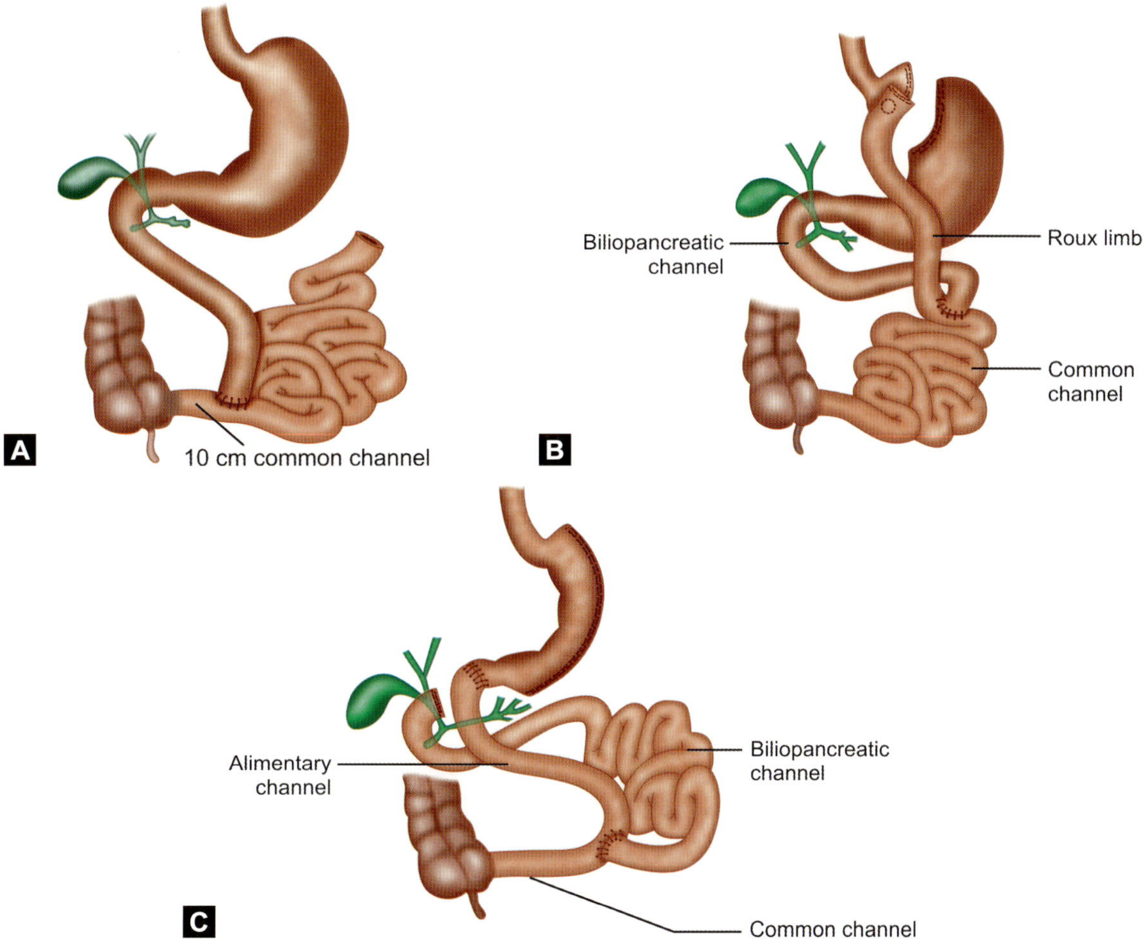

Figs. 17.2A to C: Surgical anatomy of bariatric procedures. (A) Jejunoileal bypass; (B) Roux-en-Y gastric bypass; (C) duodenal switch version of a biliopancreatic diversion.

be expected in a population with such significant derangements in urine chemistries.[97,98]

Multiple studies showed hyperoxaluria was the major lithogenic risk factor in patients with JIB. Fikri and Casella presented case reports on five JIB patients with calcium oxalate stones.[99] All had hyperoxaluria with oxalate excretion ranging from 54 to 121 mg/d. Gregory et al. reported that 12% of 543 patients who had undergone JIB had formed urolithiasis, with 94% of the stones that were analyzed being calcium oxalate.[100] They performed urine studies in 10 JIB patients with stones, 10 without stones, and 10 patients awaiting JIB surgery. Both the JIB patients with and without stones had similar levels of hyperoxaluria (mean urine oxalate 130 and 124 mg/d, respectively), markedly higher than the obese patients awaiting surgery (18 mg/d). Nordenvall et al. studied 30 JIB patients, half of whom had formed urolithiasis.[101] Hyperoxaluria was present in all patients and was of equal severity in those with and without stones. The severity of hyperoxaluria did not change with time after JIB surgery. In a study of 56 JIB patients from Sweden, 39% formed kidney stones.[102] Severe hyperoxaluria and modest hypocitraturia was noted in the patients both with and without stones. Overall, the hyperoxaluria in JIB was often severe, reaching levels seen in patients with primary hyperoxaluria. The pathophysiology of hyperoxaluria was assumed to be the same as described in patients with other forms of short gut syndrome, as described above. Prevalence of EH was very high in JIB patients, >90% in some series, with the chronic hyperoxaluria leading to recurrent calcium oxalate stone formation.[103] Hyperoxaluria was so severe that some patients developed chronic kidney disease (CKD) from oxalate nephropathy, some progressing to dialysis or transplant.[104] Requarth et al. followed 453 patients for an average of 15 years after JIB.[97] Urolithiasis were reported in 28% of patients and CKD developed in 7%, with 1.5% progressing to end-stage kidney disease. In that cohort, 138 of the 453 patients eventually had their JIB procedure reversed, with urolithiasis being the second most common reason for the reversal.

As shown in patients with small bowel resection, resolution or marked improvement of hyperoxaluria in patients placed on a very low oxalate diet confirmed the excess urine oxalate was of dietary origin.[105,106] Lindsjo measured urinary excretion of orally administered ^{14}C-oxalate in 19 patients with JIB.[107] The JIB patients excreted 29% of the oxalate load, compared to 6% in healthy subjects. The majority of the oxalate was excreted in the first 6 hours in the healthy subjects, suggesting the bulk of oxalate was absorbed in the small intestine, whereas in the JIB patients excretion of oxalate was delayed and prolonged, supporting the hypothesis of colonic oxalate absorption.

Over time, multiple complications were associated with JIB, almost all due to malabsorption.[97,108,109] Many patients required reversal of JIB due to intractable complications, most commonly liver and kidney disease. The Cleveland Clinic reported four patients who had JIB reversed for stone disease.[110] After 2 years of follow-up, urine oxalate fell from a mean of 112 to 34 mg/d. Stone formation rate dropped significantly, though the patients were also receiving alkali therapy. Kidney function remained stable. Dean et al. performed JIB reversal in 43 patients, 29 of whom received a gastroplasty at the time of the reversal procedure.[111] Both groups reported no further stone formation, but those with gastroplasty maintained a stable weight; those with only a reversal had significant weight gain during follow-up. Kirkpatirck reported two patients with JIB converted to RYGB for oxalate nephropathy requiring dialysis.[108] One was able to have a successful renal transplant and the other recovered kidney function postconversion to RYGB. In the early 1980s, a moratorium was placed on the JIB due to the many complications that had been reported.[112] Approximately 25,000 JIB procedures had been performed prior to 1980. There are still some patients with JIB anatomy intact who require care and monitoring for urolithiasis and oxalate nephropathy.[112]

Modern Bariatric Surgery

With the demise of JIB, a new procedure was needed for treatment of obesity and its complications. In 1969, the RYGB was introduced as an alternative to the JIB, after it had been noted that patients who had gastrectomy for ulcer disease frequently lost weight.[113] When the problems with JIB became increasingly evident, RYGB quickly became the preferred bariatric procedure. Initially, weight loss was thought to be due to reduced calorie consumption caused by early satiety induced by the small gastric pouch. Because of the emphasis on the restrictive nature of the procedure, RYGB became widely accepted without studies as to whether it might cause EH. When the laparoscopic RYGB was introduced in the 1990s, it quickly became the most common bariatric procedure in the United States. Over the last 20 years, bariatric surgery has become increasingly common as the obesity epidemic has spread throughout industrialized countries. In the United States, a BMI >40 kg/m^2 by itself makes a person a candidate for bariatric surgery (Table 17.6). The prevalence of severe obesity (BMI > 40) almost doubled between 1994 and 2000 and continues to rise, such that now >6% of the adult population are candidates for bariatric surgery on the basis of BMI alone (Fig. 17.3).[114-117] Approximately 15% of adults have a BMI >35, a level considered appropriate for bariatric surgery if complications of obesity such as sleep apnea, diabetes, or severe osteoarthritis are present (Table 17.6).[118] Similar trends of increasing obesity are found in children and adolescents.[119]

Table 17.6: NIH criteria for bariatric surgery.

Weight
• 100 lb or 100% above desirable weight
• BMI > 40 kg/m^2
• BMI > 35 kg/m^2 with comorbidities
Failure of nonsurgical attempts at weight loss
Absence of endocrine causes of obesity
Psychological stability
• Absence of alcohol or drug abuse
• Commitment to long-term follow-up
Acceptable operative risk

Modern bariatric surgery consists of purely restrictive procedures, such as the laparoscopic gastric banding and sleeve gastrectomy, in which food capacity is reduced but there is no disruption of intestinal flow, and mixed restrictive and malabsorptive procedures such as RYGB or BPD. Of the currently used procedures, RYGB is the most common bariatric procedure worldwide, though purely restrictive procedures are growing in popularity (Fig. 17.4).[120] The same trend of increasing utilization of the sleeve gastrectomy has also been reported in the United States.[121] In

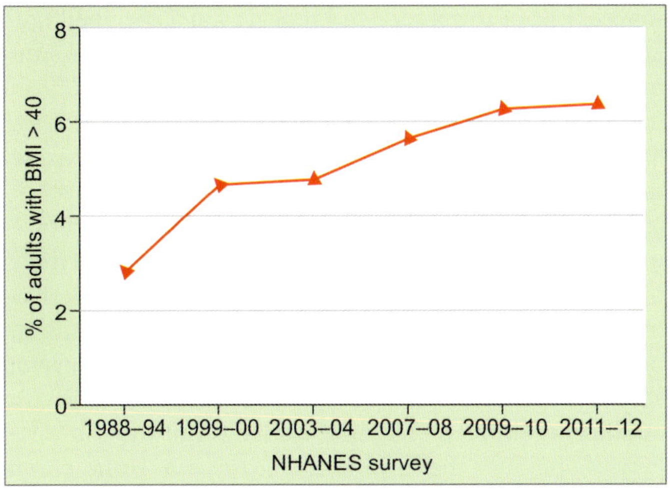

Fig. 17.3: Trend of prevalence of severe obesity (Grade 3) in the United States.
Source: Data obtained from NHANES.[114-118]

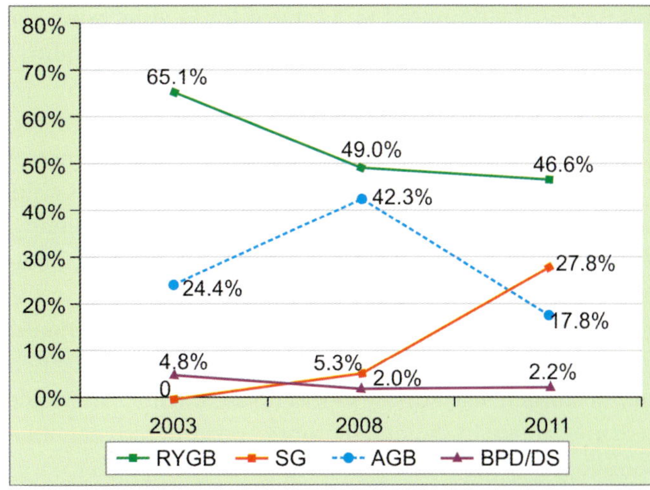

Fig. 17.4: Trends in relative utilization of bariatric procedures worldwide. (RYGB: Roux-en-Y gastric bypass; AGB: Adjustable gastric banding; SG: Sleeve gastrectomy; BPD/DS: Biliopancreatic diversion/duodenal switch).
Source: Redrawn with permission from Buchwald.[120]

the RYGB, a small stomach pouch is created and separated from the rest of the stomach and drained directly into the jejunum; the duodenum and the proximal jejunum are bypassed (Fig. 17.2B). Originally the RYGB was considered a purely restrictive procedure, but in the early 1990s, the Roux limb was lengthened from 75 to 150 cm to cause malabsorption as a second means of caloric restriction.[122] Subsequently, even longer Roux limbs came into use to promote adequate weight loss in the superobese.[123] The BPD is preferred by some surgeons for the superobese. There are a number of variations but the most popular is the duodenal switch, which includes a sleeve gastrectomy accompanied by transection of the proximal duodenum from the gastric outlet and attachment of the distal jejunum directly to the stomach outlet (Fig. 17.2C). The remaining small bowel then is anastomosed to the ileum to allow delivery of biliary and pancreatic juices to the lumen to aid in digestion. The site of the anastomoses varies from 100 to 200 cm proximal to the ileocecal valve, providing a common channel for absorption of food. The shorter the common channel, the greater the malabsorption.

The RYGB was assumed not to cause hyperoxaluria because restriction of caloric intake was presumed to be the predominant cause of weight loss, even though it was evolving into a malabsorptive procedure. In 1981, Hoffmann et al. published a paper reporting urine oxalate excretion was normal in 21 of 22 patients who had undergone BPD.[124] No details were provided about the timing of the urine collections in relation to surgery or about the diets the patients were consuming. The authors felt the common channel in the procedure was of sufficient length to prevent significant bile salt malabsorption and free fatty acids would not be in sufficient concentration to deplete intraluminal calcium. No further investigation into the risk of EH in modern bariatric procedures was performed for >20 years.

In 2005, an initial report from the Mayo Clinic suggested that hyperoxaluria and stone disease may be a problem in patients undergoing modern bariatric surgery.[123] They reported 23 patients, all of whom had had RYGB, 14 with a standard procedure and 9 with a more malabsorptive distal RYGB. Two of the patients had presented with severe kidney disease, both had oxalate nephropathy documented by kidney biopsy. The rest developed urolithiasis an average of 29 months postoperatively. On metabolic evaluation, hyperoxaluria was the prominent abnormality. They also performed a survey of 188 patients who had a very long limb RYGB, which revealed 16% had developed urolithiasis after surgery. Using data from a commercial laboratory, Asplin and Coe confirmed the association of hyperoxaluria in 132 bariatric surgery patients who had developed urolithiasis.[125] Patients were evaluated an average of 3.6 years after surgery. The specific bariatric procedure each patient had undergone was unknown, but all had procedures after 1980, thereby excluding subjects who might have had JIB surgery. Mean urine oxalate excretion was 83 mg/d, compared to 34 mg/d for healthy controls, with 23% of these patients having severe hyperoxaluria (>100 mg/d).

Both studies were retrospective and focused only on stone forming patients, so an estimate of the prevalence of hyperoxaluria in the bariatric population was not possible. Additional studies attempted to address this deficiency. Sinha et al. did a cross-sectional study of 41 patients, collecting samples from patient's prebariatric surgery, and at 6 and 12 months postoperatively (20, 8, and 13 patients, respectively).[126] One-third of the patients had a prior history of stone disease. They found no significant difference in urine oxalate in the first 6 months postoperatively but a doubling of urine oxalate at 12 months postsurgery compared to the preoperative group. Because most studies included subjects who had formed stones, Patel et al. performed a cross-sectional study of 58 patients without stone disease in order to determine the prevalence of hyperoxaluria in malabsorptive bariatric surgery.[127] All subjects were at least 6 months postsurgery; 52 patients had an RYGB and 6 had BPD. The mean oxalate for the group was markedly elevated (70 mg/d) and 10% of the subjects had a daily urine oxalate excretion above 100 mg/d. Maalouf et al. compared 19 subjects with RYGB and no history of urolithiasis, studied a mean of 3.5 years after surgery, to 19 age and gender matched obese patients.[88] They found higher urine oxalate and lower urine citrate excretion in the RYGB group. The urine oxalate was only moderately elevated (45 ± 21 mg/d), perhaps due to the relatively short bypass utilized in the study (mean Roux limb of 106 cm). Reduced urine citrate excretion was not found in the papers by Patel and Sinha; the reason for this difference is not known.

In addition to the cross-sectional studies, there have been a number of prospective studies evaluating stone risk in patients undergoing bariatric surgery.[128-131] These studies all follow the same format, urine is collected days to weeks prior to surgery and repeated at a specified time after the surgical intervention. The key findings are summarized in Table 17.7. All four studies show a significant increase in urine oxalate excretion compared to the baseline values. However, the absolute level of oxalate excretion varies between studies and is often lower than reported in the cross-sectional studies. Differences in timing of urine collections in relation to surgery likely explain much of the variation. Since the excess urine oxalate is derived from diet, it is not until patients reach their maximum postsurgical caloric intake that they are likely to develop severe hyperoxaluria.[86] In addition, differences in use of calcium supplements and the length of the intestinal bypass will alter the level of hyperoxaluria. Urine citrate fell in two of the studies and was unchanged in the others. Urine calcium fell in three of the four studies, as has been found in the cross-sectional studies as well. A fall in urine volume was also noted in three of the four studies. In total, these studies indicate that hyperoxaluria is common and at times severe in patients with RYGB or BPD. The presence of other abnormalities such as low urine flow rate and hypocitraturia contribute to stone risk when present.

The assumption that RYGB was predominantly a restrictive procedure persisted even as the Roux limb was progressively lengthened to induce malabsorption. Though hyperoxaluria was documented in RYGB and BPD and assumed to be enteric in origin, proof of intestinal fat malabsorption was lacking. Recently two separate studies showed the extent of fat malabsorption. Odstrcil et al. studied 9 patients undergoing RYGB with a 150 cm Roux limb for weight loss.[86] Patients underwent balance studies in an inpatient facility, during which time they were able to consume their usual self-selected diet. Patients were studied preoperatively and then 5 and 14 months postsurgery. Nutrient intake fell significantly at the 5-month evaluation and increased by 14 months, but not back to

Table 17.7: Urine chemistries pre- and post-RYGB.

	N	*Post-op (months)*	*Oxalate*		*Calcium*		*Citrate*	
			Pre	*Post*	*Pre*	*Post*	*Pre*	*Post*
Duffey et al.[128]	24	3	31 ± 10	41 ± 18*	146 ± 108	101 ± 74*	617 ± 399	516 ± 355
Park et al.[129]	45	9	32	40*	176	135*	675	456*
Duffey et al.[130]	19	24	33 ± 9	64 ± 30*	227 ± 115	138 ± 92*	696 ± 397	510 ± 349*
Wu et al.[131]	38	6	38 ± 15	48 ± 24*	139 ± 85	182 ± 110*	745 ± 425	844 ± 463

All urine chemistries are in mg/d. Data presented as mean ± SD except for data from Park, which provides only the median values. (RYGB: Roux-en-Y gastric bypass, *: Differs from Pre; $p < 0.05$).

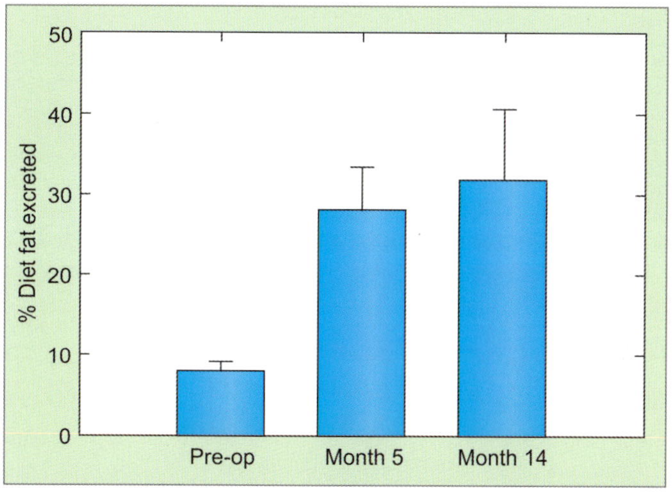

Fig. 17.5: Roux-en-Y gastric bypass surgery causes fat malabsorption. Data presented as the percentage of dietary fat that is excreted in the stool.
Source: Adapted from Odstrcil et al.[86]

baseline. Dietary intake of fat fell as well but stool fat did not, proving impaired intestinal absorption. As shown in Figure 17.5, the percentage of dietary fat excreted in the stool is considerably higher after bariatric surgery than at baseline. Fecal bile salts did not increase postoperatively, suggesting that the procedure did not cause bile acid malabsorption. A similar study was performed by Kumar et al. in which 11 patients were studied prebariatric surgery (9 RYGB, 2 BPD) and at 6 and 12 months postsurgery.[132] The RYGB was performed with a Roux limb of 100–150 cm. Fecal fat was measured and dietary composition was estimated by a food frequency questionnaire. As with the Odstricl study, fat intake fell but fecal fat increased postsurgery. Fat intake rose as time from surgery increased, and the absolute amount of fecal fat increased significantly in both studies. It is clear from these studies that there is considerable variability in the degree of fat malabsorption and that ingestion of fat is a significant variable effecting fecal fat excretion, and the risk of EH. It is not known if bile acid malabsorption is common in the very long limb RYGB or the BPD.

Whether fat malabsorption alone is a sufficient explanation for the observed hyperoxaluria in bariatric surgery is not known. Though oxalate is an end product of human metabolism, the colonic flora contains bacteria capable of breaking down oxalate. The most thoroughly studied of these oxalate degrading bacteria (ODB) is *Oxalobacter formigenes*, an anaerobic bacteria that colonizes the human colon and uses oxalate as its only energy source.[133] Other strains of bacteria have also been identified that metabolize oxalate, though most are not obligate oxalate metabolizers. A lack of colonic *O. formigenes* has been associated with increased risk of stone formation and hyperoxaluria in some studies of idiopathic calcium urolithiasis.[134,135] The role of *O. formigenes* in human metabolism is not fully understood, but it is possible that a deficiency in ODB could lead to increased net oxalate absorption by the gut. Jiang et al. compared 11 healthy subjects who were colonized with *O. formigenes* to 11 noncolonized subjects.[136] On self-selected diets urine oxalate did not differ between the groups, nor did it differ as diet oxalate was changed. However, when diet calcium was varied but oxalate kept constant (250 mg/d), the colonized subjects had a 20% lower urine oxalate excretion compared to the noncolonized group. Fecal *O. formigenes* colony counts increased as diet oxalate increased and decreased as diet calcium increased. This study highlights the complex relationship of *O. formigenes* colonization and availability of oxalate substrate. Kumar et al. determined *O. formigenes* colonization status of patients with IBD and found only 10% of them were colonized, compared to 56% of the healthy controls.[137] However, the majority of IBD patients in their study had UC and would not be considered at risk for EH. They did find urine oxalate excretion was higher in patients with IBD without *O. formigenes* colonization than those who were colonized, but it did not reach statistical significance. A study by Allison et al. investigated oxalate degradation by intestinal bacteria in humans, comparing seven normal subjects with eight patients who had undergone JIB.[138] All the JIB patients had significantly lower fecal oxalate degradation rates than any of the normal subjects, *O. formigenes* colony counts were not performed. There have not been any studies of ODB in modern bariatric surgery patients. However, a recent report showed low rates of *O. formigenes* colonization in obese patients being evaluated for bariatric surgery, raising the question as to whether altered intestinal anatomy should be implicated for a lack of colonization, even if found.[139]

Another possible explanation for hyperoxaluria in the setting of intestinal malabsorption is pyridoxine deficiency. Pyridoxal phosphate is a cofactor for the enzyme alanine:glyoxylate aminotransferase. Reduced activity of the enzyme leads to an excess of glyoxylate with subsequent conversion oxalate. Experimentally induced pyridoxine deficiency in humans has been shown to cause hyperoxaluria.[140] Small bowel disease is more likely to lead to deficiency of fat-soluble vitamins than the water-soluble vitamins such as pyridoxine. Studies of vitamin deficiencies in bariatric surgery patients show mixed results. Clements et al. found 17.6% of patients with RYGB had pyridoxine levels below the reference range 1 year after the procedure, whereas Gehrer et al. found normal pyridoxine levels in 86 patients after RYGB.[141,142] Part of this discrepancy may be due to laboratory methods and reference ranges used for pyridoxine assays. Of note, Aasheim found pyridoxine levels were frequently low in the obese population prior to surgery and improved significantly post-RYGB or duodenal switch with the use of a multivitamin.[143] If patients take multivitamins as routinely recommended as part of the bariatric procedure protocol, it is highly unlikely they would develop a pyridoxine deficit that would lead to hyperoxaluria. Even in the Clements study, the level of pyridoxine depletion was unlikely to cause an increase in oxalate production. There has not been a case of clinical pyridoxine deficiency reported in the literature in patients who have had RYGB or BPD for obesity.[144]

Though hyperoxaluria has clearly been linked to RYGB and other current malabsorptive procedures, there have only been a few studies focused on rates of stone formation with these procedures. The first study to suggest an increase rate of stones with RYGB was by Durrani et al., who performed a retrospective review of 972 patients undergoing RYGB at a single institution.[145] They found 32 subjects formed incident stones an average of 2.8 years after surgery. Of the 85 subjects who had a history of urolithiasis before surgery, 26 had a recurrence after surgery, with average time to stone formation of only 1.9 years. The incidence of stone disease post-RYGB was higher than the rate expected in the general US population. Matlaga et al. used an insurance claims database to identify 4,639 patients who had RYGB and matched them to an equal number of obese subjects who did not have bariatric surgery.[146] During 3 years of follow-up, RYGB patients had significantly more claims for stone disease than the obese controls (7.6% vs 4.6%, respectively). They also had higher rates of surgical intervention for stones. A small study from Brazil reported no urolithiasis formation in 58 subjects who had RYGB during a median follow-up of 3.5 years.[147] Of note, the RYGB had only a 100-cm Roux limb, shorter and presumably less malabsorption than the RYGB procedures routinely performed in the United States. No details of the RYGB procedure were provided in the Durrani study and no such information would be available in the claims database used in the Matlaga study. The lack of uniformity

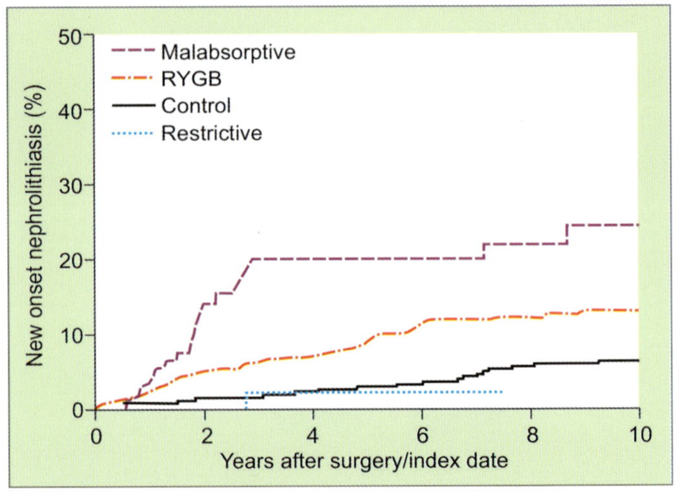

Fig. 17.6: Risk of urolithiasis in obese subjects undergoing bariatric surgery. Malabsorptive, very long limb RYGB or biliopancreatic diversion; RYGB (Roux-en-Y gastric bypass) control, obese subjects not undergoing bariatric surgery; restrictive, sleeve gastrectomy or gastric banding.
Source: Redrawn from Lieske et al.[148]

in modern bariatric procedures makes it difficult to compare data across studies. Lieske et al. reported data from 762 patients who had bariatric surgery at the Mayo Clinic.[148] Purely restrictive procedures were performed in 56 patients, RYGB in 591 and malabsorptive procedures (very long limb RYGB or BPD) in 105; mean follow-up was 6 years. Of the bariatric subjects, 11% had stones during follow-up compared to 4.3% of obese control subjects. The patients with the malabsorptive procedures had the highest rate of stone formation, followed by those with standard RYGB (Fig. 17.6). The incidence of urolithiasis secondary to bariatric surgery will be highly dependent on the types of procedures utilized.

A single study has investigated the risk of urolithiasis in patients receiving RYGB for indications other than weight loss. A paper from Japan reported the incidence of urolithiasis following surgery for gastric cancer.[149] The CT scans obtained every 6–12 months as follow-up for cancer were used to detect stone disease. With a mean follow-up of 2 years postsurgery, 9% of patients with RYGB and 25% of patients with total gastrectomy and Roux-en-Y reconstruction developed urolithiasis. In both procedures, the Roux limb was <40 cm, so fat malabsorption was not likely to have occurred. No urine chemistries were provided to document the abnormalities that contributed to stone formation. Whether the high rate of stone formation compared to the bariatric studies was due to the sensitivity of

Table 17.8: Comparison of 24 urine chemistries: restrictive versus malabsorptive bariatric surgery.

	Penniston et al.[152]		Semins et al.[151]	
	GB	RYGB	GB	RYGB
N	12	27	18	54
Volume (L/d)	1.28 ± 0.15	1.45 ± 0.10	1.73 ± 0.20	2.00 ± 0.13
Calcium (mg/d)	176 ± 22*	107 ± 14	132 ± 18	135 ± 11
Oxalate (mg/d)	34.8 ± 3.7*	50.7 ± 5.7	35.4 ± 3.1*	60.8 ± 3.5
Citrate (mg/d)	727 ± 106	477 ± 69	712 ± 120	683 ± 52

Data presented as mean ± SEM.
(GB: Gastric banding; RYGB: Roux-en-Y gastric bypass).
Values marked (*) differ significantly from RYGB, $p < 0.05$.

CT scan monitoring to detect asymptomatic stones or if there is a unique risk associated with surgical techniques and outcomes in gastric cancer is not clear. The vast majority of subjects in this study had BMIs <25 kg/m^2.

In addition to stone formation, a number of cases of oxalate nephropathy have been attributed to malabsorptive bariatric surgery. In the initial Mayo Clinic study of urolithiasis in patients with RYGB, two cases of oxalate nephropathy were included in the report.[126] Neither patient had pre-existing kidney disease, and both developed end-stage kidney disease after undergoing a standard RYGB with a 150-cm Roux limb. Nasr et al. reported 11 cases of oxalate nephropathy from a retrospective survey, a renal pathology service collected over the course of 6 years.[150] The patients presented with acute kidney injury, though a majority of the patients also had CKD at baseline. The time from RYGB to recognition of acute kidney injury ranged from 4 months to 8 years. All biopsies showed abundant intratubular CaOx crystals with signs of acute tubular injury as well as tubular atrophy. Urine oxalate excretions were not available. Eight of the patients had RYGB for obesity, while 3 had RYGB as treatment for gastric cancer. Eight of the 11 developed end-stage kidney disease and kidney function did not return to baseline levels in the remaining three. Whether the development of oxalate nephropathy in bariatric surgery requires a second event, such as severe volume depletion, in addition to hyperoxaluria is not known. Oxalate nephropathy may present as an acute event or develop over the course of years.

Despite concerns related to risk of urolithiasis and potential kidney damage, severe obesity contributes such morbidity that medical and surgical alternatives are needed for the obese population. Purely restrictive procedures such as gastric banding and sleeve gastrectomy are available as alternatives to RYGB and BPD, though weight loss tends to be less with restrictive procedures compared to the more malabsorptive procedures. Evidence obtained to this point suggests that the restrictive procedures are not associated with hyperoxaluria. Two studies have compared urine chemistries from patients with RYGB to those with gastric banding (Table 17.8).[151,152] Urine oxalate is significantly lower in the restrictive procedure group and citrate trends higher. In addition to analysis of urine risk factors, no increase in symptomatic stone events has been reported in patients with restrictive bariatric procedures. Using an insurance claims database, Semins et al. identified 201 patients who had undergone gastric banding and a control group of obese patients who did not have bariatric surgery, all with claims data for at least 2 years.[153] Fewer episodes of urinary stone disease were found in the gastric banding patients than in the controls ($p = 0.02$). Chen et al. performed a retrospective study of 417 patients who had a restrictive bariatric procedure (332 gastric banding, 85 gastric sleeve) with a mean follow-up period of 3.3 years.[154] They reported a rate of 3.4 stones per 1,000 patient-years for gastric banding and 5.2 stones per 1,000 patient-years for sleeve gastrectomy. These rates are lower than previously reported for obese subjects, but no formal control group was included in the study. One study of obese adolescents treated with gastric banding reported only one stone event in 73 patients, though follow-up was limited after the first postoperative year.[155]

Intestinal Lipase Inhibition

As would be expected from the preceding discussion, medications that induce fat malabsorption can produce EH with resultant risk of urolithiasis and/or oxalate nephropathy. Of particular interest are intestinal lipase inhibitors, which are used as a medical treatment for obesity, an alternative to bariatric surgery. Orlistat is an inhibitor of GI and

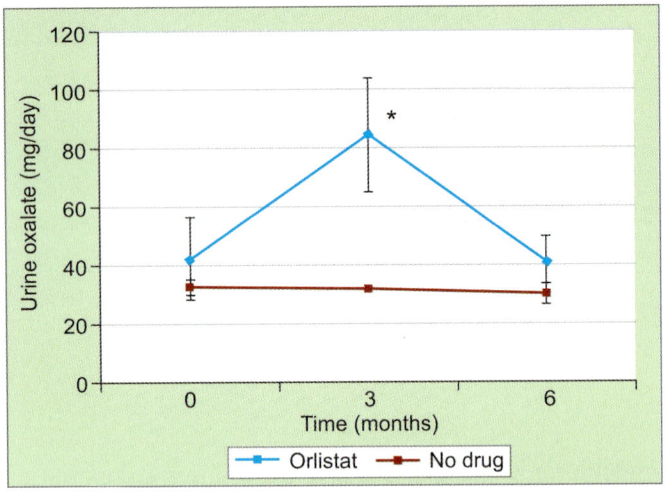

Fig. 17.7: Effect of intestinal lipase inhibition on urine oxalate excretion. Urine oxalate was measured prior to treatment and at 3 and 6 months after starting treatment with orlistat in 55 patients and 40 patients not receiving the drug.
Source: Adapted from Sarica et al.[157]

pancreatic lipase; taken orally it causes fat malabsorption in humans. It is recommended as a weight loss therapy for patients with a BMI >30. Orlistat is sold as both a prescription drug and an over-the-counter medication in the United States. The over-the-counter formulation is half the dose of the prescription version.

Ferraz et al. were the first to investigate whether orlistat might induce EH.[156] They measured urine oxalate excretion in rats fed normal chow compared to chow supplemented with either soy oil, sodium oxalate, or both. Urine oxalate increased significantly after treatment with orlistat in the rats fed oxalate or oxalate plus soy oil. The activity product of CaOx was markedly increased during orlistat administration.

In a Turkish study, Sarica et al. followed 95 patients in a weight loss program for 6 months, 55 of whom were treated with orlistat in addition to a calorie restricted diet.[157] Urinary excretion of oxalate and other urine chemistries were performed at baseline, 3 months and 6 months. Urine oxalate excretion doubled at 3 months compared to baseline (Fig. 17.7) but returned to baseline at 6 months. Of note, there were no changes in urine volume or citrate excretion. Whether the effect of orlistat on intestinal oxalate absorption is transient or whether adherence to the medication waned with time is not clear. No urolithiasis formed during the course of the study.

Case reports have implicated orlistat as a cause of EH.[158-161] The reports include kidney biopsies taken during an episode of acute kidney injury, showing tubular necrosis associated with calcium oxalate crystal deposition. Initiation of orlistat or an increase in dose was temporally related to the worsening kidney function in all three cases. In one case, hyperoxaluria was also documented while the patient was taking orlistat.[159] Though stone formation itself has not been clearly documented secondary to orlistat use, the induction of hyperoxaluria and risk of oxalate nephropathy makes it highly likely that lipase inhibitors can cause urolithiasis.

Celiac Disease

Celiac disease is a chronic inflammatory disorder of the small intestine. In susceptible people, ingestion of grains containing gluten triggers an immune response that damages the intestinal mucosa. Celiac disease affects ~1% of the population in Western societies and is the most common enteropathy causing intestinal malabsorption.[162] Overt fat malabsorption due to celiac disease has long been recognized as a cause of EH and nephrolithiasis.[163,164] However, with the advent of serologic testing, milder cases of celiac disease have been identified and improved estimates of the contribution of celiac disease to stone formation are now available.

Ciacci et al. found an increased prevalence of urolithiasis in 608 untreated adults with celiac disease compared to 3,450 subjects from the general population, adjusting for age and gender (OR 4.0, 95% CI 2.7–5.9).[165] They also noted that the clinical severity of the celiac disease did not correlate with the presence of urolithiasis. In a Swedish study, all subjects diagnosed with celiac disease by small bowel biopsy from 1969 to 2008 were included in a population-based cohort study.[166] A total of 28,735 patients with celiac disease were matched to 142,177 subjects from the general population. They found a 27% increased risk of stone disease in those with celiac disease. In addition, celiac disease patients were more likely to have stones than normal subjects even before the diagnosis of celiac disease was made. Menekse et al. investigated the prevalence of celiac disease in Turkish children who present with kidney stone disease but without a prior history of celiac disease.[167] Screening 187 children with kidney stones and 278 age- and sex-matched healthy children, they found 7 (3.7%) of the stone formers had abnormal IgA tissue transaminase compared to 1 (0.3%) control. Of the stone patients with positive serology, six had small intestinal biopsies performed and only two were abnormal. No long-term follow-up was available to see if the seropositive children eventually developed clinical

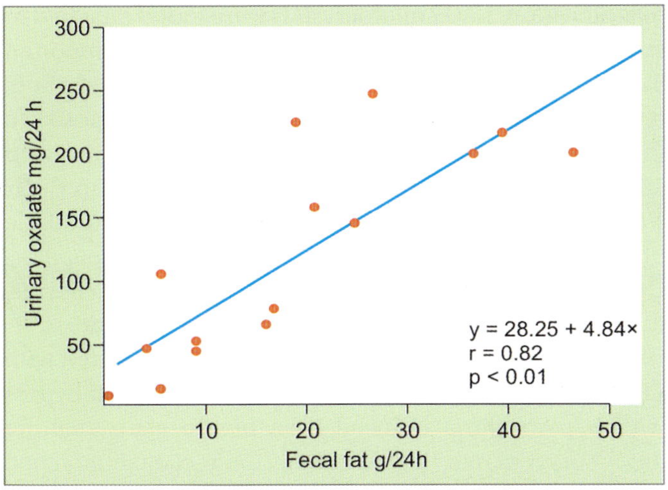

Fig. 17.8: Correlation of urine oxalate excretion with fecal fat in patients with celiac disease. The line is the least squares regression, $r = 0.82$, $p < 0.01$.
Source: Redrawn from McDonald et al.[163]

celiac disease. Though the actual risk of urolithiasis varied between studies, they all showed the same trend of higher stone rates with celiac disease.

There are only a few studies that have investigated the biochemical abnormalities that predispose to urolithiasis in celiac disease. McDonald studied six patients with celiac disease to determine the effect of steatorrhea on urine oxalate excretion.[163] Fecal fat correlated with urine oxalate, and oxalate excretion fell when steatorrhea improved with gluten-free diet (Fig. 17.8). They also noted an inverse relationship of urine Ca to fecal fat. In the Ciacci study, a subgroup of 45 patients with celiac disease performed metabolic urine studies compared to an equal number of age and gender matched healthy subjects.[165] Urine oxalate excretion was more than double that of the normal subjects and urine calcium was significantly lower. Urine citrate and flow rate were not different between the groups. Ogilvie studied oxalate excretion in children with a variety of intestinal disorders, including celiac disease, but no history of urolithiasis.[164] Of the nine patients with celiac disease, six had hyperoxaluria. In contrast, a study of 115 children with newly diagnosed celiac disease, hyperoxaluria was not found though a low urine Ca to creatinine ratio was noted in the celiac patients.[168] Whether the use of spot urine samples rather than 24-hour collections resulted in the absence of hyperoxaluria in the celiac disease subjects is not clear. None of the patients had formed kidney stones at the time of the study.

The diagnosis of celiac disease should be suspected in patients with diarrhea, cramping, and bloating.[165] Symptoms can be mild or even undetected by the clinician as the patient may not realize their bowel habits are abnormal. Asking about the particular nature of bowel habits (frequency, consistency) may provide greater insight into the probability of a patient having celiac disease. The presence of autoimmune disorders, dermatitis herpetiformis, or a family history of celiac disease increases the likelihood of celiac disease.[162] Laboratory signs of malabsorption of critical nutrients also increase the likelihood of celiac disease. In the absence of obvious causes, iron deficiency anemia, vitamin B12 deficiency, and vitamin D deficiency may be clues to the presence of celiac disease.

Historically the diagnosis of celiac disease was made using small bowel biopsy to identify the villous atrophy and crypt hyperplasia characteristic of the disease. However, serologic testing is now used to diagnose most cases of celiac disease. The most commonly recommended test is IgA anti-tissue transglutaminase which has a sensitivity of 90–95% and a specificity of 95–97%.[162] In patients who have IgA deficiency, IgG anti-tissue transglutaminase may be used for the diagnosis. Other serologic tests that may be used include IgA antiendomysial and IgA deamidated gliadin peptide. If the patient has been following a gluten-free diet prior to diagnosis, the antibody tests may turn negative. Reintroduction of gluten to the diet followed by repeat serologic testing can confirm the diagnosis if necessary. In cases where suspicion of celiac disease is high and serum antibody studies are equivocal, then consideration should be given to small bowel biopsy.

Standard therapy for celiac disease is a gluten-free diet to prevent exposure to the antigen inciting the intestinal inflammation. Metabolic derangements such as anemia and vitamin deficiencies improve with gluten restriction, as does fat malabsorption. There are limited data on the change in urine chemistries with the institution of a gluten-free diet. As noted above, MacDonald et al. found some patients had improvement in fecal fat and urine oxalate excretion when a gluten-free diet was instituted.[163] Ciacci et al. reported urine oxalate had fallen an average of 21 mg/d 1 year after starting a gluten-free diet in 45 celiac disease patients.[165] Case reports also support the effectiveness of gluten abstinence. Capolongo et al. described a woman with oxalate nephropathy diagnosed postrenal transplantation.[169] The patient had minimal GI symptoms. Urine oxalate levels were in the range of 90–130 mg/d and fell to within the normal range on a gluten-free diet. Gama and Schweitzer reported a case of a man presenting with a kidney stone and no GI symptoms.[170] His metabolic evaluation revealed hyperoxaluria with low-urine calcium. Celiac disease was diagnosed by antibody testing and intestinal biopsy. Placing the patient on a gluten-free diet reduced oxalate excretion to the normal range. The time required for hyperoxaluria to resolve is not well defined, but appears to be in the range of 3 months to 1 year.[163-165]

Pancreatitis

Malabsorption secondary to pancreatitis has been recognized as a cause of EH. Most of the case reports and series of EH associated with pancreatitis have focused on acute and chronic oxalate nephropathy. Cartery et al. reported 12 cases of oxalate nephropathy associated with pancreatitis.[171] Many of the subjects were at risk for concomitant volume depletion from either diarrhea or diuretic use. Three of the 12 required chronic dialysis. Hill et al. reported three case of oxalate nephropathy, all had diabetes mellitus as well as pancreatic insufficiency.[172] Oxalate nephropathy was confirmed at biopsy and all patients developed irreversible kidney failure requiring dialysis. There are little data concerning pancreatic insufficiency and risk of urolithiasis, though any chronic disorder that can cause hyperoxaluria, presumably, can promote stone disease.

Renal Pathology

In idiopathic calcium oxalate stone disease, the majority of stones appear to form as overgrowth on interstitial Randall's plaques, which have become exposed to the urine due to erosion of the overlying urothelium. Randall's plaques are made of hydroxyapatite, and the extent of Randall's plaques covering renal papillary surface correlates with high-urine calcium and low-urine pH and urine flow rate.[173]

In their initial report on intraoperative anatomy and biopsy studies, Evan et al. included four patients with CaOx stones secondary to intestinal bypass for obesity.[62] The bypass patients' metabolic evaluation revealed hyperoxaluria and hypocalciuria in contrast to the hypercalciuria and overall normal oxalate excretion in the idiopathic stone formers. As opposed to idiopathic stone formers, the bypass patients had no papillary Randall's plaque noted during surgery nor in the biopsies that were obtained. Crystal deposits (CaOx and apatite) were noted in the inner medullary collecting ducts with cellular injury and interstitial fibrosis at the site of the tubule deposits. At high magnification, CaOx microcrystals were found attached to collecting duct epithelia.[174] An additional study reported the histology of patients with small intestine resection, most cases secondary to Crohn's disease. As opposed to the obesity bypass patients, the resection group revealed large amounts of interstitial Randall's plaque, with CaOx stones attached to the plaque. They also displayed tubule plugging with apatite crystals and deformed papillae. Cortical disease was also noted with glomerular sclerosis, tubule atrophy, and interstitial fibrosis (*see* Chapter5).[175]

In an attempt to find the early lesions associated with EH, Worcester et al. used a rat model of intestinal bypass with hyperoxaluria induced by a high-oxalate, high-fat diet.[176] In these rats, they found tiny CaOx crystals attached to the brush border of proximal tubule cells. Cell injury was associated with some of these crystal deposits. In rats with intestinal bypass but fed normal rat chow, they found medullary collecting duct tubules plugged with CaOx crystals, though the degree of hyperoxaluria was much less than those given a high-oxalate diet. In this situation, the lesions correlated with an elevated CaOx SS, driven by both high urine Ca and oxalate excretion. Apatite could also be found in the collecting ducts in these animals, just as described in humans, but the deposition of CaOx crystals precedes the apatite formation, supporting their hypothesis that cell damage from the CaOx crystals may impair local tubule fluid acidification with subsequent deposition of apatite in a more alkaline tubule fluid.

Treatment of CaOx Stones Secondary to Small Bowel Disease

Diet

Because the excess urine oxalate is of intestinal origin, the first step in treating EH is reducing dietary oxalate intake (Table 17.9). Chadwick et al. reported the results of a low-oxalate diet in four patients with EH secondary to intestinal resection.[70] A diet with <4 mg/d oxalate normalized urine oxalate excretion in all subjects. Earnest et al. studied seven patients with extensive intestinal resection for Crohn's disease.[71] On their home diet, urine oxalate was 128 ± 13 mg/d but fell to 83 ± 10 mg/d on an oxalate intake of 30–50 mg/d. Gregory and colleagues reported that only 4 of 30 patients with JIB and kidney stones showed a reduction of urine oxalate after being instructed to avoid high oxalate foods, questioning the effectiveness of a practical low-oxalate diet in the clinical setting.[100] Pang and associates studied the effect of a controlled metabolic diet on urinary

Table 17.9: Potential therapies for enteric hyperoxaluria.
Diet
• Low oxalate*
• Low fat*
• Medium-chain triglyceride supplements
• High calcium
Oxalate binders
• Calcium*
• Magnesium
• Aluminum
• Sevelamer carbonate
• Lanthanum carbonate
Bile acid sequestrants
• Cholestyramine*
• Colestipol
• Colesevelam
• Oxalate degrading bacteria

*Best documented treatments.

oxalate excretion in nine patients with mild EH secondary to malabsorptive bariatric surgery (mean excretion of 61 mg/d on free choice diet estimated to contain 180 mg/d of oxalate).[177] The metabolic diet was low fat (<25% of calories) and contained 70–80 mg of oxalate and 1,000 mg of calcium per day. The patients continued the calcium and citrate supplements they had been prescribed by their clinicians throughout the study. There was no change in urine oxalate excretion with the metabolic diet, though there was a modest reduction in urine CaOx SS. The mild degree of hyperoxaluria and the continued use of calcium supplements may have minimized any effect of the low-oxalate diet.

An oxalate-free diet is impractical outside of a research setting. Usual diet oxalate intake in the United States is in the range of 100–200 mg/d; a goal of 50 mg seems reasonable, though still difficult for many patients to maintain over a long period of time. Another obstacle in dietary therapy is obtaining complete and accurate information on food oxalate content. Oxalate content is not provided by food manufacturers, and food oxalate lists in the literature and on the Internet provide conflicting information. These differences may be related to laboratory methods or to the variation of food oxalate content based on the age of plants when harvested, the type of soil where grown, and methods used to prepare the food. These barriers make it difficult for even a motivated patient to maintain a very low oxalate intake. A useful resource for patients trying to lower diet oxalate is https://regepi.bwh.harvard.edu/health/Oxalate/files. The website provides an extensive list of foods, all analyzed by a single laboratory, providing consistency for comparison of foods when creating menus.

Because steatorrhea is central to the etiology of EH, limiting fat intake should reduce oxalate absorption and excretion. Andersson and Jagenburg showed the effectiveness of a fat-restricted diet in study of 13 patients with ileal disease or resection.[178] In a controlled intervention, lowering dietary fat from 100 to 40 g/d significantly reduced urine oxalate in subjects with fecal fat >15 g/d at baseline (Fig. 17.9). No change in urine oxalate was noted in patients with fecal fat <15 g/d. Earnest et al. studied the effect of diet fat intake in seven patients with ileal resection.[71] They found a significant increase in urine oxalate by raising dietary fat from 40 to 100 g/d in patients with ileal resection of >100 cm, but no effect in those with resection of <50 cm (Fig. 17.9).

An alternative to a strict low-fat diet is to add medium-chain fatty acids as a substitute for the long-chain fatty acids found in an ordinary dietary. Medium-chain triglycerides do not require micelle formation to remain in solution and are more easily absorbed than long-chain fatty acids. Earnest et al. studied four patients on a controlled diet. They found that substituting 50% of the diet fat with medium-chain triglycerides reduced fecal fat from 96 to 47 g/d, while mean urine oxalate fell from 289 to 182 mg/d.[79] In patients in whom calorie intake is compromised by their bowel disease, providing fat as medium-chain triglycerides can provide calories without worsening steatorrhea and hyperoxaluria.

Nordenval et al. reported the results of a combined low-oxalate, low-fat diet in 10 patients who had undergone JIB for treatment of obesity.[179] The study was performed in an outpatient setting, with patients instructed to avoid foods of moderate to high oxalate content and to minimize dietary fat. Urine oxalate fell from 97 ± 11 mg/d on the patients' ordinary diet to 62 ± 7 mg/d on the reduced fat and oxalate diet. The study was only a week in duration but showed patients may not require special metabolic diets to control EH. Whether patients can adhere to such diets over longer periods of time was not reported.

Because inadequate free calcium in the intestinal lumen is an important factor in the genesis of EH, a high-calcium diet should lower levels of free oxalate in the gut. However, it is difficult to deliver a high-calcium diet while simultaneously limiting fat intake, since dairy products

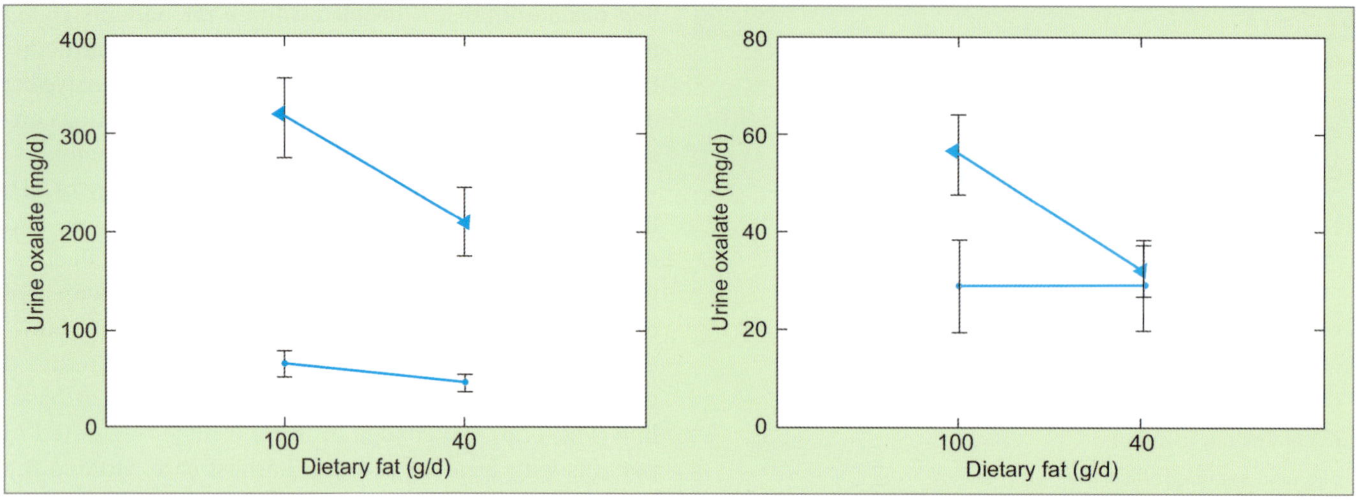

Fig. 17.9: Effect of dietary fat intake on urine oxalate excretion. (Left panel) Urine oxalate in patients with extensive (>100 cm; triangles) and minimal (<50 cm; circles) ileal resection. (Right panel) Urine oxalate in patients with small bowel disease and fecal fat >15 g/d (triangles) and <15 g/d (circles).
Source: Adapted from Earnest et al.[71] and Andersson and Jagenburg.[178]

are the most common dietary source of calcium. Most physicians depend on the use of calcium supplements to achieve a high calcium intake (*see* below).

Oxalate Binding Agents

Drugs known as phosphate binders are used to reduce intestinal phosphate absorption in patients with CKD. Calcium salts are commonly used as phosphate binders, though a number of noncalcium-based phosphate binders are available. All phosphate binders are positively charged molecules that can complex phosphate ion, limiting intestinal absorption. In theory, many of these drugs should be able to bind oxalate anion in the intestine in the same manner. Calcium is the most extensively studied oxalate binding agent in patients with EH.

The pathophysiology of EH requires a deficit of ionized calcium in the intestinal lumen, allowing a greater fraction of dietary oxalate to exist in a soluble, absorbable form. Numerous studies have shown the benefit of calcium supplementation in lowering urine oxalate excretion. Stauffer studied patients with EH on a high oxalate diet (500 mg/d) with 100 g of fat while varying dietary calcium intake.[106] Both the patients with ileal resection for Crohn's disease and the JIB patients had a significant reduction in oxalate excretion when calcium intake was increased from 250–3,000 mg/d (Fig. 17.10). He also showed that lowering diet oxalate and fat to 25 mg and 60 g/d, respectively, allowed calcium intake to be reduced to 1,000 mg/d and maintain the same level of oxalate excretion as seen with the 3,000 mg calcium intake. Earnest et al. found similar results in a study of 17 patients with malabsorption due to bowel disease or JIB.[79] Nine of the 17 were found to be hyperoxaluric on a controlled diet of 100 g fat, 500 mg Ca, and 400 mg oxalate. The nine with hyperoxaluria all had higher fecal fat excretion and lower urine calcium than the eight with normal oxalate excretion. Treatment with calcium at a dose of 3.5 g/d led to a 37% reduction in urine oxalate. Hylander et al. studied 8 patients with JIB, all of whom had steatorrhea but none had formed urolithiasis. Patients were placed on a 70-g fat, 200-mg oxalate, 800-mg Ca diet and urine oxalate excretion was measured at baseline and during treatment with 2,000 mg/d of calcium. Daily oxalate excretion fell from a median of 119 to 60 mg/d ($p < 0.01$) during calcium treatment, and they found no significant increase in urine Ca excretion.

Barilla et al. studied eight subjects with ileal resection or bypass of >100 cm, and compared them to hypercalciuric renal stone formers and normal subjects.[180] All subjects were fed a 9-mg/d oxalate, 400-mg/d calcium diet and then given an oral oxalate load; urine oxalate excretion was measured over the subsequent 2 days. This process was repeated with varying amounts of calcium being administered with the oxalate load. The patients with ileal resection excreted 35% of the oral oxalate load compared to 8% and 9% for the stone patients and normal subjects, respectively. Providing calcium with the oxalate load significantly reduced oxalate absorption in all three groups,

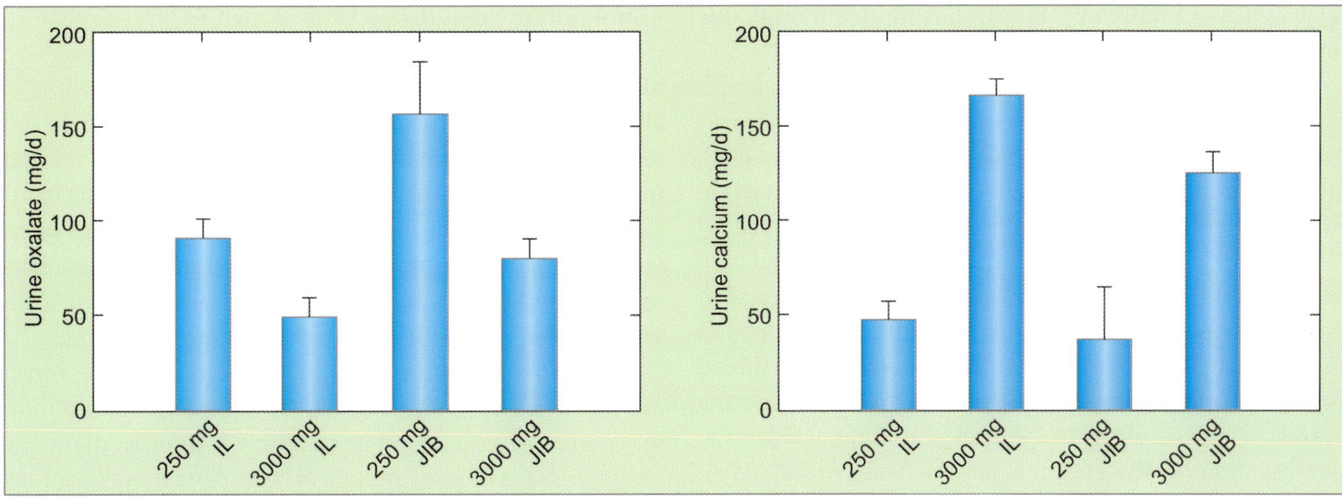

Fig. 17.10: Effect of calcium supplementation on urine oxalate and calcium excretion. Eight patients with ileectomy and partial colectomy (IL) and eight patients with jejunoileal bypass were studied on 500 mg/d oxalate diet with calcium intake varied from 250 to 3,000 mg/d. *Source*: Adapted from Stauffer.[106]

though the patients with ileal resection had greater oxalate excretion for any given intervention. They determined the effect of calcium supplementation on urine saturation of CaOx by direct measurement of the activity product ratio. Using a 400-mg Ca, 2,000-mg oxalate diet, the activity product ratio was measured with and without supplementation with 25 mmol of calcium gluconate. They found only a modest drop in urine oxalate from 79 to 68 mg/d, which was offset by an increase in urine Ca of 70–99 mg/d and an activity product ratio that did not change significantly. This paper highlights the complexity of reducing oxalate by providing a second lithogenic substance such as calcium.

Many subjects with intestinal resection have diminished intestinal calcium absorption due to reduced absorptive surface area, vitamin D deficiency, and complexation of calcium by free fatty acids. In such cases, providing extra calcium may improve overall calcium balance and reduce the risk of bone disease. However, a higher calcium intake can increase calcium absorption and urine calcium (Fig. 17.10), basically replacing one lithogenic compound for another in the urine. In general, urine calcium excretion is higher in patients with RYGB than other types of malabsorptive bariatric surgery and in EH from intestinal resection. Much of this is due to an overall higher food intake in the bariatric subjects than in those with underlying disease. Because of this, urine calcium can be quite high in RYGB patients treated with calcium supplements, so urine chemistries need to be monitored during therapy. A reasonable approach to this conundrum is to monitor CaOx saturation. If calcium rises out of proportion to the fall in oxalate, urine saturation will increase, though there are no prospective studies confirming this approach to patient management.

The choice of calcium salt used as an oxalate binder can influence the effectiveness of treatment. Calcium carbonate is commonly recommended as treatment since it is inexpensive and widely available. However, calcium carbonate is insoluble at neutral pH and requires an acidic environment to dissolve. In the setting of RYGB, where the small gastric pouch could compromise stomach acidification, a more soluble calcium salt such as calcium citrate may be preferable. Tonapu et al. compared calcium carbonate to calcium citrate supplements in a single-dose study in 18 patients with RYGB.[181] They found greater absorption of calcium with calcium citrate as reflected by the rise in serum calcium concentration and urine calcium excretion, in addition to a greater suppression of parathyroid hormone. Sakhaee et al. studied the effectiveness of a potassium-calcium citrate liquid formulation to increase calcium absorption and provide an alkali load compared to placebo in a crossover trial in 24 patients who had undergone RYGB.[182] They found significant improvements in mineral and acid-base metabolism as demonstrated by a reduction in serum parathyroid hormone, bone resorption markers, and an increase in urine citrate. There was not a significant reduction in urine oxalate, though the patients they studied had a normal mean urine oxalate. That calcium citrate is more bioavailable in patients with RYGB likely makes it a more effective oxalate binder, though this has not been specifically studied.

Magnesium is also able to bind oxalate in the gut and reduce absorption, though the ability to precipitate oxalate is not as potent as that of calcium. Zimmermann et al. showed a fall of oxalate absorption from 8.6% at baseline to 5.2% when a 50-mg oxalate load was accompanied by 10 mmol of magnesium aspartate in healthy subjects.[183] Liebman and Costa measured the effect of 12.5 mmol of magnesium oxide on absorption of a 200-mg oxalate load in 24 healthy subjects. Oxalate absorption was reduced from 13.5% at baseline to 7.6% with magnesium.[184] Barilla et al. studied the effect of calcium and magnesium supplementation on absorption of an oral oxalate load in five patients with Crohn's disease and ileal resection.[180] While consuming a 400-mg calcium, 200-mg oxalate diet, calcium or magnesium supplements at a dose of 25 mmol/d led to an equivalent fall in urine oxalate excretion. Small intestinal malabsorption is often a cause of magnesium deficiency (*see* Table 17.5), so magnesium salts may be needed to maintain body magnesium stores, in addition to their ability to lower urine oxalate. Hypomagnesuria can also contribute directly to stone risk as magnesium complexes oxalate in the urine, reducing CaOx SS.[185] Dosing of magnesium is more limited than that of calcium. Doses above 350 mg/d are associated with diarrhea in patients with normal bowel function, patients with reduced intestinal surface area may not be able to tolerate such doses. One study has reported the use of magnesium and aluminum salts in the management of EH.[186] Neither magnesium oxide at a dose of 400 mg twice daily or aluminum dihydroxide at a dose of 800 mg five times daily reduced urine oxalate excretion in seven patients with JIB. However, this study also found no response to calcium or cholestyramine which had been shown to be effective in other studies. Whether the difference in this study was due to allowing patients to have an ad lib diet or was peculiar to JIB as the etiology of the EH is not clear.

There have been limited research into the use of other phosphate binders to reduce oxalate absorption, but it seems reasonable that some of these compounds could be effective oxalate binders. There is a single trial of sevelamer in 10 patients with EH, most of whom had RYGB for weight loss.[187] Urine oxalate fell by 17%, which did not reach statistical significance. Urine phosphate fell by 44% suggesting compliance was excellent. Whether long-term phosphate depletion could be a result of this type of therapy in patients with bowel disease has not been studied. Aluminum hydroxide has been shown to bind oxalate in vitro.[188] Aluminum salts are no longer used as phosphate binders in CKD, because the reduced renal excretion of aluminum causes toxicity. In patients with EH who do not have CKD, aluminum toxicity is much less of a risk, though the long-term safety of aluminum salts has not been evaluated in patients with EH. Lanthanum carbonate has been shown to reduce oxalate excretion and nephrocalcinosis in a rat model of hyperoxaluria, but there have not been any studies of using it as an oxalate binder in humans.[189] Whether lowering diet phosphate would make the binders more effective for oxalate, by reducing competition for binding sites, has not been studied. In most diets, the molar amount of phosphate will far exceed that of oxalate, potentially limiting the effectiveness of the binders. It is the very limited solubility of the CaOx complex that appears to make calcium particularly adept as an oxalate binder; this may not apply to the other phosphate binders.

In general, calcium salts would be the preferred binder in any patient with low-urine calcium, as it indicates a deficiency in intestinal calcium absorption. The noncalcium based binders, such as sevelamer, presumably would be most beneficial in patients whose urine calcium increased excessively when calcium salts are used or who have high urine calcium even without the use of calcium supplements.

Bile Acid Sequestrants

Bile acid sequestrants are resins that bind bile acids in the intestinal lumen and prevent absorption in the ileum. They are used to treat hyperlipidemia and bile acid induced diarrhea. When used to treat bile acid malabsorption, they act by forming insoluble complexes with bile acids, lowering the free bile acid concentration of the intestinal fluid delivered to the colon. The presence of bile salts in the colon stimulates electrolyte and water secretion into the colon, producing what is known as choleretic diarrhea. Cholestyramine is the best studied of the bile acid sequestrants for treatment of bile acid malabsorption, but colestipol and colesevelam should have similar effects. Since bile salts increase colonic permeability, increasing oxalate absorption down its concentration gradient, by binding bile acids in the gut, bile acid sequestrants should normalize colonic permeability and reduce absorption of oxalate.[83] Lower levels of free bile salts will reduce secretion of water and electrolyte allowing solid stool to form, which also reduces oxalate absorption. In addition, cholestyramine has been

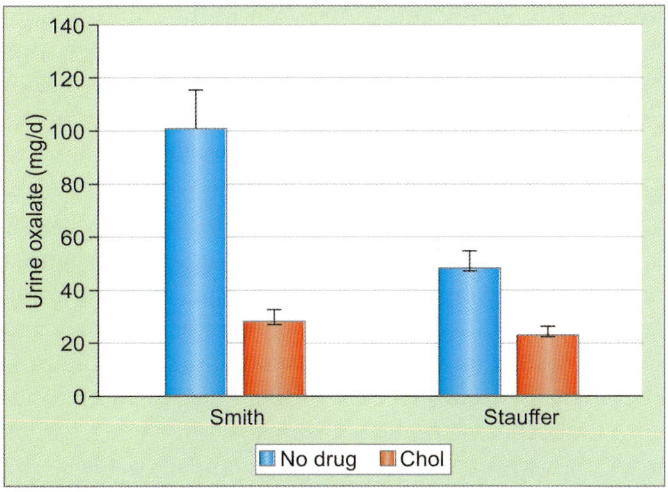

Fig. 17.11: Effect of cholestyramine on urine oxalate excretion. The dose of cholestyramine was 4 g four times per day in both studies. Smith et al., $n = 4$; Stauffer et al., $n = 6$.
Source: Adapted from Smith et al.[68] and Stauffer et al.[73]

shown to bind oxalate in vitro, providing another pathway to reduce free oxalate concentration in the colon.[83]

Smith et al. studied four patients with intestinal resection and stone formation secondary to hyperoxaluria.[68] Cholestyramine was prescribed at a dose of 4 g four times per day to reduce diarrhea and improve urine flow. In addition to a marked improvement in diarrhea, urine oxalate fell significantly in all subjects (Fig. 17.11). Stauffer et al. studied six patients with Crohn's disease with significant ileal resection (mean length of resection 68 cm) and EH.[73] The patients were maintained on stable dietary oxalate and studied at baseline and while taking 16 g of cholestyramine daily. Diarrhea rapidly improved and urine oxalate fell significantly (Fig. 17.11). Caspary et al. reported results of cholestyramine in 12 subjects, 6 of whom had steatorrhea due to pancreatic insufficiency or celiac sprue.[80] They noted no change in oxalate absorption during an oxalate load test, but urine oxalate excretion fell from 71 to 46 mg per 36 hours, which did not reach statistical significance. Unfortunately, they reported those with bowel disease with the nondisease subjects, so it is difficult to assess the effect of the drug in the patient population of interest. Nordenvall et al. studied seven subjects with EH secondary to JIB.[186] When treated with 16 g/d of cholestyramine, no reduction in urine oxalate excretion was noted; in fact, a mild increase was reported (68–80 mg/d). Patients were not on fixed diets, so whether dietary variability accounted for this difference or whether GI pathophysiology unique to JIB contributed to the surprising outcome is not clear.

It has been suggested that bile acid sequestrants are not appropriate for all patients with steatorrhea and EH. In patients with modest ileal resection (<100 cm) steatorrhea tends to be mild and bile acid delivery to the colon plays an important role in the etiology of diarrhea and increased permeability of the colon. In such patients, treatment with cholestyramine will often improve diarrhea and reduce oxalate absorption. When ileal resection or bypass is more severe (>100 cm), loss of bile acids in the stool may exceed the liver synthesis of bile, depleting the bile acid pool.[70] In this situation, use of cholestyramine will further deplete bile acids, worsening steatorrhea and diarrhea, without a beneficial effect on hyperoxaluria. In fact, in settings of severe steatorrhea and presumed bile salt depletion, bile acid supplements may be used to reduce steatorrhea.[190] Bile salts should be administered with meals. It should be noted that bile salts are not regulated by the Food and Drug Administration, so formulations and strength may not be uniform across manufacturers.[191]

The 100-cm ileal resection limit for use of bile acid sequestrants is based on a small number of studies and should be used as a rough guideline. There have been cases reported in which cholestyramine was effective in patients with more extensive resection.[68] Careful monitoring is required for patients treated with bile acid sequestrants, as they are at risk to develop deficiencies of fat-soluble vitamins and the sequestrants can alter absorption of other medications. Consultation with a gastroenterologist experienced in management of short bowel syndrome may be advisable when contemplating use of bile acid sequestrants.

Oxalate Degrading Bacteria

Whether the loss of intestinal ODB contributes to the pathogenesis of EH is not clear, but the use of ODB as a therapy is the subject of active research. Oxalate degrading bacteria are part of the normal colonic flora and contribute to regulation of oxalate traffic by degrading dietary oxalate in the intestinal lumen. In addition, there are data from animal models that *O. formigenes* can stimulate secretion of oxalate by the colon, lowering urine oxalate by diverting oxalate from renal-to-intestinal excretion.[192] Animal studies have shown that treating uncolonized animals with *O. formigenes* reduces oxalate excretion in animals given a high-oxalate diet, leading to the assumption that *O. formigenes* lowers oxalate absorption by consuming oxalate in the intestinal lumen.[193] Unfortunately, therapeutic efficacy of ODB has been difficult to prove in humans. In a study of six patients with idiopathic CaOx stones, treatment with lactic acid bacteria capable of degrading oxalate led to a significant reduction in urine oxalate.[194] Subsequently, two randomized double blind trials in idiopathic stone patients with hyperoxaluria showed no benefit from treatment with oxalate degrading lactic acid bacteria.[195,196] There is a single study of ODB for EH in which 10 patients were treated with a lactic acid bacteria probiotic.[197] In a 4-month dose escalation design, there was an overall statistically significant trend to a lower urine oxalate excretion. The maximal fall in oxalate was at month 2 of treatment, with a 25% fall of oxalate excretion from baseline. However, at 3 months, when treated with the highest dose of the drug there was no difference in oxalate excretion from baseline, leading to uncertainty regarding the effectiveness of the treatment. Additional studies are required to determine if lactic acid bacteria are clearly of benefit in patients with EH. There has not been a trial comparing *O. formigenes* and lactic acid bacteria in humans. Though an intriguing therapy, there are many issues that need to be resolved prior to ODB probiotics becoming a routine part of treatment.

General Therapy for Urolithiasis with Small Bowel Disease

In addition to treatments to lower urine oxalate, general measures common to all patients with urolithiasis need to be instituted, as described in the section on colectomy. Low urine flow tends to be more of a problem in patients with short gut due to resection of diseased bowel than in patients with bariatric surgery. Aggressive attempts to raise urine volume should be made though there is often a limit to the fluid intake a patient will tolerate due to worsening diarrhea. Frequent small boluses of fluid spread out over the day will be better tolerated than infrequent consumption of large amounts of water. Because water absorption is driven by solute uptake in the proximal small intestine, water absorption can be stimulated by providing electrolytes and sugars simultaneously with fluid loads. Oral rehydration fluids contain mixtures of amino acids, sugars and electrolytes for this purpose. For patients with bariatric surgery, providing extra calories is not advisable, but in patients with IBD and other causes of short gut, where adequate nutrition can be a problem, the extra calories may be of benefit. If diarrhea with inadequate water absorption continues, drugs to decrease intestinal motility can increase fluid absorption by prolonging contact of intestinal contents with the mucosa. Opioid receptor agonists inhibit the contraction of intestinal smooth muscle. Loperamide is usually the drug of choice, due to fewer CNS effects than other narcotic agents.[198] Loperamide also suppresses gastric, biliary, and pancreatic secretions, reducing the total fluid entering the intestinal lumen. After intestinal resection some patients develop gastric hypersecretion due to loss of endogenous gastric acid inhibitors.[198] The extra gastric fluid adds to the burden of fluid to be reabsorbed by the intestine. Suppression of gastric secretion will reduce the amount of fluid delivered to the intestine for absorption. Proton pump inhibitors or H-2 antagonists are effective in this role. For more recalcitrant diarrhea octreotide, a somatostatin analog, can be used.[191] However, the need for subcutaneous delivery, the expense, and side effects such as cholelithiasis limit its use to the most severe cases.

As for feeding, it is often useful to have multiple small meals throughout the day, to avoid large osmotic loads that overwhelm the absorptive capacity of the remaining small bowel. If the colon is intact, it can provide an important source of energy salvage, by fermenting carbohydrate that has not been absorbed by the small bowel and forming short chain fatty acids that can be utilized by the colon.[199] Thus, a diet high in carbohydrate can be beneficial for patients with short bowel syndrome with the colon in continuity. Fat malabsorption often worsens diarrhea leading to more salt and water loss, in addition to the role steatorrhea plays in overabsorption of dietary oxalate, so fat restriction is often recommended. However, fat has the greatest calorie density of the food stuffs, and many short bowel patients have calorie malnutrition. Medium-chain triglycerides can be used to supplement the diet and provide extra calories.[79] Medium-chain triglycerides remain soluble in intestinal fluid without binding bile acids and are more readily absorbed than the long-chain triglycerides that comprise the bulk of fat in the normal diet.

Hypocitraturia can be treated with alkali; the dose required will depend on the degree of acidosis caused by GI alkali loss. Since potassium depletion is common in these patients, the preferred alkali will be potassium citrate or potassium bicarbonate. Liquid forms may be preferable as the delayed release formulations may not have adequate absorption during the rapid intestinal transit time found in patients with intestinal bypass or resection. If potassium alkali cannot be tolerated, sodium bicarbonate can be used instead. Many of these patients will have chronic volume depletion, so additional sodium loads do not have the negative consequences often of concern in the general population. The dose of alkali should be titrated to increase citrate into the normal range. See the section above on treatment of colectomy for more detail regarding alkali therapy.

The most effective way to treat EH is to correct the underlying bowel disease, if possible. A low-gluten diet for patients with celiac disease or prescription of pancreatic enzyme replacement for those with pancreatic insufficiency can successfully reverse steatorrhea.[163] Any medications that cause fat malabsorption, such as the intestinal lipase inhibitors, should be discontinued. However, most causes of EH cannot be easily corrected. In patients with EH secondary to malabsorptive bariatric surgery, consideration should be given to reversing the procedure when medical and dietary therapy cannot control stone formation, or if there is progressive loss of kidney function from oxalate nephropathy.[110,200] Since there are many health benefits of weight reduction, reversing a successful weight-loss procedure to prevent kidney stones may be difficult for the patient to accept. Some surgeons will replace a malabsorptive procedure with a purely restrictive procedure such as gastric banding or sleeve gastrectomy. The restrictive procedures have not been associated with kidney stone formation or hyperoxaluria.[151,153] Restrictive procedures are not as effective at weight reduction, so there is a risk of weight gain after the surgical modification. In patients with Crohn's disease, medical therapy to minimize inflammation and improve bowel function should help control EH. However, much of the hyperoxaluria in Crohn's is related to resection of the small intestine. With improved medical therapy, surgery rates for Crohn's have fallen, which may result in fewer cases of EH due to IBD in the future.[34] In patients with established short bowel syndrome, there is little beyond medical therapy to offer them. Of interest, two cases of simultaneous kidney and intestinal transplant in patients with kidney failure due to EH have been reported.[201] The patients tolerated the procedure well with normal kidney function and normal renal excretion of oxalate at the time of last follow-up. Such aggressive therapy would only be considered in the most severe cases of short bowel syndrome.

In considering treatment, one must recognize that many of the basic studies were performed on patients who had JIB. Since the JIB was abandoned as a procedure in 1980, the RYGB and the BPD have become the more popular procedures that involve some level of malabsorption. In assessing the patient, the clinician should recognize that procedures vary in the level of malabsorption based on the lengths of the common channel in which bile salts and pancreatic enzymes mix with nutrients and the amount of intestinal surface available for absorption. The classic proximal RYGB should have much less fat malabsorption, and presumably lower risk of EH, than the distal or very long RYGB. The BPD has a common channel that may vary in length from 50 to 200 cm; one would expect risk of fat malabsorption would vary accordingly. This is in contrast to the JIB where only 10–30 cm of the ileum was left in continuity. The effectiveness of treatments such as fat restriction and bile acid sequestrants has not been well studied in patients with modern bariatric surgery. In patients with bowel resection related to underlying pathology such as IBD, management is more complex due to the need to maintain adequate calorie intake, which is generally not a problem in the bariatric population. In these patients, a thorough consideration of the relative contribution of bile salts and steatorrhea in the development of hyperoxaluria and stone is required when designing a therapeutic regimen.

AmU STONES

Ammonium acid urate stones are uncommon in industrialized societies.[202,203] In underdeveloped areas, AmU is a frequent component of endemic bladder stones. Ammonium acid urate stones may be associated with infection with urease containing bacteria, hypokalemia, or chronic diarrheal diseases.[204,205] Of particular interest is the reported association with laxative abuse. In this chapter, only AmU stones in association with bowel disease will be addressed.

Pathophysiology

Ammonium acid urate stones form in conditions of an alkaline urine pH (>6.0) in association with high ammonium levels. As noted previously, urate solubility is highly pH dependent. When pH falls below the pK_a of uric acid, most urate exists as the poorly soluble, protonated form.[41] As pH rises above the pK_a, monohydrogen urate becomes the predominant molecular species. In normal human physiology, ammonium excretion is high when dietary or metabolic acid production is high. This is accompanied by an elevated rate of proton secretion and acidic urine pH. Thus when ammonium excretion is high due to acid loading, urate tends to precipitate as uric acid and not AmU. Bowyer et al. performed in vitro studies that confirmed this phenomenon, showing only uric acid crystals in urine when pH is ≤5.7, despite high ammonium levels.[206] They determined that the optimal pH for AmU crystallization in urine is 6.3. In settings of prolonged, severe acid loads, renal ammonium production can become so elevated that ammonium will buffer enough protons in the tubule fluid so that urine pH approaches 6.0. This is particularly true when accompanied by hypokalemia, as hypokalemia is a stimulus for ammonium excretion.[207] The increasing pH reduces risk of uric acid crystallization, and increases the likelihood of AmU precipitation. In addition, extreme proximal tubule reabsorption of sodium in the setting of volume depletion, limits collecting duct proton secretion, contributing to the high urine pH.[208] Competing with ammonium to form complexes with monohydrogen urate are the other major monovalent cations in the urine, sodium, and potassium. Bowyer et al. showed the importance of cation competition for urate in a set of in vitro experiments.[206] They increased the ionic strength of a solution by adding sodium or potassium salts, and found that higher salt concentrations increased the amount of ammonium required to precipitate AmU. In the setting of chronic diarrhea, the resultant volume and potassium depletion reduces urine sodium and potassium, increasing the risk of AmU crystallization. If urine magnesium and phosphate excretion are low, as might be expected with poor nutrition and/or malabsorption, SS of AmU will be further increased because fewer magnesium-ammonium-phosphate complexes will form, increasing the free ammonium concentration and AmU SS.

Endemic Bladder Stones in Children

Endemic bladder stones, which occur mainly in young boys, are found in many nonindustrialized countries and frequently contain some component of AmU.[209,210] Diets high in grain but containing little animal protein have been associated with these stones. In addition, many of the children who develop these stones have chronic diarrhea as well.[209] Phosphate from grains is mainly in the form of phytate, which is not absorbed by humans, so if nutrition is predominantly from grains such as rice, there will be little phosphate in the diet. If the child also has a chronic diarrheal syndrome, then they will produce a concentrated urine with low levels of phosphate and electrolyte and high ammonium concentration, a situation likely to result in AmU stone formation. The impact of diet on AmU stones can be seen in the European experience. In the poorer agrarian regions, endemic bladder stones were common in the early part of the 19th century, but with improved nutrition and a broader range of available foodstuffs, AmU endemic bladder stones have largely disappeared from Europe.[210,211]

AmU and Bowel Disease

In industrialized countries, any form of chronic bowel disease may lead to AmU stone formation, as either a pure stone or mixed with uric acid or calcium oxalate.[212,213] A report by Soble et al. highlighted the role of bowel disease in the formation of Amu stones.[204] Of 44 patients with a stone containing any amount of AmU, 11 had a history of IBD and 6 had a history of laxative abuse. The mean AmU content of the stones was 37% for those with IBD and 36% for those with laxative use, higher than those with AmU stones from other causes. Dick also reported on three patients with AmU stones due to bowel disease, all of whom had ileal resections and either ileostomy or extensive colonic resection.[214] Urine chemistries showed low urine volume, Na, and citrate; urine pH and ammonium were not reported in this chapter. In contrast, Pichette et al. found only 2 cases of bowel disease in a retrospective study of 37 patients who had any AmU in their kidney stones.[205] Unfortunately, the authors provided little data on urine chemistries, nor did they report if laxative abuse had been considered during the evaluation of the patients.

Laxative Abuse

In 1990, Dick et al. reported nine case of AmU stones secondary to laxative abuse.[215] All nine patients were women and all either admitted to using laxatives or had a positive urine test for laxatives. Twenty-four-hour urine collections were performed while the patients were still taking laxatives and showed the expected electrolyte depletion and low urine flow rate. Neither 24-hour urine pH nor urine ammonium excretion was reported in the study. However, the patients had a very high urine anion gap when taking laxatives, an indirect marker of ammonium production. In three of the patients, urine chemistries were measured after laxatives were stopped and showed marked improvement (Table 17.10). Note the marked increase in urine electrolytes, citrate, and urine flow. In one patient, a renal stone dissolved in situ after discontinuation of the laxatives. Wu et al. also report a case of AmU stone formation due to laxative abuse in which discontinuation of laxatives led to stone dissolution.[216]

Laxative abuse has a lifetime prevalence of ~4%, with the majority of cases occurring in women. Laxative abuse

Table 17.10: Effect of laxative abuse on urine chemistries.

	On laxatives	*Off laxatives*
Volume (mL/d)	797 ± 279	1993 ± 1124
Uric acid (mg/d)	423 ± 172	565 ± 163
Citrate (mg/d)	125 ± 81	501 ± 208
Sodium (mmol/d)	10 ± 8	132 ± 54
Potassium (mmol/d)	24 ± 24	59 ± 28

Source: Adapted from Dick et al.[215]
Data presented as mean ± SD. *N* = 3.

may not be obvious to the clinician since most laxatives are available over the counter and many patients will actually complain of constipation, so that the extent of laxative use remains hidden.[217] The diagnosis of laxative abuse requires a high degree of clinical suspicion. A useful laboratory clue that laxative use may exist is the finding of high urine ammonium excretion as compared to sulfate excretion (both expressed as mEq/d) accompanied by a urine pH <6.5 in a patient who denies any bowel disease. Though urine anion gap is often used as an indirect measure of urine ammonium, it is not sensitive enough to detect situations where ammonium production is moderately elevated.[218] Very high urine magnesium excretion can suggest use of magnesium-containing laxatives, particularly if renal excretion of other electrolytes is low.

Treatment

Treatment should focus on correcting the unique pathophysiology associated with AmU stones due to bowel disease. If chronic diarrhea is the underlying disorder, then the primary focus of treatment is aimed at correcting the bowel disease causing diarrhea. If laxative abuse is the cause, then discontinuation of laxatives may be all that is needed to prevent future stones.[215] There are no treatment trials specifically for AmU stones, so treatment recommendations are based on physiologic principles. Correction of total body potassium deficit with potassium salts will reduce the stimulus for ammonium production. If bowel disease cannot be adequately treated, then the addition of alkali will correct any associated acidosis that is driving ammonium production. Providing adequate electrolyte in the diet or as supplements so that both urine sodium and potassium excretion are >50 mmol/d should reduce the risk of AmU crystallization. Of course, fluid intake needs to be sufficient to keep the urine flow rate >2.5 L/d in adults. Some authorities recommend acidifying urine by administration of methionine as a means of preventing AmU stone recurrence,[219] though there are little data supporting its use. Methionine loading could be dangerous in patients with chronic diarrhea and acidosis. Whether reducing urate excretion with a xanthine oxidase inhibitor is beneficial has not been studied and should probably be reserved for cases where all else fails.

REFERENCES

1. Hounnou G, Destrieux C, Desme J, et al. Anatomical study of the length of the human intestine. Surg Radiol Anat. 2002;24(5):290-4.
2. Charney AN, Donowitz M. Gastrointestinal Influences on Hydrogen Ion Balance. In: Gennari FJ, Adroogue HJ, Galla JH, et al. (Eds). Acid-Base Disorders and Their Treatment, 1st edition. Boca Raton: Taylor & Francis; 2005. pp. 209-40.
3. Christakos S, Dhawan P, Porta A, et al. Vitamin D and intestinal calcium absorption. Mol Cell Endocrinol. 2011;347(1-2): 25-9.
4. Bronner F, Pansu D. Nutritional aspects of calcium absorption. J Nutr. 1999;129(1):9-12.
5. de Baaij JH, Hoenderop JG, Bindels RJ. Regulation of magnesium balance: lessons learned from human genetic disease. Clin Kidney J. 2012;5(Suppl 1):i15-i24.
6. Walton J, Gray TK. Absorption of inorganic phosphate in the human small intestine. Clin Sci (Lond). 1979;56(5):407-12.
7. Favus MJ, Goltzman D. Regulation of calcium and magnesium. In: Rosen CJ (Ed). Primare on the Metabolic Bone Diseases and Disorders of Mineral Metabolism, 7th edition. Washington, DC: American Society for Bone and Mineral Research; 2008. pp. 104-8.
8. Bikle DD. Vitamin D insufficiency/deficiency in gastrointestinal disorders. J Bone Miner Res. 2007;22(Suppl 2):V50-V54.
9. Curhan GC, Willett WC, Speizer FE, et al. Twenty-four-hour urine chemistries and the risk of kidney stones among women and men. Kidney Int. 2001;59(6):2290-8.
10. Holmes RP, Goodman HO, Assimos DG. Contribution of dietary oxalate to urinary oxalate excretion. Kidney Int. 2001;59(1):270-6.
11. Brinkley L, McGuire J, Gregory J, et al. Bioavailability of oxalate in foods. Urology. 1981;17(6):534-8.
12. Brinkley LJ, Gregory J, Pak CYC. A further study of oxalate bioavailability in foods. J Urol. 1990;144:94-6.
13. Hess B, Jost C, Zipperle L, et al. High-calcium intake abolishes hyperoxaluria and reduces urinary crystallization during a 20-fold normal oxalate load in humans. Nephrol Dial Transplant. 1998;13(9):2241-7.
14. Hesse A, Schneeberger W, Engfeld S, et al. Intestinal hyperabsorption of oxalate in calcium oxalate stone formers: application of a new test with [13C2]oxalate. J Am Soc Nephrol. 1999;10(Suppl 14):S329-33.
15. Hautmann R. The stomach: a new and powerful oxalate absorption site in man. J Urol. 1993;149:1401-4.
16. Chen Z, Ye Z, Zeng L, et al. Clinical investigation on gastric oxalate absorption. Chin Med J (Engl). 2003;116(11):1749-51.

17. Read NW, Cammack J, Edwards C, et al. Is the transit time of a meal through the small intestine related to the rate at which it leaves the stomach? Gut. 1982;23(10):824-8.
18. Tappenden KA. Pathophysiology of short bowel syndrome: considerations of resected and residual anatomy. JPEN J Parenter Enteral Nutr. 2014;38(1 Suppl):14S-22S.
19. Bargen JA, Jackman RJ, Kerr JG. Studies on the life histories of patients with chronic ulcerative colitis, with some suggestions for treatment. Ann Intern Med. 1938;12:339-52.
20. Lindahl WW, Bargen JA. Nephrolithiasis complicating chronic ulcerative colitis after ileostomy. J Urol. 1941;46: 183-92.
21. Deren JJ, Porush JG, Levitt MF, et al. Nephrolithiasis as a complication of ulcerative colitis and regional enteritis. Ann Intern Med. 1962;56:843-53.
22. Maratka Z, Nedbal J. Urolithiasis as a complication of the surgical treatment of ulcerative colitis. Gut. 1964;5:214-7.
23. Grossman MS, Nugent FW. Urolithiasis as a complication of chronic diarrheal disease. Am J Dig Dis. 1967;12(5):491-8.
24. Gelzayd EA, Breuer RI, Kirsner JB. Nephrolithiasis in inflammatory bowel disease. Am J Dig Dis. 1968;13(12):1027-34.
25. Greenstein AJ, Janowitz HD, Sachar DB. The extra-intestinal complications of Crohn's disease and ulcerative colitis: a study of 700 patients. Medicine (Baltimore). 1976;55(5): 401-12.
26. Shield DE, Lytton B, Weiss RM, et al. Urologic complications of inflammatory bowel disease. J Urol. 1976;115(6):701-6.
27. Knudsen L, Marcussen H, Fleckenstein P, et al. Urolithiasis in chronic inflammatory bowel disease. Scand J Gastroenterol. 1978;13(4):433-6.
28. Bambach CP, Robertson WG, Peacock M, et al. Effect of intestinal surgery on the risk of urinary stone formation. Gut. 1981;22(4):257-63.
29. Bennett RC, Hughes ES. Urinary calculi and ulcerative colitis. Br Med J. 1972;2(5812):494-6.
30. Fukushima T, Ishiguro N, Matsuda Y, et al. Clinical and urinary characteristics of urolithiasis in ulcerative colitis. Am J Gastroenterol. 1982;77(4):238-42.
31. Kim MJ, Woo SY, Kim ER, et al. Incidence and risk factors for urolithiasis in patients with Crohn's disease. Urol Int. 2015;95(3):314-9.
32. Cury DB, Moss AC, Schor N. Nephrolithiasis in patients with inflammatory bowel disease in the community. Int J Nephrol Renovasc Dis. 2013;6:139-42.
33. Viana ML, Pontes RM, Garcia WE, et al. Crohn's disease and kidney stones: much more than coincidence? Arq Gastroenterol. 2007;44(3):210-4.
34. Frolkis AD, Dykeman J, Negron ME, et al. Risk of surgery for inflammatory bowel diseases has decreased over time: a systematic review and meta-analysis of population-based studies. Gastroenterology. 2013;145(5):996-1006.
35. Feagan BG, Panaccione R, Sandborn WJ, et al. Effects of adalimumab therapy on incidence of hospitalization and surgery in Crohn's disease: results from the CHARM study. Gastroenterology. 2008;135(5):1493-9.
36. Varda BK, McNabb-Baltar J, Sood A, et al. Urolithiasis and urinary tract infection among patients with inflammatory bowel disease: a review of US emergency department visits between 2006 and 2009. Urology. 2015;85(4):764-70.
37. Christl SU, Scheppach W. Metabolic consequences of total colectomy. Scand J Gastroenterol Suppl. 1997;222:20-4.
38. Parks JH, Worcester EM, O'Connor RC, et al. Urine stone risk factors in nephrolithiasis patients with and without bowel disease. Kidney Int. 2003;63(1):255-65.
39. Bennett RC, Jepson RP. Uric acid stone formation following ileostomy. Aust N Z J Surg. 1966;36(2):153-8.
40. Wilmore DW, Gots RE. The etiology of uric acid urolithiasis following ileostomy. Arch Surg. 1969;99(4):421-3.
41. Coe F, Strauss AL, Tembe V, et al. Uric acid saturation in calcium nephrolithiasis. Kidney Int. 1980;17:662-8.
42. Finlayson B, Smith A. Stability of first dissociable proton of uric acid. J Chem Eng Data. 2015;19(1):94-7.
43. Singer AM, Bennett RC, Carter NG, et al. Blood and urinary changes in patients with ileostomies and ileorectal anastomoses. Br Med J. 1973;3(5872):141-3.
44. Kennedy HJ, Al-Dujaili EA, Edwards CR, et al. Water and electrolyte balance in subjects with a permanent ileostomy. Gut. 1983;24(8):702-5.
45. Clarke AM, McKenzie RG. Ileostomy and the risk of urinary uric acid stones. Lancet 1969;2(7617):395-7.
46. Stern H, Cohen Z, Wilson DR, et al. Urolithiasis risk factors in continent reservoir ileostomy patients. Dis Colon Rectum. 1980;23(8):556-8.
47. Kennedy HJ, Fletcher EW, Truelove SC. Urinary stones in subjects with a permanent ileostomy. Br J Surg. 1982;69(11):661-4.
48. Caudarella R, Rizzoli E, Pironi L, et al. Renal stone formation in patients with inflammatory bowel disease. Scanning Microsc. 1993;7(1):371-9.
49. Leveen HH, Lyons A, Becker E. Physiologic adaptation to ileostomy. Am J Surg. 1962;103:35-41.
50. Clarke AM, Chirnside A, Hill GL, et al. Chronic dehydration and sodium depletion in patients with established ileostomies. Lancet. 1967;2(7519):740-3.
51. Hill GL, Goligher JC, Smith AH, et al. Long term changes in total body water, total exchangeable sodium and total body potassium before and after ileostomy. Br J Surg. 1975;62(7):524-7.
52. Okamoto T, Kusunoki M, Kusuhara K, et al. Water and electrolyte balance after ileal J pouch-anal anastomosis in ulcerative colitis and familial adenomatous polyposis. Int J Colorectal Dis. 1995;10(1):33-8.
53. Randall RE, Jr. Urate nephropathy following chronic ileostomy acidosis. Am J Nephrol. 2002;22(4):372-5.
54. Nicar MJ, Hill K, Pak CYC. Inhibition by citrate of spontaneous precipitation of calcium oxalate in vitro. J Bone Miner Res. 1987;2:215-20.
55. Hamm LL. Renal handling of citrate. Kidney Int. 1990; 38(4):728-35.
56. McConnell N, Campbell S, Gillanders I, et al. Risk factors for developing renal stones in inflammatory bowel disease. BJU Int. 2002;89(9):835-41.
57. Stelzner M, Phillips JD, Saleh S, et al. Nephrolithiasis and urine ion changes in ulcerative colitis patients undergoing

colectomy and endorectal ileal pull through. J Surg Res. 1990;48(6):552-6.

58. Roses RE, Rombeau JL. Recent trends in the surgical management of inflammatory bowel disease. World J Gastroenterol. 2008;14(3):408-12.
59. Christie PM, Knight GS, Hill GL. Metabolism of body water and electrolytes after surgery for ulcerative colitis: conventional ileostomy versus J pouch. Br J Surg. 1990;77(2):149-51.
60. Santavirta J, Harmoinen A, Karvonen AL, et al. Water and electrolyte balance after ileoanal anastomosis. Dis Colon Rectum. 1991;34(2):115-8.
61. Evan AP, Lingeman JE, Coe FL, et al. Intra-tubular deposits, urine and stone composition are divergent in patients with ileostomy. Kidney Int. 2009;76(10):1081-8.
62. Evan AP, Lingeman JE, Coe FL, et al. Randall's plaque of patients with nephrolithiasis begins in basement membranes of thin loops of Henle. J Clin Invest. 2003;111(5):607-16.
63. Kanaghinis T, Lubran M, Coghill NF. The composition of ileostomy fluid. Gut. 1963;4:322-38.
64. Borghi L, Meschi T, Amato F, et al. Urinary volume, water and recurrences in idiopathic calcium nephrolithiasis: a 5-year randomized prospective study. J Urol. 1996;155(3):839-43.
65. Rodman JS, Sosa E, Lopez MA. Diagnosis and treatment of uric acid calculi. In: Coe FL, Favus MJ, Pak C, et al. (Eds). Kidney Stones: Medical and Surgical Management. Philadelphia, PA: Lippincott-Raven; 1996. pp. 973-89.
66. Russinko PJ, Agarwal S, Choi MJ, et al. Obstructive nephropathy secondary to sulfasalazine calculi. Urology. 2003;62(4):748.
67. Saito M, Takahashi C, Ishida G, et al. Acute renal failure associated with sulfur calculi. J Urol. 2001;165(6 Pt 1):1985-6.
68. Smith LH, Fromm H, Hofmann AF. Acquired hyperoxaluria, nephrolithiasis, and intestinal disease. Description of a syndrome. N Engl J Med. 1972;286(26):1371-5.
69. Dowling RH, Rose GA, Sutor DJ. Hyperoxaluria and renal calculi in ileal disease. Lancet. 1971;1(7709):1103-6.
70. Chadwick VS, Modha K, Dowling RH. Mechanism for hyperoxaluria in patients with ileal dysfunction. N Engl J Med. 1973;289(4):172-6.
71. Earnest DL, Johnson G, Williams HE, et al. Hyperoxaluria in patients with ileal resection: an abnormality in dietary oxalate absorption. Gastroenterology. 1974;66(6):1114-22.
72. Froeder L, Arasaki CH, Malheiros CA, et al. Response to dietary oxalate after bariatric surgery. Clin J Am Soc Nephrol. 2012;7(12):2033-40.
73. Stauffer JQ, Humphreys MH, Weir GJ. Acquired hyperoxaluria with regional enteritis after ileal resection. Role of dietary oxalate. Ann Intern Med. 1973;79(3):383-91.
74. Admirand WH, Earnest DL, Williams HE. Hyperoxaluria and bowel disease. Trans Assoc Am Phys. 1971;84:307-12.
75. Dobbins JW, Binder HJ. Importance of the colon in enteric hyperoxaluria. N Engl J Med. 1977;296:298-301.
76. Andersson H, Filipsson S, Hulten L. Urinary oxalate excretion related to ileocolic surgery in patients with Crohn's disease. Scand J Gastroenterol. 1978;13(4):465-9.
77. Hylander E, Jarnum S, Jensen HJ, et al. Enteric hyperoxaluria: dependence on small intestinal resection, colectomy, and steatorrhoea in chronic inflammatory bowel disease. Scand J Gastroenterol. 1978;13(5):577-88.
78. Modigliani R, Labayle D, Aymes C, et al. Evidence for excessive absorption of oxalate by the colon in enteric hyperoxaluria. Scand J Gastroenterol. 1978;13(2):187-92.
79. Earnest DL, Williams HE, Admirand WH. A physicochemical basis for treatment of enteric hyperoxaluria. Trans Assoc Am Phys. 1975;88:224-34.
80. Caspary WF, Tonissen J, Lankisch PG. "Enteral" hyperoxaluria. Effect of cholestyramine, calcium, neomycin, and bile acids on intestinal oxalate absorption in man. Acta Hepatogastroenterol (Stuttg). 1977;24(3):193-200.
81. Hylander E, Jarnum S, Nielsen K. Calcium treatment of enteric hyperoxaluria after jejunoileal bypass for morbid obesity. Scand J Gastroenterol. 1980;15(3):349-52.
82. Dobbins JW, Binder HJ. Effect of bile salts and fatty acids on the colonic absorption of oxalate. Gastroenterology. 1976;70:1096-100.
83. Binder HJ. Intestinal oxalate absorption. Gastroenterology. 1974;67(3):441-6.
84. Kathpalia SC, Favus MJ, Coe FL. Evidence for size and charge permselectivity of rat ascending colon. Effects of ricinoleate and bile salts on oxalic acid and neutral sugar transport. J Clin Invest. 1984;74(3):805-11.
85. Fairclough PD, Feest TG, Chadwick VS, et al. Effect of sodium chenodeoxycholate on oxalate absorption from the excluded human colon—a mechanism for "enteric" hyperoxaluria. Gut. 1977;18(3):240-4.
86. Odstrcil EA, Martinez JG, Santa Ana CA, et al. The contribution of malabsorption to the reduction in net energy absorption after long-limb Roux-en-Y gastric bypass. Am J Clin Nutr. 2010;92(4):704-13.
87. Nightingale JM. Management of patients with a short bowel. Nutrition. 1999;15(7-8):633-7.
88. Maalouf NM, Tondapu P, Guth ES, et al. Hypocitraturia and hyperoxaluria after Roux-en-Y gastric bypass surgery. J Urol. 2010;183(3):1026-30.
89. Rudman D, Dedonis JL, Fountain MT, et al. Hypocitraturia in patients with gastrointestinal malabsorption. N Engl J Med. 1980;303(12):657-61.
90. Obialo CI, Clayman RV, Matts JP, et al. Pathogenesis of nephrolithiasis post-partial ileal bypass surgery: case-control study. The POSCH Group. Kidney Int. 1991;39(6):1249-54.
91. Elliot JS, Soles WP. Excretion of calcium and citric acid in patients with small bowel disease. J Urol. 1974;111(6):810-2.
92. Payne JH, Dewind LT, Commons RR. Metabolic observations in patients with jejunocolic shunts. Am J Surg. 1963;106:273-89.
93. Condon SC, Janes NJ, Wise L, et al. Role of caloric intake in the weight loss after jejunoileal bypass for obesity. Gastroenterology. 1978;74(1):34-7.
94. O'Leary JP, Thomas WC, Jr, Woodward ER. Urinary tract stone after small bowel bypass for morbid obesity. Am J Surg. 1974;127(2):142-7.
95. Mobley JE, Hardison W. Nephrolithiasis following intestinal bypass for obesity. Urology. 1974;3(5):639-41.

96. Dickstein SS, Frame B. Urinary tract calculi after intestinal shunt operations for the treatment of obesity. Surg Gynecol Obstet. 1973;136(2):257-60.
97. Requarth JA, Burchard KW, Colacchio TA, et al. Long-term morbidity following jejunoileal bypass. The continuing potential need for surgical reversal. Arch Surg. 1995;130(3):318-25.
98. Hocking MP, Duerson MC, O'Leary JP, et al. Jejunoileal bypass for morbid obesity. Late follow-up in 100 cases. N Engl J Med. 1983;308(17):995-9.
99. Fikri E, Casella RR. Hyperoxaluria and urinary tract calculi after jejunoileal bypass. Am J Surg. 1975;129(3):334-6.
100. Gregory JG, Park KY, Schoenberg HW. Oxalate stone disease after intestinal resection. J Urol. 1977;117(5):631-4.
101. Nordenvall B, Backman L, Larsson L, et al. Urine composition following jejunoileal bypass. Eur Urol. 1983;9(1):35-9.
102. Annuk M, Backman U, Holmgren K, et al. Urinary calculi and jejunoileal bypass operation. A long-term follow-up. Scand J Urol Nephrol. 1998;32(3):177-80.
103. Hylander E, Jarnum S, Kempel K, et al. The absorption of oxalate, calcium, and fat after jejunoileal bypass. A prospective study. Scand J Gastroenterol. 1980;15(3):343-8.
104. Drenick EJ, Stanley TM, Border WA, et al. Renal damage with intestinal bypass. Ann Intern Med. 1978;89(5 Pt 1):594-9.
105. Stauffer JQ. Hyperoxaluria and calcium oxalate nephrolithiasis after jejunoileal bypass. Am J Clin Nutr. 1977;30(1):64-71.
106. Stauffer JQ. Hyperoxaluria and intestinal disease. The role of steatorrhea and dietary calcium in regulating intestinal oxalate absorption. Am J Dig Dis. 1977;22(10):921-8.
107. Lindsjo M, Danielson BG, Fellstrom B, et al. Intestinal absorption of oxalate and calcium in patients with jejunoileal bypass. Scand J Urol Nephrol. 1989;23(4):283-9.
108. Kirkpatrick JR. Jejunoileal bypass. A legacy of late complications. Arch Surg. 1987;122(5):610-4.
109. McFarland RJ, Gazet JC, Pilkington TR. A 13-year review of jejunoileal bypass. Br J Surg. 1985;72(2):81-7.
110. Dhar NB, Grundfest S, Jones JS, et al. Jejunoileal bypass reversal: effect on renal function, metabolic parameters and stone formation. J Urol. 2005;174(5):1844-6.
111. Dean P, Joshi S, Kaminski DL. Long-term outcome of reversal of small intestinal bypass operations. Am J Surg. 1990;159(1):118-23.
112. Griffen WO, Jr, Bivins BA, Bell RM. The decline and fall of the jejunoileal bypass. Surg Gynecol Obstet. 1983;157(4):301-8.
113. Payne JH, Dewind LT. Surgical treatment of obesity. Am J Surg. 1969;118(2):141-7.
114. Flegal KM, Carroll MD, Ogden CL, et al. Prevalence and trends in obesity among US adults, 1999-2000. JAMA. 2002;288(14):1723-7.
115. Ogden CL, Carroll MD, Curtin LR, et al. Prevalence of overweight and obesity in the United States, 1999-2004. JAMA. 2006;295(13):1549-55.
116. Flegal KM, Carroll MD, Ogden CL, et al. Prevalence and trends in obesity among US adults, 1999-2008. JAMA. 2010;303(3):235-41.
117. Flegal KM, Carroll MD, Kit BK, et al. Prevalence of obesity and trends in the distribution of body mass index among US adults, 1999-2010. JAMA. 2012;307(5):491-7.
118. Ogden CL, Carroll MD, Kit BK, et al. Prevalence of childhood and adult obesity in the United States, 2011-2012. JAMA. 2014;311(8):806-14.
119. Ogden CL, Carroll MD, Kit BK, et al. Prevalence of obesity and trends in body mass index among US children and adolescents, 1999-2010. JAMA. 2012;307(5):483-90.
120. Buchwald H, Oien DM. Metabolic/bariatric surgery worldwide 2011. Obes Surg. 2013;23(4):427-36.
121. Reames BN, Finks JF, Bacal D, et al. Changes in bariatric surgery procedure use in Michigan, 2006-2013. JAMA. 2014;312(9):959-61.
122. Brolin RE, Kenler HA, Gorman JH, et al. Long-limb gastric bypass in the superobese. A prospective randomized study. Ann Surg. 1992;215(4):387-95.
123. Nelson WK, Houghton SG, Milliner DS, et al. Enteric hyperoxaluria, nephrolithiasis, and oxalate nephropathy: potentially serious and unappreciated complications of Roux-en-Y gastric bypass. Surg Obes Relat Dis. 2005;1(5):481-5.
124. Hofmann AF, Schmuck G, Scopinaro N, et al. Hyperoxaluria associated with intestinal bypass surgery for morbid obesity: occurrence, pathogenesis and approaches to treatment. Int J Obes. 1981;5(5):513-8.
125. Asplin JR, Coe FL. Hyperoxaluria in kidney stone formers treated with modern bariatric surgery. J Urol. 2007;177(2):565-9.
126. Sinha MK, Collazo-Clavell ML, Rule A, et al. Hyperoxaluric nephrolithiasis is a complication of Roux-en-Y gastric bypass surgery. Kidney Int. 2007;72(1):100-7.
127. Patel BN, Passman CM, Fernandez A, et al. Prevalence of hyperoxaluria after bariatric surgery. J Urol. 2009;181(1):161-6.
128. Duffey BG, Pedro RN, Makhlouf A, et al. Roux-en-Y gastric bypass is associated with early increased risk factors for development of calcium oxalate nephrolithiasis. J Am Coll Surg. 2008;206(3):1145-53.
129. Park AM, Storm DW, Fulmer BR, et al. A prospective study of risk factors for nephrolithiasis after Roux-en-Y gastric bypass surgery. J Urol. 2009;182(5):2334-9.
130. Duffey BG, Alanee S, Pedro RN, et al. Hyperoxaluria is a long-term consequence of Roux-en-Y gastric bypass: a 2-year prospective longitudinal study. J Am Coll Surg. 2010;211(1):8-15.
131. Wu JN, Craig J, Chamie K, et al. Urolithiasis risk factors in the bariatric population undergoing gastric bypass surgery. Surg Obes Relat Dis. 2013;9(1):83-7.
132. Kumar R, Lieske JC, Collazo-Clavell ML, et al. Fat malabsorption and increased intestinal oxalate absorption are common after Roux-en-Y gastric bypass surgery. Surgery. 2011;149(5):654-61.
133. Allison MJ, Dawson KA, Mayberry WR, et al. Oxalobacter formigenes gen. nov., sp. nov.: oxalate-degrading anaerobes that inhabit the gastrointestinal tract. Arch Microbiol. 1985;141(1):1-7.
134. Kaufman DW, Kelly JP, Curhan GC, et al. Oxalobacter formigenes may reduce the risk of calcium oxalate kidney stones. J Am Soc Nephrol. 2008;19(6):1197-203.
135. Mittal RD, Kumar R, Mittal B, et al. Stone composition, metabolic profile and the presence of the gut-inhabiting

bacterium Oxalobacter formigenes as risk factors for renal stone formation. Med Princ Pract. 2003;12(4):208-13.
136. Jiang J, Knight J, Easter LH, et al. Impact of dietary calcium and oxalate, and Oxalobacter formigenes colonization on urinary oxalate excretion. J Urol. 2011;186(1):135-9.
137. Kumar R, Ghoshal UC, Singh G, et al. Infrequency of colonization with Oxalobacter formigenes in inflammatory bowel disease: possible role in renal stone formation. J Gastroenterol Hepatol. 2004;19(12):1403-9.
138. Allison MJ, Cook HM, Milne DB, et al. Oxalate degradation by gastrointestinal bacteria from humans. J Nutr. 1986;116(3):455-60.
139. Duffey BG, Miyaoka R, Holmes R, et al. Oxalobacter colonization in the morbidly obese and correlation with urinary stone risk. Urology. 2011;78(3):531-4.
140. Faber SR, Feitler WW, Bleiler RE, et al. The effects of an induced pyridoxine and pantothenic acid deficiency on excretions of oxalic and xanthurenic acids in the urine. Am J Clin Nutr. 1963;12:406-12.
141. Clements RH, Katasani VG, Palepu R, et al. Incidence of vitamin deficiency after laparoscopic Roux-en-Y gastric bypass in a university hospital setting. Am Surg. 2006;72(12):1196-202.
142. Gehrer S, Kern B, Peters T, et al. Fewer nutrient deficiencies after laparoscopic sleeve gastrectomy (LSG) than after laparoscopic Roux-Y-gastric bypass (LRYGB)—a prospective study. Obes Surg. 2010;20(4):447-53.
143. Aasheim ET, Bjorkman S, Sovik TT, et al. Vitamin status after bariatric surgery: a randomized study of gastric bypass and duodenal switch. Am J Clin Nutr. 2009;90(1):15-22.
144. Bal BS, Finelli FC, Shope TR, et al. Nutritional deficiencies after bariatric surgery. Nat Rev Endocrinol. 2012;8(9):544-56.
145. Durrani O, Morrisroe S, Jackman S, et al. Analysis of stone disease in morbidly obese patients undergoing gastric bypass surgery. J Endourol. 2006;20(10):749-52.
146. Matlaga BR, Shore AD, Magnuson T, et al. Effect of gastric bypass surgery on kidney stone disease. J Urol. 2009;181(6):2573-7.
147. Costa-Matos A, Guidoni LR, Carvalho KA, et al. Is there an association between urolithiasis and Roux-en-Y gastric bypass surgery? Int Braz J Urol. 2009;35(4):432-5.
148. Lieske JC, Mehta RA, Milliner DS, et al. Kidney stones are common after bariatric surgery. Kidney Int. 2015;87(4): 839-45.
149. Shimizu H, Ichikawa D, Tamagaki K, et al. Evaluation of postoperative nephrolithiasis and renal dysfunction in gastric cancer patients. Gastric Cancer. 2013;16(3):338-44.
150. Nasr SH, D'Agati VD, Said SM, et al. Oxalate nephropathy complicating Roux-en-Y gastric bypass: an underrecognized cause of irreversible renal failure. Clin J Am Soc Nephrol. 2008;3(6):1676-83.
151. Semins MJ, Asplin JR, Steele K, et al. The effect of restrictive bariatric surgery on urinary stone risk factors. Urology. 2010;76(4):826-9.
152. Penniston KL, Kaplon DM, Gould JC, et al. Gastric band placement for obesity is not associated with increased urinary risk of urolithiasis compared to bypass. J Urol. 2009;182(5):2340-6.
153. Semins MJ, Matlaga BR, Shore AD, et al. The effect of gastric banding on kidney stone disease. Urology. 2009;74(4):746-9.
154. Chen T, Godebu E, Horgan S, et al. The effect of restrictive bariatric surgery on urolithiasis. J Endourol. 2013;27(2): 242-4.
155. Nadler EP, Youn HA, Ren CJ, et al. An update on 73 US obese pediatric patients treated with laparoscopic adjustable gastric banding: comorbidity resolution and compliance data. J Pediatr Surg. 2008;43(1):141-6.
156. Ferraz RR, Tiselius HG, Heilberg IP. Fat malabsorption induced by gastrointestinal lipase inhibitor leads to an increase in urinary oxalate excretion. Kidney Int. 2004;66(2):676-82.
157. Sarica K, Akarsu E, Erturhan S, et al. Evaluation of urinary oxalate levels in patients receiving gastrointestinal lipase inhibitor. Obesity (Silver Spring). 2008;16(7):1579-84.
158. Karamadoukis L, Shivashankar GH, Ludeman L, et al. An unusual complication of treatment with orlistat. Clin Nephrol. 2009;71(4):430-2.
159. Singh A, Sarkar SR, Gaber LW, et al. Acute oxalate nephropathy associated with orlistat, a gastrointestinal lipase inhibitor. Am J Kidney Dis. 2007;49(1):153-7.
160. Hinchliffe WT, Fenwick S, MacDougall K. Acute oxalate nephropathy. Clin Med (Lond). 2012;12(6):600.
161. Chaudhari D, Crisostomo C, Ganote C, et al. Acute oxalate nephropathy associated with orlistat: a case report with a review of the literature. Case Rep Nephrol. 2013;2013:124604.
162. van der Windt DA, Jellema P, Mulder CJ, et al. Diagnostic testing for celiac disease among patients with abdominal symptoms: a systematic review. JAMA. 2010;303(17):1738-46.
163. McDonald GB, Earnest DL, Admirand WH. Hyperoxaluria correlates with fat malabsorption in patients with sprue. Gut. 1977;18(7):561-6.
164. Ogilvie D, McCollum JP, Packer S, et al. Urinary outputs of oxalate, calcium, and magnesium in children with intestinal disorders. Potential cause of renal calculi. Arch Dis Child. 1976;51(10):790-5.
165. Ciacci C, Spagnuolo G, Tortora R, et al. Urinary stone disease in adults with celiac disease: prevalence, incidence and urinary determinants. J Urol. 2008;180(3):974-9.
166. Ludvigsson JF, Zingone F, Fored M, et al. Moderately increased risk of urinary stone disease in patients with biopsy-verified coeliac disease. Aliment Pharmacol Ther. 2012;35(4):477-84.
167. Menekse E, Selimoglu MA, Temel I, et al. Celiac disease in children with urolithiasis. Turk J Pediatr. 2012;54(4):382-6.
168. Saccomani MD, Pizzini C, Piacentini GL, et al. Analysis of urinary parameters as risk factors for nephrolithiasis in children with celiac disease. J Urol. 2012;188(2):566-70.
169. Capolongo G, Abul-Ezz S, Moe OW, et al. Subclinical celiac disease and crystal-induced kidney disease following kidney transplant. Am J Kidney Dis. 2012;60(4):662-7.
170. Gama R, Schweitzer FA. Renal calculus: a unique presentation of coeliac disease. BJU Int. 1999;84(4):528-9.
171. Cartery C, Faguer S, Karras A, et al. Oxalate nephropathy associated with chronic pancreatitis. Clin J Am Soc Nephrol. 2011;6(8):1895-902.

172. Hill P, Karim M, Davies DR, et al. Rapidly progressive irreversible renal failure in patients with pancreatic insufficiency. Am J Kidney Dis. 2003;42(4):842-5.
173. Coe FL, Evan AP, Lingeman JE, et al. Plaque and deposits in nine human stone diseases. Urol Res. 2010;38(4):239-47.
174. Evan AP, Coe FL, Gillen D, et al. Renal intratubular crystals and hyaluronan staining occur in stone formers with bypass surgery but not with idiopathic calcium oxalate stones. Anat Rec (Hoboken). 2008;291(3):325-34.
175. Evan AP, Lingeman JE, Worcester EM, et al. Renal histopathology and crystal deposits in patients with small bowel resection and calcium oxalate stone disease. Kidney Int. 2010;78(3):310-7.
176. Worcester E, Evan A, Bledsoe S, et al. Pathophysiological correlates of two unique renal tubule lesions in rats with intestinal resection. Am J Physiol Renal Physiol. 2006;291(5): F1061-9.
177. Pang R, Linnes MP, O'Connor HM, et al. Controlled metabolic diet reduces calcium oxalate supersaturation but not oxalate excretion after bariatric surgery. Urology. 2012;80(2):250-4.
178. Andersson H, Jagenburg R. Fat-reduced diet in the treatment of hyperoxaluria in patients with ileopathy. Gut. 1974;15(5):360-6.
179. Nordenvall B, Backman L, Burman P, et al. Low-oxalate, low-fat dietary regimen in hyperoxaluria following jejunoileal bypass. Acta Chir Scand. 1983;149(1):89-91.
180. Barilla DE, Notz C, Kennedy D, et al. Renal oxalate excretion following oral oxalate loads in patients with ileal disease and with renal and absorptive hypercalciurias. Effect of calcium and magnesium. Am J Med. 1978;64(4):579-85.
181. Tondapu P, Provost D, Adams-Huet B, et al. Comparison of the absorption of calcium carbonate and calcium citrate after Roux-en-Y gastric bypass. Obes Surg. 2009;19(9):1256-61.
182. Sakhaee K, Griffith C, Pak CY. Biochemical control of bone loss and stone-forming propensity by potassium-calcium citrate after bariatric surgery. Surg Obes Relat Dis. 2012;8(1):67-72.
183. Zimmermann DJ, Voss S, Von Unruh GE, et al. Importance of magnesium in absorption and excretion of oxalate. Urol Int. 2005;74(3):262-7.
184. Liebman M, Costa G. Effects of calcium and magnesium on urinary oxalate excretion after oxalate loads. J Urol. 2000;163(5):1565-9.
185. Kohri K, Garside J, Blacklock NJ. The role of magnesium in calcium oxalate urolithiasis. Br J Urol. 1988;61(2):107-15.
186. Nordenvall B, Backman L, Larsson L, et al. Effects of calcium, aluminium, magnesium and cholestyramine on hyperoxaluria in patients with jejunoileal bypass. Acta Chir Scand. 1983;149(1):93-8.
187. Lieske JC, Regnier C, Dillon JJ. Use of sevelamer hydrochloride as an oxalate binder. J Urol. 2008;179(4):1407-10.
188. Laker MF, Hofmann AF. Effective therapy of enteric hyperoxaluria: in vitro binding of oxalate by anion-exchange resins and aluminum hydroxide. J Pharm Sci. 1981;70(9):1065-7.
189. Robijn S, Vervaet BA, Hoppe B, et al. Lanthanum carbonate inhibits intestinal oxalate absorption and prevents nephrocalcinosis after oxalate loading in rats. J Urol. 2013; 189(5):1960-6.
190. Emmett M, Guirl MJ, Santa Ana CA, et al. Conjugated bile acid replacement therapy reduces urinary oxalate excretion in short bowel syndrome. Am J Kidney Dis. 2003;41(1):230-7.
191. Kumpf VJ. Pharmacologic management of diarrhea in patients with short bowel syndrome. JPEN J Parenter Enteral Nutr. 2014;38(1 Suppl):38S-44S.
192. Hatch M, Cornelius J, Allison M, et al. Oxalobacter sp. reduces urinary oxalate excretion by promoting enteric oxalate secretion. Kidney Int. 2006;69(4):691-8.
193. Sidhu H, Allison MJ, Chow JM, et al. Rapid reversal of hyperoxaluria in a rat model after probiotic administration of Oxalobacter formigenes. J Urol. 2001;166(4):1487-91.
194. Campieri C, Campieri M, Bertuzzi V, et al. Reduction of oxaluria after an oral course of lactic acid bacteria at high concentration. Kidney Int. 2001;60(3):1097-105.
195. Lieske JC, Tremaine WJ, De SC, et al. Diet, but not oral probiotics, effectively reduces urinary oxalate excretion and calcium oxalate supersaturation. Kidney Int. 2010;78(11): 1178-85.
196. Goldfarb DS, Modersitzki F, Asplin JR. A randomized, controlled trial of lactic acid bacteria for idiopathic hyperoxaluria. Clin J Am Soc Nephrol. 2007;2(4):745-9.
197. Lieske JC, Goldfarb DS, De Simone C, et al. Use of a probiotic to decrease enteric hyperoxaluria. Kidney Int. 2005;68(3):1244-9.
198. Bechtold ML, McClave SA, Palmer LB, et al. The pharmacologic treatment of short bowel syndrome: new tricks and novel agents. Curr Gastroenterol Rep. 2014;16(7):392.
199. Nightingale JM, Lennard-Jones JE, Gertner DJ, et al. Colonic preservation reduces need for parenteral therapy, increases incidence of renal stones, but does not change high prevalence of gall stones in patients with a short bowel. Gut. 1992;33(11):1493-7.
200. Economou TP, Cullen JJ, Mason EE, et al. Reversal of small intestinal bypass operations and concomitant vertical banded gastroplasty: long-term outcome. J Am Coll Surg. 1995;181(2):160-4.
201. Ceulemans LJ, Nijs Y, Nuytens F, et al. Combined kidney and intestinal transplantation in patients with enteric hyperoxaluria secondary to short bowel syndrome. Am J Transplant. 2013;13(7):1910-4.
202. Daudon M, Donsimoni R, Hennequin C, et al. Sex and age related composition of 10617 calculi analyzed by infrared spectroscopy. Urol Res. 1995;23:319-26.
203. Mandel NS, Mandel GS. Urinary tract stone disease in the United States veteran population. II. Geographical analysis of variations in composition. J Urol. 1989;142(6):1516-21.
204. Soble JJ, Hamilton BD, Streem SB. Ammonium acid urate calculi: a reevaluation of risk factors. J Urol. 1999;161(3): 869-73.
205. Pichette V, Bonnardeaux A, Cardinal J, et al. Ammonium acid urate crystal formation in adult North American stone-formers. Am J Kidney Dis. 1997;30(2):237-42.
206. Bowyer RC, McCulloch RK, Brockis JG, et al. Factors affecting the solubility of ammonium acid urate. Clin Chim Acta. 1979;95(1):17-22.

207. Tannen RL. Relationship of renal ammonia production and potassium homeostasis. Kidney Int. 1977;11(6):453-65.
208. Batlle DC, von RA, Schlueter W. Urinary sodium in the evaluation of hyperchloremic metabolic acidosis. N Engl J Med. 1987;316(3):140-4.
209. Thalut K, Rizal A, Brockis JG, et al. The endemic bladder stones of Indonesia—epidemiology and clinical features. Br J Urol. 1976;48(7):617-21.
210. Andersen DA. The nutritional significance of primary bladder stones. Br J Urol. 1962;34:160-77.
211. Klohn M, Bolle JF, Reverdin NP, et al. Ammonium urate urinary stones. Urol Res. 1986;14(6):315-8.
212. Buyukgebiz B, Arslan N, Ozturk Y, et al. Complication of short bowel syndrome: an infant with short bowel syndrome developing ammonium acid urate urolithiasis. Pediatr Int. 2003;45(2):208-9.
213. Ishii G, Nakajima K, Tanaka N, et al. Clinical evaluation of urolithiasis in Crohn's disease. Int J Urol. 2009;16(5):477-80.
214. Dick WH, Smith LH, Wilson DM, et al. The clinical spectrum of ammonium urate renal calculi. In: Ryall R, Bais R, Marshall VR, et al. (Eds). Urolithiasis 2. New York: Plenum Press; 1994. pp. 567-70.
215. Dick WH, Lingeman JE, Preminger GM, et al. Laxative abuse as a cause for ammonium urate renal calculi. J Urol. 1990;143(2):244-7.
216. Wu WJ, Huang CH, Chiang CP, et al. Urolithiasis related to laxative abuse. J Formos Med Assoc. 1993;92(11):1004-6.
217. Roerig JL, Steffen KJ, Mitchell JE, et al. Laxative abuse: epidemiology, diagnosis and management. Drugs. 2010;70(12):1487-503.
218. Carlisle EJ, Donnelly SM, Halperin ML. Renal tubular acidosis (RTA): recognize the ammonium defect and pHorget the urine pH. Pediatr Nephrol. 1991;5(2):242-8.
219. Skolarikos A, Straub M, Knoll T, et al. Metabolic evaluation and recurrence prevention for urinary stone patients: EAU guidelines. Eur Urol. 2015;67(4):750-63.

CHAPTER

18

Primary Hyperoxaluria

Dawn S Milliner, Jane S Matsumoto

INTRODUCTION

Primary hyperoxaluria (PH) denotes a family of inborn errors of metabolism resulting in marked overproduction of oxalate by the liver and its excretion by the kidneys. Hyperoxaluria is present from infancy in patients with this metabolic disorder and is present lifelong, leading to one of the most severe forms of kidney stone disease. Recurring stone episodes with associated pain, need for emergency medical care, repeated lithotripsy and stone removal procedures along with other stone-related problems such as obstruction and urinary tract infection are the rule. Of importance, hyperoxaluria is also injurious to the kidney, resulting in cell damage, inflammation, and scarring. Over time, kidney function is compromised and kidney failure may ensue. When that occurs, blood levels of oxalate rise markedly due to reduction in kidney capacity for oxalate excretion, leading to calcium oxalate precipitation in multiple body tissues (oxalosis). If not aggressively managed, potentially devastating multiorgan disease and ultimately death occur due to systemic oxalosis.[1]

The disease most often presents with symptoms related to nephrolithiasis in children or adolescents. However, there is marked variability in clinical expression ranging from irreversible end-stage renal disease (ESRD) in infancy or early childhood, to recurring stone episodes in patients with good kidney function well into adulthood. Due to the rarity of PH and the broad range of clinical expression, the diagnosis is often delayed and may be missed altogether until serious and irreversible clinical consequences have ensued. It is notable that despite significant advances in diagnosis, PH is recognized only after irreversible progression to advanced chronic kidney disease (CKD), or recurrence of disease in a transplanted kidney, in up to one half of the patients in some series.[2,3] The diagnosis is most often missed among those who initially present with symptoms as adults.

The diagnosis of PH should be considered in any child or adolescent with nephrocalcinosis (NC) or calcium oxalate kidney stones and any adult with recurring calcium oxalate stones or NC, especially if there is reduction in kidney function.

PRIMARY HYPEROXALURIA TYPES

Primary hyperoxaluria is a family of genetic disorders characterized by autosomal recessive inheritance. The disease occurs worldwide, with a higher prevalence in certain regions including the Canary Islands, Tunisia, and areas of the Middle East.[4] Founder effects have been suggested in individuals of Spanish North African origin and those from the Netherlands.[5] Most mutations are found in a wide variety of ethnic groups,[5] although have greater prevalence in European Americans than in African Americans.[6]

Three types of PH have been well described, each due to deficiency of a specific hepatic enzyme in the pathways leading to oxalate production. Each results in marked overproduction of oxalate by the liver. Oxalate cannot be metabolized by humans. Under physiologic conditions, nearly all of the oxalate from hepatic production or absorbed from dietary sources is eliminated by the kidneys. It is the high concentration of oxalate in the urine that results in clinical manifestations of kidney stones, NC, and loss of kidney function. A small proportion of oxalate is eliminated by the gastrointestinal (GI) tract in the stool. In CKD, GI elimination of oxalate appears to increase by adaptation.[7] The capacity for GI secretion of oxalate is of interest with respect to potential future treatments for PH (*see* Future Directions section later in this chapter).

As kidney function declines and there is reduced capacity for oxalate elimination, blood levels increase. When the concentration of oxalate in the blood exceeds the threshold for supersaturation of calcium oxalate, crystals can form in multiple organs such as the heart, blood vessels, bone marrow, retina, and nerves[1,8] (Fig. 18.1). Systemic oxalate deposition is termed oxalosis. Consequences can be severe, including infiltrative cardiomyopathy, cardiac arrhythmias, ischemic ulcers, erythropoietin-resistant anemia, neuropathy, and pathologic fractures, and ultimately are fatal.

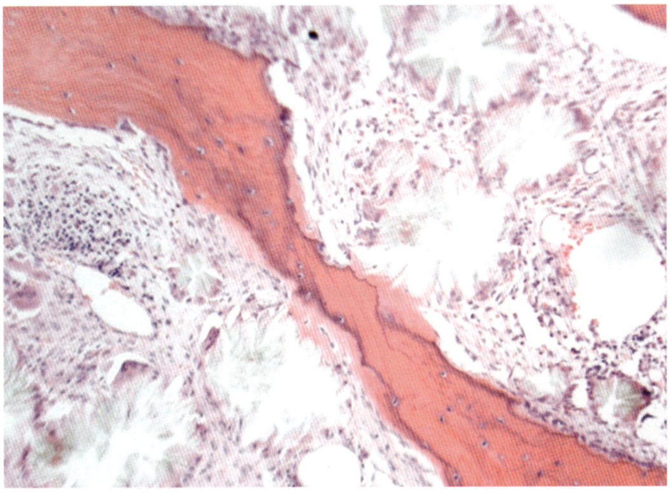

Fig. 18.1: Bone marrow biopsy in a 22-year-old patient with end-stage kidney failure and systemic oxalosis caused by primary hyperoxaluria type 1. Large calcium oxalate crystals and associated histiocytes have largely replaced normal marrow. There is marked reduction in normal hematopoietic precursors.

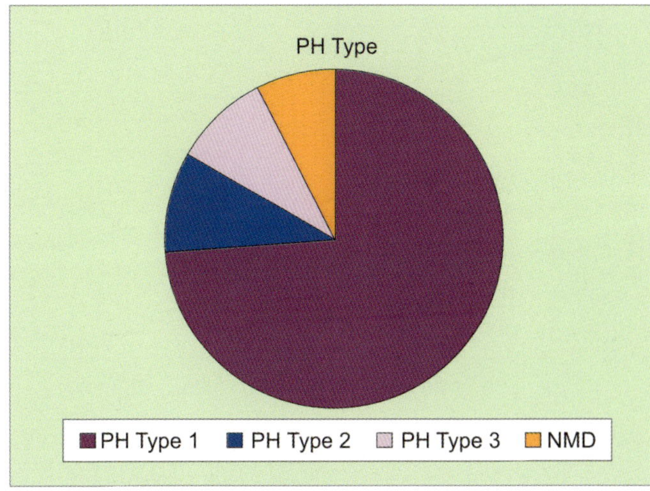

Fig. 18.2: Types of primary hyperoxaluria (PH) in 381 patients enrolled in the PH Registry of the Rare Kidney Stone Consortium. The majority have type 1 disease. No mutation detected (NMD) indicates patients who meet clinical criteria for primary hyperoxaluria, but in whom no mutations were able to be identified in *AGXT*, *GRHPR*, or *HOGA1* genes.

Type 1 PH (PH1) accounts for approximately 75–80% of cases in large registry studies from the United States and Europe (Fig. 18.2). The prevalence of PH1 has been estimated to be one to three per million population based on physician surveys in France, Switzerland, and the Netherlands.[9-11] However, recent interrogation of data from the NHBLI Exome Sequencing Project (ESP) predicted a higher prevalence of one in 152,000.[6] Underdiagnosis is also suggested by the advanced stage of CKD found in 20–75% of patients before the diagnosis is made.[2,3,12-14] Primary hyperoxaluria type 2 (PH2) accounts for 8–10% of patients enrolled in registries and has an estimated prevalence from public genome data of one in 300,000.[6] The prevalence of PH type 3 (PH3) estimated from publicly available genome sequencing data was found to be similar to that of PH1,[6] although its representation in disease registry data is much less and similar to PH2 (Fig. 18.2). Whether this discrepancy is related to underdiagnosis or incomplete penetrance is unclear.

Type 1 PH

Type 1 PH is due to mutations of the AGXT gene (PH1, OMIM 259900) that encodes for the peroxisomal enzyme alanine glyoxylate aminotransferase. The first form of PH to be described, PH1 accounts for the majority of all PH patients[13,15,16] and is the most severe form of the disease. Patients typically present with stone-related symptoms during childhood or adolescence, although there is a wide range of clinical expression. End-stage renal disease can be the first manifestation of the disease. In Europe, 11–16% of PH1 patients have been reported to present in infancy with ESRD.[2,3] Among PH1 patients in the Rare Kidney Stone Consortium (RKSC) PH Registry, 6.4% presented with kidney failure prior to 2 years of age. The diagnosis is first recognized in adulthood in approximately 25–38% of patients,[2,3,12] with some presenting in middle age or later with stones and satisfactory kidney function. Nonetheless, nearly all PH1 patients reach ESRD by the eighth decade of life (Fig. 18.3).

Alanine:glyoxylate aminotransferase (AGT) resides in the peroxisome of the hepatocyte where it detoxifies glyoxylate to form alanine and glycine. If AGT activity is reduced, glyoxylate is metabolized to oxalate. Oxalate accumulates, diffusing from the peroxisome into the hepatic cytosol and the blood stream. Although carriers of AGXT mutations may have modest reduction in AGT activity,[17] their urine oxalate excretion rates are normal. More than 190 disease-causing mutations of AGXT have been described.[18] Registry information recently available from the RKSC, OxalEurope, and a Dutch cohort confirms clinical impressions that disease outcome correlates with genotype.[3,6,19] Best established is an association of homozygosity for the G170R mutation with better long-term preservation of kidney function.[3,6,19]

The G170R mutation accounts for 24– 40% of mutant alleles[3,5,6] and is associated with mistargeting of AGT to

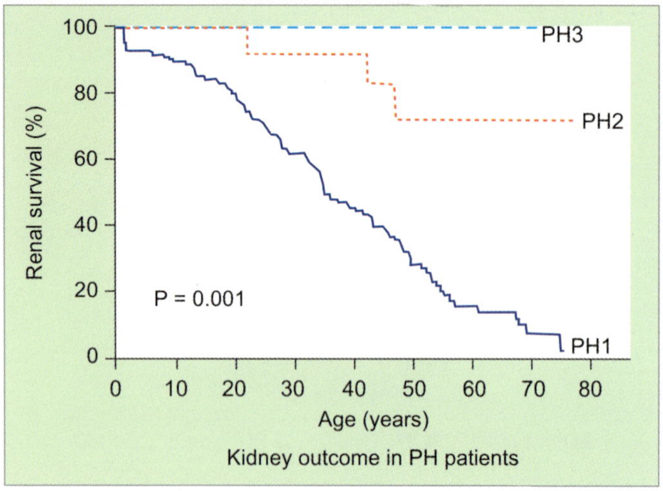

Fig. 18.3: Preservation of kidney function by age and type of primary hyperoxaluria in 301 patients from the Primary Hyperoxaluria Registry of the Rare Kidney Stone Consortium. By age 70 years, nearly all primary hyperoxaluria type 1 (PH1) patients have experienced end-stage kidney failure. Kidney outcome is more favorable in types 2 and 3 than in PH1 disease.

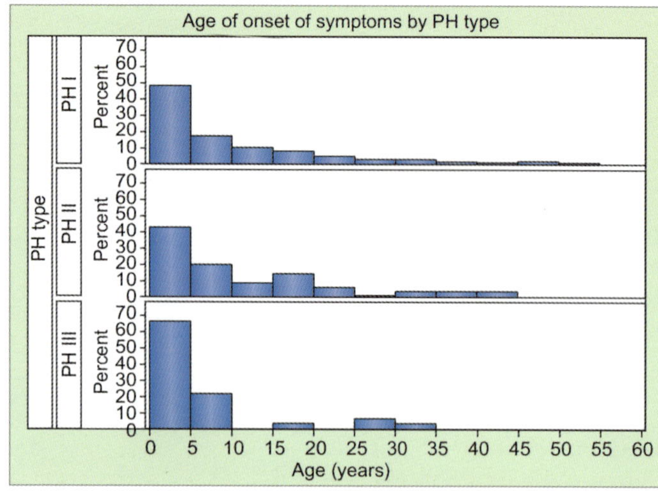

Fig. 18.4: Age at onset of symptoms by primary hyperoxaluria (PH) type. Symptom onset tends to be earlier in type 3 with a majority of patients presenting before 5 years of age. Symptoms may not be evident until well into adulthood in all types of PH.

the mitochondria, where it is ineffective for glyoxylate disposition.[20] Pyridoxine acts both as a prosthetic group that increases enzyme activity and a chemical chaperone that increases peroxisomal targeting.[21] Treatment of patients with the G170R mutation with pharmacologic doses of pyridoxine results in reduction in urine oxalate excretion, in some homozygotes to normal or near normal levels.[22,23] Three other mis-sense mutations, like G170R, alter the catalytic activity of AGT by unmasking the mitochondrial targeting sequence (F152I, I244T, G41R) and are potentially influenced by molecular chaperones.[16,24] There is evidence to suggest that PH1 patients with these mutations may also have a milder clinical course.[3,25] Type 1 PH patients with two null mutations may have worse outcomes,[3] presumably due to complete absence of functional AGT protein.

Type 2 PH

Type 2 PH (OMIM 260000) accounts for approximately 10% of patients with PH[6,15,26] and is due to mutations of the glyoxylate reductase/hydroxypyruvate reductase (GRHPR) gene encoding the enzyme GRHPR.[27] Although patients may present at any age, most often with stone-related symptoms, the overall clinical course tends to be less severe than in patients with PH1. Nephrocalcinosis is seen in a smaller proportion of patients, stone disease is less active, and kidney function is more often preserved than in PH1 (Fig. 18.3).[1,13,28]

The GRHPR enzyme is located in the cytosol and mitochondria of the hepatocyte where it catalyzes reduction of glyoxylate to glycolate.[29] Glyoxylate that accumulates due to deficiency of GRHPR is metabolized to oxalate. Accumulated hydroxypyruvate is metabolized to glycerate.[30] Increased urinary glycerate in the presence of hyperoxaluria is characteristic of PH2. Though, the liver is the primary source of oxalate production, the enzyme is widely distributed in other body tissues,[29] including kidney tubules where its expression may contribute to kidney damage in PH2.[26]

Twenty eight different mutations of the GRHPR gene have been identified to date.[18] Two mutations account for more than half the mutant alleles, with c.103delG seen primarily in Caucasians and c.430_404+2delAAGT predominantly in Asian populations.[30] Genotype phenotype correlations have not been observed, perhaps reflecting the small number of PH2 patients identified to date and marked intrafamilial heterogeneity.[6]

Type 3 PH

Mutations of the 4-hydroxy-2-glutarate aldolase (HOGA1) gene result in PH3 (OMIM 613616) and account for approximately 10% of patients (*see* Fig. 18.2).[6,13,26] This is less than would be expected based on estimates of prevalence from publicly available genome sequencing data and suggests underdiagnosis, perhaps related to a milder phenotype or lack of penetrance. Type 3 PH patients tend to have early onset, often in infancy or early childhood (Fig. 18.4), with troublesome stones with a significant requirement for urologic procedures.[6,13,31,32] Although hyperoxaluria persists, over time metabolic stone formation is more easily managed compared with PH1, and kidney function is better preserved (*see* Fig. 18.3).[31,32]

Deficiency of the mitochondrial enzyme 4-hydroxy-2-oxoglutarate (HOG) aldolase has been confirmed in PH3,[33,34] along with buildup of HOG in liver, serum, and urine in PH3 patients and a fourfold increase in oxalate in a liver sample from a patient with PH3.[34] However, the mitochondrial enzyme pathways are not fully understood, and the mechanism whereby this enzyme deficiency results in increased oxalate production is unclear. Holmes et al. have suggested inhibition of GR activity by increased HOG, resulting in a phenotype resembling PH2.[34]

Nineteen mutations of HOGA1 have been identified.[18] One (E315del) is particularly found in Ashkenazi Jews.[32,35] No genotype phenotype associations have as yet been described.

Other PH Types

There are patients who exhibit clinical features indistinguishable from PH yet do not have identifiable mutations of AGXT, GRHPR, or HOGA1.[6,31,32] These individuals have no demonstrable secondary causes of hyperoxaluria and thus likely represent as yet to be described additional types of PH.

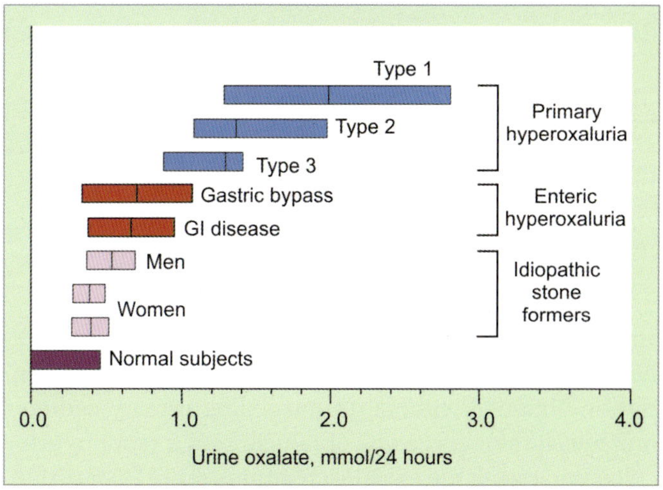

Fig. 18.5: Urine oxalate excretion rates in patients with primary hyperoxaluria types 1,2, and 3 (data from the Rare Kidney Stone Consortium PH Registry) are shown in comparison to patients with enteric hyperoxaluria related to gastrointestinal disease or gastric bypass and to urine oxalate excretion rates observed in female and male idiopathic stone formers. (GI: Gastrointestinal).
Sources: Siener R, Petzold J, Bitterlich N, et al. Determinants of urolithiasis in patients with intestinal fat malabsorption. Urology. 2013;81(1):17-24; Lieske J, Mehta R, Milliner D, et al. Kidney stones are common after bariatric surgery. Kidney Int. 2015; 87(4): 839-45.

PATHOPHYSIOLOGY

Each of these enzyme deficiencies results in marked increases in oxalate production, and the excess oxalate must be eliminated in the urine. In PH, urine oxalate excretion rates range from 0.8 to >4.0 mmol/1.73 m^2/24 hours (normal <0.5 mmol). Differences in urine oxalate excretion rates among the types of PH are seen, which may in part account for differences in clinical expression. However, there is such large overlap among types that the urine oxalate measurements cannot be relied upon to differentiate among the PH types (Fig. 18.5). By contrast, oxalate excretion associated with idiopathic stone disease is normal to mildly elevated, and generally <0.7 mmol/24 hours. The range in patients with enteric hyperoxaluria is higher, overlapping with PH, but usually not exceeding 1.5 mmol/1.73 m^2/24 hours.[36-38]

All clinical manifestations of PH, as currently understood, derive from the excess oxalate produced. High concentrations of oxalate in the urine lead to supersaturation for calcium oxalate with crystal formation and stones. Deposition of calcium oxalate in kidney tissue results in NC and damage resulting in loss of kidney function.

DIAGNOSIS

Delays in diagnosis, and thus delays in treatment, can be avoided through awareness of the disease and appropriate testing strategies. The diagnosis should be suspected in any child or adolescent presenting with stone disease, or any adult patient with multiple calcium-containing stones or recurring stone episodes. A patient of any age who has NC or an elevated serum creatinine associated with kidney stones should be evaluated for PH. A family history of calcium stone disease in a sibling or any family member with kidney failure should also heighten awareness (Table 18.1).

The algorithm shown in Figure 18.6 can be helpful to guide diagnosis. The first step is measurement of urine oxalate, ideally at a time when the patient is stable rather than during an active stone episode and when the patient is consuming his/her usual diet and fluid. There is diurnal variation in oxalate excretion,[39] such that a 24-hour timed urine collection is strongly preferred. In infants,

Table 18.1: When to suspect primary hyperoxaluria.

Calcium oxalate stones in childhood
Recurring calcium oxalate stones at any age
Nephrocalcinosis
Reduced kidney function with stones or nephrocalcinosis
Calcium oxalate tissue deposits
Family history of stones and kidney disease

young children, or other patients with urinary incontinence in whom an accurate 24-hour urine collection cannot be obtained without an indwelling urinary catheter, first measurements can be obtained from a random urine collection, using the oxalate/creatinine ratio. Hyperoxaluria should be confirmed with three separate urine collections. In patients found to have significant hyperoxaluria, placement of a catheter for a timed urine collection can be highly valuable to confirm the degree of hyperoxaluria and to guide treatment through information regarding urine volume, calcium content, as well as concentrations of citrate and magnesium that are naturally occurring inhibitors of calcium oxalate crystal formation. Full supersaturation profiles are recommended for this purpose (*see* Medical Management section of this chapter).

Urine oxalate/creatinine ratios vary continuously in childhood and to some degree until postpuberty (Fig. 18.7).[40,41] Thus, age-adjusted normal values must be used in children and adolescents (Table 18.2). Interpretation is particularly challenging in premature infants. Hyperoxaluria has been well documented related to prematurity.[42-44] Oxalate/creatinine ratios in infants who were born prematurely can reflect renal maturity rather than chronologic age and/or may reflect renal tubular damage related to NC of prematurity.[45] Similar to oxalate/creatinine ratios, timed urine oxalate measurements vary during childhood as children grow and mature and must be adjusted for meter square body surface area (BSA) in children and adolescents.[40] When adjusted for BSA, the normal range for urine oxalate excretion remains similar from early childhood through adulthood.[40]

Urine oxalate excretion rate is reduced when glomerular filtration rate (GFR) is low, although hyperoxaluria is likely to be evident in any PH patient with a GFR of >20 mL/min/1.73 m^2. In patients with very low GFR or who are oligoanuric, plasma oxalate should be measured. If the patient is on dialysis, it is important that the blood be obtained before the start of a dialysis session, as the concentration of oxalate diminishes progressively during the hours of dialysis. Patients with advanced kidney failure of any cause will have a mild-to-moderate increase in plasma oxalate concentration, due to the dependence on the kidney for elimination of this normal byproduct of body metabolism.[46] Most patients on dialysis will demonstrate plasma oxalate concentrations of 20–60 μmol/L obtained immediately before a dialysis session,[46-48] whereas in patients with PH on dialysis plasma oxalate is markedly elevated, often exceeding 60 μmol/L and may be >100 μmol/L.[48-51] Normal values and expected increases with renal failure vary by the assay used to measure plasma oxalate. Attention to method and associated reference ranges is important in interpretation.

If hyperoxaluria is confirmed on repeated testing or hyperoxalemia exceeding usual ranges for ESRD is recognized, secondary causes should be ruled out as the next step (*See* Fig. 18.6). The degree of hyperoxaluria is informative. Patients with idiopathic calcium oxalate stones may have mild increases in urine oxalate that are generally not suggestive of PH (*see* Fig. 18.5). Large intake of oxalate-containing foods is required to increase urine oxalate substantially, although absorption can be enhanced if the diet is also very low in calcium. There are reports of acute oxalate intoxication with associated kidney failure from eating large amounts of starfruit, rhubarb, and sorrel.[52-54] Toxins that are metabolized to oxalate such as ethylene glycol or xylitol have been implicated in severe hyperoxaluria and renal failure.[55,56] Patients with acute oxalate intoxication typically do not have stones on imaging studies, although it may be challenging to differentiate this clinical scenario from ESRD due to PH.

Enteric hyperabsorption of oxalate can cause moderate-to-severe hyperoxaluria (*see* Fig. 18.5). Medical and surgical causes should be considered, since any process involving the gut that leads to fat malabsorption can cause secondary hyperoxaluria. Mechanisms include complexation of calcium by fat in the lumen, thus reducing the amount of calcium available to complex with oxalate. Free oxalate is then absorbed. Fatty acids not absorbed higher in the GI tract injure colonic mucosa, leading to further increase in oxalate absorption. Inflammatory bowel disease, pancreatic insufficiency, and primary biliary cirrhosis, among other GI diseases, can result in enteric hyperoxaluria.[38] A serious and growing problem is Roux-en-Y gastric bypass or other malabsorptive procedures designed to achieve weight reduction. Patients demonstrate an increase in urine oxalate over time, following surgery, with associated stones and, in some patients, kidney failure.[36,37,57] The reader is referred to Chapter 17 for more

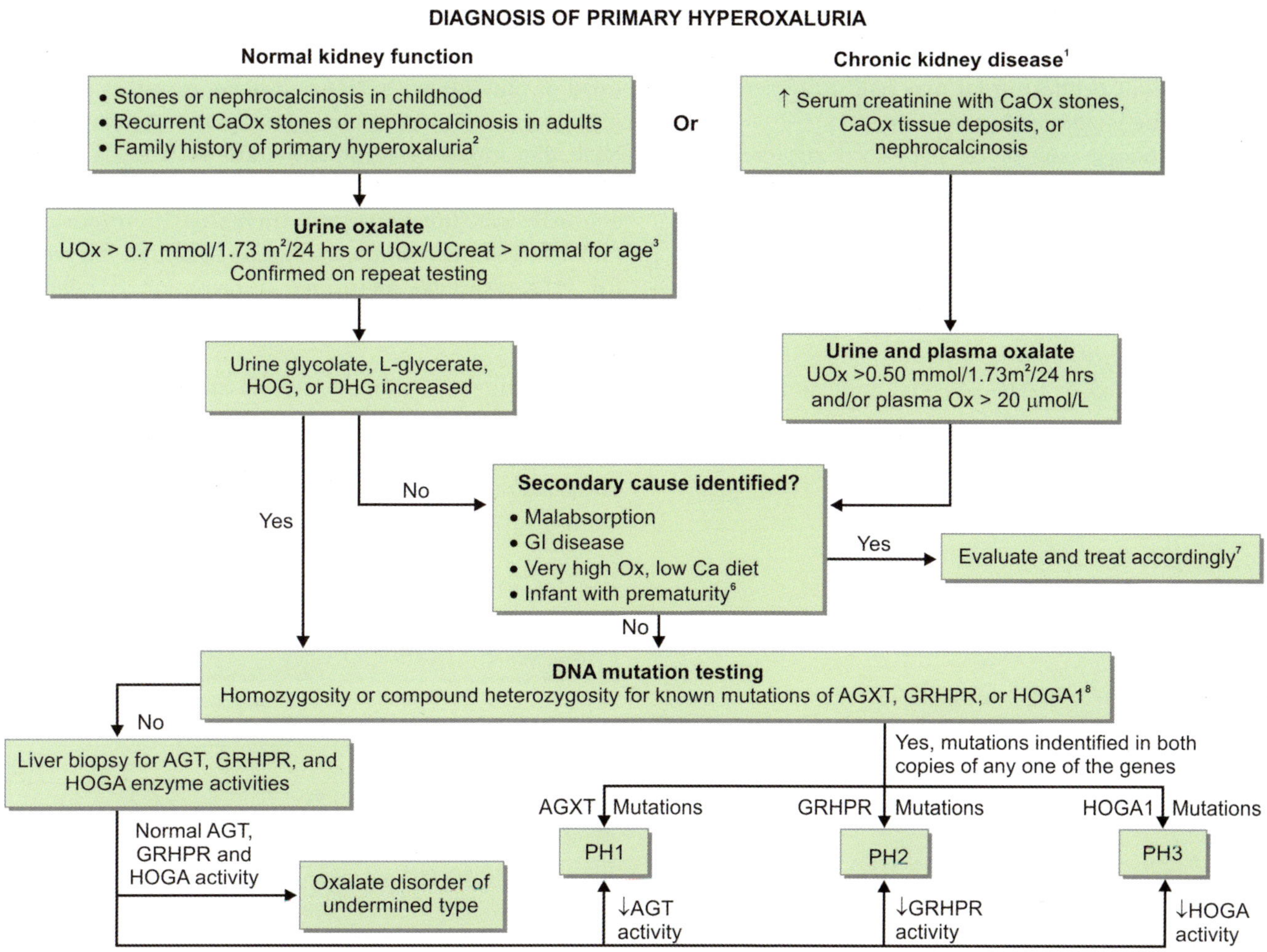

Fig. 18.6: Algorithm to guide diagnosis of primary hyperoxaluria. (Ca: Calcium; CaOx: Calcium oxalate; UOx: Urine oxalate; UCreat: Urine creatine; GI: Gastrointestinal; AGT: Alanine:glyoxylate aminotransferase; GRHPR: Glyoxylate reductase/hydroxypyruvate reductase; PH: Primary hyperoxaluria; HOGA: 4-hydroxy-2-glutarate aldolase; DNA: Deoxyribonucleic acid; DHG: Dihydroxyglutarate.

Source: Modified with permission from Edvardsson VO, Goldfarb DS, Lieske JC, Beara-Lasic L, Anglani F, Milliner DS, et al. Hereditary causes of kidney stones and chronic kidney disease. Pediatr Nephrol. 2013;28(10):1923-42.

[1]Renal insufficiency is defined as a glomerular filtration rate of <50 mL/min/1.73 m^2.

[2]The guideline does not address prenatal diagnosis.

[3]Urine and plasma oxalate and urine glycolate measurements for diagnostic testing should be obtained while the patient is receiving no pyridoxine or vitamin supplements.

[4]Increased urine glycolate in the presence of hyperoxaluria is suggestive, but not conclusive, of primary hyperoxaluria (PH) type 1. Increased urine L-glycerate in a hyperoxaluric patient suggests PH type 2. Increased HOG or DHG suggest PH type 3.

[5]Urine oxalate/creatinine ratios in healthy children vary continuously by age. Normal values tables should be consulted in interpretation of any random urine oxalate to creatinine ratio. To convert mg/mg to mmol/mmol, multiply by 1.28.

[6]Urine oxalate/creatinine ratios are higher in very premature infants than in term infants, especially when they are receiving parenteral nutrition containing amino acids.

[7]When very high oxalate or low dietary calcium is suspected as the cause of the hyperoxaluria, the diet should be corrected and the urine oxalate remeasured for verification.

[8]In some cases with firm clinical diagnosis, only one mutation is found even after analysis for large rearrangements, suggesting that regulatory or deep intronic mutations may be the second, undetected mutation. In such cases, the finding of a single disease-associated mutation in the context of a clear phenotype overall supports the clinical diagnosis of PH.

detailed information regarding enteric causes, diagnosis, and management. Medications such as orlistat that interfere with GI absorption of fat may lead to hyperoxaluria and should be systemically eliminated.[58]

If secondary causes of hyperoxaluria cannot be implicated, screening of urine for glycolate, glycerate, HOG and/or DHG is helpful to focus further testing (Table 18.3). Deoxyribonucleic acid (DNA) screening for mutations of the AGXT, GRHPR, or HOGA1 genes will provide a definitive diagnosis. Increased glycolate should prompt definitive testing for PH1, increased glycerate suggests PH2, and elevation of HOG or DHG provides indication to screen for mutations of the HOGA1 gene that cause PH3. It is important to recognize that only approximately one third of patients with PH1 will have increases in urinary glycolate. In our experience, nearly all patients with PH2 have elevations of urine glycerate as well as oxalate,[59] although one patient has been reported in whom glyceric aciduria was not present.[60] Increases in urinary HOG and DHG show promise as highly sensitive and specific for PH3, although additional information is needed to better assess their potential to obviate the need for DNA testing.[34,61]

Genetic testing for mutations of AGXT, GRHPR, and HOGA1 is highly sensitive and specific. Since, there is the potential for some mutations to escape recognition, if clinical suspicion is high, liver biopsy for enzyme analysis should be performed for measurement of AGT, GRHPR, and

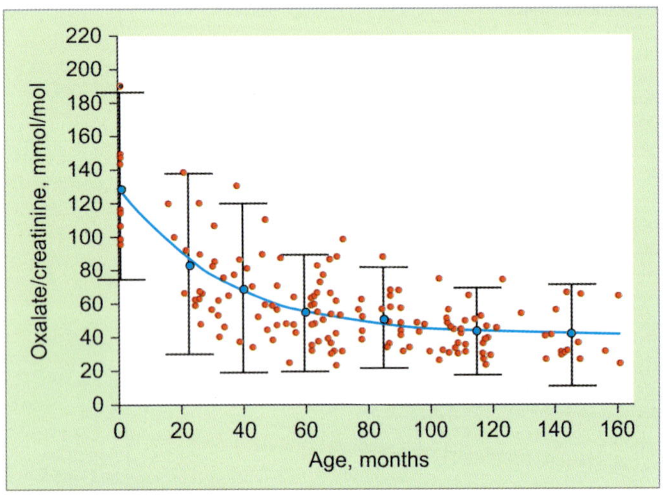

Fig. 18.7: Relationship between urinary oxalate/creatinine ratio and age in 169 healthy infants and children to 13 years of age. Regression line and bars representing means ± 2 SD are shown. Normal ranges for oxalate/creatinine vary continuously through early childhood.
Source: Reprinted with permission from von Schnakenburg C, Byrd DJ, Latta K, et al. Determination of oxalate excretion in spot urines of healthy children by ion chromatography. Eur J Clin Chem Clinic Biochem. 1994;32:27-9.

Table 18.2: Normal values for random urine oxalate-to-creatinine (Ox/Cr) ratio by age.

	Ox/Cr ratio Upper limit of normal	
Age	*(mmol/mmol)*	*(mg/mg)*
<6 months	0.37	0.29
6 months to 2 years	0.26	0.20
>2 years to 5 years	0.14	0.11
6–12 years	0.08	0.063

Sources: Gibbs DA, Watts RWE. The variation of urinary oxalate excretion with age. J Lab Clin Med. 1969;73:901-8; von Schnakenburg C, Byrd DJ, Latta K, et al. Determination of oxalate excretion in spot urines of healthy children by ion chromatography. Eur J Clin Chem Clinic Biochem. 1994;32:27-9; Morgenstern BZ, Milliner DS, Murphy ME, et al. Urinary oxalate and glycolate excretion patterns in the first year of life: a longitudinal study. J Pediatr. 1993;123:248-51; Campfield T, Braden G. Urinary oxalate excretion by very low birth weight infants receiving parenteral nutrition. Pediatrics. 1989;84:860-3.

Table 18.3: Urine organic acids in the diagnosis of primary hyperoxaluria.

		Urine Organic Acids				
PH type	*Gene*	*Oxalate*	*Glycolate*	*Glycerate*	*HOG or DHG*	*Stone composition*
Type 1	*AGXT*	↑	↑*	–	–	COM
Type 2	*GRHPR*	↑	–	↑	–	COM
Type 3	*HOGA1*	↑	–†	–†	↑	COM and COD

*Urine glycolate is increased in approximately 30% of PH1 patients.
†Slight increase in urine glycolate or glycerate may be observed in PH3.
(PH: Primary hyperoxaluria; HOG: 4-hydroxy-2-oxoglutarate; COM: Calcium oxalate monohydrate; GRHPR: Glyoxylate reductase/hydroxypyruvate reductase; HOGA: Hydroxy-2-oxoglutarate aldolase; COD: Calcium oxalate dihydrate; DHG: Dihydroxyglutarate).

HOGA. Over time, an ever-declining proportion of patients has required liver biopsy, which in our own experience is now only occasionally needed. Approximately 8% of patients who demonstrate all the clinical features of PH will have no identifiable mutations of AGXT, GRHPR, or HOGA1. It is very likely that additional types of PH will be identified over time.

All three currently known types of PH are characterized by metabolic overproduction of oxalate that is present from infancy, yet there are differences in disease expression by PH type. Although, differences in outcome are well described, their relationship to the genetics and pathophysiology is not fully understood.

All types of PH present most often in childhood, adolescence, or young adulthood with stone-related symptoms. However, there is wide variability in age at presentation, ranging from infancy to late adult life. Type 3 disease, in particular, is characterized by symptomatic stones before the age of 4 years,[31,33] even though the degree of hyperoxaluria is somewhat less than PH2 or PH1 (*see* Fig. 18.5). Other clinical features are equally variable. Nephrocalcinosis may be present, and kidney function may be normal or reduced. It is notable that a small minority of patients, typically with PH1, initially present with failure to thrive in infancy or early childhood or with symptoms of advanced CKD and are found to have irreversible loss of function requiring renal replacement therapy. Such patients are often found to have dense NC, in the absence of discrete stones.[62] Symptom onset by age and by type of PH is shown in Figure 18.4. Despite the early onset of symptomatic stone disease in most patients, the diagnosis is often delayed for years after the onset of symptoms.[1] Analysis of 322 patients in the RKSC PH Registry shows a mean (median) time from onset of symptoms to diagnosis of 7.88 (1.96) years, with the upper quartile >11 years. Since definitive diagnosis is now readily available, a lack of awareness of this disease and its manifestations appears to account for the delay.

STONES

Clinical Features

Stones are a recurring and lifelong problem for patients with PH, with stone passage or the need for a stone-removal procedure on average every few years.[13] On initial evaluation, patients with PH often have multiple stones present. Since, the stones are, for the most part, 100% calcium oxalate, it is the number of stones and their frequent association with NC that suggests PH. In patients with PH whose disease is clinically stable, renal imaging and measurement of kidney function at least annually is recommended for monitoring and management of metabolic stone-forming activity, early awareness of stones at high likelihood of causing obstruction, and to rule out subclinical hydronephrosis related to a partially obstructing stone. New symptoms should be evaluated promptly. Ultrasound imaging is sufficient for most monitoring, with computerized tomography (CT) or other modalities reserved for concerns regarding obstruction or the need for greater resolution of anatomy that cannot be met with ultrasound alone. This approach avoids repeated radiation exposure. Attention to imaging modality and frequency is of particular importance due to the young age of many of the patients and the repeated imaging studies that will be required over many decades for stone monitoring and intervention.

A number of imaging modalities can be used to identify and characterize renal stones and NC. These include plain film radiography, ultrasound, and CT. Plain film radiography is useful in detecting renal stones of significant size but there are a number of factors that limit its usefulness, including overlying bony structures, size of the patient, and variable film technique. Ultrasound, although sensitive at detecting renal stone disease in optimal conditions, is also affected by patient size, overlying bowel gas, and renal sinus fat. Computerized tomography is more sensitive than plain film or ultrasound in detecting stones, especially small ones, and accurately identifying their location in the kidney and collecting system. Computerized tomography is not usually affected by patient size or overlying structures but is affected by motion and technique. As concern has heightened over long-term exposure effects from ionizing radiation of CT, a renewed interest in the use of ultrasound has developed.

There are a number of features of renal stone disease due to PH that may suggest the diagnosis. Rather than a solitary stone, patients may present with a number of clustered stones that are relatively large in size (Fig. 18.8). Focal parenchymal scarring may be present initially or develop over time and would suggest a chronic stone disease process (Fig. 18.9). Nephrocalcinosis with or without focal renal stones is consistent with significant underlying renal stone disease (Fig. 18.10).[13] At late stages of the disease, there is diffuse calcification of the kidneys (Figs. 18.11A and B). Presentation at a relatively young age with significant stone burden is another indication that hyperoxaluria should be a consideration (Figs. 18.12A to C).

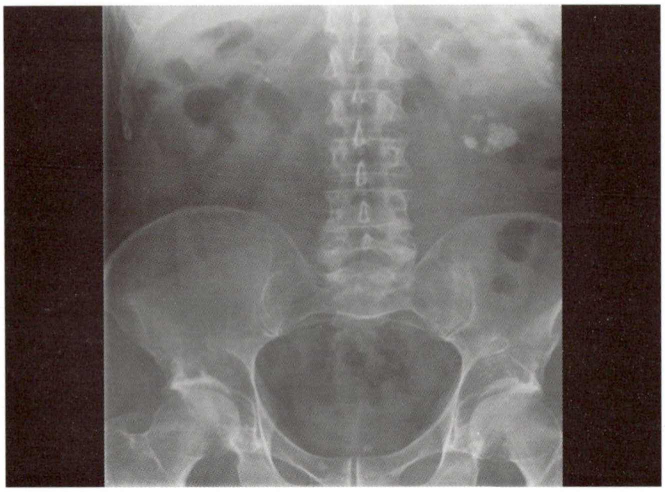

Fig. 18.8: Plain film demonstrates clusters of large stones in the left kidney, most prominently in the lower pole.

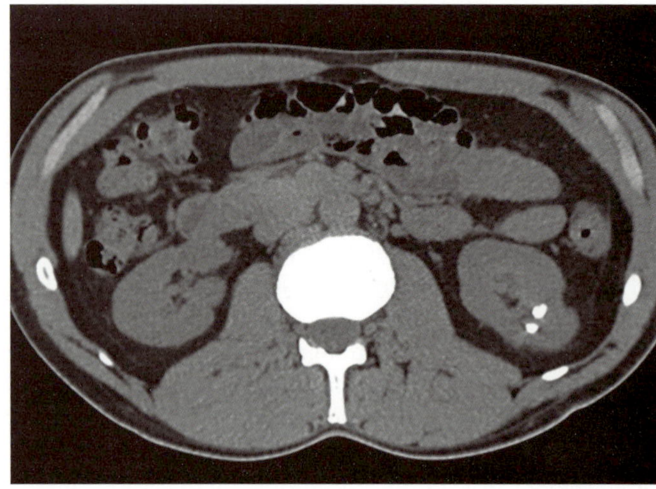

Fig. 18.9: Noncontrast computed tomography demonstrates two small stones in the lower pole of the left kidney with adjacent parenchymal focal scarring.

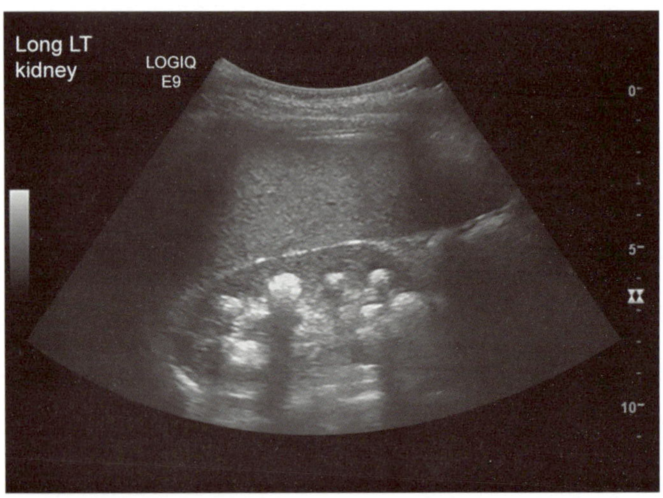

Fig. 18.10: There is focal increased echogenicity throughout the medullary pyramids consistent with nephrocalcinosis. Some of these areas have posterior acoustical shadowing consistent with dense mineralization and stone formation.

Imaging of Stones

Ultrasound

Ultrasound is an excellent imaging modality for following renal stone disease. The high acoustic density of mineralized stones results in an increased interface with the ultrasound beam and typically appears as sharp echogenic foci with posterior acoustical shadowing (Fig. 18.13). Such echogenic foci stand out compared to the adjacent relatively isoechoic renal parenchyma. Air within the collecting system can also appear as sharp echogenic foci and may demonstrate poorly defined posterior shadowing without sharp borders (Figs. 18.14A and B). If a renal stone is tiny in size and smaller than the ultrasound beam width, detection on gray-scale ultrasound and demonstration of shadowing will be difficult. Color Doppler imaging of the stones may be helpful as it can create a "twinkling" artifact that can differentiate stones from adjacent echogenic soft tissue such as fat in the renal hila (Figs. 18.15A and B). In the "twinkling" artifact, the color ultrasound beam is scattered by the highly reflective mineralized stone material, resulting in an artifact known as clock (or phase) jitter within the Doppler circuitry of the ultrasound machine.[63,64] Urate and calcium oxalate monohydrate stones may not show the twinkle artifact, likely due to the relatively smooth surface of the stone.

With ultrasound it may be difficult to discretely identify the exact number of stones if there are multiple renal stones clustered in a conglomeration (Figs. 18.16A and B). It may also be difficult to differentiate discrete stones due to adjacent dense shadowing of NC (Fig. 18.17). The size of the patient may limit ultrasound resolution of the kidneys. The greater the amount of soft tissue the ultrasound beam needs to penetrate before reaching the kidneys, the lower the image resolution. Bowel gas that obscures underlying soft tissue can also interfere with ultrasound imaging. Ultrasound is ideally suited for use in children because their

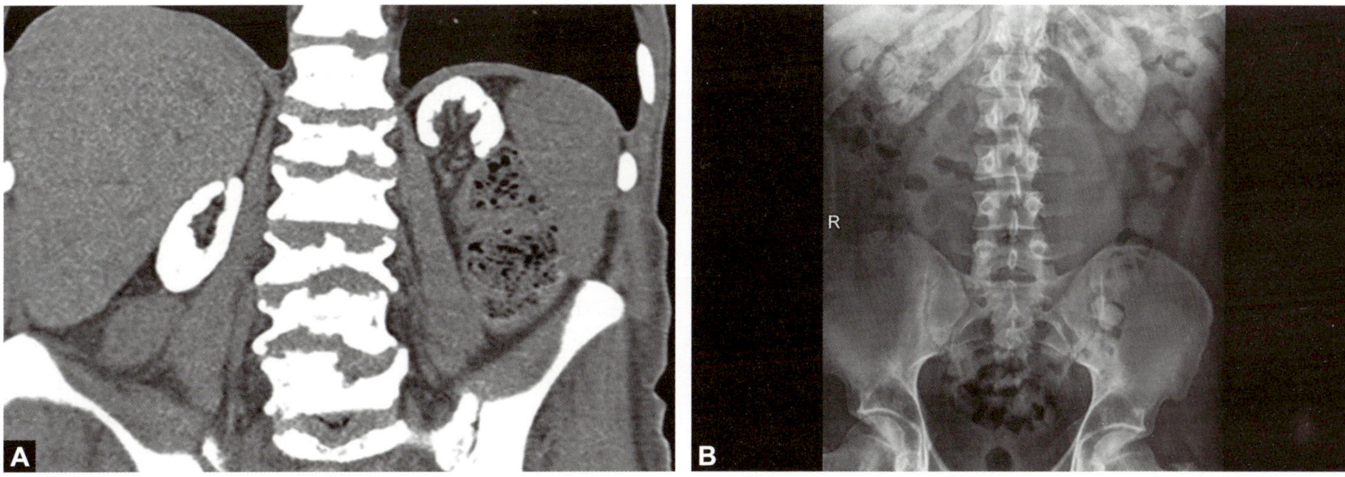

Figs. 18.11A and B: (A) Noncontrast computed tomography and (B) KUB plain film demonstrate diffuse renal calcification of end-stage hyperoxaluria.

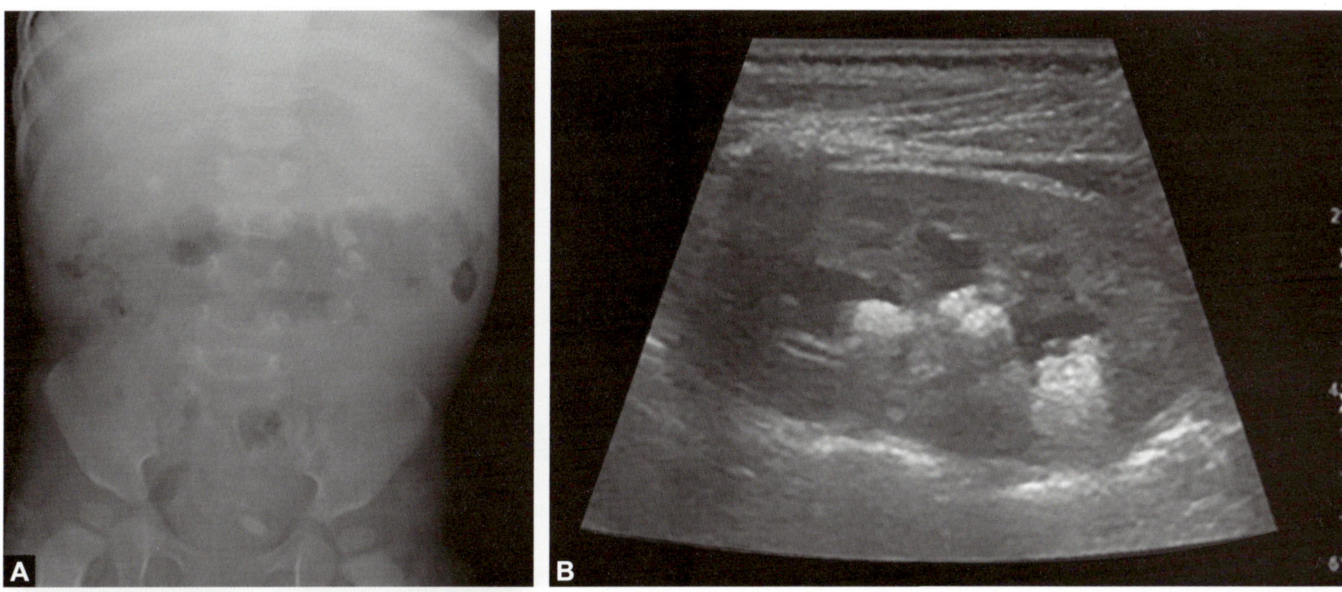

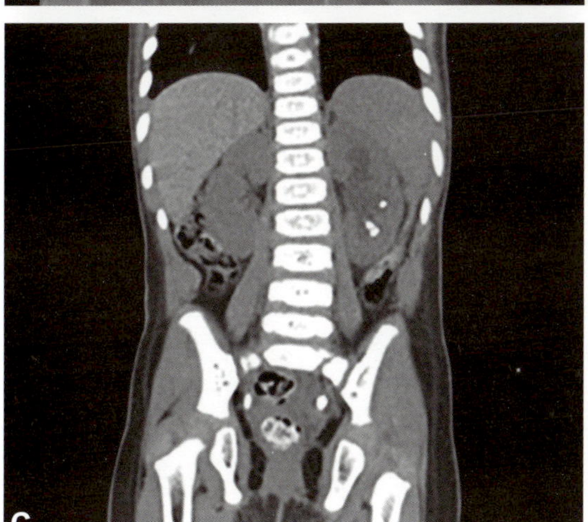

Figs. 18.12A to C: Young child presenting with obstructive hydronephrosis and significant renal stone burden. (A) KUB plain radiograph demonstrates bilateral renal stones and a large bladder stone. (B) Ultrasound demonstrating calyceal stones. The stones appear as multiple focal areas of increased echogenicity within mildly dilated calyces. (C) Noncontrast computed tomography shows stones within dilated left renal calyces as well as bilateral distal ureterovesical junction stones.

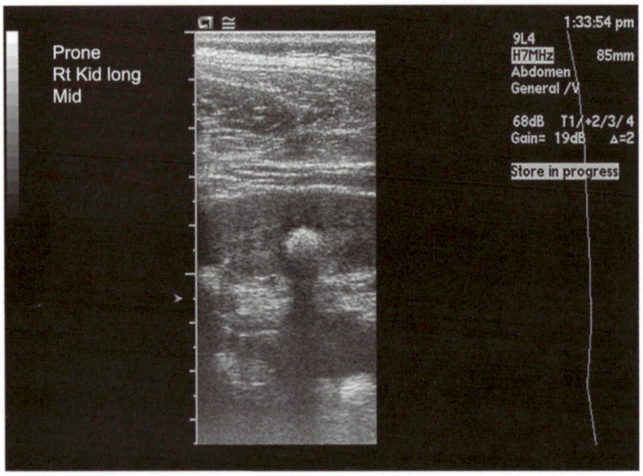

Fig. 18.13: Ultrasound image acquired in prone position demonstrates a stone with focally increased echogenicity with sharp posterior acoustically shadowing.

smaller size allows use of higher-frequency transducers, which create more detailed parenchymal resolution (Figs. 18.18A and B). Ultrasound offers other significant advantages for the imaging of children. It is a fairly sensitive imaging study with no radiation, can be done portably, and there is rarely a need for sedation.

In emergency clinical situations ultrasound is similar in sensitivity to CT as an initial imaging study for detection of obstructive hydronephrosis from renal stone disease (Figs. 18.19A and B).[65] Ultrasound is able to detect ureteral calculi, especially in the distal ureters where a full bladder can serve as an excellent acoustical window (Figs. 18.20A and B). Identification of ureteral jets is helpful for excluding the presence of ureteral obstruction. A ureteral jet will be absent in the presence of high-grade obstruction;

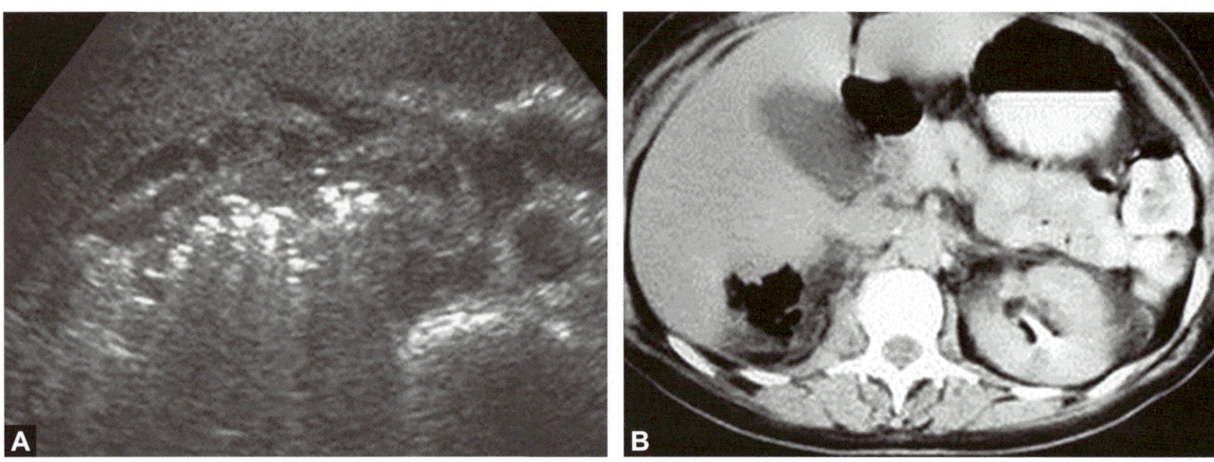

Figs. 18.14A and B: Ultrasound demonstrates echogenic material with posterior shadowing in the collecting system of the right kidney. Concurrent computed tomography shows that this represents air within the collecting system.

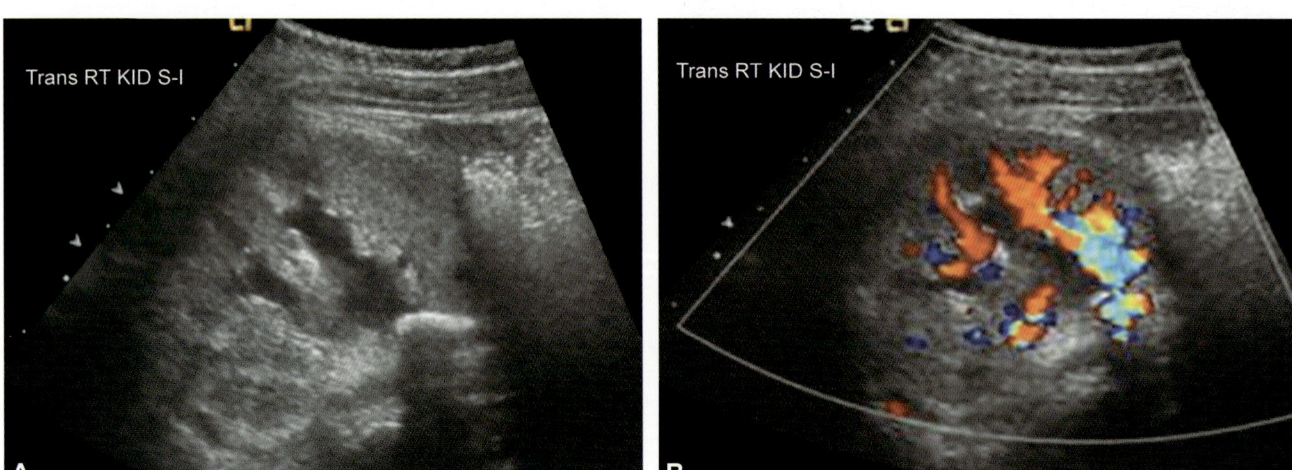

Figs. 18.15A and B: (A) Ultrasound demonstrates a focal stone with shadowing at the ureteropelvic junction resulting in hydronephrosis. (B) Color Doppler demonstrates the "twinkling artifact" with a spectrum of colors in comparison with the single color of adjacent vessels.

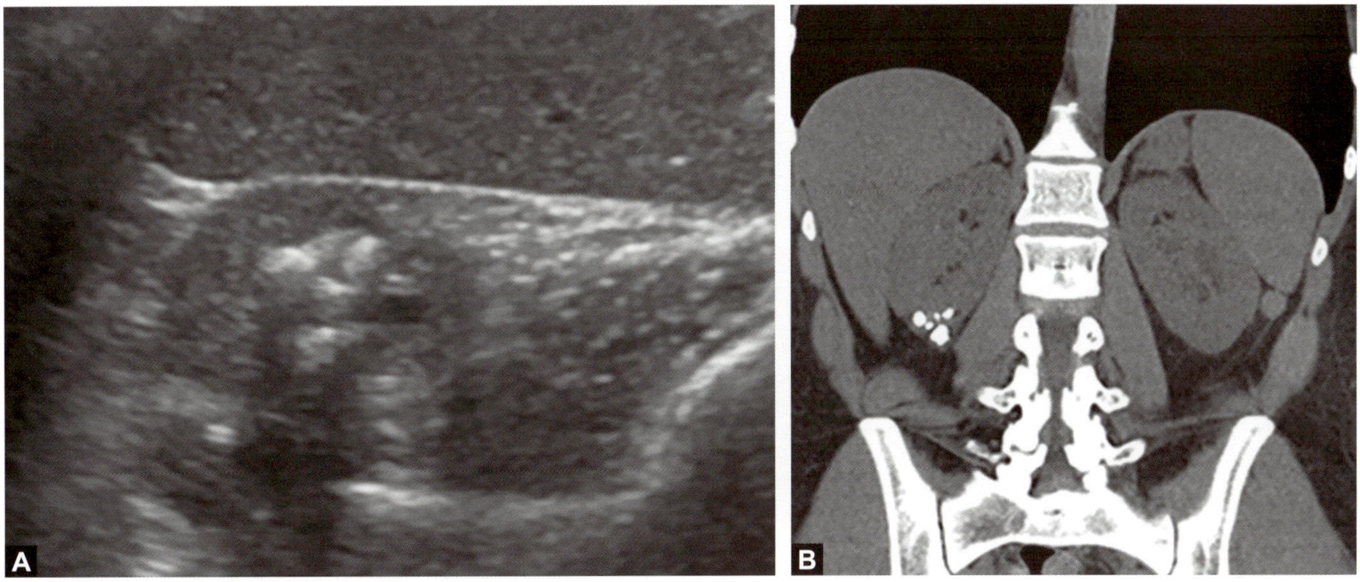

Figs. 18.16A and B: (A) Ultrasound of the lower pole of the right kidney demonstrates a cluster of echogenic stones with shadowing. It is difficult to discretely identify how many stones are present. (B) The number and size of the individual stones are more easily identified on noncontrast computed tomography.

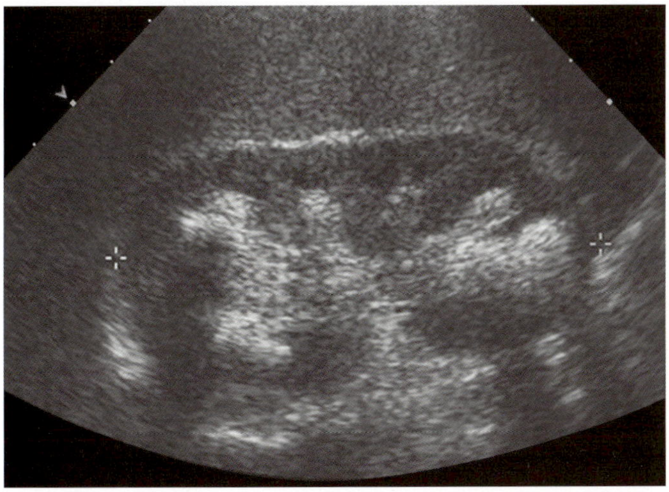

Fig. 18.17: Ultrasound demonstrates nephrocalcinosis with varying amounts of increased echogenicity within the medullary pyramids. There is some focal shadowing, but it is difficult to discretely identify the margins of stones.

however, it will be abnormal in only about one-third of patients with low-grade obstruction (Figs. 18.21A and B).

Ultrasound is very operator-dependent, which is an important factor in being able to accurately compare examinations over time and reliably follow stone burden. When performed in a systematic and thorough manner with optimal technique using standardized protocols by an experienced technologist, ultrasound is a reliable and reproducible diagnostic imaging modality to follow renal stone disease and NC. Ultrasound and CT can also be alternated in a complementary fashion with CT when clinically needed, serving to focus and direct the more frequent ultrasound evaluation. This approach is especially relevant in children with long-term stone disease and lessens the overall cumulative radiation exposure that would have been acquired using only serial CTs for following renal stone burden. Given the lack of radiation and the need for long-term imaging follow-up in children, consideration should be given to using ultrasound as the primary choice for sequential imaging for renal stones disease with CT performed when clinical questions arise that ultrasound is not able to definitively answer.

Computerized Tomography

Noncontrast CT is a more sensitive imaging modality than ultrasound for detecting renal stones.[66] Stones are composed of higher-density material than adjacent soft tissue and can be discretely localized within the kidney parenchyma, calyceal tip, and renal collecting system. The location, size, number of the stones, and overall stone burden can all be well characterized on CT (Figs. 18.22A to D). The stone burden can be quantified for each kidney, which is useful in following progression of stone disease over time (Figs. 18.23A and B).[67] Renal parenchymal thinning, focal

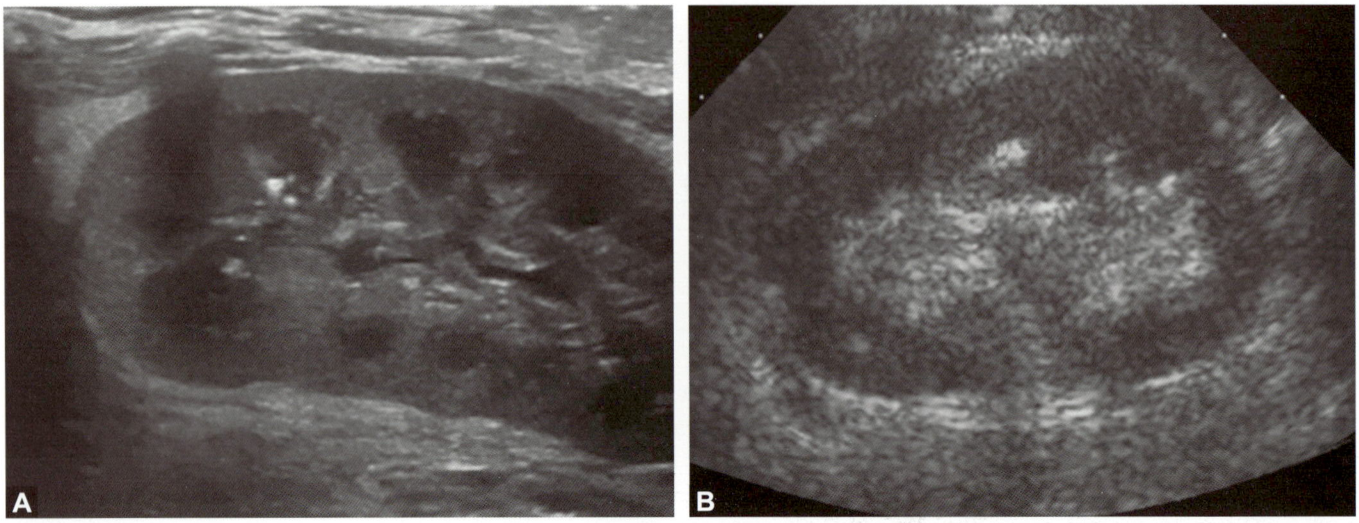

Figs. 18.18A and B: (A) Renal ultrasound of a child using a higher-frequency linear transducer demonstrates high-resolution parenchymal images. (B) Lower-frequency ultrasound transducers are generally needed to obtain images in larger, adult-size patients.

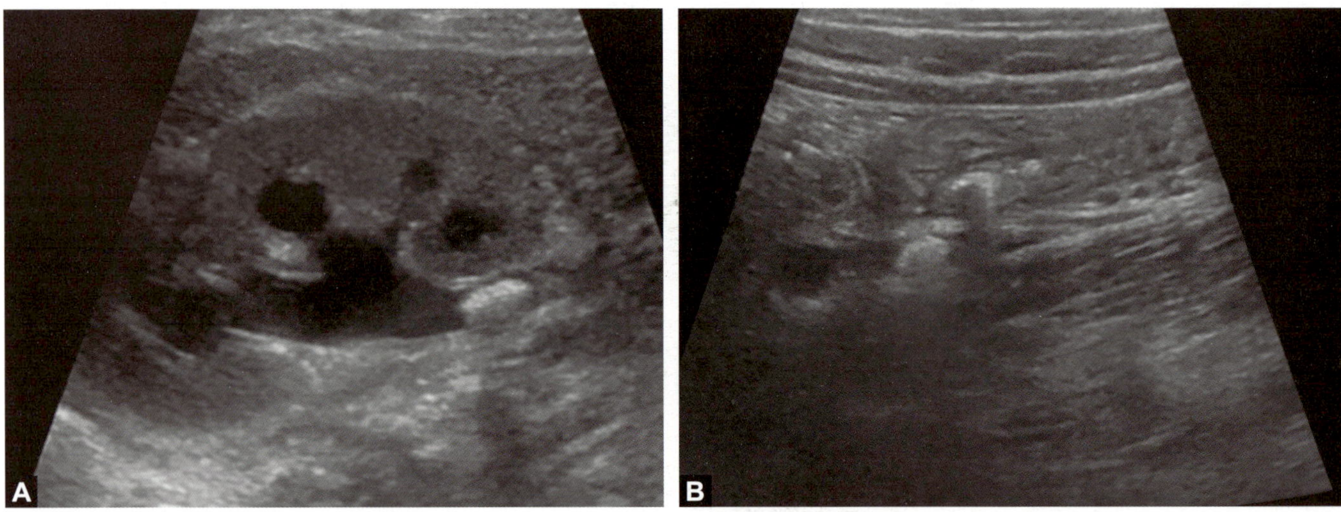

Figs. 18.19A and B: (A) Ultrasound demonstrates an obstructive stone at the ureteropelvic junction with resulting pelvocaliectasis. (B) Ultrasound demonstrates an obstructive stone in a thick-walled, mildly dilated proximal ureter.

scarring, and hydronephrosis are well demonstrated on CT (Figs. 18.24A to D). Although, ultrasound is more sensitive for early NC, the medullary calcification of NC can be identified on CT when the mineralization becomes dense (Figs. 18.25A to C).

Computerized tomography offers a global assessment of the abdomen and pelvis, which is helpful in complicated or subtle obstructive stone-related hydronephrosis. Perinephric fluid collections are well characterized on CT. The presence of fluid collections and the exact number, size, and location of stones can be evaluated. Computerized tomography can detect perinephric and periureteral inflammation and thickening of the urothelial walls (Fig. 18.26), which are helpful secondary radiographic findings of obstructive stone disease when the stones are very small or have passed and are no longer able to be visualized. These findings can help differentiate a small phlebolith in the deep pelvis from an obstructive ureteral stone when the ureter is not dilated. Computerized tomography offers additional diagnostic information in nonrenal causes of abdominal pain such as appendicitis, diverticulitis, bowel obstruction, or abscess formation.

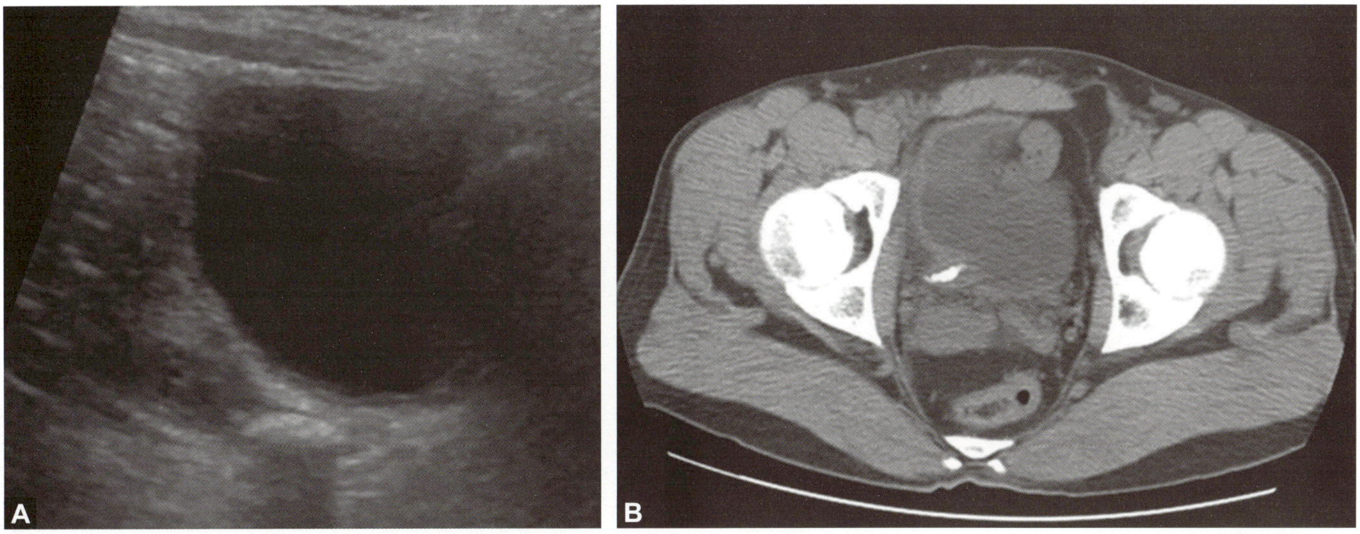

Figs. 18.20A and B: (A) Obstructing stone in the distal right ureter ureterovesical junction (UVJ) on ultrasound. (B) Noncontrast computed tomography demonstrating the same distal UVJ stone.

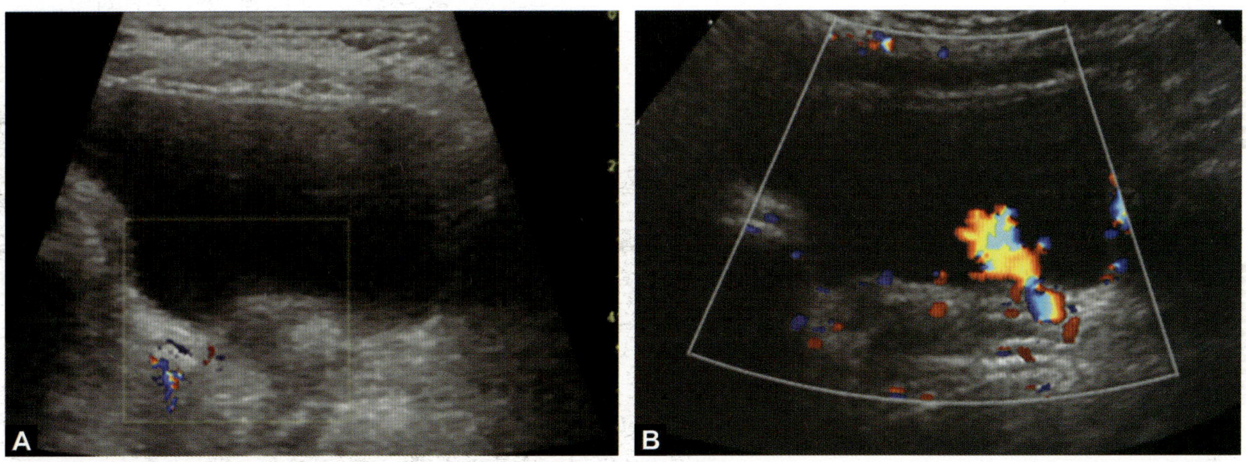

Figs. 18.21A and B: (A) Doppler evaluation demonstrates a diminished ureteral jet at the right ureterovesical junction (UVJ) consistent with diminished flow from obstruction. (B) Normal ureteral jet at the left UVJ.

Radiation Exposure Considerations

Following renal stones disease with interval CT raises concern about the accumulation of radiation exposure over the long term.[68-71] Renal stone CT protocols with reduced radiation exposure have been able to be developed because the high-density stones are able to be detected with noisier lower-dose images. These protocols have reduced radiation exposure substantially with sensitivity similar to higher-dose studies.[72-74]

Multiple variables are used to set up the parameters to optimize a CT study with the lowest radiation exposure with diagnostic accuracy for each individual patient. Computerized tomography technologies and software have been developed with the goal of decreasing radiation dose as attention has increased on the potential long-term health effects of medical radiation exposure. These technologies include automated tube current modulation or exposure control and iterative reconstruction (IR). In automated exposure, control of the radiation dose is varied according to size of the individual patient and density of body part being scanned. The X-ray exposure is automatically adjusted as the body is scanned so that the tube current is higher in the denser parts like the bony pelvis and lower in the less dense parts like the lungs. This type of exposure modulation is available on most currently manufactured CT equipment (Fig. 18.27).

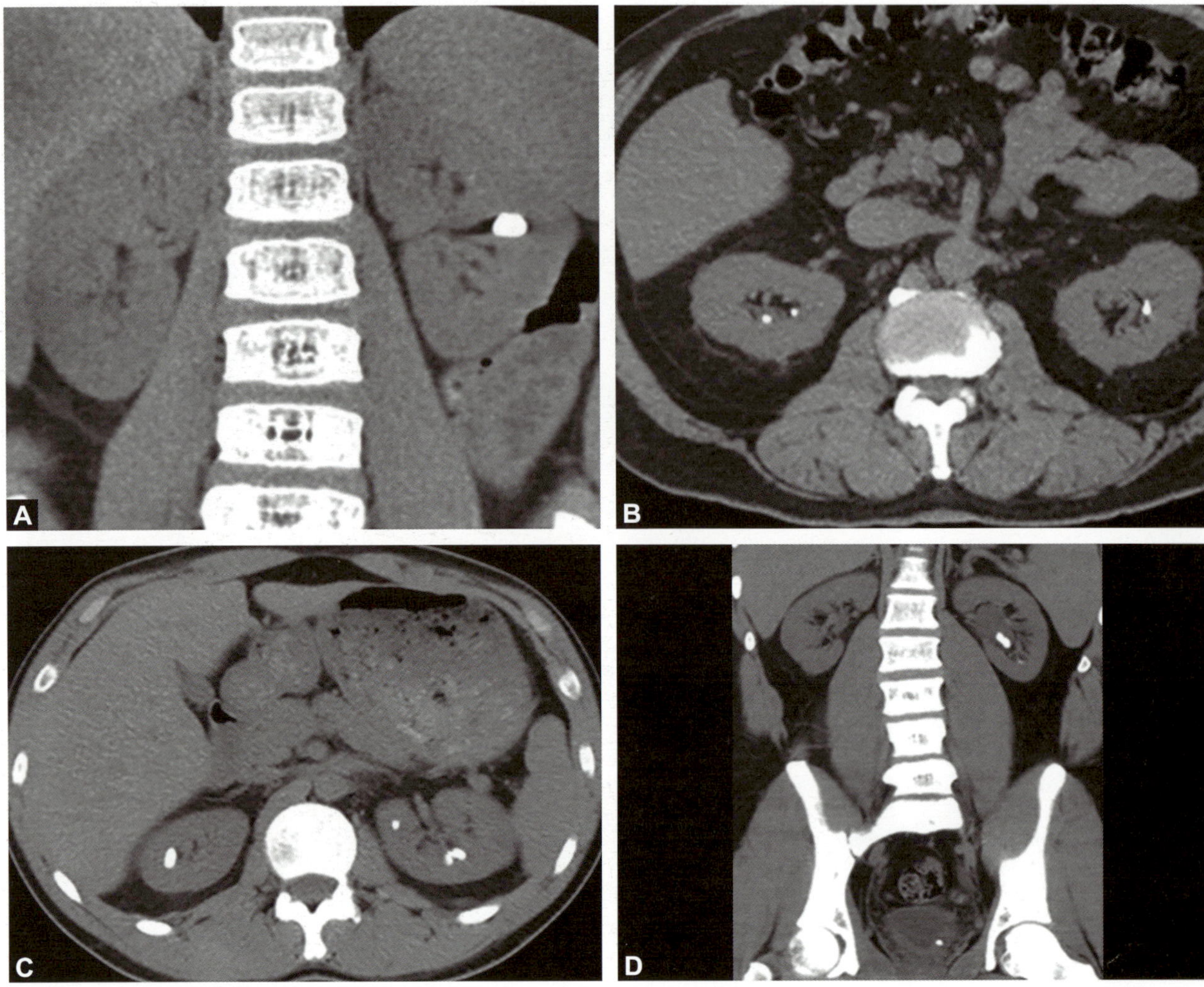

Figs. 18.22A to D: Noncontrast computed tomography demonstrates (A) a single large left intraparenchymal renal stone, (B) multiple medullary tip stones (C) larger clustered stones, (D) and stones in the renal collecting system of the left renal pelvis and distal left ureter at the ureterovesical junction.

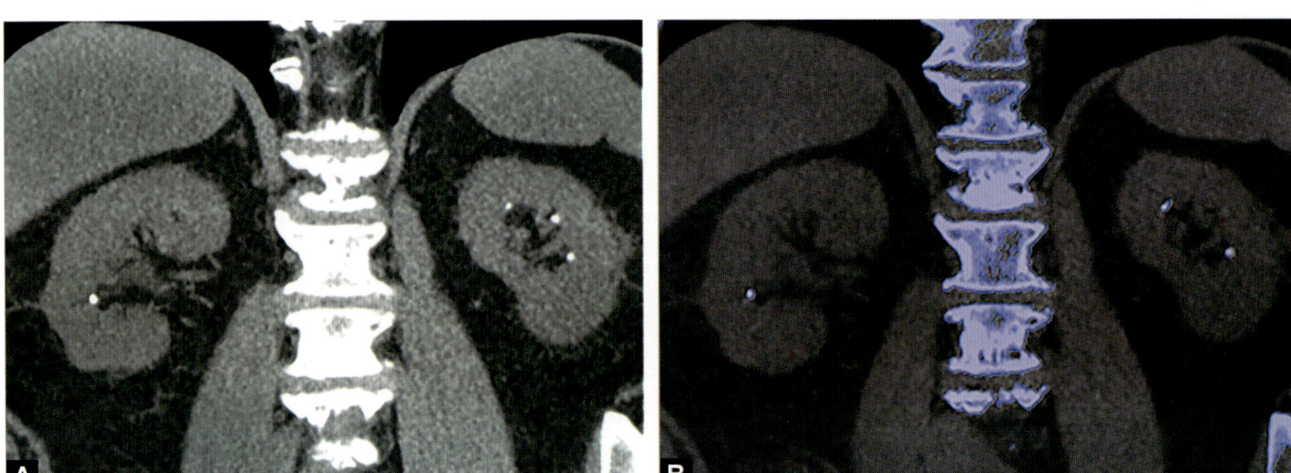

Figs. 18.23A and B: (A) Noncontrast computed tomography (CT) demonstrates multiple small bilateral medullary tip stones. (B) The total stone volume is quantified for each kidney using automated CT.

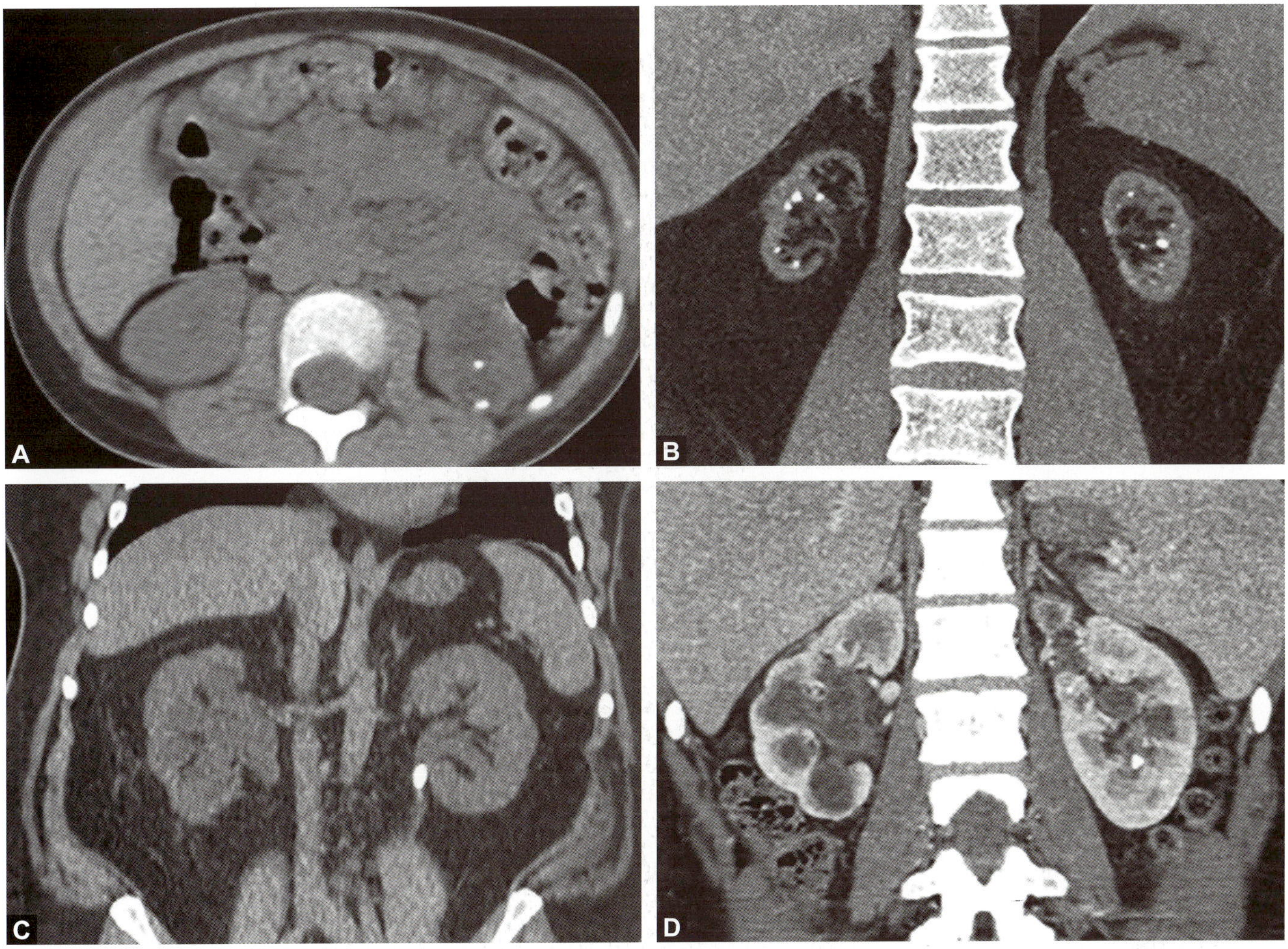

Figs. 18.24A to D: Noncontrast computerized tomography (CT) demonstrates (A) Focal scarring associated with stones in the lower pole of the left kidney, (B) Multiple medullary tip stones and diffuse bilateral renal parenchymal thinning, (C) An obstructing stone in the left ureteropelvic junction stone. (D) Contrast-enhanced CT demonstrates variable scarring of both kidneys, dilatation of the collecting systems and stones.

Iterative reconstruction is an image-reconstruction algorithm recently introduced onto commercial CT scanners. Compared to standard filtered back-projection algorithm, IR can incorporate physical models into the reconstruction to potentially improve spatial resolution and reduce image artifact.[75,76] More importantly, IR can incorporate photon statistics to substantially reduce image noise, consequently allowing lower radiation doses with the goal of diagnostic imaging at the lowest achievable radiation exposure.

Adjusting scan parameters such as increasing pitch, decreasing gantry rotation time, and lowering tube voltage all result in lower radiation dose, although noisier images.[77] The minimal radiation dose that provides sufficient clinical diagnosis varies not only based on the size of the patient but also on the type of clinical information being sought. Low-radiation-exposure CT protocols have been developed for specific clinical indications, including abdominal CT for renal stone disease, chest CT for pulmonary nodules, and head CT for ventricular dilatation.[78]

Long-term effects of low-level cumulative medical radiation exposure are difficult to ascertain due to the many complex variables and the significant length of time needed to measure effect. These variables include changing levels of radiation exposure from specific medical imaging studies, the number of examinations performed on an individual, and the age of the patient. There is also daily background radiation exposure from the natural environment. Terminology on radiation measurements is complex. Ionizing radiation deposits energy into tissue,

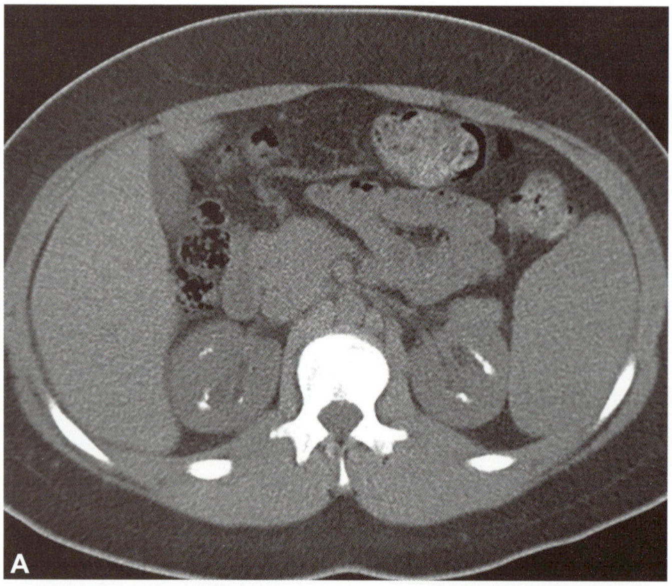

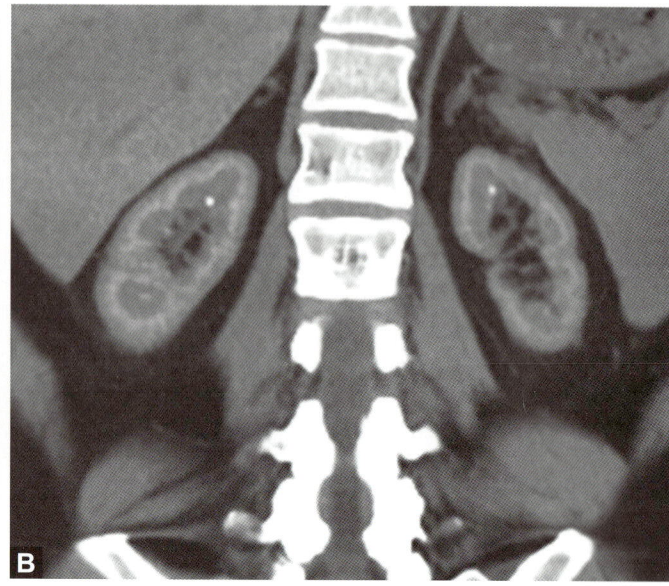

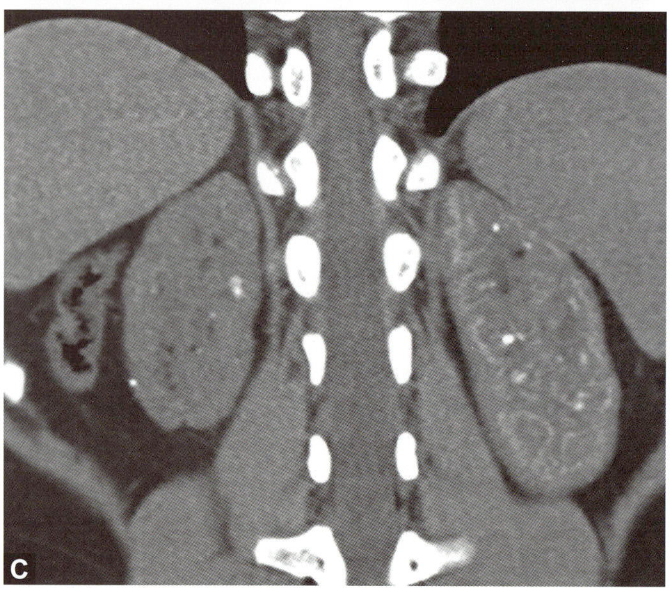

Figs. 18.25A to C: Noncontrast computerized tomography demonstrates (A) a coarse linear nephrocalcinosis and (B and C) a fine rim of nephrocalcinosis along with small focal stones in the medullary pyramids.

which is measured as the absorbed dose. The absorbed dose is the energy absorbed per unit mass and is measured in gray (Gy). The equivalent dose is obtained by multiplying the absorbed dose by a radiation-weighting factor. The equivalent dose is then multiplied by a tissue-weighting factor to obtain the effective dose. Effective dose is a calculated, not a measured, value. It is an indicator of potential detriment to various organs from ionizing radiation and is measured in Sieverts. Effective dose provides an estimate of radiation risk from partial body irradiation in terms of whole-body irradiation. It is calculated from dose to each organ weighted by tissue-weighting factor. The summation of effective doses to an individual is the cumulative effective dose.[79,80] The average yearly background radiation dose to an individual from the environment is 3.0–3.6 mSv. The average effective dose for noncontrast CT of the abdomen is 8 mSv.[80] Various low-dose noncontrast abdomen CTs for detection of renal stones have been proposed, with an average effective dose of 1–5 mSv.[72,74,81]

Ionizing radiation can result in deterministic and stochastic effects. Deterministic effects only occur after the dose exceeds a threshold that is much higher than that in routine imaging and increases with increase in radiation dose. These occur from cell damage and include cataracts and skin erythema. Stochastic effects are not associated with thresholds, but the risk of occurrence increases with

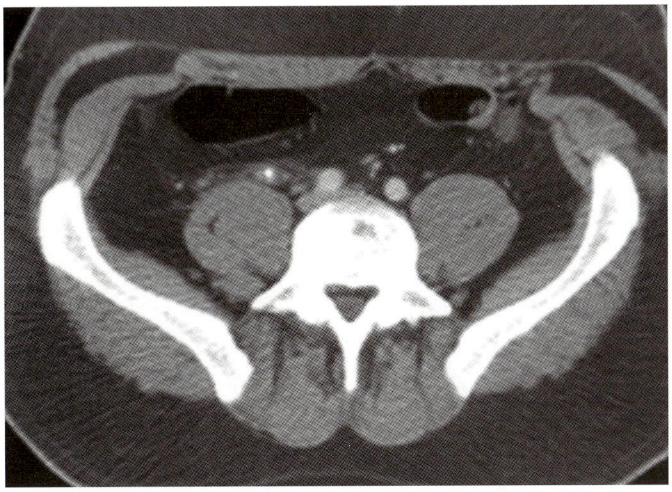

Fig. 18.26: Noncontrast computerized tomography demonstrates thickening of the wall of the right ureter with stranding perinephric edema associated with a ureteral stone.

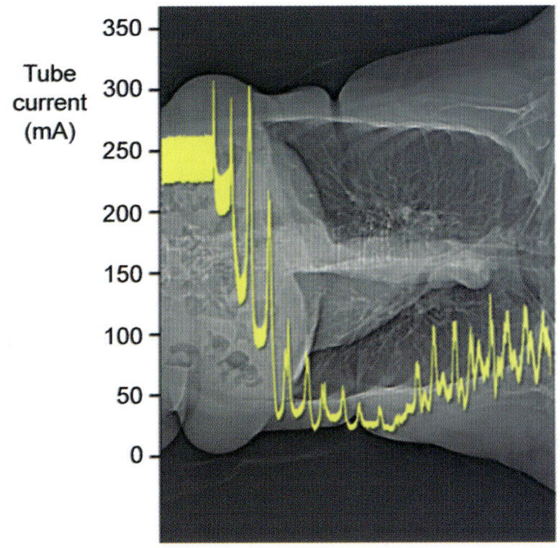

Fig. 18.27: With automated tube current modulation, the X-ray exposure is varied in a computerized tomography examination according to the density of the body part being scanned.

increasing exposure. These include cancer and genetic disorders.

There is continued debate on the extrapolation of the data on long-term health effects of radiation from historical incidents with significant exposure such as the atomic bomb explosions in Japan. The linear nonthreshold (LNT) model states that radiation effect can be extrapolated in a linear manner and that any level of radiation exposure carries increased risk. Some in the medical community feel that radiation exposure effects from high-level radiation exposure cannot be accurately extrapolated below the level of 100 mSv, which is where medical imaging takes place. They urge caution in accepting the LNT model until it can be proven or disproven with epidemiological studies. Although, there is no definite evidence of risk currently at the low levels of radiation in medical imaging, groups have developed guidelines for radiation protection.[82,83]

Increasing efforts are being focused on decreasing medical imaging radiation exposure by collaboration between the radiology and scientific community with the goal of using the radiation dose as low as reasonably achievable for acquiring the clinically needed diagnostic information.[84,85] This effort is focused on both reducing the radiation dose of current imaging examinations, advancing the development of imaging equipment with the ability to acquire diagnostic images at lower doses, educating radiology staff on best radiation practices, and ordering providers on best imaging studies for the individual patient's clinical needs.[86,87] Additional discussion of emerging techniques and radiation safety can be found in Chapter 29.

Surgical Management

Since stone-related symptoms are so often what first bring a PH patient to medical attention, management of symptomatic stones is often the first concern. Stones may be passed spontaneously. However, most patients will also require many stone removal procedures over the course of a lifetime. Principles related to stone management can be found in Section 3. However, concerns particular to patients with PH warrant consideration here.

Surgical intervention for symptomatic stone disease in patients with PH can be challenging and should be undertaken with care. A recent study by Carrasco and colleagues demonstrates the difficulties in rendering patients free of their symptomatic stone disease.[88] In this study, 14 patients underwent 54 urologic procedures with resultant primary, secondary and tertiary stone free rates of only 59%, 76%, and 78%, respectively. Percutaneous nephrolithotomy was the most successful of all surgical procedures, rendering patients clear of their symptomatic stone burden with a 70% primary and 90% secondary success rate. Ureteroscopy (URS) renders patients clear of their symptomatic stone burden with a 57% primary and 65% secondary success rate. Shock wave lithotripsy (SWL) was used to treat five patients with eight stones. Five targeted stones (63%) were treated successfully, while two patients required URS for treatment of resultant steinstrasse. A number of issues regarding SWL should be considered in patients with PH. Calcium oxalate monohydrate represents the most common stone in PH.[89] This stone composition can in some circumstances be resistant to fragmentation. Additionally,

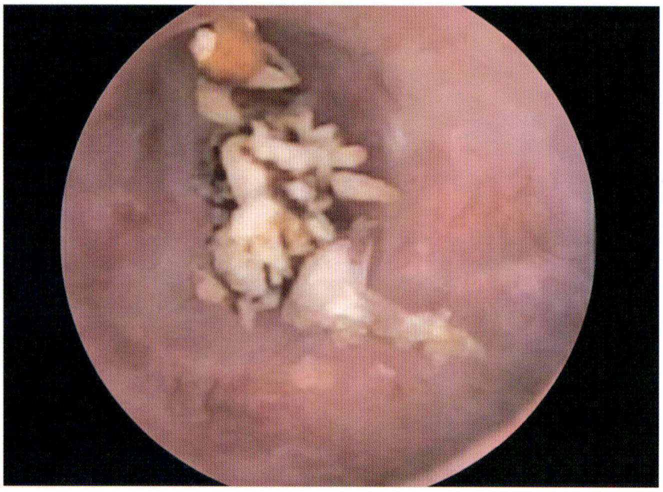

Fig. 18.28: Endoscopic evaluation of a lower pole stone in a primary hyperoxaluric patient. The stone is adherent to the papillary surface not at Randall's plaque or plug sites, but in this particular case, along the urothelial surface.
Source: A Krambeck. Department of Urology, Indiana University School of Medicine.

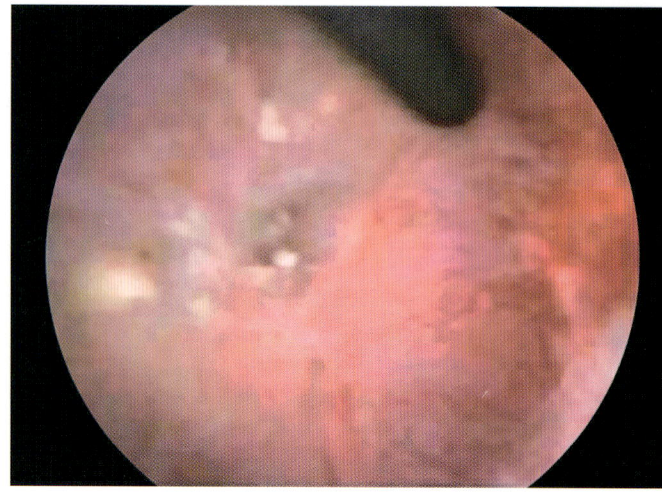

Fig. 18.29: Endoscopic evaluation of a calcified papillae in a primary hyperoxaluric patient. The dark stone material can be seen under the urothelial surface in the area of a dilated duct of Bellini. The stone is not extractable endoscopically.
Source: A Krambeck. Department of Urology, Indiana University School of Medicine.

the NC present in PH can make preoperative imaging difficult to interpret, which can lead to unnecessary shock waves delivered to the kidney.

The severe NC that occurs with PH can mislead the surgeon into believing the large calcifications noted on CT are stones that can actually be removed. However, in many circumstances the stones are adherent to the urothelium (Fig. 18.28). When such stones are extracted surgically, it can result in significant mucosal bleeding and injury to the urothelial lining. In other circumstances the calcifications can be solely within the parenchyma and not visible endoscopically from within the collecting system (Fig. 18.29). Such calcifications should not be removed since significant parenchymal damage can occur when attempting to access and extract such "stones."

In the study by Carrasco and colleagues,[88] which is the largest surgical series focusing on PH patients to date, four (29%) patients experienced >Clavien 3 grade complications, including three who developed ESRD postoperatively secondary to oxalosis crisis. Others have experienced loss of kidney function progressing to ESRD following stone removal procedures.[90-92] In an attempt to maintain oxalate homeostasis, it has become our practice to admit any surgical PH patient preoperatively for intravenous fluid hydration to avoid dehydration that may result in a change in GFR and subsequent precipitation of oxalate. Furthermore, PH patients are kept overnight for continued intravenous hydration postprocedure, even if the procedure is a simple URS.

Many PH patients require stone removal procedures in infancy or during childhood. Specific considerations for surgical management of stones in small children should be noted (*see* Chapter 36). In addition, recurring stone episodes are expected lifelong. Thus, long-term protection of kidney function is of utmost importance. Procedures with the potential to cause renal parenchymal injury or scarring should be avoided when possible.

Metabolic Aspects of Stone Formation

Stone formation in PH is a consequence of the marked hyperoxaluria and resulting supersaturation of the urine for calcium oxalate. Recurring stone formation is the rule, and multiple stones are typically present when PH patients with preserved kidney function undergo renal imaging.[13] In a group of 348 PH patients of all ages recently reported (277 with PH1), 58% had spontaneously passed stones, on average one every 3 years, and 70% required one or more urologic procedures over the course of follow-up, with an average of one procedure every 6.6 years.[13] Stone-related events (defined as stone-related symptoms, stone passage, or stone procedures) correlated inversely with urinary citrate excretion. The mean number of stones per image, however, correlated with plasma oxalate, urine oxalate, and inversely with urine calcium and citrate.[13]

Differences in metabolic stone-forming activity have been identified by PH type. Stone burden overall tends to be greater in type 1 disease, although type 3 patients not infrequently experience multiple and sometimes problematic stones in infancy or early childhood.[32,94] The frequency of stone formation in type 3 has been observed to improve with growth and maturation through childhood, although the risk of calcium oxalate stone formation persists lifelong and some adult PH3 patients have frequent stone events.[93] Type 2 patients appear to have fewer stones overall. Notably, PH1 patients frequently have low urine citrate, even when kidney function is well preserved.[13,28] A subset of PH3 patients demonstrates hypercalciuria.[32,61]

Unlike idiopathic stone formers, stones in PH1 do not form on Randall's plaque. Rather, they remain free in the tubules or collecting system or grow on calcium oxalate plugs that have formed in the medullary collecting ducts.[90] The result is a characteristic appearance on endoscopy. Specifically, the absence of Randall's plaque, widely dilated ducts of Bellini, and yellow suburothelial deposits indicative of crystals in the medullary collecting ducts.[90] A similar mechanism is presumed for PH types 2 and 3, although it has not been thoroughly studied in these patient groups. Section 1 contains additional discussion of characteristics and formation of kidney stones.

Stone composition in 74 patients with PH1 was reported by Daudon.[89] All stones were >95% calcium oxalate monohydrate (COM) (whewellite). Scanning electron microscopy demonstrated a loose crystalline structure, different from the dense radiating structure of idiopathic COM stone formers. Others have reported a mix of COM and calcium oxalate dihydrate (COD) in two of 10 type 1 patients.[94] Mixed COM and COD stones, occasionally containing calcium phosphate, are seen PH3.[32,94] Our experience has been a large predominance of COM in type 1 patients. Of six stones from three PH2 patients analyzed in our clinical stone laboratory, all were 100% COM. Composition of 15 stones from nine PH3 patients was 100% COM in 8/15, 100% COD in 2/15, and mixed COM and COD with >90% COM in 5/15. Jacob et al. speculated that differences in calcium oxalate crystal structure could be related to rapidity of stone growth and may be influenced by treatment.[94]

NEPHROCALCINOSIS

Nephrocalcinosis is deposition of calcium salts in the kidney parenchyma and is frequently observed in patients with PH. Ultrasound is more sensitive than CT in the detection of NC.[95] The medullary pyramids are relatively hypoechoic in comparison with the slightly more echogenic cortex in normal kidneys. In NC the mineralization within the tubules of the medullary pyramids creates increased acoustical interfaces, resulting in a reversed pattern of relatively increased medullary echogenicity in comparison to the cortex (Figs. 18.30A to D). Nephrocalcinosis can uniformly affect the medullary pyramids in a "rosetta" type pattern. It is fairly symmetric in both kidneys, although one kidney may be more affected if it is more diseased and/or obstructed.

This varied appearance of NC on ultrasound has been classified into four patterns of involvement.[96] The first three patterns demonstrate sequential increasing involvement from the periphery into the central portion. The fourth pattern demonstrates mineralization in the tips near the calyces. Posterior acoustical shadowing may be identified with densely mineralized NC. If present, it may be challenging to identify discrete renal stones as separate from the NC. Nephrocalcinosis may also be subtle and subject to differences of interpretation from one radiologist to another. Thus caution is warranted regarding interpretation of mild NC.

Stones and NC are both characteristic of PH, but there are differences between them with respect to pathophysiology and clinical implications. Stones are often associated with symptoms. However, the number of stones on imaging and the number of stone events do not appear to correlate with the risk of developing end stage renal disease (ESRD) over time.[13] By contrast, NC is asymptomatic yet a risk factor for future kidney failure.[11,13,14]

In a recent study of 303 PH patients in whom kidney imaging was available, NC was evident in 30% of PH1 patients at the time of initial presentation, with a progressive increase to 57% by 20 years of follow-up.[13] Among PH2 patients, 16% demonstrated this finding at presentation, increasing to 32% during follow-up. A smaller proportion of PH3 patients had NC at presentation and over time (Fig. 18.31). Thus, PH should be included in the differential diagnosis of any patient with NC. Whether prevalent at presentation, or particularly if it develops during the course of follow-up, NC is associated with later loss of kidney function.[13]

Oxalate is freely filtered by the renal glomerulus. Only the proximal tubule is known to contain oxalate transporters. Since net oxalate secretion is observed in patients with PH and since water reabsorption occurs in the S3 segment of the proximal tubule, one would expect the concentration of oxalate to be at its maximum toward the end of this segment of the nephron. Measurements in PH patients are consistent with calcium oxalate supersaturation in this segment, and calcium oxalate

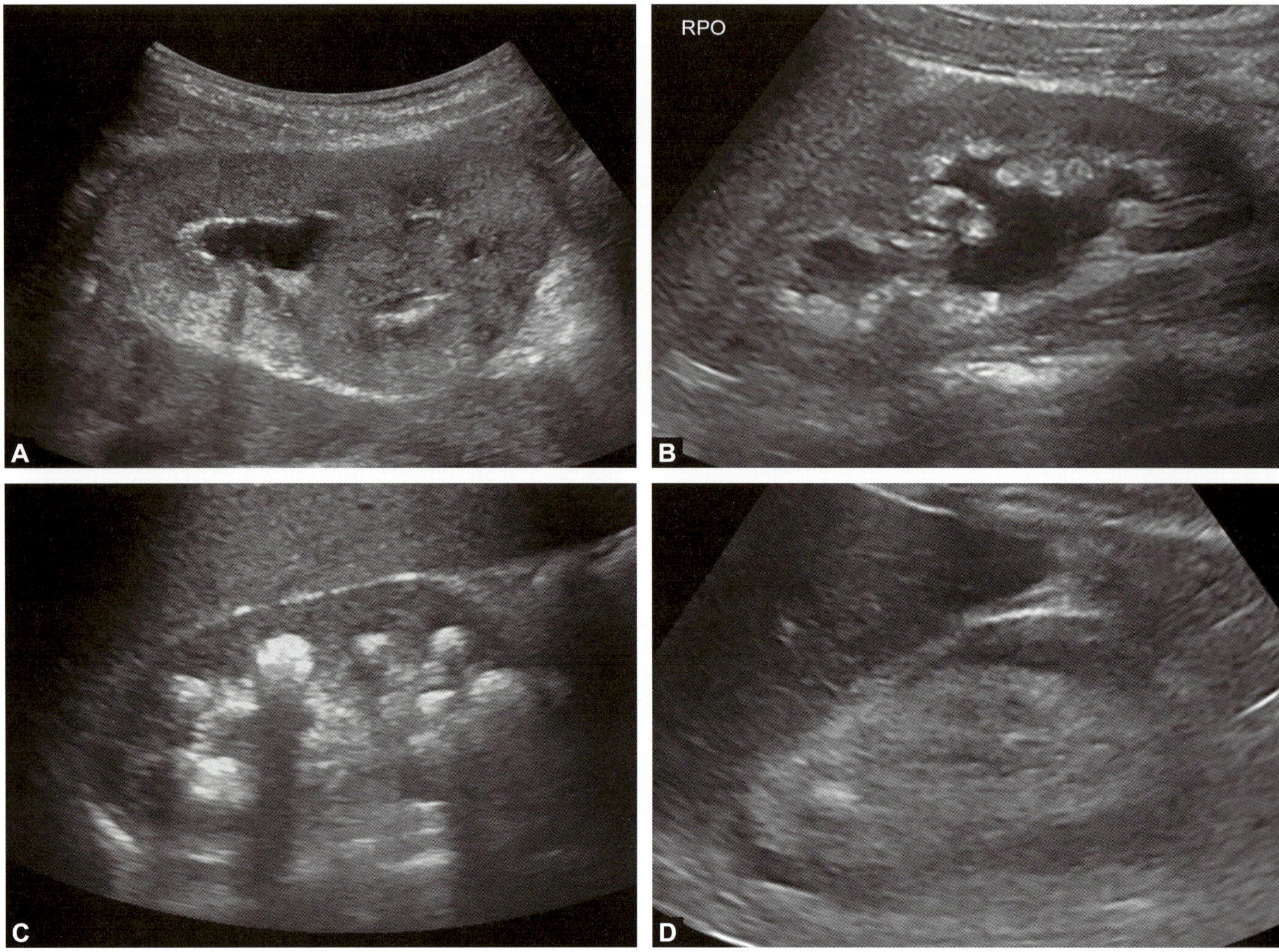

Figs. 18.30A to D: Variable appearances of nephrocalcinosis on ultrasound. The increased echogenicity may be limited to the medial rim of the medullary pyramids (A and B) or more extensively involves the medullary pyramids (C and D).

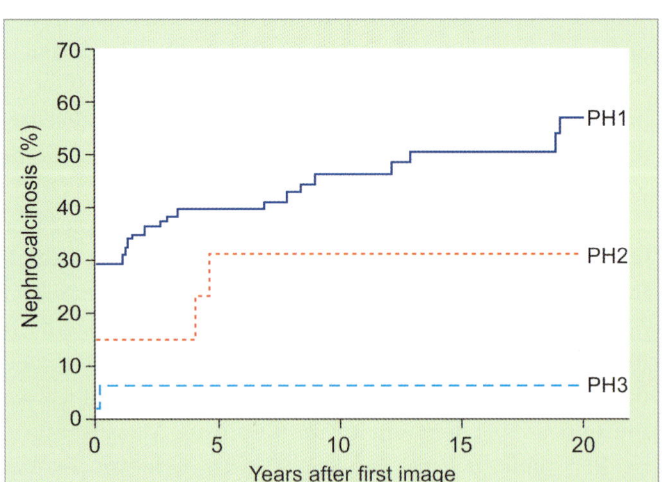

Fig. 18.31: Frequency of nephrocalcinosis at the time of diagnosis and during years of follow-up in patients with primary hyperoxaluria types 1, 2, and 3. Nephrocalcinosis is seen in 57% of primary hyperoxaluria type 1 (PH1) patients after 20 years of follow-up, and in a third of those with PH type 2, but is infrequent as a manifestation of PH type 3.
Source: Reproduced with permission from Tang X, Bergstralh EJ, Mehta RA, et al. Nephrocalcinosis is a risk factor for kidney failure in primary hyperoxaluria. Kidney Int. 2014.

crystals were demonstrated in proximal tubule cells from papillary biopsies in two PH patients with well-preserved kidney function.[90] These observations, along with crystal deposits preferentially in the S3 segments in kidneys of patients early after development of kidney failure, suggest that crystal deposition is an initiating event in renal damage in PH.[90] Of interest is an imaging study showing preferential calcification of the corticomedullary junction in a patient with kidney failure due to PH1 (*see* Figs. 18.25A to C). Kidneys examined following longer periods of dialysis show crystals scattered throughout the cortex (Figs. 18.32A to C). This pattern is distinct from other forms of stone disease.

KIDNEY DAMAGE AND KIDNEY FAILURE

Primary hyperoxaluria is notable among kidney stone diseases in causing irreversible kidney damage and ultimately ESRD. Kidney failure can occur at any age from infancy through the seventh decade of life, although is most often seen during early to mid-adulthood. There may be no identifiable inciting event, though not infrequently an episode of dehydration caused by an unrelated problem such as gastroenteritis is evident. Rapid progression to renal failure has also been observed following urologic procedures for stone removal.[90,91] Once GFR declines and serum oxalate levels begin to rise, a cycle of increasing injury can quickly become self-perpetuating. In recently published series from Europe and North America, 32–43% of patients with PH presented initially with ESRD,[1,3,19] and there is a report of 75% of Japanese patients first presenting with ESRD.[14] Patients with ESRD as the initial manifestation either have never formed stones, or stones have been present but not clinically evident prior to advanced kidney failure. Most such patients have dense NC on kidney imaging.

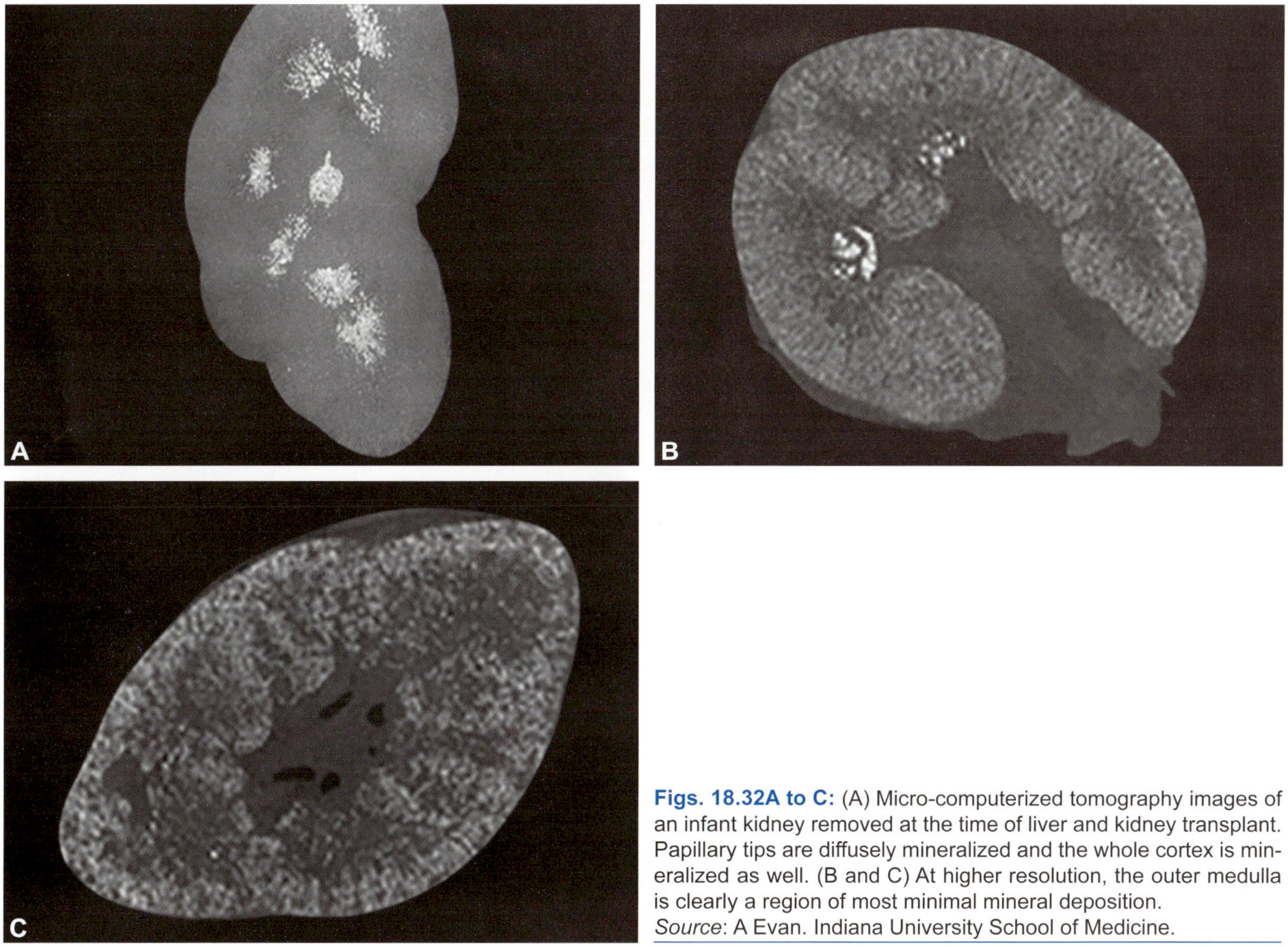

Figs. 18.32A to C: (A) Micro-computerized tomography images of an infant kidney removed at the time of liver and kidney transplant. Papillary tips are diffusely mineralized and the whole cortex is mineralized as well. (B and C) At higher resolution, the outer medulla is clearly a region of most minimal mineral deposition.
Source: A Evan. Indiana University School of Medicine.

Among patients with type 1 disease enrolled in the RKSC Primary Hyperoxaluria Registry, the median age at ESRD is 33 years.[12] Similar results have been reported by OxalEurope,[3] although another European study reported a median age of approximately 24 years.[19] Over time, nearly all patients with PH1 will eventually demonstrate kidney failure. Better preservation of kidney function is seen in PH2[28,59] and PH3[31,32] (*see* Fig. 18.3). To date only a single PH3 patient has been reported to have progressed to ESRD.[6] Although, patients with PH2 and PH3 have slightly lower urine oxalate excretion, there is sufficient overlap that this seems unlikely to fully explain the differences in outcome.

Oxalate injury to the kidney may be direct or mediated by calcium oxalate crystals. High concentrations of oxalate *in vitro* are well known to be injurious to human proximal tubule epithelial cells.[97,98] Calcium oxalate monohydrate crystals induce an inflammatory response in the kidney and specifically in renal proximal tubule cells.[99,100] *In vitro* evidence implicates COM crystals as of greater importance in pathogenesis.[101] However, it is difficult to separate the effects of oxalate ion and calcium oxalate crystals *in vivo*. By either mechanism, renal tubule cell injury or regeneration leads to upregulation and expression of hyaluronan and osteopontin at the cell surface and thus enhanced crystal adhesion.[102] Indeed, the studies of Worcester demonstrated hyaluronan in proximal tubule cells co-located with masses of calcium oxalate crystals.[90] Other forms of injury to the kidney tubules may have a similar effect, further sensitizing kidneys of PH patients to calcium oxalate crystal attachment and injury.

Attention in recent years has been directed to the mechanism of injurious effects of calcium oxalate crystals. Calcium oxalate monohydrate crystals bind to renal tubular epithelial cells, are internalized within the cells, and are associated with cell proliferation, inflammation, and formation of multinucleated giant cells.[100,103] Knauf and colleagues, using a mouse model of dietary hyperoxaluria, demonstrated that crystal-induced activity of the intrarenal inflammasome is responsible for kidney damage and loss of kidney function[104] in oxalate nephropathy. On histologic examination, intratubular calcium oxalate crystal deposition was noted along with an inflammatory response in the surrounding interstitium in kidneys of the mice. These are similar to histopathology observed in patients with PH.[105] These studies and those of other authors[106] establish a role for crystal-induced inflammation in the pathogenesis of kidney failure in PH patients.

As kidney function declines, there is less capacity to eliminate excess oxalate produced. Plasma oxalate begins to rise rapidly as GFR falls below approximately 30 mL/min/1.73 m^2 (stage 4 CKD). As plasma oxalate increases to above 30–50 μmol/L, the threshold for supersaturation of calcium oxalate in plasma is exceeded.[46,51,107] Calcium oxalate deposition then occurs in multiple body tissues (systemic oxalosis). Prominent among tissues affected are blood vessels with development of nonhealing ischemic ulcers, deposition in myocardium and the cardiac conduction system leading to infiltrative oxalate cardiomyopathy and conduction disturbances, bone marrow oxalate deposition leading to erythropoietin resistant anemia (*see* Fig. 18.1), oxalate osteodystrophy of bone resulting in pathologic fractures, and deposition in the retina of the eye.[1] The effects of systemic oxalosis are devastating and are fatal if not managed aggressively. Prevention of oxalosis should be central to clinical management of every patient with PH who has reduced kidney function.

MEDICAL MANAGEMENT

The goals of medical management are to reduce calcium oxalate crystal formation and, in so doing, minimize formation and growth of stones, as well as to protect the renal parenchyma from the injurious effects of oxalate (Table 18.4).

Fundamental to medical management of the PH patient is high oral fluid intake, thereby reducing the concentration of oxalate in the urine. In adults, a target of 4 L of oral fluid intake daily to achieve urine volume of >3 L daily is recommended. In children, oral fluid intake of >3 L/m^2 BSA is recommended.[1,15] In young children, in particular, achieving this degree of enteral fluid may require the use of a feeding tube or gastrostomy. Compliance with adequate fluid intake should be monitored periodically with timed urine collections. In CKD stages 4 and 5, the fluid prescription may require modification to avoid fluid overload and hyponatremia.

A related issue is maintenance of normal intravascular volume status at all times. For any acute illness that

Table 18.4: Medical management of stones and nephrocalcinosis.
High fluid intake
Calcium oxalate crystal inhibitor (citrate or neutral phosphate)
Pyridoxine (PH1 only)
Stones and NC monitored by imaging studies
Kidney function monitored by serum creatinine

interrupts oral fluid intake, such as severe gastroenteritis or viral illness, or if a period of fasting for >6 hours is required for a medical procedure, parenteral fluid administration is recommended. Given the role of the proximal tubule in early crystal formation and kidney injury, adequate (normal) salt intake should be maintained unless contraindicated by other health problems. This advice differs from that for other stone formers, in whom limitation of dietary salt intake is often recommended (e.g. idiopathic hypercalciuria and cystinuria).

There is little role for dietary oxalate restriction, given the hepatic origin of the large amount of excess oxalate in the urine of PH patients. Very little of the urine oxalate is of dietary origin. A practical approach is to limit intake of high oxalate foods. Calcium intake should be maintained at the recommended dietary allowances appropriate for age. In patients of all ages, but particularly in growing children, maintaining a nutritionally well-balanced diet should be the overriding consideration.

Citrate, pyrophosphate, and magnesium are naturally occurring inhibitors of calcium oxalate crystal formation in the urine.[108] In addition, citrate and other anions have been shown *in vitro* to inhibit binding of COM crystals to the surface of renal tubule epithelial cells,[109] and citrate has shown protective effects in cell cultures against calcium oxalate crystal-induced renal tubular oxidative damage.[110] All three agents have been used in the treatment of patients with PH. There has been greater experience in use of citrate and oral phosphorus,[108,111] the latter to achieve higher concentrations of urine pyrophosphate. There have been no comparative studies of effectiveness of these two agents. Both can be well tolerated over many years, although both have the disadvantage of requiring two to three times daily dosing and may have GI side effects. In patients with renal insufficiency, supplemental oral phosphorus should be avoided.

A full supersaturation profile of the urine should be obtained to guide treatment at yearly intervals or as indicated by stone-forming activity. Urine composition should be managed to minimize or avoid supersaturation for calcium oxalate.

Pyridoxine (vitamin B6) is the only medication currently available that is capable of reducing urine oxalate excretion. Pyridoxal phosphate (derived from pyridoxine) acts as a cofactor for the AGT enzyme that is deficient in PH1. When given at pharmacologic doses, urine oxalate may improve in some, but not all, patients. A favorable response is considered to be reduction in urine oxalate of ≥30%.[1] Response appears in part related to genotype[22,23,112] as discussed earlier in this chapter. Patients homozygous for the most common mutation G170R may show marked improvement with reduction in urine oxalate to normal or near normal while receiving the medication.[23,113,114] Doses of 5–8 mg/kg/day orally are usually adequate for maximum response,[113] although some have suggested higher doses.[23]

Since, pyridoxine appears to influence AGT enzyme through several different mechanisms, every patient with PH1 should receive a 3–6 month trial of the medication, with careful assessment of urine oxalate excretion before and while receiving adequate doses. If reduction in urine oxalate excretion is obtained, pyridoxine should be continued indefinitely. Pyridoxine is not effective in patients with PH2, and early evidence indicates lack of effect in PH3.[15]

Although interest in oral administration of oxalate-degrading bacteria as a potential treatment continues, an earlier double-blind, placebo-controlled clinical trial failed to confirm efficacy,[115] and its use cannot be recommended routinely pending additional well-controlled clinical studies (*see* Future Directions below).

Management of advanced CKD and ESRD is particularly challenging in PH patients due to the risks of systemic oxalosis. Renal replacement therapy in the form of dialysis or transplantation should be initiated as soon as the plasma oxalate concentration reaches 30–40 μmol/L, since that level is approaching the supersaturation threshold for calcium oxalate crystallization in the blood, and thus crystal deposition in multiple organs. Normal ranges of plasma oxalate vary by method of measurement. This threshold for calcium oxalate supersaturation assumes an assay with normal values of <5 μmol/L. Early initiation of dialysis with an intensive regimen can be effective in minimizing systemic oxalosis and achieving good transplant outcomes.[49] Hemodialysis is preferred due to better oxalate removal.[50,116] Many PH patients require daily hemodialysis or combined hemodialysis and peritoneal dialysis to manage daily oxalate production.[49,116] Individualized dialysis prescriptions are essential.[49]

Transplantation is the goal for every PH patient who reaches ESRD, and transplantation should be performed as quickly as feasible after advanced ESRD ensues. Most patients with PH type 1 require combined liver and kidney transplants to correct the metabolic defect while replacing kidney function. There is debate regarding what some have termed "pre-emptive" liver transplantation, which should be considered only in consultation with a clinician highly experienced in the management of PH. PH1 patients who are known to be fully responsive to pyridoxine may be considered for kidney-alone transplant.[114] Patients with PH2 are less likely to require renal replacement therapy, but if they do, may do well following kidney-alone transplantation. A recent case report suggests that liver transplantation can provide effective enzyme replacement in PH2. Accordingly, it may be a consideration for PH2 patients with more severe disease, pending further study.[145] There are as yet no reports of transplantation in PH3, but activity of HOGA in many body tissues and the more favorable overall clinical course would favor kidney-alone transplant pending further experience.

Urine oxalate may remain significantly elevated for up to 3–5 years or longer after combined kidney/liver transplantation due to mobilization of tissue oxalate stores[117,118] and will remain elevated indefinitely after kidney-alone transplant in patients who are not fully pyridoxine responsive. Recurrence of oxalosis in a transplanted kidney is always a concern, and in past years, outcomes of transplantation in PH patients were poor related to this problem. However, with intensive dialysis pretransplant and attentive management of PH-related risks during and after transplantation, outcomes are now similar to those of patients with other forms of kidney disease.[118]

FUTURE DIRECTIONS

Surgical and medical management of PH has advanced steadily over the years, providing better outcomes overall. However, despite these successes, recurring stone formation remains troubling, and irreversible loss of kidney function still occurs, almost universally in PH1 by the age of 70 years. Development of novel therapies to substantially improve the long-term outlook for patients with this disease will arise from improved understanding of the genetics and pathophysiology of this disease.

Oxalate Degradation by Bacteria

Unlike humans, certain bacteria are capable of enzymatic degradation of oxalate. *Oxalobacter formigenes* has captured particular attention because it uses oxalate as its primary nutrient source and also naturally inhabits the human colon.[119] These observations, followed by the demonstration that colonization of rats with *Oxalobacter* induced colonic secretion of endogenously produced oxalate,[120] stimulated interest in its potential therapeutic effect in patients with PH. Studies in animal models[121] and early clinical observations appeared promising.[122,123] However, a randomized, placebo-controlled clinical trial in patients with PH failed to show benefit in reduction in urinary oxalate.[115] Oral administration of a crystalline form of bacterial oxalate decarboxylase also has shown favorable results in AGXT deficient mice,[124] although it has not yet been studied in patients with PH.

Substrate Depletion

One strategy to reduce oxalate production has been substrate depletion. Glyoxylate is an immediate precursor of oxalate. Oxothiazolidine-4-carboxylate is converted to cysteine, which forms an adduct with glyoxylate, thus reducing conversion of glyoxylate to glycolate and oxalate. When given to animals and normal human subjects, this compound has been shown to reduce urinary oxalate excretion.[125-127] Efforts to reduce glyoxylate by administration of oxothiazolidine to PH1 patients, however, were disappointing.[128] The primary sources of glyoxylate are glycine, glycolate, and hydroxyproline.[129] Hydroxyproline has been the focus of renewed attention since recognition of HOGA1 deficiency in PH3,[34,61,130-132] although reduction of the hydroxyproline pool has not yet been tested in humans.

Selective inhibition of enzyme activity could also deplete substrate needed for glyoxylate production. Candidate enzymes are glycolate oxidase (GO), D-amino-oxidase, and hydroxyproline dehydrogenase (PRODH2).[26,133] Salido has demonstrated that genetically modified GO-deficient mice are healthy.[26] In addition, a recent report[134] describes an 8-year-old boy with asymptomatic glycolic aciduria due to a homozygous loss of function mutations of the GO gene *HAO1*. These observations provide an encouraging early step in the feasibility of this approach. Molecular modification of enzyme activity shows promise. Recent advances in ribonucleic acid interference therapy have been notable, with encouraging results in human trials of other diseases.[135] Clinical trials of GO inhibition by RNAi have recently begun in PH1 patients.

Enzyme Replacement

Orthotopic liver transplantation has to date been the only successful form of enzyme replacement. Enzyme administration, an approach that has been successful in other genetic disorders such as Fabry's disease,[136] confronts significant barriers in PH1. Alanine: glyoxylate aminotransferase enzyme must be located not only within the hepatocyte but within the peroxisome to be metabolically effective, such that its delivery is challenging. More importantly, oxalate is an end product of metabolism. Thus, in PH, all native hepatic cells that are enzyme deficient will continue to produce large amounts of oxalate. Addition of AGT competent cells does not address this problem, and elimination of most native liver cells is believed to be required in order to reduce oxalate production sufficiently to achieve clinical benefit. Thus, partial liver transplantation, where a portion of transplanted liver is placed alongside the native liver, is not a viable alternative.[137-138] Orthotopic liver transplantation is successful because complete removal of the native liver at the time of transplantation eliminates all native liver cells, replacing them with cells that contain AGT activity. Hepatocellular transplantation has been postulated as an alternative to orthotopic liver transplantation. However, the problem of native liver cells and their survival advantage over transplanted cells, poses a significant challenge. In mouse models of PH1, measures such as irradiation of native liver to destroy cells and stimulation of mitosis of transplanted hepatocytes are required.[137,139]

Molecular Chaperones

Pharmacological chaperones have been successful in correcting protein misfolding in other genetic diseases and seem a viable strategy in PH.[140,141] In PH type 1, the majority are missense mutations resulting in mitochondrial mistargeting, protein aggregation, catalytic defects, or enhanced turnover.[6,140] Studies of Mesa-Torres[142] have shown that PH1 mutations that are associated with aggregation and mistargeting share common alterations in protein folding, stability, and interaction with molecular chaperones. Stabilization of mutant forms could potentially rescue enzyme activity. An example in the case of PH1 is pyridoxal phosphate, which in pharmacologic doses administered orally as pyridoxine (vitamin B6) acts as a chaperone, favorably influencing folding and dimerization of the G170R and F152I variants, in addition to its enzyme cofactor role.[21] Urine oxalate can be reduced in patients with these variants following pyridoxine treatment.[22,112] There is reason to suspect that other mutant forms of AGT might also respond to pharmacologic chaperones.[140,142,143]

Gene Therapy

Delivery of a normal AGXT gene sequence to hepatocytes of an AGT-deficient host requires transfection of a large proportion of hepatocytes, minimal immune response, and sustained expression at sufficient levels. Nonetheless, there has been recent success in mouse models of PH1.[144] Although significant work remains before gene therapy is ready for clinical application in PH1, the progress to date is encouraging.

CONCLUSION

Outcomes for patients with PH have improved greatly over the past three decades. Stone formation and renal injury can be reduced and their consequences mitigated through knowledgeable interventions. Severe systemic oxalosis, a cause of considerable morbidity and death, can in most circumstances be avoided through early diagnosis, careful clinical management of patients who have impaired kidney function, and by aggressive approaches to transplantation. Opportunities for patients who first present with severe oxalosis are more limited.

There is even greater promise for the future. Realization of the advances of the past two decades in improved health and well-being of individuals with PH, however, requires early diagnosis. A gap remains. Thus, in addition to ongoing research, a wake-up call to physicians (particularly urologists and nephrologists) to enhance awareness of this disease is urgently needed. Education and patient advocacy groups will prepare patients and their families to partner in this work.

ACKNOWLEDGMENTS

The authors gratefully acknowledge the contribution of Amy Krambeck to the Surgical Management of patients with PH, and photographs provided by A Krambeck and A Evan. We also thank the Rare Kidney Stone Consortium (RKSC) and the Oxalosis and Hyperoxaluria Foundation for their support of the RKSC Primary Hyperoxaluria Registry. The RKSC (U54DK083908) is a part of the NIH National Center for Advancing Translational Sciences (NCATS) Rare Diseases Clinical Research Network (RDCRN), funded through a collaboration between NCATS and the NIDDK.

REFERENCES

1. Hoppe B, Beck BB, Milliner DS. The primary hyperoxalurias. Kidney Int. [Review]. 2009;75(12):1264-71.
2. van der Hoeven SM, van Woerden CS, Groothoff JW. Primary hyperoxaluria type 1, a too often missed diagnosis and potentially treatable cause of end-stage renal disease in adults: results of the Dutch cohort. Nephrol Dial Transplant. 2012;27(10):3855-62.
3. Mandrile G, van Woerden CS, Berchialla P, et al. Data from a large European study indicate that the outcome of primary

hyperoxaluria type 1 correlates with the AGXT mutation type. Kidney Int. 2014;86(6):1197-204.
4. Coulter-Mackie MB. Preliminary evidence for ethnic differences in primary hyperoxaluria type 1 genotype. Am J Nephrol. 2005;25:264-8.
5. Williams EL, Acquaviva C, Amoroso A, et al. Primary hyperoxaluria type 1: update and additional mutation analysis of the AGXT gene. Hum Mutat. [Review]. 2009;30(6):910-7.
6. Hopp K, Cogal AG, Bergstralh EJ, et al. Phenotype-genotype correlations and estimated carrier frequencies in primary hyperoxaluria. J Am Soc Nephrol. 2015;26(10): 2559-70.
7. Hatch M. Intestinal adaptations in chronic kidney disease and the influence of gastric bypass surgery. Experimental Physiology. 2014;99:1163-7.
8. Harambat J, Fargue S, Bacchetta J,et al. Primary hyperoxaluria. Int J Nephrol. 2011;2011:864580.
9. Cochat P, Deloraine A, Rotily M, et al. Epidemiology of primary hyperoxaluria type 1. Nephrol Dial Transplant. 1995;10(Suppl 8):3-7.
10. Kopp N, Leumann E. Changing pattern of primary hyperoxaluria in Switzerland. Nephrol Dial Transplant. 1995;10:2224-7.
11. Van Woerden CS, Groothoff JW, Wanders RJA, et al. Primary hyperoxaluria type 1 in the Netherlands: prevalence and outcome. Nephrol Dial Transplant. 2003;18:273-9.
12. Lieske JC, Monico CG, Holmes WS, et al. International registry for primary hyperoxaluria. Am J Nephrol. 2005;25:290-6.
13. Tang X, Bergstralh EJ, Mehta RA, et al. Nephrocalcinosis is a risk factor for kidney failure in primary hyperoxaluria. Kidney Int.2015; 87(3):623-31.
14. Takayama T, Nagata M, Ichiyama A, et al. Primary hyperoxaluria type 1 in Japan. Am J Nephrol. 2005;25(3):297-302.
15. Edvardsson VO, Goldfarb DS, Lieske JC, et al. Hereditary causes of kidney stones and chronic kidney disease. Pediatr Nephrol. 2013;28(10):1923-42.
16. Lorenzo V, Torres A, Salido E. Primary hyperoxaluria. Nefrologia. [Research Support, Non-U.S. Gov't]. 2014;34(3):398-412.
17. Danpure CJ, Jennings PR, Fryer P, et al. Primary hyperoxaluria type 1: genotypic and phenotypic heterogeneity. J Inherit Dis. 1994;17:487-99.
18. Rumsby G. Primary hyperoxaluria database. Available from http://wwwuclhnhsuk/phmd. https://www.uclh.nhs.uk/OURSERVICES/SERVICEA-Z/PATH/PATHBIOMED/CBIO/Pages/Phmdatabase.aspx. Accessed June 26, 2017.
19. Harambat J, Fargue S, Acquaviva C, et al. Genotype-phenotype correlation in primary hyperoxaluria type 1: the p.Gly170Arg AGXT mutation is associated with a better outcome. Kidney Int. 2010;77(5):443-9.
20. Danpure CJ. Targeting of alanine:glyoxylate aminotransferase in normal individuals and its mistargeting in patients with primary hyperoxaluria type 1. Ann NY Acad Sci. 1996;804:477-90.
21. Fargue S, Rumsby G, Danpure CJ. Multiple mechanisms of action of pyridoxine in primary hyperoxaluria type 1. Biochim Biophys Acta. [Research Support, Non-U.S. Gov't]. 2013;1832(10):1776-83.
22. Monico CG, Rossetti S, Olson JB, et al. Pyridoxine effect in type 1 primary hyperoxaluria is associated with the most common mutant allele. Kidney Int. 2005;67:1704-9.
23. Hoyer-Kuhn H, Kohbrok S, Volland R, et al. Vitamin b6 in primary hyperoxaluria I: first prospective trial after 40 years of practice. Clin J Am Soc Nephrol. [Research Support, Non-U.S. Gov't]. 2014;9(3):468-77.
24. Fargue S, Lewin J, Rumsby G, et al. Four of the most common mutations in primary hyperoxaluria type 1 unmask the cryptic mitochondrial targeting sequence of alanine:glyoxylate aminotransferase encoded by the polymorphic minor allele. J Biol Chem. [Research Support, Non-U.S. Gov't]. 2013;288(4):2475-84.
25. Lorenzo V, Alvarez A, Torres A, et al. Presentation and role of transplantation in adult patients with type 1 primary hyperoxaluria and the I244T AGXT mutation: single-center experience. Kidney Int. [Comparative Study]. 2006;70(6):1115-9.
26. Salido E, Pey AL, Rodriguez R, et al. Primary hyperoxalurias: disorders of glyoxylate detoxification. Biochim Biophys Acta. 2012;1822(9):1453-64.
27. Cramer SD, Ferree PM, Lin K, et al. The gene encoding hydroxypyruvate reductase (GRHPR) is mutated in patients with primary hyperoxaluria type II. Hum Mol Genet. 1999;8:2063-9.
28. Milliner DS, Wilson DM, Smith LH. Phenotypic expression of primary hyperoxaluria: comparative features of type I and II. Kidney Int. 2001;59:31-6.
29. Giafi CF, Rumsby G. Kinetic analysis and tissue distribution of human D-glycerate dehydrogenase/glyoxylate reductase and its relevance to the diagnosis of prmary hyperoxaluria type 2. Ann Clin Biochem. 1998;35:104-9.
30. Cochat P, Rumsby G. Primary hyperoxaluria. New Engl J Med. [Review]. 2013;369(7):649-58.
31. Beck BB, Baasner A, Buescher A, et al. Novel findings in patients with primary hyperoxaluria type III and implications for advanced molecular testing strategies. Eur J Hum Genet. 2013;21(2):162-72.
32. Monico CG, Rossetti S, Belostotsky R, et al. Primary hyperoxaluria type III gene HOGA1 (formerly DHDPSL) as a possible risk factor for idiopathic calcium oxalate urolithiasis. Clin J Am Soc Nephrol. 2011;6(9):2289-95.
33. Williams EL, Bockenhauer D, van't Hoff WG, et al. The enzyme 4-hydroxy-2-oxoglutarate aldolase is deficient in primary hyperoxaluria type 3. Nephrol Dial Transplant. 2012;27(8):3191-5.
34. Riedel TJ, Knight J, Murray MS, et al. 4-hydroxy-2-oxoglutarate aldolase inactivity in primary hyperoxaluria type 3 and glyoxylate reductase inhibition. Biochim Biophys Acta. [Research Support, N.I.H., Extramural]. 2012;1822(10): 1544-52.
35. Belostotsky R, Seboun E, Idelson GH, et al. Mutations in DHDPSL are responsible for primary hyperoxaluria type III. Am J Hum Genet. 2010;87(3):392-9.
36. Asplin JR, Coe FL. Hyperoxaluria in kidney stone formers treated with modern bariatric surgery. J Urol. 2007;177(2):565-9.

37. Lieske J, Mehta R, Milliner D, et al. Kidney stones are common after bariatric surgery. Kidney Int. 2015;87(4): 839-45.
38. Siener R, Petzold J, Bitterlich N, et al. Determinants of urolithiasis in patients with intestinal fat malabsorption. Urology. 2013;81(1):17-24.
39. Zarembski PM. Some factors influencing the urinary excretion of oxalic acid in man. Clinica Chimica Acta. 1969;25:1-10.
40. Gibbs DA, Watts RWE. The variation of urinary oxalate excretion with age. J Lab Clin Med. 1969;73:901-8.
41. von Schnakenburg C, Byrd DJ, Latta K, et al. Determination of oxalate excretion in spot urines of healthy children by ion chromatography. Eur J Clin Chem Clinic Biochem. 1994;32:27-9.
42. Campfield T, Braden G, Flynn-Valone P, et al. Urinary oxalate excretion in premature infants. Pediatrics. 1994;94:674-8.
43. Narendra A, White MP, Rolton HA, et al. Nephrocalcinosis in preterm babies. Arch Dis Child Fetal Neonatal Ed. 2001;85:F207-F13.
44. Ezzedeen F, Adelman RD, Ahlfors CE. Renal calcification in preterm infants: pathophysiology and long-term sequelae. J Pediatr. 1988;113:532-9.
45. Monge M, Garcia-Nieto VM, Domenech E, et al. Study of renal metabolic disturbances related to renal lithiasis at school age in very low birth weight children. Nephron. 1998;79:269-73.
46. Worcester EM, Nakagawa Y, Bushinsky DA, et al. Evidence that serum calcium oxalate supersaturation is a consequence of oxalate retention in patients with chronic renal failure. The Journal of Clinical Investigation. [Research Support, U.S. Gov't, P.H.S.]. 1986;77(6):1888-96.
47. Morgan SH, Maher ER, Purkiss P, et al. Oxalate metabolism in end stage renal disease: the effect of ascorbic acid and pyridoxine. Nephrol Dial Transplant. 1988;3:28-32.
48. Amoroso A, Pirulli D, Florian F, et al. AGXT gene mutations and their influence on clinical heterogeneity of type 1 primary hyperoxaluria. J Am Soc Nephrol. 2001;12:2072-9.
49. Tang X, Voskoboev NV, Wannarka SL, et al. Oxalate quantification in hemodialysate to assess dialysis adequacy for primary hyperoxaluria. Am J Nephrol. 2014;39(5): 376-82.
50. Watts RWE, Veall N, Purkiss P. Oxalate dynamics and removal rates during haemodialysis and peritoneal dialysis in patients with primary hyperoxaluria and severe renal failure. Clin Sci. 1984;66:591-7.
51. Hoppe B, Kemper MJ, Bokenkamp A, et al. Plasma calcium oxalate supersaturation in children with primary hyperoxaluria and end-stage renal failure. Kidney Int. 1999;56:268-74.
52. Chen C-L, Fang H-C, Chou K-J, et al. Acute oxalate nephropathy after ingestion of star fruit. Am J Kid Dis. 2001;37(2): 418-22.
53. Albersmeyer M, Hilge R, Schrottle A, et al. Acute kidney injury after ingestion of rhubarb. BMC Nephrol. 2012;13:141.
54. Farre M, Xirgu J, Salgado A, et al. Fatal oxalic acid poisoning from sorrel soup. Lancet. 1989;334:1524.
55. Hylander B, Kjellstrand CM. Prognostic factors and treatment of severe ethylene glycol intoxication. Intensive Care Med. 1996;22:546-52.
56. Meier M, Nitschke M, Perras B, et al. Ethylene glycol intoxication and xylitol infusion—metabolic steps of oxalate-induced acute renal failure. Clin Nephrol. 2005;63:225-8.
57. Nelson WK, Houghton SG, Milliner DS, et al. Enteric hyperoxaluria, nephrolithiasis, and oxalate nephropathy: potentially serious and unappreciated complications of Roux-en-Y gastric bypass. Surg Obes Relat Dis. 2005;1(5):481-5.
58. Kwan TK, Chadban SJ, Mckenzie PR, et al. Acute oxalate nephropathy secondary to orlistat-induced enteric hyperoxaluria. Nephrology. 2013;18:241-2.
59. Chlebeck PT, Milliner DS, Smith LH. Long-term prognosis in primary hyperoxaluria type II (L-glyceric aciduria). Am J Kid Dis. 1994;23:255-9.
60. Rumsby G, Sharma A, Cregeen DP, et al. Primary hyperoxaluria type 1 without L-glycericaciduria; is the disease under-diagnosed? Nephrol Dial Transplant. 2001;16:1697-9.
61. Belostotsky R, Pitt JJ, Frishberg Y. Primary hyperoxaluria type III—a model for studying perturbations in glyoxylate metabolism. J Mol Med (Berl). 2012;90(12):1497-504.
62. Latta K, Brodehl J. Primary hyperoxaluria type 1. Eur J Pediatr. 1990;149:518-22.
63. Yavuz A, Ceken K, Alimoglu E, et al. The reliability of color Doppler twinkling artifact for the diagnosis of nephrolithiasis: ROC analysis. Ultrasound Med Biol. 2006;32:226.
64. Lee JY, Kim SH, Cho JY, et al. Color and power doppler twinkling artifacts from urinary stones. Am J Roentgenol. 2001;176:1441-5.
65. Smith-Bindman R, Aubin C, Bailitz J, et al. Ultrasonography versus computed tomography for suspected nephrolithiasis. New Engl J Med. 2014;371(12):1100-10.
66. Viprakasit DP, Sawyer MD, Herrell SD, et al. Limitations of ultrasonography in the evaluation of urolithiasis: a correlation with computed tomography. J Endourol. 2012;26(3):209-13.
67. Patel SR, Stanton P, Zelinski N, et al. Automated renal stone volume measurement by noncontrast computerized tomography is more reproducible than manual linear size measurement. J Urol. 2011;1986:2275-9.
68. Huda W, Vance A. Patient radiation doses from adult and pediatric CT. Am J Roentgenol. [Research Support, N.I.H., Extramural]. 2007;188(2):540-6.
69. Council NR. Health effects of exposure to low levels of ionizing radiations (BEIR VII phase 2). Washington (DC): National Academies Press (US). 2006.
70. Mettler FA, Bhargavan M, Faulkner K, et al. Radiologic and nuclear medicine studies in the United States and worldwide: frequency, radiation dose, and comparison with other radiation sources 1950-2007. Radiology. 2009;253:520-31.
71. Westphalen AC, Hsia RY, Maselli JH, et al. Radiological imaging of patients with suspected urinary tract stones: national trends, diagnoses, and predictors. Acad Emerg Med. 2011;18(7):699-707.
72. Sung MK, Singh S, Kalra MK. Current status of low dose multi-detector CT in the urinary tract. World J Radiol. 2011;3(11):256-65.
73. Heneghan JP, McGuire KA, Leder RA, et al. Helical CT for nephrolithiasis and ureterolithiasis: comparison of

conventional and reduced radiation-dose techniques. Radiology. 2003;229:575-80.
74. Liu W, Esler SJ, Kenny BJ, et al. Low-dose enhanced helical CT of renal colic: assessment of ureteric stone detection and measurement of effective dose of equivalent. Radiology. 2000;215:51-4.
75. Frush DP, Slack CC, Hollingsworth CL, et al. Computer simulated radiation dose reduction for abdominal multidetector CT of pediatric patients. Am J Roentgenol. 2002;179:1107-13.
76. Singh S, Kalra MK, Hsieh J, et al. Abdominal CT: comparison of adaptive statistical iterative and filtered back projection reconstruction techniques. Radiology. 2010;257:373-83.
77. Kalra MK, Maher MM, Toth TL, et al. Strategies for CT radiation dose optimization. Radiology. 2004;230:619-28.
78. Gabriel S, Eckel LJ, DeLone DR, et al. Pilot study of radiation dose reduction for pediatric head CT in evaluation of ventricular size. Am J Neuroradiol. 2014;35(12): 2237-42.
79. Johnson TE, Birky BK. Centers for Disease Control and Prevention: Public Health Emergency Preparedness and Response. Health Physics and Radiological Health. 2012;4th edition: Available from http://emergency.cdc.gov/radiation/. Accessed on July 11, 2017.
80. Mettler FA, Huda W, Yoshizumi TT, et al. Effective doses in radiology and diagnostic nuclear medicine: a catalog. Radiology. 2008;248:254-63.
81. Ciaschini MW, Remer EM, Baker ME, et al. Urinary calculi: radiation dose reduction of 50% and 75% at CT–effect on sensitivity. Radiology. 2009;251:105-11.
82. Natarajan MK, Paul N, Mercuri M, et al. Canadian Cardiovascular Society position statement on radiation exposure from cardiac imaging and interventional procedures. Can J Cardiol. [Practice Guideline]. 2013;29(11):1361-8.
83. Fazel R, Krumholz HM, Wang Y, et al. Exposure to low-dose ionizing radiation from medical imaging procedures. New Engl J Med. 2009;361:849-57.
84. Strauss KJ, Goske MJ, Kaste SC, et al. Image gently: Ten steps you can take to optimize image quality and lower CT dose for pediatric patients. Am J Roentgenol. [Practice Guideline]. 2010;194(4):868-73.
85. McCollough CH, Chen GH, Kalender W, et al. Achieving routine submillisievert CT scanning: report from the Summit on Management of Radiation Dose in CT. Radiology. 2012;264:567-80.
86. Lee CI, Halms AH, Monico EP, et al. Diagnostic CT scans: assessment of patient, physician, and radiologist awareness of radiation dose and possible risks. Radiology. 2004;231: 393-8.
87. Amis ES, Jr., Butler PF, Applegate KE, et al. American College of Radiology white paper on radiation dose in medicine. J Am Coll Radiol. [Practice Guideline]. 2007;4(5):272-84.
88. Carrasco A, Granberg CF, Gettman MT, et al. Surgical management of stone disease in patient with primary hyperoxaluria. In review.
89. Daudon M, Jungers P. Peculiar morphology of stones in primary hyperoxaluria. New Engl J Med. 2008;359:100-2.
90. Worcester EM, Evan AP, Coe FL, et al. A test of the hypothesis that oxalate secretion produces proximal tubule crystallization in primary hyperoxaluria type 1. Am J Physiol Renal Physiol. 2013;305:F1574-F84.
91. Grateau G, Grunfeld JP, Beurton D, et al. Post-surgical deterioration of renal function in primary hyperoxaluria. Nephrol Dial Transplant. 1987;1:261-4.
92. Pais VM, Assimos DG. Pitfalls in the management of pts with PH. Urol Res. 2005;33:390-3.
93. Hoppe B. The enzyme 4-hydroxy-2-oxoglutarate aldolase is deficient in primary hyperoxaluria type III. Nephrol Dial Transplant. [Comment]. 2012;27(8):3024-6.
94. Jacob DE, Grohe B, Gessner M, et al. Kidney stones in primary hyperoxaluria: new lessons learnt. PLoS One. [Research Support, Non-U.S. Gov't]. 2013;8(8):e70617.
95. Boyce AM, Shawker TH, Hill SC, et al. Ultrasound is superior to computed tomography for assessment of medullary nephrocalcinosis in hypoparathyroidism. J Clin Endocrinol Metab. 2013;98(3):989-94.
96. Patriquin H, Robitaille P. Renal calcium deposition in children: sonographic demonstration of the Anderson-Carr progression. Am J Roentgenol. 1986;146:1253-6.
97. Huang MY, Chaturvedi LS, Koul S, et al. Oxalate stimulates IL-6 production in HK-2 cells, a line of human renal proximal tubular epithelial cells. Kidney Int. 2005;68:497-503.
98. Khandrika L, Koul S, Meacham RB, et al. Kidney injury molecule-1 is up-regulated in renal epithelial cells in response to oxalate in vitro and in renal tissues in response to hyperoxaluria in vivo. PLoS One. 2012;7(9):e44174.
99. Khan SR. Reactive oxygen species as the molecular modulators of calcium oxalate kidney stone formation: evidence from clinical and experimental investigations. J Urol. [Review]. 2013;189(3):803-11.
100. Schepers MSJ, van Ballegooijen ES, Bangma CH, et al. Crystals cause acute necrotic cell death in renal proximal tubule cells but not in collecting tubule cells. Kidney Int. 2005;68:1543-53.
101. Guo C, McMartin KE. The cytotoxicity of oxalate, metabolite of ethylene glycol, is due to calcium oxalate monohydrate formation. Toxicology. 2005;208(3):347-55.
102. Verhulst A, Asselman M, de Naeyer S, et al. Preconditioning of the distal tubular epithelium of the human kidney precedes nephrocalcinosis. Kidney Int. 2005;68:1643-7.
103. Lieske JC, Swift H, Martin T, et al. Renal epithelial cells rapidly bind and internalize calcium oxalate monohydrate crystals. Proc Natl Acad Sci. 1994;91:6987-91.
104. Knauf F, Asplin JR, Granja I, et al. NALP3-mediated inflammation is a principal cause of progressive renal failure in oxalate nephropathy. Kidney Int. 2013;84(5):895-901.
105. Lieske JC, Spargo BH, Toback FG. Endocytosis of calcium oxalate crystals and proliferation of renal tubular epithelial cells in a patient with type 1 primary hyperoxaluria. J Urol. 1992;148:1517-9.
106. Mulay SR, Kulkarni OP, Rupanagudi KV, et al. Calcium oxalate crystals induce renal inflammation by NLRP3-mediated IL-1β secretion. J Clin Invest. 2013;123:236-46.

107. Marangella M, Cosseddu D, Petrarulo M, et al. Thresholds of serum calcium oxalate supersaturation in relation to renal function in patients with or without primary hyperoxaluria. Nephrol Dial Transplant. 1993;8:1333-7.
108. Milliner DS, Eickholt JT, Bergstralh EJ, et al. Results of long-term treatment with orthophosphate and pyridoxine in patients with primary hyperoxaluria. New Engl J Med. 1994;331:1553-8.
109. Lieske JC, Leonard R, Toback FG. Adhesion of calcium oxalate monohydrate crystals to renal epithelial cells is inhibited by specific anions. Am J Physiol. 1995;268:F604-F12.
110. Byer K, Khan SR. Citrate provides protection against oxalate and calcium oxalate crystal induced oxidative damage to renal epithelium. J Urol. [Research Support, U.S. Gov't, P.H.S.]. 2005;173(2):640-6.
111. Leumann E, Hoppe B, Neuhaus T. Management of primary hyperoxaluria: efficacy of oral citrate administration. Pediatr Nephrol. 1993;7:207-11.
112. Van Woerden CS, Groothoff JW, Wijburg FA, et al. Clinical implications of mutation analysis in primary hyperoxaluria type 1. Kidney Int. 2004;66:746-52.
113. Monico CG, Olson JB, Milliner DS. Implications of genotype and enzyme phenotype in pyridoxine response of patients with type I primary hyperoxaluria. Am J Nephrol. 2005;25(2):183-8.
114. Lorenz EC, Lieske JC, Seide BM, et al. Sustained pyridoxine response in primary hyperoxaluria type 1 recipients of kidney alone transplant. Am J Transplant. 2014;14(6):1433-8.
115. Hoppe B, Groothoff JW, Hulton S-A, et al. Efficacy and safety of Oxalobacter formigenes to reduce urinary oxalate in primary hyperoxaluria. Nephrol Dial Transplant. 2011;26: 3609-15.
116. Illies F, Bonzel KE, Wingen AM, et al. Clearance and removal of oxalate in children on intensified dialysis for primary hyperoxaluria type 1. Kidney Int. 2006;70(9):1642-8.
117. Monico CG, Milliner DS. Combined liver-kidney and kidney-alone transplantation in primary hyperoxaluria. Liver Transplant. 2001;7(11):954-63.
118. Bergstralh EJ, Monico CG, Lieske JC, et al. Transplantation outcomes in primary hyperoxaluria. Am J Transplant. [Research Support, N.I.H., Extramural]. 2010;10(11):2493-501.
119. Allison MJ, Dawson KA, Mayberry WR, et al. Oxalobacter formigenes gen. nov., sp. nov.: oxalate-degrading anaerobes that inhabit the gastrointestinal tract. Arch Microbiol. 1985;141:1-7.
120. Hatch M, Cornelius J, Allison M, et al. Oxalobacter sp. reduces urinary oxalate excretion by promoting enteric oxalate secretion. Kidney Int. 2006;69(4):691-8.
121. Hatch M, Gjymishka A, Salido EC, et al. Enteric oxalate elimination is induced and oxalate is normalized in a mouse model of primary hyperoxaluria following intestinal colonization with Oxalobacter. Am J Physiol Gastrointest Liver Physiol. 2011;300:G461-G9.
122. Hoppe B, Beck B, Gatter N, et al. Oxalobacter formigenes: a potential tool for the treatment of primary hyperoxaluria type 1. Kidney Int. 2006;70(7):1305-11.
123. Milliner D. Treatment of the primary hyperoxalurias: a new chapter. Kidney Int. 2006;70(7):1198-200.
124. Grujic D, Salido EC, Shenoy BC, et al. Hyperoxaluria is reduced and nephrocalcinosis prevented with an oxalate-degrading enzyme in mice with hyperoxaluria. Am J Nephrol. 2009;29:86-93.
125. Baker PW, Rofe AM, Bais R. The effect of (L)cysteine and (L)-2-oxothiazolidine-4-carboxylic acid (OTZ) on urinary oxalate excretion: studies using a hyperoxaluric rat model. J Urol. 1998;159:2177-81.
126. Holmes RP, Assimos DG, Leaf CD, et al. The effects of (L)-2-oxothiazolidine-4-carboxylate on urinary oxalate excretion. J Urol. 1997;158(1):34-7.
127. Baker PW, Bais R, Rofe AM. The efficacy of (L)-2-oxothiazolidine-4-carboxylate (OTC) and (L)-cysteine in reducing urinary oxalate excretion. J Urol. 1994;152:2139-46.
128. Holmes RP, Assimos DG, Wilson DM, et al. (L)-2-oxothiazolidine-4-carboxylate in the treatment of primary hyperoxaluria type 1. BJU Int. 2001;88:858-62.
129. Coulter-Mackie MB. 4-Hydroxyproline metabolism and glyoxylate production: a target for substrate depletion in primary hyperoxaluria? Kidney Int. 2006;70(11):1891-3.
130. Riedel TJ, Johnson LC, Knight J, et al. Structural and biochemical studies of human 4-hydroxy-2-oxoglutarate aldolase: implications for hydroxyproline metabolism in primary hyperoxaluria. PLoS One. 2011;6:e26021.
131. Jiang J, Johnson LCK, John, et al. Metabolism of [13C5] hydroxyproline in vitro and in vivo: implications for primary hyperoxaluria. Am J Physiol Gastrointest Liver Physiol. 2012;302:G637-G43.
132. Knight J, Holmes R, Cramer S, et al. Hydroxyproline metabolism in mouse models of primary hyperoxaluria. Am J Physiol Renal Physiol. 2012;302:F688-F93.
133. Murray MS, Holmes RP, Lowther WT. Active site and loop 4 movements within human glycolate oxidase: implications for substrate specificity and drug design. Biochemistry. 2008;47:2439-49.
134. Frishberg Y, Zeharia A, Lyakhovetsky R, et al. Mutations in HAO1 encoding glycolate oxidase cause isolated glycolic aciduria. J Med Genet. 2014;51(8):526-9.
135. Coelho T, Adams D, Silva A, et al. Safety and efficacy of RNAi therapy for transthyretin amyloidosis. New Engl J Med. 2013;369(9):819-29.
136. Dietz HC. New therapeutic approaches to Mendelian disorders. N Engl J Med. 2010;36319:852-63.
137. Guha C, Yamanouchi K, Jiang J, et al. Feasibility of hepatocyte transplantation-based therapies for primary hyperoxalurias. Am J Nephrol. 2005;25:161-70.
138. Trotter JF, Milliner D. Auxiliary liver transplant is an ineffective treatment of primary hyperoxaluria. Am J Transplant. 2014;14(1):241.
139. Jiang J, Salido EC, Guha C, et al. Correction of hyperoxaluria by liver repopulation with hepatocytes in a mouse model of primary hyperoxaluria type-1. Transplantation. 2008;85(9):1253-60.
140. Pey AL, Albert A, Salido E. Protein homeostasis defects of alanine-glyoxylate aminotransferase: new therapeutic

strategies in primary hyperoxaluria type I. Biomed Res Int. 2013;2013:687658.

141. Cellini B, Montioli R, Oppici E, et al. The chaperone role of the pyridoxal 5'-phosphate and its implications for rare diseases involving B6-dependent enzymes. Clin Biochem. 2014;47(3):158-65.

142. Mesa-Torres N, Fabelo-Rosa I, Riverol D, et al. The role of protein denaturation energetics and molecular chaperones in the aggregation and mistargeting of mutants causing primary hyperoxaluria type I. PLoS One. [Research Support, Non-U.S. Gov't]. 2013;8(8):e71963.

143. Fodor K, Wolf J, Erdmann R, et al. Molecular requirements for peroxisomal targeting of alanine-glyoxylate aminotransferase as an essential determinant in primary hyperoxaluria type 1. PLoS Biol. 2012;10(4):e1001309.

144. Salido E, Rodriguez-Pena M, Santana A, et al. Phenotypic correction of a mouse model for primary hyperoxaluria with adeno-associated virus gene transfer. Mol Ther. 2011;19(5):870-5.

145. Dhondup T, Lorenz E, Milliner D, et al. Combined liver kidney transplant for primary hyperoxaluria type 2: A case report. Am J Trans. 2017. doi: 10.1111/ajt.14418.

CHAPTER

19 Renal Tubular Acidosis and Urolithiasis

Daniel G Fuster, Orson W Moe

INTRODUCTION

Although frequently being referred to as a single entity, renal tubular acidosis (RTA) is in fact a group of disorders with diverse congenital and acquired etiologies, and highly variable clinical presentations ranging from completely asymptomatic to serious outcomes such as end-stage renal disease or fatal hypokalemic cardiac dysrhythmias. The clinician often identifies the common thread of this group of diseases as normal anion gap (NAG) metabolic acidosis in the presence of a normal serum creatinine concentration and an alkaline urine pH. However, the true communal element is defective renal acid excretion that cannot be accounted for by reduced glomerular filtration rate (GFR). The manifestations of RTA are protean, but a very common mode that brings the patient with RTA to medical attention is the passage or incidental detection of a kidney stone. This chapter will devote due coverage of this particular aspect of RTA.

Metabolic acidosis is defined as excessive accumulation of nonvolatile acid in the body from either excessive acid production, impaired acid excretion, or a combination of both. Renal tubular acidosis is a quintessential underexcretion (as opposed to overproduction) acidosis that stems from abnormality in tubular acid secretion, which distinguishes it from underexcretion acidosis due primarily to low GFR. Increased acid load (overproduction acidosis) can of course occur concurrently and worsens the disease and conversely, a very low dietary acid intake can often mask the presentation of this disease.

The first report of RTA was attributed to the empiric description of an infant with "calcium infarction of the renal tubules," which in all likelihood was a child inflicted with distal RTA (dRTA) with calcium nephrolithiasis and nephrocalcinosis.[1] The scope of RTA is broad and the reader is referred to coverage by some excellent recent monographs that review this subject.[2-5] This chapter addresses a specific aspect of RTA: nephrolithiasis seen in association with dRTA.

BRIEF PRIMER ON RENAL ACIDIFICATION AND ACID-BASE HOMEOSTASIS

The kidney is not the sole but a principal defender of the constancy of the milieu intérieur that enables multicellular life to exist.[6] The magnitude of the homeostatic challenge can often be appreciated by consideration of the relative size of the pool to be maintained and the flux traversing that pool in unit time. With the aqueous H^+ concentration in body fluid ~40 nM yielding a total body content of free H^+ of <2 μmoles, and a daily addition of approximately 50–70 mmoles H^+ per day to this pool, it is clear that an acid defense system of enormous precision has to be installed.[7] Maintenance of body pH is a concerted effort of many concomitant physiologic homeostatic events involving the kidney, lungs and liver, and an array of buffers inside and outside cells.

ACID BUFFERING: TEMPORIZING MEASURE

As indicated, the quantity and rate of H^+ addition is colossal compared to the pool of H^+ in total body water. Even when endowed with the ultimate sensitivity in sampling, wisdom in homeostasis, and efficiency in rectification, there is no way a regulatory organ can respond with the rapidity required to correct this kind of disturbance. The first line of defense has to be buffers that sequester the invading H^+ from imparting harm.[8] A full discussion of buffering is beyond the scope of this chapter, but some features can be highlighted. Buffers can be divided into: (1) intracellular versus extracellular, (2) HCO_3^- versus non-HCO_3^-, and (3) "closed" versus "open." The concept of "buffering" by proteins deserves a brief note. All proteins can theoretically bind H^+'s but if H^+ exerts its ill effects on proteins by titrating their side chains, this process is really how H^+ imparts harm rather than "buffering."[9] Bicarbonate buffering is active in both the intracellular and extracellular space and its titration generates CO_2, which basically converts the nonvolatile acid into a volatile form, which is then eliminated by ventilation. The footprint of a nonvolatile acid is the hypobicarbonatemia, which has two impacts—buffer depletion and it sets the body fluid pH at a lower than normal level. Renal net acid excretion (see below) regenerates the decomposed bicarbonate and returns the acid-base status to normalcy.[10]

While buffering in body water forestalls an acid holocaust for the organism, urinary buffering serves a different role. To excrete 50 mEq/day of net acid in a typical urine volume of 1 L, urinary pH (UpH) will have to be <1.5. If this H^+ is to reside in UpH of 5.0, it has to be carried by 5000 L of urine; neither is possible. The majority of the H^+ excreted has to be carried by H^+ acceptors that are the "urinary buffer." The pathophysiology of RTA and kidney stones is intimately related to urinary buffer. The inability of H^+ pumping into the urine is tantamount to the inability to reabsorb luminal HCO_3^- that is normally vanishingly low in normal urine. Bicarbonaturia is the principal cause of alkaline urine that is the sine qua non for lithogenesis in RTA (see below).

RENAL ACID EXCRETION: DEFINITIVE DEFENSE

Volatile acid is basically CO_2, and its production rate far exceeds nonvolatile acids in terms of daily addition of H^+ to the body and CO_2 is cleared efficiently by ventilation, which will not be discussed in this chapter. Nonvolatile acid, on the other hand, is composed of a large group of acids, which can be inorganic or organic in nature and are excreted by the kidney.

Renal mechanisms of acid excretion consist of two parts: (1) transport H^+ into the urine from the body, which will replenish the decomposed HCO_3^- in the body fluid from buffering invading H^+ discussed above; and (2) devise ways to carry the H^+ in the urine, i.e. buffering. It is noteworthy that the magnitude of H^+ secretion into the urine far exceeds the amount of H^+ that is required to be excreted. That is because there are two components to H^+ secretion. The mammalian nephron operates on a filtration-reabsorption system to allow very high GFR to sustain high metabolic tolls. The high GFR mandates recovery of valuable low-molecular solutes that cannot be retained by the nonselective slit pores of the glomeruli. A normal GFR of 160–180 L/day will result in loss of ~4,000 mEq of HCO_3^-/day, which is clearly fatal within the hour. The reclamation of this vast amount of filtered HCO_3^- is achieved by H^+ secretion in the urine, titration of luminal HCO_3^- into

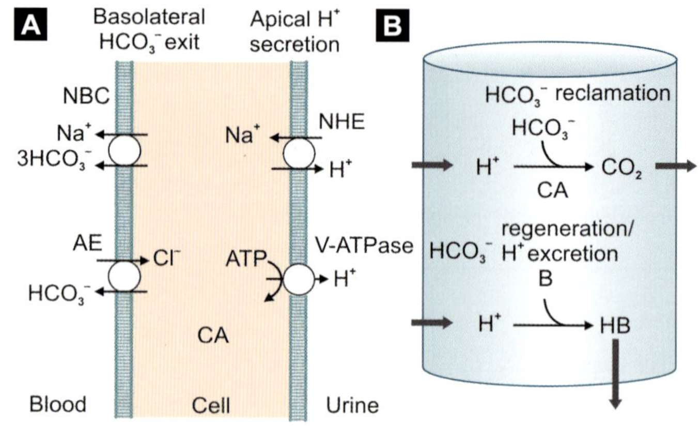

C	Normal	Metabolic acidosis
Plasma [HCO_3^-]	25 mM	18 mM
GFR	170 L	170 L
Reclamation of filtered HCO_3^-	4250 mmoles	3060 mmoles
Regeneration of decomposed HCO_3^-	70 mmoles	70 mmoles
Total H^+ secretion needed	4320 mmoles	3130 mmoles
Estimated capacity of renal secretion	>4600 mmoles	<3200 mmoles

Figs. 19.1A to C: Principles and mechanisms of renal acidification. (A) The principal transporters for apical H^+ secretion and basolateral HCO_3^- exit in renal epithelia. (B) The two fates of H^+ secreted into the urinary lumen. Titration with the filtered HCO_3^- effects reclamation of the filtered HCO_3^- and prevents loss of the valuable buffer in the body. Titration with other urinary buffers results in net acid excretion and regeneration of the decomposed HCO_3^- from buffering H+ in the body at the time of acid invasion. There are many urinary buffers, but the major ones are ammonia (pKa 9.25), phosphate (pKa1 2.1, pKa2 7.2, pKa2 12.3), citrate (pKa1 2.9, pKa2 4.3, pKa2 5.2), urate (pKa 5.3). Note that while citrate can carry H^+ and hence qualifies as a buffer, since the citrate anion is metabolizable, it itself is a base equivalent. (C) Example of renal H^+ secretory load in normal and in metabolic acidosis. (NHE: Na^+/H^+ exchanger; V-ATPase: Vacuolar or H^+ ATPase; NBC: Na-bicarbonate cotransporter; AE: Anion exchanger; CA: Carbonic anhydrase; ATP: Adenosine triphosphate. B: Non-bicarbonate buffer; HB: Titrated non-bicarbonate buffer).

CO_2, and uptake of the CO_2. The successful reclamation of filtered HCO_3^- forestalls a metabolic disaster but does not result in net acid excretion. In addition, more H^+ must be secreted into the urine to be carried by non-HCO_3^- buffers to rid the body of the 50–70 mmoles of H^+ added to the body per day (Figs. 19.1A to C). In normal adults, the daily net acid excretion can be boosted up to 300 mmoles/day.[11] This high capacity is reduced in dRTA. In addition to reduction of maximal net acid excretion, note that in a steady state of hypobicarbonatemia in dRTA, the filtered load HCO_3^- is actually much lower so the H^+ secretion dedicated and required for HCO_3^- reclamation is also reduced.

CELLULAR MECHANISMS OF H^+ EXCRETION

Regardless of whether the secreted H^+ is destined for HCO_3^- reclamation or net acid excretion, the renal tubule still has to get the H^+ into the tubular lumen. The mechanisms of H^+ secretion are summarized in Figures 19.1A to C. The organization is fairly typical for many solutes with axial heterogeneity in transport mechanisms. Apical H^+ extrusion is energetically uphill along the entire nephron and is energized by two different mechanisms: a high-capacity, low-gradient system that predominates in the more proximal segments and a low-capacity high-gradient system that predominates in the more distal segments. The former mechanism is sometimes termed entropic because it utilizes the downhill movement of Na^+ to energize the uphill movement of H^+ (Na^+/H^+ exchange); the latter mechanism is termed enthalpic because it derives its energy directly from adenosine triphosphate (ATP) hydrolysis.

The wisdom of the polarized epithelium rests in its ability to differentially eject acid on one face and base on the other, and the ability to maintain gradient (Fig. 19.2). While luminal Na^+/H^+ exchangers can sustain uphill transport of H^+ up to a maximum of a 10-fold (1 $\log_{10}$ unit) gradient,[12] the luminal vacuolar ATPase (V-ATPases) are the only transporters capable of acidifying UpH to the vicinity of 5.0,[13] which is critical not so much for trapping of urinary buffers for H^+ excretion but also to prevent precipitation of calcium phosphate (CaP).

Apical H^+ extrusion has to be accompanied by basolateral base exit or else the cell will succumb to alkaline intoxication. In the proximal tubule, this is achieved by Na^+-coupled HCO_3^- cotransporters (NBCs) and in the α-intercalated cell, this is achieved by the Cl^-/HCO_3^- anion exchanger- 1 (AE), which are all members of a much larger extended family of exchangers and cotransporters (SLC4).[14] Akin to the apical Na^+/H^+ exchanger that extrudes H^+ using the Na^+ gradient, AE1 uses the inward Cl^- gradient to transport HCO_3^- out of the cell. Any disruption of basal HCO_3^- exit will raise the cell pH, which will impair apical and transepithelial H^+ secretion.

THREE KEY ENTITIES IN DISTAL ACIDIFICATION

V-ATPase

The α-intercalated cell is the principal locale of pathology in dRTA. Apical H^+ extrusion is mediated by a multi-subunit

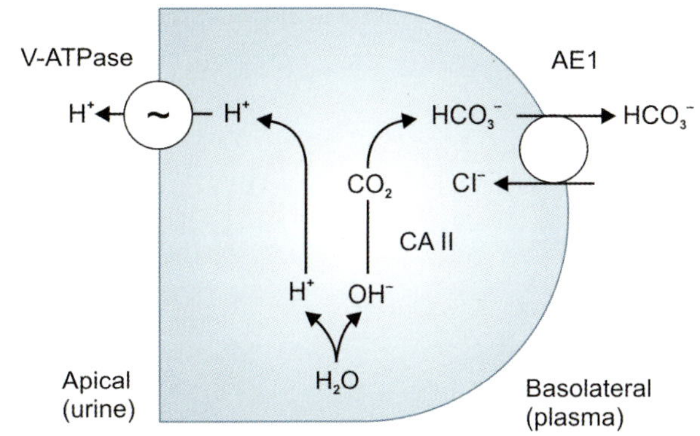

Fig. 19.2: Alpha-intercalated cell. In the collecting duct of the mammalian nephron, the α-intercalated cell secretes H^+ into the urine via the vacuolar (V) ATPase and HCO_3^- into the blood via the anion exchanger AE1. The substrates H^+ and HCO_3^- are generated from metabolic CO_2 by the catalytic action of carbonic anhydrase II (CA II). Basolateral HCO_3^- exit is crucial for sustaining apical H^+ secretion. These three proteins work in concert to mediate luminal H^+ secretion. Mutations of any one will slow down the transepithelial H^+ secretion. V-ATPase: Vacuolar or H+ ATPase; (AE: Anion exchanger).

transporter protein, V-ATPase (or H^+-ATPase), which is archaic in evolution with existence dating back to single-cell organisms. The V-ATPase is a complex multi-subunit protein containing at least 13 different proteins and is organized into two distinct functional domains: a peripheral catalytic sector 560 kDa V_1 (subunit stoichiometry of the 8 proteins: A3B3C1D1E3F1G3H1) and an intramembranous 260 kDa proteolipid V_0 (subunit stoichiometry of the 5 proteins: a1d1c″1c′1c4)—somewhat akin to the F_1F_0 complex of bacterial and mitochondrial ATP synthases[15] (Fig. 19.3A). Each of the subunits in V_0 and V_1 is coded for by specific genes and certain isoforms are expressed in tissue-specific fashion.[16] Inactivating mutations of two of these subunits in humans, B1 and a4, lead to dRTA (see below).

Anion Exchanger

The main player in distal HCO_3^- exit is the AE1 or SLC4A1 (Fig. 19.3B), which is a member of a much larger family of AEs originally identified in the erythrocyte.[17,18] The kidney version of AE1 (kAE1) differs by the lack of 65 amino acids in the N-terminus, which interacts with spectrin/ankyrin in the erythrocyte. Several lines of evidence have suggested that AE1 operate as dimers and even tetramers, but the individual units are capable of functioning independently. There is a whole host of mutations that lead to the red blood cell disorders Southeast Asian ovalocytosis

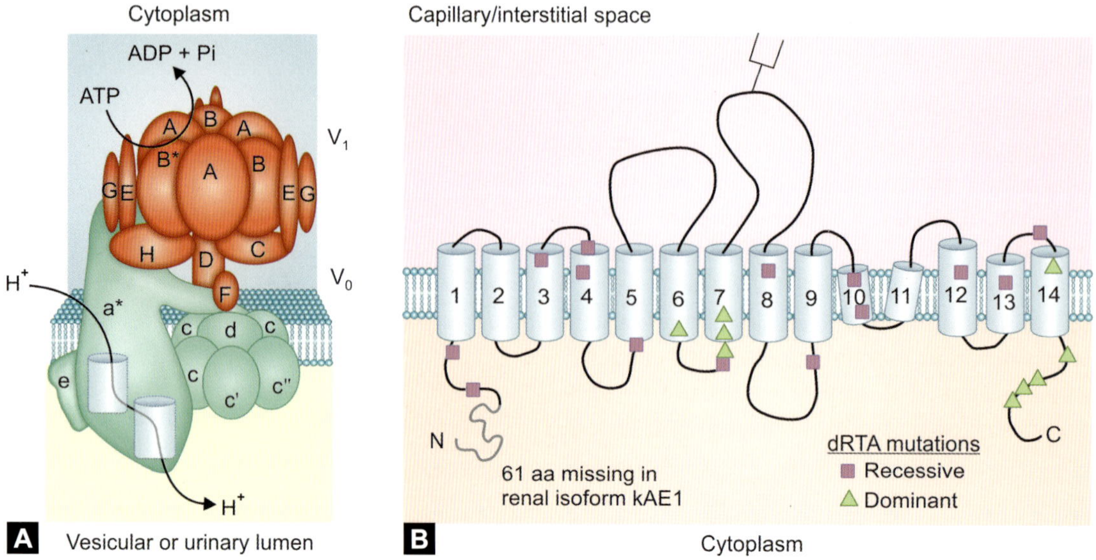

Figs. 19.3A and B: Vacuolar adenosine triphosphatase (V–ATPase) and anion exchanger— (AE) 1: (A) V-ATPase has two domains, V_1 and V_0. The peripheral cytoplasmic V_1 domain has eight different subunits (A-H, in red) that execute adenosine triphosphate (ATP) hydrolysis, whereas the membrane integral V_0 domain (a–e, in green) has six subunits and mediates H^+ translocation across the lipid bilayer. Adenosine triphosphate hydrolysis drives the rotation of a central rotor, (subunits D, F, d and proteolipid c, c′, c″). Subunit a harbors two hemichannels responsible for H^+ translocation. The V_1 and V_0 domain are connected by a central stalk (subunits D, F, and d) and three peripheral stalks (subunits C, E, G, and the N-terminal of subunit a). The peripheral stalks hold the A_3B_3 hexamer stationary with respect to subunit a. The B1 and a subunits (asterisk) harbor naturally occurring mutations in human distal renal tubular acidosis (dRTA). (B) Proposed topology of anion exchanger AE1. The documented human mutations are scattered throughout the protein. (ADP: Adenosine diphosphate; kAE1: Kidney version of AE1).

and hereditary spherocytosis, which will not be discussed here. Kidney version of AE1 interacts with an astonishing array of proteins, including carbonic anhydrase (CA) II and glyceraldehyde-3-phosphate dehydrogenase, which is likely integral to the "metabolon" that links CO_2 hydration and glycolytic H^+-producing metabolism to HCO_3^- transport. Inactivating mutations of AE1 lead to dRTA (see below).

Carbonic Anhydrase

The CO_2 that furnishes HCO_3^- and H^+ in the proximal tubule is largely from titration of filtered HCO_3^- but in the collecting duct, metabolic generation of CO_2 constitutes a significant portion. The key enzyme that allows this to transpire is the cytosolic CA.[19] This enzyme catalyzes the reversible hydroxylation of CO_2, which is of fundamental importance to carbon-based life and permeates all species on the planet. Mammals have α-CA composed of 14 different isoforms, of which CA II, CA IV, CA XII (possibly CA XIV) are expressed in the kidney. Cytosolic CA II comprises >90% of renal CA. Carbonic anhydrase II is expressed in most nephron segments. Most membrane-associated CA activity is CA IV, which is linked to the apical membrane in the proximal tubules, α-intercalated cells of collecting ducts, and all cells of initial inner medullary collecting ducts. Both CA II and CA IV are inhibited by compounds with a sulfonamide-like structure (sensitivity ~ tenths of nanomolar), but only CA II has been described in human genetic RTA (see below).

DEFINITION, CLASSIFICATION, AND CAUSES OF RTA

Definition

Metabolic acidosis can be viewed as stemming from overproduction of nonvolatile metabolic acid, inadequate excretion and/or metabolism of the same acid, or a combination of both excessive production and inadequate disposal. Renal tubular acidosis refers to the renal underexcretion of acid due to a tubular defect distinct from the generalized limitation of excretory function in acute or chronic kidney disease with marked diminution of GFR. Although this definition is sound and it excludes the metabolic acidosis of acute and chronic renal failure as "RTA,"

Table 19.1: Classification of renal tubular acidosis by nephron segment.

Tubular segment	Numeric type	Synonym(s)	Plasma chemistry	Urine chemistry	Clinical features
Proximal	II	• Proximal	• NAG metabolic acidosis • Hypokalemia (when given alkali) • Hypophosphatemia (if part of Fanconi)	Maximally acidic urine in the absence of bicarbonaturia. Alkalinuria when plasma $[HCO_3^-]$ is raised to normal	No nephrolithiasis
Distal	I	• Hypokalemic distal	• NAG metabolic acidosis • Hypokalemia	Alkaline urine, urine pH >6 Hypocitraturia	Calcium nephrolithiasis, nephrocalcinosis (frequent)
	IV	• Hyperkalemic distal	• NAG metabolic acidosis • Hyperkalemia	Urine pH < 6 Low urinary ammonium	Increased incidence of uric acid nephrolithiasis if low urinary pH (<5.3), especially if type II DM, high BMI.
Proximal and distal	III	• Juvenile RTA • Combined proximal-distal • Carbonic anhydrase deficiency or inhibition	• NAG metabolic acidosis	Alkaline urine, urine pH >6 Hypocitraturia	Calcium nephrolithiasis, nephrocalcinosis (unusual)

(BMI: Body mass index; DM: Diabetes mellitus; RTA: Renal tubular acidosis; NAG: Normal anion gap).

it is important to appreciate that the low GFR and tubular dysfunction are not mutually exclusive. In states of low GFR, there is also tubular dysfunction leading to impaired acid secretion. In a pure primary tubular disorder such as a genetic defect in a tubular transporter protein, GFR may start out as normal but with time may decline as well. Although the concept has physiologic basis and clinical distinction of tubular versus low GFR acidosis is pragmatic, it is important to appreciate that the two entities can overlap.

The clinical definition of RTA is much less pathophysiologically oriented but relies more on clinical presentation and diagnostic tests. The following cluster of laboratory findings prompt the clinician to first consider and then secure the diagnosis of RTA. This constellation includes NAG metabolic acidosis, normal or at least near normal GFR, absence of diarrhea or other alkali-losing states, high UpH, and finally a positive urinary anion gap (UAG) as a surrogate, albeit an imperfect one, for paucity of urinary ammonium.

Although this approach is practical as it utilizes readily available clinical data, it unfortunately does not probe at the primary pathophysiology of RTA. In the section below on evaluation, the caveats for some of these clinical tests will be discussed in more detail.

Classification

The traditional classification of RTA is by tubular segments of the primary lesion and by clinical chemistry. For those who are partial to numeric typing, there is the type I to IV RTA system. Although a numbering system may be convenient, and to some conveys a sense of certain mastery of knowledge, classification into numeric types really only ensures uniformity in communication between physicians but still does not imply understanding of pathophysiology. Table 19.1 summarizes the classification of the RTA.

Proximal RTA (pRTA) is only briefly discussed here because it does not pertain to the focus of the chapter. Nephrolithiasis is not a common feature of pRTA. Some of the key pathogenic features of dRTA are not present in pRTA. If a patient with pRTA wastes phosphate, the hyperphosphaturia may increase the risk of CaP precipitation. Unlike dRTA, urine pH is only high when alkali therapy is attempted to raise the plasma $[HCO_3^-]$ when the filtered load exceeds the proximal reabsorptive capacity; otherwise the urine is maximally acidic at baseline, thus negating the risk of CaP precipitation. Patients with generalized proximal dysfunction such as the Fanconi syndrome have abnormal proximal citrate reabsorption that precludes hypocitraturia. Patients with monogenic isolated pRTA from mutations of the NBC have defective basolateral

Table 19.2: Etiology of dRTA.

Type	*Etiology*	*Clinical feature/condition*
Congenital: monogenic mutations	B1	Autosomal recessive. Early onset hearing loss
	a4	Autosomal recessive. Late onset hearing loss
	AE1	Autosomal recessive or dominant forms. Hemolytic anemia
	CA	Autosomal recessive. Mixed pRTA and dRTA
Acquired conditions	Autoimmune diseases	Sjögren syndrome, systemic lupus erythematosus, cryoglubulinemia, primary biliary cirrhosis, thyroiditis
	Dysproteinemic states	Hyperglobulinemia, paraprotein states
	Endocrine hypercalciuria	Hyperparathyroidism, vitamin D intoxication, medullary sponge kidney, idiopathic hypercalciuria
	Drugs and toxins	Amphotericin B, lithium, Vanadate, Cyclamate, carbonic anhydrase inhibitors
	Tubulointerstitial disease	Interstitial nephritis, chronic pyelonephritis, obstructive uropathy, Balkan nephropathy, renal transplantation, bariatric surgery with hyperoxaluria
	Liver disease	Autoimmune hepatitis, cirrhosis.

(dRTA: Distal renal tubular acidosis; CA: Carbonic anhydrase; pRTA: Proximal renal tubular acidosis).

HCO_3^- exit, which results in intracellular alkalinization and physiologic citraturia. Regardless of the underlying mechanism, the high urinary citrate chelates calcium in a soluble complex and prevents crystallization.

Combined pRTA and dRTA, which was originally classified as type 3, was christened "juvenile RTA," a condition that was ill-defined and its existence has been questioned. However, inactivating mutations of the CA II enzyme do cause mixed pRTA and dRTA, nephrocalcinosis, and nephrolithiasis. Although this congenital disease is exceedingly rare, pharmacologic inhibition of CA causing RTA is much more common and does predispose subjects to nephrolithiasis. The main pathophysiologic factors in CA inhibition are mainly hypocitraturia and alkalinuria. Although this was originally described for acetazolamide, a much more commonly used drug nowadays against seizures, migraines, and weight loss is topiramate.[20] This condition will be discussed in more detail later.

By far the most common form of RTA is dRTA, whose features are summarized in Table 19.1. Clinically, dRTA has been categorized into hyperkalemic and hypokalemic varieties. The underlying etiology and pathophysiology of these two conditions can share some commonalities but overall, they are quite different. We will focus mostly on the hypokalemic type of dRTA, also referred to as type I.

Causes of dRTA

The etiology of dRTA can be broadly classified into congenital and acquired varieties (Table 19.2). Inactivating mutations of CA are rare but more common genetic forms of dRTA are mutations of the B1 and a4 subunit of the V-ATPase, and the AE1. Mutations of these proteins are summarized in several recent reviews[2,3,5] and will not be further elaborated upon in this chapter. A catalog of recently described mutations is provided in Table 19.3. Mutations in the B1 (V_1 peripheral domain) and a4 (V_0 transmembrane domain) lead to autosomal recessive dRTA. The basis for B1 dysfunction is primarily inability to incorporate into the holoenzyme,[21] while the mechanism of how a4 affects V-ATPase function is not known.[22] It was postulated that heterozygous carriers of mutant B1 may have idRTA due to haploinsufficiency.[23] AE1 mutations can cause nonfunctional protein, unstable protein, or defective trafficking to the cell membrane.[18] The basis for the dominant inheritance in AE1 mutations can be due to dominant negative effects of the mutant AE1 on trafficking on the heterozygous dimers and oligomers.[24] Another intriguing mechanism that was shown thus far only in vitro is loss of polarized targeting resulting in HCO_3^- transport in both the apical and basolateral membrane, resulting in nullification of net acid-base transport.[25] In CA II mutation, RTA is from inadequate generation of the H^+/HCO_3^- pair in both proximal and distal segments and is a pan-tubular RTA.[26]

More common than the congenital variety are acquired forms of dRTA, whose causes are listed in Table 19.2. The autoimmune inflammatory diseases are the most common cause of acquired dRTA. The hypokalemia can be severe, giving rise to paralysis.[27,28] The classic association with

Table 19.3: Catalog of mutations causing distal renal tubular acidosis.

Gene (protein)	*Mutation type*	*Nucleotide change*	*Amino acid change*
ATP6V1B1 (B1 subunit of V-ATPase)	Missense	227G>T	R76S
		232G>A	G78R
		242T>C	L81P
		368G>T	G123V
		370C>T	R124W
		469C>T	R157C
		481G>A	E161K
		521T>G	M174R
		823A>C	T275P
		947G>A	G316E
		988G>A	E330K
		1037C>G	P346R
		1090G>A	G364S
		1181G>A	R394Q
		1449G>A	R465H
	Nonsense	33delG	L19X
		91C>T	R31X
		1251C>G	Y417X
	Frameshift	497delC	T166fsX174
		668_683del	I223fsX509
		1155–1156delC	I386fsX395
		1155–1156insC	I386fsX441
		1401–1402dupGT	F468fsX487
	Splice-site	Intron 2	
		Intron 6	
		Intron 7	
		Intron 8	
		Intron 9	
	Insertion	978_979insGCC	A326insA
ATP6V0a4 (a4 subunit of V-ATPase)	Missense	5T>C	V2A
		524G>A	G175D
		1346G>A	R449H
		1571C>T	P524L
		1739T>C	M580T
		2420G>A	R807Q
		2458G>A	G820R
		2521T>C	X841Q

Contd...

Contd...

Gene (protein)	*Mutation type*	*Nucleotide change*	*Amino acid change*
	Nonsense	16 C>T	R6X
		322C>T	Q108X
		367G>T	E123X
		387C>A	Y129X
		571C>T	R191X
		580C>T	R194X
		727C_T	R243X
		1072C>T	Q358X
		1185_1186insC	E429X
		1350T>A	Y450X
		1506T>A	Y502X
		2257C>T	Q753X
		2308C>T	R770X
		2521T>C	X841Q
	Frameshift	105delT	V35fs
		187–188delAG	R63fsX74
		198–201delT	F67fsX77
		243–244insTC	E82fsX87
		306–307insA	L103fsX139
		337–8delA	N113fsX117
		828–831delAACA	Q276fsX301
		1181–85delC	P395fsX407
		1221delG	M408fsX410
		1647del	I549fsX850
		2137delG	E713fsX765
		2332delG	V778fsX788
		1832–1833delAGinsT	S611fsX648
	Splice-site	Intron 6	
		Intron 10	
		Intron 12	
		Intron 17	
	Deletion	709–711delAAG	K237del
		1669–1674del	I557L/558Ldel
SLC4A1 (Anion exchanger-1) Autosomal-dominant	Missense	1766G>A	R589H
		1765C>A	R589S
		1765C>T	R589C
		1825G>A	G609R
		1838C>T	S613F
		2573C>A	A858D
		2840T>C	M909T
	Nonsense	2661_2681del	A888L/D889X
		2687_2700dup	R901X
	Frameshift	2713dupG	D905fsX915

Contd...

Contd...

Gene (protein)	Mutation type	Nucleotide change	Amino acid change
SLC4A1 (Anion exchanger 1) Autosomal-recessive	Missense	268G>A	E90K
		1437C>G	C479W
		1462G>A	V488M
		1480G/A	G494S
		1564 G>A	E522K
		1805G>C	R602H
		2000C>T	S667P
		2102G>A	G701D
		2317T>C	S773P
		2277G>T	Q759H
	Deletion	1197_1224del	del400_408
		2548_2550delGTG	delV850

(V-ATPases: Vacuolar-adenosine triphosphatase).

Sjögren's syndrome was known for over four decades.[29] In a recent series of ~150 consecutive patients with dRTA and features suggestive of Sjögren's syndrome, a third of them were proven to be Sjögren's syndrome.[29] While proteinuria reflects glomerular involvement, nephrolithiasis from either complete or incomplete RTA (unmasked by acidification test) is associated with interstitial nephritis,[31] which can be present in up to 80% of patients.[32] Urinary biochemical abnormalities are present even in stone formers who are in fact at risk and idRTA is common.[33-35] In addition to dRTA, pRTA can also be present in Sjögren's syndrome.[30,36]

The nephrologist is often preoccupied with the glomerular complications of systemic lupus erythematosus (SLE), but the interstitial nephritis can also be devastating. Distal RTA was noted to occur in SLE patients with the hypokalemic variety being more common than the hyperkalemic type,[37,38] which can precede the other clinical features of SLE.[39] Subtle subclinical renal acidification defects were reported in 12 patients with SLE and normal serum bicarbonate in 1967.[40] Distal RTA can be seen in a variety of autoimmune diseases such as thyroiditis[41] and hyperglobulinemic states.[42]

Absence of the H^+-ATPase has been documented in both Sjögren's and SLE, presumably reflecting immune destruction of the tubules,[43-45] and circulating antisera against components of the α-intercalated cells has been proposed.[46-48] A model of intact pump but leakage of bicarbonate has also been proposed.[48,49] In addition to tubular lesions, upstream dysfunctional regulation, such as hyporeninemic hypoaldosteronism has also been described in autoimmune dRTA.[50]

Patients with liver disease often have distal tubule acidification defects,[51] and dRTA is well described in primary biliary cirrhosis, probably through an autoimmune mechanism.[52] In cirrhosis with portal hypertension, the reduced distal sodium delivery can also give rise to a functional defect in distal acidification.[51] The Fanconi type of pan-proximal tubular defect is often seen in paraprotein tubulopathy, but dRTA can also be encountered.[53,54] A number of endocrinopathies lead to dRTA by causing nephrocalcinosis secondary to hypercalciuria.[55,56]

EPIDEMIOLOGY OF dRTA AND UROLITHIASIS

A widely accepted belief is that urolithiasis is common in dRTA but dRTA is a rare cause of urolithiasis. Although there is some truth to this statement, the true prevalence of dRTA in kidney stone formers is actually not known. Most clinicians experienced with kidney stone patients will share their anecdotal experience of very few cases of full-blown dRTA in their practice compared to other causes of kidney stones. On closer examination, this notion may not be entirely correct. First of all, not all dRTA patients present overtly in the classical configuration of nonanion gap metabolic acidosis and alkalinuria. The late Oliver Wrong described the condition of idRTA where the abnormal renal acid excretion is subtle enough that plasma [HCO_3^-] is maintained. Although hypocitraturia is an almost universal finding in this condition, the UpH may not be frankly alkaline. This completely incapacitates the ability of the practitioner to make the diagnosis based on conventional clinical criteria, and the acid secretion defect needs to be unmasked by acid loading tests. The metabolic sequelae of chronic acid retention in idRTA are hypocitraturia and to some extent hypercalciuria, which both favor the development of calcium-containing stones.[57] The etiology of idRTA remains obscure in many cases. One report suggested that haploinsufficiency of a truncation mutation of B1 can possibly account for idRTA.[23] Furthermore, while single cases with transitions of idRTA to overt dRTA are encountered, it is unknown if these two entities represent different stages of a common disease process or not. There is currently a limited comprehensive database to define the prevalence of abnormal acidification in using provocative tests in the general calcium stone-forming population.

Although overt dRTA is uncommon in the general calcareous stone-forming population, idRTA is found more frequently. In multiple small, single-center studies, the prevalence of idRTA ranged from 2–21% in general calcium stone-forming populations. In patients with recurrent CaP stones, idRTA or even frank dRTA is even more prevalent. Some of these reports are summarized in Table 19.4.

CLINICAL MANIFESTATIONS OF dRTA

Despite the seemingly uniform final common manifestations, the underlying causes of dRTA are very diverse (Table 19.2). In addition to the dRTA, the patient can present with the features of the underlying disease.

Familial Features

For the congenital forms of Mendelian dRTA, extrarenal manifestations are common due to the presence of the V-ATPase subunits, CA II, and AE1 in extrarenal organs. Hearing loss is common in V-ATPase subunit and CA II mutations. Conductive hearing loss is typically seen in CA II mutations from osteopetrosis, whereas B1 and a4 subunit mutations cause sensorineural hearing loss. In contrast, patients with AE1 mutations usually exhibit no hearing loss. Hemolytic anemia is common in autosomal-recessive AE1 mutations, rare in autosomal-dominant AE1 mutations, and absent in V-ATPase mutations. Patients with CA II mutations typically present with cerebral calcifications, developmental delay, facial dysmorphism, and variable cognitive impairment.

Manifestations of the Underlying Diseases

The underlying diseases are summarized in Table 19.2. It is important to be cognizant of the signs and symptoms of these conditions so the right investigations can be ordered. As indicated above, abnormal renal acidification is not uncommon in patients with CaP, recurrent, or bilateral urolithiasis, so idRTA may be present in a lot of conditions listed in Table 19.2. This still comes down to the perpetually recommended approach that is enjoying waning popularity—a well-executed history and physical examination.

Urolithiasis

The classical calculus in overt dRTA is composed of CaP, coming in various flavors such as apatite [$Ca_5(F/PO_4)_3$], hydroxylapatite [$Ca_5(OH/PO_4)_3$], brushite ($CaHPO_4$*$2H_2O$), dahlite [$Ca_{10}[(PO_4,CO_3)_6(OH,CO_3)_2$], or whitlockite [β-$Ca_3$-$(PO_4)_2$]. Pure CaP calculi are rare, however, and most calculi contain some amount of calcium oxalate. In their analysis of ~50,000 stones, Daudon and colleagues found that dRTA was associated with carbonated apatite stones of characteristic morphology with an embossed and smooth shiny surface and small cracks (Figs. 19.4A to C).[76] The degree of CaP admixture is accurately reflected by magnitudes of brushite supersaturation.[77] As the stone composition changes from calcium oxalate to mixed calcium oxalate-calcium apatite, and finally to calcium apatite, the prevalence of dRTA increases from 5% to 40%.[78,79] The high urine pH promotes primarily CaP stones but the hypocitraturia, which can be marked, and hypercalciuria, can also predispose to calcium oxalate stones.

Nephrocalcinosis

The concurrent existence of RTA and nephrocalcinosis has been known since in 1950s[81,82] and the order of causality is bidirectional; nephrocalcinosis can be a result of dRTA, or alternatively dRTA can be caused by nephrocalcinosis.[83] Some have postulated that the interstitial ectopic calcification may be a variant of Randall's plaques,[84] whereas cortical nephrocalcinosis can result from nonspecific tissue damage, medullary nephrocalcinosis reflects distinct pathologies.[85] Distal RTA has been touted to account for half of the cases of medullary nephrocalcinosis.[86] The pathogenesis of nephrocalcinosis in dRTA is not well understood but likely involves the same lithogenic factors

Table 19.4: Prevalence of abnormal renal acidification in stone-formers.

Author	*Subgroup of stone-formers*	*Definition of abnormal renal acidification*	*Remarks*
Joshi et al.[58]	39 patients with first stone episode	Urinary pH >5.5 in short NH_4Cl loading test	Two of 39 patients with idRTA (5%)
Arampatzis et al.[59]	150 consecutive male idiopathic recurrent calcium stone formers	Urinary pH >5.32 in 3-day NH_4Cl loading test	Ten of 150 patients (6.7%) had idRTA. Patients with idRTA had higher 2-hour fasting and 24-hour urinary pH, 24-hour urinary calcium but lower 24-hour urinary citrate. No significant difference in bone mineral density (lumbar spine or femoral neck)
Stitchantrakul et al.[60]	86 consecutive recurrent calcium stone formers	Urinary pH >5.5 in short NH_4Cl loading test	Seven of 86 patients (8.1%) with idRTA. Patients with idRTA tended to have less urinary citrate and higher calcium/citrate ratio than idiopathic calcium stone formers, but hypercalciuria was uncommon
Ito et al.[61]	474 consecutive recurrent calcium stone formers	Urinary pH >5.4 in short NH_4Cl loading test	11 of 474 patients (2.3%) with RTA (10 incomplete, 1 complete)
Gault et al.[62]	30 recurrent calcium oxalate and 24 recurrent calcium phosphate stone formers. 15 healthy volunteers	Urinary pH >5.25 in short NH_4Cl loading test	All patients with recurrent calcium oxalate stones and nonstone-formers acidified urine to pH <5.25. Eight of 23 (34%) calcium phosphate stone formers failed to acidify urinary pH below 5.25
Osther et al.[63]	90 recurrent calcium stone formers	Urinary pH >5.4 in short NH_4Cl loading test	15 patients (16.6%) with dRTA (14 incomplete, 1 complete)
Osther et al.[64]	110 recurrent calcium stone formers	Urinary pH >5.4 in short NH_4Cl loading test	14 patients (12.7%) with dRTA (13 incomplete, 1 complete)
Osther et al.[65]	40 consecutive patients with first stone episode	Urinary pH >5.4 in short ammonium chloride loading test	Two of 40 patients had idRTA (2%)
Mateos Antón et al.[66]	50 consecutive recurrent stone formers	Urinary pH >5.5 in arginine chloride loading test	Two patients (4%) with dRTA (1 incomplete, 1 complete)
Wikström et al.[67]	389 consecutive stone formers	Urinary pH >5.4 in short NH_4Cl loading test	26 (6 males, 20 female) of 389 (275 male, 114 females) patients with idRTA (7%)
Backman et al.[68]	318 consecutive recurrent stone formers	Urinary pH >5.5 in short NH_4Cl loading test	26 of 310 patients with idRTA (8.3%)
Cintron-Nadal et al.[69]	120 recurrent calcium stone formers	Urinary pH >5.3 in short NH_4Cl loading test	Eight of 120 patients with idRTA (6.7%)
D'Angelo et al.[70]	28 patients with bilateral recurrent calcium-containing staghorn calculi and chronic pyelonephritis. 14 had normal renal function, 14 had mild renal insufficiency	Urinary pH >5.3 in short NH_4Cl loading test	(9/14) 64% of patients with normal GFR and (10/14) 71.4% of patients with reduced GFR had idRTA
Backman et al.[71]	51 idiopathic recurrent calcium stone formers	Urinary pH >5.4 in short NH_4Cl loading test	Three patients (5.9%) with dRTA (2 incomplete, 1 complete)
Williams et al.[72]	120 patients with symptomatic or asymptomatic nephrolithiasis	Urinary pH >5.3 in short NH_4Cl loading test	34 patients (21%) with RTA (30 incomplete, 4 complete)
Tannen et al.[73]	17 recurrent calcium stone formers	Urinary pH >5.35 in short NH_4Cl loading test	One patient with idRTA (5.9%)
Sommerkamp et al.[75]	15 patients with recurrent bilateral calcium phosphate calculi	Urinary pH >5.4 in short NH_4Cl loading test	Six patients with idRTA (40%)

(idRTA: Incomplete distal renal tubular acidosis; RTA: Renal tubular acidosis; dRTA: Distal renal tubular acidosis; GFR: Glomerular filtration rate).

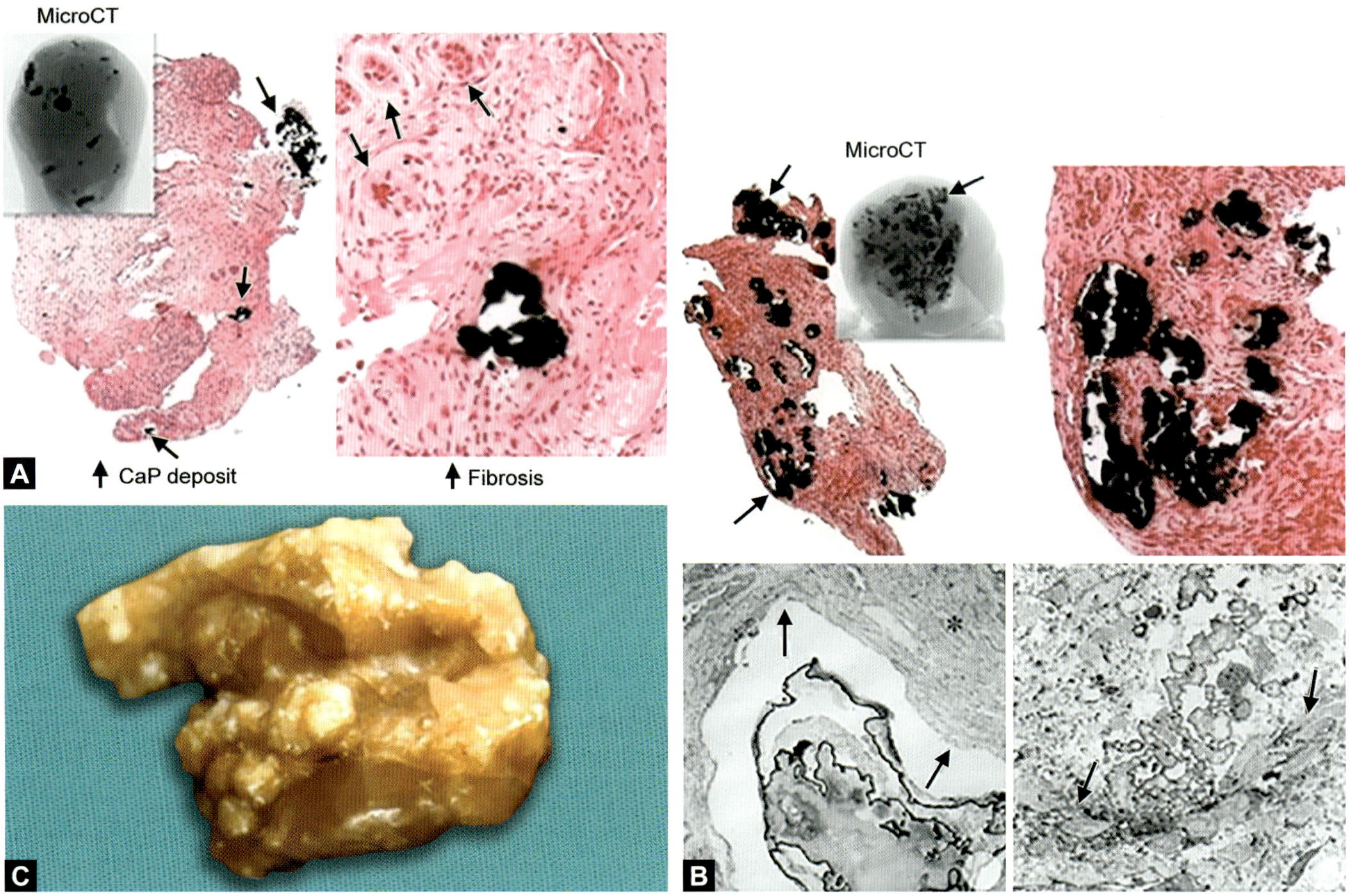

Figs. 19.4A to C: Histopathological abnormalities and a representative stone in distal renal tubular acidosis (dRTA). (A) Biopsy from a patient with minimal inner medullary collecting duct (IMCD) plugging (arrows); the micro-computed tomography (CT) (inset) shows the intratubular location and the infrequent crystal deposits. At higher magnification (right panel) diffuse interstitial fibrosis is present (arrows). (B) Biopsy from another patient with more diffused IMCD plugging with fibrosis. Deposits (arrows) are also seen on micro-CT (inset). Transmission electron microscopy: The bottom panels show tissue from the same patient showing complete loss of cells (arrows) and interstitial fibrosis (asterisk). (C) Example of a calcium phosphate (CaP) stone from a patient with dRTA showing the smooth surface with glazed appearance and small cracks. Daudon et al. proposed that this morphology is almost exclusively found in stones associated with dRTA.
Source: (B) Adapted with permission from Evan et al.[80]
Source: (C) With permission from Daudon et al.[76]

that also foster the development of stones. The prevalence typically depends on the severity of the disease, with late occurrence in autosomal-dominant AE1 mutations but early and severe occurrence in autosomal-recessive AE1 and V-ATPase mutations. In contrast, in patients with CA II mutations, nephrocalcinosis seems to be rare.[87]

Bone Disease

Acidification of resorption pits requires functional CA II in osteoclasts, hence patients with CA II mutations typically present with osteopetrosis. The most detailed studies using bone mineral density and histomorphometry in dRTA patients are from Thailand.[87-90] With the exception of RTA from CA II deficiency, patients with dRTA typically present with low bone mass primarily due to reduced bone formation and turnover rates, and to some extent defective mineralization, and reduced noncollagenous proteins. The low bone density and formation rate was not associated with hypercalciuria but with metabolic acidosis, and both of these parameters improved with alkali therapy.[89] Overt osteomalacia is rare in dRTA,[88] but dRTA from Sjögren's syndrome can be concomitant with proximal tubule phosphate wasting and secondary osteomalacia.[91,92]

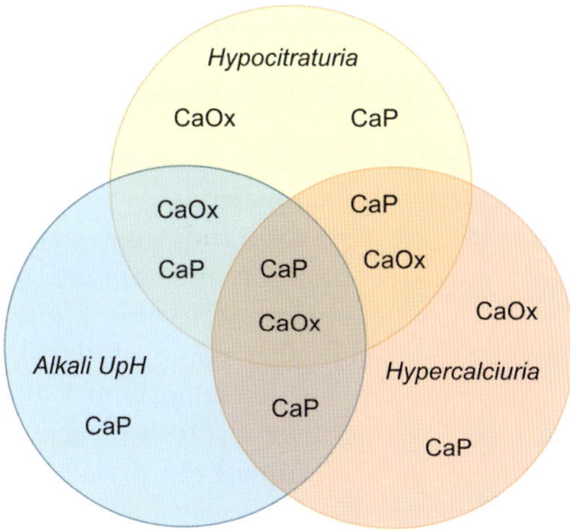

Fig. 19.5: Three fundamental urine biochemical abnormalities in distal renal tubular acidosis (dRTA). Urinary abnormalities predispose to both calcium oxalate (CaOx) or calcium phosphate (CaP) stone formation. A given individual may have a combination of the three risk factors in different degrees. Alkalinuria and hypocitraturia are more prevalent and more severe than hypercalciuria in dRTA.

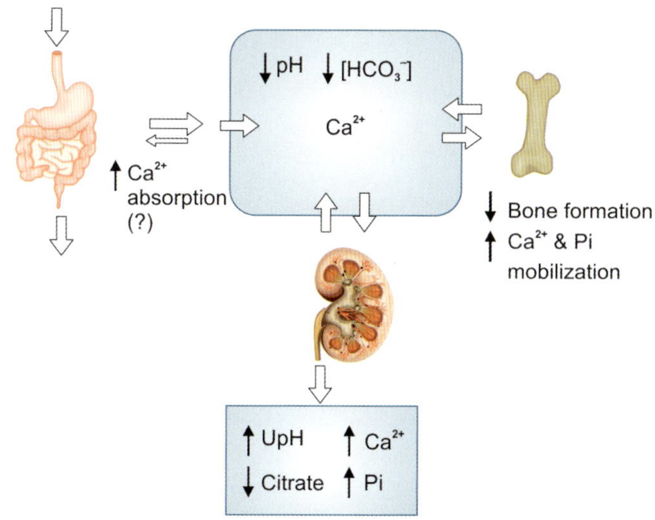

Fig. 19.6: Multisystem pathophysiology in distal renal tubular acidosis (dRTA). The urinary abnormalities are generated by three organs: (1) There is an ill-defined but possible contribution from increased gut absorption; (2) systemic acidosis decreases bone formation and increases calcium and phosphate release. (3) Alkalinuria and hypocitraturia are the two primary pathogenic factors in lithogenesis. Alkalinuria is from inadequate H^+ secretion and failure to reabsorb HCO_3^-. The systemic acidosis causes avid proximal tubule citrate reabsorption, resulting in hypocitraturia. The increased calcium load from bone and direct effects of acidosis on the tubule both lead to hypercalciuria. Increased phosphate release from bone as well as suppression of proximal tubule phosphate reabsorption by acidosis also contribute to a modest degree of hyperphosphaturia in some patients, which can be a contributor to calcium phosphate kidney stone formation.

PATHOPHYSIOLOGY OF UROLITHIASIS IN dRTA

How does an acid-base disorder present itself with kidney stone formation? To dissect out the pathology, one needs to examine the principal urinary abnormalities, which are hypocitraturia, alkalinuria, and hypercalciuria, and one needs to investigate three organs for origins of these abnormalities. The overall scheme is summarized in Figure 19.5 and discussed below.

Anatomic Abnormality

Abnormal urinary chemistry alone, as in the case of an imbalance of promoters and inhibitors of crystallization-agglomeration-growth, can cause crystalluria but is unlikely to be sufficient to cause urolithiasis. There are epithelial factors that may promote adhesion and growth. Evan and colleagues performed intraoperative papillary and cortical biopsies in five patients with dRTA (one with Sjögren's syndrome and the others with undefined etiologies), all of whom had multiple lithotrypsies and normal renal function.[80] The main abnormalities were plugging of inner medullary collecting ducts and ducts of Bellini with mainly apatite along with epithelial cell injury. Obliterated ducts were surrounded by interstitial fibrosis, along with general interstitial fibrosis even away from the plugs (*see* Fig. 19.4). In five patients, the radiographic, surgical, and histologic abnormalities were quite variable in severity. The parenchymal damage and fibrosis may be a result of the underlying disease, a reaction to the CaP precipitate, trauma from repeated lithotripsy, or all of the above.

Intestine

The gut affects acid-base homeostasis by absorbing sources of nonvolatile acid (sulfur-containing and cationic amino acids in proteins) but also base in the form of metabolizable organic anions. Unlike bone and kidney, intestinal absorption likely plays a minor role in the adaptation to metabolic acidosis.[93] However, in patients with idRTA and healthy subjects on an acidogenic high-protein diet, increased intestinal absorption of calcium and thus involvement of the gut in the development of acid-induced hypercalciuria was shown (Fig. 19.6),[94,95] although nonacid-related hypercalciuric effects of protein also exist.[97] It is intriguing and puzzling that the correction of metabolic acidosis by alkali therapy in patients with incomplete RTA caused increased intestinal fractional absorption of calcium from 45% to 60% without changes in 25(OH) or $1,25(OH)_2$ vitamin D, arguing against acidosis causing increased intestinal calcium absorption.[94] The mechanism by which calcium absorption is modulated by dRTA is unknown.

Bone

Bone disease and hypercalciuria are complexly linked in idiopathic hypercalciuria,[97] but in dRTA the bone lesion has been described in the absence of hypercalciuria.[88] There is likely a relationship between the acid load and an osteogenic source of calcium. During metabolic acidosis, acid is buffered by the largest alkali reservoir of the body, the bony skeleton, which releases ample amounts of cations, mainly calcium, into the circulation via physicochemical as well as cell-mediated mechanisms.[98] It is most likely that bone buffering of the acid load is contributing to the hypercalciuria as alkali therapy significantly reduces the hypercalciuria.[94,99]

Kidney

The kidney plays a central role in promoting stone formation. The inability to secrete H^+ leads to high urine pH and higher divalent phosphate concentration, thus, promoting CaP precipitation. In addition to alkalinuria, the kidney also contributes to hypercalciuria. Acid inhibits paracellular calcium reabsorption in the proximal tubule, the thick ascending limb and transcellular reabsorption in the distal convoluted tubule,[100] thus superimposing an added renal calcium leak to the hypercalciuria.

Although hypercalciuria is an important prolithogenic factor in the setting of dRTA, it is not the only one. In the setting of acid retention or frank acidosis, the proximal tubule avidly retains citrate, leading to hypocitraturia. This response makes sense physiologically to defend systemic pH, but it leaves less citrate in the urine to chelate calcium and thus inhibits nucleation and growth of calcium crystals. Whereas hypercalciuria and hypocitraturia are always observed in the setting of metabolic acidosis, the unduly alkaline urine is peculiar to distal tubular acidosis. Supersaturation of CaP is highly dependent on UpH. Virtually no urine is supersaturated below pH 5.3; above pH 6.5 almost all urines are supersaturated for CaP. Thus, alkaline urine represents the third important prolithogenic factor in the setting of dRTA.

Special Scenario with CA Inhibitors

Strictly speaking, inhibition of CA produces combined proximal and distal acidification defects and hence is not a pure form of dRTA. It is discussed here because it does predispose the subject to kidney stones.

In human kidney, both CA II and IV play a critical role for renal H^+ and HCO_3^- transport and both are subject to inhibition by acetazolamide.[101] Carbonic anhydrase II resides in the cytosol of tubular cells, with the exception of the loop of Henle and thin ascending limb.[102] The membrane-associated, extracellular CA IV is present on both apical and basolateral membranes in proximal, and on the apical membrane of α-intercalated cells in the distal nephron. A mixed proximal/dRTA develops with CA inhibition. Chronic treatment regimens with acetazolamide are not commonly employed today except for glaucoma. Much more frequently used is topiramate, which has multiple pharmacologic actions, among them inhibition of CA. Indications for topiramate include seizure disorders, migraine, and weight loss. Treatment with topiramate causes systemic metabolic acidosis with a reduction in urinary citrate, increased fractional excretion of HCO_3^-, a rise in UpH and Ca excretion, which is identical to dRTA. These changes increase the supersaturation for CaP significantly and predispose the subject to CaP stones.[20,103] In short-term studies that led to approval of the drug by the FDA, the claim was that 1–2% of patients developed kidney stones; however, this is an underestimate due to short duration of follow-up and also many asymptomatic stone formers. In chronic topiramate users, the incidence and prevalence of symptomatic nephrolithiasis are variable but much higher than the initial estimate. This is summarized in Table 19.5. In a cohort of chronic topiramate users without symptomatic nephrolithiasis, the prevalence of asymptomatic stones by CT scan was as high as 20%.[74] Thus, chronic topiramate is a risk factor for the development of calcareous stones and physicians prescribing the drug must be aware of it.

EVALUATION AND TREATMENT OF DRTA AND DRTA-ASSOCIATED UROLITHIASIS

As should be evident from the diverse causes of secondary dRTA, a carefully executed history and physical examination by an internist is a critical first step in the evaluation. All the basic tests one orders for evaluation of calcium stones still apply. The issue is what specific tests one should use if dRTA is suspected as the cause of urolithi-

Table 19.5: Occurrence of kidney stones in topiramate users.

Study	*Number of patients*	*Mean age (years)*	*Average dose (per day)*	*Average treatment duration (months)*	*Stone occurrence*
Symptomatic stones					
Stephen[104]	170	46.5	250–450 mg	6	1.8%
Coppola[105]	45	15.9	4 mg/kg	15.8	4.5%
Corbin Bush[106]	41	9.2	8 mg/kg	27	4.9%
Coppola[107]	18	9.0	5 mg/kg	11.9	5.6%
Cudkowicz[108]	197	57.8	400–800 mg	12	9.1%
Maalouf[74]	75	40	300 mg	48	10.7%
Goyal[109]	24	20	7.9 mg/kg	36	54%
Stones by imaging					
Mahmoud[110]	96	6.0	NA	10–23	5% incident
Corbin Bush[106]	41	9.2	8 mg/kg	27	4.8% prevalent
Maalouf[74]	75	40	300 mg	48	20% prevalent

(NA: Not available).

asis. There are tests that are clearly available in every routine clinical practice and laboratory; one just has to know how to interpret the results. Other tests may be harder to come by but are still available in some facilities. Here, one needs to know when they need to be used and seek referral. Finally, there are tests that are performed solely in a research setting. One needs to know how to use them when contemplating investigative work and how to interpret the literature.

When dRTA is present in its full-blown form, the diagnosis is obvious. This is the classical NAG metabolic acidosis of hypobicarbonatemia with high urinary pH. As stated above, incomplete forms exist that are not readily detected in routine clinical tests and need to be searched by provocative tests.

Baseline Tests

- *Serum chemistry:* The classic nonanion gap metabolic acidosis is very helpful when present, but the serum [HCO_3^-] can be very mildly depressed or even normal in idRTA. Part of this is due to some ability to excrete acid and a low dietary acid or high dietary alkali load.
- *Urinary pH:* dRTA is characterized by inability to pump H^+ into the urine so UpH. In complete dRTA, random UpH is often 7.0 or higher and almost never below 6.5. Alkali UpH per se is not abnormal, particularly when serum [HCO_3^-] is not low, because the high UpH may be appropriate for a high alkali intake. Urinary pH can be diagnostic in the setting of an acid load (see below).
- *Urinary citrate:* Hypocitraturia is an invariant finding in dRTA.[111] Although citrate handling is exclusively a proximal tubule event, the systemic acidosis and, when present, hypokalemia will both acidify the proximal tubule cell and stimulate citrate uptake and metabolism (*see* Chapter 10). It is highly unusual to have dRTA and normal citrate excretion except when a patient consumes a high alkali (surrogate high 24 hour K^+ excretion >70 mEq/day) and low acid diet (surrogate low 24 hour SO_4^{2-} <20 mEq/day).
- *Urinary anion gap:* The UAG defined as urine $Na^+ + K^+ - Cl^-$.[112] This number is numerically equal to (all anions that not are Cl^-) - (all cations that not Na^+ or K^+). The original purpose was to have a quick way to estimate urine [NH_4^+], which is critical for diagnosing dRTA,[113] but for unjustified reasons this test is not readily available to clinicians. Abundance of NH_4Cl in the urine will render the UAG more negative. When comparing two conditions with very high (intestinal base loss) or very low (dRTA) urinary NH_4Cl, the UAG segregates clearly and has led to the arbitrary cut-off of "positive versus negative" UAG to assess renal acidification.[114] There are several caveats that the clinician must be cognizant of when using the UAG. Even when the UAG is zero, there is still 80 mEq/L of NH_4^+ in the urine, which is not a trivial amount of acid.[112,114] Urinary anion gap is really an estimate of NH_4Cl, so when ample amounts of NH_4SO_4 (high protein intake) or NH_4 hippurate (toluene

toxicity) are being excreted, both NH_4^+ and the anion are unaccounted for in the UAG equation; thus, UAG grossly underestimates urinary NH_4^+. This led to the use of the urinary osmolar gap (UOG).

- *Urinary osmolar gap:* While NH_4^+ with an anion other than Cl^- will not render the UAG more negative, it will introduce osmoles that are not Na^+, K^+, urea, and glucose—the most abundant osmoles.[115] Therefore, the urine osmolal gap (UOG), which is measured in osmoles - estimated osmoles [2(Na^+) + 2[K^+] + glucose + urea; all in mmoles), will be elevated beyond its normal value of ~ 80–100 mOsm.
- *Urine-blood PCO_2:* The CO_2 tension of urine is usually higher than blood and its magnitude is determined by the quantity of HCO_3^- in the lumen as well as all factors that stimulate collecting H^+ secretion.[116,117] While parameters such as UpH reflect the ability of the collecting duct to mount and sustain a H^+ gradient, it does not assess H^+ flux.[118,119] In order for the urine PCO_2 to increase, there has to be adequate H^+ transport into the urine.

Provocative Acid-Loading Tests

Provocative tests are employed to unmask subtle urinary acidification deficits. The gold standard is the short ammonium chloride loading test as described by Oliver Wrong in 1959.[120] Absence of a systemic acidosis (prior to the administration of ammonium chloride) and failure to acidify the urine below a pH of 5.3 are diagnostics for idRTA. The main problems with this test are nausea and emesis, which occur in a portion of patients. In our experience, premedication with an antiemetic and allowing the patient enough time (30 minutes) to swallow the capsules in divided doses greatly alleviate the problem. Alternative tests with improved tolerability have been described, including the furosemide/fludrocortisone test[121] and administration of $CaCl_2$.[122] However, due to a lack of rigorous comparative studies, the validity of the different provocative test protocols in patients with nephrolithiasis is currently unknown.

Genotyping

In the case of positive family history, early onset of disease or presence of extrarenal symptoms (hearing loss, hemolytic anemia), a genetic cause of the dRTA should be sought. Currently, the leading candidates are B1, a4, and AE1 (Table 19.2). CA II deficiency is exceeding rare and the clinical manifestations are more characteristic, so routine clinical genotyping may not be necessary.

Treatment of dRTA

The management of dRTA needs to be directed at the treatment of the underlying cause, if such can be identified. This cannot be overemphasized. For example, the interstitial nephritis and the dRTA of Sjögren syndrome respond favorably to immunosuppressive therapy.[32,123] If treating the primary disease is not possible, therapy should be directed at the chemical abnormalities, i.e. the metabolic acidosis, hypokalemia, and urinary lithogenic chemistry.

The main therapeutic option is alkali, usually administered as a potassium salt. Treatment with alkali for bone and somatic growth in children has been well established for a long time.[124,125] High doses of alkali may be needed in children, especially if there is accompanying proximal HCO_3^- wasting. Alkali therapy for 1 year was enough to show improvement in both weight and height in children with dRTA.[126] In grown adults, treatment with alkali is a little less established. There are no randomized controlled trials for the treatment of nephrolithiasis in adults with dRTA. Even treatment trials for calcium stones in the absence of dRTA have not addressed specifically the outcomes in patients with CaP stones.

One feature that remains unexplained is the discrepancy between the dose of alkali, such as potassium citrate, administered and the urinary citraturic response. It is not unusual that doses > 60 mEq/day are needed to achieve a detectable increase in urinary citrate excretion. Although the increase in 24-hour urinary K^+ may be exactly 60 mEq, thus reflecting compliance and complete gut absorption, the increase in 24-hour urinary citrate is far from 60 mEq. The reason for this poor citraturic response is unclear. Thus very high doses may be required, which can be limited by gastric irritation and in patients with impaired renal function, the dangers of a K^+ load.

If the lithogenicity stems from the metabolic acidosis, neutralizing the excess acid with alkali therapy makes the most sense. However, there is a downside to alkali therapy. Such treatment may raise UpH, thereby worsening urinary CaP supersaturation (Figs. 19.7A to C). There is also an empirical observation without clear mechanism that alkali therapy increases intestinal calcium absorption; an effect that may be counterproductive.[94] Treatment with alkali in adults with dRTA decreases skeletal calcium mobilization and hypercalciuria, increases citraturia, and reduces stone formation.[89,99,127,128] In a related condition, RTA associated with medullary sponge kidney, alkali therapy also led to decrease in stone passage and improvement of the associated bone disease.[129–131] Urinary pH, calcium, citrate, and relative supersaturation of CaP should be monitored

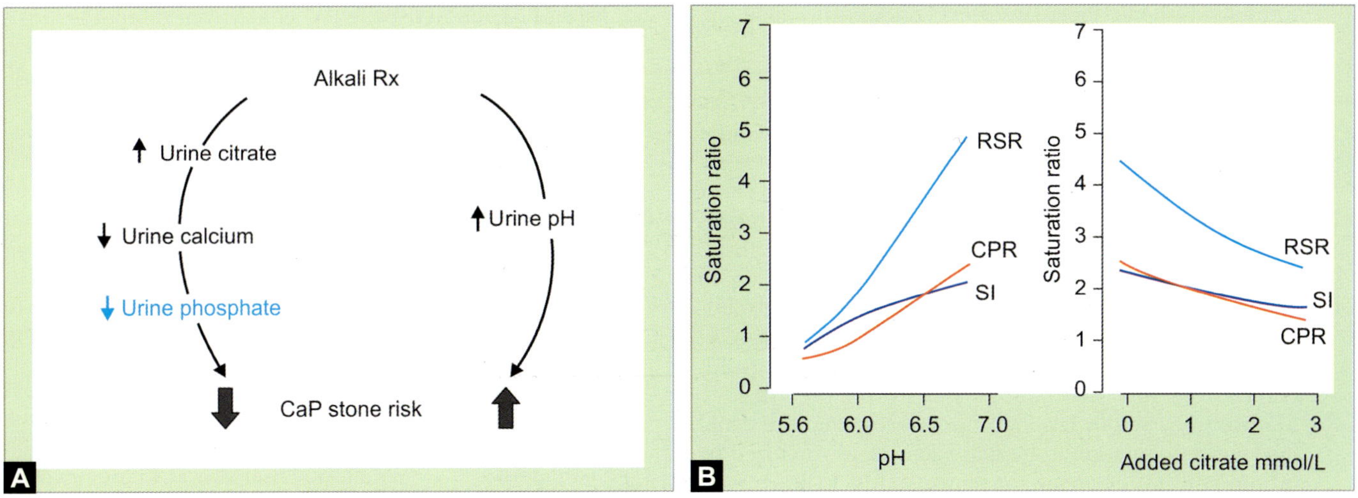

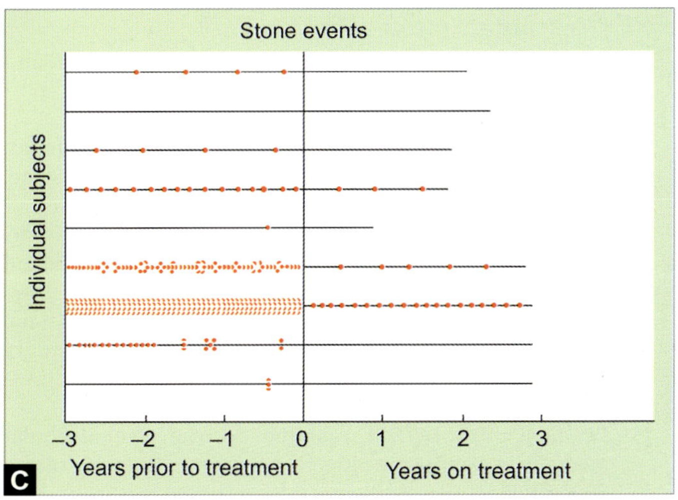

Figs. 19.7A to C: Treating distal renal tubular acidosis (dRTA) with potassium alkali. (A) Comparing the beneficial and deleterious effects of potassium alkali on calcium phosphate (CaP) stone risk. (B) Three predictors of brushite saturation were determined as a function of varying urine pH or citrate. Relative supersaturation ratio (RSR)[132] and saturation index (SI)[133] are computer generated, and concentration-to-product ratio (CPR) is an empirically determined parameter by physicochemical methods.[134]
Source: Data are taken from Pak et al.[135,136] (C) Actual clinical outcome data from Preminger et al.[99] Nine subjects with dRTA were treated with potassium citrate with significant decrease in stone events. Rx, reaction.

repeatedly upon initiation of treatment (Figs. 19.7A to C). If urinary CaP supersaturation rises, the treatment may not be of benefit and even be harmful. There are no definite clinical guidelines regarding target UpH, but a general opinion-based guideline is around 6.8–7.0, although this may be individualized. Computer-based predictive programs can also be used (Figs. 19.7A to C) to assess the composite effect of changes in calciuria, citraturia, and UpH secondary to alkali therapy.

ACKNOWLEDGMENT

The authors are supported by the National Institute of Health (R01-DK081423, R01-DK091392, R01-DK092461, P30 DK-079328, U01-HL111146), the Charles and Jane Pak Foundation, the Simmon Family Foundation, the Swiss National Science Foundation (#3100A0_135503, #3100A0_152829, NCCR Kidney.CH, NCCR TransCure), and by a Medical Research Position Award by the Prof. Dr Max Cloëtta Foundation. We thank Ms Ashlei Johnson for her assistance in the preparation of the chapter.

REFERENCES

1. Lightwood R. Calcium infarction of the kidneys. Arch Dis Child. 1935;10:205-6.
2. Fry AC, Karet FE. Inherited renal acidoses. Physiology. 2007;22:202-11.
3. Batlle D, Haque SK. Genetic causes and mechanisms of distal renal tubular acidosis. Nephrol Dial Transplant. 2012;27:3691-704.
4. Golembiewska E, Ciechanowski K. Renal tubular acidosis—underrated problem? Acta biochimica Polonica. 2012;59: 213-7.
5. Rodriguez Soriano J. Renal tubular acidosis: the clinical entity. J Am Soc Nephrol. 2002;13:2160-70.
6. Moe OW GG, Seldin DW. The logic of the kidney. In: Lifton R SS, Seldin DW, Giebisch G (Eds). Genetic Diseases of the

Kidney. Academic Press (Elsevier) London, UK. 2009. pp. 33-76.

7. Curthoys NM, Moe OW. Proximal tubule function and response to acidosis. Clin J Am Soc Nephrol. 2014;9(9):1627-38.
8. Forster R. Buffering in blood. In: Seldin DW GG (Ed). Seldin and Giebisch's the Kidney: Physiology and Pathophysiology, 1st edition. New York: Raven Press; 1985. pp. 137-48.
9. Gowrishankar M, Kamel KS, Halperin ML. A brain protein centered view of H^+ buffering. J Am Soc Nephrol. 2007;18:2278-80.
10. Hamm LL AR, Preisig PA. Cellular mechanisms of renal tubular acidification. In: Alpern RJ CM, Moe OW (Eds). Seldin and Giebisch's The Kidney: Physiology and Pathophysiology, 5th edition. New York: Academic Press; 2014. pp. 1917-78.
11. Madison LL, Seldin DW. Ammonia excretion and renal enzymatic adaptation in human subjects, as disclosed by administration of precursor amino acids. J Clin Invest. 1958;37:1615-27.
12. Bobulescu IA, Moe OW. Luminal Na^+/H^+exchange in the proximal tubule. Pflugers Archiv Eur J Physiol. 2009;458:5-21.
13. Breton S, Brown D. Regulation of luminal acidification by the V-ATPase. Physiology. 2013;28:318-29.
14. Romero MF, Chen AP, Parker MD, et al. The SLC4 family of bicarbonate (HCO_3^-) transporters. Mol Aspects Med. 2013;34:159-82.
15. Muench SP, Trinick J, Harrison MA. Structural divergence of the rotary ATPases. Q Rev Biophys. 2011;44:311-56.
16. Toei M, Saum R, Forgac M. Regulation and isoform function of the V-ATPases. Biochemistry. 2010;49:4715-23.
17. Bonar PT, Casey JR. Plasma membrane Cl^-/HCO_3^- exchangers: structure, mechanism and physiology. Channels. 2008;2:337-45.
18. Cordat E, Reithmeier RA. Structure, function, and trafficking of SLC4 and SLC26 anion transporters. Curr Top Membr. 2014;73:1-67.
19. Becker HM, Klier M, Deitmer JW. Carbonic anhydrases and their interplay with acid/base-coupled membrane transporters. Subcell Biochem. 2014;75:105-34.
20. Welch BJ, Graybeal D, Moe OW, et al. Biochemical and stone-risk profiles with topiramate treatment. Am J Kid Dis. 2006;48:555-63.
21. Fuster DG, Zhang J, Xie XS, et al. The vacuolar-ATPase B1 subunit in distal tubular acidosis: novel mutations and mechanisms for dysfunction. Kid Int. 2008;73:1151-8.
22. Ochotny N, Van Vliet A, Chan N, et al. Effects of human a3 and a4 mutations that result in osteopetrosis and distal renal tubular acidosis on yeast V-ATPase expression and activity. J Biol Chem. 2006;281:26102-11.
23. Zhang J, Fuster DG, Cameron MA, et al. Incomplete distal renal tubular acidosis from a heterozygous mutation of the V-ATPase B1 subunit. Am J Physiol Renal physiol. 2014;307(9):F1063-71.
24. Quilty JA, Li J, Reithmeier RA. Impaired trafficking of distal renal tubular acidosis mutants of the human kidney anion exchanger kAE1. Am J Physiol Renal Physiol. 2002;282:F810-20.
25. Fry AC, Su Y, Yiu V, et al. Mutation conferring apical-targeting motif on AE1 exchanger causes autosomal dominant distal RTA. J Am Soc Nephrol. 2012;23:1238-49.
26. Nagai R, Kooh SW, Balfe JW, et al. Renal tubular acidosis and osteopetrosis with carbonic anhydrase II deficiency: pathogenesis of impaired acidification. Pediatr Nephrol. 1997;11:633-6.
27. Christensen KS. Hypokalemic paralysis in Sjögren's syndrome secondary to renal tubular acidosis. Scand J Rheumatol. 1985;14:58-60.
28. Poux JM, Peyronnet P, Le Meur Y, et al. Hypokalemic quadriplegia and respiratory arrest revealing primary Sjögren's syndrome. Clin Nephrol. 1992;37:189-91.
29. Kaltreider HB, Talal N. Impaired renal acidification in Sjögren's syndrome and related disorders. Arthritis Rheum. 1969;12:538-41.
30. Ram R, Swarnalatha G, Dakshinamurty KV. Renal tubular acidosis in Sjögren's syndrome: A case series. Am J Nephrol. 2014;40:123-30.
31. Siamopoulos KC, Mavridis AK, Elisaf M, et al. Kidney involvement in primary Sjögren's syndrome. Scand J Rheumatol Suppl. 1986;61:156-60.
32. Ren H, Wang WM, Chen XN, et al. Renal involvement and followup of 130 patients with primary Sjögren's syndrome. J Rheumatol. 2008;35:278-84.
33. Eriksson P, Denneberg T, Tiselius HG. Risk factors of calcium stone formation in patients with primary Sjögren's syndrome. Urol Res. 1996;24:39-43.
34. Eriksson P, Denneberg T, Larsson L, et al. Biochemical markers of renal disease in primary Sjögren's syndrome. Scand J Urol Nephrol. 1995;29:383-92.
35. Nishinarita S, Kinoshita S, Kaneko M, et al. Subclinical renal tubular acidosis in patients with primary and secondary Sjögren's syndrome: a possible marker of disease progression. Mod Rheumatol. 2002;12:318-22.
36. Pessler F, Emery H, Dai L, et al. The spectrum of renal tubular acidosis in paediatric Sjögren syndrome. Rheumatology. 2006;45:85-91.
37. Caruana RJ, Barish CF, Buckalew VM, Jr. Complete distal renal tubular acidosis in systemic lupus: clinical and laboratory findings. Am J Kidney Dis. 1985;6:59-63.
38. Li SL, Liou LB, Fang JT, et al. Symptomatic renal tubular acidosis (RTA) in patients with systemic lupus erythematosus: an analysis of six cases with new association of type 4 RTA. Rheumatology. 2005;44:1176-80.
39. Bagga A, Jain Y, Srivastava RN, et al. Renal tubular acidosis preceding systemic lupus erythematosus. Pediatrc Nephrol. 1993;7:735-6.
40. Tu WH, Shearn MA. Systemic lupus erythematosus and latent renal tubular dysfunction. Ann Int Med. 1967;67:100-9.
41. Mason AM, Golding PL. Renal tubular acidosis and autoimmune thyroid disease. Lancet. 1970;2:1104-7.
42. Mason AM, Golding PL. Hyperglobulinaemic renal tubular acidosis: a report of nine cases. Br Med J. 1970;3:143-6.
43. DeFranco PE, Haragsim L, Schmitz PG, et al. Absence of vacuolar H^+-ATPase pump in the collecting duct of a patient with hypokalemic distal renal tubular acidosis and Sjögren's syndrome. J Am Soc Nephrol. 1995;6:295-301.
44. Cohen EP, Bastani B, Cohen MR, et al. Absence of H^+-ATPase in cortical collecting tubules of a patient with Sjögren's syndrome and distal renal tubular acidosis. J Am Soc Nephrol. 1992;3:264-71.

45. Joo KW, Jeon US, Han JS, et al. Absence of H^+-ATPase in the intercalated cells of renal tissues in classic distal renal tubular acidosis. Clin Nephrol. 1998;49:226-31.
46. Inagaki Y, Jinno-Yoshida Y, Hamasaki Y, et al. A novel autoantibody reactive with carbonic anhydrase in sera from patients with systemic lupus erythematosus and Sjögren's syndrome. J Dermatol Sci. 1991;2:147-54.
47. Takemoto F, Hoshino J, Sawa N, et al. Autoantibodies against carbonic anhydrase II are increased in renal tubular acidosis associated with Sjögren syndrome. Am J Med. 2005;118:181-4.
48. Bastani B, Underhill D, Chu N, et al. Preservation of intercalated cell H^+-ATPase in two patients with lupus nephritis and hyperkalemic distal renal tubular acidosis. J Am Soc Nephrol. 1997;8:1109-17.
49. Zawadzki J. Permeability defect with bicarbonate leak as a mechanism of immune-related distal renal tubular acidosis. Am J Kidney Dis. 1998;31:527-32.
50. Otabe S, Muto S, Asano Y, et al. Selective hypoaldosteronism in a patient with Sjögren's syndrome: insensitivity to angiotensin II. Nephron. 1991;59:466-70.
51. Ahya SN, Jose Soler M, Levitsky J, et al. Acid-base and potassium disorders in liver disease. Sem Nephrol. 2006;26:466-70.
52. Komatsuda A, Wakui H, Ohtani H, et al. Tubulointerstitial nephritis and renal tubular acidosis of different types are rare but important complications of primary biliary cirrhosis. Nephrol Dial Transplant. 2010;25:3575-9.
53. Lazar GS, Feinstein DI. Distal renal tubular acidosis in multiple myeloma. Arch Int Med. 1981;141:655-6.
54. Smithline N, Kassirer JP, Cohen JJ. Light-chain nephropathy. Renal tubular dysfunction associated with light-chain proteinuria. New Engl J Med. 1976;294:71-4.
55. Muthukrishnan J, Hari Kumar KV, Jha R, et al. Distal renal tubular acidosis due to primary hyperparathyroidism. Endocr Prac. 2008;14:1133-6.
56. Liborio AB, Nasserala JC, Gondim AS, et al. The case: renal failure in a bodybuilder athlete. Diagnosis: nephrocalcinosis secondary to exogenous vitamin D intoxication. Kidney Int. 2014;85:1247-8.
57. Buckalew VM, Jr. Nephrolithiasis in renal tubular acidosis. J Urol. 1989;141:731-7.
58. Joshi A, Gupta SK, Srivastava A. Metabolic evaluation in first-time renal stone formers in North India: a single center study. Saudi J Kidney Dis Transpl. 2013;24:838-43.
59. Arampatzis S, Ropke-Rieben B, Lippuner K, et al. Prevalence and densitometric characteristics of incomplete distal renal tubular acidosis in men with recurrent calcium nephrolithiasis. Urol Res. 2012;40:53-9.
60. Stitchantrakul W, Kochakarn W, Ruangraksa C, et al. Urinary risk factors for recurrent calcium stone formation in Thai stone formers. J Med Assoc Thai. 2007;90:688-98.
61. Ito H, Kotake T, Suzuki F. Incidence and clinical features of renal tubular acidosis-1 in urolithiasis. Urol Int. 1993;50:82-5.
62. Gault MH, Chafe LL, Morgan JM, et al. Comparison of patients with idiopathic calcium phosphate and calcium oxalate stones. Medicine. 1991;70:345-59.
63. Osther PJ, Hansen AB, Rohl HF. Distal renal tubular acidosis in recurrent renal stone formers. Dan Med Bull. 1989;36:492-3.
64. Osther PJ, Hansen AB, Rohl HF. Screening renal stone formers for distal renal tubular acidosis. Br J Urol. 1989;63:581-3.
65. Osther PJ, Hansen AB, Rohl HF. Renal acidification defects in patients with their first renal stone episode. Scand J Urol Nephrol Suppl. 1988;110:275-8.
66. Mateos Antón F, Garcia Puig J, Gaspar G, et al. Renal tubular acidosis in recurrent renal stone formers. Eur Urol. 1984;10:55-9.
67. Wikstrom B, Backman U, Danielson BG, et al. Ambulatory diagnostic evaluation of 389 recurrent renal stone formers. A proposal for clinical classification and investigation. Klin Wochenschr. 1983;61:85-90.
68. Backman U, Danielson BG, Johansson G, et al. Incidence and clinical importance of renal tubular defects in recurrent renal stone formers. Nephron. 1980;25:96-101.
69. Cintron-Nadal E, Lespier LE, Roman-Miranda A, et al. Renal acidifying ability in subjects with recurrent stone formation. J Urol. 1977;118:704-6.
70. D'Angelo A, Pagano F, Ossi E, et al. Renal tubular defects in recurring bilateral nephrolithiasis. Clin Nephrol. 1976;6: 352-60.
71. Backman U, Danielson BG, Sohtell M. Urine acidification capacity in renal stone formers. Scand J Urol Nephrol. 1976;Suppl 35:49-61.
72. Williams G, Chisholm GD. Stone screening and follow-up are necessary? Br J Urol. 1975;47:745-50.
73. Tannen RL, Falls WF, Jr, Brackett NC, Jr. Incomplete renal tubular acidosis: some clinical and physiological features. Nephron. 1975;15:111-23.
74. Maalouf NM, Langston JP, Van Ness PC, et al. Nephrolithiasis in topiramate users. Urol Res. 2011;39:303-7.
75. Sommerkamp H, Schwerk WB. Incomplete tubular acidosis in recurrent urinary phosphate calculi. Der Urologe Ausg A. 1973;12:167-72.
76. Daudon M, Bouzidi H, Bazin D. Composition and morphology of phosphate stones and their relation with etiology. Urol Res. 2010;38:459-67.
77. Parks JH, Coward M, Coe FL. Correspondence between stone composition and urine supersaturation in nephrolithiasis. Kidney Int. 1997;51:894-900.
78. Pak CY, Poindexter JR, Adams-Huet B, et al. Predictive value of kidney stone composition in the detection of metabolic abnormalities. Am J Med. 2003;115:26-32.
79. Pak CY, Poindexter JR, Peterson RD, et al. Biochemical and physicochemical presentations of patients with brushite stones. J Urol. 2004;171:1046-9.
80. Evan AP, Lingeman J, Coe F, et al. Renal histopathology of stone-forming patients with distal renal tubular acidosis. Kidney Int. 2007;71:795-801.
81. Farrell RH. Hyperchloraemic renal acidosis of infants (nephrocalcinosis infantum): report of a case and review of literature. Guy's Hosp Rep. 1953;102:234-9.
82. Mortensen J, Baggenstoss AH. Nephrocalcinosis: a review. Am J Clin Pathol. 1954;24:45-63.
83. Moutsopoulos HM, Cledes J, Skopouli FN, et al. Nephrocalcinosis in Sjögren's syndrome: a late sequela of renal tubular acidosis. J Int Med. 1991;230:187-91.

84. Gambaro G, Abaterusso C, Fabris A, et al. The origin of nephrocalcinosis, Randall's plaque and renal stones: a cell biology viewpoint. Arch Ital Urol Androl. 2009;81:166-70.
85. Sayer JA, Carr G, Simmons NL. Nephrocalcinosis: molecular insights into calcium precipitation within the kidney. Clin Sci. 2004;106:549-61.
86. Mantan M, Bagga A, Virdi VS, et al. Etiology of nephrocalcinosis in northern Indian children. Pediatr Nephrol. 2007;22: 829-33.
87. Ismail EA, Abul Saad S, Sabry MA. Nephrocalcinosis and urolithiasis in carbonic anhydrase II deficiency syndrome. Eur J Pediatr. 1997;156:957-62.
88. Domrongkitchaiporn S, Pongsakul C, Stitchantrakul W, et al. Bone mineral density and histology in distal renal tubular acidosis. Kidney Int. 2001;59:1086-93.
89. Domrongkitchaiporn S, Pongskul C, Sirikulchayanonta V, et al. Bone histology and bone mineral density after correction of acidosis in distal renal tubular acidosis. Kidney Int. 2002;62:2160-6.
90. Disthabanchong S, Domrongkitchaiporn S, Sirikulchayanonta V, et al. Alteration of noncollagenous bone matrix proteins in distal renal tubular acidosis. Bone. 2004;35: 604-13.
91. Fulop M, Mackay M. Renal tubular acidosis, Sjögren syndrome, and bone disease. Arch Int Med. 2004;164:905-9.
92. Cherif E, Ben Hassine L, Kaoueche Z, et al. Osteomalacia as inaugural manifestation of Sjögren syndrome. BMJ Case Rep. 2013;2013.
93. Lennon EJ, Lemann J, Jr, Litzow JR. The effects of diet and stool composition on the net external acid balance of normal subjects. J Clin Invest. 1966;45:1601-7.
94. Preminger GM, Sakhaee K, Pak CY. Hypercalciuria and altered intestinal calcium absorption occurring independently of vitamin D in incomplete distal renal tubular acidosis. Metabolism. 1987;36:176-9.
95. Kerstetter JE, O'Brien KO, Caseria DM, et al. The impact of dietary protein on calcium absorption and kinetic measures of bone turnover in women. J Clin Endocrinol Metab. 2005;90:26-31.
96. Maalouf NM, Moe OW, Adams-Huet B, et al. Hypercalciuria associated with high dietary protein intake is not due to acid load. J Clin Endocrinol Metab. 2011;96:3733-40.
97. Sakhaee K, Maalouf NM, Kumar R, et al. Nephrolithiasis-associated bone disease: pathogenesis and treatment options. Kidney Int. 2011;79:393-403.
98. Bushinsky DA. Net calcium efflux from live bone during chronic metabolic, but not respiratory, acidosis. Am J Physiol. 1989;256:F836-42.
99. Preminger GM, Sakhaee K, Skurla C, et al. Prevention of recurrent calcium stone formation with potassium citrate therapy in patients with distal renal tubular acidosis. J Urol. 1985;134:20-3.
100. Moe OW, Huang CL. Hypercalciuria from acid load: renal mechanisms. J Nephrol. 2006;19 Suppl 9:S53-61.
101. Sly WS, Whyte MP, Krupin T, et al. Positive renal response to intravenous acetazolamide in patients with carbonic anhydrase II deficiency. Pediatr Res. 1985;19:1033-6.
102. Purkerson JM, Schwartz GJ. The role of carbonic anhydrases in renal physiology. Kidney Int. 2007;71:103-15.
103. Lamb EJ, Stevens PE, Nashef L. Topiramate increases biochemical risk of nephrolithiasis. Ann Clin Biochem. 2004;41:166-9.
104. Stephen LJ, Sills GJ, Brodie MJ. Topiramate in refractory epilepsy: a prospective observational study. Epilepsia. 2000;41:977-80.
105. Coppola G, Caliendo G, Veggiotti P, et al. Topiramate as add-on drug in children, adolescents and young adults with Lennox-Gastaut syndrome: an Italian multicentric study. Epilepsy Res. 2002;51:147-53.
106. Corbin Bush N, Twombley K, Ahn J, et al. Prevalence and spot urine risk factors for renal stones in children taking topiramate. J Pediatr Urol. 2013;9:884-9.
107. Coppola G, Capovilla G, Montagnini A, et al. Topiramate as add-on drug in severe myoclonic epilepsy in infancy: an Italian multicenter open trial. Epilepsy Res. 2002;49:45-8.
108. Cudkowicz ME, Shefner JM, Schoenfeld DA, et al. A randomized, placebo-controlled trial of topiramate in amyotrophic lateral sclerosis. Neurology. 2003;61:456-64.
109. Goyal M, Grossberg RI, O'Riordan MA, et al. Urolithiasis with topiramate in nonambulatory children and young adults. Pediatr Neurol. 2009;40:289-94.
110. Mahmoud AA, Rizk T, El-Bakri NK, et al. Incidence of kidney stones with topiramate treatment in pediatric patients. Epilepsia. 2011;52:1890-3.
111. Norman ME, Feldman NI, Cohn RM, et al. Urinary citrate excretion in the diagnosis of distal renal tubular acidosis. J Pediatr. 1978;92:394-400.
112. Hilton JG, Vandenbroucke AC, Josse RG, et al. The urine anion gap: the critical clue to resolve a diagnostic dilemma in a patient with ketoacidosis. Diabetes Care. 1984;7:486-90.
113. Halperin ML, Richardson RM, Bear RA, et al. Urine ammonium: the key to the diagnosis of distal renal tubular acidosis. Nephron. 1988;50:1-4.
114. Batlle DC, Hizon M, Cohen E, et al. The use of the urinary anion gap in the diagnosis of hyperchloremic metabolic acidosis. New Engl J Med. 1988;318:594-9.
115. Halperin ML, Margolis BL, Robinson LA, et al. The urine osmolal gap: a clue to estimate urine ammonium in "hybrid" types of metabolic acidosis. Clin Invest Med. 1988;11: 198-202.
116. Aubert E, Guignard JP. Urinary-blood delta PCO_2 in renal tubular acidosis (author's transl). J Physiol. 1980;76:881-3.
117. Tam SC, Goldstein MB, Stinebaugh BJ, et al. Studies on the regulation of hydrogen ion secretion in the collecting duct in vivo: evaluation of factors that influence the urine minus blood PCO_2 difference. Kidney Int. 1981;20:636-42.
118. Strife CF, Clardy CW, Varade WS, et al. Urine-to-blood carbon dioxide tension gradient and maximal depression of urinary pH to distinguish rate-dependent from classic distal renal tubular acidosis in children. J Pediatr. 1993;122:60-5.
119. Lin JY, Lin JS, Tsai CH. Use of the urine-to-blood carbon dioxide tension gradient as a measurement of impaired distal tubular hydrogen ion secretion among neonates. J Pediatr. 1995;126:114-7.

120. Wrong O, Davies HE. The excretion of acid in renal disease. Q J Med. 1959;28:259-313.
121. Walsh SB, Shirley DG, Wrong OM, et al. Urinary acidification assessed by simultaneous furosemide and fludrocortisone treatment: an alternative to ammonium chloride. Kidney Int. 2007;71:1310-6.
122. Oster JR, Hotchkiss JL, Carbon M, et al. A short duration renal acidification test using calcium chloride. Nephron. 1975;14:281-92.
123. Goules AV, Tatouli IP, Moutsopoulos HM, et al. Clinically significant renal involvement in primary Sjogren's syndrome: clinical presentation and outcome. Arthritis Rheum. 2013;65:2945-53.
124. Nash MA, Torrado AD, Greifer I, et al. Renal tubular acidosis in infants and children. Clinical course, response to treatment, and prognosis. J Pediatr. 1972;80:738-48.
125. McSherry E, Morris RC, Jr. Attainment and maintenance of normal stature with alkali therapy in infants and children with classic renal tubular acidosis. J Clin Invest. 1978;61: 509-27.
126. Santos F, Chan JC. Renal tubular acidosis in children. Diagnosis, treatment and prognosis. Am J Nephrol. 1986;6: 289-95.
127. Preminger GM, Sakhaee K, Pak CY. Alkali action on the urinary crystallization of calcium salts: contrasting responses to sodium citrate and potassium citrate. J Urol. 1988;139:240-2.
128. Greenberg AJ, McNamara H, McCrory WW. Metabolic balance studies in primary renal tubular acidosis: effects of acidosis on external calcium and phosphorus balances. J Pediatr. 1966;69:610-8.
129. Higashihara E, Nutahara K, Niijima T. Renal hypercalciuria and metabolic acidosis associated with medullary sponge kidney: effect of alkali therapy. Urol Res. 1988;16:95-100.
130. Fabris A, Lupo A, Bernich P, et al. Long-term treatment with potassium citrate and renal stones in medullary sponge kidney. Clin J Am Soc Nephrol. 2010;5:1663-8.
131. Fabris A, Bernich P, Abaterusso C, et al. Bone disease in medullary sponge kidney and effect of potassium citrate treatment. Clin J Am Soc Nephrol. 2009;4:1974-9.
132. Werness PG, Brown CM, Smith LH, et al. EQUIL2: a BASIC computer program for the calculation of urinary saturation. J Urol. 1985;134:1242-4.
133. Rodgers A, Allie-Hamdulay S, Jackson G. Therapeutic action of citrate in urolithiasis explained by chemical speciation: increase in pH is the determinant factor. Nephrol Dial Transpl. 2006;21:361-9.
134. Pak CY. Physicochemical basis for formation of renal stones of calcium phosphate origin: calculation of the degree of saturation of urine with respect to brushite. J Clin Invest. 1969;48:1914-22.
135. Pak CY, Moe OW, Maalouf NM, et al. Comparison of semi-empirical and computer derived methods for estimating urinary saturation of brushite. J Urol. 2009;181:1423-8.
136. Pak CY, Rodgers K, Poindexter JR, et al. New methods of assessing crystal growth and saturation of brushite in whole urine: effect of pH, calcium and citrate. J Urol. 2008;180:1532-7.

CHAPTER

20 Medullary Sponge Kidney and Human Monogenic Hypercalciurias

Giovanni Gambaro

INTRODUCTION

This chapter discusses pathological conditions associated with nephrolithiasis that, though rare, are intriguing. It is important to know about them because many are systemic in nature, carry a risk of progressing to renal failure, and demand specific treatments.

MEDULLARY SPONGE KIDNEY

Medullary sponge kidney (MSK) is a renal malformation. Its presenting signs are usually nephrocalcinosis and recurrent renal stones, though there may also be evidence of renal acidification and concentration defects, precalyceal duct ectasias often called cysts. Medullary sponge kidney is considered a sporadic condition and, although it is not easy to establish its prevalence in the general population, it is generally assumed to be quite rare. When a sizable, unselected radiological series[1] was checked for more or less obvious radiological evidence of MSK, only 0.5–1% of cases appeared to be involved. Renal stone patients are more likely to be affected, and as many as 20% of patients suffering from recurrent calcium stones have reportedly revealed MSK;[2] in the author's personal experience, about 12% of such patients carry the condition.[3]

Its pathogenesis is by no means clear, with theories focusing on abnormal developmental and genetic mechanisms, or on a condition acquired secondary to calcium crystals obstructing the collecting ducts, with a role being attributed to hyperparathyroidism too.[4] The natural history and clinical phenotype of MSK likewise remain to be thoroughly explained. To compound this hazy picture, the fact that urography is no longer routinely used to investigate kidney and urinary tract disorders make the chances of MSK being diagnosed rather slim nowadays.

MSK as a Malformation

Patients with MSK have been described as having a variety of renal and extrarenal malformations (Table 20.1).

Table 20.1: Renal and extrarenal malformations seen in MSK patients.

- Congenital hemihypertrophy
- Beckwith-Wiedemann syndrome
- Rabson-Mendenhall syndrome
- Wilms' tumor
- Cakut' syndrome
- ADPKD
- Congenital hepatic fibrosis
- Caroli's disease
- Young's syndrome (obstructive azoospermia and chronic sinopulmonary infections)
- Renal artery fibromuscular dysplasia
- Ehlers–Danlos syndrome
- Marfan's syndrome
- Congenital pyloric stenosis
- Anodontia

(MSK: Medullary sponge kidney; ADPKD: Autosomal dominant polycystic kidney disease).

The condition may be associated with renal developmental anomalies and neoplasms like Wilms' tumor, horseshoe kidney, contralateral congenital small kidney, and pyeloureteral abnormalities,[5-7] or it may coincide with hypertrophic disorders such as Beckwith–Wiedemann syndrome or congenital hemihypertrophy. It has also been reported in associations with hepatic fibrosis, congenital dilation of the intrahepatic bile ducts (Caroli's disease), and other liver conditions. When 72 unrelated MSK renal stone formers were systematically assessed to identify any concurrent renal and urinary tract malformations, six of them revealed unilateral small kidneys and one had a unilateral bifid renal pelvis (Fig. 20.1).[7] This cohort had a higher prevalence of developmental anomalies of the kidney and urinary tract than in the general population,[7] giving the impression that the same pathogenic mechanisms might be behind MSK and certain renal developmental anomalies.

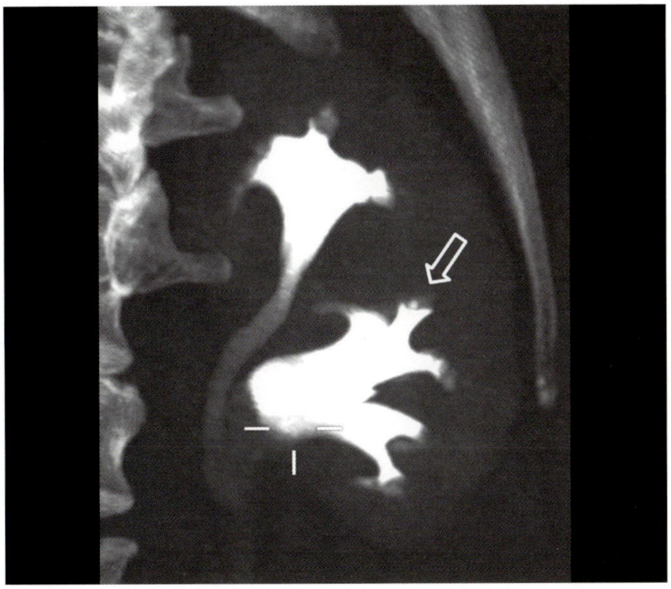

Fig. 20.1: UroCT in medullary sponge kidney. During the urographic phase some papillae disclose a flamed aspect; one small papillary "cyst" is evident (arrow). Bifid renal pelvis.
Courtesy: Prof FM Danza. A Gemelli University Hospital, Catholic University, Rome.

Assuming that MSK is a malformation, we can classify the condition as a developmental disorder and seek the pathogenic mechanisms responsible for it among the many and highly complex stages that characterize the kidney's morphogenesis. To clarify the pathogenesis of MSK, we need to account both for the alterations, such as "cysts," nephrocalcinosis and acidification, and concentration defects, that occur in the "lower nephron" (the ureteric bud-derived precalyceal and collecting ducts), and for the proximal tubular defects and other changes occurring in the metanephric blastema-derived nephron, or "upper nephron."

During the process of renal organogenesis, reciprocal inductive interactions take place between two different primordial epithelial and mesenchymal tissues—the ureteric bud and the metanephric blastema (Fig. 20.2). It is essential for differentiation, signals to be triggered at the interface between the ureteric bud and the metanephric blastema in order for the mesenchymal cells to transit from the metanephros to the nephronic cells, for the latter to be correctly polarized, for the different tubular segments of the nephron to become specialized, and for the ureteric bud to grow and its epithelium to ramify (Fig. 20.2). As the process of renal morphogenesis proceeds, numerous transcription factors, growth factors, receptors, and matrix proteins are involved in controlling cell proliferation, apoptosis, migration, and differentiation; the glial cell line derived neurotrophic factor (GDNF) and its receptor tyrosine kinase (RET) are among them.

Glial cell line derived neurotrophic factor is a member of the transforming growth factor-β family. It plays an indispensable part in the development of the parasympathetic, enteric, and motor neuron systems. Moreover, GDNF has a non-neuronal function as well, particularly in the development of the kidney and urinary tract.[8]

Glial cell line derived neurotrophic factor is synthesized by the metanephric blastema during nephrogenesis, and this prompts ureteric bud outgrowth and branching from Wolff's duct. Glial cell line derived neurotrophic factor requires a RET and a coreceptor GDNF family receptor (Gfr) α1 for the signaling pathway downstream (Fig. 20.2). In the initial stages of a kidney's development, RET and Gfrα1 are expressed along Wolff's duct, while GDNF is only expressed in the metanephric mesenchyme alongside the caudal portion of Wolff's duct, from where the ureteric bud subsequently sprouts.

Later on in the process, RET and Gfrα1 are only expressed in the distal tips of the branches, while the peripheral and undifferentiated mesenchyme surrounding these tips reveal GDNF expression. One of the main outcomes of GDNF/RET signaling involves the transcriptional activation of a set of target genes, including the RET gene itself plus, Wnt11 and Sprouty1.[9-11]

In vivo experiments involving the homozygous inactivation of GDNF or RET gave rise to renal agenesia because the ureteric bud failed to develop from Wolff's duct, and the experimental animals died soon after birth, whereas animals heterozygous for a GDNF or RET null allele were both fertile and viable.[12-14] The GDNF heterozygotes showed a number of different renal phenotypes that varied from smaller kidneys (many of which revealed cortical cysts) to unilateral renal dysgenesia. These findings go to show that GDNF levels affect renal development, and loss of one allele is enough to give rise to a significant renal phenotype. Small cystic kidneys were identified as a result of the ectopic expression of RET in transgenic mice[15] and, more recently, RET mutations were found in 37% of fetuses with bilateral renal agenesis and in 20% of those with unilateral renal agenesis,[16] associated with a GDNF mutation too in one case.

Glial cell line derived neurotrophic factor-RET interactions thus have a fundamental role in the development of the kidney and urinary tract, and in nephron genesis.

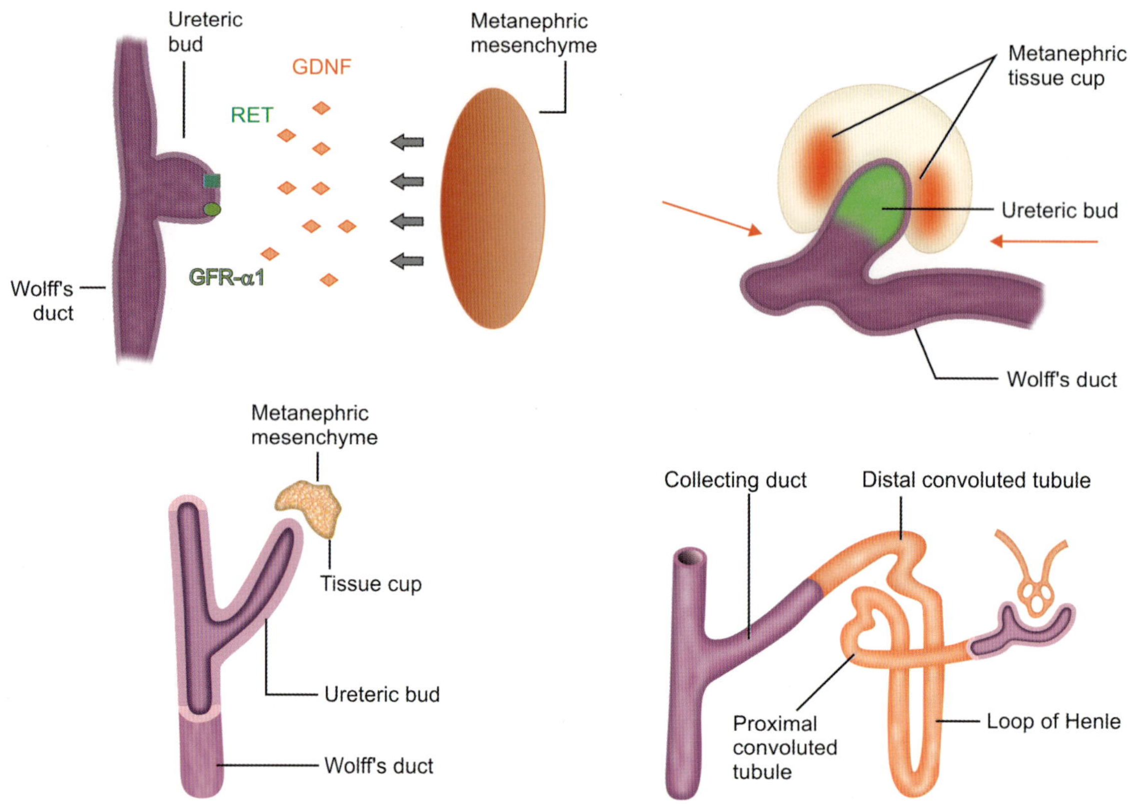

Fig. 20.2: Renal organogenesis is triggered by reciprocal inductive interactions between the ureteric bud and the metanephric blastema. It is essential for differentiation signals to be triggered at the interface between the ureteric bud and the metanephric blastema in order for the mesenchymal cells to transit from the metanephros to the nephronic cells, for the latter to be correctly polarized, for the different tubular segments of the nephron to become specialized, and for the ureteric bud to grow and its epithelium to ramify. If such a complex developmental phase goes wrong someway it may explain why abnormalities of the whole nephron coexist in medullary sponge kidney (MSK) (papillary "cysts," and several functional defects in the proximal tubule and the collecting ducts) and the association of MSK with kidney and urinary tract abnormalities.
(GDNF: Glial cell line derived neurotrophic factor; RET: Receptor tyrosine kinase; GFR: GDNF family receptor).

Any anomalies involving them could therefore plausibly be responsible for a disorder such as MSK, in which both the lower and the upper nephrons are affected, and has often urinary tract developmental anomalies too. It is worth mentioning here the case of a woman described as having MSK associated with multiple endocrine neoplasia (MEN 2A) due to a RET mutation.[17]

Medullary Sponge Kidney as a Genetic Disease

Medullary sponge kidney (MSK) is considered a sporadic disease, despite a handful of reports of familial MSK, in which the condition segregated as an autosomal dominant trait,[18-20] having said that, it is not unusual for nephrologists to encounter cases of MSK in familial clusters. Assuming that MSK is a developmental disorder, then we should seek the culprit among the genes governing renal development. Medullary sponge kidney might presumably result from the interface between the "ureteric bud and the metanephric mesenchyme" being disrupted by mutations or specific GDNF and RET gene polymorphisms, or particular GDNF/RET genotype interactions. When apparently sporadic MSK cases and healthy controls were analyzed, 12% of MSK patients were found heterozygous for two rare and previously unknown variants of the GDNF gene located in a putative binding domain for PAX2 (the c.-45G>C and c.-27+18G>A variants)[21] and the R93W low-penetrance GDNF mutation (Anglani F, unpublished). In five investigated families the GDNF mutations were inherited and segregated with the MSK phenotype in an apparently autosomal dominant pattern.[21]

The two variants are located in the 5'UTR region of the gene, and they could be responsible for quantitative changes in messenger ribonucleic acid expression and/or an altered response to regulatory factors because both the GDNF variants are located in a domain binding the transcription factor PAX2, which has a well-known crucial role in nephrogenesis.[22] An altered GDNF response to PAX2 could feasibly interfere with the nephric ducts' growth, giving rise to "cysts" and disrupting renal cell polarization by the metanephric tubules, leading to a mistargeting of carriers involved in acidification and ion handling, and to the consequent anatomical and functional abnormalities seen in the patients involved.[21] The known GDNF upregulation in dysplastic/cystic renal disorders is a clear sign of this factor's involvement in these developmental disorders.[23] Finding MSK patients with no GDNF alterations, and patients with no family history of MSK, suggests a genetic heterogeneity.

Two cases of syndromic autosomal recessive distal renal tubular acidosis (dRTA) that seemed to be associated with MSK have been described,[24] and it was suggested that MSK might be part of the clinical phenotype of autosomal recessive dRTA, being caused by the same gene. But recessive dRTA typically has quite a different clinical phenotype from adult MSK. Distal RTA is common in MSK, albeit in its incomplete form most of the time. Medullary sponge kidney patients generally do not fail to thrive; and there have been no reports of typical MSK patients having sensorineural hearing loss. In addition, the line of inheritance seen in familial cases of MSK is more suggestive of an autosomal dominant than of a recessive trait. Having said that, patients with multiple renal calcifications (as in full-blown dRTA) are quite often diagnosed as having MSK—but then the urographic diagnosis of MSK is easier said than done.

MSK and Ciliopathies

Since MSK has been reported in association with conditions caused by nonmotile cilia disorders, it was suggested quite recently that MSK might be a ciliopathy.[25] Medullary sponge kidney has been found associated with autosomal dominant polycystic kidney disease,[26] and with congenital hepatic fibrosis.[27] Gunay-Aygun et al.[25] also found medullary echogenicity enhanced in some obligate heterozygotes for PKHKD1 mutations that in the homozygous state are responsible for autosomal recessive polycystic kidney disease (ARPKD). A connection has also been made between MSK and Young's syndrome:[28] This is an intriguing hypothesis, but for the time being there is nothing to link the medullary echogenicity seen in the parents of ARPKD patients with nephrocalcinosis or dilated papillary collecting ducts. Besides, it is only the precalyceal collecting ducts that are dilated in MSK, unlike the picture encountered in ARPKD.

Clinical Issues

Medullary sponge kidney may go unnoticed, although its anatomical features and its association with tubular dysfunctions account for the most often-encountered signs of the condition, which are nephrolithiasis and pyelonephritis, while macro- and microhematuria, renal failure, and hyperparathyroidism are less common.

Medullary sponge kidney has no predilection for either gender. The diagnosis is usually established when patients are already adults, after recurrent episodes of calcium nephrolithiasis and nephrocalcinosis. These are the dominant manifestations in most patients' clinical history. When MSK emerges already in children, it is likely to be more severe and the bone-related consequences of dRTA are the most obvious signs of the condition, with failure to thrive, short stature, and rickets-like symptoms.[29,30] It is probably the progressive nature of MSK that leads to it almost always being diagnosed in adulthood. The "cysts" and nephrocalcinosis give the impression of becoming worse with time. Anecdotal reports support this idea—see the case shown by Cameron[31] or the case of Figure 20.3.

Although nephrocalcinosis is very common in MSK, some cases without this finding (despite a typical papillary pattern at urography) have been observed. Hypercalciuria and hypocitraturia are very common too. In the author's case series, all typical MSK patients had hypercalciuria and 83% of them had hypocitraturia.[3] Other researchers have reported lower rates, however, with 58% and 19%, respectively, for hypercalciuria and hypocitraturia.[32] These two conditions—combined with urinary stasis in the dilated papillary duct—trigger the formation of calcium phosphate and/or calcium oxalate stones. Chemical analyses on stones from the author's MSK case series revealed mainly calcium phosphate in 67% of cases and mainly calcium oxalate in 33%.[3]

The MSK patients in the author's cohort frequently suffered from recurrent stones (averaging a new episode every couple of years), but <3% of these patients needed urological procedures (involving extracorporeal shock wave lithotripsy in all cases). This would mean that MSK is associated with the frequent formation of small stones that pass spontaneously, as reported elsewhere.[3]

Medullary sponge kidney may also remain completely silent; however, or it may follow an indolent course with only few stone episodes. This was the case for 25% of the

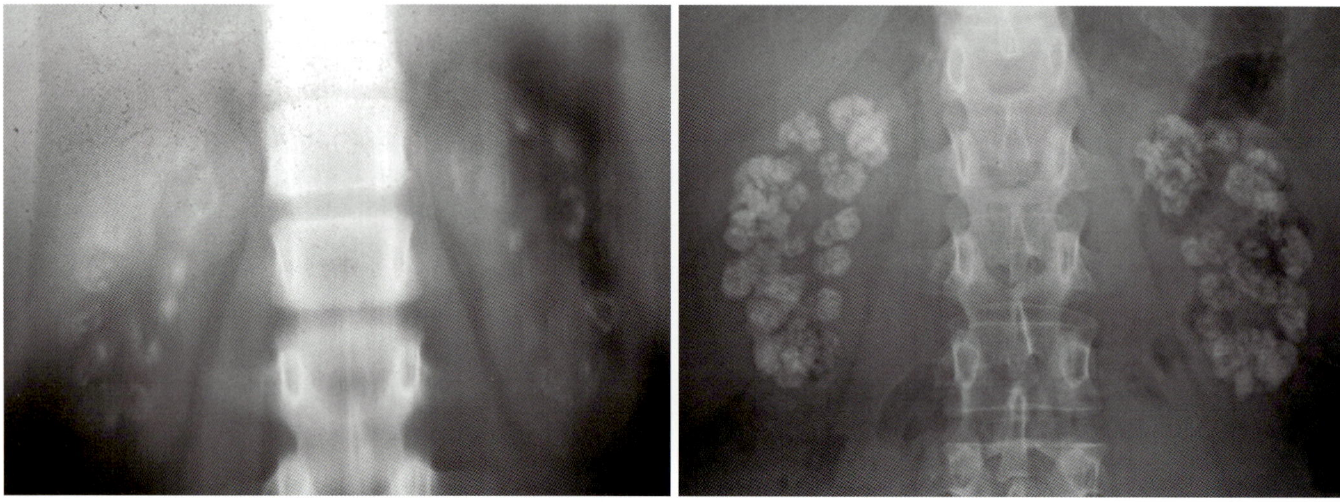

Fig. 20.3: Plain kidney X-ray in medullary sponge kidney (MSK). Severe papillary nephrocalcinosis in a familial MSK case. The young lady was 24-year-old in 1994. Progression of nephrocalcinosis in 20 years (left panel 1994; right panel 2013).

author's series of MSK patients.[3] These patients were diagnosed with MSK because they complained of other symptoms, including hematuria, a vague pain or burning sensation in the loin, etc., or their MSK was found incidentally during diagnostic tests for other purposes. A recent report from the Mayo Clinic indicated that 32% of their MSK patients were diagnosed during tests for more or less severe hematuria, urinary tract infections, or renal masses.[32] The follow-up of such patients with "silent/indolent" MSK is also reportedly uneventful in terms of any stone formation.[3] These patients notably had none of the urinary metabolic abnormalities typically predisposing to stone formation—neither hypercalciuria or hypocitraturia, nor a biochemical profile suggestive of dRTA.[3]

The clinical course in MSK patients may very occasionally involve pain, which is not necessarily associated with the passage of a stone or macrohematuria. They can sometimes experience an occasional sharp, shooting pain that proves difficult to treat, often with a constant background dullness in the loin that does not irradiate to the groin. This picture is suggestive of "loin-pain hematuria syndrome", which should really only be diagnosed after excluding other conditions (one of which is MSK). Such patients often gain little from any pre-emptive treatment for stones.

Urinary tract infections are considered the second most common clinical problem associated with MSK—after renal stones—but they are actually quite rare, with 0.1 episodes per patient-year.[3] Some patients are found to have MSK after presenting with pyelonephritis,[33] the onset of which is bound to be facilitated by the anatomical derangement typical of the disorder.

Infectious episodes may influence the findings relating to renal stones, giving rise to secondary struvite stones and/or pyelonephritis. This is probably the most common reason for MSK patients experiencing renal failure—but such an end result is relatively rare.[34] Some MSK patients with severe nephrocalcinosis and more severe kidney development derangement may suffer from a functional impairment. A mildly reduced GFR has been reported in MSK patients with contralateral congenital small kidney,[7] but this is an uncommon combination and such patients account for less than one in ten of the author's case series.[7] Renal failure and end-stage renal disease (ESRD) are rare in MSK patients and, when they do occur, other causes should be suspected. Renal disease with nephrocalcinosis, stones, and a risk of ESRD is characteristic of complete dRTA and Dent's disease—among other, much rarer conditions.

There is a reported association between MSK and hyperparathyroidism (which was also seen in a handful of the author's patients[7]). It has even been suggested that hyperparathyroidism is a cause of MSK and that it triggers nephrolithiasis in these patients.[35] In the author's experience, however, hyperparathyroidism develops after the onset of hypercalciuria, nephrocalcinosis, and renal stones. Dlabal et al. suggested that the negative calcium balance caused by renal hypercalciuria would stimulate the parathyroids and thus give rise to hyperplasia.[36] While such an effect of the negative calcium balance is convincing, its suggested cause is more doubtful. More than 40% of MSK patients have incomplete and overt dRTA,[37-39] but a prevalence of the overt form has been reported in only 2.9% of cases.[40] Daudon studied a large series of stones from MSK patients[41] and their prevalently carbapatite and brushite content would support the conviction that distal acidification defects must be very common in MSK. For >80% of the MSK patients seen by the present author, the biochemical profile pointed to incomplete dRTA.[42] Dual-energy X-ray absorptiometry revealed osteopenia and osteoporosis in 58% and 14% of these MSK patients respectively, but these conditions could not be attributed to any of the most common causes of bone demineralization (such as hyperparathyroidism and menopause, in particular).[42]

Since treatment with alkaline citrate reduced calciuria and improved bone mineral density,[42] we speculated that a defective acidification presumably has an essential part to play in MSK, triggering a cascade of events that would include a decreased bone mineralization, hypercalciuria, hypocitraturia, and stone formation. Osther et al. also suggested a pivotal role for distal renal acidification defects in the genesis of hypercalciuria in MSK,[43] and Higashihara et al. demonstrated that these patients' calciuria could be reduced by correcting their acidosis with bicarbonate.[44] On the other hand, it could be that this acidification defect is secondary to recurrent episodes of stones causing "microobstructions", but MSK patients carrying the previously-described GDNF variants have a more severe acidification defect,[21] and this would support the impression that the acidification is a primary phenomenon. Either way, published data indicate that, once acidosis has set in, it has a marked, highly prevalent impact on bone mineralization and the patient's urinary stone risk profile.[3,42] That is why it seems most likely that the hypercalciuria seen in MSK is all, or almost all, bone related.

Tubular Abnormalities

Medullary sponge kidney is associated with other tubular defects of the lower and upper nephron, as well as with the previously-described morphological abnormalities and dRTA. Those affecting the lower nephron reportedly include a defective urinary concentration.[31] It is highly likely that hypocitraturia is an epiphenomenon of dRTA. Among the several dysfunctions of the upper nephron (of the proximal tubule) reportedly associated with MSK, there are changes affecting maximum glucose reabsorption and maximum P-amino hippurate secretion.[45] In the present author's experience, 40% of MSK patients have low molecular weight (LMW) proteinuria and low plasma phosphate levels due to a reduced maximum transport for phosphate (unpublished data).

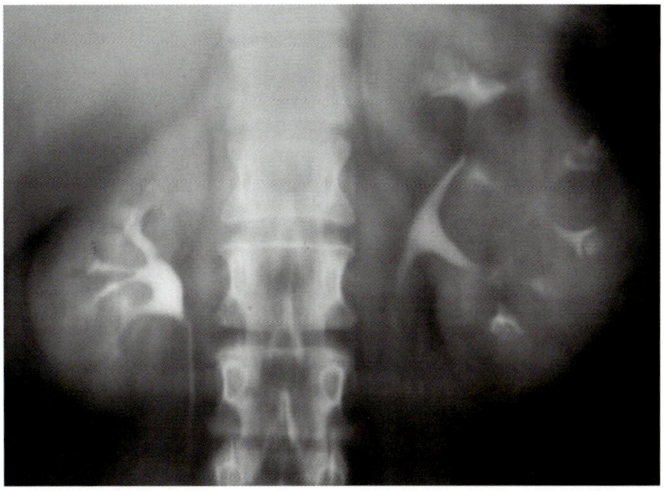

Fig. 20.4: Typical flamed aspects of renal papillae in medullary sponge kidney. Urography.

That MSK patients should have such proximal tubular abnormalities goes to show that the whole nephron is deranged in this condition. This comes as no surprise, given our assumption that MSK is a developmental embryological disorder involving the interface between the ureteral bud and the metanephric blastema.[4] Differentiation "messages" originating from the interface between the ureteric bud and the metanephric blastema are needed for mesenchymal cells to transit from the metanephros to the nephronic cells, and for renal tubular cells to be correctly polarized and become suitably specialized.[9,46] It is not hard to imagine that any disruption at this interface would lead to the concomitant occurrence of alterations in both the distal and the proximal nephron.

Diagnosis

Medullary sponge kidney is diagnosed radiographically. Up until not long ago the gold standard method was intravenous (IV) urography, which typically showed contrast medium pooling in dilated papillary ducts, giving the impression of a blush or linear striations in very mild cases, or of bunches of flowers if the cystic dilation of the collecting ducts was severe (Fig. 20.4).

Medullary nephrocalcinosis is a common (Figs. 20.5A to C), but not constant finding, so it is not necessary to confirm the diagnosis. Generally speaking, MSK affects all

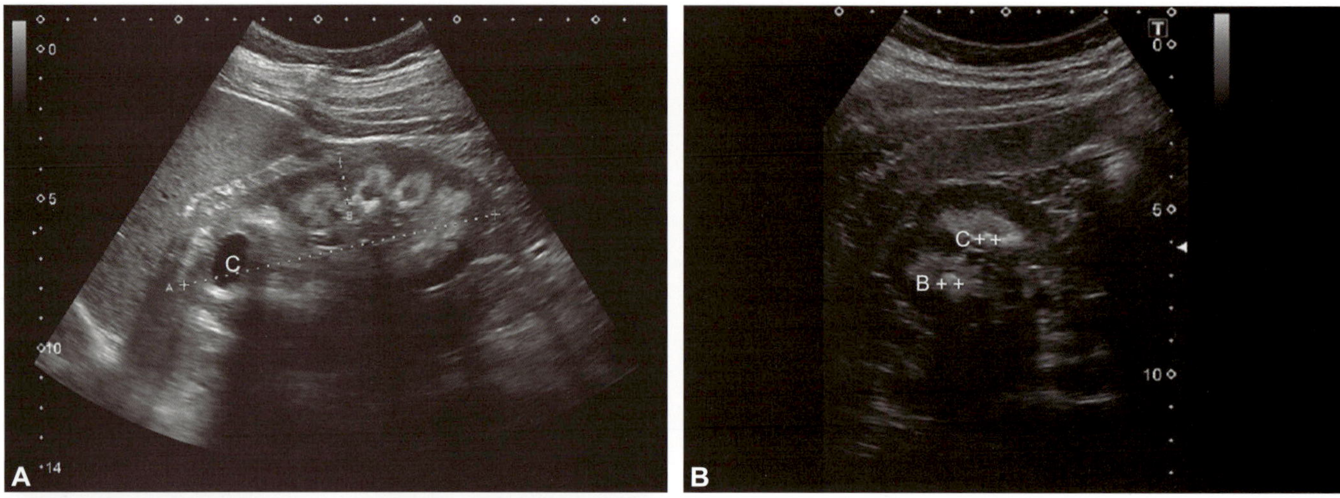

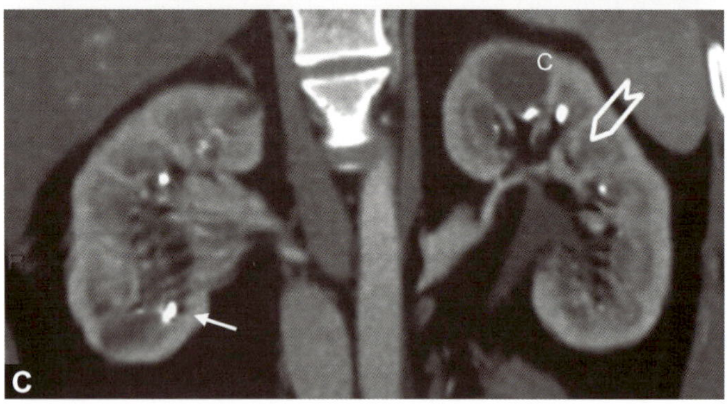

Figs. 20.5A to C: A severe case of medullary sponge kidney (MSK). (A) Wreath images depicting the papillae contour due to nephrocalcinosis in MSK. (B) Detail of two flanked papillae: They are diffusely hyperechoic. The markers identify two small stones (same case as A). (C) UroCT in MSK (same case as A and B): In the pyelographic phase typical features of MSK can be recognized: Papillary concretions (nephrocalcinosis) (empty arrow), small renal stones (white arrow) attached to the papillae and "cysts" (C).
Courtesy: Prof FM Danza, A Gemelli University Hospital, Catholic University, Rome.

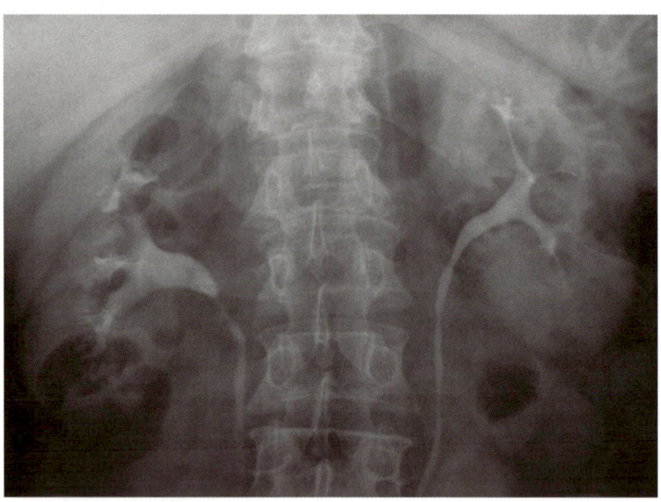

Fig. 20.6: Unilateral medullary sponge kidney. Typical blushes are visible only in the right kidney in all papillae (urography).
Courtesy: Prof FM Danza. A Gemelli University Hospital, Catholic University, Rome.

renal papillae in both kidneys (*see* Figs. 20.4 and 20.5), but it may be unilateral (Fig. 20.6) or involve only a few papillae (Fig. 20.7), making the diagnostic process rather more difficult. The extent of the evidence on urography correlates with the severity of a patient's condition in terms of symptomatic stone rates, hospitalizations, and procedures required.[47]

Nowadays, spiral computed tomography (CT) (with no IV contrast agent) has practically replaced urography in the diagnostic workup for patients with renal stones because it performs better in cases of renal colic.[48] This has led to a reduction in the number of cases of MSK being diagnosed; however, because spiral CT is unable to show the "cysts" typical of MSK and, in patients with nephrocalcinosis, it is also generally incapable of revealing its distribution in spots, tending instead to present an image of gross calcifications.[49] Although a comparison drawn 20 years ago between urography and CT (with and without IV contrast medium) indicated a considerably lower sensitivity of CT for detecting MSK,[50] modern CT scanners have become much more sensitive and uroCT can identify cystic dilations of the prepapillary collecting ducts[51-53] (Figs. 20.1 and 20.5C). The downside of this approach is that patients are exposed to far more radiation than in the

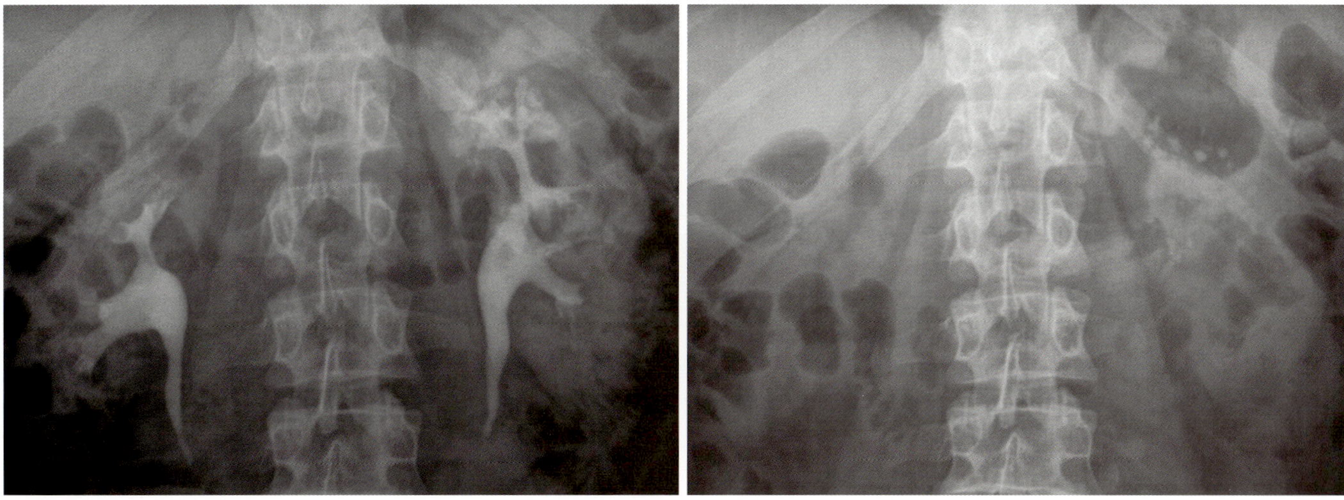

Fig. 20.7: Partial medullary sponge kidney. Only the upper papillae in the left kidney are involved. The typical flamed aspect can be observed (left panel) (urography). Concurrently, nephrocalcinosis was only present in the upper left pole (right panel) (plain X-ray). *Courtesy*: Prof FM Danza. A Gemelli University Hospital, Catholic University, Rome.

case of urography, but dose reduction protocols have been suggested to reduce their exposure to lower levels than those needed for urography.[53]

Some authors[54] have claimed that MSK can be diagnosed using renal ultrasound (US), but this method is unable to show the typical urographic signs characteristic of the disorder. On renal US, we can only find nonspecific evidence of hyperechoic medulla caused by nephrocalcinosis and stones[55,56] (*see* Figs. 20.5A and B).

Nuclear magnetic resonance imaging (MRI) lacks the sensitivity needed to reveal the typical signs of MSK and nephrocalcinosis,[57] which would only be suspected in sporadic cases with a particularly extensive ectasia. A diagnosis of MSK was suggested on MR urography in a recent case report,[58] prompted by a remarkable hyperintensity on fat-saturated T_2-weighted MRI and a clustering of cystic structures.

Treatment

It is difficult to diagnose MSK reliably nowadays, and there is no specific treatment for the condition, but it is undeniably useful to ascertain whether recurrent stone formers have MSK in order to customize their treatment for the purposes of stone prevention.

Metabolic abnormalities in urine (hypercalciuria and hypocitraturia, together with a relatively high urinary pH) play a fundamental part in lithogenesis and it is wise to administer alkaline citrate treatment, based on the assumption that the primary functional defect in MSK is an incomplete dRTA. In the author's experience, this treatment has led to a marked reduction in patients' stone recurrence rates,[3] and had a positive effect on their bone mineral density.[42] It is also a good idea to recommend general prophylactic measures, which include drinking more water, limiting dietary sodium and proteins, and eating more fruit and vegetables. Thiazides have been used to reduce calciuria, but they can give rise to a reduced citraturia.

Laser papillotomy has been used successfully to vaporize small stones in the prepapillary "cysts" for the purposes of pain control in some symptomatic MSK patients and stone-formers with frequent recurrences.[59] Kidney autotransplantation with a modified pyelovesicostomy proved effective in one MSK patient with intractable metabolic stone disease who had become dependent on narcotics.[60]

HUMAN MONOGENIC HYPERCALCIURIA

Is Idiopathic Hypercalciuria Monogenic?

Based on the pattern of inheritance of hypercalciuria observed in a number of pedigrees, many research groups have suggested an autosomal dominant transmission of this condition.[61-64] Both renal and absorptive forms of hypercalciuria have been seen to be inherited with this pattern and both types have sometimes been found in different members of the same family.[62-64] The authors suggested that primary hypercalciuria must be a monogenic trait with a Mendelian transmission, but this may not be the case. Quantitative traits, such as calcium excretion, are generally assumed to be caused by multiple genes and their interaction with the environment.[65,66] Data from different groups and geographical areas support the idea that calciuria is governed by a polygenic background for at least 50% of its variance.[67-69] On the other hand, recent results from whole genome sequencing and association studies (GWAS), and the application of next-generation sequencing in families with inherited disorders previously believed to be polygenic have opened a new perspective, supporting the impression that private or rare mutations might also cause disorders that were previously assumed to be polygenic.[70] In fact, rare functional genetic variants of still unknown genes could be responsible in some pedigrees of specific disorders, and hypercalciuria might well be among them.

The above paragraph concerns idiopathic hypercalciuria, but there are also a few known truly monogenic disorders occasionally found associated with hypercalciuria (Table 20.2).

Autosomal Dominant Hypocalcemia with Hypercalciuria

Activating mutations of the gene for the calcium sensing receptor (CaSR) extracellular domain lead to autosomal dominant hypocalcemia with hypercalciuria (ADHH).[71] Patients have a clinical syndrome mirroring hypoparathyroidism, given their mild and usually asymptomatic hypocalcemia and marginally high phosphatemia but with low-normal serum parathyroid hormone (PTH) concentrations. Since CaSR inhibits active and passive calcium reabsorption in the thick ascending limb of Henle's loop these patients have hypercalciuria (Fig. 20.8).

It is important to recognize that these patients have ADHH and not hypoparathyroidism to avoid the therapeutic use of vitamin D that would worsen hypercalciuria, and cause nephrocalcinosis, nephrolithiasis, and renal impairment.[71]

Inherited Hyperparathyroidism

Familial isolated primary hyperparathyroidism (FIHP), multiple endocrine neoplasia type 1 (MEN1), MEN type 2 (MEN2), and the hyperparathyroidism-jaw tumor (HPT-JT) syndrome are autosomal dominant inherited disorders in which hypercalcemia is associated with hypercalciuria and sometimes kidney stones. Twenty percent of patients with HPT-JT have renal cysts and more rarely renal hamartomas, Wilms' tumor, or papillary renal carcinoma.

Although in a minority of patients with FIHP mutations of the MEN1 (Menin, 11q13), HPT-JT (parafibromin/HRPT2, 1q31.2) and CaSR genes have been found, in the majority the gene(s) involved is not known.[72]

Because of the high risk of primary tumors occurring even at younger ages, an early diagnosis of these conditions is important for the clinical management of patients and their families and in life-planning decisions of affected patients.

MEN 1: Approximately, 10% of cases are caused by *de novo* mutations. Direct sequencing of the MEN1 gene coding region and intron–exon junctions is generally performed looking for known mutations. When no MEN1 mutation in a MEN 1 family is identified, the genetic confirmation can be achieved by haplotype or linkage analysis of at least two generations of affected members.[73] Prenatal diagnosis is possible if the disease-causing mutation in the family is known.

MEN 2: de novo mutations are possible. c-RET gene mutation screening, for instance by high resolution melting analysis can be done for germ-line and sporadic mutations.[74] Prenatal testing is possible.

HPT-JT: Although *de novo* mutations are possible most patients have an affected parent. Prenatal diagnosis is possible if the disease-causing mutation in the family is known.

Idiopathic Infantile Hypercalcemia from Inactivating Mutations of Vitamin D 24-Hydroxylase

CYP24A1 gene inactivating mutations can cause idiopathic infantile hypercalcemia (IIH) (Lightwood's syndrome), a rare autosomal recessive disease that develops in the first few months after birth.[75] CYP24A1 is the gene that encodes vitamin D 24-hydroxylase, which degrades 1,25-$(OH)_2$ vitamin D_3 and thereby regulates plasma calcitriol concentrations; if defective it gives rise to higher levels of 1,25-$(OH)_2$ vitamin D_3 (Fig. 20.9). This leads to severe hypercalcemia, nephrocalcinosis, nephrolithiasis and, ultimately, renal failure. Despite their hypercalcemia, patients with this condition have inappropriately high serum 25-OH vitaminD_3 and 1,25-$(OH)_2$ vitamin D_3 levels, and low 24,25-$(OH)_2$ vitamin D_3 and PTH levels. 1,25-$(OH)_2$ vitamin D-24-hydroxylase deficiency may become clinically evident as osteopenia because 1,25-$(OH)_2$

Table 20.2: Monogenic disorders of tubular function with hypercalciuria.

	Defective gene	*Chromosome*	*Inheritance*	*Clinical manifestations*	*Treatment of stone disease and nephrocalcinosis*
Familial hypocalcemia with hypercalciuria (Bartter's syndrome type V)	Calcium sensing receptor	3q13.3-21	Autosomal dominant	Nephrocalcinosis, Bartter's syndrome phenotype, hypocalcemia, hypercalciuria	No specific measure
Dent's disease TP 1	Chloride channel 5	Xp 11.22	X-linked	Hypercalciuria, LMW proteinuria, low serum phosphate, renal stones, nephrocalcinosis, ESRD, metabolic bone disease/rickets	Thiazides, potassium citrate
Dent's disease TP 2	OCRL1 [PIP(2) 5-phosphatase]	Xq26.1	X-linked	Dent's disease phenotype, possible association with mild impaired cognitive function (mild variant of Lowe s.)	No specific measure
Hereditary hypophosphatemic rickets with hypercalciuria	Sodium-phosphate cotransporter NaPi-2c	9a34.3	Autosomal recessive	Hypophosphatemia, elevated 1,25-$(OH)_2D_3$ levels, suppressed PTH, absorptive hypercalciuria, nephrocalcinosis, renal stones, rickets or osteomalacia, short stature	Oral phosphate
Hypophosphatemic nephrolithiasis and osteoporosis	Sodium-phosphate cotransporter NaPi-2a	5q35	Autosomal-dominant	Nephrolithiasis, osteoporosis	No specific measure
Bartter's syndrome TP 1 TP 2 TP 3	Bumetanide sensitive Na-K-2Cl cotransport K channel ROMK1 Cl channel CLC-kb	15q15-21 11q21-25 1p36	Autosomal-recessive	Fasting hypercalciuria, nephrocalcinosis, Bartter's syndrome phenotype	No specific measure
Distal renal tubular acidosis	Anion exchanger AE1 Vacuolar H^+-ATPase α4 subunit Vacuolar H^+-ATPase ss1 (β1) subunit	17q21 7q33-34 2p13	Autosomal dominant Autosomal recessive Autosomic recessive	Hyperchloremic metabolic acidosis, failure to thrive, rickets/osteomalacia, hypercalciuria, hypocitraturia, inappropriately high urinary pH nephrocalcinosis, stones, CKD, episodes of hypokalemic paralysis and early sensorineural deafness	Alkali citrate
Hereditary hypomagnesemia-hypercalciuria syndrome	Claudin 16, Claudin 19	3q27 1p34.2	Autosomal-recessive	Magnesium and calcium wasting, polyuria, dRTA, hypocitraturia, nephrocalcinosis, stones, ESRD and sensorineural hearing loss, ocular abnormalities	High dose magnesium, hydrochlorothiazide, indomethacin
Familial hyperkalemic hypertension (with hypercalciuria)	WNK4 kinase	17q21	Autosomal dominant	Hyperkalemia, acidosis, arterial hypertension, low renin, serum calcium levels mildly reduced, hypercalciuria	Thiazides

(LMW: Low molecular weight; ESRD: End-stage renal disease; PTH: Parathyroid hormone; ROMK: Renal outer medullary potassium; Cl: Chloride; CLC: Chloride channel; CKD: Chronic kidney disease; dRTA: Distal renal tubular acidosis).

vitamin D_3 stimulates osteoclastic bone resorption,[76] although a high bone mineral content has been reported too in some cases.[77]

The phenotypic spectrum of IIH has recently become broader as new cases have been described, in which the disease became apparent from recurrent nephrolithiasis beginning in young adults who were hypercalciuric, but their serum calcium levels were only mildly or intermittently higher than normal.[77,78] Carriers of the mutated CYP24A1 gene may tend to have high 1,25-$(OH)_2$ vitamin D_3 levels, hypercalciuria, and renal stones.[77] CYP24A1 mutations increase an individual's sensitivity to vitamin D,[75] so IIH has to be considered in the differential diagnosis of adult hypercalciuric nephrolithiasis, especially now that adults are often prescribed oral vitamin D supplements.

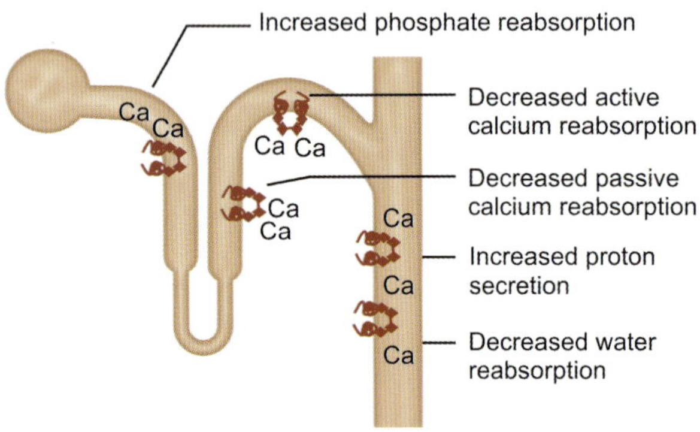

Fig. 20.8: Possible activities of calcium sensing receptor (CaSR) in renal lithogenesis and in hypercalciuria. In the proximal tubule, CaSR is expressed on the luminal side where, by limiting PTH activity decreases the urinary loss of phosphate. In the thick ascending limb of the Henle's loop, it is basolateral where, by interfering with the activity of renal outer medullary potassium channel and Na-K-2Cl, it dissipates the electrical driving gradient necessary for the passive calcium reabsorption. In the distal convoluted tubule, CaSR is on the basolateral side where it inhibits active calcium reabsorption. In the principal and intercalated cells of the collecting duct CaSR is luminal; in the principal cells, it modulates the trafficking of aquaporin 2 and, as a consequence, the activity of vasopressin and the urine concentration. In the intercalated cells CaSR enhances proton secretion in urine.

It has been estimated that the rate of homozygosity for CYP24A1 gene mutations is in the range of 420–1960 per 100,000 population,[76] suggesting that many cases of nephrolithiasis considered as sporadic, or induced by vitamin D supplementation, are really phenotypic variants of IIH. Although the above-mentioned rate seems hard to credit on the strength of day-to-day clinical experience, it would be wise to bear this possibility in mind.

The treatment for IIH includes a low-calcium diet and a low intake of vitamin D and sodium cellulose phosphate in order to contain the calcium load, plus ketoconazole (a 25-OH vitamin D-1α-hydroxylase inhibitor).

Dent's Disease

Dent's disease[79] is a rare X-linked disease that appears in children and young adults. It is more severe in males (who are hemizygous) than in females, who carry the disease. One in 10 patients is *de novo* case. Dent's disease involves medullary nephrocalcinosis, nephrolithiasis, hypercalciuria, LMW proteinuria and other tubular dysfunctions, and progressive renal failure. Male patients may sometimes have hypophosphatemic rickets or osteomalacia too. The disease's genetic features can vary and it is associated with numerous CLCN5 (Dent's disease 1) and ORCL1 (Dent's disease 2) mutations. No genotype-to-phenotype correlations have been identified and the signs and symptoms of the disease can also differ considerably, even in individuals belonging to the same family.

The chloride channel CLCN5 gene encodes a 746-amino acid protein, CIC-5, that is expressed in the renal proximal tubules, the thick ascending limb of Henle's loop, and the α-intercalated cells of the collecting ducts.[80,81] ClC-5 is located in the subapical endosomes of proximal

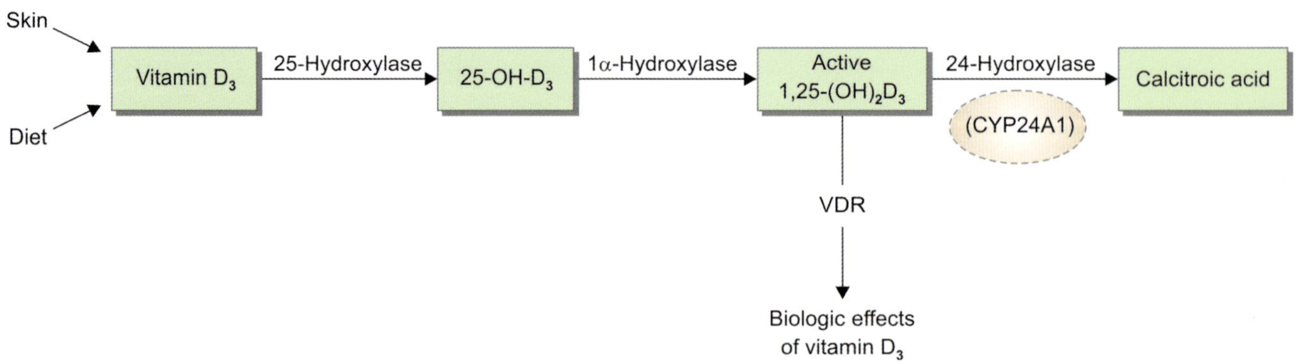

Fig. 20.9: Vitamin D metabolism and role of the CYP24A1 gene and its codified protein 24-hydroxylase. Vitamin D 24-hydroxylase degrades 1,25-$(OH)_2$ vitamin D_3 and thereby regulates plasma calcitriol concentrations; if defective, it gives rise to higher levels of 1,25-$(OH)_2$ vitamin D_3.

tubule cells where it colocalizes with vacuolar H^+-ATPases and endocytosed β2-microglobulin.[80,81] Intracellular ClC-5 is involved in LMW protein endocytosis,[80] in endosomal acidification and sorting, and in lysosomal trafficking.[82-84] ClC-5 knock-out mice have a phenotype resembling Dent's disease, revealing an impaired proximal tubule reabsorption of LMW proteins,[82,83] and confirming the crucial role of ClC-5 in proximal tubule endocytosis. The mechanisms that lead to CLCN5 mutations resulting in hypercalciuria and other tubule abnormalities are still not clear. Piwon et al.[82] suggested that hypercalciuria might derive from the stimulation of luminal PTH receptors increasing as a result of a reduction in PTH endocytosis. A greater luminal PTH concentration should stimulate 25-OH vitamin D_3 hydroxylation and conversion into its active form, but this would be counteracted by the precursor 25-OH vitamin D_3 bound to the vitamin D binding protein being lost in the urine due to tubular proteinuria. Whether a patient develops hypercalciuria or kidney stones probably depends on the balance between these two opposite effects. According to Piwon et al.[82] the mouse model strongly points to hormonal changes being involved in calcium homeostasis as indirect effects of a defective apical endocytosis of PTH and 25-OH vitamin D_3. This could explain how a chloride channel defect might give rise to kidney stones and nephrocalcinosis. Patients with Dent's disease may also have other issues that influence calcium excretion, possibly enhanced by sodium and chloride wastage in the proximal tubules and the ascending limb of Henle's loop, and by the hypophosphatemia-activated 1α-hydroxylation of 25-OH vitamin D_3.

The ORCL1 gene encodes a phosphatidylinositol bisphosphate 5-phosphatase. Mutations of this gene are associated with Lowe's syndrome too, but there is no overlap between the mutations seen in patients with Dent's disease 2 and those causing Lowe's syndrome. OCRL1 mutations probably give rise to OCRL1 protein deficiencies and, in much the same way as for CLCN5 mutations, this probably interferes with endosomal and/or lysosomal trafficking.[85]

Almost all patients with Dent's disease have LMW proteinuria and hypercalciuria, and they usually have nephrocalcinosis and nephrolithiasis too (with prevalence rates of 75% and 50%, respectively, in males). Dent's disease progresses to ESRD in 30–80% of male sufferers by the time they are 30–50 years old. Low molecular weight proteinuria and hypercalciuria are seen in >50% of females carrying the mutated gene, while these women rarely suffer from nephrolithiasis/nephrocalcinosis and only one case of ESDR has been reported.

Dent's disease patients may have very mild intellectual impairments, hypotonia, and subclinical cataracts in no more than 20% of cases; these are cases of Dent's disease 2 (with OCRL1 mutations).

Dent's disease is diagnosed on evidence of LMW proteinuria, hypercalciuria, and at least one of the following: Nephrocalcinosis, kidney stones, hypophosphatemia, microhematuria, and renal failure. A history of X-linked inheritance of nephrolithiasis and renal failure supports the diagnosis, which is confirmed on identifying mutations in the CLCN5 or ORCL1 genes, although up to one in five patients with the clinical phenotype of Dent's disease reveal no such mutations. On the other hand, just one of the above-listed clinical conditions suffices to establish the diagnosis in individuals carrying CLCN5 or ORCL1 mutations. Very occasionally, we encounter hypercalciuric stone-formers who carry CLCN5 gene base mutations without any other clinical criteria of Dent's disease, so CLCN5 mutations may occasionally be responsible for primary hypercalciuria.[86] No disease-specific lesions are detectable on renal biopsies.

Antenatal diagnosis and preimplantation genetic testing for Dent's disease is not recommended, given that there are no known genotype-to-phenotype correlations and the disease also varies considerably within the same family, and the vital prognosis is good for most patients.[87]

No treatments targeting the molecular defects are available, but thiazide diuretics can be used to treat Dent's patients' hypercalciuria.[88] Judging from research conducted on ClC-5-deficient mice, a diet high in citrates can slow the renal disease's progression.[89]

Hereditary Hypophosphatemic Rickets with Hypercalciuria

Hereditary hypophosphatemic rickets with hypercalciuria (HHRH) is a very rare autosomal recessive disorder and most reported cases have occurred in Bedouin kindreds. It is characterized by tubular phosphate wasting due to an impaired activity of the sodium-phosphate cotransporter NaPi-2c (codified by gene SLC34A3, on chromosome 9a34.3).[90] This tubular phosphate leakage results in hypophosphatemia, stimulated 1-α hydroxylation and elevated 1,25-$(OH)_2$ vitamin D_3 levels, suppressed PTH, absorptive hypercalciuria, rickets or osteomalacia, and short stature. Unlike other forms of hypophosphatemia, in HHRH increased 1,25-$(OH)_2$ vitamin D_3 levels result in hypercalciuria, nephrocalcinosis, and renal stones. In the original Bedouin kindred,[91] and also in other kindreds identified afterwards,[92,93] the clinical phenotype may be only partially expressed in the individuals affected, some of whom are apparently healthy, but exhibit "idiopathic" hypercalciuria, while others have only the renal phenotype (nephrocalcinosis and stones) with normal serum phosphate levels. The magnitude of the hypophosphatemia, which regulates 1,25-$(OH)_2$ vitamin D_3 levels, appears to determine which individuals have hypercalciuria and which ones have bone disease too. Heterozygous subjects may have less severe biochemical changes and look like cases of idiopathic hypercalciuria.

An autosomal recessive proximal tubulopathy was recently described in two families due to mutations in GLUT2, the gene encoding the glucose transporter 2. This gene is mutated in Fanconi–Bickel syndrome, a rare condition characterized by mild proximal renal tubulopathy, impaired glucose homeostasis, and hepatomegaly. These two pedigrees revealed no Fanconi–Bickel syndrome; however, one had severe hypercalciuria with normal phosphate handling, the other a severe urinary phosphate wasting and hypophosphatemic rickets, possibly due to an impaired expression of the sodium-phosphate cotransporter NaPi-2c in the proximal tubule.[94]

Mutations of the *NPT2A* (also known as SLC34A1) encoding the sodium-phosphate cotransporter 2a in the proximal tubules have been accused of causing chronic hypophosphatemia in two unrelated, heterozygous patients, one with stones and the other with osteoporosis.[95] The issue remains controversial, however.[96]

Treating HHRH with oral phosphate reverses patients' hypophosphatemia and hypercalciuria, and cures their bone disease. Oral phosphate could be a reasonable treatment for patients with NPT2A and GLUT2 gene mutations too. A correct diagnosis of the above vitamin D-resistant forms of rickets is important to avoid any unnecessary vitamin D supplementation, which can cause nephrocalcinosis, renal stones, and kidney failure.

PRIMARY dRTA

Primary dRTA is a heterogeneous hereditary tubular disorder characterized by impaired renal acid secretion resulting in metabolic acidosis, failure to thrive, rickets/osteomalacia, nephrocalcinosis, nephrolithiasis, and episodes of hypokalemic paralysis. The biochemical changes consist of hyperchloremic metabolic acidosis, hypokalemia, hypercalciuria, hypocitraturia, and an inappropriately high urinary pH. The hypercalciuria is probably the consequence of an increased bone demineralization due to the buffering activity of the bone on the proton tide. Combined with hypocitraturia and inappropriately high urinary pH, hypercalciuria leads to nephrocalcinosis and apatite nephrolithiasis. Patients with overt dRTA have a significant risk of developing chronic kidney disease (CKD).[97]

Distal RTA may be caused by heritable defects in any of the several transporters of the type α-intercalated cells needed for transepithelial acid secretion and bicarbonate reabsorption. Autosomal dominant and rare forms of recessive dRTA are known to be caused by mutations in the gene SLC4A1 for the anion exchanger AE1.[98] Some patients with this condition may have erythrocytosis[99] and South West Asia ovalocytosis.[100] Mutations in the ATP6B1 (or ATP6V1B1) gene coding for the ss1 subunit of the vacuolar H^+-ATPase (located in chromosome 2p13) have proved responsible for recessive dRTA with sensorineural deafness,[101,102] while an autosomal recessive dRTA with preserved hearing is caused by mutations of the ATP6N1B (or ATP6V0A4) gene in chromosome 7q33-34, which encodes another proton-pump accessory subunit. This is generally believed to cause no sensorineural deafness, although early-onset hearing loss has been described in association with mutations of this gene too.[103]

Identifying the mutations that cause the disease enables antenatal or postnatal diagnoses in affected families and improves prognosis. The treatment of choice is potassium citrate because it is converted into bicarbonate and restores the body's potassium and citrate levels, and cures acidosis, increasing citraturia and reducing calciuria. Sodium bicarbonate can be used too, but the consequent increase in natriuresis could aggravate calciuria.

Bartter's Syndrome

Bartter's syndrome is a rare renal tubular disorder caused by defects in one of the molecules involved in transepithelial NaCl transport across the thick ascending limb of Henle's loop. This genetically heterogeneous syndrome is characterized by hypokalemia, metabolic alkalosis, renal salt wasting possibly leading to hypotension, and secondary hyperaldosteronism. Five different types have been recognized, depending on the mutated gene involved. Fasting hypercalciuria leading to medullary nephrocalcinosis is seen in Bartter type 1 (gene SLC12A1, locus 15q15-q21.1, encoding the luminal bumetanide-sensitive Na^+-K^+-$2Cl^-$ cotransporter; autosomal recessive), Bartter type 2

(KCNJ1, locus 11q21-25, which encodes the luminal potassium channel, renal outer medullary potassium; autosomal recessive),[104] and some patients with Bartter type 3 (CLCNKB gene encoding the basolateral renal chloride channel CLC-kb, locus 1p36; autosomal recessive).[105] The Bartter phenotype has also been described in patients with autosomal hypoparathyroidism (familial hypocalcemia with hypercalciuria) due to activating mutations of the CaSR gene capable of generating a conspicuous gain of function (Bartter type 5; autosomal dominant). In addition to the classical features of the syndrome, these patients develop hypocalcemia (which may be symptomatic with carpopedal spasm) and hypercalciuria, possibly associated with nephrocalcinosis.[106-108]

Activation of the renal CaSR is thought to inhibit paracellular divalent cation reabsorption in the cortical ascending limb, both directly and indirectly via a decrease in NaCl transport. While there is generally no defective tubular reabsorption of NaCl, and no renal loss of NaCl has been reported in patients with familial hypocalcemia with hypercalciuria caused by CaSR gain-of-function mutations, the potent gain-of-function mutation of the CaSR observed in Bartter type 5 patients is probably capable of reducing NaCl reabsorption in the cortical ascending limb, giving rise to renal loss of NaCl with secondary hyperaldosteronism and hypokalemia.[107] Given the heterogeneity of Bartter's syndrome and the common clinical phenotype involved, genetic testing is needed for a definite diagnosis of this disease.

Familial Hypomagnesemia with Hypercalciuria and Nephrocalcinosis

Familial hypomagnesemia with hypercalciuria and nephrocalcinosis (FHHNC) is a rare autosomal recessive disease of infancy that was first described in 1995.[109] About a hundred such patients have been described to date. Familial hypomagnesemia with hypercalciuria and nephrocalcinosis is characterized by magnesium and calcium wasting, resulting in persistent hypomagnesemia and hypocalcemia, which may cause seizures and tetany when severe. Marked hypercalciuria and nephrocalcinosis, nephrolithiasis, incomplete dRTA, hypocitraturia, urinary tract infections, polyuria and polydipsia, failure to thrive and progressive renal failure are generally observed, although less severe phenotypes have also been described. In two families, for instance, the missense mutation Thr233Arg of CLDN16 caused childhood hypercalciuria, which improved with age and was not associated with renal failure.[110] Mutations in Claudin16 mapping to 3q27, or in Claudin 19 on chromosome 1p34.2, have been reported in FHHNC families.[111,112]

Claudins 16 and 19 are tight junction proteins. They mediate cell-cell adhesion and form paracellular ion channels in the thick ascending limb of Henle's loop, and in the same segment of the nephron and retinal pigment epithelium, respectively. This explains why >90% of FHHNC patients due to CLDN19 mutations have ocular abnormalities (pigmentary retinitis, macular coloboma, nystagmus, visual loss).[112] Patients with CLDN19 mutations also seem to develop CKD earlier than those with CLDN16 mutations.[112] Interestingly, a large percentage of heterozygous relatives of FHHNC patients have hypercalciuria and stones without any other traits of the disease.[113]

High-dose magnesium is the treatment of choice. Hydrochlorothiazide is effective in reducing hypercalciuria due to CLDN16 mutations. Indomethacin is also used for this purpose. The efficacy of these two drugs in slowing disease progression is unclear, however.[112,114]

Absorptive Hypercalciuria and Low Spinal Bone Density

Absorptive hypercalciuria in linkage with chromosome 1q23-24 was first described in three families, seemingly with an autosomal dominant inheritance.[115] Mutations of a ubiquitously-expressed soluble adenylate cyclase (sAC) gene located on 1q23-24 were suggested as the putative cause of the condition. These individuals had an increased intestinal calcium uptake, normocalcemia, normal circulating PTH levels, and a low spinal bone density. Whether sAC causes absorptive hypercalciuria remains to be demonstrated.[116,117]

Familial Hyperkalemic Hypertension (With Hypercalciuria)

Mutations in the lysine-deficient protein kinase 4 (WNK4) gene on chromosome 17a21 cause a rare autosomal dominant disease with hyperkalemia, acidosis, arterial hypertension (pseudohypoaldosteronism type 2B), low renin levels, and hypercalciuria. Serum calcium levels are mildly reduced, suggesting a renal calcium leak.[118] Renal function is normal.[119] The mechanism underlying hypercalciuria in these patients is unclear. WNK4 is a kinase of the distal tubule, but the increased calcium excretion may be due to downregulation of the calcium channel TRPV5 with calcium reabsorption in the distal tubule, and an upregulated sodium-chloride cotransport activity in the same tubular segment.[120] A study on the WNK4 knock-in mouse model suggested that decreased Ca^{2+} reabsorption in the thick ascending loops of Henle, with a secondary adaptive increase in the calcium channel TRPV6 and calbindin-D28k expression in the distal tubules, might be responsible for the hypercalciuria in this condition.[121]

These findings open a new window on the relationship between calcium handling, renal stones and hypertension, which remains to be explained.[122] In the few families described in the literature, nephrolithiasis and/or nephrocalcinosis were apparently not observed. In the family described by Mayan et al, the affected members had a lower bone mineral density,[119] a finding supported by a recent study in a Portuguese cohort that disclosed a tendency for osteoporosis in association with the rare WNK4 allelic variant rs56116165.[123] Thiazide diuretics correct all the abnormalities in this condition, including hypercalciuria and it has been estimated that patients' sensitivity to these agents is 6–7 times higher than in control.[119]

REFERENCES

1. Palubinskas AJ. Renal pyramidal structure opacification in excretory urography and its relation to medullary sponge kidney. Radiology. 1963;81:963-70.
2. Thomas E, Witte Y, Thomas J, et al. Maladie de Cacchi et Ricci: remarques radiologiques, epidémiologiques et biologiques. Progrès en Urologie. 2000;10:29-35.
3. Fabris A, Lupo A, Bernich P, et al. Long-term treatment with potassium citrate and renal stones in medullary sponge kidney. Clin J Am Soc Nephrol. 2010;5:1663-8.
4. Gambaro G, Feltrin GP, Lupo A, et al. Medullary sponge kidney (Lenarduzzi-Cacchi-Ricci disease): a Padua medical school discovery in the 1930s. Kidney Int. 2006;69:663-70.
5. Lambrianides AL, John DR. Medullary sponge disease in horseshoe kidney. Urology. 1987;29:426-7.
6. Iwig J, Thiemann KJ. Medullary sponge kidney with megapyelon and primary congenital megaureter in unilateral renal aplasia. Fortschr Geb Rontgenstr Nuklearmed. 1969;111: 137-40.
7. Gambaro G, Fabris F, Citron L, et al. An unusual association of contralateral congenital small kidney, reduced renal function and hyperparathyroidism in sponge kidney patients: on the track of the molecular basis. Nephrol Dial Transplant. 2005;20:1042-7.
8. Sariola H, Saarma M. Novel functions and signalling pathways for GDNF. J Cell Sci. 2003;1:3855-62.
9. Schedl A, Hastie ND. Cross-talk in kidney development. Curr Opin Genet Dev. 2000;10:543-9.
10. Michos O. Kidney development: From ureteric bud formation to branching morphogenesis. Curr Opin Genet Dev. 2009;19:484-90.
11. Michos O, Cebrian C, Hyink D, et al. Kidney development in the absence of Gdnf and Spry1 requires Fgf10. PLoS Genet. 2010;6:e1000809.
12. Sánchez MP, Silos-Santiago I, Frisén J, et al. Renal agenesis and the absence of enteric neurons in mice lacking GDNF. Nature. 1996;382:70-3.
13. Schuchardt A, D'Agati V, Larsson-Blomberg L, et al. Defects in the kidney and enteric nervous system of mice lacking the tyrosine kinase receptor RET. Nature. 1994;367:380-3.
14. Manie S, Santoro M, Fusco A, et al. The RET receptor: Function in development and dysfunction in congenital malformation. Trends Genet. 2001;17:580-9.
15. Srinivas S, Wu Z, Chen CM, et al. Dominant effects of RET receptor misexpression and ligand-independent RET signaling on ureteric bud development. Development. 1999;126:1375-86.
16. Diouf B, Ka EH, Calender A, et al. Association of medullary sponge kidney disease and multiple endocrine neoplasia type IIA due to RET gene mutation: Is there a causal relationship? Nephrol Dial Transplant. 2000;15:2062-6.
17. Skinner MA, Safford SD, Reeves JG, et al. Renal aplasia in humans is associated with RET mutations. Am J Hum Genet. 2008;82:344-51.
18. Kuiper JJ. Medullary sponge kidney in three generations. N Y State J Med. 1971;71:2665-9.
19. Copping GA. Medullary sponge kidney: its occurrence in a father and daughter. Can Med Assoc J. 1967;96:608-11.
20. Klemme LA, Fish AJ, Rich S, et al. Familial ureteral abnormalities syndrome: genomic mapping, clinical findings. Pediatr Nephrol. 1998;12:349-56.
21. Torregrossa R, Anglani F, Fabris A, et al. Identification of GDNF gene sequence variations in patients with medullary sponge kidney disease. Clin J Am Soc Nephrol. 2010;5:1205-10.
22. Brophy PD, Ostrom L, Lang KM, et al. Regulation of ureteric bud outgrowth by Pax2-dependent activation of the glial derived neurotrophic factor gene. Development. 2001;128:4747-56.
23. El-Ghoneimi A, Berrebi D, Levacher B, et al. Glial cell line derived neurotrophic factor is expressed by epithelia of human renal dysplasia. J Urol. 2002;168:2624-8.
24. Carboni I, Andreucci E, Caruso MR, et al. Medullary sponge kidney associated with primary distal renal tubular acidosis and mutations of the H+-ATPase genes. Nephrol Dial Transplant. 2009;24:2734-38.
25. Gunay-Aygun M, Turkbey BI, Bryant J, et al. Hepatorenal findings in obligate heterozygotes for autosomal recessive polycystic kidney disease. Mol Genet Metab. 2011;104:677-81.
26. Torres VE, Erickson SB, Smith LH, et al. The association of nephrolithiasis and autosomal dominant polycystic kidney disease. Am J Kidney Dis. 1988;11:318-25.
27. Kerr D, Warrick C, Hart-Mercer J. A lesion resembling medullary sponge kidney in patients with congenital hepatic fibrosis. Clin Radiol. 1962;13:85-91.
28. Handelsman DJ, Conway AJ, Boylan LM, et al. Young's syndrome: obstructive azoospermia in chronic sinopulmonary infections. New Eng J Med. 1984;310:3-9.

29. Sluysmans T, Vanoverschelde JP, Malvaux P. Growth failure associated with medullary sponge kidney, due to incomplete renal tubular acidosis type 1. Eur J Pediatr. 1987;146:78-80.
30. Kasap B, Soylu A, Oren O, et al. Medullary sponge kidney associated with distal renal tubular acidosis in a 5-year-old girl. Eur J Pediatr. 2006;165:648-51.
31. Cameron S. Medullary sponge kidney. In: Davison AM, Cameron JS, Grunfeld J-P, (Eds). Oxford Textbook of Clinical Nephrology, 3rd edition. Oxford, UK: Oxford University Press; 2004.
32. McPhail EF, Gettman MT, Patterson DE, et al. Nephrolithiasis in medullary sponge kidney: evaluation of clinical and metabolic features. Urology. 2012;79:277-81.
33. Chu HY, Yan MT, Lin SH. Recurrent pyelonephritis as a sign of "sponge kidney." Cleve Clin J Med. 2009;76:479-80.
34. Gambaro G, Favaro S, D'Angelo A. Risk for renal failure in nephrolithiasis. Am J Kidney Dis. 2001;37:233-43.
35. Maschio G, Tessitore N, D'Angelo A, et al. Medullary sponge kidney and hyperparathyroidism—a puzzling association. Am J Nephrol. 1982;2:77-84.
36. Dlabal PW, Jordan RM, Dorfman SG. Medullary sponge kidney and renal-leak hypercalciuria. A link to the development of parathyroid adenoma? JAMA. 1979;241:1490-1.
37. Granberg PO, Lagergren C, Theve NO. Renal function studies in medullary sponge kidney. Scand J Urol Nephrol. 1971;5:177-80.
38. Lahme S, Bichler K-H, Lang F, et al. Metabolic evaluation of patients suffering from medullary sponge kidney In: Borghi L (Ed). 8th European Symposium on Urolithiasis, Parma, Italy. Bios, Italy; 1999.
39. Higashihara E, Nutahara K, Tago K, et al. Medullary sponge kidney and renal acidification defect. Kidney Int. 1984;25:453-9.
40. Ginalski JM, Portmann L, Jaeger P. Does medullary sponge kidney cause nephrolithiasis? Am J Roentgenol. 1990;155:299-302.
41. Daudon M, Cohen-Solal F, Lacour B, et al. Urinary stones and urinary tract abnormalities. Is the stone composition independent of the anatomical abnormality? Prog Urol. 2003;13:1320-9.
42. Fabris A, Bernich P, Abaterusso C, et al. Bone disease in medullary sponge kidney and effect of potassium citrate treatment. Clin J Am Soc Nephrol. 2009;4:1974-9.
43. Osther PJ, Mathiasen H, Hansen AB, et al. Urinary acidification and urinary excretion of calcium and citrate in women with bilateral medullary sponge kidney. Urol Int. 1994;52:126-30.
44. Higashihara E, Nutahara K, Niijima T. Renal hypercalciuria and metabolic acidosis associated with medullary sponge kidney: effect of alkali therapy. Urol Res. 1988;16:95-100.
45. Pabico RC, McKenna BA, Freeman RB. Renal tubular dysfunction in patients with cystic disease of the kidneys. Urology. 1998;51(5A Suppl):156-60.
46. Huber SM, Braun GS, Segerer S, et al. Metanephrogenic mesenchyme-to-epithelium transition induces profound expression changes of ion channels. Am J Renal Physiol. 2000;279:F65-F76.
47. Forster JA, Taylor J, Browning AJ, et al. A review of the natural progression of medullary sponge kidney and a novel grading system based on intravenous urography findings. Urol Int. 2007;78:264-9.
48. Teichman JM. Clinical practice. Acute renal colic from ureteral calculus. N Engl J Med. 2004;350:684-93.
49. Raynal G, Dugardin F, Hassani H, et al. Maladie de Cacchi et Ricci et tomodensitométrie sans injection. Presse Med. 2010;39:524-5.
50. Ginalski JM, Schnyder P, Portmann L, et al. Medullary sponge kidney on axial computed tomography: comparison with excretory urography. Eur J Radiol. 1991;12:104-7.
51. Lang EK, Macchia RJ, Thomas R, et al. Improved detection of renal pathologic features on multiphasic helical CT compared with IVU in patients presenting with microscopic hematuria. Urology. 2003;61:528-32.
52. Maw AM, Megibow AJ, Grasso M, et al. Diagnosis of medullary sponge kidney by computed tomographic urography. Am J Kidney Dis. 2007;50:146-50.
53. Koraishy FM, Ngo TT, Israel GM, et al. CT urography for the diagnosis of medullary sponge kidney. Am J Nephrol. 2014;39:165-70.
54. Patriquin HB, O'Regan S. Medullary sponge kidney in childhood. AJR. 1985;145:315-9.
55. Toyoda K, Miyamoto Y, Ida M, et al. Hyperechoic medulla of the kidneys. Radiology. 1989;173:431-4.
56. Dick PT, Shuckett BM, Tang B, et al. Observer reliability in grading nephrocalcinosis on ultrasound examinations in children. Pediatr Radiol. 1999;29:68-72.
57. Schepens D, Verswijvel G, Kuypers D, et al. Renal cortical nephrocalcinosis. Nephrol Dial Transplant. 2000;15:1080-2.
58. Hida T, Nishie A, Asayama Y, et al. MR imaging of focal medullary sponge kidney: case report. Magn Reson Med Sci. 2012;11:65-9.
59. Taub DA, Suh RS, Faerber GJ, et al. Ureteroscopic laser papillotomy to treat papillary calcifications associated with chronic flank pain. Urology. 2006;67:683-7.
60. Flechner SM, Noble M, Tiong HY, et al. Renal autotransplantation and modified pyelovesicostomy for intractable metabolic stone disease. J Urol. 2011;186:1910-5.
61. Coe FL, Parks JH, Moore ES. Familial idiopathic hypercalciuria. N Engl J Med. 1979;300:337-40.
62. Pak CY, McGuire J, Peterson R, et al. Familial absorptive hypercalciuria in a large kindred. J Urol. 1981;126:717-9.
63. Lerolle N, Coulet F, Lantz B, et al. No evidence for point mutations of the calcium-sensing receptor in a familial idiopathic hypercalciuria. Nephrol Dial Transplant. 2001;16:2317-22.
64. Harangi F, Mehes K. Family investigations in idiopathic hypercalciuria. Eur J Pediatr. 1993;152:64-8.
65. Goodman HO, Holmes RP, Assimov DG. Genetic factors in calcium oxalate stone disease. J Urol. 1995;153:301-7.
66. Colhoun HM, McKeigue PM, Davey Smith G. Problems of reporting genetic association with complex outcomes. Lancet. 2003;361:865-72.
67. Falchetti A, Vezzoli G, Gambaro G. Genetics of primary hypercalciuria. Clin Cases Miner Bone Metab. 2004;1:27-33.

68. Hunter D, De Lange M, Snieder H, et al. Genetic contribution to bone metabolism, calcium excretion, and vitamin D and parathyroid hormone regulation. J Bone Miner Res. 2001;16:371-8.
69. Loredo-Osti JC, Roslin NM, Tessier J, et al. Segregation of urine calcium excretion in families ascertained for nephrolithiasis: evidence for a major gene. Kidney Int. 2005;68:966-71.
70. Zuk O, Hechter E, Sunyaev SR, et al. The mystery of missing heritability: genetic interactions create phantom heritability. Proc Natl Acad Sci. 2012;109:1193-98.
71. Pearce SH, Williamson C, Kifor, et al. A familial syndrome of hypocalcemia with hypercalciuria due to mutations in the calcium-sensing receptor. New Engl J Med. 1996;335:1115-22.
72. Stechman MJ, Loh NY, Thakker RV. Genetic causes of hypercalciuric nephrolithiasis. Pediatr Nephrol. 2009;24:2321-32.
73. Falchetti A, Marini F, Giusti F, et al. DNA-based test: when and why to apply it to primary hyperparathyroidism clinical phenotypes. J Intern Med. 2009;266:69-83.
74. Benej M, Bendlova B, Vaclavikova E, et al. Establishing high resolution melting analysis: method validation and evaluation for c-RET proto-oncogene mutation screening. Clin Chem Lab Med. 2011;50:51-60.
75. Schlingmann KP, Kaufmann M, Weber S, et al. Mutations in CYP24A1 and idiopathic infantile hypercalcemia. N Engl J Med. 2011;365:410-21.
76. Nesterova G, Malicdan MC, Yasuda K, et al. 1,25-(OH)2D-24 hydroxylase (CYP24A1) deficiency as a cause of nephrolithiasis. Clin J Am Soc Nephrol. 2013;8:649-57.
77. Colussi G, Ganon L, Penco S, et al. Chronic hypercalcaemia from inactivating mutations of vitamin D 24-hydroxylase (CYP24A1): implications for mineral metabolism changes in chronic renal failure. Nephrol Dial Transplant. 2014;29: 636-43.
78. Wolf P, Müller-Sacherer T, Baumgartner-Parzer S, et al. A case of "late onset" idiopathic infantile hypercalcemia secondary to mutations in the CYP24A1 gene. Endocr Pract. 2014:1-14. [Epub ahead of print].
79. Lloyd SE, Pearce SH, Fisher SE, et al. A common molecular basis for three inherited kidney stone diseases. Nature. 1996;379:445-9.
80. Gunther W, Luchow A, Cluzeaud F, et al. ClC-5, the chloride channel mutated in Dent's disease, colocalizes with the proton pump in endocytically active kidney cells. Proc Natl Acad Sci USA. 1998;95:8075-80.
81. Devuyst O, Christie PT, Courtoy PJ, et al. Intra-renal and subcellular distribution of the human chloride channel, ClC-5, reveals a pathophysiological basis for Dent's disease. Hum Mol Genet. 1999;8:247-57.
82. Piwon N, Gunther W, Schwake M, et al. ClC-5 Cl-channel disruption impairs endocytosis in a mouse model for Dent's disease. Nature 2000;408:369-373.
83. Wang SS, Devuyst O, Courtoy PJ, et al. Mice lacking renal chloride channel, ClC-5, are a model for Dent's disease, a nephrolithiasis disorder associated with defective receptor-mediated endocytosis. Hum Mol Genet. 2000;9:2937-45.
84. Christensen EI, Devuyst O, Dom G, et al. Loss of chloride channel ClC-5 impairs endocytosis by defective trafficking of megalin and cubilin in kidney proximal tubules. Proc Natl Acad Sci USA. 2003;100:8472-7.
85. Erdmann KS, Mao Y, McCrea HJ, et al. A role of the Lowe syndrome protein OCRL in early steps of the endocytic pathway. Dev Cell. 2007;13:377-90.
86. Scheinmn SJ, Cox JPD, Lloyd SE, et al. Isolated hypercalciuria with mutation in CLCN5: relevance to idiopathic hypercalciuria. Kidney Int. 2000;57:232-9.
87. Devuyst O, Thakker RV. Dent's disease. Orphanet J Rare Dis. 2010;5:28.
88. Blanchard A, Vargas-Poussou R, Peyrard S, et al. Effect of hydrochlorothiazide on urinary calcium excretion in Dent disease: an uncontrolled trial. Am J Kidney Dis. 2008;52:1084-95.
89. Cebotaru V, Kaul S, Devuyst O, et al. High citrate diet delays progression of renal insufficiency in the ClC-5 knockout mouse model of Dent's disease. Kidney Int. 2005;68:642-52.
90. Lorenz-Depiereux B, Benet-Pages A, Eckstein G, et al. Hereditary hypophosphatemic rickets with hypercalciuria is caused by mutations in the sodium-phosphate cotransporter gene SLC34A3. Am J Hum Genet. 2006;78:193-201.
91. Tieder M, Modai D, Shaked U, et al. "Idiopathic" hypercalciuria and hereditary hypophosphatemic rickets. Two phenotypical expressions of a common genetic defect. N Engl J Med. 1987;316:125-9.
92. Tieder M, Arie R, Bab I, et al. A new kindred with hereditary hypophosphatemic rickets with hypercalciuria: implications for correct diagnosis and treatment. Nephron. 1992;62:176-81.
93. Tencza AL, Ichikawa S, Dang A, et al. Hypophosphatemic rickets with hypercalciuria due to mutation in SLC34A3/ type IIc sodium-phosphate cotransporter: presentation as hypercalciuria and nephrolithiasis. Clin Endocrinol Metab. 2009;94:4433-8.
94. Mannstadt M, Magen D, Segawa H, et al. Fanconi-Bickel syndrome and autosomal recessive proximal tubulopathy with hypercalciuria (ARPTH) are allelic variants caused by GLUT2 mutations. J Clin Endocrinol Metab. 2012;97: E1978-1986.
95. Prie D, Huart V, Bakouh N, et al. Nephrolithiasis and osteoporosis caused by mutations in the type 2a sodium-phosphate cotransporter. N Engl J Med. 1992;347:983-91.
96. Virkki LV, Forster IC, Hernando N, et al. Functional characterization of two naturally occurring mutations in the human sodium-phosphate cotransporter type IIa. J Bone Miner Res. 2003;18:2135-41.
97. Gambaro G, Favaro S, D'Angelo A. Risk for renal failure in nephrolithiasis. Am J Kidney Dis. 2001;37:233-43.
98. Devonald MA, Smith AN, Poon JP, et al. Non-polarized targeting of AE1 causes autosomal dominant distal renal tubular acidosis. Nat Genet. 2003;33:125-7.
99. Bruce LJ, Cope DL, Jones GK, et al. Familial distal renal tubular acidosis is associated with mutations in the red cell anion exchanger (Band 3, AE1) gene. J Clin Invest. 1997;100:1693-707.
100. Wrong O, Bruce LJ, Unwin RJ, et al. Band 3 mutations, distal renal tubular acidosis, and Southeast Asian ovalocytosis. Kidney Int. 2002;62:10-9.

101. Karet FE, Finberg KE, Nelson RD, et al. Mutations in the gene encoding B1 subunit of H^+-ATPase cause renal tubular acidosis with sensorineural deafness. Nat Genet. 1999;21:84-90.
102. Ruf R, Rensing C, Topaloglu R, et al. Confirmation of the ATP6B1 gene as responsible for distal renal tubular acidosis. Pediatr Nephrol. 2003;18:105-9.
103. Vargas-Poussou R, Houillier P, Le Pottier N, et al. Genetic investigation of autosomal recessive distal renal tubular acidosis: evidence for early sensorineural hearing loss associated with mutations in the ATP6V0A4 gene. J Am Soc Nephrol. 2006;17:1437-43.
104. Karolyi L, Koch MC, Grzeschik KH, et al. The molecular genetic approach to "Bartter's syndrome." J Mol Med. 1998;76:317-25.
105. Simon DB, Bindra RS, Mansfield TA, et al. Mutations in the chloride channel gene, CLCNKB, cause Bartter's syndrome type III. Nature Genet. 1997;17:171-8.
106. Watanabe S, Fukumoto S, Chang H, et al. Association between activating mutations of calcium-sensing receptor and Bartter's syndrome. Lancet. 2002;360:692-4.
107. Vargas-Poussou R, Huang C, Hulin P, et al. Functional characterization of a calcium-sensing receptor mutation in severe autosomal dominant hypocalcemia with a Bartter-like syndrome. J Am Soc Nephrol. 2002;13:2259-66.
108. Vezzoli G, Arcidiacono T, Paloschi V, et al. Autosomal dominant hypocalcemia with mild type 5 Bartter syndrome. J Nephrol. 2006;19:525-8.
109. Praga M, Vara J, Gonzalez-Parra E, et al. Familial hypomagnesemia with hypercalciuria and nephrocalcinosis. Kidney Int. 1995;47:1419-25.
110. Muller D, Kausalya PJ, Clavierie-Martin F, et al. A novel claudin 16 mutation associated with childhood hypercalciuria abolishes binding to ZO-1 and results in lysosomal mistargeting. Am J Hum Genet. 2003;73:1293-301.
111. Weber S, Hoffmann K, Jeck N, et al. Familial hypomagnesaemia with hypercalciuria and nephrocalcinosis maps to chromosome 3q27 and is associated with mutations in the PCLN-1 gene. Eur J Hum Genet. 2000;8:414-22.
112. Godron A, Harambat J, Boccio V, et al. Familial hypomagnesemia with hypercalciuria and nephrocalcinosis: phenotype-genotype correlation and outcome in 32 patients with CLDN16 or CLDN19 mutations. Clin J Am Soc Nephrol. 2012;7:801-9.
113. Weber S, Schneider L, Peters M, et al. Novel paracellin-1 mutations in 25 families with familial hypomagnesemia with hypercalciuria and nephrocalcinosis. J Am Soc Nephrol. 2001;12:1872-81.
114. Zimmermann B1, Plank C, Konrad M, et al. Hydrochlorothiazide in CLDN16 mutation. Nephrol Dial Transplant. 2006;21:2127-32.
115. Reed BY, Gitomer WL, Heller HJ, et al. Identification and characterization of a gene with base substitutions associated with the absorptive hypercalciuria phenotype and low spinal bone density. J Clin Endocrinol Metab. 2002;87:1476-85.
116. Geng W, Wang Z, Zhang J, et al. Cloning and characterization of the human soluble adenylyl cyclase. Am J Physiol Cell Physiol. 2005;288:C1305-C1316.
117. Econs MJ, Foroud T. The genetics of absorptive hypercalciuria—a note of caution. J Clin Endocrinol Metab. 2002;87:1473-5.
118. Mayan H, Munter G, Shaharabany M, et al. Hypercalciuria in familial hyperkalemia and hypertension accompanies hyperkalemia and precedes hypertension: description of a large family with the Q565E WNK4 mutation. J Clin Endocrinol Metab. 2004;89:4025-30.
119. Mayan H, Vered I, Mouallem M, et al. Pseudohypoaldosteronism type II: marked sensitivity to thiazides, hypercalciuria, normomagnesemia, and low bone mineral density. J Clin Endocrinol Metab. 2002;87:3248-54.
120. Jiang Y, Ferguson WB, Peng JB. WNK4 enhances TRPV5-mediated calcium transport: potential role in hypercalciuria of familial hyperkalemic hypertension caused by gene mutation of WNK4. Am J Physiol Renal Physiol. 2007;292:F545-F554.
121. Yang SS, Hsu YJ, Chiga M, et al. Mechanisms for hypercalciuria in pseudohypoaldosteronism type II-causing WNK4 knock-in mice. Endocrinology. 2010;151:1829-36.
122. Resnick L. Calcium metabolism, renin activity, and the antihypertensive effects of calcium channel blockade. Am J Med. 1986;81:6-14.
123. Mendes AI, Mascarenhas MR, Matos S, et al. A WNK4 gene variant relates to osteoporosis and not hypertension in the Portuguese population. Mol Genet Metab. 2011;102:465-9.

CHAPTER 21

Cystine and Uncommon Organic Stones

David S Goldfarb

INTRODUCTION

As the result of mutations in a handful of genes, relatively insoluble molecules appear in the urine at levels beyond their supported supersaturation. Precipitation and stone formation result. In this chapter I have described three consequential, if relatively rare, disorders: cystinuria; adenine phosphoribosyltransferase deficiency (APRTd), which causes 2,8-dihydroxyadenine (DHA) stones; and xanthinuria. Other genetic diseases that cause stones, such as primary hyperoxaluria and Dent disease, cause the more common calcium oxalate and calcium phosphate stones. These three disorders themselves constitute an important indication for determining kidney stone composition in all patients at least once, as failure to make these diagnoses can lead to important missed opportunities.

CYSTINURIA

The amino acid cystine is a dimer composed of two molecules of cysteine, linked by a disulfide bridge as seen in Figure 21.1.[1] Its loss in the urine is the major disorder characterizing cystinuria. Cystinuria is said to account for approximately 1% of all stones and 7% of stones in children.[1] It is a hereditary kidney disorder that impairs the proximal tubule's ability to reabsorb filtered cystine and dibasic amino acids. It is the result of a mutation in an amino acid transporter (AT) particularly expressed in the proximal tubule. While the transporter is also expressed in the small intestine, the mutation that causes cystinuria and the resulting impaired absorption of amino acids are not presently considered a cause of any clinical manifestations. Cystinuria was among the first inborn errors of metabolism recognized by Sir Archibald Garrod in 1908.[2] Normally, there is near-complete reabsorption of filtered cystine and the dibasic amino acids ornithine, arginine, and lysine (mnemonic for affected amino acids: COAL); the amino acids are instead not reabsorbed. They reach high concentrations in the urine of affected individuals. Only the abnormal excretion of cystine results in a

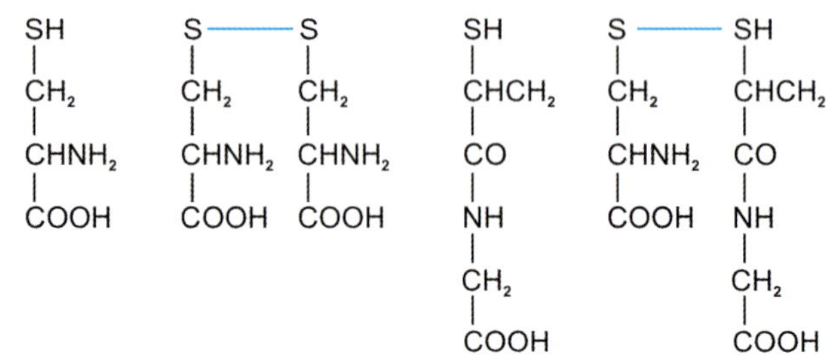

Cysteine Cystine Tiopronin Tiopronin-cysteine

Fig. 21.1: Chemical structures of cystine, cysteine, and drug-cysteine complex.

clinically significant effect due to its low solubility at urine pH values <6.5. At more acid urine pH values and at high concentrations, cystine crystals form and stones in the urinary tract result. These stones can be frequent, recurrent, and large. Urolithiasis causes renal colic, hematuria, urinary obstruction, chronic kidney disease (CKD) and, rarely, renal failure. Loss of the dibasic amino acids ornithine, arginine, and lysine does not cause any recognized phenotypic traits.

Physiology and Pathophysiology of Cystine Transport

Mutations in two genes account for almost all cases of cystinuria. These two genes encode two proteins, which together are responsible for normal amino acid reabsorption in the proximal tubule and intestine. Both genes are included in the class of solute carriers (SLCs). The catalytic AT, a protein with 487 amino acids, is itself called $b^{0,+}$AT and is the product of gene SLC7A9. Amino acid transport system $b^{0,+}$ is responsible for transport of both neutral and dibasic amino acids. The product of SLC3A1 is rBAT (for related to $b^{0,+}$ AT), a type II membrane N-glycoprotein with 685 amino acids, which traffics $b^{0,+}$AT properly to the apical membrane of the epithelial cells in which they are both expressed.[3] The two proteins are linked by a disulfide bridge. The dimer is an example of a heteromeric AT (HAT), a class that has both a heavy subunit, in this case rBAT, and a light component, in this case $b^{0,+}$AT.[4] The light component is considered a glycoprotein-associated protein, as its association with the glycoprotein rBAT is required for it to reach the apical membrane. Without rBAT, $b^{0,+}$ AT remains in the endoplasmic reticulum.[5] Expression of both proteins is required for cystine transport to proceed in vivo, but when reconstituted in proteoliposomes, $b^{0,+}$ AT functions successfully as an AT in the absence of rBAT.[6] rBAT, like other heavy subunits of HATs, has a single transmembrane domain, an intracellular N terminus, and a large extracellular C-terminus. $b^{0,+}$ AT, like other light subunits of HATs is highly hydrophobic and not glycosylated. Current models suggest that it has 12 transmembrane domains.[7]

The luminal cystine transporter functions as an exchanger, transporting cystine and cationic amino acids (0,+) into the proximal tubular epithelial cells in a 1:1 exchange for neutral amino acids (but not imino acids) from within the cells. This high affinity process has a K_m of 100 μmol/L. There are three driving forces for the action of the cystine transporter. The cell interior has a negative potential difference relative to the lumen; the intracellular concentration of neutral amino acids is high; and one molecule of cystine is reduced to two molecules of cysteine within the cell. All of these maintain a favorable electrochemical gradient to allow cystine and dibasic amino acid transport to proceed. The transport process is electrogenic, generating a change in charge across the membrane. At the pH of the tubular fluid the amino groups of cystine and dibasic amino acids are protonated and carry a positive charge. The effect of cystine absorption then is to depolarize the relatively negative cell interior, making it relatively more positive. This transport process is itself independent of sodium.[8] However, the intracellular amino acids exchanged for cystine, ornithine, arginine, and lysine were themselves taken up from the tubular lumen by a sodium-dependent amino acid cotransporter.

While cystine reabsorption at the apical membrane is well characterized, the exit step for cysteine across the basolateral membrane is not as well understood. At least one L-type amino acid transport system (LAT, members of the SLC7 family) probably participates.[9]

In normal humans, >99% of amino acids filtered by the glomerulus is reabsorbed by the end of the proximal tubule. In cystinuria, the fractional excretion of cystine can be slightly >100% of the filtered load, implying a tubular cystine secretory pathway that has not been identified. There remain some uncertainties about the exact location of normal cystine transport in the proximal tubule, and how cystine transport is affected in cystinuria. There is a high-affinity–low-capacity system mediating the uptake of cystine and dibasic amino acids, found almost exclusively in the S3 segment of the proximal tubule. About 10% of the filtered cystine is reabsorbed via this transporter. The S3 location of this high-affinity–low-capacity system coincides with the location of the majority of expression of rBAT. About 90% of the filtered load of cystine is reabsorbed in the more proximal S1 and S2 segments of the proximal tubule through a low affinity–high-capacity transport system.[10] The transporting protein $b^{0,+}$ AT protein is expressed in all three segments of the proximal tubule, highest in S1 and lesser amounts in S2 and then S3 segments. Its role in the more proximal low-affinity–high capacity transport process had been suggested but has been shown to associate exclusively with rBAT. That low-affinity–high capacity transport remains uncharacterized to date. rBAT, on the other hand, does not exclusively form heterodimers with $b^{0,+}$ AT, suggesting the existence of another unknown light subunit for it to bind to.

The high-affinity cystine transporter, composed of the heavy (rBAT) and light ($b^{0,+}$ AT) subunits, is also present in the apical brush border membranes of the jejunum where it mediates absorption of cystine, dibasic amino acids, and some neutral amino acids as well. Although cystine absorption by the intestine following an oral cystine feeding is impaired in most patients with cystinuria, cystine deficiency or amino acid malnutrition are not clinically significant. This is because the intestine's absorption of oligopeptides, specifically di- and tripeptides, mediated by PEPT1 (encoded by gene SLC15A1), is intact.[11] Adequate cystine, as well as the affected dibasic amino acids (ornithine, lysine, and arginine), can be absorbed in this form, combined with other amino acids. Plasma levels of these amino acids may be normal or slightly reduced. Dietary methionine, the absorption of which is not affected by cystinuria, serves as a precursor for the body's cystine requirement. One study of sulfur-containing compounds and sulfate balance in cystinurics demonstrated decreased urinary excretion of sulfates and decreased glutathione in white blood cells, suggesting a deficiency in intracellular cystine and cysteine.[12] Although glutathione is an important antioxidant, no clinically significant consequence of the abnormal sulfur metabolism and loss of urinary amino acids has been demonstrated in people with cystinuria.

Genetics

Most studies of genotype in patients with cystinuria demonstrate nearly equal contributions of SLC3A1 and SLC7A9 mutations. SLC3A1 is located on the short arm of chromosome 2 (2p16.3-21) and contains 10 exons.[13] Mutations in SLC3A1 are associated with autosomal recessive mode of inheritance. The parents of an affected child with cystinuria due to SLC3A1 mutations are obligate heterozygotes and do not have abnormal urinary excretion of amino acids. In such families, on average 25% of the offspring of those heterozygotic parents would be expected to have cystinuria, 50% would be unaffected heterozygotic carriers, and 25% would be unaffected, noncarriers.

The pattern of inheritance for SLC7A9 mutations is different. The gene is located on chromosome 19 and contains 13 exons. SLC7A9 variants result in incompletely dominant inheritance, as heterozygous individuals do have abnormal urinary amino acid excretion. This pattern may also be called autosomal dominant inheritance with incomplete penetrance. These terms arise because some, but not all, of these heterozygotic individuals will have enough cystine in the urine to have kidney stones. One estimate is that 86–90% of SLC7A9 heterozygotes have increased urinary cystine excretion and 2–18% of such cases have kidney stones. Therefore the great majority of patients with cystinuria have two mutated alleles in either of the known genes. With this mode of inheritance, 75% of the offspring of two parents with SLC7A9 mutations, 25% homozygous, and 50% heterozygous, would have abnormal cystine excretion, with the homozygous individual much more likely to have stones.

While detailed studies of SLC7A9 heterozygotic stone formers have not been performed, stone disease would presumably be most often associated with low urine volume or ingestion of more dietary protein.[14] It is also possible that the stone-forming tendency of patients with cystinuria, whether homozygous or heterozygous for mutations in either gene, is affected by specific polymorphisms in the two known genes or that it is influenced by other yet-unidentified modifier genes.

More than 100 pathogenic variants in both SLC3A1 and SLC7A9 have been reported. The observed variants cover the full spectrum of mutations, ranging from nonsense, missense, splicing, and frameshift mutations to whole- and multi-exon imbalances. One of the most common mutations in SLC3A1 is Met467Thr, coding for a substitution of threonine for methionine at position 467. This mutation is relatively common in Mediterranean populations, accounting for 40% of the abnormal genes in a Spanish cohort of families with cystinuria. On the other hand, it is relatively rare in patients studied in Quebec. The M467T mutation leads to an impaired protein glycosylation after synthesis in the endoplasmic reticulum.[15] The most common mutation in the population of Libyan Jews with SLC7A9 mutations leads to a methionine replacing the expected valine amino acid residue at position 170 (V170 M) in the protein. About 6% of patients with cystinuria have no mutations in the two currently known relevant genes. The explanatory genotype of such individuals has not yet been revealed but presumably leads to changes in reabsorption of cystine by other unspecified cystine transporters in the nephron's proximal tubule.

At present genotyping patients with cystinuria does not affect therapy. The lack of therapeutic implications of genotype may change as study of the pathophysiology of cystinuria-causing mutations could lead to the development of drugs specifically targeted to various etiologies, as has been the case in cystic fibrosis.[16] As the cost of genotyping individuals continues to fall, there will be less impediment to performing the test and it will likely become a more routine component of the evaluation of affected patients.

Cystinuria was originally divided into three types depending on the amount of cystine excreted by the obligate heterozygous parents of affected children. In this phenotypic classification, the parents of type I patients excreted normal amounts of cystine, while the heterozygous parents of types 2 and 3 had abnormal excretion of cystine, indicating that the disease is transmitted in a dominant mode with incomplete penetrance.[17] The distinction between type 2 and type 3 was in part based on the appearance of cystine in the urine following an orally administered cystine load, suggesting that differences in intestinal transport of amino acids led to varying phenotypes. This classification preceded knowledge of the relevant genes and the ability to genotype affected individuals.

Once genotyping could be performed on a wider scale, the International Cystinuria Consortium (ICC) recognized that there was a poor genotype–phenotype correlation. Although type I cystinuria was largely caused by mutations in SLC3A1, a small proportion of the patients classified that way had two mutated SLC7A9 alleles.[18] In contrast, almost all cases of nontype I (types 2 and 3) cystinuria were caused by mutations in SLC7A9, with the exception of a few cases with a complex, in-frame duplication of SLC3A1.[18] Type 2 and type 3 phenotypes were genetically indistinguishable.

Some heterozygotes for SLC7A9 mutations did not have abnormal urinary amino acid excretion.

The result of these studies was a new genotype-based classification that is currently in use. Type A cystinuria is the designation for individuals with mutations in both SLC3A1 alleles (genotype AA). Type B cystinuria is the designation for disease attributed to mutations in both SLC7A9 alleles (genotype BB).[19] There are rare individuals who are compound heterozygotic with one mutated allele in each gene. These people with digenic inheritance (type AB) do not produce stones. Other digenic individuals who did produce stones were shown to have ABB or AAB patterns; in other words, they were homozygous for mutations in one of the two genes and heterozygous in the other.

Little difference is seen between the phenotypes of patients with cystinuria caused by SLC3A1 and SLC7A9 mutations. Both equally affected boys and girls (boys were somewhat more significantly affected) and had similar ages of onset of clinically recognized stones.[19] While about 94% of people homozygous for SLC3A1 or SLC7A9 mutations will develop kidney stones in their lives, the age of onset of kidney stone formation is difficult to predict and shows broad intrafamilial variability.[18,20]

Another syndrome that includes cystinuria results from rearrangements and deletions of genes in close proximity on chromosome 2p21 to SLC3A1. The result is hypotonia-cystinuria syndrome (HCS) and atypical HCS. Recessive deletion of alleles for SLC3A1 and PREPL, which codes for prolyl endopeptidase-like, leads to neonates affected by cystinuria as well as hypotonia and growth retardation due to growth hormone deficiency.[21] Chromosome 2p21 deletions can also occur without cystinuria if SLC3A1 is spared. A worse prognosis is associated with deletion of additional genes in that area.

Prevalence, Clinical Features, and Presentation

The prevalence of cystinuria has been estimated to vary from 1:2,500 in a group of Libyan Jews to 1:100,000 in Sweden.[22] Screening of 110,000 Japanese students for cystinuria identified six patients. None of them had clinically evident stone formation after 7 years of follow-up.[23] The incidence of persistent cystinuria was 562 cases per million infants, a rate seven times higher than that for clinically manifested cystinuria in the adult population of Quebec. This confirms that many cystinurics will not form kidney stones. The relative rarity of cystinuria accounts for the scarcity of data involving large databases.

The median age of onset of stones was 12 years in a cohort of over 200 patients.[24] Males appear to be more significantly affected than females, but the reasons for this difference are unknown. That onset most often occurs in teenage years suggests that sex hormones could influence stone formation. Substantial variability existed in the age of onset of stones, as 40% of patients had their first stone between 11 and 20 years, while 14% of females and 28% of males formed calculi before the age of 3 years.[25] In a database of 224 patients from 150 families, there were no clinical differences in urinary amino acid excretion patterns between cystinuria type A and B.[19] Stone formation did not correlate with amino acid urinary excretion, suggesting the importance of other modifiers of stone formation such as fluid intake, diet, and modifier genes.

Like noncystine stone formers, cystinuria presents with symptoms related to stone formation, such as renal colic and hematuria. However, people with cystinuria are almost five times as likely to have undergone a nephrectomy compared with noncystine stone formers, as they may present with a nonfunctioning kidney containing a large staghorn calculus that failed to produce other symptoms that would have led to earlier recognition.[26] As the result of more frequent stones, patients with cystinuria have reduced health-related quality of life in both mental and physical health domains.[27] Quality of life improved following stone episodes as in noncystine stone formers, but more frequent stones led to an overall greater effect on these symptoms.

Cystinuria is associated with reduced glomerular filtration rates (GFR). In the ICC data, GFR was reduced in 17% of those patients. Factors that might contribute to reduced GFR include the need for multiple urological procedures such as extracorporeal shock wave lithotripsy (SWL) and repeated episodes of urinary tract obstruction. Intranephronal crystal formation has been noted on biopsies of renal papillae obtained at the time of ureteroscopy or percutaneous nephrostolithotomy.[28] These crystals may cause obstruction of the nephron or perhaps induce a degree of inflammation, leading to tubulointerstitial atrophy.

Diagnosis

An algorithm for the diagnosis of cystinuria is presented in Figure 21.2. Cystinuria is most often diagnosed when kidney stone composition is shown to be cystine. For this reason, kidney stone composition, whether determined by infrared spectroscopy or by X-ray crystallography, should

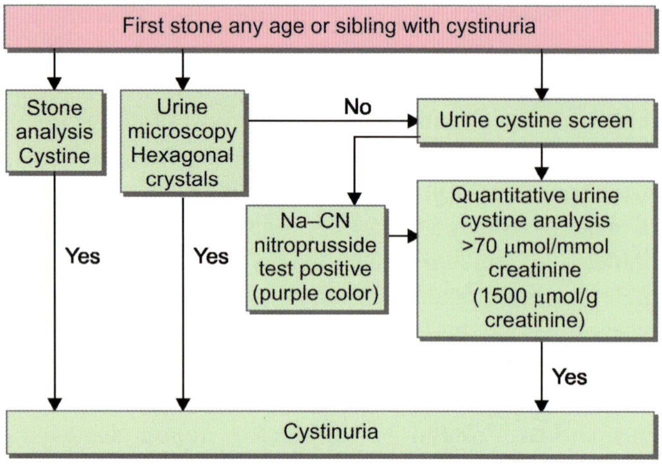

Fig. 21.2: Diagnosis algorithm for cystinuria.
Source: Redrawn with permission from Edvardsson VO, Goldfarb DS, Lieske JC, et al. Hereditary causes of kidney stones and chronic kidney disease. Pediatr Nephrol. 2013;28:1923-42. Springer Science + Business Media.

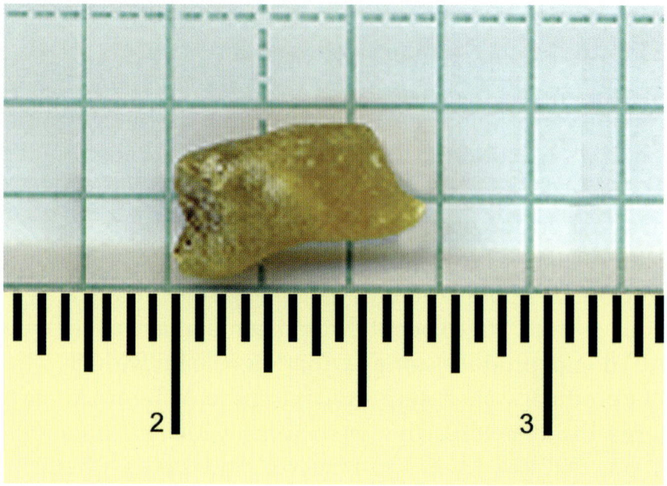

Fig. 21.3: Spontaneously passed cystine stone. Scale is in inches.

be performed at least once in every individual presenting with kidney stones at any age.[29] It is a very inexpensive test with real potential to influence therapy. Some cases have finally been diagnosed at age 50–80 years, either after presenting with a first stone or after multiple surgical interventions. The stone may have been passed spontaneously or obtained during a urologic intervention. The stones are typically lemon yellow in color as seen in Figure 21.3.

A positive family history of cystinuria may lead to screening of urine, or perhaps genotyping, of asymptomatic siblings of a family's first affected individual. Given the risk of asymptomatic stones causing kidney dysfunction and the ability of simple therapies to affect the course of the disease, we do recommend screening of siblings. Screening can most easily be accomplished by the collection of urine for 24 hours with measurement of the cystine and dibasic amino acid content.

Diagnosis can also be accomplished by the inexpensive and sensitive addition of sodium nitroprusside to the urine. Laboratories specializing in determining kidney stone risk factors in urine perform this test in all individuals whose urine appears at the lab for the first time. A purple color results when sodium nitroprusside and cystine are present together.[30] The test may therefore detect some asymptomatic heterozygotes with a single mutated SLC7A9 allele, who themselves may very infrequently form a stone. Some affected heterozygotic children may have higher levels of cystine excretion only in their 1st year of life. As they mature, their cystine excretion often falls, and they are much less likely to form stones.[22]

Cystinuria can also be first diagnosed when the pathognomonic hexagonal crystals are seen on careful urinalysis. Crystalluria is seen on initial urinalysis in about 25% of patients. Cystinuria should particularly be suspected in younger children who present with large branched (staghorn) calculi, which fill the collecting system and require surgical management. While stones of any composition can present with staghorn formation, in the absence of urinary tract infection with urease-producing bacteria, cystinuria should be considered.

Cystine has been shown to reduce the solubility of calcium oxalate in vitro.[31] In a search for monogenic mutations causing kidney stones, several patients who were heterozygous for SLC7A9 mutations were found to have calcium oxalate or calcium phosphate stones.[32] Whether this finding was a coincidence, since calcium stones are highly prevalent in the general population, or whether increased urinary cystine excretion was a causative factor in these stones is not clear.

Laboratory Studies

Once cystinuria is diagnosed, quantitative testing of urinary cystine excretion should be performed. Measurement of dibasic amino acid excretion does not have clear clinical value. The sodium nitroprusside test detects concentrations of >75 mg/L; normal cystine excretion is not >30 mg/day (0.13 mmol/day). Homozygous patients with cystinuria generally excrete >400 mg/day (1.7 mmol/day). However, the accuracy of cystine testing will be inaccurate if the cystine in the urine is not solubilized. At urine pH below 6.5, cystine is relatively insoluble and remains in nonmeasurable, crystalline form. The result is artifactually low values if urine samples are not alkalinized and crystals not dissolved after voiding before measurement of cystine.[33] One factor that mitigates this problem is that patients with cystinuria tend to have higher urine pH without treatment, so that more acid urine pH values are not as common as in the noncystine stone forming population.[34]

Thiol drugs tiopronin and d-penicillamine are commonly used to manage cystinuria (see below). Another potential problem in the quantitation of urinary cystine excretion is that the usual colorimetric cystine assays cannot reliably distinguish cystine from soluble thiol drug-cysteine complexes, as the tests actually detect the thiol groups present in thiol drugs tiopronin and d-penicillamine and the amino acids.[35] Thiol-cysteine bonds can be broken by sample preparation, releasing the amino acid monomer cysteine, which recombines with itself to form the insoluble dimer cystine. The result can be inaccurate measurement in patients taking thiol drugs with an inability to judge drug efficacy.

These problems led to the development of an alternative methodology, a solid-phase assay that is reliable in the presence of thiol drugs.[35] Preformed cystine crystals are added to the patient's non-alkalinized urine and incubated for 48 hours. The urine is spun down and the crystals collected. In urine supersaturated for cystine, the added crystals, the solid phase, grow. The urine is said to have a "negative cystine capacity" in that the urine could take up none of the added cystine. If the urine is undersaturated for cystine, the added cystine crystals can give up cystine and shrink. Such urine has a "positive cystine capacity", meaning that it has the capacity to hold additional cystine.[36] The assay is not widely available currently but is performed in the United States by Litholink Corp (Chicago, IL).

This assay also addresses the lack of a formula or nomogram that can be used to estimate cystine supersaturation. For calcium oxalate stones, the iterative program EQUIL2 can estimate supersaturation, a value that reflects overall risk of stone formation.[37] Development of such a program was not possible for cystine, as cystine solubility varied widely at any given pH.[33] The solid phase assay for cystine generates a measured, rather than an estimated, supersaturation. The result is affected by urine volume, cystine concentration, and urine pH and is a way of integrating all the relevant variables that affect cystine solubility.[36] It may be a better predictor of the stone-forming activity, and a more reliable estimate of cystine solubility when thiol drugs are prescribed. The value of the test for these purposes has not yet been established but is a topic of study by the Rare Kidney Stone Consortium.[38]

The collection of 24-hour urine samples also is useful for determining other variables relevant to cystine stone formation. These samples reveal total urine volume, although this value can be easily determined by patients at home. Adherence to dietary prescriptions (see below) can be assessed as well.[36] Restriction of dietary sodium should lead to reductions in urine sodium excretion, while reduced animal protein ingestion should reduce urinary urea excretion and contribute to an increase in urine pH. Prescriptions of potassium citrate should lead to increases in urine potassium, citrate and pH, while decreasing urinary ammonium excretion. Serial collections are invaluable in judging changes in stone risk that result from modifications of diet and prescribed pharmaceutical regimens.

Pathology

Renal papillae can be biopsied in patients undergoing ureteroscopy or percutaneous nephrostolithotomy. In well-characterized cystine stone formers, histopathological findings vary from normal in some people to plugging, dilatation, and injury of the ducts of Bellini.[28] Inner medullary collecting ducts are also frequently affected. The large plugs of crystals in the ducts of Bellini were composed of cystine, while crystal deposits in the inner medulla and thin loop of Henle were composed of hydroxyapatite. Since higher urine pH is usually a prerequisite for precipitation of calcium phosphate, the etiology of such a finding could be attributed to the higher urine pH often seen in cystinuria. Prescription of potassium citrate or other urinary alkalinizers apparently did not correlate with this finding.

Patients with cystinuria often have some reduction in GFR.[26] The pathology of cystinuria, with crystal deposits in the nephron and interstitium, suggests that this reduction is not simply the result of repeated episodes of obstructive uropathy or SWL, although such factors certainly play a role in some patients. Microscopic obstruction could cause upstream nephronal injury with interstitial reaction, loss of glomeruli, and tubulointerstitial fibrosis. An additional mechanism of crystal-induced inflammation with tissue remodeling has recently been recognized in models of calcium oxalate nephropathy.[39,40] Activation of the NLRP3 inflammasome leads to secretion of the proinflammatory cytokine IL-1β, while ablating that complex ameliorates progressive renal injury.[41] While these studies suggest possible pathways for the therapy of calcium oxalate stones, cystine has not yet been shown to stimulate these inflammatory pathways.

Animal Models

Cystinuria occurs in other mammalian species, including some dogs, such as mastiffs and Newfoundlands, and in the maned wolf.[42,43] Three mouse models have also been developed by knocking out both of the murine analogs of the human genes. The first was a knock-out of Slc7a9, which led to only 42% of homozygous animals developing stones.[44] The fact that some mice developed cystine calculi from an early age while others did not suggested that there were modifier genes affecting the stone phenotype. Exposure of mice to the mutagen N-ethyl-N-nitrosourea led to identification of a missense mutation in Slc3a1 leading to an amino acid exchange in the extracellular domain of the rBAT protein.[45] An additional Slc3a1 knock-out was produced and has recently been useful in testing the efficacy of cystine dimethylester (CDME, see below).[46,47] More recently, to study digenic inheritance of cystinuria, and interactions of mutations in Slc7a9 and Slc3a1, double heterozygotes were produced. This pattern of genetic mutation has not been seen to cause cystinuria in people. In the mice, double heterozygous mice (Slc7a9: ± Slc3a1±) presented lower expression of system $b^{0,+}$ and higher excretion of cystine than single heterozygotes (Slc7a9± Slc3a1+/+ and Slc7a9+/+ Slc3a1±). Stones occurred in 4% of the mice, suggesting that digenic inheritance may produce a clinically evident phenotype.[48] It is interesting that the knockout mouse models feature prominent bladder stone formation and bladder outlet obstruction, relatively rare occurrences in humans with cystinuria. These animal models are helpful in confirming our understanding of the genetics of cystinuria and will likely be useful in demonstrating the efficacy and safety of new treatments.

Management

Surgical management of obstructing cystine stones is not substantially different than the strategies addressing noncystine stones. The exception is that cystine stones are generally considered less amenable to fragmentation with extracorporeal shock wave lithotripsy (ESWL).[49,50] One small study suggested that rough cystine stones are more amenable to fragmentation by ESWL than stones with a smoother crystalline structure.[51] This finding had some clinical correlation in another study that showed that helical computed tomography (CT) could distinguish the stones most likely to be successfully fragmented by lithotripsy.[52] Stones with areas of low X-ray attenuation required lower intensity of shock waves than those that did not show CT-visible internal variation. In general, however, endoscopic management with ureteroscopy, or for larger stones, percutaneous nephrostolithotomy, are now considered the preferred modalities for urologic interventions. This is true for cystinuria because of the resistance of many stones but also because SWL has been less frequently deployed in kidney stone disease of any composition.[53]

Both percutaneous nephrostolithotomy and ureteroscopy may be followed by chemolysis, the direct infusion of alkalinizing buffers into the urinary tract, to dissolve residual fragments.[54] If patients undergo successful lithotripsy, they and their urologist might reasonably regard it as a useful therapy for the future when stones recur. But if unsuccessful, repeating the procedure is not advised. In rare instances, construction of an ileal ureter, a loop of bowel replacing the native ureter, and extending from renal pelvis to bladder, could be useful.[55] Kidney failure necessitating dialysis or renal transplantation is exceedingly unusual in an era of outstanding endourology, but patients with cystinuria are prone to nephrectomy, especially at presentation, and may have additional adverse events affect the contralateral kidney. Transplantation can be thought of as "curative" and is not associated with recurrence of cystinuria, assuming the donor is not a related heterozygous carrier for cystinuria-related mutations.

Prevention of Recurrence

Prevention of stone recurrence is focused on both a reduction of the absolute amount of cystine in the urine and an increase of the solubility of cystine. The initial prescription for all patients with cystinuria and stone formation consists of increasing fluid intake and urine pH. Decreasing cystine excretion by limiting dietary sodium and animal protein is also appropriate. If these measures fail, cystine-binding thiol drugs (CBTDs) are appropriate.[56] In rare instances of cystinuria, stone disease may be so severe that both kidneys could be damaged irreparably, leading to renal failure. With current techniques, devastating renal failure is nearly always avoidable. Should renal failure occur, treatment with renal transplantation would be appropriate after the institution of dialysis. Cystinuria would not be expected to recur after renal transplantation since the tubular transport of cystine in the transplanted kidney would be normal.

Increasing Oral Fluid Intake

Increasing oral fluid intake to increase urine volume and dilute cystine concentration is an essential measure in cystinuria. The goal should be to reduce urine cystine supersaturation to <1.0 at a urine pH above 7.0. At this pH, most patients will need to drink 3–4 L per day to achieve undersaturated urine, with a urine cystine concentration of <243 mg/L (1 mmol/L).[36] Fluid intake should be spaced out throughout the day. Drinking fluids at bedtime is important as sleep leads to reduced urine volume and higher urinary concentrations. Similarly augmenting fluid intake to achieve higher urine volumes with higher ambient temperatures or exercise should be stressed. The choice of fluids is left to the patient to find something palatable that can lead to adherence to this prescription. Citrus juices, such as lemon and orange juice, lead to net urinary alkalinization after metabolism of their organic anions by the liver.[57] Folk lore states that coffee and alcohol lead to "dehydration" but no data suggest that they have led to more stones, whether cystine or calcium.

This level of fluid intake may be difficult to accomplish for many people, particularly younger children. Some patients have benefitted from placement of a gastric tube or a peripherally inserted central catheter line in order to reliably receive adequate volumes. Prescription of an antidiuretic hormone (ADH, or vasopressin) antagonist to stimulate thirst has also been proposed.[58] In two reported cases, tolvaptan 15 mg once daily was administered for 5 days. Thirst was provoked, resulting in urinary dilution without significant adverse effects. The drug is extremely costly and currently has a black box warning associated with its use in treatment of polycystic kidney disease because of some cases of hepatotoxicity.[59] This modality of increasing urine volume does not currently appear to be safe or cost-effective.

Urinary Alkalinization

Increasing urine pH to 7.0 or more increases cystine solubility and is best achieved with oral administration of potassium citrate.[60] A starting dose of 20 mEq twice daily might or might not be sufficient with increases based on periodic pH testing, which patients should be encouraged to accomplish at home. Hyperkalemia is unusual unless GFR is reduced, in which case serum potassium concentration should be measured in 2–4 weeks. Taking the supplements after meals reduces the risk of gastrointestinal complaints, which are most common in older patients. Potassium bicarbonate sometimes causes fewer adverse gastrointestinal effects but does not come in a sustained-release preparation. Sodium citrate or sodium bicarbonate may also be tolerated by some patients but are not first-line agents as increased urinary sodium excretion leads to increased cystine excretion.

A frequently stated concern of physicians is the possibility of higher urine pH leading to the formation of calcium phosphate stones. This is extremely rare in the management of cystinuria, since patients are generally successful at maintaining higher urine volumes. In addition, citrate inhibits calcium phosphate, as well as calcium oxalate stone formation.[61] Finally, it would be unusual for a patient with cystinuria to also have hypercalciuria or other urinary risk factors for noncystine stones. These urinary variables can be measured in order to assess risk, if desired. Without a prior history of calcium phosphate stone formation, recurrent cystine stone formation can be managed with a plan to increase urine pH to values as high as 8.0.

Treatment with acetazolamide has sometimes been recommended, as carbonic anhydrase inhibitors increase urinary pH.[62] This option has not been shown to be superior to citrate. The resulting metabolic acidosis would be presumed to cause risk to bone mineral density, making carbonic anhydrase inhibition less than an ideal method to raise urine pH.

Dietary Manipulation

Two dietary prescriptions are generally made for management of recurrent cystine stones. Cystine excretion is reduced by decreasing dietary sodium, thereby reducing urinary sodium.[36,63] The physiology of this effect is not known since the tubular reabsorption of cystine in the proximal tubule occurs via a sodium-independent transporter. Restricting salt intake to about 2 g, or <100 mEq, of sodium per day may be achievable for people who can control their dietary sodium intake.

Reduction of animal protein intake to 1 g/kg of body weight may also be useful. First, animal protein is a major source of dietary cystine and its precursor, methionine. Less animal protein ingestion is then associated with a reduction in urinary cystine excretion.[64] Perhaps more importantly, animal protein is also a major source of nonvolatile acid and protons in the Western diet. Restricting protein intake leads to an increase in urine pH and should cause a reduction in the dose of potassium citrate required to achieve therapeutic urinary alkalinization.[65] Although the evidence that protein and salt restriction lead to less cystine excretion is robust, there are no long-term studies demonstrating that these dietary manipulations actually reduce formation of cystine stones.

Cystine-Binding Thiol Drugs

In patients who continue to form stones after prescription of higher fluid intake, alkali, and modification of diet, CBTDs are recommended. Currently two are available in the United States: D-penicillamine and α-mercaptopropionylglycine, also known as tiopronin. Both drugs are organic thiols, meaning that they contain a sulfhydryl (-SH) group. The thiol reduces the disulfide bond of cystine, substituting for one cysteine to form a new drug-cysteine disulfide as shown in Figure 21.1. The drug-cysteine complexes are more soluble than cystine. For example, the solubility of the cysteine-penicillamine complex is 50-fold higher than that of cystine.[66] Both drugs are associated with increases in urine cystine capacity, with a greater effect in those whose cystine capacity was most negative off thiol therapy.[67] No randomized trials have compared the two drugs head-to-head, but anecdotal reports suggest that tiopronin may be more effective in reducing cystine excretion and in producing cysteine-drug disulfides.[68,69] In some studies in Europe, doses were determined by maintaining low urinary levels of free cystine, the molecule not bound to thiol drugs.[70]

Both drugs have significant adverse effects, some of which are serious, but rash, fever, and gastrointestinal effects including vomiting are not uncommon.[71] Many of these effects resolve with continued therapy. Infrequent but serious adverse effects include abnormal liver function tests, hematological abnormalities including thrombocytopenia, agranulocytosis and aplastic anemia, and nephrotic syndrome. The renal lesion seen on kidney biopsy in thiol-associated nephrotic syndrome is membranous nephropathy.[72] Dermatologic manifestations include skin wrinkling, pemphigus, and elastosis perforans serpiginosa (Fig. 21.4).[73] The incidence of adverse effects such as allergy is lower with tiopronin, making it the usual first-line agent today. D-penicillamine is reserved for people with adverse events related to tiopronin and for those who have taken it for prolonged periods with success and without adverse effects. Adverse events may be less frequent if one starts with low doses. Monitoring of liver enzymes, complete blood count, and urinary protein excretion is recommended at 4- to 6-month intervals. Cystine-binding thiol drugs should not be used in pregnant or breastfeeding women.

Captopril, the first angiotensin converting enzyme inhibitor, is also a thiol molecule and increases the solubility of cystine in vitro. However, its appearance in the urine even at the highest recommended dose may not be adequate to meaningfully change cystine solubility.[36]

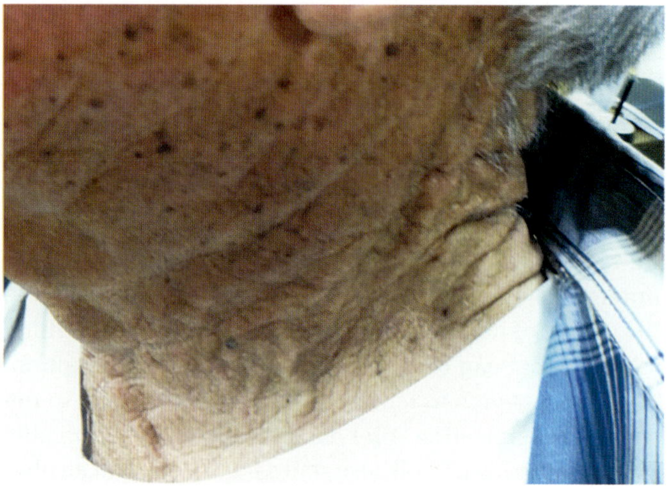

Fig. 21.4: Elastosis perforans serpiginosa on the neck of a patient with cystinuria who took d-penicillamine for many years.

A recent in vitro study showed that increasing urine pH was associated with increased efficacy of thiol drugs to increase cystine solubility.[74] No study has shown that thiol drugs are not useful in the absence of alkali, but using CBTDs without alkali would not be recommended based on this nonclinical study.

Prospects for New Drugs

The velocity of crystal growth can be measured with atomic force microscopy. Candidate molecules for inhibition of cystine crystallization were selected and studied using this technique.[75] The most effective inhibitor of cystine crystal growth was L-CDME, a structural analog of cystine. The protruding methyl groups may provide steric inhibition of cystine crystal growth. Cystine dimethylester was then administered to Slc3a1 knock-out mice, which had a significant reduction in the total weight of cystine stones, although the number of stones increased.[76] There was no evidence of hepatic or renal toxicity. While these results are encouraging, CDME has been used to produce an animal model of cystinosis, a disorder in which intracellular lysosomal cystine accumulation occurs.[77] That effect requires a higher concentration than inhibition of cystine crystallization and has not yet been noted in mice with cystinuria. Other diamides that may have superior stability and ability to inhibit cystine crystallization are now being studied.[78a]

An older thiol drug, bucillamine, used in the treatment of rheumatoid arthritis, may be useful in the treatment of cystinuria.[78] Unlike monothiols d-penicillamine and tiopronin, it is a dithiol. The drug may therefore offer greater potency than the currently available CBTDs. To the extent that the adverse effects of thiols are dose dependent, lower toxicity would be expected when half as much drug is prescribed.

Another possible strategy for the treatment of cystinuria might be chaperone therapy, which has led to important clinical benefit in some diseases caused by mutations that lead to misfolded proteins, such as cystic fibrosis.[79,16] Such chaperones may stabilize folded proteins against proteolytic degradation or thermal denaturation. The result is facilitating the escape of abnormal proteins from the endoplasmic reticulum-associated protein degradation pathway, leading to increased expression of functional protein activity.[80,81] This pharmacologic effect would apply only to some and not all proteins produced from mutated genes. As some mutations affecting rBAT do cause protein misfolding, chaperone therapy might be worth investigating as a treatment strategy for cystinuria.

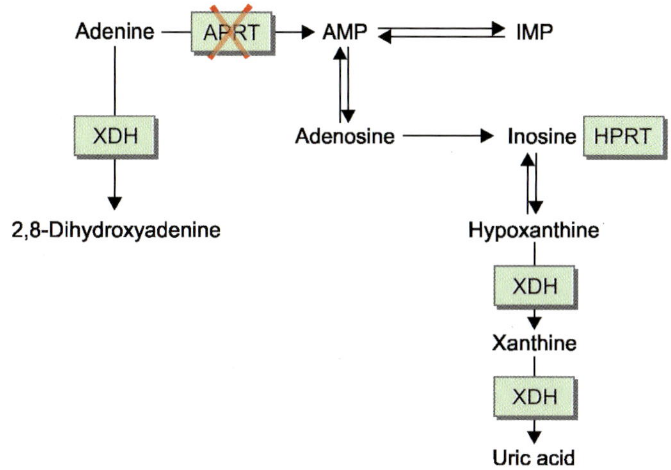

Fig. 21.5: Overview of adenine metabolism. In APRTd, adenine cannot be converted to AMP and is instead converted by xanthine dehydrogenase to 2,8-dihydroxyadenine. (APRT: Adenine phosphoribosyltransferase; AMP: Adenosine monophosphate; HPRT: Hypoxanthine-guanine phosphoribosyltransferase; IMP: Inosine monophosphate; XDH: Xanthine dehydrogenase).
Source: Redrawn with permission from Edvardsson VO, Goldfarb DS, Lieske JC, et al. Hereditary causes of kidney stones and chronic kidney disease. Pediatr Nephrol. 2013;28:1923-42. Springer Science + Business Media.

APRT DEFICIENCY

Pathophysiology

Deficiency of APRT activity (APRTd, OMIM 614723) is the only cause of 2,8-DHA stones and 2,8-dihydroxyadeninuria. Adenine phosphoribosyl transferase deficiency was first described in 1968 in a report of partial enzymatic deficiency in four asymptomatic people.[82] The enzyme activity is normally present throughout the body, including in liver, intestine, and red blood cells. The disorder's inheritance is as an autosomal recessive error in purine metabolism. The result is abnormal production of the poorly soluble DHA leading to urinary tract stones with the potential for CKD and renal failure. Most of the well-characterized cohorts have been reported from Iceland, France, and Japan.[83]

Adenine phosphoribosyl transferase is expressed in the cytoplasm of most somatic cells where it catalyzes the synthesis of 5′-adenosine monophosphate (AMP) from adenine and 5-phosphoribosyl-1-pyrophosphate (Fig. 21.5).[84] Enzyme activity is magnesium dependent. Two subunits of 179 amino acids form a homodimer and comprise the active enzyme. Absence of cytoplasmic enzyme activity prevents the usual pathway leading to recycling of adenine and the formation of uric acid. Instead, the lack of APRT obligates the conversion of the 8-hydroxy intermediate, by xanthine dehydrogenase (XDH), to the highly insoluble DHA.

Genetics

The human gene APRT is 2,466 base pairs long, has five exons, and is located on chromosome 16q24.[85] At least 40 mutations in APRT have been reported to date, with the three well-characterized populations all possessing a unique genotype. The white populations and the Japanese populations have different manifestations in vitro, leading to a classification of two types. Type I APRTd, demonstrated in white patients, including the well-characterized cohorts in Iceland and France, is caused by a diverse set of mutations, with the mutated alleles classified as APRT*Q0. The patients have complete enzyme deficiency both in vivo and in vitro. Patients with type I deficiency may be homozygous or compound heterozygous for APRT*Q0 mutations. In Iceland, all patients are homozygous for a missense mutation, which involves an A→T transversion at position 1,350 in exon 3, resulting in the replacement of aspartic acid by valine at position 65 (p.Asp65Val).[83] In the French population, the most prevalent mutation was a single T insertion in an intron splice donor site named IVS4 + 2insT, which accounted for 40.3% of mutated chromosomes.[86] Aberrant splicing at that site leads to a deletion of exon 4 from mRNA, causing a frame shift and a truncated protein of 109 amino acids instead of 180, named Ala108GluX3.

The Japanese patients are classified as type II APRTd, with mutant allele APRT*J; they demonstrate complete enzymatic deficiency in vivo and only partial deficiency in vitro. The most common mutation in Japanese people with APRTd, known as APRT*J, is a missense mutation in exon 5, c.407T>C, which leads to the amino acid change in the enzyme of threonine replaced by methionine at position 136 (p.Thr136Met).[87] This single mutation is responsible for at least 70% of clinically detected individuals in Japan.[88] Most patients are homozygous for APRT*J, but some are heterozygous with the designation APRT*J/APRT*Q0. Two other mutations account for nearly all of the other 30% of affected cases in Japan.[88]

Animal Model

Mice with APRTd were produced using targeted homologous recombination in embryonic stem cells.[89] Mice that are homozygous for a null APRT allele excrete both adenine and DHA crystals in the urine. Histopathology of the kidneys shows tubular dilation, inflammation, necrosis, and fibrosis, the severity of which varies with different mouse backgrounds. Male mice are earlier and more significantly affected with CKD than females for unclear reasons, possibly due to differences in the rate of adenine or DHA production or because of sex-determined responses of the kidneys.[90] Demonstrating the utility of the model in mimicking the human disease, allopurinol has an important beneficial effect on renal pathology, although it does not lead to a recovery of lost GFR.[91]

Prevalence

Estimates of prevalence of the carrier state for mutated APRT genes range from 0.4% to 1.2%, which would be associated with a prevalence of the homozygous genotype of 1:50,000–100,000.[84] In that case, there would be 70–80,000 APRTd cases worldwide, with about 3,000 cases in the United States alone. These numbers far exceed the number of cases reported in the medical literature. Among >43,000 stones analyzed at the Mayo Clinic in 2010, only one was composed of DHA.[92] These values suggest that the diagnosis of APRTd is being missed as a cause of kidney stones, CKD, and end stage renal disease (ESRD).[93,94] It is also possible that many patients remain relatively asymptomatic for prolonged periods, perhaps having no or only occasional small stones that clinicians fail to send for determination of composition. This notion is supported by the fact that the age at diagnosis extends from 0.5 to 78.0 years with a median age of 36.3 years.[86]

Clinical Manifestations

The clinically significant manifestations of APRTd are kidney stones and reduced GFR. Other than the kidneys, no organs are affected. Stones composed of DHA are radiolucent and in older people may be mistaken for uric acid stones. These stones do not appear on plain radiographs, but can be visualized by ultrasound and CT. They may appear as filling defects if intravenous radiocontrast agents are administered. Since uric acid nephrolithiasis is rare in children, radiolucent stones presenting in the pediatric population should be suspected to be DHA (though cystine stones are sometimes radiolucent as well). Furthermore, since uric acid stones are generally associated with acidic urine pH, the finding of radiolucent stones with urine pH >6.0, especially in children, should heighten suspicion for DHA stones. As with any stones in the urinary tract, renal colic, hematuria, and urinary tract infection are typical presenting signs.

A second presentation of APRTd is otherwise unexplained and unsuspected acute kidney injury (AKI) or CKD. Either of these causes of reduced GFR has been attributed to bilateral kidney obstruction or to crystalline nephropathy, with precipitation of DHA in tubules and renal interstitium. Most of these latter patients have not had, and will not have, stones.[95] Reduced GFR may occur in individuals, both children and adults, who are entirely asymptomatic. In the extreme, at least 20% of adults with ESRD may present with end stage kidney disease (ESKD).[93] In some cases, the diagnosis was not suspected, and not confirmed, until after patients received renal transplantation.[93,96] Unlike the case in cystinuria, in which transplantation is "curative" of disease manifestations, that is not the case for APRTd as DHA over-production is not largely from the kidney.[97] In children, reddish diaper stains may be the first manifestation.[83]

Diagnosis

Adenine phosphoribosyltransferase deficiency is a highly treatable disorder, the most severe manifestation of which, ESKD, is preventable. It is therefore incumbent upon all pediatricians, nephrologists, and urologists to maintain a high level of alertness for potential patients. If an appropriate level of awareness of the disorder is maintained by

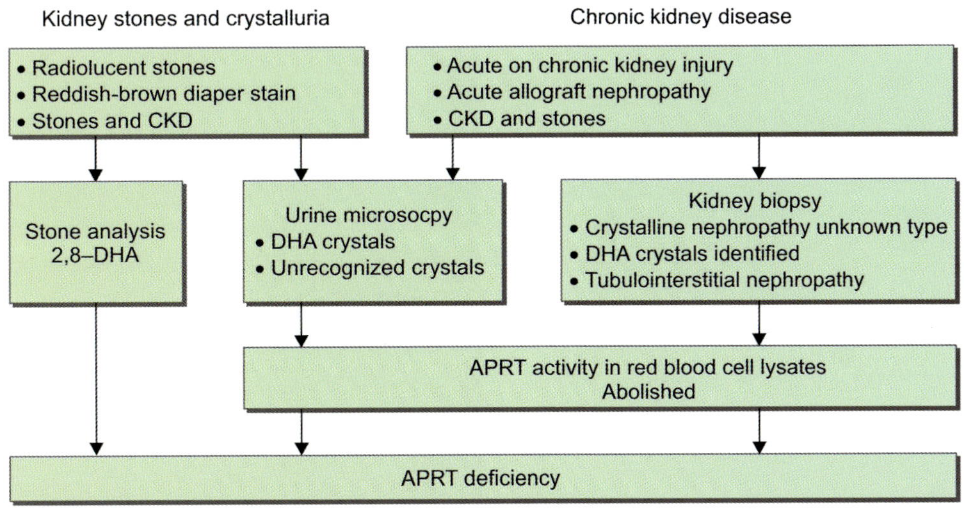

Fig. 21.6: Algorithm for diagnostic evaluation of adenine phosphoribosyltransferase (APRT) deficiency and 2,8-dihydroxyadeninuria. *Source*: Redrawn with permission from Edvardsson VO, Goldfarb DS, Lieske JC, et al. Hereditary causes of kidney stones and chronic kidney disease. Pediatr Nephrol. 2013;28:1923-42. Springer Science + Business Media.

those who see stones and reduced kidney function, fewer patients may present with irreversible kidney failure and recurrent stones. An algorithm developed by the Rare Kidney Stone Consortium for the diagnosis of APRTd is shown in Figure 21.6.

The diagnosis of APRTd is most easily made by the demonstration of DHA as the relevant molecule comprising a kidney stone, whether spontaneously passed or obtained in the operating room. Every patient should have kidney stone composition determined at least once by either infrared spectroscopy or by X-ray crystallography, in part so that unusual stones, such as those composed of cystine and DHA, can be detected.[29] There may, however, be both false-positive and false-negative reports for DHA stones, but the rates for such events are not known. The author, in fact, has twice seen reports of DHA stones in patients who clearly did not have APRTd. Biochemical analysis of stones is an archaic technique that cannot distinguish DHA from uric acid and therefore should be abandoned by clinical laboratories.

Microscopic examination of the urine may also lead to the correct diagnosis. Dihydroxyadenine crystals are typically round and brown and frequently visualized in patients with stones or reduced GFR. Using polarized light, these crystals demonstrate a Maltese cross pattern, shown in Figures 21.7A and B. Urine microscopy is an important manner of screening asymptomatic siblings of affected index cases.[84] However, crystalluria may become less frequently noted as CKD progresses.[98] The distinctive crystals may also be seen in kidney biopsies of patients with CKD or AKI whether stones are present or not.[93,99] The crystals are seen in the renal tubules, interstitium, and epithelial cells, accompanied by tubular degenerative changes and tubulointerstitial scarring (Figs. 21.8A and B).[100] The pathologist unfamiliar with this diagnosis may misdiagnose the biopsy as uric acid or oxalate nephropathy. If available, the preferred method for accurate identification of crystals on kidney biopsy is Fourier transform infrared spectroscopy.[101]

The enzymatic activity of APRT should be absent from red blood cell lysates.[102] This test, which measures the conversion of ^{14}C-labeled adenine to AMP, is performed by a limited number of specialty laboratories and is used to confirm the diagnosis when stone composition is shown to be DHA or when appropriate crystalline deposits are seen on renal biopsies. In the United States, the test is done by the University of California at San Diego Biochemical Genetics and Metabolomics Laboratory (see http://www.ucsdbglab.org). In red blood cell lysates from healthy people, APRT activity is from 16 to 32 nmol/h/mg. Affected individuals with homozygotic and compound heterozygotic APRT*Q0 mutations have no measurable enzyme activity. Heterozygotes for APRT*Q0 (unaffected parents and siblings) have activity variably reduced to approximately 25%.[83,103] Heterozygotes for APRT*J cannot be distinguished from normal people because of significant overlap. Recent transfusion of red blood cells may falsely elevate APRT enzymatic activity. An assay for DHA using

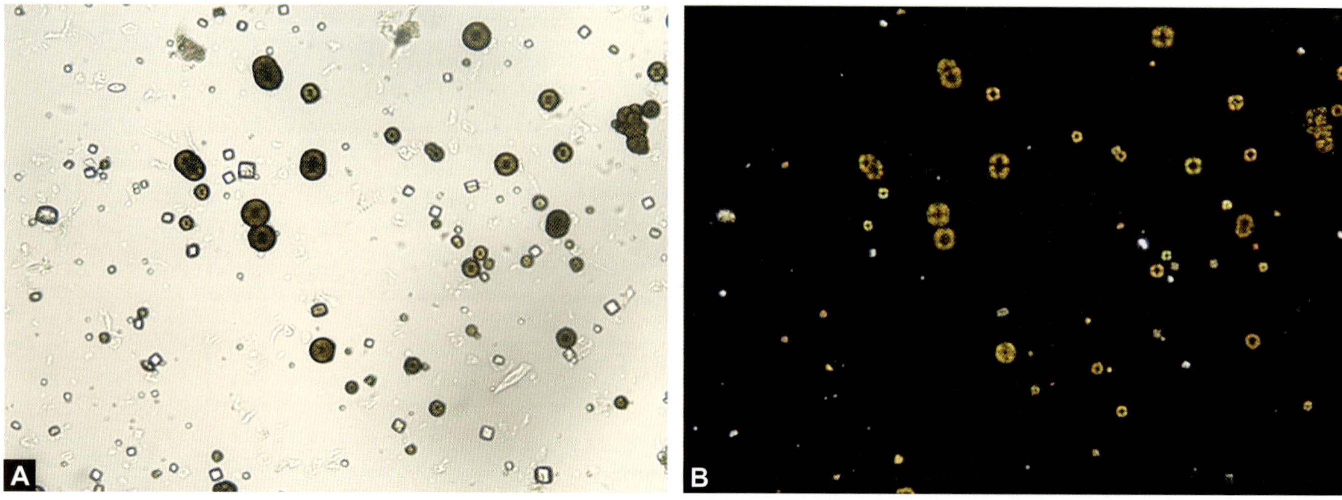

Figs. 21.7A and B: 2,8-dihydroxyadenine crystals. (A) The crystals are seen under normal light. (B) Using a conventional polarizer, the same crystals demonstrate the Maltese cross pattern.
Courtesy: Hrafnhildur Linnet Runolfsdottir, Resident in Internal Medicine, Landspitali-The National University Hospital of Iceland, Reykjavik, Iceland.

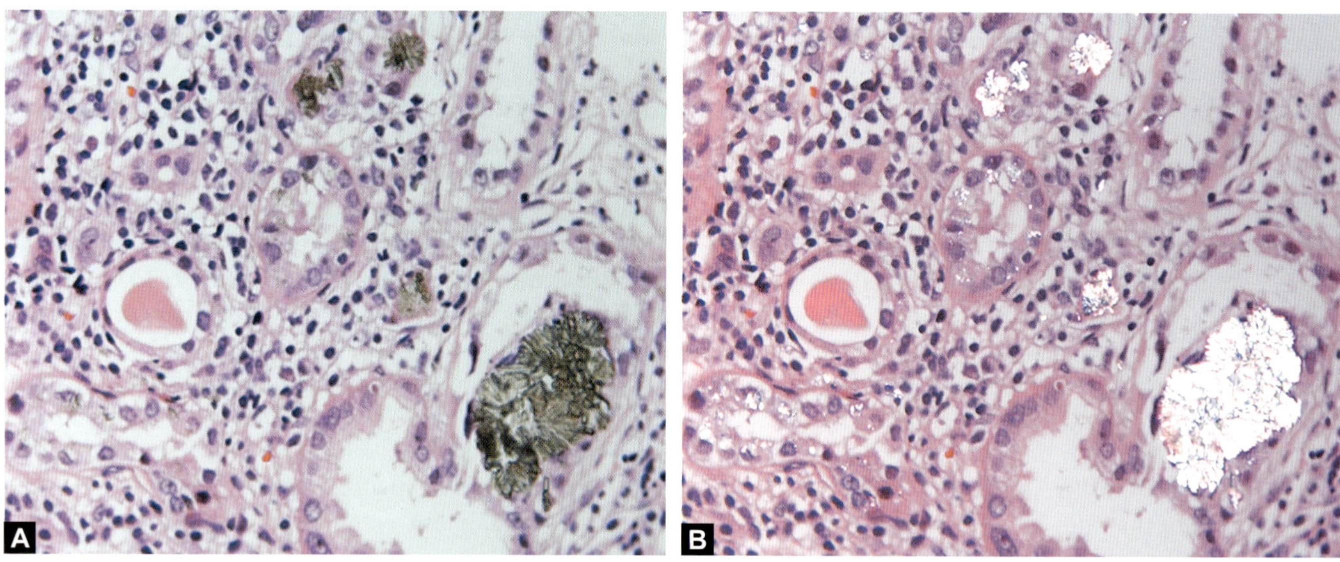

Figs. 21.8A and B: Kidney biopsy in adenine phosphoribosyltransferase deficiency (APRTd). (A) A kidney biopsy from a patient with APRTd, with hematoxylin and eosin stain. Brownish crystals typical of 2,8-dihydroxyadenine deposits are seen in the tubules and interstitium. (B) The same field is viewed with polarized light demonstrating the refractile properties of the crystals.
Courtesy: Dr Sverrir Hardarson, Landspitali-The National University Hospital of Iceland, Reykjavik, Iceland.

ultra performance liquid chromatography-tandem mass spectrometer has now been developed by the group in Iceland. Sending urine to Landspitali—The National University Hospital of Iceland in Reykjavik can confirm the presence of DHA in urine.[104]

A definitive diagnosis can also be made by genotyping the patient for APRT and demonstrating two mutant alleles. Only about 90% of cases will be detected, however. As the cost of genotyping falls and its availability continues to broaden, it can be predicted to become the leading and most reliable means of confirming the diagnosis in appropriately affected individuals. In the absence of APRT activity, genotyping is not considered necessary, but genotyping may eventually supplant the measure of the enzyme's activity.

Since APRTd has autosomal recessive inheritance, each sibling of an affected individual has a 25% chance of being affected, a 50% chance of being an asymptomatic carrier, and a 25% chance of being genetically normal for APRT. Given that early diagnosis has important implications for prevention of stones, CKD and consequential loss of kidney function, screening of siblings is recommended. Screening should include measurement of serum creatinine, urine microscopy and either measurement of APRT activity in red cell lysates or by genotyping potentially affected individuals.[105]

Treatment

Inhibition of XDH with allopurinol or febuxostat prevents the formation of DHA and therefore is very effective therapy. The usual recommended dose is 5–10 mg/kg per day in children and 200–600 mg in adults. The maximal daily dose approved by the US Food and Drug Administration for the treatment of gout is 800 mg. Whether such higher doses are required or beneficial in APRTd has not been studied. These drugs are generally effective and well tolerated in most patients with APRT deficiency.[83,86] In fact, XDH inhibition can lead to dissolution of kidney stones and significant improvements in GFR even in people with advanced CKD.

The caveat about the use of allopurinol is the incidence of hypersensitivity with manifestations as mild as maculopapular rash and drug reaction with eosinophilia and systemic symptoms to the rare but potentially life-threatening Stevens–Johnson syndrome/toxic epidermal necrolysis.[106] These adverse effects are more frequent in, but not limited to, people with the HLA-B*58:01 allele, a genotype more common in Asians, if not exclusively so.[107] For patients with CKD, some studies, but not all, suggest an increase in toxicity and allergy with CKD. The drug is thought to be safer when dosing is started low and adjusted slowly.[108] The consensus (regarding the therapy of gout, not APRTd) is that adequate results can be achieved with higher doses.[109,110]

Febuxostat, significantly more expensive, has usually been reserved for people who are allergic or intolerant to allopurinol.[111] As its elimination is largely performed by the liver, febuxostat is not thought to require dose adjustment in CKD, although the drug is not well studied in patients with GFR <30 mL/min.[112,113] It may therefore be a preferred agent in patients with CKD. In addition, in both in vitro and in vivo animal studies, febuxostat was a more potent inhibitor of XDH than allopurinol.[114] It may therefore not be surprising that febuxostat appears to be a more potent inhibitor of urinary DHA excretion than allopurinol in paired studies in patients with APRTd. Two adult patients from among those in the Icelandic cohort had significant reductions of DHA crystalluria, determined by microscopy, when treated with 80 mg of febuxostat.[84] In a crossover study, 80 mg of febuxostat reduced urinary DHA excretion substantially more than 400 mg allopurinol.[104] Whether these observations of superior efficacy will lead to better prevention and resolution of stones or CKD has not yet been determined, but the treatment is promising. If an assay for urinary DHA excretion becomes more readily and widely available, it would become an attractive tool to measure the efficacy of treatment and determine appropriate drug dosages. At present, without the assay, drug dosages must be titrated to achieve a resolution of crystalluria and radiographically determined stone burden.

Nonspecific treatment for stone prevention and progressive CKD is prescribed, although data demonstrating clinical benefit are lacking. Adequate fluid intake of up to 3 L per day is usually recommended, as it is for all causes of kidney stones, as long as GFR is not advanced. If it is, hyponatremia would be an expected adverse effect. A reduction in animal protein ingestion will limit purine intake and possibly reduce production of DHA. However, given the potential adverse effects, well-tolerated XDH inhibition is almost always recommended.

XANTHINURIA

Deficiency of xanthine oxidoreductase (XOR) leads to hereditary xanthinuria (HX, MIM 607633) and xanthine stones. Xanthine oxidoreductase has two different forms, with different enzymatic activities and substrates: XDH, which preferentially utilizes nicotinamide adenine dinucleotide (NAD^+), and xanthine oxidase (XO), which prefers O_2.[115] The mammalian XOR exists in the XDH form within the cell and is converted to XO during purification. This is the reason that XO is familiar as the enzyme inhibited by allopurinol and febuxostat, drugs commonly used in the management of gout. Xanthine oxidoreductase catalyzes two hydroxylation steps in purine degradation: Hypoxanthine to xanthine, and then xanthine to uric acid. Xanthine oxidoreductase is a homodimer with each subunit containing a molybdenum center, a flavin adenine dinucleotide (FAD) cofactor, and two iron sulfur centers.[115]

Type I xanthinuria (OMIM 278300) is an extremely rare cause of kidney stones with fewer than 200 patients reported worldwide. It was first reported in 1954.[116] The incidence of XOR deficiency, including type II (below), has been reported to be 1/69,000, but analysis of single nucleotide polymorphisms suggests a higher frequency of mutations, demonstrating that not all mutations lead to absence of function.[117] Various levels of XOR function are seen with various mutations. The heredity of HX is autosomal recessive, with the gene found at chromosome 2p23.1.[118] Because XOR is the enzyme responsible for the production of uric acid from xanthine, affected patients are characterized as extremely hypouricemic with no detectable uric acid in the serum or urine.[119] When uric acid is detectable in the serum, its appearance is attributed to metabolism of xanthine by intestinal bacteria.

The presentation of HX is with the typical manifestations of stone disease or crystalluria: hematuria, renal colic, and, when severe, AKI or CKD.[120] More than 50% of cases present before 10 years of age. Occasionally the disorder becomes manifest after an episode of diarrhea, causing urinary concentration and precipitation of xanthine crystals. Athletic activity may also be associated with onset of crystalluria and stones for the same reason. With time, and in older, affected people, xanthine may accumulate in other organs and cause duodenal ulcers, myopathy and myositis, and arthropathy. Screening of siblings of affected cases demonstrates that 20% of patients are asymptomatic, with males symptomatic more often than females.

The diagnosis is most often made when kidney stone composition, by X-ray crystallography or infrared spectroscopy, demonstrates xanthine. Patients should also have hypouricemia, hypouricosuria, and elevated blood and urine xanthine levels. Xanthine oxidoreductase activity can be assayed in cells obtained by biopsy of liver, duodenum or jejunum, the only organs expressing the enzyme complex. Today, however, genotyping is more likely to be the diagnostic test of choice.[119]

There is no specific treatment for prevention of xanthine stones due to xanthinuria. Increased fluid intake in order to dilute urinary xanthine excretion is the most effective maneuver that can help prevent these stones. Restricted dietary purine intake, achieved by reducing ingestion of animal protein and thereby purine precursors of xanthine, may also be useful. Urinary alkalinization is not effective as xanthine solubility is not pH-responsive. Measurement of urine volume and the urinary excretion of xanthine and hypoxanthine may be performed periodically in order to judge responses to these therapies. Serial microscopic examination of a first morning urine sample for crystalluria may also be correlated with response to treatment. In severe cases, in very young children who are unable to maintain higher fluid intake, placement of a gastric tube for administration of water may be necessary.

Type II xanthinuria (OMIM 603592) is rarer than type I. It is caused by deficiency of activity of XOR and of the enzyme aldehyde oxidase (AOX). Both enzymes fail to function when individuals are affected by mutations in the necessary molybdenum cofactor sulfurase gene (MOCOS, previously known as HMCS for human MOCOS), found on chromosome 18q12.2.[121] The AOX enzyme is responsible for metabolism of allopurinol, the XOR inhibitor commonly used in the management of gout and APRTd. As a result, distinguishing type I from type II xanthinuria was done by the allopurinol loading test, which is not performed when genotyping is available.[119] The active metabolite of allopurinol, oxypurinol, can be demonstrated in patients with type I xanthinuria as the result of the successful metabolism of the prodrug by AOX. Oxypurinol is not detected in patients with defective AOX function.

Type III xanthinuria is the result of deficiency of the molybdenum cofactor for XOR. When the synthesis of molybdopterin, a precursor of the molybdenum cofactor, is defective, three enzymes have impaired function: XOR, AOX, and sulfite oxidase.[115] In addition to the manifestations of type I xanthinuria, affected patients have severe neurological disorders including mental retardation, lens dislocations, facial dysmorphism, and feeding disorders.[122] They have reduced urinary excretion of inorganic sulfate and increased excretion of sulfite and other sulfur metabolites.

ACKNOWLEDGMENTS

The author gratefully acknowledges the support of the Rare Kidney Stone Consortium (U54KD083908), a part of National Institutes of Health (NIH) Rare Diseases Clinical Research Network (RDCRN), funded by the National Institute of Diabetes and Digestive and Kidney Diseases (NIDDK) and the NIH Office of Rare Diseases Research (ORDR).

REFERENCES

1. Milliner DS. Cystinuria. Endocrinol Metab Clin North Am. 1990;19:889-907.
2. Garrod A. The Croonian lectures on inborn errors of metabolism. Lancet. 1908;172:1-7.
3. Bertran J, Werner A, Moore ML, et al. Expression cloning of a cDNA from rabbit kidney cortex that induces a single transport system for cystine and dibasic and neutral amino acids. Proc Natl Acad Sci USA. 1992;89:5601-5.
4. Fotiadis D, Kanai Y, Palacin M. The SLC3 and SLC7 families of amino acid transporters. Mol Aspects Med. 2013;34:139-58.

5. Broer S. Amino acid transport across mammalian intestinal and renal epithelia. Physiol Rev. 2008;88:249-86.
6. Reig N, Chillaron J, Bartoccioni P, et al. The light subunit of system b(o,+) is fully functional in the absence of the heavy subunit. EMBO J. 2002;21:4906-14.
7. Chillaron J, Font-Llitjos M, Fort J, et al. Pathophysiology and treatment of cystinuria. Nat Rev Nephrol. 2010;6:424-34.
8. Verrey F, Singer D, Ramadan T, et al. Kidney amino acid transport. Pflugers Arch. 2009;458:53-60.
9. Fernandez E, Torrents D, Chillaron J, et al. Basolateral LAT-2 has a major role in the transepithelial flux of L-cystine in the renal proximal tubule cell line OK. J Am Soc Nephrol. 2003;14:837-47.
10. Silbernagl S. The renal handling of amino acids and oligopeptides. Physiol Rev. 1988;68:911-1007.
11. Daniel H. Molecular and integrative physiology of intestinal peptide transport. Ann Rev Physiol. 2004;66:361-84.
12. Martensson J, Denneberg T, Lindell A, et al. Sulfur amino acid metabolism in cystinuria: a biochemical and clinical study of patients. Kidney Int. 1990;37:143-9.
13. Calonge MJ, Gasparini P, Chillaron J, et al. Cystinuria caused by mutations in rBAT, a gene involved in the transport of cystine. Nat Genet. 1994;6:420-5.
14. Goodyer P, Boutros M, Rozen R. The molecular basis of cystinuria: an update. Exp Nephrol. 2000;8:123-7.
15. Chillaron J, Estevez R, Samarzija I, et al. An intracellular trafficking defect in type I cystinuria rBAT mutants M467T and M467K. J Biol Chem. 1997;272:9543-9.
16. Accurso FJ, Rowe SM, Clancy JP, et al. Effect of VX-770 in persons with cystic fibrosis and the G551D-CFTR mutation. N Engl J Med. 2010;363:1991-2003.
17. Rosenberg LE, Downing S, Durant JL, et al. Cystinuria: biochemical evidence for three genetically distinct diseases. J Clin Invest. 1966;45:365-71.
18. Font-Llitjos M, Jimenez-Vidal M, Bisceglia L, et al. New insights into cystinuria: 40 new mutations, genotype-phenotype correlation, and digenic inheritance causing partial phenotype. J Med Genet. 2005;42:58-68.
19. Dello Strologo L, Pras E, Pontesilli C, et al. Comparison between SLC3A1 and SLC7A9 cystinuria patients and carriers: a need for a new classification. J Am Soc Nephrol. 2002;13:2547-53.
20. Eggermann T, Venghaus A, Zerres K. Cystinuria: an inborn cause of urolithiasis. Orphanet J Rare Dis. 2012;7:19.
21. Regal L, Shen XM, Selcen D, et al. PREPL deficiency with or without cystinuria causes a novel myasthenic syndrome. Neurology. 2014;82:1254-60.
22. Goodyer PR, Clow C, Reade T, et al. Prospective analysis and classification of patients with cystinuria identified in a newborn screening program. J Pediatr. 1993;122:568-72.
23. Ito H, Murakami M, Miyauchi T, et al. The incidence of cystinuria in Japan. J Urol. 1983;129:1012-4.
24. Lambert EH, Asplin JR, Herrell SD, et al. Analysis of 24-hour urine parameters as it relates to age of onset of cystine stone formation. J Endourol. 2010;24:1179-82.
25. Harnevik L, Fjellstedt E, Molbaek A, et al. Mutation analysis of SLC7A9 in cystinuria patients in Sweden. Genet Test. 2003;7:13-20.
26. Assimos DG, Leslie SW, Ng C, et al. The impact of cystinuria on renal function. J Urol. 2002;168:27-30.
27. Modersitzki F, Pizzi L, Grasso M, et al. Health-related quality of life (HRQoL) in cystine compared with non-cystine stone formers. Urolithiasis. 2014;42:53-60.
28. Evan AP, Coe FL, Lingeman JE, et al. Renal crystal deposits and histopathology in patients with cystine stones. Kidney Int. 2006;69:2227-35.
29. Pearle MS, Goldfarb DS, Assimos DG, et al. Medical management of kidney stones: AUA guideline. J Urol. 2014;192:316-24.
30. Nakagawa Y, Coe FL. A modified cyanide-nitroprusside method for quantifying urinary cystine concentration that corrects for creatinine interference. Clin Chim Acta. 1999;289:57-68.
31. Martins MC, Meyers AA, Whalley NA, et al. Cystine: a promoter of the growth and aggregation of calcium oxalate crystals in normal undiluted human urine. J Urol. 2002;167:317-21.
32. Halbritter J. Fourteen monogenic genes account for 15% of nephrolithiasis/nephrocalcinosis. J Am Soc Nephrol. 2014;26:543-51.
33. Nakagawa Y, Asplin JR, Goldfarb DS, et al. Clinical use of cystine supersaturation measurements. J Urol. 2000;164:1481-5.
34. Sakhaee K, Poindexter JR, Pak CY. The spectrum of metabolic abnormalities in patients with cystine nephrolithiasis. J Urol. 1989;141:819-21.
35. Coe FL, Clark C, Parks JH, et al. Solid phase assay of urine cystine supersaturation in the presence of cystine binding drugs. J Urol. 2001;166:688-93.
36. Goldfarb DS, Coe FL, Asplin JR. Urinary cystine excretion and capacity in patients with cystinuria. Kidney Int. 2006;69:1041-7.
37. Finlayson B. Calcium stones: some physical and clinical aspects. In: David DS, (ed). Calcium Metabolism in Renal Failure and Nephrolithiasis. New York: John Wiley & Sons; 1977. pp. 337-82.
38. Sumorok N, Goldfarb DS. Update on cystinuria. Curr Opin Nephrol Hypertens. 2013;22:427-31.
39. Mulay SR, Evan A, Anders HJ. Molecular mechanisms of crystal-related kidney inflammation and injury. Implications for cholesterol embolism, crystalline nephropathies and kidney stone disease. Nephrol Dial Transplant. 2014;29:507-14.
40. Knauf F, Asplin JR, Granja I, et al. NALP3-mediated inflammation is a principal cause of progressive renal failure in oxalate nephropathy. Kidney Int. 2013;84:895-901.
41. Mulay SR, Kulkarni OP, Rupanagudi KV, et al. Calcium oxalate crystals induce renal inflammation by NLRP3-mediated IL-1beta secretion. J Clin Invest. 2013;123:236-46.
42. Bovee KC, Bush M, Dietz J, et al. Cystinuria in the maned wolf of South America. Science. 1981;212:919-20.
43. Brons AK, Henthorn PS, Raj K, et al. SLC3A1 and SLC7A9 mutations in autosomal recessive or dominant canine cystinuria: a new classification system. J Vet Intern Med. 2013;27:1400-8.
44. Feliubadalo L, Font M, Purroy J, et al. Non-type I cystinuria caused by mutations in SLC7A9, encoding a subunit (bo,+AT) of rBAT. Nat Genet. 1999;23:52-7.

45. Peters T, Thaete C, Wolf S, et al. A mouse model for cystinuria type I. Hum Mol Genet. 2003;12:2109-20.
46. Ercolani M, Sahota A, Schuler C, et al. Bladder outlet obstruction in male cystinuria mice. Int Urol Nephrol. 2009;42: 57-63.
47. Sahota A, Parihar JS, Capaccione KM, et al. Novel cystine ester mimics for the treatment of cystinuria-induced urolithiasis in a knockout mouse model. Urology. 2014;84:1249 e9-15.
48. Espino M, Font-Llitjos M, Vilches C, et al. Digenic inheritance in cystinuria mouse model. PLoS One. 2015;10:e0137277.
49. Cranidis AI, Karayannis AA, Delakas DS, et al. Cystine stones: the efficacy of percutaneous and shock wave lithotripsy. Urol Int. 1996;56:180-3.
50. Ringden I, Tiselius HG. Composition and clinically determined hardness of urinary tract stones. Scand J Urol Nephrol. 2007;41:316-23.
51. Bhatta KM, Prien EL Jr, Dretler SP. Cystine calculi—rough and smooth: a new clinical distinction. J Urol. 1989;142:937-40.
52. Kim SC, Burns EK, Lingeman JE, et al. Cystine calculi: correlation of CT-visible structure, CT number, and stone morphology with fragmentation by shock wave lithotripsy. Urol Res. 2007;35:319-24.
53. Ordon M, Urbach D, Mamdani M, et al. The surgical management of kidney stone disease: a population based time series analysis. J Urol. 2014;192:1450-6.
54. Bernardo NO, Smith AD. Chemolysis of urinary calculi. Urol Clin North Am. 2000;27:355-65.
55. Kvarstein B, Mathisen W. Total replacement of ureter with a segment of ileum. Scand J Urol Nephrol. 1977;11:249-51.
56. Mattoo A, Goldfarb DS. Cystinuria. Semin Nephrol. 2008;28:181-91.
57. Odvina CV. Comparative value of orange juice versus lemonade in reducing stone-forming risk. Clin J Am Soc Nephrol. 2006;1:1269-74.
58. de Boer H, Roelofsen A, Janssens PM. Antidiuretic hormone antagonist to reduce cystine stone formation. Ann Intern Med. 2012;157:459-60.
59. Torres VE, Chapman AB, Devuyst O, et al. Tolvaptan in patients with autosomal dominant polycystic kidney disease. N Engl J Med. 2012;367:2407-18.
60. Fjellstedt E, Denneberg T, Jeppsson JO, et al. A comparison of the effects of potassium citrate and sodium bicarbonate in the alkalinization of urine in homozygous cystinuria. Urol Res. 2001;29:295-302.
61. Goldfarb DS. A woman with recurrent calcium phosphate kidney stones. Clin J Am Soc Nephrol. 2012;7:1172-8.
62. Sterrett SP, Penniston KL, Wolf JS Jr, et al. Acetazolamide is an effective adjunct for urinary alkalization in patients with uric acid and cystine stone formation recalcitrant to potassium citrate. Urology. 2008;72:278-81.
63. Jaeger P, Portmann L, Saunders A, et al. Anticystinuric effects of glutamine and of dietary sodium restriction. N Engl J Med. 1986;315:1120-3.
64. Rodman JS, Blackburn P, Williams JJ, et al. The effect of dietary protein on cystine excretion in patients with cystinuria. Clin Nephrol. 1984;22:273-8.
65. Meschi T, Maggiore U, Fiaccadori E, et al. The effect of fruits and vegetables on urinary stone risk factors. Kidney Int. 2004;66:2402-10.
66. Lotz M, Bartter FC. Stone dissolution with D-penicillamine in cystinuria. Br Med J. 1965;2:1408-9.
67. Dolin DJ, Asplin JR, Flagel L, et al. Effect of cystine-binding thiol drugs on urinary cystine capacity in patients with cystinuria. J Endourol. 2005;19:429-32.
68. Remien A, Kallistratos G, Burchardt P. Treatment of cystinuria with Thiola (alpha-mercaptopropionyl glycine). Eur Urol. 1975;1:227-8.
69. Harbar JA, Cusworth DC, Lawes LC, et al. Comparison of 2-mercaptopropionylglycine and D-penicillamine in the treatment of cystinuria. J Urol. 1986;136:146-9.
70. Dello Strologo L, Laurenzi C, Legato A, et al. Cystinuria in children and young adults: success of monitoring free-cystine urine levels. Pediatr Nephrol. 2007;22:1869-73.
71. Pak CY, Fuller C, Sakhaee K, et al. Management of cystine nephrolithiasis with alpha-mercaptopropionylglycine. J Urol. 1986;136:1003-8.
72. Zheng Z, Xue Y, Jia J, et al. Tiopronin-induced membranous nephropathy: a case report. Ren Fail. 2014;36:1455-60.
73. Ishak R, Abbas O. Penicillamine revisited: historic overview and review of the clinical uses and cutaneous adverse effects. Am J Clin Dermatol. 2013;14:223-33.
74. Asplin DM, Asplin JR. The Interaction of thiol drugs and urine pH in the treatment of cystinuria. J Urol. 2013;189:2147-51.
75. Rimer JD, An Z, Zhu Z, et al. Crystal growth inhibitors for the prevention of L-cystine kidney stones through molecular design. Science. 2010;330:337-41.
76. Sahota A, Parihar JS, Yang M, et al. Novel cystine ester mimics for the treatment of cystinuria-induced urolithiasis in a knockout mouse model. Urology. 2014;84:1249.e9-15.
77. Wilmer MJ, Willems PH, Verkaart S, et al. Cystine dimethylester model of cystinosis: still reliable? Pediatr Res. 2007;62:151-5.
78. Koide TYS, Utsonomiya M, Yoshioka T. A new therapeutic agent for cystinuria. VII International Symposium on Urolithiasis. Cairns, Australia: Plenum Press; 1992. p. 168.
78a. Hu L, Yang Y, Aloysius H, et al. I-Cystine Diamides as I-Cystine Crystallization Inhibitors for Cystinuria. J Med Chem. 2016 Aug 11;59(15):7293-8.
79. Ringe D, Petsko GA. What are pharmacological chaperones and why are they interesting? J Biol. 2009;8:80.
80. Fan JQ, Ishii S. Active-site-specific chaperone therapy for Fabry disease. Yin and Yang of enzyme inhibitors. FEBS J. 2007;274:4962-71.
81. Bartoccioni P, Rius M, Zorzano A, et al. Distinct classes of trafficking rBAT mutants cause the type I cystinuria phenotype. Hum Mol Genet. 2008;17:1845-54.
82. Kelley WN, Levy RI, Rosenbloom FM, et al. Adenine phosphoribosyltransferase deficiency: a previously undescribed genetic defect in man. J Clin Invest. 1968;47:2281-9.
83. Edvardsson V, Palsson R, Olafsson I, et al. Clinical features and genotype of adenine phosphoribosyltransferase deficiency in iceland. Am J Kidney Dis. 2001;38:473-80.

84. Edvardsson VO, Goldfarb DS, Lieske JC, et al. Hereditary causes of kidney stones and chronic kidney disease. Pediatr Nephrol. 2013;28:1923-42.
85. Broderick TP, Schaff DA, Bertino AM, et al. Comparative anatomy of the human APRT gene and enzyme: nucleotide sequence divergence and conservation of a nonrandom CpG dinucleotide arrangement. Proc Natl Acad Sci U S A. 1987;84:3349-53.
86. Bollee G, Dollinger C, Boutaud L, et al. Phenotype and genotype characterization of adenine phosphoribosyltransferase deficiency. J Am Soc Nephrol. 2010;21:679-88.
87. Hidaka Y, Tarle SA, Fujimori S, et al. Human adenine phosphoribosyltransferase deficiency. Demonstration of a single mutant allele common to the Japanese. J Clin Invest. 1988;81:945-50.
88. Kamatani N, Hakoda M, Otsuka S, et al. Only three mutations account for almost all defective alleles causing adenine phosphoribosyltransferase deficiency in Japanese patients. J Clin Invest. 1992;90:130-5.
89. Engle SJ, Stockelman MG, Chen J, et al. Adenine phosphoribosyltransferase-deficient mice develop 2,8-dihydroxyadenine nephrolithiasis. Proc Natl Acad Sci U S A. 1996;93:5307-12.
90. Tzortzaki EG, Glass D, Yang M, et al. Gender- and age-dependent changes in kidney androgen protein mRNA expression in a knockout mouse model for nephrolithiasis. J Histochem Cytochem. 2002;50:1663-9.
91. Stockelman MG, Lorenz JN, Smith FN, et al. Chronic renal failure in a mouse model of human adenine phosphoribosyltransferase deficiency. Am J Physiol. 1998;275:F154-63.
92. Lieske JC, Rule AD, Krambeck AE, et al. Stone composition as a function of age and sex. Clin J Am Soc Nephrol. 2014;9:2141-6.
93. Nasr SH, Sethi S, Cornell LD, et al. Crystalline nephropathy due to 2,8-dihydroxyadeninuria: an under-recognized cause of irreversible renal failure. Nephrol Dial Transplant. 2010;25:1909-15.
94. Fye KH, Sahota A, Hancock DC, et al. Adenine phosphoribosyltransferase deficiency with renal deposition of 2,8-dihydroxyadenine leading to nephrolithiasis and chronic renal failure. Arch Intern Med. 1993;153:767-70.
95. Harambat J, Bollee G, Daudon M, et al. Adenine phosphoribosyltransferase deficiency in children. Pediatr Nephrol. 2012;27:571-9.
96. Zaidan M, Palsson R, Merieau E, et al. Recurrent 2,8-dihydroxyadenine nephropathy: a rare but preventable cause of renal allograft failure. Am J Transplant. 2014;14:2623-32.
97. Bollee G, Cochat P, Daudon M. Recurrence of crystalline nephropathy after kidney transplantation in APRT deficiency and primary hyperoxaluria. Can J Kidney Health Dis. 2015;2:31.
98. Rule AD, Krambeck AE, Lieske JC. Chronic kidney disease in kidney stone formers. Clin J Am Soc Nephrol. 2011;6:2069-75.
99. Greenwood MC, Dillon MJ, Simmonds HA, et al. Renal failure due to 2,8-dihydroxyadenine urolithiasis. Eur J Pediatr. 1982;138:346-9.
100. Gelb AB, Fye KH, Tischfield JA, et al. Renal insufficiency secondary to 2,8-dihydroxyadenine urolithiasis. Hum Pathol. 1992;23:1081-5.
101. Estepa-Maurice L, Hennequin C, Marfisi C, et al. Fourier transform infrared microscopy identification of crystal deposits in tissues: clinical importance in various pathologies. Am J Clin Pathol. 1996;105:576-82.
102. Auler K, Broock R, Nyhan WL. Determination of activity of the enzymes hypoxanthine phosphoribosyl transferase (HPRT) and adenine phosphoribosyl transferase (APRT) in blood spots on filter paper. Curr Protoc Hum Genet.
103. Bollee G, Harambat J, Bensman A, et al. Adenine phosphoribosyltransferase deficiency. Clin J Am Soc Nephrol. 2012;7:1521-7.
104. Edvardsson VO RH, Oddsdottir S, Agustsdottir IM, et al. Comparison of allopurinol and febuxostat in APRT deficiency: effect on urinary 2,8-dihydroxyadenine excretion. J Am Soc Nephrol. 2014;25:176A.
105. Edvardsson VO, Palsson R, Sahota A. Adenine phosphoribosyltransferase deficiency. In: Pagon RA, Adam MP, Ardinger HH et al., (eds.). GeneReviews. Seattle (WA), 1993.
106. Stamp LK, Day RO, Yun J. Allopurinol hypersensitivity: investigating the cause and minimizing the risk. Nat Rev Rheumatol. 2015 doi: 10.1038/nrrheum.2015.132. [Epub ahead of print].
107. Saito Y, Stamp LK, Caudle KE, et al. Clinical Pharmacogenetics Implementation Consortium (CPIC) guidelines for human leukocyte antigen B (HLA-B) genotype and allopurinol dosing: 2015 update. Clin Pharmacol Ther. 2015;99(1):36-7.
108. Becker MA, Fitz-Patrick D, Choi HK, et al. An open-label, 6-month study of allopurinol safety in gout: The LASSO study. Semin Arthritis Rheum. 2015;45:174-83.
109. Dalbeth N, Kumar S, Stamp L, et al. Dose adjustment of allopurinol according to creatinine clearance does not provide adequate control of hyperuricemia in patients with gout. J Rheumatol. 2006;33:1646-50.
110. Dalbeth N, Stamp L. Allopurinol dosing in renal impairment: walking the tightrope between adequate urate lowering and adverse events. Semin Dial. 2007;20:391-5.
111. Becker MA, Schumacher HR Jr, Wortmann RL, et al. Febuxostat, a novel nonpurine selective inhibitor of xanthine oxidase: a twenty-eight-day, multicenter, phase II, randomized, double-blind, placebo-controlled, dose-response clinical trial examining safety and efficacy in patients with gout. Arthritis Rheum. 2005;52:916-23.
112. Mayer MD, Khosravan R, Vernillet L, et al. Pharmacokinetics and pharmacodynamics of febuxostat, a new non-purine selective inhibitor of xanthine oxidase in subjects with renal impairment. Am J Ther. 2005;12:22-34.
113. Beara-Lasic L, Pillinger MH, Goldfarb DS. Advances in the management of gout: critical appraisal of febuxostat in the control of hyperuricemia. Int J Nephrol Renovasc Dis. 2010;3:1-10.
114. Osada Y, Tsuchimoto M, Fukushima H, et al. Hypouricemic effect of the novel xanthine oxidase inhibitor, TEI-6720, in rodents. Eur J Pharmacol. 1993;241:183-8.
115. Ichida K, Amaya Y, Okamoto K, et al. Mutations associated with functional disorder of xanthine oxidoreductase and hereditary xanthinuria in humans. Int J Mol Sci. 2012;13:15475-95.

116. Dent CE, Philpot GR. Xanthinuria, an inborn error (or deviation) of metabolism. Lancet. 1954;266:182-5.
117. Kudo M, Moteki T, Sasaki T, et al. Functional characterization of human xanthine oxidase allelic variants. Pharmacogenet Genomics. 2008;18:243-51.
118. Minoshima S, Wang Y, Ichida K, et al. Mapping of the gene for human xanthine dehydrogenase (oxidase) (XDH) to band p23 of chromosome 2. Cytogenet Cell Genet. 1995;68:52-3.
119. Mraz M, Hurba O, Bartl J, et al. Modern diagnostic approach to hereditary xanthinuria. Urolithiasis. 2015;43:61-7.
120. Bradbury MG, Henderson M, Brocklebank JT, et al. Acute renal failure due to xanthine stones. Pediatr Nephrol. 1995;9:476-7.
121. Ichida K, Matsumura T, Sakuma R, et al. Mutation of human molybdenum cofactor sulfurase gene is responsible for classical xanthinuria type II. Biochem Biophys Res Commun. 2001;282:1194-200.
122. Beemer FA, Duran M, Wadman SK, et al. Absence of hepatic molybdenum cofactor. An inborn error of metabolism associated with lens dislocation. Ophthalmic Paediatr Genet. 1985;5:191-5.

CHAPTER

22

Drug-Induced Stones

Lama Nazzal, David S Goldfarb

INTRODUCTION

The first drug-induced stones, attributed to treatment with sulfonamides, were described as early as the 1940s. Since then, multiple medications have been recognized as etiologic factors for nephrolithiasis, representing 1–2% of all cases.[1,2] Drug-induced stone formation can be explained by two different mechanisms: (1) the drug or its metabolites are lithogenic and form the main component of the stone; (2) the drug causes metabolic alterations in purine or calcium oxalate metabolism, predisposing to uric acid or calcium-based kidney stone formation.

DIAGNOSIS OF DRUG-INDUCED NEPHROLITHIASIS

The diagnosis of a new renal calculus following the start of a new drug in a patient with no history of kidney stones should raise the possibility of a drug-induced stone. Complexity arises when the patient is on multiple, potentially lithogenic drugs at the time of stone formation or when the timing of the development of a stone does not coincide with starting of a new drug. Establishing the causal link between drug consumption and formation of kidney stones requires a careful evaluation of the patient's medical history, comorbidities, and timing of drug initiation.

Most drug-induced calculi are radiolucent but detectable by echography. To identify drug-containing calculi, it is essential to analyze the calculi by physical methods to help identify all inorganic compounds. X-ray diffraction,[3] mass spectroscopy, or infrared spectroscopy with optic examination can be used to examine the stone.[4] Rarely, the infrared spectrum of new lithogenic drugs or supplements may not be available in the laboratory, which may imply that the stone is of unknown composition. In emergency cases and/or when the calculus is not available, examination of the urine for crystalluria can be very helpful.[5-8]

EPIDEMIOLOGY

True prevalence of drug-induced calculi is likely underestimated because the rate is extracted from published data from a large series of calculi analyzed at specialized laboratories. This evaluation will only identify renal calculi composed of the drug or its metabolites and would miss calcium oxalate, uric acid, and calcium phosphate calculi, which are metabolically induced by the drugs.

Drug-induced stones were first described as a complication of poorly soluble sulfonamide therapy.[1] The epidemiology of drug-induced stones has varied considerably since then. Between 1977 and 1986, the most common culprits were glafenine and triamterene; from 1987 to 1996 these were triamterene and sulfonamides; and from 1997 to 2002 they were indinavir and triamterene.[1] In the last two decades, the most common causes of drug-induced stones have been carbonic anhydrase inhibitors, protease inhibitors, and calcium or vitamin D supplements.[9]

Although a few case reports and small case series of drug-induced stones were published before 1980s, Ettinger et al. were the first to publish a large-scale epidemiological study of drug-induced calculi.[10] They reported that 0.4% of calculi analyzed by the crystallographic method over a 6-month period contained triamterene. This study did not report any other drug-induced stones. In 1986, another study from Switzerland analyzed the stone composition of >14,000 calculi analyzed between 1982 and 1985, and observed an incidence of drug-induced stones of 0.1%.[11] Several large epidemiological studies have reported the incidence and prevalence of drug-induced stones since then.[12] The incidence varied between 0.1 and 1.45%, and prevalence was about 1% of all stones. From 1995 to 2012, Daudon et al. analyzed >49,000 stones and reported that the most common types of drug-containing stones were protease inhibitors (166 stones, 0.3%) followed by sulfonamides (25 stones, 0.06%). The most common metabolically induced calculi were secondary to carbonic anhydrase inhibitors such as acetazolamide, vitamin D, and calcium supplements (32, 27, and 27 stones, respectively).[9]

Triamterene

Triamterene is a widely used drug in the treatment of hypertension. It is often prescribed with hydrochlorothiazide to counteract the potassium wasting effect of thiazides. Triamterene blocks the epithelial sodium channel, offering a mild blood pressure lowering effect while minimizing electrogenic sodium reabsorption, which, in turn, limits potassium wasting. Triamterene has been used since 1961, but the first triamterene-associated stone was reported in 1979.[13] Since then, triamterene has been well known for its lithogenic potential.[14-16] Earlier reports estimated the prevalence of triamterene-containing stones at 0.4%[1,10,17] of total kidney stones, but its incidence has been declining in recent decades secondary to the use of less lithogenic potassium-sparing drugs such as amiloride and spironolactone.[1,9] The solubility of triamterene and its metabolite is low in the urine, especially at a low pH, where 30–70% of the ingested dose is excreted within 2–3 hours after oral ingestion. In fact, more than half of the healthy volunteers ingesting the drug form urinary crystals. However, predisposition for kidney stone formation is present in only a few patients taking the drug. A high daily dose of the medication and low urinary pH are among the factors that increase the risk for crystallization.[18] Triamterene stones are usually mixed stones containing triamterene, calcium oxalate, calcium phosphate, or uric acid with a minority containing exclusively triamterene.[10] To prevent the formation of kidney stones, this therapy should be avoided in patients with a history of nephrolithiasis. The use of thiazides to reduce urine calcium excretion in calcium stone formers should be accompanied by potassium citrate or potassium chloride supplements, or by amiloride or spironolactone; all are preferable to prescription of thiazide–triamterene combination pills. Triamterene should also be avoided in patients who form uric acid stones, which are often caused by acidic urine. Other preventive measures include daily dose of triamterene not exceeding 100 mg and achieving urine pH above 6 with administration of alkali.[1,9]

Human Immunodeficiency Virus Medications

As new and more effective retroviral therapy for human immunodeficiency virus (HIV) treatment expanded, patients developed complications of the drug therapy. Drug-induced calculi are a common complication that occasionally leads to the discontinuation of drugs.

Protease Inhibitors

Protease inhibitors have been the mainstay of the treatment of HIV since their introduction in 1995.[19] Shortly after their first use, various agents in this class have been associated with radiolucent renal calculi. They are the only common stones not visualized by computed tomography (CT). Patients presenting with renal colic and hydronephrosis who undergo noncontrast CT scanning that fails to demonstrate an obstructing stone will have the correct diagnosis made if their drug history reveals the use of a protease inhibitor. For the last 15 years, protease inhibitors have replaced sulfonamides as the leading cause of drug-induced nephrolithiasis where HIV is prevalent.[9]

Indinavir

Indinavir was a widely prescribed protease inhibitor for HIV patients associated with kidney stones,[1] asymptomatic crystalluria, and reduced glomerular filtration rate.[20,21] It is less frequently used today because of its toxic profile. It induced the formation of calculi in 7–12% of treated patients.[22-26] Pure indinavir calculi are radiolucent on plain abdominal radiograph and CT.[27] To be visualized, ultrasonography, intravenous pyelography, or contrast-enhanced CT needs to be used. When contrast is administered, these stones may appear as filling defects in the stream of contrast. In addition to obstructive renal calculi, indinavir has also been implicated in acute renal failure secondary to interstitial nephritis because of indinavir crystal deposition in the cortical and medullary collecting ducts.[20,21,28] The renal failure is usually reversible after drug discontinuation. In the stone, indinavir is usually present as indinavir monohydrate crystals identified by Infrared spectroscopy.[29] The drug's pharmacokinetics can explain the high incidence of renal calculi at the commonly prescribed dose of 800 mg every 8 hours; ~20% of the oral dose is excreted in the urine where indinavir solubility is highly pH dependent. At the usual urine pH, indinavir reaches the limit of solubility 3 hours following the oral dose making crystal formation common.[23,29-31] The incidence of crystalluria in 54 indinavir-treated patients was reported to be 67% when their urine was examined monthly for 1 year.[32]

Many indinavir-induced stones pass spontaneously (>80%) with no need for urological intervention.[23]

Management is usually conservative, including pain control, monitoring of renal function, and temporary discontinuation of the drug. Extracorporeal shock-wave lithotripsy is often ineffective secondary to the loose, highly proteinaceous structure of the stones;[33] therefore, ureteric stenting or ureteroscopy might be needed.[23,34] Five of 29 symptomatic indinavir stones required removal by ureteroscopy in one study.[29]

Prevention of renal complications of indinavir focuses on increasing fluid intake to at least 1.5L per day since prolonged urine acidification to a pH <5.5 would be difficult to tolerate and increases the risk of uric acid stones. The recommendation is to ingest 150 mL of fluids every 2 hours when taking the drug. Lightly acidic beverages such as cola soft drinks may reduce formation of crystals and stones.[1] The development of new therapeutic protocols consisting of coadministration of indinavir and ritonavir, a potent inhibitor of P4503A4, resulted in increasing the half-life of indinavir and decreasing its lithogenic potential. Only 9.2% of participants had to discontinue therapy.[24]

Atazanavir

Atazanavir, an azapeptide inhibitor of HIV protease, was introduced in 2003 and is also recognized to induce kidney stone formation.[35] The combination of atazanavir and ritonavir (ATV/r), acting as its booster, is currently one of the key first-line drugs for the treatment of HIV because it is dosed once daily, is highly efficacious, and is tolerated with a favorable lipid profile. Epidemiological data described a higher incidence of calculi in patients treated with atazanavir compared with other protease inhibitor-based regimens.[36,37] In a retrospective study from 2004 to 2007 including 1,134 patients treated with atazanavir, the overall prevalence of symptomatic atazanavir-associated calculi was 0.97%.[38] The mean time for stone formation since starting therapy was about 2 years. The diagnosis of stone was determined by infrared spectrophotometry and revealed that stones contained atazanavir crystals without metabolites. The US Food and Drug Administration's (FDA) Adverse Event Reporting System identified 30 cases of kidney stones from December 2002 to January 2007 in HIV-infected patients treated with atazanavir.[39] The median time between atazanavir treatment initiation and the onset of nephrolithiasis was 1.7 years. The incidence of atazanavir-associated calculi was 23.7 cases per 1,000 patient-years in the ATV/r treated group compared to 2.2 cases per 1,000 patient years in the other protease inhibitor group.[37] The calculi were diagnosed clinically and no chemical composition was performed. Of the patients who continued ATV/r despite the diagnosis of nephrolithiasis, 33% experienced recurrence while no recurrence was reported in patients who discontinued the drug.[37] The stones are radiolucent and yellow–orange in color, composed of thin atazanavir needles without metabolites.

Although ritonavir-boosted atazanavir crystalluria is present in 8.9% of asymptomatic patients, the number of crystals is lower than in indinavir-treated patients and they form smaller aggregates.[40] The development of interstitial nephropathy secondary to ATV/r has been reported in only six cases in the literature.[41-44] The mechanism of formation of atazanavir stones is unknown but several risk factors have been suggested, including pre-existing renal and hepatic diseases, history of kidney stones, high serum bilirubin, alkaline urine, longer duration of therapy, and chronic active hepatitis C.[36-39,45] Similar to indinavir-induced stones, prevention of crystallization is achieved by increasing fluid intake. For patients who develop atazanavir stones, discontinuation of the drug is important because of high-risk for recurrence.[37]

Darunavir

Darunavir is a novel protease inhibitor with broad activity against drug-resistant clinical isolates. Its lithogenic potential was evaluated in the study by Rockwood et al. of HIV-infected patients treated with ATZ/r, efavirenz, ritonavir-boosted lopinavir, and ritonavir-boosted darunavir over a 45-month period.[36] They showed that the incidence of renal stones in patients exposed to ATZ/r is greater than that with other commonly utilized antiretroviral therapy. A recent study by de Lastours et al. examined the urine for crystals of patients treated with atazanavir, darunavir, and lopinavir. Atazanavir crystals were detected in 7/78 patients receiving ATV300/r and darunavir crystals were found in 4/52 patients receiving darunavir; no crystals were found in any patients receiving lopinavir.[40]

Nelfinavir

Engeler et al. reported the first case of nelfinavir stones in a 37-year-old HIV-infected patient with hepatitis C coinfection. The stone contained 99% nelfinavir and indinavir.[46] Her antiretroviral treatment was changed to fosamprenavir with ritonavir and delavirdine, but she subsequently developed bilateral nephrolithiasis 6 years later. The stones were composed of 95% amprenavir and 5% ritonavir.[47]

Other Protease Inhibitors

Urolithiasis has been associated with nonindinavir or atazanavir protease inhibitors, including saquinavir, lopinavir, and lopinavir/ritonavir, but all are considered rare.[48,49]

Nonprotease Inhibitor Antiretroviral-based Treatment

Several nonprotease inhibitor antiretroviral drugs have been reported to induce renal calculi. Raltegravir and its metabolites are excreted in the urine and have been reported to cause stones in one patient.[50]

Efavirenz, a nonnucleoside reverse transcriptase inhibitor, can rarely cause kidney stones.[51,52] It is metabolized to hydroxylated metabolites and glucuronidated, then excreted in the urine. The stone was composed of 50–60% efavirenz metabolites and the rest of unspecified proteins.

Sulfonamides

Sulfonamides have been used for >60 years to treat multiple conditions. They are known to cause kidney stones and renal injury secondary to intratubular crystallization of the drugs.[53,54] They are mainly metabolized in the liver to *N*-acetyl metabolites, then excreted in the urine where they are poorly soluble at physiological pH.[1,55] Even though the incidence of sulfonamide calculi has decreased since 1980s because of the development of more soluble sulfonamides and the use of other antibiotics, sulfadiazine continues to be used for the treatment of toxoplasma encephalitis in acquired immune deficiency syndrome patients and transplant recipients on long-term immunosuppressive therapy. The fact that sulfadiazine crosses the blood–brain barrier makes it an important drug for the treatment of cerebral toxoplasmosis requiring very high doses of the drug. This high dose induces heavy intratubular crystallization of the poorly soluble *N*-acetylsulfadiazine,[56] which forms a needle-shaped crystal that aggregates readily, resulting in the rapid formation of bilateral nephrolithiasis[57] and tubular obstruction that can lead to acute renal failure. Daudon et al. reported that, over the period spanning from 1987 to 1996, 16% of the drug-containing stones analyzed in their laboratory were mainly composed of sulfadiazine metabolite *N*-acetylsulfadiazine. They also noted that the incidence of these stones was trending down.[9]

High daily dose sulfadiazine and quick liver acetylation of sulfadiazine to N-acetylsulfadiazine, coupled with high urinary excretion and low urinary pH are the main risk factors of sulfadiazine stone formation.[1] Sulfadiazine stones are usually radiolucent and give a weak attenuation (<100 Hounsfield units, HU) with unenhanced helical CT. However, they are detectable by ultrasonography. Identification of large agglomerates of the needle-shaped crystals on urinary sediment examination can expedite the diagnosis. Prevention of stone formation relies on increasing urinary solubility of the sulfadiazine metabolite by increasing urine volume and urine pH over the duration of the treatment.[9]

Sulfasalazine

Sulfasalazine, a sulfonamide used for the treatment of ulcerative colitis, has been reported to cause bilateral kidney stones.[57-59] Sulfasalazine is composed of sulfapyridine linked to 5-aminosalicylic acid by an azo bond. The colonic bacteria cleave the azo bond and form 5-ASA and sulfapyridine, which are absorbed from the colon, acetylated in the liver, and excreted into the urine. The acetylated metabolite is poorly soluble and crystallizes easily.

Sulfamethoxazole

Sulfamethoxazole is a widely used sulfonamide as a component of the antibiotic cotrimoxazole. It frequently causes crystalluria in the form of *N*-acetylsulfamethoxazole hydrochloride, a smooth rhomboid-shaped crystal, but rarely causes nephrolithiasis.[54,60,61] The prevention of this complication is similar to sulfonamides and requires increased fluid intake and urine alkalinization.

Amino-4-quinoleines

Glafenine, a potent analgesic, was associated with multiple cases of drug-induced calculi until its withdrawal in 1992.[62] Calculi mainly contained free glafenic acid around a preformed calculus.[63] The main metabolite of glafenine, glafenic acid glucoronide, is very soluble but its deconjugated metabolite, free glafenic acid, is poorly soluble.[1] The calculi contain high protein concentrations; hence they are radiolucent.[64] There might be a role of bacteria in deconjugation of the glafenic acid glucoronide and the resulting lithogenic process.

Silica

Silica-induced kidney stones are common in grazing animals.[65] In humans, calculi develop following long-term consumption of magnesium trisilicate as an antacid for gastrointestinal symptoms.[66,67] Patients taking these agents usually have high levels of silica in their plasma resulting in high rates of excretion in the urine.[1] This effect is thought to be secondary to the change of magnesium trisilicate into various silicic acid metabolites (orthosilicic and metasilicic acids) within the stomach at low pH, which can be absorbed in the gut and secreted in the urine. The calculi are composed, usually, entirely of amorphous silicon dioxide (silica).[68] Colloid silica was once added to babies' milk to thicken it and prevent regurgitation. Several children developed calculi that contained a nucleus of opaline silica, often surrounded by calcium oxalate and/or calcium phosphate. These stones were discovered years after the drug was stopped.[1,69] Studies to establish the urinary conditions that predispose to crystallization showed conflicting results. There might be a relationship between silica precipitation and protein level in the urine.[70] Crystalline forms of silica α-quartz can be associated with spurious calculi collected from the environment and submitted for analysis as renal calculi by patients who complain of pain.[71,72]

Antibacterials

Different classes of antibacterial drugs including (1) the quinolones flumequine,[73] oxolinic acid,[74] and ciprofloxacin;[75] (2) the aminopenicillins amoxicillin[76] and ampicillin;[1] and (3) the cephalosporins including ceftriaxone[77-79] and 4) phenazopyridine[80] have been reported to induce calculi. Formation of calculi composed of these drugs is favored when the urine output is low; the urine pH is low; and high doses of medications are used. However, more recent fluoroquinolones, particularly ciprofloxacin, cause crystalluria in high urine pH.

Ciprofloxacin

Ciprofloxacin has been reported to cause toxic tubulointerstitial nephritis while patients were given therapeutic doses.[81-83] Urinary crystallization of ciprofloxacin and norfloxacin is secondary to their magnesium salts, which form large needle-shaped crystals, and rarely lead to calculus formation.[75,84,85]

Amoxicillin

Amoxicillin and ampicillin can crystallize in the urine in the trihydrate form and induce renal failure or hematuria but rarely nephrolithiasis.[86-89]

Ceftriaxone

The third-generation cephalosporin ceftriaxone is widely used for the treatment of community-acquired pneumonia, meningitis, and pyelonephritis, especially in children. Shortly after its introduction in 1980s, it was reported to cause nephrolithiasis.[90] We now know that it causes nephrolithiasis in 1.4–7.8%[91,92] of treated subjects and accounts for a large proportion of drug-induced stones in children. Stones can form in the first 10 days of therapy.[93] The stones are composed of ceftriaxone calcium salt since ceftriaxone induces an increase in urinary calcium excretion.[94] Timely pharmacological and surgical intervention can correct the associated acute kidney injury.[95,96]

Guaifenesin, Ephedrine, and Pseudoephedrine

Guaifenesin

Guaifenesin is a popular over-the-counter (OTC) expectorant drug that was approved in 1989 by the FDA and soon thereafter reported to cause renal calculi. Ephedrine prescription was limited as of 1994, so the OTC ephedrine was combined with guaifenesin in a 8:1 ratio and given to patients previously on ephedrine. Hence, the patients were exposed to very high doses of guaifenesin, increasing their risk for calculus formation. The stones are mostly made of the renally eliminated main metabolite of guaifenesin, the calcium salt of β-(2-methoxy-phenoxy)-lactic acid, identifiable by infrared spectroscopy.[97,98] It was found in 0.05% of all stones analyzed by Daudon et al.[1] Stones are radiolucent, but can be visualized on unenhanced helical CT scan. Because of its weak density on CT, it is often confused with uric acid stones. Some stones can also contain ephedrine. Guaifenesin calculi are usually multiple, bilateral and recurrent. Shock wave lithotripsy can be used to treat the calculi since these stones fragment easily. In addition, urinary alkalinization is useful.[9]

Ephedrine and Pseudoephedrine

Ephedrine and pseudoephedrine are naturally occurring alkaloids widely used as decongestants and bronchodilators. However, they are commonly used as stimulants, or in herbal preparations. They are available over the counter, which raises their abuse potential.[99] With guaifenesin, ephedrine stones make up to one-third of drug-induced stones in the United States.[100] The Herring Lab identified

106 ephedrine metabolite specimens from a total of 166,466 stones yielding an incidence of 0.06%. Most of the identified patients with ephedrine metabolite stones reported significant ephedrine and pseudoephedrine consumption.[101] Similar to guaifenesin-induced stones, ephedrine calculi are radiolucent and often confused with uric acid calculi but differentiated by CT scan. Stones are easily fragmented by shock wave lithotripsy and are treated with alkalinization.[9,102]

Stimulants

Commonly used stimulants like Ma-Huang extracts containing ephedrine are known to cause calculi composed of ephedrine, norephedrine and pseudoephedrine.[101]

Allopurinol

Allopurinol is an inhibitor of xanthine dehydrogenase (also known as xanthine oxidase) generally used for the treatment of hyperuricemia and gout. Very high doses of allopurinol are used to treat Lesh-Nyhan syndrome. Landgrebe et al. reported that the drug and its active and poorly soluble metabolites are excreted in the urine where they can form calculi containing either pure oxypurinol or oxypurinol with allopurinol.[103] Inhibition of adenine metabolism to uric acid leads to higher urinary excretion of xanthine. In children with Lesh-Nyhan syndrome receiving normal to moderately high doses of allopurinol, calculi are composed of xanthine mixed with oxypurinol. Only two cases have been described of allopurinol-induced stones in patients being treated with high dose of allopurinol for hyperuricemia not caused by Lesh-Nyhan syndrome.[104,105] Allopurinol-induced calculi respond to urine alkalinization and reduction in the allopurinol dosage.[1]

Metabolically Induced Stones

Metabolically induced stones are produced as a result of the metabolic effect of the drug and not the crystallization of the drug or its metabolites. These stones can be radiopaque or radiolucent depending on the metabolic pathway affected. Carbonic anhydrase inhibitors and calcium-vitamin D supplements are the most important drugs leading to metabolically induced stones.

Carbonic Anhydrase

Acetazolamide: Acetazolamide inhibits carbonic anhydrase activity, an effect implicated in the development of renal calculi. It is frequently prescribed to treat glaucoma and more recently epilepsy. Like all carbonic anhydrase inhibitors (CAI), it acts on the proximal tubule to block the reabsorption of bicarbonate and sodium and inhibit the excretion of hydrogen ions. This results in intracellular acidosis enhancing tubular reabsorption of citrate, thus causing hypocitraturia.[106] Other CAIs in addition to acetazolamide, such as methazolamide, dorzolamide and diclofenamide, are frequently associated with nephrolithiasis.[107-109] The incidence was reported as 10% in 51 patients treated with acetazolamide for juvenile myoclonic epilepsy.[110]

The urine of patients treated with carbonic anhydrase inhibitors contains low citrate concentrations and has a high pH, both of which are lithogenic factors favoring the precipitation of calcium phosphate.[111] Hence, carbapatite was the predominant component of the 30 calculi from patients treated with CAI examined by Daudon et al.[1] In addition to the effects of the drug, a history of kidney stones or underlying hypercalciuria increases the risk for stone development.[1] For these complications, locally administered CAI was developed for patients with glaucoma. Intraophthalmic administration does not change urine chemistry. In the case of epilepsy, newer anticonvulsants such as topiramate and zonisamide have CAI properties; hence they can also induce calcium phosphate calculi. To prevent stone formation, high fluid intake and addition of a thiazide diuretic to reduce hypercalciuria are recommended. The efficacy of potassium citrate supplementation in risk reduction of renal calculi during acetazolamide therapy has not been studied but is rational, as the use of the drug frequently leads to metabolic acidosis and hypokalemia.[112]

Topiramate : Topiramate is a neuromodulatory drug synthesized in 1979. It was originally FDA approved to treat epilepsy in 1996, but since then it has often been prescribed for multiple neurological and psychological disorders. Soon thereafter, it was recognized to commonly induce calcium phosphate and, less so, calcium oxalate stones when patients are on long-term therapy.[113] The incidence of kidney stones not requiring surgery was reported at 1.5% in long-term treated epileptic patients. The prevalence of symptomatic stones was estimated at 10.7% in 75 topiramate-treated people with a median daily dose of 300 mg and a median treatment duration of 48 months. When CT scan was used to diagnose nephrolithiasis, the prevalence of asymptomatic stones was 20%.[114] In a similar study of neurologically impaired, nonambulatory and institutionalized children on topiramate for a mean duration of 3 years, thirteen of 24 (54%) individuals developed symptomatic stones.[115] In a recent nationwide population-based cohort study investigating the association of topiramate and urolithiasis, Shen et al. evaluated 1,377 patients receiving topiramate and 1,377 age-and gender-matched controls. They showed that 3.3% of patients receiving topiramate developed urolithiasis, similar to the 2.4% of controls that developed renal calculi ($p = 0.14$).[116] Potassium citrate supplementation does increase urinary citrate excretion in people taking topiramate but whether that prevents stones is not clear.[117]

Zonisamide: Zonisamide is a weak inhibitor of carbonic anhydrase licensed in the United States and Europe as adjunctive treatment for refractory partial seizures and is recognized for its lower incidence of renal calculi compared with other CAI.[118] In a study examining 1296 patients treated with zonisamide at varying doses (<100 to 1,400 mg/day) for up to 8.7 years, 15/1,296 patients (1.2%) developed symptomatic stones. Following ultrasound, CT or intravenous pyelography screening, an additional 34 (2.6%) renal calculi were identified.[118] The stone events were not related to dose, age or duration of treatment. This complication appeared more commonly in the United States and Europe than in Japan. Crystalluria increased when zonisamide treatment was initiated in 27 patients and crystalluria decreased after stopping the drug.[119]

The incidence in these studies suggests that the true incidence of stones is often underappreciated when the diagnosis is based only on clinical manifestations with no CT imaging.

Furosemide

In contrast to the hypocalciuric effects of thiazides, furosemide induces an increase in urinary calcium excretion. In premature neonates, it is a commonly used drug in the medical management of pulmonary and cardiac disease. A complication of this treatment in neonates is the formation of renal calcifications composed of calcium oxalate alone or mixed with calcium phosphate.[120,121] Urinary calcium excretion is greatly increased (up to 20X) and reduced by the addition of thiazide diuretic, which results in the resolution of the calcifications.[122] In adults, no case of furosemide-associated calculi has been reported.

Antibiotics

The gut microbiota is known for its oxalate-degrading capacity, decreasing the absorption of oxalate, hence reducing the risk for calcium oxalate kidney stones.[123] Antibiotic treatment is thought to cause perturbations of this community, increasing the risk for kidney stones. In recent years, *Oxalobacter formigenes* was recognized as the most efficient intestinal oxalate degrader. Its absence was associated with hyperoxaluria and recurrent kidney stones in humans.[124,125] *O. formigenes* is sensitive to commonly used antibiotics.[126] Following a single course of antibiotics for the treatment of *Helicobacter pylori*, mostly amoxicillin and clarithromycin, >60% of *O. formigenes*-positive subjects lost their colonization and the majority remained negative at 6 months.[127] However, to date, treatment of *H. pylori* has not been shown to predispose to stone formation. The role of other facultative oxalate-degraders remains to be elucidated.

Vitamin C

Daily consumption of high doses of OTC ascorbic acid (vitamin C) often exceeding the recommended daily dose by 10–20 times is not uncommon. Since ascorbic acid is metabolized in vivo to oxalate, ascorbic acid overdosing (>2 g/day) can cause hyperoxaluria and calcium oxalate nephrolithiasis. Traxer et al. demonstrated in a double-blind, randomized, crossover study that ingestion of 2 g of ascorbic acid daily results in a significant increase in urinary oxalate in normal individuals and stone formers. Hyperoxaluria was more pronounced in stone formers.[128] When calcium stone-forming patients and nonstone forming controls were given 1 or 2 g of vitamin C supplements for 3 days, urinary oxalate excretion increased, even in urine immediately acidified, in order to prevent ex vivo conversion of ascorbate to oxalate.[129] Initial large observational studies by Curhan et al. examined the association between the intake of vitamin C and the incidence of kidney stones in 45,251 men and 85,557 women followed prospectively and showed no significant increase in the risk of stone formation with increasing vitamin C intake.[130,131] However, the same group later demonstrated, in the Health Professionals Follow-up Study, that the multivariate relative risk for stone formation for men who consumed >1,000 mg of vitamin C per day compared with those who consumed <90 mg/day, the recommended dietary allowance, was

1.41 [95% confidence interval (CI), 1.11–1.80]. This was the first prospective study to show a significant association between the intake of vitamin C and the development of nephrolithiasis.[132]

Uricosuric Drugs

Uricosuric drugs such as benziodarone, benzbromarone, lesinurad or tienilic acid are treatments for hyperuricemia when allopurinol or febuxostat is not tolerated or contraindicated. They inhibit tubular reabsorption of urate and increase the urinary excretion of uric acid. They can thereby increase the risk of uric acid stones, especially in patients with a history of gout or hyperuricosuria.[133,134] If necessary, the drugs can presumably be continued safely if urinary alkalinization is achieved with potassium citrate supplementation.[1]

Laxatives

Anorexic females occasionally abuse laxatives to enhance their weight loss. Dick et al. reported 9 cases of women with laxative abuse and predominantly radiolucent ammonium acid urate stones. Lithogenicity is secondary to chronic diarrhea, leading to a low urine volume coupled with the loss of bicarbonate and other electrolytes (magnesium, potassium, sodium) and intracellular acidosis. These factors stimulate an increase in urinary ammonia, which is titrated to ammonium. Urate anion that would normally be excreted in urine accompanied by sodium, instead combines with ammonium because of low urinary sodium and high urinary ammonium.[135] A few cases of calcium oxalate stones in the setting of laxative abuse have also been described.[136] Since bowel sodium losses should lead to reduced urine sodium and therefore urine calcium, this association appears to be quite unusual.

Calcium/Vitamin D Supplements

Supplemental calcium is commonly used by adults in the United States, and large doses have been recommended for the prevention of osteoporosis. Calcium supplements, especially when combined with vitamin D, can result in hypercalciuria leading to calcium nephrolithiasis. The risk is augmented with the coexistence of underlying idiopathic hypercalciuria.[137] In the Women's Health Initiative, which evaluated 36,282 postmenopausal women randomly assigned to either receive 1000 mg of elemental calcium citrate with 400 IU of vitamin D3 daily or placebo, the risk for renal calculi increased with calcium and vitamin D (hazard ratio, 1.17; 95% CI, 1.02–1.34).[138,139]

Calcium: Curhan et al. studied the association between intake of dietary and supplemental calcium and the incidence of kidney stones among 91,731 women in a 12-year prospective analysis. Whereas a high-calcium diet was strongly associated with a reduced risk for kidney stones (the relative risk of kidney stone was 0.65 (95% CI, 0.5, 0.83) among women in the highest quintile of intake of dietary calcium compared with women in the lowest quintile), daily supplementation with oral calcium and vitamin D significantly increased the risk of stones by 20%.[140] In men, dietary calcium was also protective, but there was a nonsignificant increase in stone risk with calcium supplements.[132] These findings suggest that increasing dietary calcium intake is superior to pharmacological formulations for prevention of nephrolithiasis and osteoporosis.[141] The subjects receiving calcium and vitamin D supplements should be monitored for hypercalciuria, particularly if they have a history of nephrolithiasis or hypercalciuria. If calcium supplements are considered necessary, the preferred supplement is calcium citrate as it should be associated with at least a small increase in citraturia. It should be administered during or within an hour after meals, so that the calcium can also serve as an oxalate binder.

Vitamin D: In recent years, vitamin D supplements are increasingly being prescribed for the treatment of vitamin D deficiency, a very common condition.[142] Leaf et al. examined the effect of vitamin D repletion on urinary calcium among 29 stone formers in an unblinded study. They showed that although overall 24-hour urinary calcium excretion did not change with vitamin D repletion, 11 subjects had an increase in urinary calcium excretion of >20 mg/day.[143] Although supplementation can induce the formation of calcium calculi, prudent repletion in healthy postmenopausal women, the elderly, and kidney stone formers was not associated with increased urinary calcium excretion.[143-145] However, excessive and uncontrolled vitamin D and/or calcium supplementation can contribute to the increase in prevalence of papillary calcium oxalate stones observed recently in young and postmenopausal women.[147] It is possible that the people most at risk for developing hypercalciuria with vitamin D supplementation are those with CYP24A1 mutations, which reduces the activity of 24-hydroxylase, the enzyme that inactivates 1,25-OH-vitamin D.[148]

MANAGEMENT OF PATIENTS WITH DRUG-INDUCED CALCULI

Diagnosis of Drug-induced Stones

The identification of an offending drug resulting in drug-induced stones is essential for designing the appropriate treatment strategy. The diagnosis relies on a careful review of the clinical information, imaging characteristics and stone analysis. The clinical information focusing on medical history, co-morbidities, and current therapy can be essential for the fast diagnosis of common drug-induced stones. For example, a patient with HIV and a diagnosis of nephrolithiasis should raise the possibility of antiretroviral-induced calculi and or sulfadiazine. In patients suffering from epilepsy, glaucoma, migraines or other neuropathologies, the current or previous use of drugs with carbonic anhydrase inhibitor activity should be investigated. Children with recent or past bacterial infection and kidney stones suggest an effect of antibacterial agents. The diagnosis of guaifenesin and/or ephedrine calculi might be more difficult to recognize. On conventional X-ray, all drug-containing stones are radiolucent and often confused with uric acid, cystine, dihydroxyadenine or xanthine stones. Noncontrast helical CT can help visualize all these stones, except protease inhibitor stones. Stone analysis by physical methods, comprising X-ray diffraction or infrared spectroscopy, are the most powerful, rapid and inexpensive methods to identify all organic compounds constituting the stone including the suspected drug and its metabolites. Metabolically induced stones are similar in molecular composition and morphology to usual stones. Therefore the diagnosis is made based on clinical data and the composition of the calculi. Crystalluria examination by urinalysis and infrared spectroscopy might be helpful if no stone is available for analysis.

Treatment of Drug-induced Stones

Drug-induced nephrolithiasis is usually managed medically. Urinary dilution with increased fluid intake can help prevent and, rarely, dissolve the calculi. In addition, the solubility of most of the drug-induced calculi is pH dependent, so that adjustment of urinary pH can be an important part of the therapy. Shock wave lithotripsy is effective in fragmenting most of the drug-induced stones except protease inhibitor-induced stones. In the case of acute obstruction, ureteral stents are therapeutic and ureteroscopy may be appropriate to extract the causative stones.

In conclusion, the most important preventive measure for drug-induced calculi is based on early and adequate identification of the culprit agent.

REFERENCES

1. Daudon M, Jungers P. Drug-induced renal calculi: epidemiology, prevention and management. Drugs. 2004;64(3):245-75.
2. Lehr D. Clinical toxicity of sulfonamides. Ann N Y Acad Sci. 1957;69(3):417-47.
3. Watson RA, Ettinger B, Deshon GE Jr, et al. Triamterene stone: advantage of crystallographic analysis. Urology. 1981;18(3):238-40.
4. Daudon M, Bader CA, Jungers P. Urinary calculi: review of classification methods and correlations with etiology. Scanning Microsc. 1993;7(3):1081-104; discussion 104-6.
5. Daudon M, Reveillaud RJ. Drug-induced crystalluria: myths and realities. Ann Biol Clin (Paris). 1986;44(1):25-34.
6. Perazella MA. Crystal-induced acute renal failure. Am J Med. 1999;106(4):459-65.
7. Gagnon RF, Tsoukas CM, Watters AK. Light microscopy of indinavir urinary crystals. Ann Intern Med. 1998;128(4):321.
8. Daudon M. Crystalluria. Nephrol Ther. 2015;11(3):174-90. [Article in French]
9. Daudon M, Jungers P. Drug-induced stones. In: Grasso M, Goldfarb DS (Eds). Urinary Stones: medical and Surgical Management, 1st edition. Hoboken, NJ: John Wiley and Sons, Ltd.; 2014. pp. 106-19.
10. Ettinger B, Oldroyd NO, Sorgel F. Triamterene nephrolithiasis. J Am Med Assoc. 1980;244(21):2443-5.
11. Asper R. Iatrogenic urinary calculi: detection and identification by X-ray diffraction. Clin Chem. 1986;24:767-8.
12. Rapado A, Traba ML, Caycho C, et al. Drug-induced renal stones: incidence, clinical expression and stone analysis. Contrib Nephrol. 1987;58:25-9.
13. Ettinger B, Weil E, Mandel NS, et al. Triamterene-induced nephrolithiasis. Ann Intern Med. 1979;91(5):745-6.
14. Socolow EL. Triamterene-induced nephrolithiasis. Ann Intern Med. 1980;92(3):437.
15. Baudin S, Rodrigue H. Drug induced nephrolithiasis: observation of an oxalate and hydroxylated triamterene stone (author's transl). Nephrologie. 1980;1(4):183-5.
16. Carey RA, Beg MM, McNally CF, et al. Triamterene and renal lithiasis: a review. Clin Ther. 1984;6(3):302-9.
17. Daudon M, Protat MF, Reveillaud RJ. Triamterene and renal calculi. Nephrologie. 1982;3(3):119-23.
18. Fairley KF, Birch DF, Haines I. Abnormal urinary sediment in patients on triamterene. Lancet. 1983;1(8321):421-2.
19. Lv Z, Chu Y, Wang Y. HIV protease inhibitors: a review of molecular selectivity and toxicity. HIV AIDS (Auckl).. 2015;7:95-104.
20. Kopp JB, Falloon J, Filie A, et al. Indinavir-associated interstitial nephritis and urothelial inflammation: clinical and cytologic findings. Clin Infect Dis. 2002;34(8):1122-8.
21. Berns JS, Cohen RM, Silverman M, et al. Acute renal failure due to indinavir crystalluria and nephrolithiasis: report of two cases. Am J Kidney Dis. 1997;30(4):558-60.

22. Herman JS, Ives NJ, Nelson M, et al. Incidence and risk factors for the development of indinavir-associated renal complications. J Antimicrob Chemother. 2001;48(3):355-60.
23. Kopp JB, Miller KD, Mican JA, et al. Crystalluria and urinary tract abnormalities associated with indinavir. Ann Intern Med. 1997;127(2):119-25.
24. Piroth L, Grappin M, Waldner A, et al. Discontinuing protease inhibitor treatment of HIV-1 patients for intolerance. Longitudinal study of 309 patients. Presse Med. 1999;28(8):381-7.
25. Boubaker K, Sudre P, Bally F, et al. Changes in renal function associated with indinavir. AIDS. 1998;12(18):F249-54.
26. Reiter WJ, Schon-Pernerstorfer H, Dorfinger K, et al. Frequency of urolithiasis in individuals seropositive for human immunodeficiency virus treated with indinavir is higher than previously assumed. J Urol. 1999;161(4):1082-4.
27. Schwartz BF, Schenkman N, Armenakas NA, et al. Imaging characteristics of indinavir calculi. J Urol. 1999;161(4):1085-7.
28. Tashima KT, Horowitz JD, Rosen S. Indinavir nephropathy. N Engl J Med. 1997;336(2):138-40.
29. Daudon M, Estepa L, Viard JP, et al. Urinary stones in HIV-1-positive patients treated with indinavir. Lancet. 1997;349(9061):1294-5.
30. Salahuddin S, Kok DJ, Buchholz NN. Influence of body temperature on indinavir crystallization under loop of Henle conditions. J Antimicrob Chemother. 2007;59(1):114-7.
31. Polhemus ME, Aronson NE. Persistent nephrolithiasis after discontinuation of indinavir therapy. Clin Infect Dis. 1998;27(6):1536-7.
32. Gagnon RF, Tecimer SN, Watters AK, et al. Prospective study of urinalysis abnormalities in HIV-positive individuals treated with indinavir. Am J Kidney Dis. 2000;36(3):507-15.
33. Gentle DL, Stoller ML, Jarrett TW, et al. Protease inhibitor-induced urolithiasis. Urology. 1997;50(4):508-11.
34. Bruce RG, Munch LC, Hoven AD, et al. Urolithiasis associated with the protease inhibitor indinavir. Urology. 1997;50(4):513-8.
35. Chang HR, Pella PM. Atazanavir urolithiasis. N Engl J Med. 2006;355(20):2158-9.
36. Rockwood N, Mandalia S, Bower M, et al. Ritonavir-boosted atazanavir exposure is associated with an increased rate of renal stones compared with efavirenz, ritonavir-boosted lopinavir and ritonavir-boosted darunavir. AIDS. 2011;25(13):1671-3.
37. Hamada Y, Nishijima T, Watanabe K, et al. High incidence of renal stones among HIV-infected patients on ritonavir-boosted atazanavir than in those receiving other protease inhibitor-containing antiretroviral therapy. Clin Infect Dis. 2012;55(9):1262-9.
38. Couzigou C, Daudon M, Meynard JL, et al. Urolithiasis in HIV-positive patients treated with atazanavir. Clin Infect Dis. 2007;45(8):e105-8.
39. Chan-Tack KM, Truffa MM, Struble KA, et al. Atazanavir-associated nephrolithiasis: cases from the US Food and Drug Administration's Adverse Event Reporting System. AIDS. 2007;21(9):1215-8.
40. de Lastours V, Ferrari Rafael De Silva E, Daudon M, et al. High levels of atazanavir and darunavir in urine and crystalluria in asymptomatic patients. J Antimicrob Chemother. 2013;68(8):1850-6.
41. Brewster UC, Perazella MA. Acute interstitial nephritis associated with atazanavir, a new protease inhibitor. Am J Kidney Dis. 2004;44(5):e81-4.
42. Izzedine H, M'Rad MB, Bardier A, et al. Atazanavir crystal nephropathy. AIDS. 2007;21(17):2357-8.
43. Schmid S, Opravil M, Moddel M, et al. Acute interstitial nephritis of HIV-positive patients under atazanavir and tenofovir therapy in a retrospective analysis of kidney biopsies. Virchows Arch. 2007;450(6):665-70.
44. Viglietti D, Verine J, De Castro N, et al. Chronic interstitial nephritis in an HIV type-1-infected patient receiving ritonavir-boosted atazanavir. Antivir Ther. 2011;16(1):119-21.
45. Lafaurie M, De Sousa B, Ponscarme D, et al. Clinical features and risk factors for atazanavir (ATV)-associated urolithiasis: a case-control study. PloS one. 2014;9(11):e112836.
46. Engeler DS, John H, Rentsch KM, et al. Nelfinavir urinary stones. J Urol. 2002;167(3):1384-5.
47. Feicke A, Rentsch KM, Oertle D, et al. Same patient, new stone composition: amprenavir urinary stone. Antivir Ther. 2008;13(5):733-4.
48. Doco-Lecompte T, Garrec A, Thomas L, et al. Lopinavir-ritonavir (Kaletra) and lithiasis: seven cases. AIDS. 2004;18(4):705-6.
49. Green ST, McKendrick MW, Schmid ML, et al. Renal calculi developing de novo in a patient taking saquinavir. Int J STD AIDS. 1998;9(9):555.
50. Vassallo M, Dunais B, Naqvi A, et al. Raltegravir-induced nephrolithiasis: a case report. AIDS. 2012;26(10):1323-4.
51. Izzedine H, Valantin MA, Daudon M, et al. Efavirenz urolithiasis. AIDS. 2007;21(14):1992.
52. Wirth GJ, Teuscher J, Graf JD, et al. Efavirenz-induced urolithiasis. Urol Res. 2006;34(4):288-9.
53. Schreiner GE, Maher JF. Toxic nephropathy. Am J Med. 1965;38:409-49.
54. Albala DM, Prien EL Jr, Galal HA. Urolithiasis as a hazard of sulfonamide therapy. J Endourol. 1994;8(6):401-3.
55. Daudon M, Protat MF, Reveillaud RJ. Detection and diagnosis of drug induced lithiasis. Ann Biol Clin (Paris). 1983;41(4):239-49.
56. Cuervo C, Gonzalez J, Rives V, et al. Characterization of a sulfadiazine-induced lithiasis calculus by physicochemical techniques. AAPS PharmSciTech. 2013;14(1):128-32.
57. Erturk E, Casemento JB, Guertin KR, et al. Bilateral acetylsulfapyridine nephrolithiasis associated with chronic sulfasalazine therapy. J Urol. 1994;151(6):1605-6.
58. Russinko PJ, Agarwal S, Choi MJ, et al. Obstructive nephropathy secondary to sulfasalazine calculi. Urology. 2003;62(4):748.
59. Saito M, Takahashi C, Ishida G, et al. Acute renal failure associated with sulfur calculi. J Urol. 2001;165(6 Pt 1):1985-6.
60. Dorfman LE, Smith JP. Sulfonamide crystalluria: a forgotten disease. J Urol. 1970;104(3):482-3.
61. Siegel WH. Unusual complication of therapy with sulfamethoxazole-trimethoprim. J Urol. 1977;117(3):397.

62. Reveillaud RJ, Daudon M, Protat MF, et al. Renal pelvis stones made of glafenic acid in two patients under prolonged treatment with analgesics (author's transl). Nephrologie. 1980;1(1):3-8.
63. Daudon M, Protat MF, Reveillaud RJ. Renal toxicity of glafenine in man: renal stones and acute renal failure. Ann Biol Clin (Paris). 1983;41(2):105-11.
64. Pasquier B, Griffa N, Heritier P, et al. Urinary calculi caused by glaphenine. Role of radiology in diagnosis. Apropos of a case. J Radiol. 1989;70(6-7):423-5.
65. Whiting F, Connell R, Forman SA. Silica urolithiasis in beef cattle the incidence on different rations and on range. Can J Comp Med Vet Sci. 1958;22(10):332-7.
66. Herman JR, Goldberg AS. New type of urinary calculus caused by antacid therapy. J Am Med Assoc. 1960;174:1206-7.
67. Farrer JH, Rajfer J. Silicate urolithiasis. J Urol. 1984;132(4): 739-40.
68. Lipworth E, Bloomberg BM, Reid FP. Urinary Calculi Containing Silica: a Case Report. S Afr Med J. 1964;38:50-1.
69. Augusti M, Mikaelian JC, Monsaint H, et al. A silica urinary calculus secondary to the absorption of gelopectose in a child. Prog Urol. 1993;3(5):812-5.
70. Bailey CB. The precipitation of polymerized silicic acid by urine protein: a possible mechanism in the etiology of silica urolithiasis. Can J Biochem. 1972;50(3):305-11.
71. Gault MH, Campbell NR, Aksu AE. Spurious stones. Nephron. 1988;48(4):274-9.
72. Sabot JF, Bornet CE, Favre S, et al. The analysis of peculiar urinary (and other) calculi: an endless source of challenge. Clin Chim Acta. 1999;283(1-2):151-8.
73. Rince C, Daudon M, Moesch C, et al. Identification of flumequine in a urinary calculus. J Clin Chem Clin Biochem. 1987;25(5):313-4.
74. Daudon M, Reveilland RJ, Laurence C, et al. Drug-induced oxolinic acid crystalluria and nephrolithiasis. Clin Nephrol. 1987;28(3):156.
75. Chopra N, Fine PL, Price B, et al. Bilateral hydronephrosis from ciprofloxacin induced crystalluria and stone formation. J Urol. 2000;164(2):438.
76. Daudon M, Estepa L. Drug induced lithiases. Presse Med. 1998;27(14):675-83.
77. Daudon M. Drug-induced urinary calculi in 1999. Prog Urol. 1999;9(6):1023-33.
78. Cochat P, Cochat N, Jouvenet M, et al. Ceftriaxone-associated nephrolithiasis. Nephrol Dial Transplant. 1990;5(11):974-6.
79. de Moor RA, Egberts AC, Schroder CH. Ceftriaxone-associated nephrolithiasis and biliary pseudolithiasis. Eur J Pediatr. 1999;158(12):975-7.
80. Mulvaney WP, Beck CW, Brown RR. Urinary phenazopyridine stones. A complication of therapy. J Am Med Assoc. 1972;221(13):1511-2.
81. Rippelmeyer DJ, Synhavsky A. Ciprofloxacin and allergic interstitial nephritis. Ann Intern Med. 1988;109(2):170.
82. Hootkins R, Fenves AZ, Stephens MK. Acute renal failure secondary to oral ciprofloxacin therapy: a presentation of three cases and a review of the literature. Clin Nephrol. 1989;32(2):75-8.
83. Allon M, Lopez EJ, Min KW. Acute renal failure due to ciprofloxacin. Arch Intern Med. 1990;150(10):2187-9.
84. Thorsteinsson SB, Bergan T, Oddsdottir S, et al. Crystalluria and ciprofloxacin, influence of urinary pH and hydration. Chemotherapy. 1986;32(5):408-17.
85. Thorsteinsson SB, Bergan T, Johannesson G, et al. Tolerance of ciprofloxacin at injection site, systemic safety and effect on electroencephalogram. Chemotherapy. 1987;33(6):448-51.
86. Rafat C, Haymann JP, Gaudry S, et al. The case: a crystal-clear diagnosis: acute kidney injury in a patient with suspected meningoencephalitis. Diagnosis: Amoxicillin-induced crystal nephropathy. Kidney Int. 2014;86(5):1065-6.
87. Moesch C, Rince M, Raby C, et al. Aminopenicillin crystalluria: identification by infrared spectrophotometry. Ann Biol Clin (Paris). 1985;43(3):227-31.
88. Fogazzi GB, Cantu M, Saglimbeni L, et al. Amoxycillin, a rare but possible cause of crystalluria. Nephrol Dial Transplant. 2003;18(1):212-4.
89. Boursas M, Benhassine L, Kempf J, et al. Obstructive renal insufficiency caused by amoxicillin crystalluria. Ann Fr Anesth Reanim. 1997;16(7):908-10.
90. Lopez AJ, O'Keefe P, Morrissey M, et al. Ceftriaxone-induced cholelithiasis. Ann Intern Med. 1991;115(9):712-4.
91. Mohkam M, Karimi A, Gharib A, et al. Ceftriaxone associated nephrolithiasis: a prospective study in 284 children. Pediatr Nephrol. 2007;22(5):690-4.
92. Avci Z, Koktener A, Uras N, et al. Nephrolithiasis associated with ceftriaxone therapy: a prospective study in 51 children. Arch Dis Child. 2004;89(11):1069-72.
93. Fesharakinia A, Ehsanbakhsh AR, Ghorashadizadeh N. Ceftriaxone-associated nephrolithiasis in children. Iran J Pediatr. 2013;23(6):643-7.
94. Kimata T, Kaneko K, Takahashi M, et al. Increased urinary calcium excretion caused by ceftriaxone: possible association with urolithiasis. Pediatr Nephrol. 2012;27(4):605-9.
95. Shen X, Liu W, Fang X, et al. Acute kidney injury caused by ceftriaxone-induced urolithiasis in children: a single-institutional experience in diagnosis, treatment and follow-up. Int Urol Nephrol. 2014;46(10):1909-14.
96. Li N, Zhou X, Yuan J, et al. Ceftriaxone and acute renal failure in children. Pediatrics. 2014;133(4):e917-22.
97. Assimos DG, Langenstroer P, Leinbach RF, et al. Guaifenesin- and ephedrine-induced stones. J Endourol. 1999;13(9):665-7.
98. Pickens CL, Milliron AR, Fussner AL, et al. Abuse of guaifenesin-containing medications generates an excess of a carboxylate salt of beta-(2-methoxyphenoxy)-lactic acid, a guaifenesin metabolite, and results in urolithiasis. Urology. 1999;54(1):23-7.
99. Blau JJ. Ephedrine nephrolithiasis associated with chronic ephedrine abuse. J Urol. 1998;160(3 Pt 1):825.
100. Bennett S, Hoffman N, Monga M. Ephedrine- and guaifenesin-induced nephrolithiasis. J Altern Complement Med. 2004;10(6):967-9.
101. Powell T, Hsu FF, Turk J, et al. Ma-huang strikes again: ephedrine nephrolithiasis. Am J Kidney Dis. 1998;32(1):153-9.
102. Hoffman N, McGee SM, Hulbert JC. Resolution of ephedrine stones with dissolution therapy. Urology. 2003;61(5):1035.

103. Landgrebe AR, Nyhan WL, Coleman M. Urinary-tract stones resulting from the excretion of oxypurinol. N Engl J Med. 1975;292(12):626-7.
104. Stote RM, Smith LH, Dubb JW, et al. Oxypurinol nephrolithiasis in regional enteritis secondary to allopurinol therapy. Ann Intern Med. 1980;92(3):384-5.
105. Potter JL, Silvidi AA. Xanthine lithiasis, nephrocalcinosis, and renal failure in a leukemia patient treated with allopurinol. Clin Chem. 1987;33(12):2314-6.
106. Ahlstrand C, Tiselius HG. Urine composition and stone formation during treatment with acetazolamide. Scand J Urol Nephrol. 1987;21(3):225-8.
107. Ellis PP. Urinary calculi with methazolamide therapy. Doc Ophthalmol. 1973;34(1):137-42.
108. Carlsen J, Durcan J, Zabriskie N, et al. Nephrolithiasis with dorzolamide. Arch Ophthalmol. 1999;117(8):1087-8.
109. Wallace MR, MacDiarmid J, Reeder J. Exacerbation of nephrolithiasis by a carbonic anhydrase inhibitor. N Z Med J. 1974;79(509):687-90.
110. Resor SR Jr, Resor LD. Chronic acetazolamide monotherapy in the treatment of juvenile myoclonic epilepsy. Neurology. 1990;40(11):1677-81.
111. Paisley KE, Tomson CR. Calcium phosphate stones during long-term acetazolamide treatment for epilepsy. Postgrad Med J. 1999;75(885):427-8.
112. Goldfarb DS. A woman with recurrent calcium phosphate kidney stones. Clin J Am Soc Nephrol. 2012;7(7):1172-8.
112a. Jhagroo RA, Wertheim ML, Penniston KL. Alkali replacement raises urinary citrate excretion in patients with topiramate-induced hypocitraturia. Br J Clin Pharmacol. 2016;81(1): 131-6.
113. Kuo RL, Moran ME, Kim DH, et al. Topiramate-induced nephrolithiasis. J Endourol. 2002;16(4):229-31.
114. Maalouf NM, Langston JP, Van Ness PC, et al. Nephrolithiasis in topiramate users. Urol Res. 2011;39(4):303-7.
115. Goyal M, Grossberg RI, O'Riordan MA, et al. Urolithiasis with topiramate in nonambulatory children and young adults. Pediatr Neurol. 2009;40(4):289-94.
116. Shen AL, Lin HL, Tseng YF, et al. Topiramate may not increase risk of urolithiasis: a nationwide population-based cohort study. Seizure. 2015;29:86-9.
117. Jhagroo RA, Wertheim ML, Penniston KL. Alkali replacement raises urinary citrate excretion in patients with topiramate-induced hypocitraturia. Br J Clin Pharmacol. 2016;81(1): 131-6.
118. Wroe S. Zonisamide and renal calculi in patients with epilepsy: how big an issue? Curr Med Res Opin. 2007;23(8): 1765-73.
119. Go T. Zonisamide induces crystalluria without urinary pH changes in children and young adults. ISRN Neurol. 2013;2013:841902.
120. Hufnagle KG, Khan SN, Penn D, et al. Renal calcifications: a complication of long-term furosemide therapy in preterm infants. Pediatrics. 1982;70(3):360-3.
121. Alon US, Scagliotti D, Garola RE. Nephrocalcinosis and nephrolithiasis in infants with congestive heart failure treated with furosemide. J Pediatr. 1994;125(1):149-51.
122. Noe HN, Bryant JF, Roy S 3rd, et al. Urolithiasis in preterm neonates associated with furosemide therapy. J Urol. 1984;132(1):93-4.
123. Abratt VR, Reid SJ. Oxalate-degrading bacteria of the human gut as probiotics in the management of kidney stone disease. Adv Appl Microbiol. 2010;72:63-87.
124. Siener R, Bangen U, Sidhu H, et al. The role of Oxalobacter formigenes colonization in calcium oxalate stone disease. Kidney Int. 2013;83(6):1144-9.
125. Kaufman DW, Kelly JP, Curhan GC, et al. Oxalobacter formigenes may reduce the risk of calcium oxalate kidney stones. J Am Soc Nephrol. 2008;19(6):1197-203.
126. Lange JN, Wood KD, Wong H, et al. Sensitivity of human strains of Oxalobacter formigenes to commonly prescribed antibiotics. Urology. 2012;79(6):1286-9.
127. Kharlamb V, Schelker J, Francois F, et al. Oral antibiotic treatment of Helicobacter pylori leads to persistently reduced intestinal colonization rates with *Oxalobacter formigenes*. J Endourol. 2011;25(11):1781-5.
128. Traxer O, Huet B, Poindexter J, et al. Effect of ascorbic acid consumption on urinary stone risk factors. J Urol. 2003;170(2 Pt 1):397-401.
129. Baxmann AC, De OGMC, Heilberg IP. Effect of vitamin C supplements on urinary oxalate and pH in calcium stone-forming patients. Kidney Int. 2003;63(3):1066-71.
130. Curhan GC, Willett WC, Rimm EB, et al. A prospective study of the intake of vitamins C and B6, and the risk of kidney stones in men. J Urol. 1996;155(6):1847-51.
131. Curhan GC, Willett WC, Speizer FE, et al. Intake of vitamins B6 and C and the risk of kidney stones in women. J Am Soc Nephrol. 1999;10(4):840-5.
132. Taylor EN, Stampfer MJ, Curhan GC. Dietary factors and the risk of incident kidney stones in men: new insights after 14 years of follow-up. J Am Soc Nephrol. 2004;15(12):3225-32.
133. Navas P, Grasset D. Anuria due to bilateral ureteral uric acid lithiasis during a treatment with Amplivix. J Urol Nephrol (Paris). 1973;79(12 Pt 2):466-9.
134. McLain DA, Garriga FJ, Kantor OS. Adverse reactions associated with ticrynafen use. J Am Med Assoc. 1980;243(8):763-4.
135. Dick WH, Lingeman JE, Preminger GM, et al. Laxative abuse as a cause for ammonium urate renal calculi. J Urol. 1990;143(2):244-7.
136. Leaf DE, Bukberg PR, Goldfarb DS. Laxative abuse, eating disorders, and kidney stones: a case report and review of the literature. Am J Kidney Dis. 2012;60(2):295-8.
137. Pak CY, Sakhaee K, Hwang TI, et al. Nephrolithiasis from calcium supplementation. J Urol. 1987;137(6):1212-3.
138. Wallace RB, Wactawski-Wende J, O'Sullivan MJ, et al. Urinary tract stone occurrence in the Women's Health Initiative (WHI) randomized clinical trial of calcium and vitamin D supplements. Am J Clin Nutr. 2011;94(1):270-7.
139. Jackson RD, LaCroix AZ, Gass M, et al. Calcium plus vitamin D supplementation and the risk of fractures. N Engl J Med. 2006;354(7):669-83.
140. Curhan GC, Willett WC, Speizer FE, et al. Comparison of dietary calcium with supplemental calcium and other nutri-

ents as factors affecting the risk for kidney stones in women. Ann Intern Med. 1997;126(7):497-504.
141. Favus MJ. The risk of kidney stone formation: the form of calcium matters. Am J Clin Nutr. 2011;94(1):5-6.
142. Visser M, Deeg DJ, Puts MT, et al. Low serum concentrations of 25-hydroxyvitamin D in older persons and the risk of nursing home admission. Am J Clin Nutr. 2006;84(3):616-22; quiz 71-2.
143. Leaf DE, Korets R, Taylor EN, et al. Effect of vitamin D repletion on urinary calcium excretion among kidney stone formers. Clin J Am Soc Nephrol. 2012;7(5):829-34.
144. Penniston KL, Jones AN, Nakada SY, et al. Vitamin D repletion does not alter urinary calcium excretion in healthy postmenopausal women. BJU Int. 2009;104(10):1512-6.
145. Demontiero O, Herrmann M, Duque G. Supplementation with vitamin D and calcium in long-term care residents. J Am Med Dir Assoc. 2011;12(3):190-4.
146. Daudon 2011: Daudon M, Traxer O, Williams JC, Bazin DC. Randall's plaques. In: Rao PN, Preminger GM, Kavanagh JP, eds. Urinary Tract Stone Disease. London: Springer, 2011, pp.103–12.
147. Daudon 2011: Daudon M, Traxer O, Williams JC, Bazin DC. Randall's plaques. In: Rao PN, Preminger GM, Kavanagh JP, eds. Urinary Tract Stone Disease. London: Springer, 2011, pp.103–12.
148. Goldfarb DS. Does Vitamin D Supplementation Cause Kidney Stones? J Urol. 2017;197(2):280-281.

CHAPTER

23 Uric Acid Stones: Epidemiology, Pathophysiology and Treatment

Khashayar Sakhaee

EPIDEMIOLOGY OF URIC ACID NEPHROLITHIASIS AND ITS LINK TO THE METABOLIC SYNDROME

Globally, there are wide variations in the prevalence of uric acid (UA) stones. The highest prevalence has been reported in the Middle East, certain South East Asian countries, and a few European countries.[1-5] Although UA stones comprise only 8–10% of all kidney stones in the United States, their prevalence has increased over the past three decades with the increasing prevalence of obesity (Fig. 23.1).[6] The incidence of UA stones in Southeast Asia, and descendants from Japan and China who live in the United States were reported to be 15–16%. However, the prevalence of (UA) nephrolithiasis and gout among Hmong population who immigrated from their homeland Laos to the United States was reported to be significantly high.[7,8] The high prevalence of UA stones in this population is novel as a significantly low incidence of UA stones is reported in Northeastern Thailand, which is a geographically adjacent to Laos.[9] At this time, it has not been fully explored without such a diverse prevalence of UA stones.

Stone formers with type 2 diabetes mellitus (T2DM) have a higher prevalence of UA stones than nondiabetic stone formers.[10-13] Moreover, a higher prevalence of UA stones has also been shown among obese stone formers.[14,15] It has been shown that greater body mass index (BMI) and T2DM are independent risk factors for UA nephrolithiasis[16] (Fig. 23.2).

In most mammals, ingested purines are converted to UA and then further to soluble allantoin through a series of enzymatic reactions that occur primarily in the peroxisomes of hepatic cells. Humans are higher primates that lack functional uricase, the enzyme that converts UA to allantoin, making UA the final product of purine metabolism in these species.[17] Urinary UA solubility is limited to 96 mg/L. In an average human being with approximately 600–800 mg of UA excretion per day, which exceeds the limit of solubility, a higher risk for UA precipitation and UA

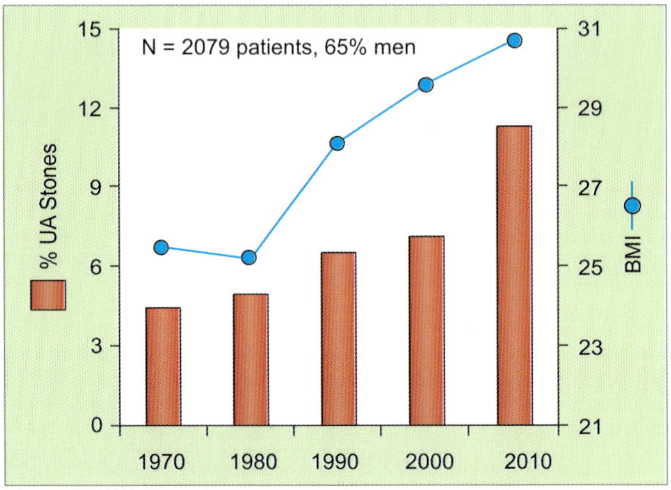

Fig. 23.1: Proportion of uric acid stones and BMI by decade. UA, uric acid; BMI, body mass index.

stone formation is posed.[18,19] Urinary pH has a significant role in UA solubility, as UA is a weak organic acid with dissociation constant (pK_a 5.35 at 37°C).[20] Unduly acidic urine pH (urine pH ≤5.5) is an invariable feature in UA nephrolithiasis that leads to precipitation of the sparingly soluble UA, which increases the risk of UA nephrolithiasis.[21] With limited solubility of 96 mg/L at urinary pH ranging between 4.5 and 5.5, a total UA concentration (comprising undissociated plus urate) of 110–200 mg/L exceeds the solubility limit. However, at a urinary pH of 6.2–6.4 the total UA concentration should exceed 1,100 mg/L to precipitate (Fig. 23.3). However, under normal physiologic states, it is not expected that urinary UA excretion displays such a wide variation between 110 and 1,100 mg/L per day; variation in urinary pH between 4.6 and 6.6 is highly anticipated in normal subjects.

Despite the dominant role of urine pH in UA precipitation, normal urine is frequently metastably supersaturated with respect to UA. This implies that the presence of a urinary inhibitor or promoter of uric crystallization

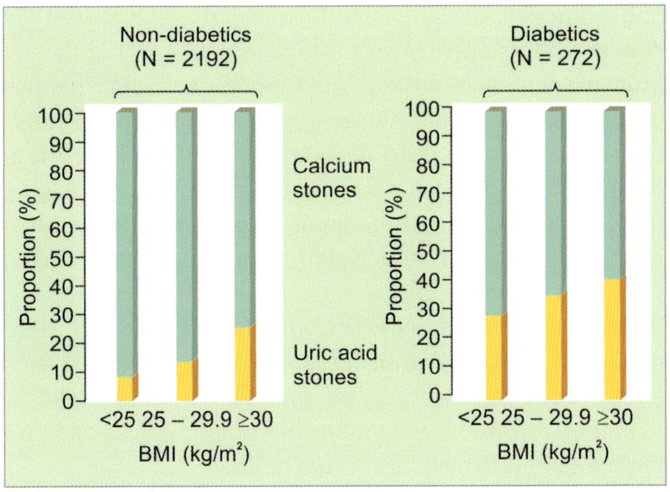

Fig. 23.2: Distribution of stone type with respect to BMI and diabetes status. BMI, body mass index.
Source: Adapted from Daudon M, Traxer O, Conort P, et al. Type 2 diabetes increases the risk for uric acid stones. J Am Soc Nephrol. 2006;17(7):2026-33.

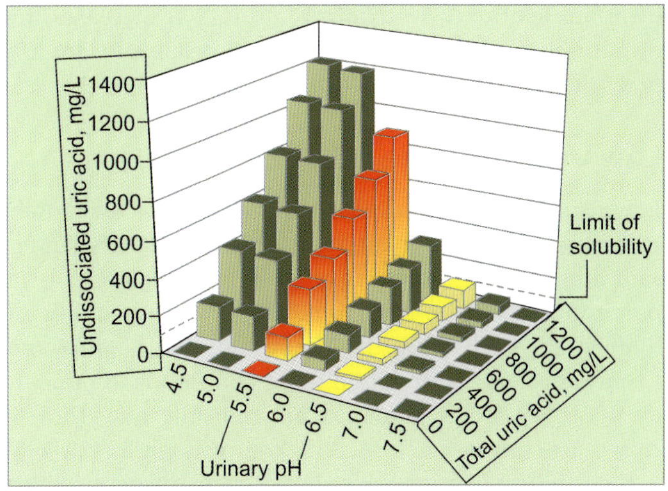

Fig. 23.3: Significance of urinary pH in uric acid solubility.
Source: Adapted with permission from Maalouf NM, Cameron MA, Moe OW, et al. Novel insights into the pathogenesis of uric acid nephrolithiasis. Curr Opin Nephrol Hypertens. 2004;13(2):181-9.

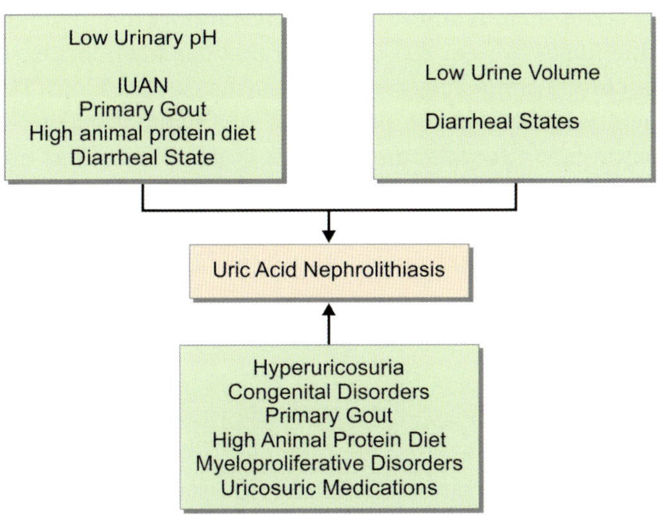

Fig. 23.4: Pathophysiologic mechanisms and etiologic causes of uric acid nephrolithiasis. (IUAN: Idiopathic uric acid nephrolithiasis).

may participate in UA precipitation. There is a sparsity of data clearly identifying the presence of modulators, which inhibit adhesion of UA to renal epithelial cells. One experimental study has supported the inhibitory role of such a micromolecule against UA precipitation.[22]

Furthermore, the solubility of UA in the urinary environment is influenced by urinary electrolyte constituents. It has been shown that the abundance of potassium urate increases while sodium urate reduces solubility.[23,24] The thermodynamic solubility product of sodium urate at 2.79×10^{-5} M^2 was found to be 3.5-fold lower than potassium urate at 9.63×10^{-5} M^2.[25] The latter physicochemical characteristic has a significant clinical impact in the treatment of UA stone formers, demonstrating the advantage[26,27] of potassium-alkali over sodium-alkali therapy. Both sodium and potassium alkali treatments were equally effective in raising urinary pH and lowering the risk for UA stone formation. However, potassium-alkali therapy was superior to sodium-alkali therapy in attenuating the risk of calcium precipitation without raising urinary supersaturation of monosodium urate.[26]

ETIOLOGIC CAUSES: ACQUIRED, CONGENITAL AND IDIOPATHIC

Multiple etiologic mechanisms, including congenital,[12,18,28-41] are known to participate in UA stone formation (Fig. 23.4). However, idiopathic UA nephrolithiasis (IUAN), a pathogenically distinct entity with features of metabolic syndrome (MS), has been increasingly recognized as the most common cause of UA stone formation.

Pathophysiologic Mechanisms of UA Nephrolithiasis

The following significant urinary abnormalities have been described in patients with UA nephrolithiasis: low urine volume, hyperuricosuria and low urinary pH (Fig. 23.4). However, in IUAN patients, the most important and invariant feature is overly acidic urine that increases the urinary content of undissociated UA propensity for UA precipitation.[12,40-44.]

Low Urine Volume

Low urine volume is a recognized risk factor for kidney stone formation due to an increase in the urinary supersaturation of stone-forming salt.[42] This mechanism is in part important in the development of UA stones in inflammatory bowel diseases, including ulcerative colitis and Crohn's disease. Although in these conditions the majority of stones are calcium stones, and only one third of stones are composed of UA. A higher incidence of 8.5–10% is reported in a general population with UA nephrolithiasis.[33-35] Moreover, UA stones can commonly occur following ileostomy and comprise two thirds of all stones in this condition.[33] Low urinary volume and overly acidic urine have been commonly encountered in this population. Nonetheless, the underlying pathophysiologic mechanisms have not yet been fully explored.[36,37,43] Despite the high prevalence of low urinary pH, urinary UA excretion has been reported to be normal in this population.[39]

Hyperuricosuria

The underlying pathogenic mechanisms in the development of hyperuricosuria are genetic and/or acquired. In patients with primary gout, both dietary and genetic factors contribute to hyperuricemia and consequently hyperuricosuria.[44] In addition to hyperuricosuria, patients with primary gout have low urinary pH.[45] Early studies proposed that defective ammoniagenesis is responsible for abnormally low urine pH in patients with gout. Ammoniagenic defect was attributed to dysfunctional enzymatic metabolism with abnormalities in either glutaminase or glutamate dehydrogenase.[46,47] This scheme implied that defective conversion of glutamine to α-ketoglutarate is associated with impaired ammonium production but an increase in purine synthesis. The result of this study using radioactive tracer (^{15}N) glycine showed the role of diminished enzymatic activities in gout patients, but this was later disputed by investigators.[46,48,49] Since these studies, there have been no additional investigations exploring the potential role of enzymatic defects in this population. Despite a familial occurrence of approximately 30% in patients with primary gout, the molecular genetic basis has not yet been identified.[44,45]

Limited monogenic enzymatic abnormalities in purine metabolism demonstrate elevated UA production and ultimately a highly significant increase in serum UA concentration and UA excretion. Due to the highly significant increase in urinary acid excretion, more than two thirds of this population develops UA stones early in childhood or before the third decade of life.[50] The three established enzymatic disorders in UA metabolism include: (1) X-linked hypoxanthine guanine phosphoribosyltransferase deficiency (Lesch–Nyhan syndrome), (2) X-linked phosphoribosylpyrophosphate synthetase overactivity, and (3) autosomal recessive glucose-6-phosphate deficiency.[51] In Lesch–Nyhan syndrome, hematuria and crystalluria may be present in the first months of life, leading to kidney injury,[51] but its neurological complications may appear later during the first year of life.

Uric acid transporter URAT1 (encoded by SLC22A12) has been identified to have a major role in renal tubular UA reabsorption.[52,53] A genetic mutation localized in chromosomes 11q13 encoding URAT1 has been demonstrated to show evidence of hyperuricosuria, hypouricemia, increased UA kidney stone formation, and exercise in acute renal failure.[54,55] A protein product identified as zinc finger protein 365 (ZNF365) that has been localized in chromosome 10q21–q22 has been associated with UA nephrolithiasis in the population of Talana, a village in Sardinia.[55,56] To date, the function of this protein has not been fully explored. However, one significant finding was the presence of low urinary pH (5.55) in this population without significantly low urinary NH_4^+.[56]

Acquired Causes of Hyperuricosuria

An increased tissue breakdown occurs in numerous diseases, such as myeloproliferative disorders and hemolytic anemia. Additionally, chemotherapy may cause hyperuricemia and hyperuricosuria, and consequently increase the risk of development of secondary gout associated with recurrent UA stone and UA nephropathy.[57] Moreover, uricosuric medications, including high doses of salicylates, probenecid, radiocontrast agents, and losartan, have been shown to increase UA excretion and increase the risk of UA stone formation.[18,58]

Acidic Urinary pH

Clinical Basis

Idiopathic UA nephrolithiasis has been increasingly recognized as the most prevalent cause of UA stone cases.[40,41,59,60] In this population, the identifiable underlying key factor in the development of UA stones is low urinary pH.

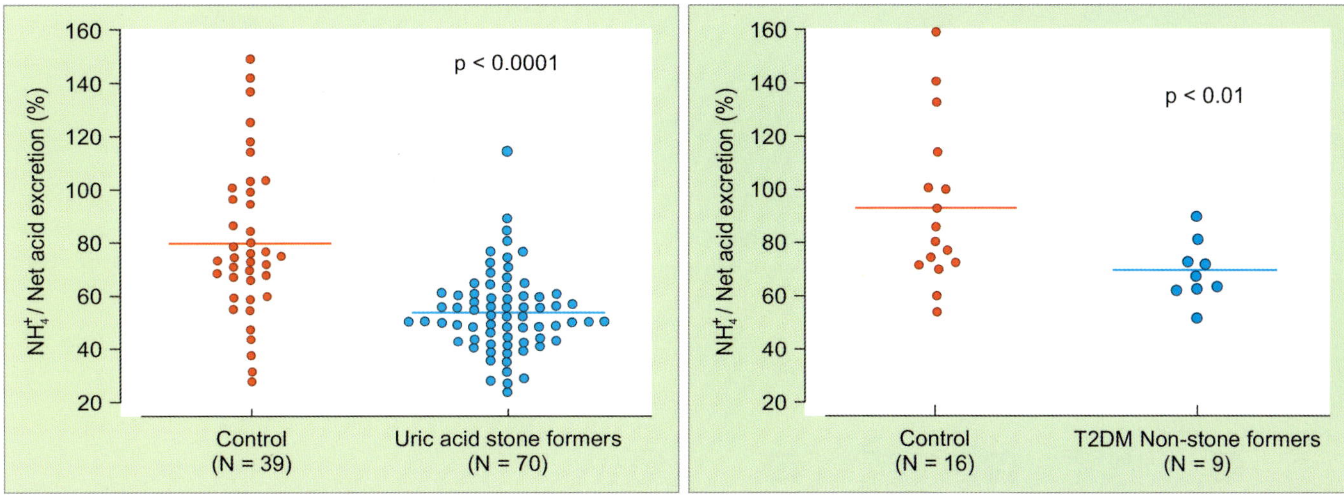

Fig. 23.9: NH_4^+ excretion in idiopathic uric acid nephrolithiasis and type 2 diabetes mellitus (T2DM) nonstone-formers under controlled metabolic diet.

Source: Redrawn with permission from Maalouf NM, Cameron MA, Moe OW, et al. Metabolic basis for low urine pH in type 2 diabetes. Clin J Am Soc Nephrol. 2010;5(7):1277-81.

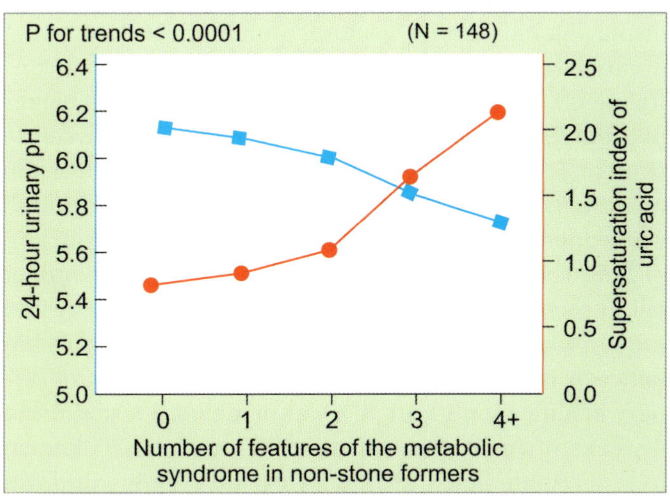

Fig. 23.10: Urinary pH and supersaturation index of uric acid and features of metabolic syndrome in normal nonstone-forming subjects.

Source: Adapted from Maalouf NM, Cameron MA, Moe OW, et al. Low urine pH: a novel feature of the metabolic syndrome. Clin J Am Soc Nephrol. 2007;2(5):883-8.

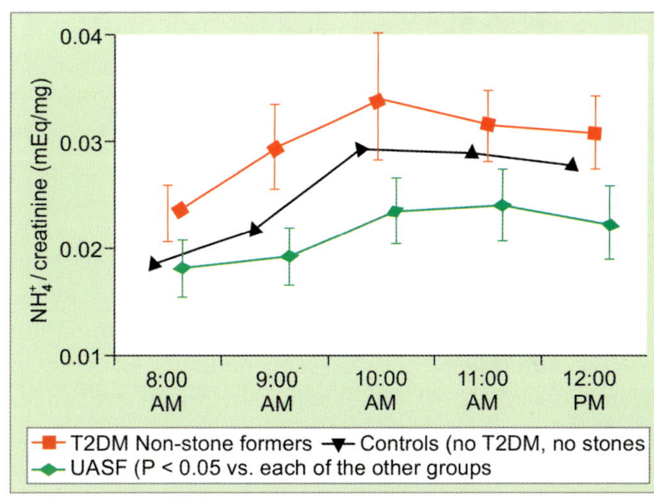

Fig. 23.11: NH_4^+ excretion after an acute acid load (50 mEq NH_4Cl at 8:00 AM) in body mass index-matched subjects. (UASF: Uric acid stone formers; T2DM: Type 2 diabetes mellitus).

has been shown on a fixed metabolic diet and on an ad-lib diet in IUAN, T2DM patients without kidney stones (Fig. 23.9). Additionally, it has been demonstrated that in normal subjects, urinary pH increases with increased features of the MS urinary supersaturation index UA increases (Fig. 23.10).[12,40,60-62,68] Although both T2DM and obesity are associated with low basal 24-hour urinary pH and increased risk of UA stones, IUAN patients were specifically shown to have a blunted renal NH_4^+ excretory response to acid challenges compared to normal subjects and those with T2DM without kidney stones[60] (Fig. 23.11). This magnitude difference in NH_4^+ excretory response may suggest that the same alteration may occur in the urinary environment in these patients after ingestion of meals rich in acid content, thereby predisposing them to UA precipitation and increasing the risk of UA stone formation. The selection of acute acid load using ammonium chloride instead of a large acid-producing meal was appropriate to

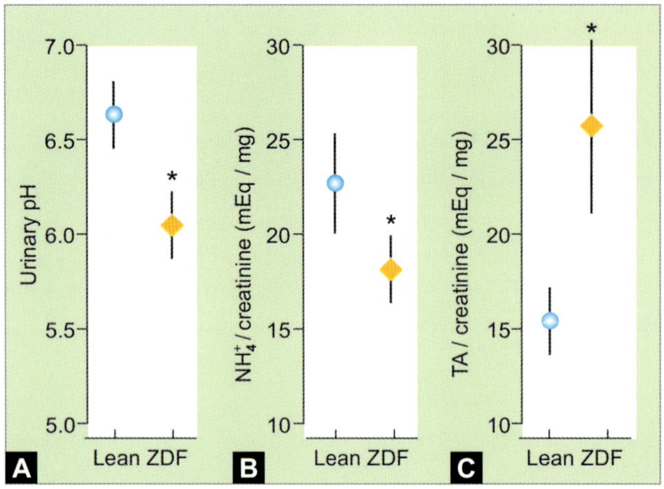

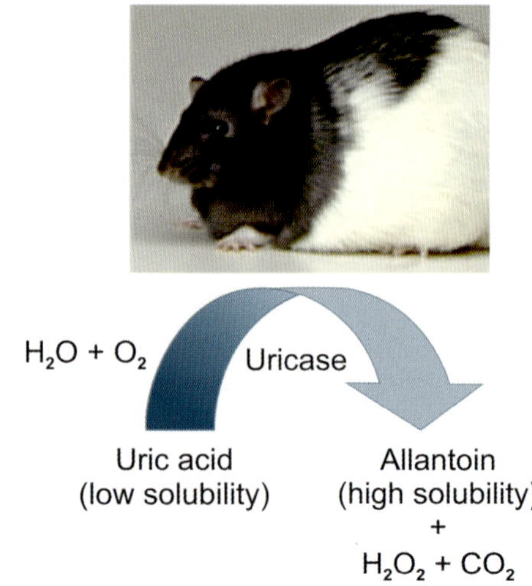

Figs. 23.12A to C: Urinary acidification defects in Zucher diabetic fatty (ZDF) rats. (A) Urinary pH, (B) urinary ammonium, (C) urinary titratable acidity (TA) in ZDF rat compared with lean control littermates $P < 0.05$.
Source: With permission from Bobulescu IA, Dubree M, Zhang J, et al. Effect of renal lipid accumulation on proximal tubule Na^+/H^+ exchange and ammonium secretion. Am J Physiol Renal Physiol. 2008;294(6):F1315-22.

uncover the acidification defect in IUAN subjects. Meals rich in acid load due to variability from individual alterations in digestion, absorption, and difference in insulin response to caloric load may pose potential experimental errors.

Role of Lipotoxicity

Renal production of NH_4^+occurs principally in the renal proximal tubular cell following the delivery of a major precursor, L-glutamine, by the process of deamination as NH_3 buffering protons are subsequently excreted in the urine as NH_4^+.[90-92] The sodium-hydrogen exchanger (NHE3) plays an important role in this process, acting both as Na^+/ NH_4^+ exchanger or by trapping diffused ammonium (NH_3) in the renal proximal tubular lumen.[93-96] In obesity, diabetes, and MS, there is a disequilibrium between caloric intake and caloric utilization. This imbalance process leads to fat redistribution to nonadipocyte tissues or "steatosis," and consequently to cellular tissue damage or "lipotoxicity."[77] Previous studies have supported that this mechanism is operative in cellular damage influencing myocardial cells, pancreatic β-cells, skeletal myocytes, and hepatocytes.[77-81,97] With increased plasma free fatty acid concentration and an increased filtered load of free fatty acid, the proximal renal tubular cells are specifically vulnerable to lipotoxicity.[84,98] The pathophysiologic link of renal lipotoxicity to the pathogenesis of impaired urinary acidification has been demonstrated in studies performed in Zucher diabetic fatty (ZDF) rats[99,100] (Figs. 23.12A to C),which are an established animal model displaying biochemical features similar to IUAN showing diminished urinary pH and NH_4^+ compared to lean control rats.[40,100,101] These changes were associated with higher plasma free fatty acid level and renal cortical triglyceride content (Figs. 23.13A to C).[100] In order to establish the direct effect of fat accumulation, a study was performed using opossum kidney cell lines incubating with a mixture of long-chain free fatty acid showing a dose-dependent fall in secretion of NH_4^+, expression of NHE3 activity and protein decrease.[100] Furthermore, the causal relationship between renal fat accumulation and impairment of urinary acidification in the ZDF rat model was tested using 4 weeks of treatment with thiazolidinediones,[102] known to redistribute lipids to adipocytes and thereby diminish nonadipose tissue lipotoxicity (Figs. 23.14A to C).[103,104] This treatment was associated with changes in urinary profiles comparable to lean control rats as well as a reduction in renal triglyceride accumulation.[102] To further establish the direct effects of fat, it was shown that in a cell culture model of proximal tubule steatosis and lipid toxicity, both can be reversed by fat removal but not by TZD alone.

Role of Substrate Competition

Under normal physiological circumstances, the kidney uses glutamine as a source of energy and produces NH_3.[90-92] However, the kidney may utilize a variety of metabolic substrates instead of glutamine to produce ATP through a mechanism called "substrate inhibition."[105-107] In a previous

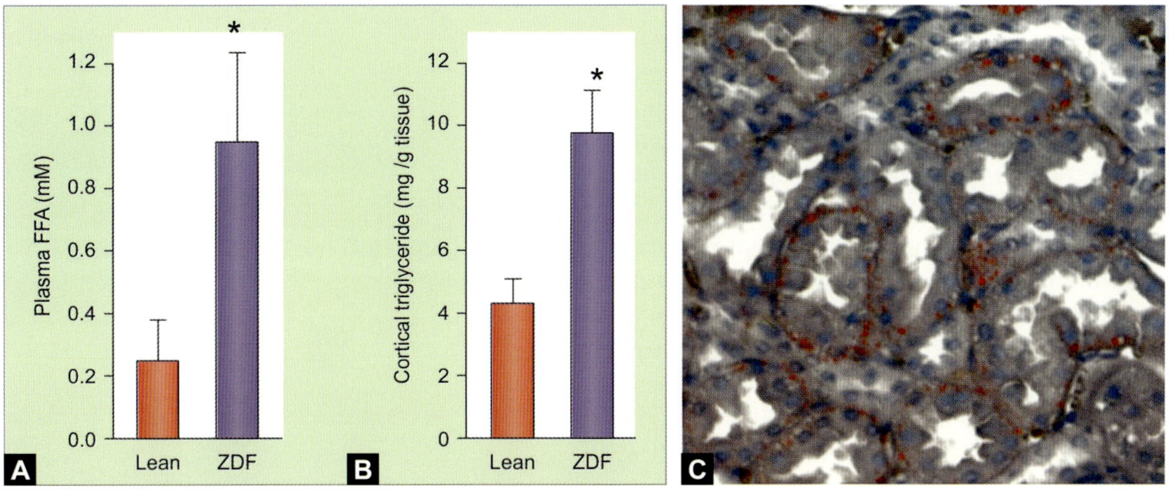

Figs. 23.13A to C: (A) Comparison of plasma free fatty acid (FFA) and (B) renal cortical triglyceride in Zucher diabetic fatty (ZDF) rats and lean control littermates. *$P < 0.001$, and (C) oil red O lipid staining of ZDF rat kidney cortex.
Source: With permission from Bobulescu IA, Dubree M, Zhang J, et al. Effect of renal lipid accumulation on proximal tubule Na^+/H^+ exchange and ammonium secretion. Am J Physiol Renal Physiol. 2008;294(6):F1315-22.

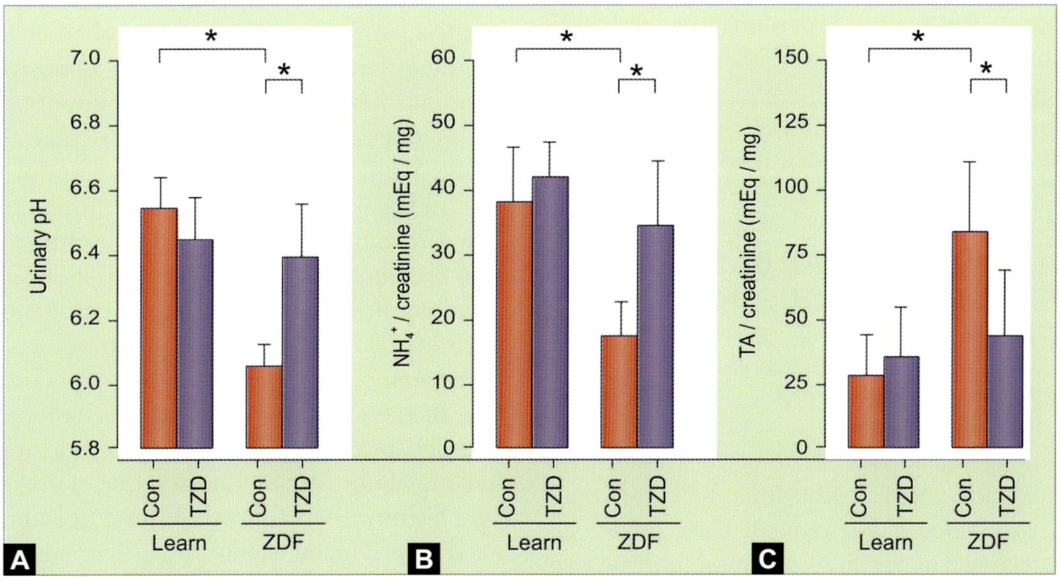

Figs. 23.14A to C: Thiazolidinedione (TZD) treatment in Zucher diabetic fatty (ZDF) rats and lean littermates: (A) urinary pH, (B) urinary ammonium, (C) urinary titratable acidity (TA); * $P < 0.05$. Con, controls.
Source: With permission from Bobulescu IA, Dubree M, Zhang J, et al. Reduction of renal triglyceride accumulation: effects on proximal tubule Na+/H+ exchange and urinary acidification. Am J Physiol Renal Physiol. 2009;297(5):F1419-26.

in vivo study in female mongrel dogs as well as an *in vitro* study using kidney cortical slices, it was demonstrated that addition of fatty acids, including octanoate or palmitate, may interfere with ammoniagenesis and glucose production during metabolic acidosis caused by ammonium chloride[108] since fatty acids are a significant nutritional supply for the kidney.[109-111]

It is anticipated but not yet fully elucidated that with an increased level of plasma free fatty acids as occurs in obesity, T2DM, MS, and IUAN, the proximal renal tubule will potentially utilize free fatty acid over glutamine via the process of "substrate inhibition," thereby reducing NH_3 synthesis, which buffers protons and limits NH_4^+ excretion in the urine.[112-114]

Role of Insulin

There are limited data regarding the role of insulin in the kidney beyond glucose metabolism.[115] Insulin receptors are expressed in various segments of the kidney. In two in vitro studies, it was demonstrated that insulin stimulates renal ammoniagenesis in renal tubular cells from L-glutamine.[112,113] It has also been shown that insulin stimulates the proximal tubular NHE3, which plays a significant role in either direct transport or ionic trapping of NH_4^+ in the proximal tubular lumen.[114,116-120] The causal role of peripheral insulin resistance and its association with defective ammonium excretion and low urinary pH has been supported in only one study in human subjects with IUAN using hyperinsulinemic euglycemic clamps.[101] In this study, 55 healthy nonstone formers with a various range of BMI and 13 patients with IUAN underwent hyperinsulinemic euglycemic clamp procedures. Patients with IUAN were found to be significantly insulin resistant and had lower urinary pH compared to normal nonstone-forming subjects. Moreover, IUAN subjects demonstrated a significantly low urinary pH for the degree of insulin resistance. This result suggested that in IUAN patients, there may be unidentified mechanisms responsible for abnormally acidic pH, which is not totally accounted for by insulin resistance.

CLINICAL AND CELLULAR BASIS OF INCREASED ENDOGENOUS ACID PRODUCTION

Another important pathophysiologic mechanism in development of abnormally acid urine in IUAN and obese nonstone-forming subjects has been demonstrated to be increased endogenous acid production.[40,41,60-62] Since all these studies were conducted under a fixed metabolic diet and in a steady state, an increased NAE in these two populations is suggestive of increased endogenous acid production (Fig. 23.15). In addition, NAE for any given urinary sulfate (a surrogate marker of acid intake) tends to be higher in obese and T2DM nonstone-forming subjects.[12,61,68] Supporting evidence for these findings in clinical studies has demonstrated a correlation between increased organic acid excretion, higher body weight, and higher body surface area.[121,122]

At the present time, the source and nature of these putative acid anions have not been fully explored. One potential underlying mechanism may be through an increase in organic acid production by intestinal micro-

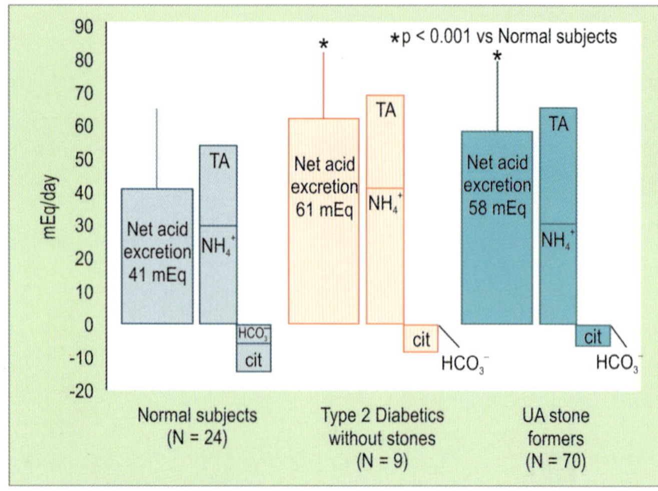

Fig. 23.15: Net acid excretion (NAE) under fixed metabolic diet. (TA: Titratable acidity; Cit: Citrate; NAE = NH_4 + TA- (HCO_3^-+ Cit); NSF: Nonstone formers).

flora mediated by anaerobic metabolism.[123-125] The human intestine contains trillions of microbial cells that constitute the gut microbiota. Alterations in normal gut microbiota have been shown to play an important pathogenic role in obesity, T2DM,[126] cardiovascular disease[127] and chronic kidney disease.[128,129] In one unpublished preliminary study conducted in IUAN and normal subjects under a fixed metabolic diet, increased production of key bacterial metabolites in UA stone formers was shown using metabolomics data using gas chromatography-mass spectrometric analysis. These preliminary results demonstrated an increased amount of bacterial metabolites in UA stone formers. These metabolites include microbial products such as 3-hydroxy-3-methyglutarate, which is a principal metabolite of butyrate and one of the main products of gut bacteria. Pyruvate results from hepatic conversion of bacterial-produced lactate and 4-hydroxyphenylacetate, a key bacterial metabolite of tyrosine in IUAN stone formers more than nonstone-formers.

DIAGNOSIS

General Aspects

The initial step in the diagnosis of UA stone is stone analysis. If a stone composition is documented, one of them should exclude the acquired causes of UA nephrolithiasis including intestinal diseases associated with diarrheal state, heavy physical exercise, increased animal protein consumption, myeloproliferative disorders, cancer chemotherapy, and the use of uricosuric medications (*see* Fig. 23.4).[32-39] Commonly, patients with a hereditary enzymatic UA pathway mutation present with robust hyperuricemia (serum urine acid >10 mg/dL), hyperuricosuria (>1,000 mg/day), high stone burden, and renal failure.[50,51,130] The disease presentation commonly occurs in early childhood and very rarely in early adulthood. The association of hypouricemia, hyperuricosuria, increased risk of kidney stones, and exercise-induced acute kidney injury may indicate a genetic mutation in the URAT1 transporter.[54,131]

A full metabolic evaluation including 24-hour urine profiles should include total volume, pH determined by electrode, creatinine, sodium, potassium, calcium, magnesium, oxalate, citrate, sulfate, and chloride. This metabolic evaluation will distinguish between the contributions of dietary and metabolic abnormalities. Urinary sulfate is a marker of consumption of an acid-ash diet found in meat and meat products known to significantly lower urinary pH and increase urinary UA with increased purine levels.[132] Urinary biochemical profiles will also allow determination of net gastrointestinal alkali absorption, showing contribution of dietary alkali compared to dietary acid. The assessment of urinary NH_4^+ is optional due to its instability in urine, which is not collected under mineral oil and could be utilized to assess adequacy of alkali treatment. Commonly a 50% reduction in urinary NH_4^+ suggests sufficient alkali treatment. Additionally, CT examination is required to monitor stone burden.

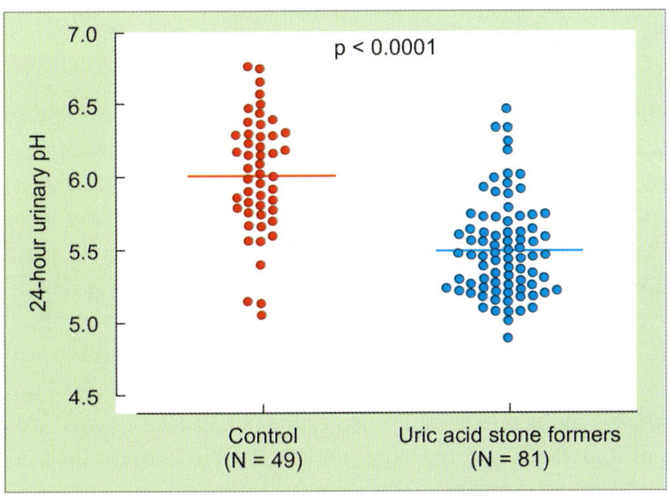

Fig. 23.16: 24-hour urinary pH in IUAN versus control under fixed metabolic diet.

Differential Diagnosis

Urinary pH is the most distinctive diagnostic test to distinguish between hyperuricosuric calcium stone formers and IUAN stone formers,[133] since an abnormally low urinary pH ≤5.5 is an invariable feature of IUAN (Fig. 23.16).[40,41,59] Urinary pH >5.5 in conjunction with hyperuricosuria commonly occurs in hyperuricosuric calcium stone formers[24,134] (Table 23.1). Ammonium urate stones are radiolucent and comprise a very small fraction of stones in the Western world.[135] This stone is encountered in those with diarrheal conditions due to inflammatory bowel disease, following ileostomy and with laxative abuse.[136] The pathogenesis of these stones is related to an increased abundance of urinary NH_4^+ associated with significantly low urinary sodium and potassium, making the urine supersaturated with respect to highly insoluble ammonium urate.[25]

Table 23.1: Differential diagnosis of UA stones.

		Urinary findings					
Stone type	*Radiographic findings*	*pH*	*UA*	*FE uric acid*	*Calcium*	*Serum UA findings*	*Response to alkali therapy*
UA stones	Radiolucent	≤5.5	Normal	Decreased	Normal	Increased	Positive
Ammonium urate stones	Radiolucent	Variable	Normal	Normal	Normal	Normal	Unknown
Hyperuricosuric calcium stones		Normal to or ≥5.5	Increased	Normal	Normal to Increased	Radiopaque	Positive
Mixed UA/ calcium oxalate stones	Mixed Radiolucent Radiopaque	Normal to or ≤5.5	Normal	Normal	Normal	Normal	Positive
2,8-DHA stones	Radiolucent	Normal	Normal	Normal	Normal	Normal	Negative
Xanthine stones	Radiolucent	Normal	Decreased	Normal	Normal	Decreased	Negative

(UA: Uric acid; FE: Fractional excretion; 2,8-DHA: 2,8-dihydroxyadenine).

On rare occasions, other radiolucent kidney stones should be ruled out. 2,8-dihydroxyadenine (DHA) and xanthine stones are rare causes of radiolucent stones. 2,8-dihydroxyadenine stones are caused by excessive urinary excretion of DHA as a result of a deficiency of adenine phosphoribosyltransferase deficiency (APRT), an inherited autosomal recessive disorder.[137] 2,8-dihydroxyadenine, which is significantly insoluble in the urinary environment, is responsible for crystal aggregation and kidney stone formation.[138,139] This diagnosis can be made by the microscopic appearance of round DHA crystals in the urine (central maltese cross pattern). The definitive diagnosis is made by the absence of APRT enzyme activity in red cells[137] (Table 23.1).

Xanthine stones occur as the result of an inherited autosomal recessive trait involving mutation in the gene encoding xanthine, dehydrogenase, leading to significant production of excessive excretion of xanthine in the urine and ultimately xanthine stones and hypouricemia.[137] Xanthinuria is suspected by a significant degree of hypouricemia and hypouricosuria.

TREATMENT APPROACH

Physicochemical Basis of Alkali Treatment

Low urinary pH is the most invariable feature in IUAN.[26,40,41,59,60,62] However, normal uricosuria and low fractional urinary acid excretion have been studied under both constant metabolic diet and ad lib diet.[26,27,40,59,60,62] These studies underpin the dominant role of the lower urinary pH in the development of UA stones.

At low urinary pH, ranging from 4.4 to 5.5, a total UA concentration (consisting of undissociated + urate) of 110–200 mg/L is needed to exceed the limited solubility of approximately 96 mg/L. However, at a normal urinary pH of 6.2–6.4, the total UA concentration should exceed 1,100 mg/L to initiate precipitation (Fig. 23.3). Under normal physiological circumstances, such a wide variation in urinary UA excretion is not anticipated. However, urinary pH changes and variations between 4.6 and 6.6 in human subjects are not unlikely. These physicochemical features have an important clinical implication in the treatment of patients with UA nephrolithiasis.

The effectiveness of alkali treatment in reducing UA stone incidence in a large randomized, placebo-controlled study is lacking. However, in one open-ended trial that included 18 patients with UA nephrolithiasis, six patients with pure UA stones and 12 with mixed UA and/or

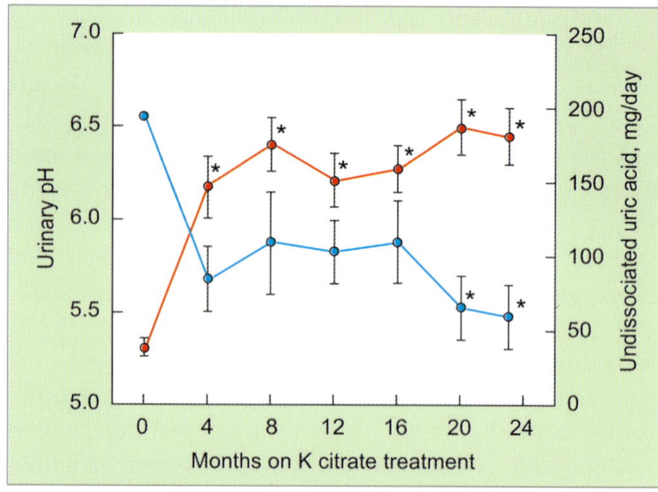

Fig. 23.17: Changes in urinary pH and urinary undissociated uric acid content with long-term potassium citrate. (K: Citrate treatment; *: $P < 0.05$)

calcium oxalate stones subjects were treated for a mean of 2.7–8 years with potassium alkali doses of approximately 60 mEq/day. A rise in urinary pH and significant fall in urinary content of undissociated UA (Fig. 23.17) was associated with a significant decline in stone incidence from 1.20 ± 1.68 stones per year to 0.01 ± 0.04 stones per year.[27] Another study explored this treatment with sodium alkali in a limited number of patients with pure UA stones and associated this treatment with stone transformation from UA to calcium oxalate and calcium phosphate stones. This clinical finding was expected since the metabolic balance study compared the effects of potassium citrate and sodium citrate treatment in UA stone formers, and demonstrated that both alkali therapies significantly increase urinary pH. However, potassium alkali treatment lowered urinary calcium significantly, thereby lowering the risk for calcium stone formation[26] (Table 23.2). It has been shown that UA solubility in the urine is affected by ambient cation concentration.[24] The thermodynamic solubility product of sodium urate at 2.79×10^{-5} M^2 was found to be 3.5-fold lower than potassium urate at 9.63×10^{-5} M^2.[24,140] The monosodium urate has been shown to participate in calcium oxalate crystallization, but its physicochemical basis has not been fully agreed upon.[141-144]

Clinical Basis of Alkali Treatment

On the basis of the aforementioned, physicochemical potassium alkali therapy is used commonly in the treatment of UA nephrolithiasis. The common alkali treatment dosage ranges from 30 to 60 mEq/day. This selection is

Table 23.2: Comparison of potassium alkali treatment versus sodium alkali treatment in UA nephrolithiasis.

	Potassium alkali	*Sodium alkali*
Urinary pH	↑	↑
Urinary citrate	↑	↑
Urinary calcium	↓	↑ ↔
Inhibitory effect against CaOx	↑↑	↑ ↔
Prevention of UA stones	↑↑	↑↑
Prevention of calcium stones	↑↑	↑

(UA: Uric acid; CaOx: Calcium oxalate. ↑: Increased; ↑↑: Highly significant increase; ↓: Decreased; ↔: Normal/no change).

based on the principle that optimal intake of protein (acid-ash diet) in the population is 0.8 g/kg body weight per day. Since approximately 1 mEq of proton is produced by 1 g of dietary protein, this amount of alkali will be sufficient to neutralize acid load introduced by protein. Furthermore, the metabolic study has shown this amount of alkali to be sufficient to raise urinary pH from 5.30 to a normal value of 6.19–6.46, lower urinary content of undissociated UA to normal range (64–108 mg/day) (*see* Fig. 23.17),[27] and reduce stone incidence. The diurnal variation in urinary acidification has been demonstrated to be different among normal individuals and UA stone formers.[62] Although both normal and UA stone formers showed significant variation in urinary pH throughout the day, the urinary pH remained significantly lowered in UA stone formers compared to normal subjects. In both populations, urinary pH increased in the morning, peaked at noon, fell after lunch, rose again in the afternoon, and fell again after an evening meal. However, during the night, urinary pH decreased at 6 AM before rising again in the morning. Therefore, it is prudent to suggest that a single dose of alkali treatment be given at bedtime to overcome abnormal acidic urine during the night and potentially reduce the propensity for UA precipitation.[145] In rare instances, carbonic anhydrase inhibitors (Diamox) have been used as an alternative alkalinizing agent. This treatment must be used carefully since metabolic acidosis can be encountered with this agent by producing significant hypocitraturia, and highly alkaline urine poses the potential risk for the development of calcium phosphate stones.[146,147] Alkali treatment has been used in patients with inflammatory bowel disease since UA stones comprise two thirds of stones in this population,[33,34,36] with abnormally acidic urine pH (<5.5) highly prevalent.[36,37,39,43]

Treatment with Hypouricosuric Agents

The two hypouricosuric agents available for the treatment of hyperuricosuric conditions are allopurinol and febuxostat. Treatment with a hypouricosuric agent is necessary in those with monogenic enzymatic disorders in purine metabolism, of whom more than two-thirds were demonstrated to have UA stones before the third decade of life.[50] The primary treatment tested in these disorders today is allopurinol, which has been shown to improve and stabilize renal function. In these genetic disorders, alkalization of the urine is not indicated, since impaired urinary acidification has not been reported. Treatment with a hypouricosuric agent may be necessary in patients with primary gout since the disposition is directly proportional to the amount of urinary acid excretion in addition to low urinary pH.[44,45]

In those with evidence of an increased tissue turnover, including myeloproliferative disorders and hemolytic anemia, significant hyperuricemia and hyperuricosuria may ensue from increased tissue breakdown.[57] In these subjects, secondary gout is prevalent and associated with recurrent UA stones and UA nephropathy, with consequent significant mobility and mortality. Treatment with allopurinol has been shown to be effective in such populations, and in one study this treatment aborted new kidney stone formation.[57]

ACKNOWLEDGMENTS

The author is supported by NIH R01-DK081423 and by the Office of Naval Research N000141110203 grants. He would like to acknowledge Valeria Rodela and Ashlei Johnson for their role in the preparation of this chapter.

REFERENCES

1. Frank M, Atsmon A, Sugar P, et al. Epidemiological investigation of urolithiasis in the hot arid Southern region of Israel. Urologia Int. 1963;15:65-76.
2. Hesse A, Schneider HJ, Berg W, et al. Uric acid dihydrate as urinary calculus component. Invest Urol. 1975;12(5):405-9.
3. Rafique M, Bhutta RA, Rauf A, et al. Chemical composition of upper renal tract calculi in Multan. J Pak Med Assoc. 2000;50(5):145-8.
4. Herbstein FH, Kleeberg J, Shalitin Y, et al. Chemical and X-ray diffraction analysis of urinary stones in Israel. Isr J Med Sci. 1974;10(12):1493-9.
5. Hossain RZ, Ogawa Y, Hokama S, et al. Urolithiasis in Okinawa, Japan: a relatively high prevalence of uric acid stones. Int J Urol. 2003;10(8):411-5.
6. Sakhaee K. Uric acid metabolism and uric acid stones. In: Rao NP PG, Kavanaugh J, (eds). Urinary Tract Stone Disease.

London: BC Decker Publishing, Springer-Verlag; 2011. pp. 185-93.
7. Portis AJ, Hermans K, Culhane-Pera KA, et al. Stone disease in the Hmong of Minnesota: initial description of a high-risk population. J Endourol. 2004;18(9):853-7.
8. Portis AJ, Laliberte M, Tatman P, et al. High prevalence of gouty arthritis among the Hmong population in Minnesota. Arthritis Care Res. 2010;62(10):1386-91.
9. Prasongwatana V, Sriboonlue P, Suntarapa S. Urinary stone composition in North-East Thailand. Br J Urol. 1983;55(4):353-5
10. Pak CY, Sakhaee K, Moe O, et al. Biochemical profile of stone-forming patients with diabetes mellitus. Urology. 2003;61(3):523-7.
11. Daudon M, Lacour B, Jungers P. High prevalence of uric acid calculi in diabetic stone formers. Nephrol Dial Transplant. 2005;20(2):468-9.
12. Cameron MA, Maalouf NM, Adams-Huet B, et al. Urine composition in type 2 diabetes: predisposition to uric acid nephrolithiasis. J Am Soc Nephrol. 2006;17(5):1422-8.
13. Lieske JC, de la Vega LS, Gettman MT, et al. Diabetes mellitus and the risk of urinary tract stones: a population-based case-control study. Am J Kidney Dis. 2006;48(6):897-904.
14. Ekeruo WO, Tan YH, Young MD, et al. Metabolic risk factors and the impact of medical therapy on the management of nephrolithiasis in obese patients. J Urol. 2004;172(1):159-63.
15. Daudon M, Lacour B, Jungers P. Influence of body size on urinary stone composition in men and women. Urol Res. 2006;34(3):193-9.
16. Daudon M, Traxer O, Conort P, et al. Type 2 diabetes increases the risk for uric acid stones. J Am Soc Nephrol. 2006;17(7):2026-33.
17. Bobulescu IA, Moe OW. Renal transport of uric acid: evolving concepts and uncertainties. Adv Chronic Kidney Dis. 2012;19(6):358-71.
18. Maalouf NM, Cameron MA, Moe OW, et al. Novel insights into the pathogenesis of uric acid nephrolithiasis. Curr Opin Nephrol Hypertens. 2004;13(2):181-9.
19. Asplin JR. Uric acid stones. Semin Nephrol. 1996;16(5):412-24.
20. Finlayson AJ. Stability of first dissociable proton of uric acid. J Chem Eng Data. 1974;19(1):94-7.
21. Riese RJ, Sakhaee K. Uric acid nephrolithiasis: pathogenesis and treatment. J Urol. 1992;148(3):765-71.
22. Koka RM, Huang E, Lieske JC. Adhesion of uric acid crystals to the surface of renal epithelial cells. Am J Physiol Renal Physiol. 2000;278(6):F989-98.
23. Wilcox WR, Khalaf A, Weinberger A, et al. Solubility of uric acid and monosodium urate. Med Biol Eng. 1972;10(4): 522-31.
24. Pak CY, Waters O, Arnold L, et al. Mechanism for calcium urolithiasis among patients with hyperuricosuria: supersaturation of urine with respect to monosodium urate. J Clin Invest. 1977;59(3):426-31.
25. Pak C, Britton F, Peterson R, et al. Assessment of pathogenic role of uric acid, monopotassium urate, monoammonium urate, monosodium urate in hyperuricosuric calcium, nephrolithiasis. Miner Electrolyte Metab. 1980;4(3):130-6.
26. Sakhaee K, Nicar M, Hill K, et al. Contrasting effects of potassium citrate and sodium citrate therapies on urinary chemistries and crystallization of stone-forming salts. Kidney Int. 1983;24(3):348-52.
27. Pak CY, Sakhaee K, Fuller C. Successful management of uric acid nephrolithiasis with potassium citrate. Kidney Int. 1986;30(3):422-8.
28. Lai CM, Lai YK, Rakoczy PE. Adenovirus and adeno-associated virus vectors. DNA Cell Biol. 2002;21(12):895-913.
29. Sakhaee K. Uric acid metabolism and uric acid stones. In: Rao NP, Preminger G, Kavanaugh J (Eds). Urinary Tract Stone Disease. BC Decker Publishing, Springer-Verlag. London, UK. Ch 15. 2011.
30. Sakhaee K. Medical management: Uric acid and cystine stones. In: Rao NP, Preminger G, Kavanaugh J (Eds). Urinary Tract Stone Disease. BC Decker Publishing, Springer-Verlag. London, UK. 2011. pp 673-80.
31. Sakhaee K. Uric acid nephrolithiasis: Uric acid or urine pH?. In: Pearle MS, Nakada SY (Eds). Practical Controversies in Medical Management of Stone Disease. Springer Publishing, Springer Science + Business Media. New York, NY. 2014. pp 91-103.
32. Grossman MS, Nugent FW. Urolithiasis as a complication of chronic diarrheal disease. Am J Dig Dis. 1967;12(5):491-8.
33. Deren JJ, Porush JG, Levitt MF, et al. Nephrolithiasis as a complication of ulcerative colitis and regional enteritis. Ann Int Med. 1962;56:843-53.
34. Gelzayd EA, Breuer RI, Kirsner JB. Nephrolithiasis in inflammatory bowel disease. Am J Dig Dis. 1968;13(12):1027-34.
35. Knudsen L, Marcussen H, Fleckenstein P, et al. Urolithiasis in chronic inflammatory bowel disease. Scand J Gastroenterol. 1978;13(4):433-6.
36. Bambach CP, Robertson WG, Peacock M, et al. Effect of intestinal surgery on the risk of urinary stone formation. Gut. 1981;22(4):257-63.
37. Fukushima T, Yamazaki Y, Sugita A, et al. Prophylaxis of uric acid stone in patients with inflammatory bowel disease following extensive colonic resection. Gastroenterol Jpn. 1991;26(4):430-4.
38. Fixed-dose antibiotic combinations. Lancet. 1969;2(7616):365-6.
39. Obialo CI, Clayman RV, Matts JP, et al. Pathogenesis of nephrolithiasis post-partial ileal bypass surgery: case-control study. The POSCH Group. Kidney Int. 1991;39(6):1249-54.
40. Sakhaee K, Adams-Huet B, Moe OW, et al. Pathophysiologic basis for normouricosuric uric acid nephrolithiasis. Kidney Int. 2002;62(3):971-9.
41. Sakhaee K. Recent advances in the pathophysiology of nephrolithiasis. Kidney Int. 2009;75(6):585-95.
42. Pak CY, Skurla C, Harvey J. Graphic display of urinary risk factors for renal stone formation. J Urol. 1985;134(5):867-70.
43. Clarke AM, McKenzie RG. Ileostomy and the risk of urinary uric acid stones. Lancet. 1969;2(7617):395-7.
44. Yu T, Gutman AB. Uric acid nephrolithiasis in gout. Predisposing factors. Ann Int Med. 1967;67(6):1133-48.

45. Gutman AB, Yu TF. Uric acid nephrolithiasis. Am J Med. 1968;45(5):756-79.
46. Gutman AB, Yue TF. An abnormality of glutamine metabolism in primary gout. Am J Med. 1963;35:820-31.
47. Pagliara AS, Goodman AD. Elevation of plasma glutamate in gout. Its possible role in the pathogenesis of hyperuricemia. New Engl J Med. 1969;281(14):767-70.
48. Pollak VE, Mattenheimer H. Glutaminase activity in the kidney in gout. J Lab Clin Med. 1965;66(4):564-70.
49. Sperling O, Wyngaarden JB, Starmer CF. The kinetics of intramolecular distribution of 15N in uric acid after administration of (15N) glycine. A reappraisal of the significance of preferential labeling of N-(3+9) of uric acid in primary gout. J Clin Invest. 1973;52(10):2468-85.
50. Stanbury JB, Wyngaarden JB, Fredrickson DS (Eds). The Metabolic Basis of Inherited Disease, 3rd edition. McGraw-Hill, New York. 1778 pp. 1972.
51. Roche A, Perez-Duenas B, Camacho JA, et al. Efficacy of rasburicase in hyperuricemia secondary to Lesch-Nyhan syndrome. Am J Kidney Dis. 2009;53(4):677-80.
52. Enomoto A, Kimura H, Chairoungdua A, et al. Molecular identification of a renal urate anion exchanger that regulates blood urate levels. Nature. 2002;417(6887):447-52.
53. Hediger MA, Johnson RJ, Miyazaki H, et al. Molecular physiology of urate transport. Physiology. 2005;20:125-33.
54. Ichida K, Hosoyamada M, Hisatome I, et al. Clinical and molecular analysis of patients with renal hypouricemia in Japan-influence of URAT1 gene on urinary urate excretion. J Am Soc Nephrol. 2004;15(1):164-73.
55. Gianfrancesco F, Esposito T, Ombra MN, et al. Identification of a novel gene and a common variant associated with uric acid nephrolithiasis in a Sardinian genetic isolate. Am J Human Genet. 2003;72(6):1479-91.
56. Ombra MN, Forabosco P, Casula S, et al. Identification of a new candidate locus for uric acid nephrolithiasis. Am J Human Genet. 2001;68(5):1119-29.
57. Yu T, Weinreb N, Wittman R, et al. Secondary gout associated with chronic myeloproliferative disorders. Semin Arthritis Rheum. 1976;5(3):247-56.
58. Shahinfar S, Simpson RL, Carides AD, et al. Safety of losartan in hypertensive patients with thiazide-induced hyperuricemia. Kidney Int. 1999;56(5):1879-85.
59. Pak CY, Sakhaee K, Peterson RD, et al. Biochemical profile of idiopathic uric acid nephrolithiasis. Kidney Int. 2001;60(2):757-61.
60. Bobulescu IA, Maalouf NM, Capolongo G, et al. Renal ammonium excretion after an acute acid load: blunted response in uric acid stone formers but not in patients with type 2 diabetes. Am J Physiol Renal Physiol. 2013;305(10):F1498-503.
61. Maalouf NM, Cameron MA, Moe OW, et al. Metabolic basis for low urine pH in type 2 diabetes. Clin J Am Soc Nephrol. 2010;5(7):1277-81.
62. Cameron M, Maalouf NM, Poindexter J, et al. The diurnal variation in urine acidification differs between normal individuals and uric acid stone formers. Kidney Int. 2012;81(11): 1123-30.
63. Vega GL, Adams-Huet B, Peshock R, et al. Influence of body fat content and distribution on variation in metabolic risk. J Clin Endocrinol Metab. 2006;91(11):4459-66.
64. Larsson B, Bengtsson C, Bjorntorp P, et al. Is abdominal body fat distribution a major explanation for the sex difference in the incidence of myocardial infarction? The study of men born in 1913 and the study of women, Goteborg, Sweden. Am J Epidemiol. 1992;135(3):266-73.
65. Kissebah AH, Vydelingum N, Murray R, et al. Relation of body fat distribution to metabolic complications of obesity. J Clin Endocrinol Metab. 1982;54(2):254-60.
66. Pigna F, Sakhaee K, Adams-Huet B, et al. Body fat content and distribution and urinary risk factors for nephrolithiasis. Clin J Am Soc Nephrol. 2014;9(1):159-65.
67. Taylor EN, Curhan GC. Body size and 24-hour urine composition. Am J Kidney Dis. 2006;48(6):905-15.
68. Maalouf NM, Cameron MA, Moe OW, et al. Low urine pH: a novel feature of the metabolic syndrome. Clin J Am Soc Nephrol. 2007;2(5):883-8.
69. Sakhaee K, Capolongo G, Maalouf NM, et al. Metabolic syndrome and the risk of calcium stones. Nephrol Dial Transplant. 2012;27(8):3201-9.
70. Sinha R, Dufour S, Petersen KF, et al. Assessment of skeletal muscle triglyceride content by (1)H nuclear magnetic resonance spectroscopy in lean and obese adolescents: relationships to insulin sensitivity, total body fat, and central adiposity. Diabetes. 2002;51(4):1022-7.
71. Thomas EL, Hamilton G, Patel N, et al. Hepatic triglyceride content and its relation to body adiposity: a magnetic resonance imaging and proton magnetic resonance spectroscopy study. Gut. 2005;54(1):122-7.
72. Lingvay I, Esser V, Legendre JL, et al. Noninvasive quantification of pancreatic fat in humans. J Clin Endocrinol Metab. 2009;94(10):4070-6.
73. Unger RH, Clark GO, Scherer PE, et al. Lipid homeostasis, lipotoxicity and the metabolic syndrome. Biochim Biophys Acta. 2010;1801(3):209-14.
74. Wende AR, Abel ED. Lipotoxicity in the heart. Biochim Biophys Acta. 2010;1801(3):311-9.
75. Muoio DM. Intramuscular triacylglycerol and insulin resistance: guilty as charged or wrongly accused? Biochim Biophys Acta. 2010;1801(3):281-8.
76. Suganami T, Tanaka M, Ogawa Y. Adipose tissue inflammation and ectopic lipid accumulation. Endocrine J. 2012;59(10):849-57.
77. Lee Y, Hirose H, Ohneda M, et al. Beta-cell lipotoxicity in the pathogenesis of non-insulin-dependent diabetes mellitus of obese rats: impairment in adipocyte-beta-cell relationships. Proc Natl Acad Sci USA. 1994;91(23):10878-82.
78. Szczepaniak LS, Nurenberg P, Leonard D, et al. Magnetic resonance spectroscopy to measure hepatic triglyceride content: prevalence of hepatic steatosis in the general population. Am J Physiol Endocrinol Metab. 2005;288(2):E462-8.
79. Bachmann OP, Dahl DB, Brechtel K, et al. Effects of intravenous and dietary lipid challenge on intramyocellular lipid content and the relation with insulin sensitivity in humans. Diabetes. 2001;50(11):2579-84.

80. McGavock JM, Victor RG, Unger RH, et al. The American Physiological S. Adiposity of the heart, revisited. Ann Int Med. 2006;144(7):517-24.
81. Szczepaniak LS, Dobbins RL, Metzger GJ, et al. Myocardial triglycerides and systolic function in humans: in vivo evaluation by localized proton spectroscopy and cardiac imaging. Magn Reson Med. 2003;49(3):417-23.
82. McGarry JD. Banting lecture 2001: dysregulation of fatty acid metabolism in the etiology of type 2 diabetes. Diabetes. 2002;51(1):7-18.
83. Schaffer JE. Lipotoxicity: when tissues overeat. Curr Opin Lipidol. 2003;14(3):281-7.
84. Weinberg JM. Lipotoxicity. Kidney Int. 2006;70(9):1560-6.
85. Browning JD, Szczepaniak LS, Dobbins R, et al. Prevalence of hepatic steatosis in an urban population in the United States: impact of ethnicity. Hepatology. 2004;40(6):1387-95.
86. Bobulescu IA. Renal lipid metabolism and lipotoxicity. Current opinion in nephrology and hypertension. 2010;19(4):393-402.
87. Bobulescu IA, Lotan Y, Sakhaee K et al. Triglycerides in the human kidney cortex: Relationship with body size. PLoS ONE.2014;9(8):e101285. doi: 10.1371/journal.pone.0101285.
88. Niv Y. Pentagastrin-induced urinary alkaline tide—a repeatable phenomenon that is abolished after vagotomy. Isr J Med Sci. 1992;28(2):97-8.
89. DuBose TD Jr, Good DW, Hamm LL, et al. Ammonium transport in the kidney: new physiological concepts and their clinical implications. J Am Soc Nephrol. 1991;1(11):1193-203.
90. Atkinson DE, Camien MN. The role or urea synthesis in the removal of metabolic bicarbonate and the regulation of blood pH. Curr Top Cell Regul. 1982;21:261-302.
91. Halperin ML, Jungas RL. Metabolic production and renal disposal of hydrogen ions. Kidney Int. 1983;24(6):709-13.
92. Vinay P, Lemieux G, Gougoux A, et al. Regulation of glutamine metabolism in dog kidney in vivo. Kidney Int. 1986;29(1): 68-79.
93. Bobulescu IA, Di Sole F, Moe OW. Na^+/H^+ exchangers: physiology and link to hypertension and organ ischemia. Curr Opin Nephrol Hypertens. 2005;14(5):485-94.
94. Bobulescu IA, Moe OW. Na^+/H^+ exchangers in renal regulation of acid-base balance. Semin Nephrol. 2006;26(5):334-44.
95. Kinsella JL, Aronson PS. Interaction of $NH4^+$ and Li^+ with the renal microvillus membrane Na^+-H^+ exchanger. Am J Physiol. 1981;241(5):C220-6.
96. Nagami GT. Ammonia production and secretion by the proximal tubule. Am J Kidney Dis. 1989;14(4):258-61.
97. Unger RH. Lipotoxic diseases. Ann Rev Med. 2002;53:319-36.
98. Birn H, Christensen EI. Renal albumin absorption in physiology and pathology. Kidney Int. 2006;69(3):440-9.
99. Clark JB, Palmer CJ, Shaw WN. The diabetic Zucker fatty rat. Proc Soc Exp Biol Med. 1983;173(1):68-75.
100. Bobulescu IA, Dubree M, Zhang J, et al. Effect of renal lipid accumulation on proximal tubule Na^+/H^+ exchange and ammonium secretion. Am J Physiol Renal Physiol. 2008;294(6):F1315-22.
101. Abate N, Chandalia M, Cabo-Chan AV Jr, et al. The metabolic syndrome and uric acid nephrolithiasis: novel features of renal manifestation of insulin resistance. Kidney Int. 2004;65(2):386-92.
102. Bobulescu IA, Dubree M, Zhang J, et al. Reduction of renal triglyceride accumulation: effects on proximal tubule Na^+/H^+ exchange and urinary acidification. Am J Physiol Renal Physiol. 2009;297(5):F1419-26.
103. Shulman GI. Cellular mechanisms of insulin resistance. J Clin Invest. 2000;106(2):171-6.
104. Yki-Jarvinen H. Thiazolidinediones. New Engl J Med. 2004;351(11):1106-18.
105. Balaban RS, Mandel LJ. Metabolic substrate utilization by rabbit proximal tubule. An NADH fluorescence study. Am J Physiol. 1988;254(3 Pt 2):F407-16.
106. Dies F, Herrera J, Matos M, et al. Substrate uptake by the dog kidney in vivo. Am J Physiol. 1970;218(2):405-10.
107. Nieth H, Schollmeyer P. Substrate-utilization of the human kidney. Nature. 1966;209(5029):1244-5.
108. Vinay P, Lemieux G, Cartier P, et al. Effect of fatty acids on renal ammoniagenesis in in vivo and in vitro studies. Am J Physiol. 1976;231(3):880-7.
109. Gold M, Spitzer JJ. Metabolism of free fatty acids by myocardium and kidney. Am J Physiol. 1964;206:153-8.
110. Goldstein L. Relation of glutamate to ammonia production in the rat kidney. Am J Physiol. 1966;210(3):661-6.
111. Hohenleitner F. Changes in plasma free fatty acid concentrations on passage through the dog kidney. Am J Physiol Endocrinol Metab. 1965;200:1095-8.
112. Krivosikova Z, Spustova V, Dzurik R. Participation of P-dependent and P-independent glutaminases in rat kidney ammoniagenesis and their modulation by metabolic acidosis, hippurate and insulin. Physiol Res. 1998;47(3):177-83.
113. Chobanian MC, Hammerman MR. Insulin stimulates ammoniagenesis in canine renal proximal tubular segments. Am J Physiol. 1987;253(6 Pt 2):F1171-7.
114. Klisic J, Hu MC, Nief V, et al. Insulin activates Na^+/H^+exchanger 3: biphasic response and glucocorticoid dependence. Am J Physiol Renal Physiol. 2002;283(3):F532-9.
115. Cersosimo E, Garlick P, Ferretti J. Insulin regulation of renal glucose metabolism in humans. Am J Physiol. 1999;276(1 Pt 1): E78-84.
116. Gesek FA, Schoolwerth AC. Insulin increases Na^+-H^+ exchange activity in proximal tubules from normotensive and hypertensive rats. Am J Physiol. 1991;260(5 Pt 2):F695-703.
117. Baum M. Insulin stimulates volume absorption in the rabbit proximal convoluted tubule. J Clin Invest. 1987;79(4):1104-9.
118. Nagami GT. Luminal secretion of ammonia in the mouse proximal tubule perfused in vitro. J Clin Invest. 1988;81(1):159-64.
119. Meezan E, Freychet P. Specific insulin receptors in rat renal glomeruli. Renal Physiol. 1980;3(1-6):72-8.
120. Nakamura R, Emmanouel DS, Katz AI. Insulin binding sites in various segments of the rabbit nephron. J Clin Invest. 1983;72(1):388-92.
121. Remer T, Berkemeyer S, Rylander R, et al. Muscularity and adiposity in addition to net acid excretion as predictors of 24-h urinary pH in young adults and elderly. Eur J Clin Nutr. 2007;61(5):605-9.

122. Remer T, Dimitriou T, Manz F. Dietary potential renal acid load and renal net acid excretion in healthy, free-living children and adolescents. Am J Clin Nutr. 2003;77(5):1255-60.
123. Halperin ML, Kamel KS. D-lactic acidosis: turning sugar into acids in the gastrointestinal tract. Kidney Int. 1996;49(1):1-8.
124. Larsen N, Vogensen FK, van den Berg FW, et al. Gut microbiota in human adults with type 2 diabetes differs from non-diabetic adults. PloS one. 2010;5(2):e9085.
125. Iber FL, Parveen S, Vandrunen M, et al. Relation of symptoms to impaired stomach, small bowel, and colon motility in long-standing diabetes. Dig Dis Sci. 1993;38(1):45-50.
126. Ley RE, Turnbaugh PJ, Klein S, et al. Microbial ecology: human gut microbes associated with obesity. Nature. 2006;444(7122):1022-3.
127. Wang Z, Klipfell E, Bennett BJ, et al. Gut flora metabolism of phosphatidylcholine promotes cardiovascular disease. Nature. 2011;472(7341):57-63.
128. Hida M, Aiba Y, Sawamura S, et al. Inhibition of the accumulation of uremic toxins in the blood and their precursors in the feces after oral administration of Lebenin, a lactic acid bacteria preparation, to uremic patients undergoing hemodialysis. Nephron. 1996;74(2):349-55.
129. Vaziri ND, Wong J, Pahl M, et al. Chronic kidney disease alters intestinal microbial flora. Kidney Int. 2013;83(2):308-15.
130. Moe OW, Abate N, Sakhaee K. Pathophysiology of uric acid nephrolithiasis. Endocrinol Metab Clin North Am. 2002;31(4):895-914.
131. Tanaka M, Itoh K, Matsushita K, et al. Two male siblings with hereditary renal hypouricemia and exercise-induced ARF. Am J Kidney Dis. 2003;42(6):1287-92.
132. Reddy ST, Wang CY, Sakhaee K, et al. Effect of low-carbohydrate high-protein diets on acid-base balance, stone-forming propensity, and calcium metabolism. Am J Kidney Dis. 2002;40(2):265-74.
133. Zerwekh JE, Reed-Gitomer BY, Pak CY. Pathogenesis of hypercalciuric nephrolithiasis. Endocrinol Metab Clin North Am. 2002;31(4):869-84.
134. Pak CY, Britton F, Peterson R, et al. Ambulatory evaluation of nephrolithiasis. Classification, clinical presentation and diagnostic criteria. Am J Med. 1980;69(1):19-30.
135. Daudon M, Donsimoni R, Hennequin C, et al. Sex- and age-related composition of 10,617 calculi analyzed by infrared spectroscopy. Urol Res. 1995;23(5):319-26.
136. Soble JJ, Hamilton BD, Streem SB. Ammonium acid urate calculi: a reevaluation of risk factors. J Urol. 1999;161(3):869-73.
137. Bollee G, Harambat J, Bensman A, et al. Adenine phosphoribosyltransferase deficiency. Clin J Am Soc Nephrol. 2012;7(9):1521-7.
138. Van Acker KJ, Simmonds HA, Potter C, et al. Complete deficiency of adenine phosphoribosyltransferase. Report of a family. New Engl J Med. 1977;297(3):127-32.
139. Hesse A, Miersch WD, Classen A, et al. 2,8-dihydroxyadeninuria: laboratory diagnosis and therapy control. Urol Int. 1988;43(3):174-8.
140. Pak C, Holt K, Britton F, et al. Assessment of pathogenetic role of uric acid, monopotassium urate, monoammonium urate, monosodium urate in hyperuricosuric calcium oxalate nephrolithiasis. Miner Electrolyte Metab. 1980;4:130-60.
141. Pak CY, Arnold LH. Heterogeneous nucleation of calcium oxalate by seeds of monosodium urate. Proc Soc Exp Biol Med. 1975;149(4):930-2.
142. Lonsdale K. Epitaxy as a growth factor in urinary calculi and gallstones. Nature. 1968;217(5123):56-8.
143. Zerwekh JE, Holt K, Pak CY. Natural urinary macromolecular inhibitors: attenuation of inhibitory activity by urate salts. Kidney Int. 1983;23(6):838-41.
144. Grover PK, Ryall RL. Urate and calcium oxalate stones: from repute to rhetoric to reality. Miner Electrolyte Metab. 1994;20(6):361-70.
145. Cameron MA, Baker LA, Maalouf NM, et al. Circadian variation in urine pH and uric acid nephrolithiasis risk. Nephrol Dial Transplant. 2007;22(8):2375-8.
146. Gordon EE, Sheps SG. Effect of acetazolamide on citrate excretion and formation of renal calculi. New Engl J Med. 1957;256(26):1215-9.
147. Kuo RL, Moran ME, Kim DH, et al. Topiramate-induced nephrolithiasis. J Endourol. 2002;16(4):229-31.

CHAPTER 24

Pediatric Kidney Stone Disease

David J Sas

INTRODUCTION

Kidney stones in children are becoming more common.[1,2] While some portion of this increase may be due to a combination of increased awareness and better diagnostic modalities, the increasing impact of nephrolithiasis in children is not in dispute as the clinical, social, and financial significance of this disease is well documented. [2-5] The impact of each individual pediatric patient with kidney stones is actually quite broad, given that acute episodes and scheduled appointments to address the condition cause not only school absence for the child but also work absence for one or both parents. Children present other special considerations as well. They are more likely to have an identifiable underlying abnormality predisposing to kidney stones. Developmental and cognitive limitations may hinder the ability to perform certain evaluative tests. Similarly, their treatment strategies must take into account their limitations regarding diet and medication intake. Lastly, but perhaps most importantly, the fact that the diagnosis of nephrolithiasis is occurring so early in life means that the lifelong impact will be greater as they will be living with the condition far longer.

Although the volume of literature on pediatric nephrolithiasis represents only a small percentage of the literature in adult stone disease, more work has been done in recent years, improving our fund of knowledge and, hopefully, improving our care for these unfortunate young patients. This chapter will cover epidemiology, pathophysiology, evaluation, and medical treatment of pediatric nephrolithiasis. Since other chapters in this book will explore rare and genetic causes of kidney stones as well as surgical considerations, these topics will not be discussed in this chapter.

EPIDEMIOLOGY

The true incidence and prevalence of pediatric nephrolithiasis are uncertain as there has not yet been a study performed to determine this on a large scale. Studies using smaller regions or data meant to reflect relative incidence have been performed in recent years. Using a data set that captures the population of an entire county in Minnesota, Dwyer et al. determined that the incidence of pediatric kidney stones increased from 13 per 100,000 person-years to 36 per 100,000 person-years between 1984 and 2008.[1] Interestingly, the increase was seen almost exclusively in the adolescent population, which experienced a 6% yearly rate increase during that time period. Two other studies detail the increasing proportion of pediatric inpatient admissions due to nephrolithiasis.[6,7] These studies by Bush and Routh show that admissions to children's hospitals due to kidney stones have increased to 1 in 685. Both of these studies also show that girls are more likely than boys to be admitted to the hospital for stones and that these admissions most commonly occur in the summer months.

Lastly, data from South Carolina reveal that the estimated incidence of kidney stones in children was 18.5 per 100,000 children in 2007, increasing steadily from 7.9 per 100,000 in 1996.[2] Studies on adult stone-forming populations identify the Southeastern region of the United States as having the highest prevalence of kidney stones.[8,9] Since no large-scale data have been collected in the pediatric population, the same conclusion cannot be drawn regarding geographic distribution. We are left only to speculate that the same distribution is likely. Similarly, although studies regarding the costs associated with kidney stones have been published in the adult literature,[3,5] no similar nationwide studies have been published in the pediatric literature to date. The aforementioned data from South Carolina reveal charges of about $4.2 million per year for nephrolithiasis for a population of 1.12 million children in 2007. If one were to extrapolate that to the entire pediatric population of the United States, the nationwide charges for childhood nephrolithiasis would equal about $277 million, keeping in mind that such a simple extrapolation may not be valid; only considers charges, not actual costs; and these data are from emergency department databases, which would not include costs from inpatient and other outpatient sources.

In adults, nephrolithiasis has historically been a predominantly male disease, although more recent studies are showing a shrinking male predilection.[4,10] Older studies in the pediatric population document a similar male predominance for nephrolithiasis.[11,12] More recent publications, however, show a small but consistent predisposition among female pediatric stone patients, particularly in the adolescent population.[1,2,7,13] The reasons for the different gender predisposition both between the adult and pediatric populations and over time are not clear. Regarding the significant predisposition for kidney stones in adolescent females, pubertal hormonal changes may play a role along with differences in dietary intake within this group. This area is ripe for further investigation.

Race and ethnicity appear to play a role in stone formation as well. Recent studies examining pediatric stone formers reveal that between 72 and 88% are white (incidence 26.2 per 100,000), 11 and 15% are Hispanic, 6 and 9% are black (incidence 4.2 per 100,000), and 1% are Asian.[6,7,14] Although studies in adults show that blacks have lower calcium excretion than whites, likely accounting for the lower incidence of nephrolithiasis; similar studies have not been done in children. As such, the reasons for racial and ethnic differences in risk for stone formation remain uncertain in children.

The age of the child presenting with kidney stones can affect the clinician's approach to evaluation and management. Similar to hypertension, the younger the nephrolithiasis patient is, the more likely that he will have an identifiable secondary cause for kidney stones as the impact of underlying genetics is greater than environmental contributions earlier in life (excepting the tragedy involving melamine-induced stones in China[15], the discussion of which is beyond the scope of this text). The incidence of nephrolithiasis increases throughout childhood and the peak age of initial presentation ranges from 11 to 13-year-old.[1,13,16] The mean age for hospitalization of pediatric patients for stones follows a similar pattern, with older patients more likely to require hospital admission.[6,7] Age, however, does not appear to predict likelihood of spontaneous stone passage, which depends more simply on the size of the stone, regardless of age.[17,18]

Regarding the recurrence rate for kidney stones in children, there are few data. A study by Pietrow et al. published in 2002 reported an overall recurrence rate of 19% in all pediatric stone formers. Further analysis revealed a recurrence rate of 38% among those pediatric patients with an identified metabolic abnormality across all pediatric age groups and a 45% recurrence rate when limited to those 10 years old and younger with an identified metabolic abnormality.[18] Lao et al. reported a recurrence rate of 55% over 5 years among pediatric patients who required surgical intervention.[19] Not surprisingly, DeFoor et al. found that hypercalciuria and hypocitraturia were independent risk factors for recurrence in children.[20] To better understand recurrence rates among the pediatric stone-forming population along with the relevant risk factors, further studies in larger populations must be performed.

PATHOPHYSIOLOGY

The pathophysiology of kidney stone formation has been expertly covered in previous chapters of this text. The basic elements that lead to stone formation in adults are the same in children: Solute supersaturation, crystal formation and aggregation, followed by retention in the collecting system and continued growth. Although the biophysics of nephrolithiasis is undifferentiated between adult and pediatric patients, there are differences between the two related to how the urine chemistry arrives at such a lithogenic state.

Even more so than adults, children with kidney stones overwhelmingly form calcium-based stones. Whereas adult data suggest that 10% of adult stones are uric acid, uric acid stones in children are exceedingly rare.[1,21,22] The reasons for this are not completely certain, but are likely related to the slightly higher pH of children's urine. There has also been a shift away from struvite (magnesium ammonium phosphate) stone formation, which used to account for up to 25% of pediatric nephrolithiasis, presumably due to earlier identification and treatment of urinary tract infection (UTI), which predisposes to struvite stones.[1,23,24] Indeed, concomitant UTI was a common feature of pediatric kidney stone disease in decades past.[11,12] Since uric acid and struvite stones have become so rare, pediatricians are most focused on calcium oxalate and calcium phosphate stone formation.

It is not surprising that infants are the age group least likely to form kidney stones, given that the vast majority of their nutritional intake is derived from hypo-osmotic fluid. Despite having considerably higher urinary calcium excretion, otherwise normal infants rarely form stones. One exception can be infants with chronic respiratory or cardiac conditions who take furosemide regularly. Furosemide increases calcium excretion and chronic administration can lead to nephrocalcinosis or nephrolithiasis. This effect is generally transient, with the urinary chemistry normalizing once the diuretic is discontinued.[25-27]

In potty-trained toddlers and young school-aged children with kidney stones, one must consider dysfunctional elimination syndrome (DES) as a contributing factor. Dysfunctional elimination syndrome is a behaviorally derived condition that includes infrequent voiding and urine withholding, incomplete bladder emptying, constipation, and poor water intake. Children with this condition can be at higher risk for stone formation due to irregular urine flow, stasis, and greater presence of bacteriuria. Fortunately, implementation of a strategy to address DES is typically successful and results in normal voiding habits, eliminating the aforementioned risk factors.[28]

As children move from school-age to adolescence, external environmental factors play a larger role in their health status and these include risk factors for stone formation. It is no secret that adolescents commonly make poor dietary choices when given the freedom, and this often includes foods that are lithogenic. These children typically eat a diet higher in sodium and sugar (including high-fructose corn syrup) and lower in calcium.[29,30] Additionally, they eat fewer vegetables. They often participate in more intense athletics, resulting is more volume depletion. Based on this more lithogenic lifestyle, it is not surprising that adolescents represent the fastest-growing age group among our pediatric population.

Examining this age group more closely, we find that adolescent females are at particularly high-risk for kidney stone formation.[1,7] The reasons for this are not clear. It may be that there is some relationship between female pubertal hormones and stone formation, although no research has yet been performed to address this question. Alternatively, there may be some different environmental interactions typical of adolescent females that also contribute to their risk. Further investigation is warranted.

Although the urine chemistry and kinetics that lead to stone formation in children are the same as in adults, there are some differences worth discussing. There is wide variation regarding the percentage of pediatric stone formers who have an identifiable metabolic abnormality predisposing to kidney stone formation (ranging from 44 to 93%), but it is generally agreed that children are more likely to have an abnormality than adult stone formers.[1,16-18,31-33] Children have a higher excretion rate for calcium and oxalate as well as higher supersaturation of calcium phosphate than adults.[34] Why, then, would children form kidney stones less frequently? There is some evidence that children's urine contains more potent inhibitors of crystallization and aggregation, including more commonly described inhibitors citrate and magnesium, as well as less well-known urinary macromolecules and proteins.[35,36] Although it is presumed that children form Randall's plaque like adult idiopathic calcium stone formers, it is interesting to note that there is not a single mention of Randall's plaque in a child in the published literature. Further investigation into inhibitors of stone formation as well as the mechanism of plaque and stone formation is warranted.

Table 24.1: Typical urine chemistry abnormalities identified in 24-hour urine collections from pediatric kidney stone formers.

24-hour urine abnormality	*% Abnormal in pediatric stone formers*
Low urine volume	5–81
Hypocitraturia	8–62
Hypercalciuria	19–58
Hyperoxaluria	3–52

Studies of urinary chemistry in children vary with regards to the prevalence of specific abnormalities.[1,16-18,31-33] This wide variation is likely a direct result of the data originating from multiple single-institution data sets with varying reference ranges and populations. In addition, some studies also show differences in urine chemistry abnormalities within smaller age ranges among children.[17,18] The heterogeneity of this data confirms that further research to establish normal ranges in children of varying ages is required before we can dependably assess urine chemistry in the pediatric stone-forming population. With that in mind, Table 24.1 summarizes the common 24-hour urine abnormalities seen in pediatric kidney stone formers.

MEDICAL EVALUATION

Unlike adults, in whom a comprehensive evaluation is limited to those with recurrent disease or red flags for an underlying metabolic disorder, expert consensus recommends that all children with nephrolithiasis deserve a complete evaluation.[37]

Controversy exists regarding the most appropriate imaging modality to use for initial evaluation of a child suspected of having nephrolithiasis. Computed tomography (CT) scans are the most sensitive for positively identifying stones, but are more expensive, expose children disproportionately to radiation increasing their cancer risk, and require the child to stay completely still.[38-41] In fact, nephrolithiasis is the diagnosis that accounts for most repeat

CT scans in pediatric emergency departments.[42] Renal ultrasound (RUS) is less expensive and does not expose the child to radiation, but is very operator-dependent and may miss smaller stones. The operator-dependence of RUS is reflected in the wide range of sensitivity between published studies, with sensitivity ranging from 24 to 76%, though with specificities typically >90%.[43,44] Despite the lower sensitivity of RUS compared to CT, studies also show that stones missed by RUS are usually not clinically significant.[44,45] A recent large, well-designed study by Smith-Bindman and colleagues concluded that, for initial imaging, ultrasonography was associated with lower cumulative radiation exposure than CT, without significant differences in high-risk diagnoses with complications, serious adverse events, pain scores, return emergency department visits, or hospitalizations.[46] There are significant regional and institutional differences regarding preference for CT scan versus RUS. Comparing data from two sets of single-institution data in the pediatric literature, one report revealed that CT scan confirmed stone presence in 82% of patients, while another institution used CT scan in 27%, with the remainder in each diagnosed by RUS.[1,13] Another recent study examining emergency department imaging practices found that 71% of pediatric stone formers had a CT scan performed as their initial imaging modality, despite published guidelines recommending RUS for initial evaluation.[47,48] In practice, it may be reasonable to rely on RUS when the healthcare provider is confident that his patients will be evaluated by pediatric-trained ultrasonographers and radiologists, and rely on CT scan otherwise. Additionally, CT is indicated in patients in whom RUS was negative, but there is a high clinical suspicion for nephrolithiasis.

Regardless of which imaging modality is used to diagnose kidney stones in a child, once the diagnosis is made, an appropriate comprehensive evaluation including history, physical examination, blood testing, urine testing, and stone composition (when available) is warranted. The overall goal of the evaluation is to identify any underlying metabolic abnormality that may predispose the child to kidney stone formation and, perhaps more importantly, provide focus for a strategy for prevention.

The history should focus on circumstances under which the stone was formed, dietary habits, past medical history (including medication history), previous history of renal colic, recurrent UTIs, anatomical anomalies or hematuria, DES, and family history for stones. The circumstances under which the stone was formed may provide clues regarding the likelihood that the child has an underlying metabolic abnormality predisposing to stone formation. For instance, a child who formed a stone while eating his usual diet in a state of adequate hydration is more likely to have an underlying predisposition for stone formation compared to a child who formed a stone in August after a week of twice-a-day football practices with limited water breaks and a high-salt diet.

Medical conditions revealed in the past medical history may be related to kidney stone formation, either directly in the case of vesicoureteral reflux or recurrent UTI or indirectly due to the interventions implemented to address a condition. For instance, a patient with an underlying seizure disorder may form stones due to a ketogenic diet used to reduce seizure frequency or the use of topiramate.[49,50] Additionally, children with a history of prematurity, congenital cardiac disease, or chronic lung disease may have nephrolithiasis or nephrocalcinosis secondary to chronic furosemide use.[25,51,52] Other conditions such as short stature, bone fractures, or developmental delay may point to an underlying syndrome or metabolic disorder associated with nephrolithiasis.

A careful diet history is most useful for identifying areas for improvement, especially once the laboratory evaluation is complete, and urinary chemistry reveals the patient's lithogenic characteristics. Additionally, one may identify children whose diet falls well out of the normal spectrum for the given age, providing exogenous factors predisposing to stone formation. For example, the care provider may discover a child who eats a diet very high in oxalate, leading to enteric hyperoxaluria. More commonly, though, one will discover the typical pediatric diet is high in sodium, low in calcium, and includes low fluid volume intake.[29,30,53-55]

The physical examination findings in pediatric stone formers are generally unremarkable. Blood pressure percentiles should be closely monitored because there is evidence in adults that nephrolithiasis increases the risk for hypertension,[56] although this has not been investigated in pediatric populations. The patient's body mass index (BMI) is also worth noting, given the interest in the relationship between obesity and nephrolithiasis. Although increased BMI does appear to be a risk factor for nephrolithiasis in adults (particularly uric acid stones),[57,58] evidence is mounting that overweight and obesity do not increase the risk for kidney stones in children.[59,60] Appropriate height and weight are also noteworthy to ensure no growth delay that may suggest an underlying genetic syndrome or metabolic abnormality associated with kidney stones. Lastly, careful abdominal palpation may reveal a mass consistent with stool in the colon suggestive of constipation, which should be addressed.

The initial laboratory evaluation of a child with nephrolithiasis should include blood and urine testing. The purpose of the blood work is to identify more severe metabolic derangements or decrease in renal function. Urine tests more subtly reveal the urinary environment in which the stone are formed; it is then up to the clinician to determine which of these factors are based on genetics and which are based on environmental interactions.

The basic blood work for all new pediatric stone formers should include a basic metabolic panel (sodium, potassium, chloride, bicarbonate, blood urea nitrogen, creatinine, and glucose), calcium, phosphorus, magnesium, parathyroid hormone, vitamin D (both 25- and 1,25-vitamin D), serum pH, alkaline phosphatase, and uric acid. This provides ample screening for major underlying metabolic/genetic abnormalities that would lead to kidney stones. Of note, a normal pH under normal conditions does not rule out a so-called partial renal tubular acidosis, which can only be properly evaluated using an ammonium chloride challenge; this is rather invasive for a child and, therefore, rarely performed in children.

Initial urine testing should include a urinalysis with microscopy and a 24-hour urine stone risk profile. Additional urine testing including random creatinine, protein, calcium, citrate, oxalate, or other metabolites may be useful. There is some evidence that following serial urine calcium-to-creatinine or calcium-to-citrate ratios may be useful in the management of hypercalciuria when 24-hour urine collections are less convenient.[61,62] Certainly, for infants and toddlers who are not continent of urine, random samples will be the only source of urine chemistry information short of invasive measures. As such, random urine test results may be used to identify underlying metabolic abnormalities, although the limitations of this testing must be taken into consideration.[61]

Ultimately, though, an analysis of an appropriately collected 24-hour urine collection is the most useful tool for evaluating underlying urinary chemistry. The 24-hour urine should be analyzed using a reputable laboratory for supersaturation of calcium oxalate, calcium phosphate, and uric acid, as well as calcium, citrate, oxalate, phosphorus, magnesium, pH, sodium, uric acid, potassium, creatinine, and volume. Cystine should also be measured if there is clinical suspicion for cystine stones. All of these should be carefully reviewed in the context of the patient's weight/body surface area and reference ranges appropriate for the patient's age. It is important that the clinician be aware of the different reference ranges for children compared to adults to avoid misdiagnosis and inappropriate therapy. It should also be noted that the available data supporting reference ranges for children are limited by the size and quality of many of the studies used to establish these norms.

For children who are not yet continent of urine, obviously, a 24-hour urine sample cannot be collected without placement of a bladder catheter, which is quite invasive and requires hospitalization. However, for severe cases in which the 24-hour urine data are vital, it is worth considering. Every 24-hour urine collection for stone risk analysis should be evaluated for adequacy of collection to confirm validity of the data as mistakes in collection technique are not uncommon. Although there is not one universally agreed-upon range for creatinine per kilogram bodyweight to define an adequate sample, reasonable ranges are found in Table 24.2. It should be noted that there is evidence to suggest that using this method to assess adequacy of urine collection may not be valid.[63,64] Keeping that in mind, it is still useful to analyze 24-hour urine results in the context of expected creatinine excretion.

Supersaturation, as described in other chapters in the text, has been shown to be a valid predictor of kidney stone formation and recurrence in children.[31,34,65,66] In the absence of a stone for composition analysis, supersaturation data from a 24-hour urine collection can be used to predict stone type.[67] There are discrepancies in the literature regarding whether or not supersaturation values are age-dependent, particularly with regard to supersaturation of calcium oxalate. DeFoor et al. found similar calcium oxalate supersaturation values between adults and children, whereas Hoppe et al. found them to be age-dependent (as well as gender-dependent).[34,68] While we are waiting for the establishment of more uniform supersaturation reference ranges for children, the intrapatient trends can be useful to determine the efficacy of our treatment.[69]

Additionally, excretion rates of calcium, oxalate, and citrate are age- and size-dependent. As such, physicians must rely on available reference ranges if the laboratory performing the analysis does not provide them (Table 24.2).

Kidney stone composition analysis is also very useful for determining the underlying metabolic underpinnings of nephrolithiasis in a child, but is frequently unavailable as the patients often do not or are unable to collect a stone for analysis. As healthcare providers who care for children

Table 24.2: Normal urine values in children for kidney stone risk factors.

Risk factor	*Age*	*Random*	*Timed*	*References*
Calcium		mg/mg creatinine:		(70, 71)
	<7 months	<0.86	<4 mg/kg/24 h	
	7–18 months	<0.60		
	19 months–6 years	<0.42		
	7+ years	<0.22		
Calcium-to-citrate ratio		mg calcium/mg citrate:		(62, 72)
	Boys:	Boys:		
	2–6 years	0.05		
	7–12 years	0.05		
	13+ years	0.06		
	Girls:	Girls:		
	2–6 years	0.03		
	7–12 years	0.04		
	13+ years	0.05		
Citrate		mg/mg creatinine:		(62, 72)
	Boys:	Boys:	Boys: (in mg/1.73m^2/24 h	
	2–6 years	0.242	177	
	7–12 years	0.139	162	
	13+ years	0.090	130	
	Girls:	Girls:	Girls:	
	2–6 years	0.290	218	
	7–12 years	0.261	253	
	13+ years	0.216	248	
Creatinine	Prepubertal		10–15 mg/kg/24 h	
	Postpubertal girls		15–20 mg/kg/24 h	
	Postpubertal boys		28–24 mg/kg/24 h	
Cystine		<100 µmoles/g creatinine	<100 µmoles/g creatinine	(73, 74)
Magnesium		mg/mg creatinine:	>88 mg/1.73 m^2/24 h	(75)
	<1 year	>0.10		
	1–2 years	>0.09		
	2–5 years	>0.07		
	5–7 years	>0.06		
	7+ years	>0.05		
Oxalate		mg/mg creatinine:	<52 mg/1.73 m^2/24 h	(13, 76)
	<6 months	<0.18		
	6 months–1 year	<0.14		
	1–2 years	<0.10		
	2–3 years	<0.08		
	3–7 years	<0.06		
	7+ years	<0.0.5		
Phosphorus		mg/mg creatinine:		(75)
	<1 year	<5.24		
	1–2 years	<3.95		
	2–3 years	<3.13		
	3–5 years	<2.17		
	5–7 years	<1.49		
	7–10 years	<0.97		
	10–14 years	<0.86		
	14+ years	<0.75		

Contd...

Contd...

Risk factor	Age	Random	Timed	References
Potassium			>3 mEq/kg/24 h	(77)
Sodium			<3 mEq/kg/24 h	(77)
Uric acid		mg/mg creatinine:		(76, 78)
	<6 months	<2.38	<815 mg/1.73 m^2/24 h	
	6 months–1 year	<2.23		
	1–2 years	<2.08		
	2–3 years	<1.93		
	3–5 years	<1.64		
	5–7 years	<1.19		
	7–10 years	<0.83		
	10–14 years	<0.65		
	14+ years	<0.59		
Volume			>1.0 mL/kg/h	

with kidney stones, we should educate our colleagues in emergency departments, urgent care centers, and primary care offices to provide strainers for patients when they present with renal colic and stone passage is possible. When a stone is made available, it is important that it be sent to a credible laboratory for analysis. It is also worth noting that chemical composition can change for stones from the same patient over time.[79]

Based on the results of this evaluation, the skilled clinician should be able to compose a strategy for prevention for the child as well as identify patients for whom further investigation is warranted for precise diagnosis of a rare or genetic cause for kidney stones. Further investigation is warranted when laboratory results suggest substantial underlying metabolic derangement, recurrent disease, or suggestive positive family history.

TREATMENT AND FOLLOW-UP

Careful consideration must be given to the optimal treatment strategy for children with kidney stones, given the developmental and nutritional needs of a growing child. Although the results of the laboratory evaluation will guide therapy just as they do in adults, the healthcare professional caring for pediatric stone formers must also take into account the impact of medication options and dietary restrictions on growth and development. The goal of preventive therapy is to minimize crystallization leading to new stones while stopping expansion of stones already formed. Whereas dissolution therapy may have a role in adults with uric acid stones, it is rarely applicable in pediatric populations with overwhelmingly predominant calcium-based stones.

Table 24.3: Suggested water intake for children with nephrolithiasis based in age.

Age	Water (liters per day)
Infant	0.75
Preschool	1
School-age	1.5
Adolescent	2
Adult	2.5-4

The mainstay of therapy for all types of stone formers is increased water intake to achieve dilute urine. This can be challenging in younger children and adolescents, who may not accept the rational explanation for the increased water intake. Additional barriers include common school-enforced restrictions on water and limited trips to the restroom during the school day, but this can typically be over-ruled by a note from the physician indicating that this patient must have free access to water and the restroom throughout the day due to a medical condition. General guidelines for water intake are listed in Table 24.3.

Inevitably, the question will arise regarding drinking fluids other than water, as parents will sometimes declare that their child finds water unpalatable. Fruit juice may be acceptable as an adjunct to water if a young child truly will not drink enough water to reduce stone formation, although the risk of exogenous overweight and obesity from excessive calories is increased. Additionally, beverages with high fructose corn syrup contribute to stone disease, although the evidence for this is not strong.[80] Excessive milk intake should be avoided to limit overconsumption of calcium and vitamin D. Generally, the United States Recommended Daily Allowances (USRDA) recommendation for calcium intake should be followed as there is no evidence to suggest that divergence might be beneficial.[81]

Limiting salt intake is also important as sodium intake is directly related to urinary calcium excretion and contributes to stone formation.[69,82,83] Recent evidence supports the notion that children are getting too much salt,[30] and this may be a contributing factor to the rise in pediatric nephrolithiasis. Table 24.4 lists recommended sodium intake adapted from guidelines from the Institute of Medicine on Adequate Intake as published by the Centers for Disease Control (CDC).[84]

It is important to discuss with parents how to reduce salt intake. Many parents are not aware of how or where their children are getting excessive salt. Reviewing the major contributors to sodium intake in a child's diet is required in order for parents to minimize their child's stone-forming propensity.

Beyond telling patients to drink more water and eat less salt, other dietary modifications depend on the results of the 24-hour urine collection. Dietary recommendations should be based on the abnormalities identified in the context of a growing and developing child.

Table 24.4: Suggested sodium intake for children with nephrolithiasis based on age.

Age (years)	*Sodium intake (mg per day)*
1–3	1,000
4–8	1,200
9–14	1,500
14+	2,000

Hypocitraturia

Hypocitraturia is one of the most common risk factors for kidney stone formation in children and can be directly addressed with enteral citrate supplementation[85] (for a complete discussion on how citrate supplementation interferes with stone formation *see* Chapter 10). Caution should be used when contemplating citrate supplementation for CaP stone formers, as urine alkalinization may counteract the benefit from citrate-calcium binding.[86] Despite the paucity of data providing evidence-based support for the use of citrate therapy in pediatric stone disease, citrate supplementation is often employed to treat pediatric stone formers. The results from three studies from Turkey suggest that citrate therapy may benefit children with calcium-based nephrolithiasis.[87-89] Citrate can be supplemented pharmacologically using potassium citrate tablets, powder for mixing into solution, or premixed solution (Table 24.5). Alternatively, sodium bicarbonate may be a less expensive way to improve urinary citrate and increase urine pH.[86]

Citrate supplementation can also be achieved through dietary means. The two most common beverages used to increase urinary citrate are lemonade and orange juice. There are a number of studies that have evaluated the effects of drinking these and other beverages (though none in pediatric patients), which are nicely summarized

Table 24.5: Medications commonly used in pediatric nephrolithiasis.[77,101]

Medication	*Indication*	*Formulations*	*Dose*	*Comments*
Allopurinol	Hyperuricosuria	Tablet: 100, 300 mg Oral solution can be made from tablets	10 mg/kg per day divided QD-TID	
Chlorothiazide	Hypercalciuria refractory to dietary modifications	Tablets: 250 and 500 mg Suspension: 250 mg/5 mL	10–20 mg/kg per day divided QD or BID	
Hydrochlorothiazide	Hypercalciuria refractory to dietary modifications	Tablets: 25 and 50 mg Suspension: 50 mg/5 mL	0.5–2 mg/kg/day divided QD-BID	Monitor electrolytes
Potassium citrate	Hypocitraturia, Hypercalciuria	Tablets: 5, 10, and 15 mEq Crystals: 1,002 mg citric acid/3,300 mg potassium citrate per packet (= 30 mEq/packet) Solution: 334 mg citric acid/1,100 mg potassium citrate per 5 mL (= 10 mEq/5 mL)	0.5–1.5 mEq/kg/day divided BID or TID	Crystals: mix with at least 6 oz cool water or juice Solution: dilute solution with 4 oz water to minimize gastrointestinal injury

(QD: Once a day; BID: Twice a day; TID: Thrice a day).

in a review by Kurtz and Eisner.[90] Overall, there is evidence that orange juice best improves urinary citrate levels with the added benefit of citrate complexed with potassium, compared with lemon-based beverages, which had mixed results. The variety of results from studies examining the use of fruit juices for stones reminds us that interventions with enteral foods may not be as simple as measuring citrate in a given juice and measuring citrate in the urine; many more complex interactions may be in play. Citrate-containing juices may optimally be used in patients who prefer not to take medications and/or struggle to drink an adequate volume of water. Getting a child to drink two glasses a day of orange juice is often preferred by both the parents and the child. However, this approach is suboptimal for overweight or obese patients due to the large quantity of sugar that comes with fruit juice. For overweight and obese children with hypocitraturia, sugar-free powdered lemonade products may be used to provide citrate supplementation without added calories from sugar.[91,92]

Although a diet high in acid load can contribute to hypocitraturia, protein restriction is not recommended in growing children. However, encouraging intake of more fruits and vegetables is probably, overall, a healthy recommendation and may help correct hypocitraturia.[93]

Hypercalciuria

The most important strategy for addressing hypercalciuria as a contributing factor to nephrolithiasis is increasing water intake and decreasing salt intake as outlined above. Limiting salt intake will decrease calcium excretion, and increasing water intake will dilute the calcium concentration. Calcium intake should be maintained at the RDA to ensure adequate bone health in a growing skeleton and, potentially, curb enteric oxalate absorption.

Citrate supplementation as described above may be helpful in treating hypercalciuric stone formers as citrate binds with calcium, interrupting crystallization.[94,95] Hydrochlorothiazide has been shown to reduce calciuria and reduce the risk of stone recurrence in adults,[96] but no randomized controlled trials have been performed in children. Two studies in pediatrics suggest that hydrochlorothiazide may be helpful in reducing calciuria in children.[97,98] Although hydrochlorothiazide has been used safely for years in children, they are more susceptible to unwanted side effects such as hypotension and electrolyte abnormalities. As such, more careful monitoring of serum electrolytes and blood pressure is recommended. It is also important to educate the family regarding the clinical signs of hypotension, hypokalemia, and hyponatremia. Lastly, the family must be counseled regarding the need for even more fluid intake given that hydrochlorothiazide is, first, a diuretic. Given the risk for significant side effects, it may be prudent to reserve use of hydrochlorothiazide for hypercalciuric stone-forming children in whom more conservative measures have failed to prevent recurrence.

The role of evaluating bone density in children with hypercalciuria and nephrolithiasis using dual-energy X-ray absorptiometry (DEXA) scans is controversial. Although there is evidence that children with hypercalciuria have lower bone density,[99,100] there is no evidence that the results of this test benefit the children or change management. Given the increased risk for untoward side effects in children with hydrochlorothiazide use, it may be reasonable to perform a DEXA scan prior to starting the medication to support its use and quantify any progress. Otherwise, empiric treatment of hypercalciuria with dietary modification without a DEXA scan may be the most rational and efficient approach.

Hyperoxaluria

Here, the discussion will focus on enteric hyperoxaluria rather than one of the forms of primary hyperoxaluria, which have been covered in Chapter 22. Once primary hyperoxaluria has been ruled out in a child with excessive oxalate in the urine, enteric hyperoxaluria is the likely diagnosis. The separation is warranted as the approach to therapy for enteric hyperoxaluria is very different from that of primary hyperoxaluria. Although further research is needed to elucidate mechanisms of excessive enteric oxalate absorption, we know that conditions causing malabsorption (inflammatory bowel disease, bowel resection) lead to increased oxalate absorption, and emerging research continues to reveal genetic differences related to intestinal oxalate transporters leading to increased oxalate absorption.[102,103] Since calcium is far more abundant than oxalate in the urine, managing increased intestinal absorption in hyperoxaluria is thought to be the principal factor in calcium oxalate stone formation.[104] As such, limiting enteric absorption of oxalate is the logical approach to therapy, along with the aforementioned increase in fluid intake, decreased sodium intake, and, possibly, increased citrate supplementation.

Since there is no pharmacological way to block oxalate transport from the gut to the bloodstream, decreased intake of oxalate is the only way to reduce urine oxalate excretion. For most families, oxalate is not a familiar component of food, so the help of a skilled dietitian is ideal. Unfortunately, many foods that contain a significant amount of oxalate are otherwise healthy foods, so limiting oxalate intake while still promoting an overall healthy diet for a growing, active child can be a challenge. One must weigh the severity of the child's stone disease with the importance of maintaining other aspects of health and well-being. For some, starting with avoiding foods that are very high in oxalate, rechecking a 24-hour urine to monitor the efficacy of dietary changes and adjusting appropriately can be a reasonable approach. Aside from using data from the published medical literature regarding lists of food and their oxalate content, practitioners can simply perform an Internet search to find information for families regarding which foods to avoid and which to encourage based on oxalate content, although there are discrepancies in this information.[105]

Other Factors

The 24-hour urine analysis may reveal other modifiable risk factors besides urine volume, sodium intake, hypocitraturia, hypercalciuria, and hyperoxaluria, although these are the most common. Potassium and magnesium are thought to be inhibitors of stone formation, and may be found to be low in the urine of stone formers. This can be addressed through recommendation of foods with ample amounts of these nutrients (again, ideally with the help of a skilled dietitian) or (less optimally) supplementation with oral tablets. If results reveal excessive phosphaturia, one may wish to revisit the child's diet to see if there is excessive dietary intake of phosphorus or else look for other metabolic cause for phosphorus wasting.

In children, it is also important to address other factors that could be predisposing to kidney stone formation. Although there is no published literature examining the relationship between DES and nephrolithiasis, research does suggest DES as a risk factor for recurrent UTIs.[106,107] Dysfunctional elimination syndrome is a constellation of urinary withholding, incomplete bladder emptying, poor fluid intake, and constipation. It is commonly seen in preschool-aged children just after toilet training. Without correction, it often persists into the elementary school years. For the same reasons that DES predisposes to UTI, the condition likely increases risk for kidney stone formation. Patients with DES have abnormal urine flow with stasis and turbulence, which can lead to bacterial proliferation and, presumably, crystal and stone formation. Screening for DES is easily accomplished during the history by asking parents questions consistent with each of the features of DES. If any of the features are identified, they should be addressed through behavioral modification to reduce the risk of UTIs and kidney stones and for overall genitourinary health.

One special population of children with a high-risk for kidney stones who can be difficult to manage is patients with severe seizure disorder who are on a strict ketogenic diet. Patients on a ketogenic diet are at high-risk for developing kidney stones due to the acidogenic nature of their diet.[50] They typically have low urine pH, hypocitraturia, and hypercalciuria. As one would expect, they can form uric acid stones but also calcium oxalate stones. The challenge for this population is manipulation of the diet and citrate supplementation that still fits with their ketogenic diet. Dietary manipulation is virtually impossible aside from increasing water intake and possibly decreasing salt intake. Given the different options available for citrate supplementation, citrate crystals (Cytra-K Crystals, Cypress Pharmaceutical, Inc., Madison, MS) are best for patients on a ketogenic diet as they provide only 4.2 mg of carbohydrate per milliliter of solution when mixed, compared to 100–300 mg/mL carbohydrate in other formulations. Alternatively, sodium bicarbonate can also be used to alkalinize the urine.[86] One last consideration is that if the child receives most of his nutrition through enteral tube feeds, increasing free-water intake should be considered with close electrolyte monitoring, although the resultant increase in urine output may put a further burden on the patient's caregivers.

Once pharmacologic and dietary changes are implemented along with increased fluid and decreased sodium intake, one must monitor the plan for efficacy. One can monitor efficacy in three ways: (1) recurrent episodes of renal colic, (2) stone burden as seen on imaging tests, and (3) changes in urinary chemistry. For patients, obviously, the first facet is most important as families most desperately want to avoid painful stone episodes for their child. The family should be given clear instructions (or an "action plan") regarding what to do in case of an acute episode of renal colic and be reminded that an episode of renal colic with concomitant fever is a true urological emergency. The nephrologist should be made aware of each episode.

Regarding the second facet, follow-up imaging for patients regardless of painful episodes, there are no clear guidelines. Repeat imaging studies can be helpful to assess the efficacy of therapy in asymptomatic patients as stone burden may be worsening without any clinical signs.

A reasonable starting point is to check yearly RUS for children with no symptomatic recurrence or complications. These results can help the practitioner follow the number and size of calculi with an awareness of the aforementioned limitations of ultrasound versus CT scan. Computed tomography scans should be limited to patients with more complicated situations and for whom ultrasound has missed calculi in the past.

The third facet, following urine chemistry via 24-hour urine collection, is the most sophisticated tool of the three. Although the 24-hour urine collection can provide the most nuanced information for the team, it is not without flaws. There is the risk of "collection bias" in which the family makes a particularly heroic effort to adhere to the agreed-upon strategy for prevention only on the days just prior to the urine collection, leading to falsely optimistic results. For that reason, it is important to stress to the family that the goal of the 24-hour urine collection is to best reflect their usual dietary and pharmacological habits to get an accurate picture of the urine chemistry on a day-to-day basis. The results of this testing will reveal to the practitioner whether or not the interventions suggested are changing the urine chemistry for the better or whether further intervention is needed. The importance of this step cannot be overemphasized as the main goal is to correct the urine chemistry using this information so that the patient does not experience abnormalities in facets one or two of this approach, i.e. end up with symptomatic stones or increased stone burden on imaging. Changes in urine chemistry are seen in short order after making dietary or pharmacologic modifications, so repeat 24-hour urine collections can be done a few weeks after the changes are implemented.[108]

In summary, the keys to success in pediatric nephrolithiasis are evaluations that include age- and size-appropriate interpretation of chemistry findings combined with developmentally appropriate strategy for management. Children are not just small adults; their urinary chemistry can be very different depending on tubular maturation. Dietary and pharmacological interventions must take into account the special needs of a growing and developing child. A multidisciplinary approach including pediatric specialists in nephrology, urology, laboratory services, and nutrition is required for optimal management.

REFERENCES

1. Dwyer ME, Krambeck AE, Bergstralh EJ, et al. Temporal trends in incidence of kidney stones among children: a 25-year population based study. J Urol. 2012;188(1):247-52.
2. Sas DJ, Hulsey TC, Shatat IF, et al. Incidence of kidney stones in children evaluated in the ER is increasing. J Pediatr. 2010. Jul;157(1):132-7.
3. Lotan Y. Economics and cost of care of stone disease. Adv Chronic Kidney Dis. 2009;16(1):5-10.
4. Pearle MS, Calhoun EA, Curhan GC. Urologic diseases in America project: urolithiasis. J Urol. 2005;173(3):848-57.
5. Saigal CS, Joyce G, Timilsina AR. Direct and indirect costs of nephrolithiasis in an employed population: opportunity for disease management? Kidney Int. 2005;68(4):1808-14.
6. Bush NC, Xu L, Brown BJ, et al. Hospitalizations for pediatric stone disease in United States, 2002–2007. J Urol. 2010;183(3):1151-6.
7. Routh JC, Graham DA, Nelson CP. Epidemiological trends in pediatric urolithiasis at United States freestanding pediatric hospitals. J Urol. 2010;184(3):1100-4.
8. Breyer BN, Sen S, Aaronson DS, et al. Use of Google Insights for Search to track seasonal and geographic kidney stone incidence in the United States. Urology. 2011;78(2):267-71.
9. Soucie JM, Coates RJ, McClellan W, et al. Relation between geographic variability in kidney stones prevalence and risk factors for stones. Am J Epidemiol. 1996;143(5):487-95.
10. Scales CD, Jr, Curtis LH, Norris RD, et al. Changing gender prevalence of stone disease. J Urol. 2007;177(3):979-82.
11. Malek RS, Kelalis PP. Pediatric nephrolithiasis. J Urol. 1975;113(4):545-51.
12. Wenzl JE, Burke EC, Stickler GB, et al. Nephrolithiasis and nephrocalcinosis in children. Pediatrics. 1968;41(1):57-61.
13. Penido MG, Srivastava T, Alon US. Pediatric primary urolithiasis: 12-year experience at a Midwestern Children's Hospital. J Urol. 2013;189(4):1493-7.
14. Sas DJ. An update on the changing epidemiology and metabolic risk factors in pediatric kidney stone disease. Clin J Am Soc Nephrol. 2011;6(8):2062-8.
15. Langman CB. Melamine, powdered milk, and nephrolithiasis in Chinese infants. New Engl J Med. 2009;360(11):1139-41.
16. VanDervoort K, Wiesen J, Frank R, et al. Urolithiasis in pediatric patients: a single center study of incidence, clinical presentation and outcome. J Urol. 2007;177(6):2300-5.
17. Kalorin CM, Zabinski A, Okpareke I, et al. Pediatric urinary stone disease—does age matter? J Urol. 2009;181(5):2267-71; discussion 71.
18. Pietrow PK, Pope JCt, Adams MC, et al. Clinical outcome of pediatric stone disease. J Urol. 2002;167(2 Pt 1):670-3.
19. Lao M, Kogan BA, White MD, et al. High recurrence rate at 5-year followup in children after upper urinary tract stone surgery. J Urol. 2014;191(2):440-4.
20. DeFoor WR, Jackson E, Minevich E, et al. The risk of recurrent urolithiasis in children is dependent on urinary calcium and citrate. Urology. 2010;76(1):242-5.
21. Moe OW. Kidney stones: pathophysiology and medical management. Lancet. 2006;367(9507):333-44.
22. Wood KD, Stanasel IS, Koslov DS, et al. Changing stone composition profile of children with nephrolithiasis. Urology. 2013;82(1):210-3.
23. Milliner DS, Murphy ME. Urolithiasis in pediatric patients. Mayo Clin Proc. 1993;68(3):241-8.

24. Polinsky MS, Kaiser BA, Baluarte HJ. Urolithiasis in childhood. Pediatr Clin North Am. 1987;34(3):683-710.
25. Hufnagle KG, Khan SN, Penn D, et al. Renal calcifications: a complication of long-term furosemide therapy in preterm infants. Pediatrics. 1982;70(3):360-3.
26. Osorio AV, Alon MM, Nichols MA, et al. Effect of age on furosemide-induced nephrocalcinosis in the rat. Biol Neonate. 1998;73(5):306-12.
27. Saarela T, Lanning P, Koivisto M, et al. Nephrocalcinosis in full-term infants receiving furosemide treatment for congestive heart failure: a study of the incidence and 2-year follow up. Eur J Pediatr. 1999;158(8):668-72.
28. Feldman AS, Bauer SB. Diagnosis and management of dysfunctional voiding. Curr Opin Pediatr. 2006;18(2):139-47.
29. Clark MA, Fox MK. Nutritional quality of the diets of US public school children and the role of the school meal programs. J Am Diet Assoc. 2009;109(2 Suppl):S44-56.
30. Reducing sodium in children's diets. In: Prevention CDC, editor. Atlanta, GA 2014. Available: https://www.cdc.gov/vitalsigns/children-sodium/index.html
31. Battino BS, De FW, Coe F, et al. Metabolic evaluation of children with urolithiasis: are adult references for supersaturation appropriate? J Urol. 2002;168(6):2568-71.
32. Perrone HC, dos Santos DR, Santos MV, et al. Urolithiasis in childhood: metabolic evaluation. Pediatr Nephrol. 1992;6(1):54-6.
33. Spivacow FR, Negri AL, del Valle EE, et al. Metabolic risk factors in children with kidney stone disease. Pediatr Nephrol. 2008;23(7):1129-33.
34. Defoor W, Asplin J, Jackson E, et al. Results of a prospective trial to compare normal urine supersaturation in children and adults. J Urol. 2005;174(4 Pt 2):1708-10.
35. Miyake O, Kakimoto K, Tsujihata M,et al. Strong inhibition of crystal-cell attachment by pediatric urinary macromolecules: a close relationship with high urinary citrate secretion. Urology. 2001;58(3):493-7.
36. Miyake O, Yoshimura K, Yoshioka T, et al. High urinary excretion level of citrate and magnesium in children: potential etiology for the reduced incidence of pediatric urolithiasis. Urol Res. 1998;26(3):209-13.
37. Pearle MS, Goldfarb DS, Assimos DG, et al. Medical management of kidney stones: AUA guideline. J Urol. 2014;192(2):316-24.
38. Paterson A, Frush DP, Donnelly LF. Helical CT of the body: are settings adjusted for pediatric patients? Am J Roentgenol. 2001;176(2):297-301.
39. Brenner D, Elliston C, Hall E, et al. Estimated risks of radiation-induced fatal cancer from pediatric CT. Am J Roentgenol. 2001;176(2):289-96.
40. Katz SI, Saluja S, Brink JA, et al. Radiation dose associated with unenhanced CT for suspected renal colic: impact of repetitive studies. Am J Roentgenol. 2006;186(4):1120-4.
41. Kuhns LR, Oliver WJ, Christodoulou E, et al. The predicted increased cancer risk associated with a single computed tomography examination for calculus detection in pediatric patients compared with the natural cancer incidence. Pediatr Emerg Care. 2011;27(4):345-50.
42. Hahn B, Dima J, Hirschorn D, et al. Incidence and pathology of repeat computed tomography of the abdomen and pelvis in a pediatric emergency department population. Pediatr Emerg Care. 2013;29(7):822-5.
43. Fowler KA, Locken JA, Duchesne JH, et al. US for detecting renal calculi with nonenhanced CT as a reference standard. Radiology. 2002;222(1):109-13.
44. Passerotti C, Chow JS, Silva A, et al. Ultrasound versus computerized tomography for evaluating urolithiasis. J Urol. 2009;182(4 Suppl):1829-34.
45. Johnson EK, Faerber GJ, Roberts WW, et al. Are stone protocol computed tomography scans mandatory for children with suspected urinary calculi? Urology. 2011;78(3):662-6.
46. Smith-Bindman R, Aubin C, Bailitz J, et al. Ultrasonography versus computed tomography for suspected nephrolithiasis. New Engl J Med. 201418;371(12):1100-10.
47. Fulgham PF, Assimos DG, Pearle MS, et al. Clinical effectiveness protocols for imaging in the management of ureteral calculous disease: AUA technology assessment. J Urol. 2013;189(4):1203-13.
48. Ziemba JB, Canning DA, Lavelle J, et al. Patient and institutional characteristics associated with initial CT use for children presenting to the emergency department with kidney stones. J Urol. 2014. May;193(5 Suppl):1848-53.
49. Maalouf NM, Langston JP, Van Ness PC, et al. Nephrolithiasis in topiramate users. Urol Res. 2011;39(4):303-7.
50. Sampath A, Kossoff EH, Furth SL, et al. Kidney stones and the ketogenic diet: risk factors and prevention. J Child Neurol. 2007;22(4):375-8.
51. Ali SKM. Renal calculi complicating short-term furosemide therapy after congenital heart surgery. Congenit Heart Dis. 2006;1(5):251-3.
52. Alon US, Scagliotti D, Garola RE. Nephrocalcinosis and nephrolithiasis in infants with congestive heart failure treated with furosemide. J Pediatr. 1994;125(1):149-51.
53. Youth Risk Behavior Surveillance System. National Center for Chronic Disease Prevention and Health Promotion; 2008 Available from http://apps.nccd.cdc.gov/yrbss/SelQuestyear.asp?cat=5&desc=Dietary%20Behaviors&loc=SC [Accessed May 2008].
54. Keller KL, Kirzner J, Pietrobelli A, et al. Increased sweetened beverage intake is associated with reduced milk and calcium intake in 3- to 7-year-old children at multi-item laboratory lunches. J Am Diet Assoc. 2009;109(3):497-501.
55. Rajeshwari R, Yang SJ, Nicklas TA, et al. Secular trends in children's sweetened-beverage consumption (1973 to 1994): the Bogalusa Heart Study. J Am Diet Assoc. 2005;105(2):208-14.
56. Madore F, Stampfer MJ, Rimm EB, et al. Nephrolithiasis and risk of hypertension. Am J Hypertens. 1998;11(1 Pt 1):46-53.
57. Negri AL, Spivacow R, Del Valle E, et al. Clinical and biochemical profile of patients with "pure" uric acid nephrolithiasis compared with "pure" calcium oxalate stone formers. Urol Res. 2007;35(5):247-51.
58. Taylor EN, Stampfer MJ, Curhan GC. Obesity, weight gain, and the risk of kidney stones. JAMA. 2005;293(4):455-62.

59. Kieran K, Giel DW, Morris BJ, et al. Pediatric urolithiasis—does body mass index influence stone presentation and treatment? J Urol. 2010;184(4 Suppl):1810-5.
60. Kim SS, Luan X, Canning DA, et al. Association between body mass index and urolithiasis in children. J Urol. 2011;186(4 Suppl):1734-9.
61. Mir S, Serdaroglu E. Quantification of hypercalciuria with the urine calcium osmolality ratio in children. Pediatr Nephrol. 2005;20(11):1562-5.
62. Srivastava T, Winston MJ, Auron A, et al. Urine calcium/citrate ratio in children with hypercalciuric stones. Pediatr Res. 2009;66(1):85-90.
63. Remer T, Neubert A, Maser-Gluth C. Anthropometry-based reference values for 24-h urinary creatinine excretion during growth and their use in endocrine and nutritional research. Am J Clin Nutr. 2002;75(3):561-9.
64. Sawyer MD, Dietrich MS, Pickens RB, et al. Adequate or not? A comparison of 24-hour urine studies for renal stone prevention by creatinine to weight ratio. J Endourol. 2013;27(3):366-9.
65. Sikora P, Zajaczkowska M, Hoppe B. Assessment of crystallization risk formulas in pediatric calcium stone-formers. Pediatr Nephrol. 2009;24(10):1997-2003.
66. DeFoor W, Minevich E, Jackson E, et al. Urinary metabolic evaluations in solitary and recurrent stone forming children. J Urol. 2008;179(6):2369-72.
67. Asplin J, Parks J, Lingeman J, et al. Supersaturation and stone composition in a network of dispersed treatment sites. J Urol. 1998;159(6):1821-5.
68. Hoppe B, Jahnen A, Bach D, et al. Urinary calcium oxalate saturation in healthy infants and children. J Urol. 1997;158(2):557-9.
69. Borghi L, Schianchi T, Meschi T, et al. Comparison of two diets for the prevention of recurrent stones in idiopathic hypercalciuria. New Engl J Med. 2002;346(2):77-84.
70. Ghazali S, Barratt TM. Urinary excretion of calcium and magnesium in children. Arch Dis Child. 1974;49(2):97-101.
71. Sargent JD, Stukel TA, Kresel J, et al. Normal values for random urinary calcium to creatinine ratios in infancy. J Pediatr. 1993;123(3):393-7.
72. Kirejczyk JK, Porowski T, Konstantynowicz J, et al. Urinary citrate excretion in healthy children depends on age and gender. Pediatr Nephrol. 2014;29(9):1575-82.
73. Edvardsson VO, Goldfarb DS, Lieske JC, et al. Hereditary causes of kidney stones and chronic kidney disease. Pediatr Nephrol. 2013;28(10):1923-42.
74. Knoll T, Zollner A, Wendt-Nordahl G, et al. Cystinuria in childhood and adolescence: recommendations for diagnosis, treatment, and follow-up. Pediatr Nephrol. 2005;20(1):19-24.
75. Matos V, van Melle G, Boulat O, et al. Urinary phosphate/creatinine, calcium/creatinine, and magnesium/creatinine ratios in a healthy pediatric population. J Pediatr. 1997;131(2):252-7.
76. Matos V, Van Melle G, Werner D, et al. Urinary oxalate and urate to creatinine ratios in a healthy pediatric population. Am J Kidney Dis. 1999;34(2):e1.
77. Alon US. Medical treatment of pediatric urolithiasis. Pediatr Nephrol. 2009;24(11):2129-35.
78. Stapleton FB, Linshaw MA, Hassanein K, et al. Uric acid excretion in normal children. J Pediatr. 1978;92(6):911-4.
79. Lee TT, Elkoushy MA, Andonian S. Are stone analysis results different with repeated sampling? Can Urol Assoc J. 2014;8(5-6):E317-22.
80. Taylor EN, Curhan GC. Fructose consumption and the risk of kidney stones. Kidney Int. 2008;73(2):207-12.
81. Calcium: dietary supplement fact sheet. National Institutes of Health; 2013. Available from http://ods.od.nih.gov/factsheets/Calcium-HealthProfessional/#en1 [updated November 21, 2013; cited 2014 October 29, 2014]
82. Osorio AV, Alon US. The relationship between urinary calcium, sodium, and potassium excretion and the role of potassium in treating idiopathic hypercalciuria. Pediatrics. 1997;100(4):675-81.
83. Sakhaee K, Harvey JA, Padalino PK, et al. The potential role of salt abuse on the risk for kidney stone formation. J Urol. 1993;150(2 Pt 1):310-2.
84. Dietary Guidelines for Americans, 2010. In: Services. USDoAaUSDoHaH, editor. 7th edition. Washington, DC: US Government Printing Office; 2010.
85. Kovacevic L, Wolfe-Christensen C, Edwards L, et al. From hypercalciuria to hypocitraturia--a shifting trend in pediatric urolithiasis? J Urol. 2012;188(4 Suppl):1623-7.
86. Pinheiro VB, Baxmann AC, Tiselius HG, et al. The effect of sodium bicarbonate upon urinary citrate excretion in calcium stone formers. Urology. 2013;82(1):33-7.
87. Oguz U, Unsal A. The efficacy of medical prophylaxis in children with calcium oxalate urolithiasis after percutaneous nephrolithotomy. J Endourol. 2013;27(1):92-5.
88. Sarica K, Erturhan S, Yurtseven C, et al. Effect of potassium citrate therapy on stone recurrence and regrowth after extracorporeal shockwave lithotripsy in children. J Endourol. 2006;20(11):875-9.
89. Tekin A, Tekgul S, Atsu N, et al. Oral potassium citrate treatment for idiopathic hypocitruria in children with calcium urolithiasis. J Urol. 2002;168(6):2572-4.
90. Kurtz MP, Eisner BH. Dietary therapy for patients with hypocitraturic nephrolithiasis. Nat Rev Urol. 2011;8(3):146-52.
91. Haleblian GE, Leitao VA, Pierre SA, et al. Assessment of citrate concentrations in citrus fruit-based juices and beverages: implications for management of hypocitraturic nephrolithiasis. J Endourol. 2008;22(6):1359-66.
92. Penniston KL, Nakada SY, Holmes RP, et al. Quantitative assessment of citric acid in lemon juice, lime juice, and commercially-available fruit juice products. J Endourol. 2008;22(3):567-70.
93. Meschi T, Maggiore U, Fiaccadori E, et al. The effect of fruits and vegetables on urinary stone risk factors. Kidney Int. 2004;66(6):2402-10.
94. Barcelo P, Wuhl O, Servitge E, et al. Randomized double-blind study of potassium citrate in idiopathic hypocitraturic calcium nephrolithiasis. J Urol. 1993;150(6):1761-4.
95. Hallson PC, Rose GA, Sulaiman S. Raising urinary citrate lowers calcium oxalate and calcium phosphate crystal formation in whole urine. Urol Int. 1983;38(3):179-81.

96. Reilly RF, Peixoto AJ, Desir GV. The evidence-based use of thiazide diuretics in hypertension and nephrolithiasis. Clin J Am Soc Nephrol. 2010;5(10):1893-903.
97. Choi JN, Lee JS, Shin JI. Low-dose thiazide diuretics in children with idiopathic renal hypercalciuria. Acta Paediatr. 2011;100(8):e71-4.
98. Reusz GS, Dobos M, Tulassay T, et al. Hydrochlorothiazide treatment of children with hypercalciuria: effects and side effects. Pediatr Nephrol. 1993;7(6):699-702.
99. Penido MG, Lima EM, Marino VS, et al. Bone alterations in children with idiopathic hypercalciuria at the time of diagnosis. Pediatr Nephrol. 2003;18(2):133-9.
100. Schwaderer AL, Cronin R, Mahan JD, et al. Low bone density in children with hypercalciuria and/or nephrolithiasis. Pediatr Nephrol. 2008;23(12):2209-14.
101. Micromedex 2.0. Truven Health Analytics Inc.; October 22, 2014. Available from http://www.micromedexsolutions.com/micromedex2/librarian/.
102. Knauf F, Ko N, Jiang Z, et al. Net intestinal transport of oxalate reflects passive absorption and SLC26A6-mediated secretion. J Am Soc Nephrol. 2011;22(12):2247-55.
103. Hatch M, Freel RW. The roles and mechanisms of intestinal oxalate transport in oxalate homeostasis. Semin Nephrol. 2008;28(2):143-51.
104. Sikora P, von Unruh GE, Beck B, et al. [13C2]oxalate absorption in children with idiopathic calcium oxalate urolithiasis or primary hyperoxaluria. Kidney Int. 2008;73(10):1181-6.
105. Attalla K, De S, Monga M. Oxalate content of food: a tangled web. Urology. 2014;84(3):555-60.
106. Combs AJ, Van Batavia JP, Chan J, et al. Dysfunctional elimination syndromes--how closely linked are constipation and encopresis with specific lower urinary tract conditions? J Urol. 2013;190(3):1015-20.
107. Dias CS, Silva JM, Diniz JS, et al. Risk factors for recurrent urinary tract infections in a cohort of patients with primary vesicoureteral reflux. Pediatr Infect Dis J. 2010;29(2):139-44.
108. Siener R, Schade N, Nicolay C, et al. The efficacy of dietary intervention on urinary risk factors for stone formation in recurrent calcium oxalate stone patients. J Urol. 2005;173(5):1601-5.

CHAPTER

25

Chronic Kidney Disease and Stone Disease

Andrew D Rule, John C Lieske

In the past few decades, there has been much interest in identifying and potentially modifying risk factors for chronic kidney disease (CKD). Kidney stones are common, and it would not seem surprising if they were in some manner associated with an increased risk of CKD. However, until recently the data linking these two conditions have been fairly limited. Much of the increased CKD risk among those with kidney stones has been attributed to shared features of the metabolic syndrome such as obesity, hypertension, and diabetes.[1] Although these metabolic derangements are common to both kidney stones and CKD, there is also an independent relationship between the two conditions. In this chapter, studies will be reviewed that have advanced our understanding of kidney stone disease and how stones might potentially associate with renal function loss and end-stage renal disease (ESRD). We will specifically review and discuss risk factors for CKD that are enriched among patients with kidney stones.

KIDNEY STONES AS RISK FACTORS FOR CKD

There are several important methodological concerns that need consideration when assessing the relationship between kidney stones and CKD. Most studies have been retrospective. This is of particular concern because the diagnostic evaluation for kidney stones can detect previously unrecognized CKD, and conversely the diagnostic evaluation of CKD can detect previously unrecognized kidney stones, thus inflating the strength of the association between these two conditions.[2] Furthermore, a decline in glomerular filtration rate (GFR), the principal component of a CKD diagnosis, may in fact be protective against kidney stones because low GFR leads to lower urine calcium, and hence decreases calcium oxalate and calcium phosphate supersaturation,[3] although the lower urine pH associated with CKD could increase uric acid supersaturation.[4] However, urine metabolic abnormalities, frequency of stone events, symptomatic versus asymptomatic stones, and stone composition are often not available in reports associating kidney stones and CKD. Finally, the high prevalence of comorbid conditions (such as diabetes, obesity, and hypertension) in stone formers who portend a higher risk for CKD can make the independent contribution of kidney stones to CKD difficult to detect. Many, but not all, of these concerns have been addressed in investigations on the relationship between kidney stones and CKD as described in the next sections.

A population-based historical cohort study assessed the risk of CKD among those with kidney stones using the Rochester Epidemiologic Project to match all 4,066 stone formers in Olmsted County, Minnesota to 10,150 controls.[5] Kidney stones and CKD were detected by diagnostic codes, and in a subset, a newly sustained (>3 months) elevated serum creatinine was also analyzed to detect CKD. Stone formers were more likely to have CKD risk factors such as diabetes, hypertension, and obesity. However, after adjusting for these comorbidities, stone formers had a 51–68% higher risk of CKD by diagnostic codes and 25–44% higher risk by chronically elevated serum creatinine levels. Whether diagnostic codes overestimate the risk of CKD due to detection bias, or instead better capture all CKD cases by detecting proteinuria among patients with normal serum creatinine levels, was unclear. The study found that the increased CKD risk among those with kidney stones was detected whether all subjects were followed for CKD events (to minimize selection bias), or only those with serum creatinine measurements were studied (to minimize detection bias).

Other recent studies are consistent with this report. In a large (N = 1,574,749) population-based cohort in England and Wales, a prediction model was developed that included kidney stones as a candidate predictor to estimate risk of pre-ESRD CKD.[6] The adjusted relative risk for CKD was 1.27 (1.11, 1.46) among women with history of kidney stones, although an association was not detected in men. Notably, only 0.68% of the subjects were identified as having a kidney stone, which is substantially lower than the

7–9% known prevalence of kidney stone disease,[7] raising concern about the accuracy of data where most kidney stone patients are missed. When 548 chart-confirmed cases of newly diagnosed CKD (defined by diagnostic codes and creatinine >1.5 mg/dL) were matched to community controls, after adjusting for comorbid conditions the odds ratio for CKD was 1.9 times higher among those with a self-reported history of kidney stones.[8] In a cross-sectional study of the Third National Health and Nutrition Examination Survey (NHANES III), 15,005 adult patients were included who completed a survey that included kidney stone history and whom also had a serum creatinine measurement.[9] A history of stones was associated with a 3.4 mL/min/1.73 m^2 lower estimated GFR. A population-based survey in Thailand also detected an increased adjusted risk of CKD in the 5% with a reported history of kidney stones [odd ratio (OR) = 2.7].[10]

Besides identifying kidney stones by their symptomatic passage events, other investigations have assessed the risk of CKD with radiographic presence of stones. A population-based Chinese study assessed predictors of prevalent CKD. All 2554 participants underwent a renal ultrasound that detected kidney stones in 56 (2.2%). These sonographic stones were associated with CKD (OR = 2.6).[11]

KIDNEY STONES AS RISK FACTORS FOR ESRD

The clinical relevance of mild-moderate CKD in many kidney stone formers is itself uncertain. Furthermore, the prognosis of CKD may differ among patients with CKD, primarily from their kidney stones rather than from other conditions (such as diabetes). Of particular interest is whether there is a risk of progression to ESRD among patients with kidney stones.

To address this question, a cohort study of the Olmsted County general population evaluated the risk of ESRD in stone formers compared to matched controls with up to 25 years of follow-up.[2] Not only were stone formers identified by diagnostic codes ($N = 6{,}911$), but in subset manual chart review was used to validate symptomatic stone formers ($N = 2{,}457$) and exclude those miscoded or who had merely incidental, asymptomatic stones. The risk of ESRD was about twofold higher in symptomatic stone formers (Fig. 25.1), and this risk remained even after adjustment for comorbidities and baseline presence of CKD. Stone formers who developed ESRD were, as expected, more likely to have ESRD attributed to stones, but also were more likely to have ESRD that was attributed to other urological conditions. For example, stone formers with ESRD had more recurrent urinary tract infections, ileal conduits, neurogenic bladders, and documented hydronephrosis compared to controls who developed ESRD (Table 25.1). Another cohort study, this time in Canada, utilized the Alberta Kidney Disease Network database to identify stone formers by diagnostic codes in a limited time window.[12] Only 0.8% of the sample were identified as stone formers rather than the expected 7–9%, raising a question regarding the sensitivity of the codes for identifying stone formers over a short period. Nevertheless, in this large sample

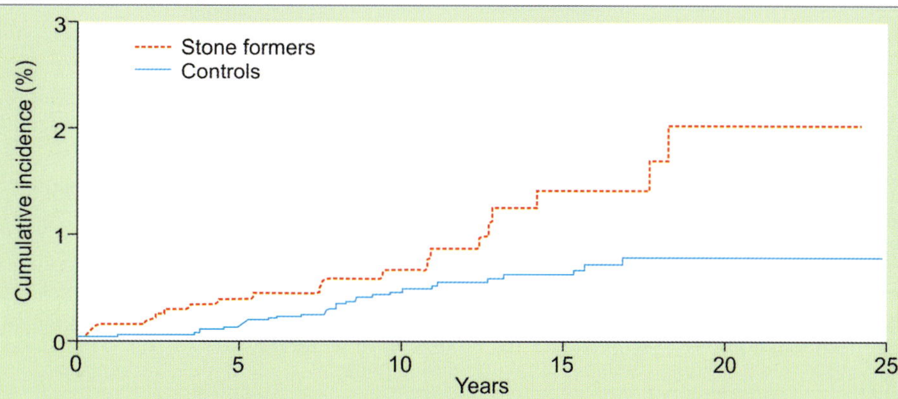

Incidence (no. at risk)						
Controls	0 (8,711)	0.1 (6,797)	0.4 (3,904)	0.6 (2,069)	0.8 (808)	0.8 (7)
Stone formers	0 (2,453)	0.4 (2,004)	0.6 (1,177)	1.2 (639)	2 (250)	2 (4)

Fig. 25.1: The cumulative end-stage renal disease incidence in symptomatic stone formers compared to controls.
Source: Reproduced from El-Zoghby ZM, Lieske JC, Foley RN, et al. Urolithiasis and the risk of ESRD. Clin J Am Soc Nephrol. 2012; 7:1409-15.

Table 25.1: Characteristics of incident ESRD among validated symptomatic stone formers compared to ESRD among control subjects in Olmsted County, MN.

	Stone formers who developed ESRD (n = 34)	*Controls who developed ESRD (n = 75)*	*P-value (Fischer's exact test)*
Primary cause of ESRD			
Diabetes mellitus	6 (18%)	22 (29%)	0.24
Hypertension	6 (18%)	13 (17%)	1.0
Glomerulonephritis	4 (12%)	10 (13%)	1.0
Cystic kidney disease	2 (6%)	3 (4%)	0.64
Urolithiasis	4 (12%)	0 (0)	0.008
Other urologic disease	6 (18%)	3 (4%)	0.03
Other known cause	4 (12%)	19 (25%)	0.13
Unknown cause	2 (6%)	5 (7%)	1.0
Comorbidities present prior to onset of ESRD			
Diabetes mellitus	11 (32%)	37 (49%)	0.14
Hypertension	15 (44%)	39 (52%)	0.54
Recurrent urinary tract infections	9 (26%)	3 (4%)	0.001
Acquired single kidney	5 (15%)	2 (3%)	0.03
Ileal conduit	3 (9%)	0 (0%)	0.03
Neurogenic bladder	4 (12%)	1 (1%)	0.03
Hydronephrosis	15 (44%)	3 (4%)	<0.001

(ESRD: End-stage renal disease).

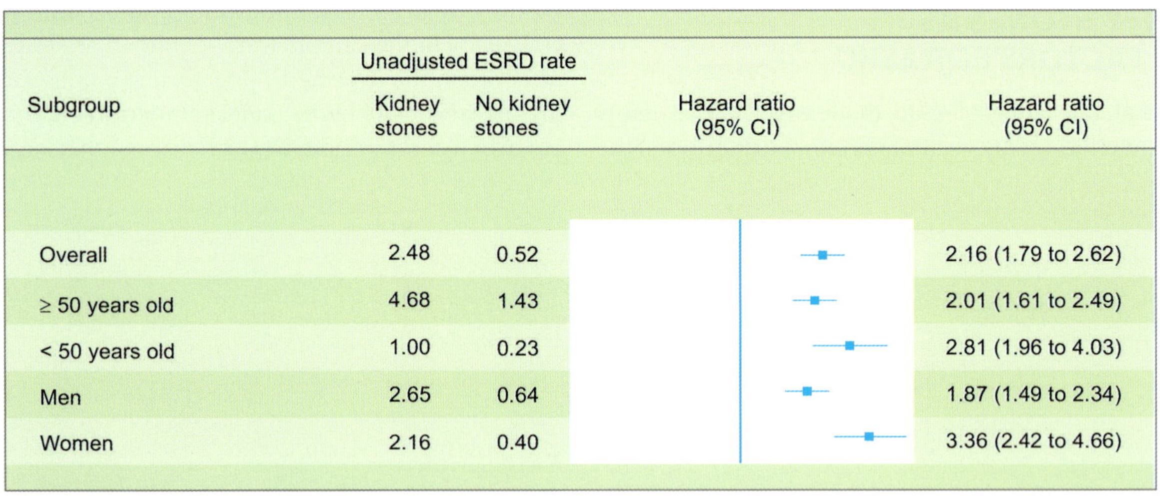

Fig. 25.2: Forest plot of multivariable adjusted hazard ratios for end-stage renal disease (ESRD) risk with nephrolithiasis overall and in age and gender subgroups. (CI: Confidence interval).
Source: Modified from Alexander RT, Hemmelgarn BR, Wiebe N, et al. Kidney stones and kidney function loss: a cohort study. BMJ. 2012;345:e5287

size (N = 3,089,194), the risk of ESRD among stone formers was about twofold higher than nonstone formers, and these associations were independent of other comorbid conditions (Fig. 25.2).

When 300 African American hemodialysis patients in a Chicago network were surveyed, 8% reported a history of kidney stones, more than double of that reported by the 5,341 African Americans who participated in the NHANES

III survey (3%).[13] Only two of the 25 stone formers with ESRD had it attributed to kidney stones. A more recent NHANES survey (2007–2010) found a higher risk of CKD and ESRD in stone formers compared to nonstone formers, although these associations were only statistically significant in women.[14]

To put the public health relevance of stone-related ESRD into perspective, the attributable risk ESRD from kidney stones is 5%,[2] which represents a small but relevant contribution to the burden of ESRD. End-stage renal disease thought to be due primarily to kidney stones is less. A study in France carefully evaluated the cause of ESRD in a cohort of 1,391 patients with ESRD starting hemodialysis.[15] The authors identified 45 patients (3.2%) with nephrolithiasis as the exclusive or primary cause of ESRD. Another study found that 2.1% of ESRD patients could primarily attribute their kidney failure to the kidney stones.[16] Interestingly, the United States Renal Data System (USRDS) survey found only 0.2% of ESRD cases were attributed primarily to kidney stones.[17] This suggests that while kidney stones contribute to the risk of ESRD, they may not be always recognized as a primary or even important contributor to ESRD. Stone recurrence rates appear to be lower in stone formers with a reduced GFR.[18] Indeed, among 25 stone formers who developed ESRD, only five had a stone episode within 5 years of starting dialysis.[13]

It should also be noted that several studies have found the risk of CKD and ESRD with kidney stones appears to be stronger in women than in men. [6,12,14,15] The reasons for this are not clear but may be related to parenchymal-damaging urinary tract infections that are more common in women and are associated with kidney stones, particularly struvite stones.

RISK OF CKD BY STONE CHARACTERISTICS

Few studies have characterized the stone-specific CKD risk factors among symptomatic stone formers. Indeed, symptomatic stone formers appear to be at higher risk for CKD, whereas the presence of asymptomatic stones does not clearly increase CKD risk.[19] A nested case-control study in Olmsted County, Minnesota identified 53 community stone formers who developed CKD matched to 106 controls who did not develop CKD. Hypertension, diabetes, frequent urinary tract infections, allopurinol therapy, and struvite stone composition were risk factors for CKD. However, the phenotype of the stone formers was incompletely defined since only half had ever had stone composition analysis and even fewer had urinary studies for stone risk factors.[20] When 24-hour creatinine clearance of 1,856 stone formers seen in a stone clinic was compared to 153 normal subjects, cystine stone formers had the lowest kidney function.[21] Uric acid, calcium oxalate, apatite, and struvite stone formers also had a lower creatinine clearance than normal subjects. Patient groups with specific comorbidities that increase stone risk, including bowel disease, surgical bypass for obesity, and renal tubular acidosis, were also more likely to have a lower creatinine clearance than normal subjects.[21]

Certain stone compositions are thought to more strongly associate with CKD. A retrospective study found CKD to be more common among stone formers with lower urine pH and uric acid stones, and less common among stone formers with calcium phosphate stones.[22] Whether the association with uric acid stone composition relates to presence of the metabolic syndrome, since hyperuricemia is a risk factor for CKD, or perhaps parenchymal injury from uric acid stones and/or crystals, is unclear. Infected struvite stones can also grow into large staghorn calculi and may present with CKD, likely due to obstruction and inflammation. A study in Taiwan further found that patients with both struvite and uric acid kidney stones were more likely to have CKD.[23] Another study identified both struvite and calcium as the most common compositions among stone formers who developed ESRD.[15] Since calcium stones are also much more common than any other stone composition, this should not be interpreted as calcium stones being more associated with ESRD.

About 40% of stone formers who developed ESRD had a solitary functioning kidney prior to developing ESRD.[15] The top three characteristics that lead to a solitary functioning kidney among stone formers are staghorn calculi or very high stone burden (29%), infection (23%), and ureteral obstruction (21%).[24] However, stone surgery was not a major cause of a solitary functioning kidney. Several studies have noted renal function deterioration after surgical intervention for kidney stones, but it is not clear whether the extent of the surgery versus the underlying CKD from the stone disease contributes to loss of renal function.[25] Furthermore, analysis from a tertiary stone clinic did not suggest that those with a solitary kidney had accelerated stone disease or loss of function.[26]

ACUTE KIDNEY INJURY WITH KIDNEY STONES

Few studies have defined the incidence and/or prevalence of kidney stone-associated acute kidney injury (AKI). Among 100 patients with community-acquired

AKI, obstruction from any cause was implicated in 17.[27] The Madrid acute renal failure study group also noted that obstruction from any cause accounted for 10% of community-acquired AKI, which translated to 23 cases per million population per year.[28] These data suggest that obstruction is more common than typically appreciated as a cause of AKI in the community. However, only a small subset (approximately 10–12%) of these community-acquired obstructive uropathy cases is deemed secondary to urolithiasis.[28,29] In a retrospective analysis of approximately 2,000 adults presenting with ureteral stones, AKI was evident upon presentation in only 0.72%.[30] Those with AKI were more likely to have bilateral ureteral stones that were larger (1.05 ± 0.34 cm *vs* 0.82 ± 0.40 cm), pre-existing CKD, or the presence of a solitary kidney.[30] In a group of pediatric AKI patients, obstructing stones were cited as a contributing cause in up to 30%, suggesting that urolithiasis may be a particularly important factor in community-acquired AKI that occurs in children.[31]

Urolithiasis-associated AKI appears to have a relatively good prognosis as long as the obstruction is promptly relieved. In a group of 93 children who presented with obstruction attributed to stones, full recovery of kidney function was observed in 57% with significant improvement in another 38%.[32] This study suggested that kidney function is more likely to recover if it is relieved quickly, since significant improvement was observed within 72 hours after relief of the obstruction in the vast majority (84%).[32] Many patients who present with obstructive uropathy may require short-term dialysis, although aggressive measures to relieve the obstruction can minimize this outcome. Even so, the ultimate extent of renal functional recovery appears to be determined by the completeness and duration of the obstruction, rather than the baseline level of kidney function on presentation, although infection is also an important comorbidity.[33,34] Diabetes and urinary tract infection appear to be the most highly predictive factors of renal function decline after a surgical intervention on a stone.[35]

Data from animal studies suggest that the severity of tubular atrophy and interstitial fibrosis increases in a linear fashion in relation to the length of time an obstruction is present.[33] However, some damage may occur even with brief obstruction, since even a 24-hour unilateral obstruction of a rat kidney leads to irreversible loss of 15% of the affected nephrons.[36] The kidney responds to increased intratubular pressure with vasoconstriction and inflammation.[37-39] In turn, increasing renal perfusion leads to ischemia,[40] with the long-term result being nephrosclerosis (glomerulosclerosis, tubular atrophy, and interstitial fibrosis). Renal biopsies of patients with large staghorn stones reveal extensive inflammation with macrophage infiltration and mesenchymal epithelial cell transition.[41] It is unclear if infection and/or ischemia drive the inflammatory response. To some extent, the remaining functional nephrons can hyperfilter to compensate for this nephrosclerosis, leading to no detectable GFR decline in the short term, but in longer term this process can itself promote nephrosclerosis and worsening CKD.[42]

Clinical features can be used to predict the likelihood of renal recovery after obstruction-associated AKI. In a cohort of 76 patients followed for a mean of 61 months after iatrogenic ureteral obstruction, multivariable models suggested that the time between onset of obstruction and its relief was the only significant predictor of outcome.[34] Furthermore, if the obstruction was relieved within 2 weeks there was no evidence of any long-term renal damage.[34] Conversely, if repair was delayed for >2 weeks, the renal outcome became progressively worse the longer this time became. In this study, the ratio of epidermal growth factor to monocyte chemotactic peptide-1 in the urine measured just 4 weeks after the obstruction was relieved correlated with long-term outcome.[34] These results suggest that biological events in the obstructive kidney that determine long-term outcome are activated quite early in the process. Data from a recent study were used to develop a model that projects the likelihood of recovery after relief of obstructive uropathy. In a cohort of 167 patients, ureteroscopy or percutaneous nephrolithotomy (PCNL) was used to treat patients with bilateral obstruction due to stones. Creatinine was quite elevated (7.3 ± 4.4 mg/dL) at presentation. Even so, only 20% progressed to kidney failure within 1 year. In a multiple logistic stepwise progression model, significant predictors of kidney function loss during the first year included renal cortical thinning, the presence of proteinuria, a lower estimated GFR within 5 days after relief of obstruction, and the presence of a positive urine culture.[43]

Pyelonephritis associated with infected struvite stones can also damage the renal parenchyma and favor eventual ESRD.[44,45] Large staghorn calculi in struvite stone formers can cause papillary necrosis.[46] Besides ongoing damage from bacteria and the response to them, the high urine pH caused by urea-splitting organisms could also potentially injure the kidney.

LONG-TERM EFFECTS OF STONE REMOVAL PROCEDURES

Open nephrolithotomy has long been associated with long-term kidney damage. However, newer, less-invasive treatments are not thought to be associated with permanent renal injury. In particular, PCNL has not been associated with adverse renal outcome, either long or short term.[47] Patients who receive ureteroscopic or percutaneous procedures for stone removal are at higher risk for CKD,[48] but this likely reflects a severe stone burden that in turn influences the choice of surgical intervention. Conversely, the presence of underlying CKD appears to impact the course when stones are surgically removed, since the length of hospitalization and complication rates were both increased in PCNL patients with baseline stage 4 or 5 CKD.[49]

The long-term effects of shockwave lithotripsy (SWL) on the kidney are more controversial. Studies in animals and patients clearly demonstrate short-term structural and functional changes to kidneys. Indeed, hematoma development is universally observed.[50-52] However, there appears to be little evidence of lasting kidney damage when reexamined 1–3 months later.[50,53,54] One study actually found that removing nonobstructing stones in stone formers with extracorporeal SWL delayed the rate of kidney function decline.[55] Previously, SWL was associated with new onset hypertension, exacerbation of stone disease, or even the development of diabetes.[56] However, these findings were not confirmed in larger and more recent population-based cohort studies in which neither hypertension[57] nor diabetes[58] was more common in kidney stone patients who received SWL.

Patients occasionally require nephrectomy for management of large obstructing stones. There has been concern about the effect that kidney loss might have on the remaining kidney, and whether or not ongoing damage and obstruction from stones might potentially predispose such individuals to ESRD. Not surprisingly, 24-hour creatinine clearance was significantly lower in a recent study of 20 stone patients who underwent nephrectomy.[59] Women comprised the vast majority of the nephrectomy patients (17/20), perhaps because concurrent pyelonephritis is an indication for nephrectomy.[59] A retrospective analysis of outcomes covering three decades of clinical experience in a tertiary kidney stone clinic did not reveal evidence that stone patients with a solitary kidney continued to lose kidney function or develop increased metabolic stone-forming activity.[26] In this series, women were also overrepresented in the nephrectomized group (50%) compared to the overall stone clinic population (34%).

Many studies have been performed to delineate the mechanism of renal damage associated with urinary tract obstruction, which appears to be related to changes in renal perfusion. Unilateral obstruction of the ureter increases pressure in renal tubules; intense vasoconstriction and a rapid fall in renal blood flow and GFR ensue.[60] If this obstruction persists, interstitial fibrosis and loss of nephrons follow with the long-term outcome of chronic kidney disease.[61]

CRYSTALLINE NEPHROPATHY

Acute kidney injury among those with nephrolithiasis is most commonly attributed to mechanical obstruction. However, crystalline nephropathy can occur under certain circumstances where rapid and extensive crystallization occludes the nephron. Examples include acute uric acid nephropathy, most commonly observed in the setting of tumor lysis;[62] acute phosphate nephropathy observed after use of phosphate containing cathartics;[63-65] and precipitation of certain poorly soluble drugs (e.g. triamterene, acyclovir, and indinavir).[66-68] Crystalline nephropathy has also been observed in certain genetic disorders associated with overproduction of poorly soluble metabolites, including cystine (cystinuria)[69] and dihydroxyadenine (adenine phosphoribosyltransferase) deficiency.[70]

Acute oxalate nephropathy, manifested by tubular plugging with calcium oxalate crystals, can also occur under conditions of marked overproduction of oxalate (primary hyperoxaluria),[71] overabsorption of oxalate in association with chronic fat malabsorption (enteric hyperoxaluria),[72] overdose of vitamin C,[73] overingestion of oxalate-rich foods,[74] or intoxication with ethylene glycol.[75] Patients with pre-existing CKD may be more likely to develop superimposed oxalate nephropathy under the right circumstances.[76] Once it develops, oxalate nephropathy in the setting of baseline CKD often leads to irreversible kidney damage. In this recent series only about one quarter of patients experienced significant functional recovery after the initial injury.[76]

Acute uric acid nephropathy is most commonly observed after initiation of chemotherapy for lymphoproliferative disorders.[77,78] Uric acid nephropathy has also been reported in association with the inborn error of metabolism hypoxanthine guanine phosphoribosyltransferase deficiency (Lesch–Nyhan syndrome)[79] or in the setting of genetic or acquired impairment of urate in the proximal tubule.[62] Among those individuals with familial renal hypouricemia, vigorous exercise is often a precipitating factor.[62] Acute uric acid nephropathy often has a better outcome than oxalate nephropathy and resolves when treated by aggressive volume expansion, alkalinization of the urine, and xanthine oxidase inhibitors (allopurinol, febuxostat).[77,78] Somewhat paradoxically, it is important to note that high doses of xanthine oxidase inhibitors can increase levels of xanthine, which is also poorly soluble and can crystallize in the kidney.[80,81] Uric acid stone formers may also have a subacute crystalline nephropathy with uric acid deposits within the medulla associated with an inflammatory reaction and eventual interstitial fibrosis.[82] Hyperuricemia is also an independent CKD risk factor that may involve other noncrystal-mediated mechanisms, but whether or not this is along the same pathway as uric acid stone-induced CKD is unclear.[83,84]

A select group of medications are both excreted via the urinary tract and relatively poorly soluble in urine. Examples include acyclovir, sulfonamide antibiotics, methotrexate, and indinavir. More recently, melamine-induced AKI was reported in animals exposed to tainted pet food and babies exposed to tainted baby formula.[85] In children, the mean time from initial exposure to the tainted formula to onset of renal disease was 9 months, and acidic urine pH appeared to be an important cofactor that favored melamine crystallization, deposition in the urinary tract, and resulting AKI.[85] More analogous to uric acid nephropathy than oxalate nephropathy, melamine-induced renal damage appears to be relatively reversible and long-term renal outcomes have been reported to be good.[86]

A body of literature suggests that renal tubular cells interact with urinary crystals, and these events might also precipitate chronic renal damage. For example, renal tubular cells avidly bind calcium oxalate crystals, both in cell culture[87] and in animal models.[88] Once adherent, the cells phagocytose these crystals to eventually lie within endosomes.[89] Smaller crystals may dissolve in endosomes.[90] Exposure of cells to crystals is associated with altered gene expression,[91] proliferation,[90] and possibly apoptotic cell death.[92] These earlier observations had been recently extended to demonstrate that calcium oxide crystals can activate the innate immunity response in the intracellular inflammasome.[93,94] In a mouse model of acute oxalate poisoning, resulting intrajugular and interstitial calcium oxalate crystals triggered a diffuse interstitial neutrophilic infiltration and surrounding tubular necrosis.[93] Strong evidence implicates a role for the NLPR3 inflammasome in this response, including secretion of the inflammatory cytokines interleukin (IL)-1β and IL-18. Furthermore, use of an IL-1 antagonist markedly abated tubular injury and neutrophil accumulation with a resulting improvement in kidney function. These studies suggest novel potential pathways to block oxalate and potentially other crystalline nephropathies.[93]

Exposure of renal cells to soluble oxalate can also trigger similar reactions.[92,95,96] Within the kidney in vivo, it remains unanswered whether pathologic changes associated with marked hyperoxaluria are the result of oxalate ion or calcium oxalate crystals. Similar renal tubular cell responses (adhesion internalization and altered gene expression) have been observed with hydroxyapatite crystals.[97] It remains equally unclear whether or not crystallization, adhesion, and internalization are occurring in the nephron frequently, or only in pathologic states of marked supersaturation. Interestingly, proximal tubular cells appear more susceptible to crystal adhesion than distal nephron cells.[98] Thus, cells most likely to encounter crystals (collecting duct cells) are least likely to bind them, while those that are more prone to crystal adhesion (proximal tubular cells) are only rarely exposed to supersaturated fluid and crystals. Recent studies suggest that the proximal tubule of patients with marked hyperoxaluria, namely patients with primary hyperoxaluria, might favor ongoing crystallization,[99] and indeed response to those calcium oxalate crystals that deposit there (as described above) might be an underlying mechanism that drives chronic kidney damage in this select population.

Aside from acute or chronic crystalline nephropathy, plugging at the level of ducts of Bellini could potentially cause a regional obstructive nephropathy. Certain types of stone formers, such as brushite and gastric bypass stone formers, appear more prone to such plugs.[100-102] Prominent ductal plugging has even been documented in a subset of idiopathic calcium oxalate stone formers.[103,104] Given that only 100 ducts of Bellini are available to drain each kidney, it is plausible that obstructive injury to these ducts can induce chronic parenchymal injury to substantial zones of a kidney, as has been suggested by one study of brushite stone formers.[102]

CONCLUSION

Multiple studies suggest that patients with nephrolithiasis have a higher incidence of both CKD as well as ESRD (Table 25.2). Many factors contribute to this association (Fig. 25.3). Certainly, the population of kidney stone

Table 25.2: Studies that associate CKD or ESRD with nephrolithiasis.

Study	*Design*	*Stone detection*	*Main results*
Rule et al.[5]	Population-based historical cohort in Olmsted County, MN, USA	Past and recent diagnostic codes	HR of 1.51–1.68 for CKD
Hippisley-Cox et al.[6]	Population-based historical cohort in UK	Recent diagnostic code	Relative risk of 1.27 for CKD among women; no association in men
Vupputuri et al.[8]	Case-control of newly diagnosed CKD in North Carolina, USA	Telephone interview	OR of 1.9 for CKD
Gillen et al.[9]	Cross sectional analysis of Third National Health and Nutrition Examination Survey (NHANES III), USA	Survey	eGFR lower by 3.4 mL/min/1.73 m^2 with stones
Ingsathit et al.[10]	Population-based Survey in Thailand	Survey	OR of 2.7 for CKD
Chen et al.[11]	Population-based cross-sectional study in China	Ultrasound	OR of 2.6 for CKD
El-Zhoghby et al.[2]	Population-based historical cohort in Olmsted County, MN, USA	Chart-validated	HR of 2.0 for ESRD
Alexander et al.[12]	Population based cohort in Alberta, Canada	Recent diagnostic code	HR of 2.2 for ESRD HR of 1.7 for CKD
Shoag et al.[14]	Cross-sectional analysis of NHANES 2007–2012, USA	Survey	HR of 2.4 for ESRD HR of 1.5 for CKD
Stankus et al.[13]	Survey of African American dialysis patients, Chicago, IL, USA; compared to NHANES III	Survey	Past stones in 8% of dialysis patients versus 3% in general population

(CKD: Chronic kidney disease; ESRD: End-stage renal disease; HR: Hazard ratio; OR: Odds ratio; eGFR: Estimated glomerular filtration rate; NHANES: National Health and Nutrition Examination Survey).

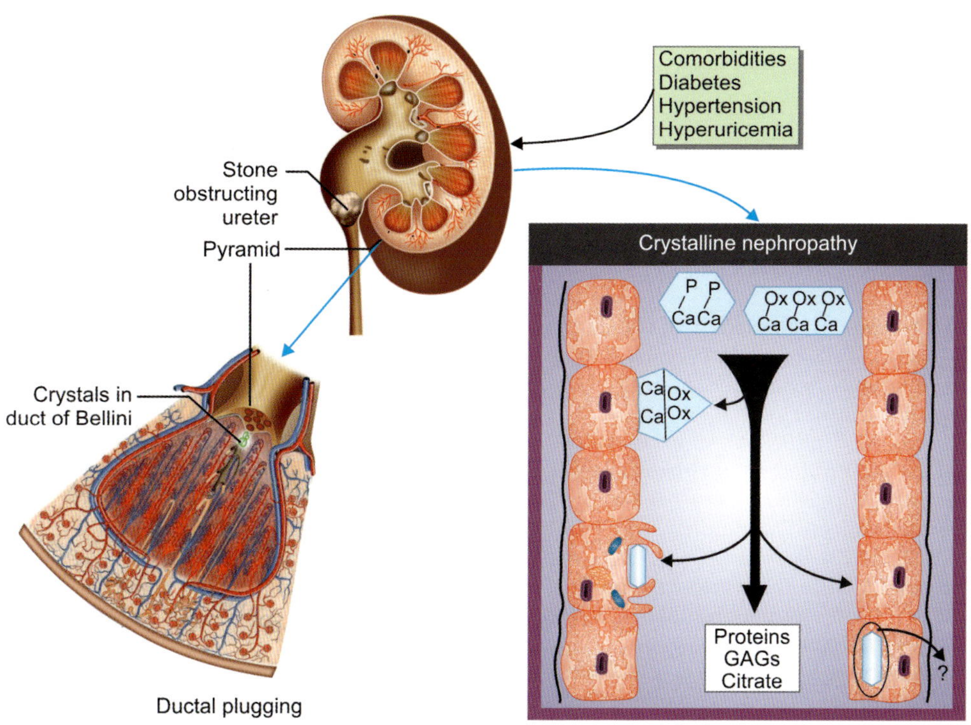

Fig. 25.3: Putative factors that contribute to chronic kidney disease (CKD) in stone formers. Comorbidities that are commonly associated with CKD are also enriched in stone formers, including diabetes, hypertension, and hyperuricemia. Obstructive uropathy from larger stones in the renal pelvis or ureter can damage kidneys, if not promptly relieved. Duct of Bellini plugging has also been described in certain populations of stone formers (e.g. brushite stone formers; patients with enteric hyperoxaluria), and could produce localized obstructive damage to populations of nephrons. A large literature describes the interaction of renal epithelial cells and urinary crystals, and recently it has been observed that crystal internalization could activate the inflammasome pathways. Whether ongoing crystalline nephropathy in the proximal tubule could be a factor and/or cofactor in CKD progression in certain populations of stone formers remains to be determined. (GAGs: Glycosaminoglycans).

formers is enriched with regard to known CKD risk factors such as diabetes and hypertension. Increased medical care and disease detection among the stone-forming population could also be a factor. However, studies that control for these potential confounders still report a significant and independent association between nephrolithiasis and CKD. Certain stone formers (e.g. those with brushite stones or enteric hyperoxaluria) may have pathology that favors duct of Bellini plugging, which results in kidney damage. Surgical treatment of stones, particularly open nephrolithotomy, could be a factor in some. Stone-associated urinary tract infection could be a factor in others. Crystalluria and the response of the kidney to crystal deposition appear to be important in certain circumstances (e.g. primary hyperoxaluria and uric acid nephropathy). Whether similar processes are ongoing within the kidney of more common stone formers remains to be seen.

REFERENCES

1. Sakhaee K. Nephrolithiasis as a systemic disorder. Curr Opin Nephrol Hypertens. 2008;17:304-09.
2. El-Zoghby ZM, Lieske JC, Foley RN, et al. Urolithiasis and the risk of ESRD. Clin J Am Soc Nephrol. 2012;7:1409-15.
3. Gershman B, Sheth S, Dretler SP, et al. Relationship between glomerular filtration rate and 24-hour urine composition in patients with nephrolithiasis. Urology. 2012;80:38-42.
4. Lush DJ, King JA, Fray JC. Pathophysiology of low renin syndromes: sites of renal renin secretory impairment and prorenin overexpression. Kidney Int. 1993;43:983-99.
5. Rule AD, Bergstralh EJ, Melton LJ, 3rd, et al. Kidney stones and the risk for chronic kidney disease. Clin J Am Soc Nephrol. 2009;4:804-11.
6. Hippisley-Cox J, Coupland C. Predicting the risk of chronic kidney disease in men and women in England and Wales: prospective derivation and external validation of the QKidney Scores. BMC Fam Pract. 2010;11:49.
7. Scales CD Jr, Smith AC, Hanley JM, et al. Prevalence of kidney stones in the United States. Eur Urol. 2012;62:160-5.
8. Vupputuri S, Soucie JM, McClellan W, et al. History of kidney stones as a possible risk factor for chronic kidney disease. Ann Epidemiol. 2004;14:222-8.
9. Gillen DL, Worcester EM, Coe FL. Decreased renal function among adults with a history of nephrolithiasis: a study of NHANES III. Kidney Int. 2005;67:685-90.
10. Ingsathit A, Thakkinstian A, Chaiprasert A, et al. Prevalence and risk factors of chronic kidney disease in the Thai adult population: Thai SEEK study. Nephrol Dial Transplant. 2010;25:1567-75.
11. Chen N, Wang W, Huang Y, et al. Community-based study on CKD subjects and the associated risk factors. Nephrol Dial Transplant. 2009;24:2117-23.
12. Alexander RT, Hemmelgarn BR, Wiebe N, et al. Kidney stones and kidney function loss: a cohort study. BMJ. 2012;345:e5287.
13. Stankus N, Hammes M, Gillen D, et al. African American ESRD patients have a high pre-dialysis prevalence of kidney stones compared to NHANES III. Urol Res. 2007;35:83-7.
14. Shoag J, Halpern J, Goldfarb DS, Eisner BH. Risk of chronic and end stage kidney disease in patients with nephrolithiasis. J Urol. 2014;192:1440-5.
15. Jungers P, Joly D, Barbey F, et al. ESRD caused by nephrolithiasis: prevalence, mechanisms, and prevention. Am J Kidney Dis. 2004;44:799-805.
16. Tosetto E, Graziotto R, Artifoni L, et al. Dent's disease and prevalence of renal stones in dialysis patients in Northeastern Italy. J Human Genet. 2006;51:25-30.
17. Collins AJ, Foley RN, Herzog C, et al. US renal data system 2010 annual data report. Am J Kidney Dis. 2011;57:A8, e1-526.
18. Marangella M, Bruno M, Cosseddu D, et al. Prevalence of chronic renal insufficiency in the course of idiopathic recurrent calcium stone disease: risk factors and patterns of progression. Nephron. 1990;54:302-6.
19. Lorenz EC, Lieske JC, Vrtiska TJ, et al. Clinical characteristics of potential kidney donors with asymptomatic kidney stones. Nephrol Dial Transplant. 2011;26:2695-700.
20. Saucier NA, Sinha MK, Liang KV, et al. Risk factors for CKD in persons with kidney stones: a case-control study in Olmsted County, Minnesota. Am J Kidney Dis. 2010;55:61-8.
21. Worcester EM, Parks JH, Evan AP, et al. Renal function in patients with nephrolithiasis. J Urol. 2006;176:600-03; discussion 603.
22. Kadlec AO, Greco KA, Fridirici ZC, et al. Effect of renal function on urinary mineral excretion and stone composition. Urology. 2011;78:744-7.
23. Chou YH, Chou WP, Liu ME, et al. Comparison of secondary signs as shown by unenhanced helical computed tomography in patients with uric acid or calcium ureteral stones. Kaohsiung J Med Sci. 2012;28:322-6.
24. Worcester E, Parks JH, Josephson MA, et al. Causes and consequences of kidney loss in patients with nephrolithiasis. Kidney Int. 2003;64:2204-13.
25. Kuzgunbay B, Gul U, Turunc T, et al. Long-term renal function and stone recurrence after percutaneous nephrolithotomy in patients with renal insufficiency. J Endourol. 2010;24:305-8.
26. Worcester E, Parks JH, Josephson MA, et al. Causes and consequences of kidney loss in patients with nephrolithiasis. Kidney Int. 2003;64:2204-13.
27. Kaufman J, Dhakal M, Patel B, et al. Community-acquired acute renal failure. Am J Kidney Dis. 1991; 17: 191-198.
28. Liano F, Pascual J. Epidemiology of acute renal failure: a prospective, multicenter, community-based study. Madrid Acute Renal Failure Study Group. Kidney Int. 1996;50:811-8.
29. Organ M, Norman RW. Acute reversible kidney injury secondary to bilateral ureteric obstruction. Can Urol Assoc J. 2011;5:392-6.
30. Wang SJ, Mu XN, Zhang LY, et al. The incidence and clinical features of acute kidney injury secondary to ureteral calculi. Urol Res. 2012;40:345-8.
31. Jamal A, Ramzan A. Renal and post-renal causes of acute renal failure in children. J Coll Physicians Surg Pak. 2004; 14:411-5.

32. Ziada AM, Sarhan OM, Habib EI, et al. Assessment of recoverability of kidney function in children with obstructive calcular anuria: multicenter study. J Pediatr Urol. 2011;7:252-6.
33. Chevalier RL, Thornhill BA, Chang AY. Unilateral ureteral obstruction in neonatal rats leads to renal insufficiency in adulthood. Kidney Int. 2000;58:1987-95.
34. Lucarelli G, Ditonno P, Bettocchi C, et al. Delayed relief of ureteral obstruction is implicated in the long-term development of renal damage and arterial hypertension in patients with unilateral ureteral injury. J Urol. 2013;189:960-5.
35. Ozden E, Mercimek MN, Bostanci Y, et al. Long-term outcomes of percutaneous nephrolithotomy in patients with chronic kidney disease: a single-center experience. Urology. 2012;79:990-4.
36. Bander SJ, Buerkert JE, Martin D, et al. Long-term effects of 24-hr unilateral ureteral obstruction on renal function in the rat. Kidney Int. 1985;28:614-20.
37. Klahr S. New insights into the consequences and mechanisms of renal impairment in obstructive nephropathy. Am J Kidney Dis. 1991;18:689-99.
38. Hwang SJ, Haas M, Harris HW Jr, et al. Transport defects of rabbit medullary thick ascending limb cells in obstructive nephropathy. J Clin Invest. 1993;91:21-8.
39. Ophascharoensuk V, Giachelli CM, Gordon K, et al. Obstructive uropathy in the mouse: role of osteopontin in interstitial fibrosis and apoptosis. Kidney Int. 1999;56:571-80.
40. Gaudio KM, Siegel NJ, Hayslett JP, et al. Renal perfusion and intratubular pressure during ureteral occlusion in the rat. Am J Physiol. 1980;238:F205-9.
41. Boonla C, Krieglstein K, Bovornpadungkitti S, et al. Fibrosis and evidence for epithelial-mesenchymal transition in the kidneys of patients with staghorn calculi. BJU Int. 2011;108:1336-45.
42. Brenner BM, Chertow GM. Congenital oligonephropathy: an inborn cause of adult hypertension and progressive renal injury? Curr Opin Nephrol Hypertens. 1993;2:691-5.
43. Mishra S, Sinha L, Ganesamoni R, et al. Renal deterioration index: preoperative prognostic model for renal functional outcome after treatment of bilateral obstructive urolithiasis in patients with chronic kidney disease. *Journal of endourology / Endourological Society* 2013; 27:1405-10.
44. Larsson PA, Cano M, Grenabo L, et al. Morphological lesions of the rat urinary tract induced by inoculation of mycoplasmas and other urinary tract pathogens. Urol Int. 1989; 44:210-7.
45. Gupta M, Bolton DM, Gupta PN, et al. Improved renal function following aggressive treatment of urolithiasis and concurrent mild to moderate renal insufficiency. J Urol. 1994;152:1086-90.
46. Gambaro G, Favaro S, D'Angelo A. Risk for renal failure in nephrolithiasis. Am J Kidney Dis. 2001;37:233-43.
47. Kartha G, Calle JC, Marchini GS, et al. Impact of stone disease: chronic kidney disease and quality of life. Urol Clin North Am. 2013;40:135-47.
48. Keller JJ, Chen YK, Lin HC. Association between chronic kidney disease and urinary calculus by stone location: a population-based study. BJU Int. 2012;110:E1074-8.
49. Sairam K, Scoffone CM, Alken P, et al. Percutaneous nephrolithotomy and chronic kidney disease: results from the CROES PCNL Global Study. J Urol. 2012;188:1195-200.
50. Fahmy N, Sener A, Sabbisetti V, et al. Urinary expression of novel tissue markers of kidney injury after ureteroscopy, shockwave lithotripsy, and in normal healthy controls. J Endourol. 2013;27:1455-62.
51. McAteer JA, Evan AP, Williams JC Jr, et al. Treatment protocols to reduce renal injury during shock wave lithotripsy. Curr Opin Urol. 2009;19:192-5.
52. Evan AP, Willis LR, Lingeman JE, et al. Renal trauma and the risk of long-term complications in shock wave lithotripsy. Nephron. 1998;78:1-8.
53. Sheir KZ, Gad HM. Prospective study of the effects of shock wave lithotripsy on renal function: role of post-shock wave lithotripsy obstruction. Urology. 2003;61:1102-6; discussion 1106.
54. Eassa WA, Sheir KZ, Gad HM, et al. Prospective study of the long-term effects of shock wave lithotripsy on renal function and blood pressure. J Urol. 2008;179:964-8; discussion 968-9.
55. Yoo DE, Han SH, Oh HJ, et al. Removal of kidney stones by extracorporeal shock wave lithotripsy is associated with delayed progression of chronic kidney disease. Yonsei Med J. 2012;53:708-14.
56. Krambeck AE, Gettman MT, Rohlinger AL, et al. Diabetes mellitus and hypertension associated with shock wave lithotripsy of renal and proximal ureteral stones at 19 years of followup. J Urol. 2006;175:1742-7.
57. Krambeck AE, Rule AD, Li X, et al. Shock wave lithotripsy is not predictive of hypertension among community stone formers at long-term followup. J Urol. 2011;185:164-9.
58. de Cogain M, Krambeck AE, Rule AD, et al. Shock wave lithotripsy and diabetes mellitus: a population-based cohort study. Urology. 2012;79:298-302.
59. Carvalho M, Martin RL, Passos RC, et al. Nephrectomy as a cause of chronic kidney disease in the treatment of urolithiasis: a case-control study. World J Urol. 2013;31:1141-5.
60. Hsu CH, Kurtz TW, Rosenzweig J, et al. Intrarenal hemodynamics and renal function in postobstructive uropathy. Invest Urol. 1978;15:348-51.
61. Tanner GA, Evan AP. Glomerular and proximal tubular morphology after single nephron obstruction. Kidney Int. 1989;36:1050-60.
62. Fathallah-Shaykh SA, Cramer MT. Uric acid and the kidney. Pediatric nephrology. 2014;29:999-1008.
63. Markowitz GS, Perazella MA. Acute phosphate nephropathy. Kidney Int. 2009;76:1027-34.
64. Patel V, Emmett M, Santa Ana CA, et al. Pathogenesis of nephrocalcinosis after sodium phosphate catharsis to prepare for colonoscopy: intestinal phosphate absorption and its effect on urine mineral and electrolyte excretion. Hum Pathol. 2007;38:193-4; author reply 194-5.

65. Beloosesky Y, Grinblat J, Weiss A, et al. Electrolyte disorders following oral sodium phosphate administration for bowel cleansing in elderly patients. Arch Int Med. 2003;163:803-8.
66. Nasr SH, Milliner DS, Wooldridge TD, et al. Triamterene crystalline nephropathy. Am J Kidney Dis. 2014;63:148-52.
67. Jao J, Wyatt CM. Antiretroviral medications: adverse effects on the kidney. Adv Chronic Kidney Dis. 2010;17:72-82.
68. Fleischer R, Johnson M. Acyclovir nephrotoxicity: a case report highlighting the importance of prevention, detection, and treatment of acyclovir-induced nephropathy. Case Rep Med. 2010;2010:602783.
69. Evan AP, Coe FL, Lingeman JE, et al. Renal crystal deposits and histopathology in patients with cystine stones. Kidney Int. 2006;69:2227-35.
70. Bollee G, Dollinger C, Boutaud L, et al. Phenotype and genotype characterization of adenine phosphoribosyltransferase deficiency. J Am Soc Nephrol. 2010;21:679-88.
71. Lieske JC, Spargo B, Toback FG. Endocytosis of calcium oxalate crystals and proliferation of renal tubular epithelial cells in a patient with type 1 primary hyperoxaluria. JUrol. 1992;148:1517-9.
72. Canos HJ, Hogg GA, Jeffery JR. Oxalate nephropathy due to gastrointestinal disorders. Can Med Assoc J. 1981;124:729-33.
73. Auer BL, Auer D, Rodgers AL. Relative hyperoxlauria, crystalluria and haematuria after megadose ingestion of vitamin C. Eur J Clin Invest. 1998;28:695-700.
74. Getting JE, Gregoire JR, Phul A, et al. Oxalate nephropathy due to 'juicing': case report and review. Am J Med. 2013;126:768-72.
75. Poldelski V, Johnson A, Wright S, et al. Ethylene glycol-mediated tubular injury: identification of critical metabolites and injury pathways. Am J Kidney Dis. 2001;38:339-48.
76. Nasr SH, D'Agati VD, Said SM, et al. Oxalate nephropathy complicating Roux-en-Y gastric bypass: an underrecognized cause of irreversible renal failure. Clin J Am Soc Nephrol. 2008;3:1676-83.
77. Locatelli F, Rossi F. Incidence and pathogenesis of tumor lysis syndrome. Contrib Nephrol. 2005;147:61-8.
78. Suh WM, Wainberg ZA, de Vos S, et al. Acute lymphoblastic leukemia presenting as acute renal failure. Nat Clin Pract Nephrol. 2007;3:106-10.
79. Pela I, Donati MA, Procopio E, et al. Lesch-Nyhan syndrome presenting with acute renal failure in a 3-day-old newborn. Pediatr Nephrol. 2008;23:155-8.
80. Sikora P, Pijanowska M, Majewski M, et al. Acute renal failure due to bilateral xanthine urolithiasis in a boy with Lesch-Nyhan syndrome. Pediatr Nephrol. 2006;21:1045-7.
81. LaRosa C, McMullen L, Bakdash S, et al. Acute renal failure from xanthine nephropathy during management of acute leukemia. Pediatr Nephrol. 2007;22:132-5.
82. Johnson RJ, Kivlighn SD, Kim YG, et al. Reappraisal of the pathogenesis and consequences of hyperuricemia in hypertension, cardiovascular disease, and renal disease. Am J Kidney Dis. 1999;33:225-34.
83. Weiner DE, Tighiouart H, Elsayed EF, Griffith JL, Salem DN, Levey AS. Uric acid and incident kidney disease in the community. Journal of the American Society of Nephrology : JASN. 2008;19:1204-11.
84. Obermayr RP, Temml C, Gutjahr G, et al. Elevated uric acid increases the risk for kidney disease. J Am Soc Nephrol. 2008;19:2407-13.
85. Bhalla V, Grimm PC, Chertow GM, et al. Melamine nephrotoxicity: an emerging epidemic in an era of globalization. Kidney Int. 2009;75:774-9.
86. Shang P, Chang H, Yue ZJ, et al. Acute kidney injury caused by consumption of melamine-contaminated infant formula in 47 children: a multi-institutional experience in diagnosis, treatment and follow-up. Urol Res. 2012;40:293-8.
87. Lieske JC, Swift HS, Martin T, et al. Renal epithelial cells rapidly bind and internalize calcium oxalate monohydrate crystals. Proc Natl Acad Sci USA. 1994;91:6987-91.
88. Khan SR. Calcium oxalate crystal interaction with renal tubular epithelium, mechanism of crystal adhesion and its impact on stone development. Urol Res. 1995;23:71-9.
89. Lieske JC, Walsh-Reitz MM, Toback FG. Calcium oxalate monohydrate crystals are endocytosed by renal epithelial cells and induce proliferation. Am J Physiol. 1992;262:F622-F630.
90. Lieske JC, Norris R, Swift H, et al. Adhesion, internalization and metabolism of calcium oxalate monohydrate crystals by renal epithelial cells. Kidney Int. 1997;52:1291-301.
91. Hammes MS, Lieske JC, Pawar S, et al. Calcium oxalate monohydrate crystals stimulate gene expression in renal epithelial cells. Kidney Int. 1995;48:501-9.
92. Khan SR, Byer KJ, Thamilselvan S, et al. Crystal-cell interaction and apoptosis in oxalate-associated injury of renal epithelial cells. J Am Soc Nephrol. 1999;10 Suppl 14:S457-463.
93. Mulay SR, Evan A, Anders HJ. Molecular mechanisms of crystal-related kidney inflammation and injury. Implications for cholesterol embolism, crystalline nephropathies and kidney stone disease. Nephrology, dialysis, transplantation : official publication of the European Dialysis and Transplant Association - European Renal Association. 2014;29:507-14.
94. Knauf F, Asplin JR, Granja I, Schmidt IM, Moeckel GW, David RJ, et al. NALP3-mediated inflammation is a principal cause of progressive renal failure in oxalate nephropathy. Kidney international. 2013;84:895-901.
95. Joshi S, Peck AB, Khan SR. NADPH oxidase as a therapeutic target for oxalate induced injury in kidneys. Oxid Med Cell Longev. 2013;2013:462361.
96. Koul H, Kennington L, Nair G, et al. Oxalate-induced initiation of DNA synthesis in LLC-PK1 cells, a line of renal epithelial cells. Biochem Biophys Res Commun. 1994;205:1632-7.
97. Lieske JC, Norris R, Toback FG. Adhesion of hydroxyapatite crystals to anionic sites on the surface of renal epithelial cells. Am J Physiol. 1997;273:F224-F233.
98. Verkoelen CF, van der Boom BG, Kok DJ, et al. Cell type-specific acquired protection from crystal adherence by renal tubule cells in culture. Kidney Int. 1999;55:1426-33.

99. Worcester EM, Evan AP, Coe FL, et al. A test of the hypothesis that oxalate secretion produces proximal tubule crystallization in primary hyperoxaluria type I. Am J Physiol Renal Physiol. 2013;305:F1574-1584.
100. Evan AP, Lingeman JE, Worcester EM, et al. Renal histopathology and crystal deposits in patients with small bowel resection and calcium oxalate stone disease. Kidney Int. 2010;78:310-7.
101. Evan AP, Coe FL, Gillen D, et al. Renal intratubular crystals and hyaluronan staining occur in stone formers with bypass surgery but not with idiopathic calcium oxalate stones. Anat Rec (Hoboken). 2008;291:325-34.
102. Evan AP, Lingeman JE, Coe FL, et al. Crystal-associated nephropathy in patients with brushite nephrolithiasis. Kidney Int. 2005;67:576-91.
103. Linnes MP, Krambeck AE, Cornell L, Williams JC, Jr., Korinek M, Bergstralh EJ, et al. Phenotypic characterization of kidney stone formers by endoscopic and histological quantification of intrarenal calcification. Kidney Int. 2013;84:818-25.
104. Wang X, Krambeck AE, Williams JC, Jr., Tang X, Rule AD, Zhao F, et al. Distinguishing characteristics of idiopathic calcium oxalate kidney stone formers with low amounts of Randall's plaque. Clinical journal of the American Society of Nephrology : CJASN. 2014;9:1757-63.

Section 3

Surgical Management of Kidney Stones

—James E Lingeman

CHAPTER

26

The Natural History of Kidney Stones

Jubilee Tan, Dean G Assimos

The prevalence of kidney stones is increasing. Some individuals have asymptomatic stones located in the kidney and are interested in the implications of harboring such calculi. Others have ureteral stones that make it important to predict the likelihood of spontaneous stone passage. Patients subjected to stone-removing procedures may have residual stones, and these smaller fragments have been classified as "clinically insignificant". However, this classification may be misleading, based on the natural history of such stones. In this chapter, we will discuss the aforementioned issues to provide the practitioner with guidance for management of patients with urolithiasis.

NATURAL HISTORY OF UNTREATED CALYCEAL STONES

A number of studies have assessed the natural history of asymptomatic calyceal stones in adults. Glowacki and associates followed 107 such patients over a mean follow-up of 31.6 months. Thirty-four (31.8 %) had a symptomatic stone event. A Kaplan Meier analysis demonstrated that the risks of developing a symptomatic event were 7.8%, 20.4%, 33.8%, 40.6% and 48.5% at 1, 2, 3, 4 and 5 years, respectively. Eighteen of these 34 subjects (53%) required a stone-removing intervention. Gender, age, and urinary risk factors for stones were not found to be predictive. When the linear progression was extrapolated to 10 years, the probability of a stone event approached 90-100%.[1] Keeley and colleagues undertook a prospective, randomized study in which 228 patients with asymptomatic stones less than 15 mm in diameter were randomized to either observation or shock wave lithotripsy (SWL). Two-hundred patients returned for at least one annual follow-up with a KUB x-ray. The mean follow-up was 2.2 years. A higher percentage of patients in the treatment group were stone-free at the time of last follow-up, 28% versus 17%, respectively. However after adjusting for confounding variables, this was not statistically significant. There was no significant difference in the need for additional treatment in the form of analgesics, antibiotics, or stone-removing procedures between the groups—15% for the SWL cohort and 21% for the observational group. [2] Burgher and associates performed a retrospective study of 300 males with asymptomatic renal stones, mean age 62.8 years. The average cumulative stone diameter was 10.8 mm. Most were evaluated with annual nephrotomograms. The mean period of follow-up was 3.26 years. They considered disease progression as any one of the following: stone growth, need for surgical intervention, or renal colic. Seventy-seven percent of patients progressed, with 26% requiring a surgical intervention. Larger stones, ≥4 mm, had a higher likelihood of disease progression. Kaplan-Meier analysis predicted a 50% risk of intervention at 7.25 years.[3] Koh and colleagues performed a retrospective study in which 50 patients with stones a mean size of 5.7 mm were followed for a mean of 46 months. Twenty percent spontaneously passed their stones, 45.9% had stone growth, while only 7.1% required a surgical intervention. Stones less than 5 mm were more prone to pass.[4] Kang and associates undertook a retrospective study of 347 patients with asymptomatic stones; mean age was 47.9 years and average stone size was 4.39 mm. Spontaneous passage occurred in 29.1%, 24.5% underwent an intervention, but only 4.6% required surgery. Stone-related events were more common in males.[5] Two groups have analyzed the natural history of lower pole stones in a prospective fashion. Inci and colleagues followed 24 such patients for a mean of 52.3 months. Three of the group had bilateral lower pole stones. The mean stone size was 8.8 mm; cumulative diameters were used in those with multiple stones. Stone growth was seen in one third of the kidneys containing stones. However, a stone-removing procedure was undertaken in only 3 (11%) of the renal units. The stones spontaneously passed from 5 renal units (18.5%).[6] Yuruk and associates randomized 31 patients with lower pole stones to percutaneous nephrolithotomy (PCNL), 31 to SWL and 32 to observation. They were followed with computerized tomography (CT) and dimercapto-succinic acid renal scans (DMSA). All of the patients undergoing PCNL were rendered stone-free and a renal scar was demonstrated in one (3.2%). The stone-free rate with SWL was 54.8% with scarring in 7(18.7%). Seven (18.7%) required intervention in the observation cohort and none developed scarring. The median time to intervention was 22.5 months.[7]

These studies suggest that patients harboring asymptomatic calyceal stones are at moderate risk for having a symptomatic stone event. A significant number will also have stone growth over time. Patients with smaller stones may pass them spontaneously, while a few will require stone-removing interventions. More information is required regarding the impact of asymptomatic stones on quality of life and economics.

NATURAL HISTORY OF UNTREATED STAGHORN STONES

There is little contemporary information defining the impact of untreated staghorn renal calculi. This is due to the availability of minimally invasive treatment approaches such as PCNL that are endorsed by treatment guidelines.[8] PCNL allows for stone removal in patients with substantial comorbidities, who previously would have been considered poor candidates for open surgical interventions. A number of older studies demonstrated the significant renal damage that a staghorn stone could cause, as well as its impact on patient mortality, if left untreated. In 1949, Priestly and Dunn reported on 382 patients at the Mayo clinic with staghorn stones. Thirty-two percent had no symptoms. Sixty-three had bilateral staghorn stones. Management approaches included stone removal, nephrectomy, and observation. The survival at 15 years for those with unilateral staghorn stones was 81% for those undergoing stone removal, 76% for those undergoing nephrectomy, and only 41% in those observed. In those with bilateral staghorn stones, the five-year survival was 95% for those undergoing stone removal and only 50% for the observation cohort. Thirty percent succumbed to renal failure or sepsis.[9] In 1973, Singh and Blandy reported on 185 patients with staghorn stones, 60 in an observational cohort and 125 subjected to surgery. The 10-year mortality rate was 28% in those observed and 7.2% in those whom stones were surgically removed.[10] Rous and Turner described similar outcomes in 95 patients with staghorn calculi. Of those patients treated with a nonoperative approach, 30% died of renal failure and/or sepsis.[11] Libertino and colleagues reported on 15 patients with solitary kidneys harboring staghorn stones. Of the 8 who were observed, 2 died from renal failure, 4 died from non-renal causes, and 2 were alive at 7 and 25 years of follow-up.[12] Vargas and associates profiled the structural and histologic consequences of staghorn stones. Of 88 kidneys analyzed, they noted hydronephrosis in 26%, xanthogranulomatous pyelonephritis in 7%, severe pyelonephritis in 13%, and perinephric abscess in 5%.[13] These reports from the older literature demonstrate the morbid consequences of untreated staghorn stones. However, this may have been accentuated due to selection bias. The profile of today's staghorn stone patient is somewhat different in that the majority harbor metabolic stones, as opposed to infectious stones, and thus the morbidity may be less severe if the stone is not removed.[14]

NATURAL HISTORY OF RESIDUAL FRAGMENTS AFTER STONE-REMOVING PROCEDURES

Shortly after SWL was introduced into clinical practice, the term "clinically insignificant fragments" (CISF) was introduced. Various thresholds for defining CISF have been used, including < 4 mm, ≤ 4 mm, and < 5 mm. Several studies suggest that this term is actually a misnomer. Streem and associates prospectively followed 160 patients with <4 mm fragments after SWL who were initially asymptomatic. The mean follow-up period was 23 months. Ninety-one (56.9%) remained without symptoms, while 43.1% had a symptomatic stone event or required an intervention. Thirty-eight (23.8%) became stone free, 26 (16.3%) reduced their stone burden, 67 (41.9%) had no change in their stones, and 29 (18.1%) had stone growth.[15] Candau and colleagues followed 83 subjects with <4 mm fragments after SWL with a mean follow-up of 40.6 months. Twenty-seven (33%) became stone free, 1 (1%) had reduction in stone size, 24 (29%) had no change in stone burden, while 31 (37%) demonstrated stone growth. Eighteen (22%) eventually required another stone-removing procedure.[16] Khaitan and associates followed 75 patients with < 4 mm fragments after SWL with a mean follow-up of 15 months. Twenty-four percent became stone-free, 16% had no change and 60% had stone growth or new stone formation. Fifty-nine percent had a symptomatic stone event, including 32% who needed another procedure.[17] Osman and colleagues reported on 173 patients with ≤ 4 mm residual fragments after SWL with a mean follow-up of 4.9 years. Thirty-seven patients (21%) required another procedure for symptoms or stone growth.[18] El-Nahas and associates assessed 154 patients with ≤ 5 mm after SWL with a mean follow-up of 31 months. Twenty-one

(13.6%) became stone-free, 52 (33.8%) had stone growth, and 81 (52.6%) had a stable stone burden. Seventy-five (48.7%) had a symptomatic stone event with 52 (33.8%) requiring a surgical intervention. Recurrent kidney stone formers were more likely to have a subsequent symptomatic event.[19] The majority of patients in these studies were adults. However, similar outcomes with persistent residual fragments after SWL have been reported in children. Afshar and colleagues followed 25 children with fragments ≤5 mm in 26 renal units after SWL with a mean follow-up of 46 months. Stone growth ensued in 9 renal units (34.5%), stones remained stable in 8 kidneys (30.8%), and the fragments caused symptoms in 9 (34.5%). A procedural intervention was undertaken in 11 renal units (42.3%).[20] Dincel and associates reported on 85 children subjected to stone-removing procedures, the majority being SWL, who had residual fragments <4 mm after treatment. After a 22-month median follow-up, 22 (25.8%) passed the fragments, 18 (21.2%) had stone growth, and 45 (53%) remained unchanged. Thirty-four children (40%) had a symptomatic stone event and 25 (29.4%) required further stone-removing procedures.[21] Beck and Riehle reported on the fate of stone fragments <5 mm in 17 patients with infection stones (struvite and carbonate apatite) subjected to SWL with a mean follow-up of 26.6 months. Seven (41.2%) eventually passed these fragments, eight (47.1%) had stone growth, and stone size remained stable in 2 (1.2%).[22] Only one study has reported an inconsequential effect of small residual fragments. Buchholz and colleagues followed 44 patients with residual fragments ≤5 mm after SWL for a mean of 2.5 years. Thirty-eight (87.5%) subsequently passed all fragments over a 16-month period while only 2% of those with residual fragments had stone growth. There were no subsequent stone events or stone-removing procedures.[23]

The preponderance of evidence indicates that small residual fragments after SWL may grow, incite future stone events, or both. This may ultimately require further stone-removing procedures. However, preemptive procedures in asymptomatic patients with small stone fragments are not necessarily justified. Patients should be informed about the natural history of these fragments, which may prompt some to undergo another stone-removing procedure. Metabolic evaluation, dietary modifications, and preventive medical therapy should also be considered. The latter is justified by a study by Fine and associates, who reported that patients with residual fragments after SWL prescribed selective medical therapy for stone prevention were less at risk for stone growth compared to those who were not treated—23.1% compared to 63.9%. The mean follow-up interval was 43.2 months. These investigators also reported an economic benefit to medical therapy in this setting.[24] In addition, others have shown that the administration of potassium citrate to both children and adults with stone fragments after SWL facilitates eventual stone clearance and limits stone regrowth.[25-27] Although most would endorse the removal of residual stone fragments in those with infection stones, Michaels and Fowler reported that administration of antibiotics for 2-4 weeks in those with small residual stone fragments after SWL may eradicate recurrent urinary tract infections and limit stone progression.[28]

Patients can certainly have residual stones after PCNL and ureteroscopic stone removal (URS). Ganpule and Desai reported on 187 such patients who were subjected to PCNL and noted that 65% passed these fragments spontaneously within 3 months of the procedure, particularly those with stone fragments <25 mm^2 in the renal pelvis[29] Altunrende and associates reported on 38 post-PCNL patients who had residual fragments ≤4 mm with a median follow-up of 28.4 months. Ten (26.3%) had a symptomatic stone event, 8 (21.1%) had stone growth, 27 (71.1%) had stable or reduced stone burden, and 3 (7.9%) spontaneously passed the remaining stones.[30] Raman and associates reported on 42 patients with residual fragments after PCNL with a median follow-up of 41 months. The median residual fragment size was 2 mm. Eighteen patients (43%) had a symptomatic stone event at a median of 32 months. Stone fragments >2 mm and the location of the fragments in the renal pelvis were predictors of a stone event.[31] There is limited information regarding the natural history of renal stone fragments following URS. Rebuck and colleagues reported on 46 patients with fragments ≤ 4 mm on initial postoperative CT scans following URS of calcium stones with a mean follow-up of 1.6 years. Nine (19.6%) had a stone event, 6 (13%) required another URS intervention, 10 (21.7%) spontaneously eliminated the fragments, and the others had no growth of the stone fragments over time.[32] Therefore, small stone fragments remaining after PCNL and URS may not be innocent bystanders and provoke problems for the patient. The approach should be similar for that of patients with small stone fragments after SWL, where at minimum periodic follow-up imaging is obtained. In addition, metabolic evaluation, prescription of dietary modifications, and preventive medical therapy are also advised and have proven beneficial in this setting.[33]

SPONTANEOUS URETERAL STONE PASSAGE

Patients with ureteral stones in whom pain is controlled and without pressing indications for immediate or urgent stone removal often inquire about the likelihood of spontaneous passage, expected time for passage, and methods to facilitate this process. Hubner and associates reviewed a series of articles published between 1954 and 1991 regarding spontaneous ureteral stone passage. Overall, spontaneous passage occurred in 38% (1023 out of 2,704 cases). As expected, stone size impacted passage (56.9% for < 4 mm, 35.2% for 4-6 mm, 8.3% for > 6 mm).[34] In 2007 the American Urological Association and European Association of Urology (AUA/EAU) Nephrolithiasis Guidelines Panel performed a meta-analysis to assess the rate of spontaneous ureteral stone passage using the control arms of MET trials. The median probability of stone passage was 68% for stones ≤ 5 mm (n=224) and 47% for those > 5 mm and ≤10 mm (n=104).[35] Coll and associates assessed the relationship between ureteral stone size measured on CT and the rate of spontaneous passage. They used the maximum axial diameter in their investigation and reported that 87% of 1 mm, 76% of 2-4 mm, 60% of 5-7 mm, 48% of 7-9 mm and 25% of stones > 9 mm passed spontaneously.[36]

Stone location also influences passage: the more distal the stone, the higher the likelihood of elimination. Morse and Resnick reported that 71% of distal, 46% of middle and 22% of proximal ureteral stones passed spontaneously.[37] Coll and colleagues found a similar relationship (79% for ureterovesical junction, 75% for distal, 60% for middle, and 48% for proximal stones).[36]

Miller and Kane evaluated the impact of both stone size and location on spontaneous stone passage. They reported a mean passage time of 8.2 days for stones ≤ 2 mm, 12.2 days for 2-4 mm, and 22.1 days for > 4 mm. A multivariate analysis demonstrated that the more distal the stone, the faster the rate of elimination. They also calculated length of time required for 95% of the cohort to expel their stones: 31 days for stones ≤ 2 mm, 40 days for 2-4 mm, and 39 days for 4-6 mm.[38]

Other factors may influence ureteral stone passage. Cummings and associates used an artificial neural network to predict the probability of spontaneous stone passage. They reported that duration of symptoms prior to manifestation and degree of hydronephrosis were the most influential factors for accurately predicting stone passage.[39]

The majority of the patients included in the aforementioned studies were, again, adults. There have been scattered reports regarding spontaneous passage of stones in children; the size of the cohorts in these studies is small. Mokhless and colleagues reported on 72 children with ureteral stones 2–10 mm in size with a mean age of 7 years. At approximately 6 weeks, 100% of 1–2 mm (mean time to passage 12 days), 92% of 2–4 mm (mean time to passage 18 days), and 68% of 4-6 mm stones spontaneously passed (mean time to passage 35 days). When stratified by location, 45% of proximal (mean time to passage 32 days), 70% of middle (mean time to passage 21 days) and 94% of distal (mean time to passage 19 days) spontaneously passed. The degree of hydronephrosis was inversely correlated with stone passage.[40] Pietrow and associates stratified spontaneous ureteral stone passage in 87 children based on age. The stone passage rates were quite similar (63% for 0-5 years, 61% for 6-10 years, and 64% for 11-18 years). The rates of spontaneous stone passage in their series precipitously declined when stone size was > 4 mm for all age cohorts.[41] Van Savage and colleagues reported that 58% of 1 mm, 67% of 2 mm and 33% of 3 mm distal ureteral stones passed spontaneously in a group of 33 children with a mean age of 11 years. None of the stones ≥4 mm passed.[42]

Although a number of investigators have reported on spontaneous stone passage during pregnancy, the majority did not specify whether the stones were located in the kidney or ureter.[43-45] Adreoiu and MacMahon found that the 3 of 11 (27.3%) pregnant women with proximal ureteral stones passed them spontaneously, whereas this occurred in 15 of 34 (44.1%) harboring distal calculi.[46] These investigators did not provide an analysis of the impact of ureteral stone size. However, they noted that among those with renal and/or ureteral stones, 12 of 22 (54.5%) with 0-4 mm, 14 of 33 (42.4%) with 5-8 mm and none of the 8 individuals with > 8 mm stones experienced spontaneous passage.

These studies suggest that spontaneous ureteral stone passage is influenced by stone size and location in both children and adults. Other factors such as the degree of hydronephrosis may have an impact. The latter parameter may serve as an index of stone impaction or threat to renal function and thus prompt surgical stone removal. Additionally, the majority of ureteral stones that will pass do so within a 30-day period.

REFERENCES

1. Glowacki LS, Beecroft ML, Cook RJ, et al. The natural history of asymptomatic urolithiasis. The Journal of urology. 1992;147:319-21.
2. Keeley FX, Jr. et al. Preliminary results of a randomized controlled trial of prophylactic shock wave lithotripsy for

small asymptomatic renal calyceal stones. BJU international. 2001;87:1-8.
3. Burgher A, Beman M, Holtzman JL, et al. Progression of nephrolithiasis: long-term outcomes with observation of asymptomatic calculi. Journal of endourology/Endourological Society. 2004;18:534-9.
4. Koh LT, Ng FC, Ng KK. Outcomes of long-term follow-up of patients with conservative management of asymptomatic renal calculi. BJU International. 2012;109:622-5.
5. Kang HW, et al. Natural history of asymptomatic renal stones and prediction of stone related events. The Journal of Urology. 2013;189:1740-6.
6. Inci K, et al. Prospective long-term follow-up of patients with asymptomatic lower pole caliceal stones. The Journal of Urology. 2007;177:2189-92.
7. Yuruk E, et al. A prospective, randomized trial of management for asymptomatic lower pole calculi. The Journal of Urology. 2010;183:1424-8.
8. Preminger GM, et al. Chapter 1: AUA guideline on management of staghorn calculi: diagnosis and treatment recommendations. The Journal of Urology. 2005;173:1991-2000.
9. Priestly JT, Dunn JH. Branched renal stones. Journal of Urology. 1949;61:194-203.
10. Blandy JP, Singh M. The case for a more aggressive approach to staghorn stones. The Journal of Urology. 1976;115:505-6.
11. Rous SN, Turner WR. Retrospective study of 95 patients with staghorn calculus disease. The Journal of Urology. 1977;118:902-4.
12. Libertino JA, Newman HR, Lytton B, et al. Staghorn calculi in solitary kidneys. The Journal of Urology. 1971;105:753-7.
13. Vargas AD, Bragin SD, Mendez R. Staghorn calculis: its clinical presentation, complications and management. The Journal of Urology. 1982;127:860-2.
14. Viprakasit DP, Sawyer MD, Herrell SD, et al. Changing composition of staghorn calculi. The Journal of Urology. 2011;186:2285-90.
15. Streem SB, Yost A, Mascha E. Clinical implications of clinically insignificant store fragments after extracorporeal shock wave lithotripsy. The Journal of Urology. 1996;155:1186-90.
16. Candau C, et al. Natural history of residual renal stone fragments after ESWL. European urology. 2000;37:18-22.
17. Khaitan A, et al. Post-ESWL, clinically insignificant residual stones: reality or myth? Urology. 2002;59:20-4.
18. Osman M, M, et al. 5-year-follow-up of patients with clinically insignificant residual fragments after extracorporeal shockwave lithotripsy. European Urology. 2005;47:860-4.
19. El-Nahas AR, El-Assmy AM, Madbouly K, et al. Predictors of clinical significance of residual fragments after extracorporeal shockwave lithotripsy for renal stones. Journal of endourology/Endourological Society. 2006;20:870-4.
20. Afshar K, et al. Outcome of small residual stone fragments following shock wave lithotripsy in children. The Journal of Urology. 2004;172:1600-3.
21. Dincel N, et al. Are small residual stone fragments really insignificant in children? Journal of Pediatric Surgery. 2013;48:840-4.
22. Beck EM, Riehle RA, Jr. The fate of residual fragments after extracorporeal shock wave lithotripsy monotherapy of infection stones. The Journal of Urology. 1991;145:6-9; discussion 9-10.
23. Buchholz NP, Meier-Padel S, Rutishauser G. Minor residual fragments after extracorporeal shockwave lithotripsy: spontaneous clearance or risk factor for recurrent stone formation? Journal of Endourology/Endourological Society. 1997;11:227-32.
24. Fine JK, Pak CY, Preminger GM. Effect of medical management and residual fragments on recurrent stone formation following shock wave lithotripsy. The Journal of Urology. 1995;153:27-32; discussion 32-23.
25. Sarica K, Erturhan S, Yurtseven C, et al. Effect of potassium citrate therapy on stone recurrence and regrowth after extracorporeal shockwave lithotripsy in children. Journal of Endourology/Endourological Society. 2006;20:875-9.
26. Cicerello E, et al. Effect of alkaline citrate therapy on clearance of residual renal stone fragments after extracorporeal shock wave lithotripsy in sterile calcium and infection nephrolithiasis patients. The Journal of Urology. 1994;151:5-9.
27. Soygur T, Akbay A, Kupeli S. Effect of potassium citrate therapy on stone recurrence and residual fragments after shockwave lithotripsy in lower caliceal calcium oxalate urolithiasis: a randomized controlled trial. Journal of Endourology/Endourological Society. 2002;16:149-52.
28. Michaels EK, Fowler JE, Jr, Mariano M. Bacteriuria following extracorporeal shock wave lithotripsy of infection stones. The Journal of Urology. 1988;140:254-6.
29. Ganpule A, Desai M. Fate of residual stones after percutaneous nephrolithotomy: a critical analysis. Journal of Endourology/Endourological Society. 2009;23:399-403.
30. Altunrende F, et al. Clinically insignificant residual fragments after percutaneous nephrolithotomy: medium-term follow-up. Journal of Endourology/Endourological Society. 2011;25:941-5.
31. Raman JD, et al. Natural history of residual fragments following percutaneous nephrostolithotomy. The Journal of Urology. 2009;181:1163-8.
32. Rebuck DA, Macejko A, Bhalani V, et al. The natural history of renal stone fragments following ureteroscopy. Urology. 2011;77:564-8.
33. Kang DE, et al. Effect of medical management on recurrent stone formation following percutaneous nephrolithotomy. The Journal of Urology. 2007;177:1785-8; discussion 1788-9.
34. Hubner WA, Irby P, Stoller ML. Natural history and current concepts for the treatment of small ureteral calculi. European Urology. 1993;24:172-6.
35. Preminger GM, et al. 2007 guideline for the management of ureteral calculi. The Journal of Urology. 2007;178:2418-34.
36. Coll DM, Varanelli MJ, Smith RC. Relationship of spontaneous passage of ureteral calculi to stone size and location as revealed by unenhanced helical CT. American Journal of Roentgenology (AJR). 2002;178:101-3.
37. Morse RM, Resnick MI. Ureteral calculi: natural history and treatment in an era of advanced technology. The Journal of Urology. 1991;145:263-5.

38. Miller OF, Kane CJ. Time to stone passage for observed ureteral calculi: a guide for patient education. The Journal of Urology. 1999;162:688-90; discussion 690-681.
39. Cummings JM, Boullier JA, Izenberg SD, et al. Prediction of spontaneous ureteral calculous passage by an artificial neural network. The Journal of Urology. 2000;164:326-8.
40. Mokhless I, Zahran AR, Youssif M, et al. Factors that predict the spontaneous passage of ureteric stones in children. Arab Journal of Urology. 2012;10:402-7.
41. Pietrow PK, Pope JC IV, Adams MC, et al. Clinical outcome of pediatric stone disease. The Journal of Urology. 2002;167: 670-3.
42. Van Savage JG, Palanca LG, Andersen RD, et al. Treatment of distal ureteral stones in children: similarities to the American Urological Association Guidelines in adults. The Journal of urology. 2000;164:1089-93.
43. Parulkar BG, Hopkins TB, Wollin MR, et al. Renal colic during pregnancy: a case for conservative treatment. The Journal of Urology. 1998;159:365-8.
44. Burgess KL, Gettman MT, Rangel LJ, et al. Diagnosis of urolithiasis and rate of spontaneous passage during pregnancy. The Journal of Urology. 2011;186:2280-4.
45. Meria P, Hadjadj H, Jungers P, et al. & Members of the French Urological Association Urolithiasis, C. Stone formation and pregnancy: pathophysiological insights gained from morphoconstitutional stone analysis. The Journal of Urology. 2010;183:1412-6.
46. Andreoiu M, MacMahon R. Renal colic in pregnancy: lithiasis or physiological hydronephrosis? Urology. 2009;74:757-61.

CHAPTER

27

Stone Factors Affecting Treatment Choices (Anatomy, Composition, etc.)

Aaron D Benson, Nicole L Miller

INTRODUCTION

Kidney stone disease is relatively common and affects ~10% of the American population, with an increasing incidence and prevalence.[1,2] The recurrence rate for kidney stones in industrialized countries has been reported at ~25%[3] but as high as 50% at 10 years and 75% by 20 years.[4] Historically, nephrolithiasis has demonstrated male predominance, especially for the most common calcium-containing stones, with a male-to-female ratio of 2.7:1.[5] A significant proportion of nephrolithiasis patients require surgical intervention for resolution of their renal stone burden.[6] The significance of appropriate surgical treatment is demonstrated in the various morbidities and mortality of untreated nephrolithiasis. The most important outcomes to consider in untreated nephrolithiasis are long-term renal function, infection in the setting of renal/ureteral obstruction, and associated mortality.

The various surgical modalities for treatment of nephrolithiasis have inherent advantages and disadvantages, each of which may be more pronounced depending on the characteristics of the stone burden. In addition, many stone-related factors influence the treatment option. These factors include stone size, location, conformation, number, composition, density, and fragility. Without proper consideration of these aspects, surgical stone treatment may result in suboptimal outcomes.

SURGICAL TREATMENT OPTIONS

The primary goal of surgical intervention is complete stone removal. There are many factors to consider when determining the appropriate surgical treatment for a renal stone burden. When choosing between surgical options, the associated techniques, available instruments, advantages, disadvantages, contraindications, and potential complications of each procedure must be considered. The possible treatment options include extracorporeal shockwave lithotripsy (SWL), ureteroscopy (URS) with laser lithotripsy (with or without stone fragment removal), percutaneous nephrolithotomy (PCNL), and open or laparoscopic surgery. These procedures are discussed briefly in this chapter (and, in more detail, in other Chapters 30 and 35 of this publication) for a basic understanding in order to relate these surgical options to different stone factors.

Shockwave Lithotripsy

Extracorporeal SWL is the least invasive and most frequently utilized surgical treatment for nephrolithiasis. The popularity of SWL can be attributed to this procedure's perceived lack of invasiveness and ease of use. For certain stone burdens, SWL has demonstrated good success with a relatively low complication rate. The systematic review of the literature on management of ureteral calculi by the American Urological Association (AUA)/European Association of Urology (EAU) Nephrolithiasis Panel indicated a 90% stone-free rate for SWL used to treat proximal ureteral stones that were <10 mm in diameter (Table 27.1).[7] There are reports of newer-generation SWL machines demonstrating nephrolithiasis treatment efficacy comparable to the Dornier HM3 lithotripter. Neisius et al. reported a 91% stone-free rate at 3 months postoperatively using a third-generation standard lithotripter in 183 patients with a 0.5% major complication rate.[8] Compared to the Dornier HM3, the popularity of the newer-generation lithotripters centers on the portable, more compact design with dry head coupling and increased power settings. Despite the increase in power, some studies have demonstrated lower success and higher complication rates with newer lithotripter models, likely related to the narrower focal zone and higher peak positive pressure.[9-11]

The mechanism by which SWL treats nephrolithiasis involves stone localization with fluoroscopy. Localization can also be performed with ultrasound, but is less common. Lithotripters generate shock waves by different mechanisms. Electrohydraulic lithotripters have a spark source, which generates a shock wave that is focused by

Table 27.1: Stone-free rates for shockwave lithotripsy and ureteroscopy in overall population.

	AUA/EAU Ureteral Stones Guideline Panel			
	Stone-free rate—Primary treatments or first treatment			
	SWL		URS	
Overall population	G/P	Med/95% CI	G/P	Med/95% CI
Distal Ureter	50 6981	74% (73–75)%	59 5952	94% (93–95)%
• Distal ureter < 10 mm	17 1684	86% (80–91)%	13 1622	97% (96–98)%
• Distal ureter > 10 mm	10 966	74% (57–87)%	8 412	93% (88–96)%
Mid Ureter	31 1607	73% (66–79)%	30 1024	86% (81–89)%
• Mid ureter < 10 mm	5 44	84% (65–95)%	5 80	91% (81–96)%
• Mid ureter > 10 mm	2 15	76% (36–97)%	5 73	78% (61–90)%
Proximal Ureter	41 6428	82% (79–85)%	46 2242	81% (77–85)%
• Proximal ureter < 10 mm	14 886	90% (85–93)%	9 243	80% (73–85)%
• Proximal ureter > 10 mm	11 293	68% (55–79)%	8 230	79% (71–87)%

G – Number of groups/treatment arms extracted; P – Number of patients in those groups.

(SWL: Shockwave lithotripsy; URS: Ureteroscopy; AUA/EAU: American Urological Association/European Association of Urology).

an ellipsoid reflector. Electromagnetic lithotripters use an electrical coil to generate a short electrical pulse that interacts with a metal plate to generate an acoustic (shock) wave. Piezoelectric lithotripters use piezoelectric crystals to form an ultrasonic wave. The shockwave source is coupled to the patient via a water bath (Dornier HM3) or via a dry "therapy" head where the shock wave source is mounted in the head filled with water and capped by a thin rubber membrane. The generated pressure or shock waves propagate through the patient's tissue, which has density similar to water. The shock waves are focused and delivered to a focal zone surrounding the focal point of the lithotripter. The focal zone is the zone of highest pressure and ideally where the stone is placed for fragmentation. Focal zones vary among lithotripsy machines. Lithotripters with the narrowest focal zones have the highest peak pressure, which may sound advantageous but this has not been shown to correlate with better stone fragmentation and may actually result in increased adverse tissue effects such as subcapsular hematoma. Based on reported SWL stone fragmentation and success, the EAU 2008 guideline recommends a shock wave frequency of 1.0–1.5 Hz for treatment.[12] The maximum number of shockwaves applied depends upon the lithotripter type and shock wave power.

Shockwaves may negatively affect tissues and organ structures between the lithotripter head and the stone or adjacent to the stone (due to the cigar-shaped energy path). Thus, there are various absolute and relative contraindications that may preclude SWL as a treatment option. The absolute contraindications include large abdominal aortic or renal artery aneurysm (especially if ≥4 cm), vascular calcifications near the target stone to which shock waves could be applied inadvertently or mistakenly, coagulopathy, pregnancy, and active urinary tract infection (UTI).[12] These absolute contraindications are related to the potential surrounding tissue injury that could occur with SWL, the resulting complications of which would be magnified secondary to the patient's pathology or pregnancy. The relative contraindications include chronic pancreatitis (especially with an existing pancreatic calcification), obstruction distal to the targeted stone (e.g. ureteral stricture), and a history of urolithiasis resistant to SWL. Except for chronic pancreatitis, the relative contraindications emphasize potential failure or postoperative stone-related complications rather than tissue injury. Both absolute and relative contraindications should be considered in order to avoid major complications and maximize success.

Despite its noninvasiveness, complications may still occur with SWL. Stone-related complications include steinstrasse or "stone street," which refers to multiple stone fragments forming a column in the ureter and causing ureteral obstruction. The rate of steinstrasse has traditionally been reported as 5–6%, but may be as high as 27%.[13] Other stone-related complications include residual stone fragments (especially >4–5 mm), which may lead to acute stone episodes or act as a nidus for continued stone growth/recurrence, and UTI, which may be related to treatment of infection-related stones. Post-SWL sepsis rates are historically low (<1%) but may be higher for treatment of staghorn renal calculi or infection-related nephrolithiasis. Adjacent tissue injury and post-SWL UTI may also lead to further negative sequelae, such as abscesses of the retroperitoneum, kidney, or other associated structures. Adjacent tissue injury can also result in immediate or possibly long-term complications. The most common immediate result of tissue injury is bleeding, which most often presents as ecchymosis/petechiae at the lithotripter coupling site, hematuria, and renal/retroperitoneal hematoma. Renal subcapsular hematoma occurs in 4.1% of cases overall, with increasing risk in older patients.[11] Most post-SWL renal or retroperitoneal hematomas are clinically insignificant and likely underdiagnosed;[14] however, large post-SWL hematomas or significant gross hematuria warrant further evaluation to treat any continued active bleeding. Other immediate tissue injury-related complications include injury to adjacent organ structures, such as bowel, spleen, and kidney. Cardiovascular complications can occur, and are primarily related to dysrhythmias. Gating the shock wave firing to the cardiac cycle was common practice with the Dornier HM3, but was found to be unnecessary for most patients, so most lithotripters now run in ungated mode. Shockwave lithotripsy is not contraindicated for patients with pacemakers, but pacemakers may require reprogramming prior to treatment.

Lastly, there may be long-term adverse effects related to SWL that are likely dose dependent. Those that have been described include renal insufficiency, new onset hypertension, diabetes mellitus, and conversion of stone composition to dicalcium phosphate (brushite). Animal studies suggest that acute hemorrhagic lesions from SWL may develop into renal scar with eventual loss of renal cortical function. A prospective study by Janetschek et al. showed an increase in intrarenal resistance index in patients over 60 years of age.[15] The question of the potential for the development of diabetes mellitus following SWL is unanswered. Conflicting data have been reported from various studies, all of which suffer from limitations in experimental design or long-term followup. Strategies to reduce potential adverse effects from SWL have been described, including utilization of a pretreatment protocol delivering a priming dose of ~100 low-amplitude (12 kV) shock waves before delivery of higher amplitude pulses, inclusion of a brief 3–4 minute pause following the priming dose of shock waves, and slowing the shock wave firing rate to 60 shock waves per minute.[16]

In addition to its relative safety, traditionally high success rates, and relatively low technical difficulty, there are several benefits of SWL that add to its popularity. Since no incisions or even endoscopy is required, SWL is noninvasive. Given the noninvasiveness, general anesthesia is not required (though often utilized to minimize respiratory movement), and anesthesia may be limited to conscious sedation. Shockwave lithotripsy may also be accompanied by less postoperative pain. Thus, the potential success and noninvasive nature of SWL makes this procedure an appealing option in appropriate cases.

Ureteroscopy

Ureteroscopy is a minimally invasive approach to urolithiasis treatment. Ureteroscopy may offer the most flexibility in its ability to treat a wide variety of renal and ureteral stone burdens. Modern ureteroscopes are produced in both semirigid and flexible forms, which enable differing approaches to stone burdens in different locations of the urinary tract. The AUA/EAU nephrolithiasis Panel indicated 81%, 86%, and 94% stone-free rates for URS used to treat proximal, mid-, and distal ureteral stones (Table 27.1).[7] These high success rates likely can be attributed to improved optics of modern ureteroscopes, increased flexibility and maneuverability of flexible ureteroscopes, and the wide assortment of auxiliary equipment (e.g. baskets and lasers) that can be used through the ureteroscope to fragment and remove stones. These physical advantages minimize invasiveness while allowing effective treatment of both small and relatively large upper urinary tract stones.

The mechanism of function varies regarding semirigid and flexible URS (also termed ureterorenoscopy when involving use in the renal collecting system). However, both types of ureteroscopes require the same basic components for use, which include a light source, a camera and video system, and pressurized irrigation. The latest ureteroscopes utilize digital imaging systems. Both semirigid and flexible ureteroscopes vary in size and maneuverability depending on the brand and model. Semirigid ureteroscopes generally measure ~330–430 mm in length (for "short" and "long" versions) with a beak diameter range of 4.5–9.0 French (F) and a shaft base diameter range of 6.5–15.0 F. Unlike semirigid ureteroscopes, flexible ureteroscopes are designed to access and treat pathologies in the more proximal portions of the upper urinary tract, which requires maneuvering around anatomic angulations and narrowing in the ureter and renal collecting system. Flexible ureteroscopes generally measure ~640–700 mm in length with a tip diameter range of 5.3–8.7 F and a shaft diameter range of 7.4–9.9 F. The main advantages of flexible ureteroscopes are the maneuverability that allows access around acute angles and direct visualization of the stone burden. In the end, the compact design and variety of ureteroscopes provides a minimally invasive, direct-vision option for treatment of upper tract urolithiasis.

Unlike many surgical procedures, there are few absolute or relative contraindications other than untreated infection to consider with URS. Clinical scenarios that might remove URS as a treatment option are due to increased possibility of failure rather than increased risk of complications. Such scenarios include large stone burdens (especially >2 cm), lower urinary tract diversion, and lower urinary tract reconstruction. The lack of contraindications is a significant advantage to URS as a surgical treatment.

Despite a few contraindications, there is still a risk of complications in URS. The most feared complication, but also the rarest, is ureteral avulsion, which occurs most frequently in the proximal ureter. The mechanism of ureteral avulsion can almost exclusively be attributed to overly aggressive attempts to remove stone fragments that are too large down the ureter rather than avulsion by the ureteroscope itself. Ureteral avulsion requires treatment with a long-term ureteral stent and/or ureteral repair. Ureteral perforation is a more common complication, but also occurs most frequently in the proximal ureter. Ureteral perforation generally occurs from guidewire use but can be caused by the ureteroscope and requires an indwelling ureteral stent for a minimum of 6 weeks. Ureteral stone extrusion may occur by pushing a ureteral stone through the wall of the ureter and into the periureteral tissue with the ureteroscope or balloon ureteral dilator. The treatment for ureteral stone extrusion is placement of an indwelling ureteral stent without any attempt to remove the extruded stone. Ureteral strictures may occur following URS. Contemporary studies report stricture rate of <1.5% for uncomplicated cases, but the risk increases in cases with impacted stones or ureteral perforation.[17] Similar to other surgical procedures, URS can be complicated by infection, pain, and bleeding. However, the risk for perioperative bleeding is low, so patients with coagulopathy, bleeding diatheses or whose anticoagulation cannot be discontinued may still be safely treated with URS. In most cases, URS for the treatment of nephrolithiasis carries a low complication risk.

In addition to the few contraindications, low complication risk, and high stone-free rates, URS has several other advantages. The compact design of ureteroscopes enables a completely endoscopic approach to nephrolithiasis to remain minimally invasive. The two types, semirigid and flexible, enable access, control, and maneuverability around anatomic variables in the ureter and renal collecting system. Ureteroscopy also allows real-time direct visualization of the stone during treatment as well as the renal papillae, which may provide insight into the stone composition and pathogenesis of the patient's stone disease. Other benefits of URS are the many auxiliary instruments/equipment (e.g. guidewires and lasers), which enable ureteroscopes to be more than image-producing instruments. The primary disadvantage of URS is the frequent need for a ureteral stent postoperatively to prevent obstruction from ureteral edema, as stents increase the postoperative pain associated with the procedure.

Percutaneous Nephrolithotomy

Percutaneous nephrolithotomy is a more invasive form of endoscopic nephrolithiasis treatment. The increased invasiveness is due to the percutaneous approach and dilation of the nephrostomy tract through the renal parenchyma directly into the renal collecting system. Such access provides not only a shorter and more direct approach to a renal stone burden, but also enables the use of larger-caliber instruments for stone fragmentation. Likewise, the direct percutaneous approach and larger-diameter access allow for efficient removal of larger renal stones. A Cochrane review reported better effectiveness of PCNL versus SWL in the treatment of large lower pole renal stones among 214 patients in two randomized, controlled trials.[18] The review reported a higher success rate for PCNL at 3 months by risk ratio (RR) 0.39, fewer retreatments (RR = 1.81), fewer additional procedures (RR = 9.06), and a higher efficiency quotient.

Percutaneous nephrolithotomy requires percutaneous access to the renal collecting system, which is dilated sufficiently (most commonly to 30 F) to accommodate a rigid nephroscope. The nephrostomy tract is ideally created along the axis of a posterior renal calyx. Lower pole renal access is generally thought to be the safest approach since there is low associated risk of traversing the pleural space compared to upper pole renal access. However, a lower pole nephrostomy tract typically provides more limited access, with a direct path only to the calyx of puncture, adjacent lower pole calyces and the renal pelvis. Despite higher associated risk, upper pole percutaneous access is typically the shortest route to the kidney and provides greater overall access to the renal collecting system and proximal ureter due to less acute angles into the lower/interpolar calices, renal pelvis, uretero-pelvic junction (UPJ), and proximal ureter. Posterior interpolar calices may also be accessed, but provide the least amount of access to the renal collecting system beyond the entry calyx itself. Once the nephrostomy tract is established and dilated, a rigid nephroscope (diameter range: 24–28 F) with an offset eyepiece is placed through the tract into the renal collecting system. Through the rigid nephroscope, a variety of instruments can be utilized to fragment the target renal stone burden, including rigid probes for electrohydraulic lithotripsy (EHL), pneumatic lithotripsy, and most commonly, ultrasonic lithotripsy, and combined ultrasonic and pneumatic devices. Ultrasonic lithotripsy utilizes ultrasonic vibration of a hollow metal probe (up to 12 F) to fragment and simultaneously evacuate the stone burden. As with the EHL and pneumatic lithotripsy probes, the ultrasonic lithotripsy probe is limited by its rigid design, but there is less concern for collecting system injury since it does not function via a ballistic mechanism. Thermal injury is possible due to the heat generated by the ultrasonic vibration of the metal probe; however, effective fluid irrigation and suction during the procedure mitigate this risk. The major advantage of ultrasonic lithotripsy is efficiency of stone treatment provided by simultaneous stone fragmentation and evacuation. When rigid devices for stone fragmentation and evacuation cannot be utilized due to unfavorable anatomy, stone location, or other deterring factors, the large caliber of the nephrostomy tract allows for the use of flexible nephroscopes, laser fibers, and endoscopic basket removal/relocation of stone fragments. Thus, the direct, short, and generally large-caliber access to the renal collecting system provides several options for effective and efficient treatment of large renal stone burdens.

Contraindications to PCNL, such as concurrent UTI and coagulopathy, are similar to contraindications for other less invasive urologic stone procedures. However, since PCNL requires creation of renal access that traverses the flank and posterior abdominal wall to the kidney, the location of adjacent structures must be considered. Location of percutaneous access, while often dictated by the location of the stone to be treated, is also very dependent on patient anatomy. Computed tomography (CT) imaging is required to define adjacent structures such as the liver, spleen, and colon. Although the presence of a retrorenal colon is rare (historic rate of 1%), it would be considered a contraindication to PCNL. Upper pole percutaneous access may also be less desirable in more superiorly located kidneys that would require supracostal access (especially above the 11th rib), as the risk of violating the pleural space with resultant hemothorax, hydrothorax, and/or pneumothorax is increased. Likewise, in the setting of the rare thoracic kidney, PCNL may have an increased risk of pleural space violation or pleural injury since accurate localization of the diaphragm may be difficult under fluoroscopy. Percutaneous nephrolithotomy may also be contraindicated in malrotated kidneys if there are no posteriorly oriented calices and infundibula.

Serious complications are more common with PCNL than URS or SWL. The risk of bleeding is understandably greater as the kidney is a highly vascular organ and the percutaneous access traverses the renal cortex. Recently, the PCNL Global Study, which included over 5,800 patients prospectively observed from over 90 centers worldwide, reported bleeding complications in 7.8% of procedures, 5.7% of which required transfusion.[19] Nephrostomy access directly into the renal pelvis and not through a posterior calyx can result in significant bleeding secondary to adjacent renal vasculature injury. Delayed hemorrhage can also occur following PCNL and is most commonly secondary to the development of a pseudoaneurysm or arteriovenous fistula along the site of percutaneous access. Fortunately, the rate of occurrence is rare at 1%, but angioembolization is usually necessary. Other complications that can occur as a result of percutaneous access include pneumohydrothorax (historic rate of 10% supracostal access) and injury to adjacent organs such as spleen, liver, and colon. Complications occurring during actual stone treatment include renal pelvis perforation and duodenal injury, which is most often a consequence of right renal pelvis perforation. Postoperative sepsis (historic rate of 1–2%) can occur in patients with an untreated UTI or with stones harboring bacteria not completely eradicated by perioperative antibiotics. In a retrospective review of >1,000 patients who underwent PCNL, the overall complication rate was reported to be as high as 83%. Fortunately, these complications mostly consisted of contrast extravasation (7.2%), transfusion (11.2–17.5%), and fever (21–32.1%), whereas major complications were rare and included urosepsis (0.3–4.7%), colonic injury (0.2–0.8%), and pleural injury (up to 3.1%).[20]

Despite the possible complications, the benefits of PCNL make it a highly utilized option for the treatment of large renal stones. The large-caliber and direct renal collecting system access leads to efficient and thorough removal of large stone burdens with high stone-free rate. In patients with lower urinary tract reconstruction or diversion, percutaneous renal access may be the only feasible approach for treatment of renal or ureteral stones. Although serious complications are possible, PCNL performed with an understanding of the possible complications can be accomplished safely and effectively in appropriate cases.

Open or Laparoscopic Urologic Stone Surgery

Urologic stone surgery through an open or laparoscopic approach primarily includes ureterolithotomy, pyelolithotomy, and anatrophic nephrolithotomy. However, the success of SWL, URS, and PCNL has essentially minimized the role of open surgery for urologic stone treatment. The challenge with the laparoscopic approach is the high degree of technical difficulty, which generally limits its application to those surgeons with specific training. Presently, in the age of robotic surgery, laparoscopy is more broadly utilized by surgeons with less laparoscopic experience or training, and stone treatments, such as pyelolithotomy and anatrophic nephrolithotomy, are not entirely extinct. In some cases, these procedures may be the best option for urologic stone treatment, such as laparoscopic pyelolithotomy for a large stone in a malrotated kidney not amenable to PCNL. Anatrophic nephrolithotomy using robotic-assisted laparoscopy is an option for treatment of complete staghorn calculi to minimize the number of treatments required for a single renal stone burden. Other indications for choosing these types of procedures over less invasive options include inability to position patients due to anatomic abnormalities (e.g. contractures), renal anatomic abnormalities (e.g. UPJ obstruction, infundibular stenosis, and calyceal diverticulum), and previous renal surgery. Regardless of the approach, these procedures are the most invasive of urologic stone surgical treatments, which generally limit their application.

Ureterolithotomy and pyelolithotomy are limited to circumstances in which other less invasive urologic stone treatments would be ineffective or contraindicated. The laparoscopic approach, with or without robotic assistance, is generally transperitoneal. Once the kidney or ureter is exposed from under the overlying peritoneal contents, the stone is localized. For pyelolithotomy, an incision in the renal pelvis is made, generally in a transverse orientation. For ureterolithotomy, an incision over the stone is made, generally in a longitudinal orientation. In both procedures, the whole stone is removed through the incision, following which a ureteral stent is placed prior to closure of the incision. The ureteral stent allows passage of urine down to the bladder without extravasation through the closed incision. Overall, these procedures are effective for stone removal, but are more invasive.

Anatrophic nephrolithotomy is the most invasive procedure for renal stone removal. While anatrophic nephrolithotomy may be performed through an open approach, robotic-assisted laparoscopy is making the procedure relatively more appealing. Although less invasive with robotic surgery, anatrophic nephrolithotomy still requires a longitudinal incision through the renal parenchyma along the length of the kidney in order to remove the staghorn calculus en bloc. The nephrotomy incision is made through the theoretically avascular plane of Brödel. Despite the nephrotomy incision through an avascular plane, the renal hilar vessels are generally clamped to prevent excessive bleeding. The incision is extended through the renal collecting system in order to expose and remove the staghorn calculus. In other circumstances, such as calyceal stones, the nephrotomy incision is not so extensive. Following stone removal, the nephrotomy incision is closed in layers, beginning with the renal collecting system and concluding with the renal capsule covered by Gerota's fascia or omentum.

Complications in these procedures are generally related to the specific approach. Overall, ureterolithotomy, pyelolithotomy, and anatrophic nephrolithotomy all risk injury to adjacent organs during laparoscopic access and dissection. Specifically, ureterolithotomy risks subsequent ureteral stricture, while both ureterolithotomy and pyelolithotomy may be complicated by urine leak or urinoma. The primary concern for anatrophic nephrolithotomy is bleeding due to the nephrotomy incision, even with renal

Table 27.2: Summary of algorithm for surgical nephrolithiasis treatment.

	Stone factors					
Treatment options	*Single; <1 cm*	*Multiple; <1 cm*	*Single; 1–2 cm*	*Multiple; 1–2 cm*	*Single; >2 cm*	*Multiple/complex; >2 cm*
Observation	Yes*	No	No	No	No	No
SWL	Yes	Yes†	Yes	No	No	No
URS	Yes	Yes	Yes	Yes	Yes‡	Yes‡
PCNL	No§	No	Yes	Yes	Yes	Yes
Open or laparoscopic	No	No	No	Yes‖	Yes‖	Yes‖

(SWL: Shockwave lithotripsy; URS: Ureteroscopy; PCNL: Percutaneous nephrolithotomy).
*Observation is not recommended for most ureteral stones >5 mm.
†Shockwave lithotripsy is an option for multiple small stones if stone composition is known to fragment well.
‡Ureteroscopy is an option for these cases when there are contraindications to PCNL or open/laparoscopic surgery, but may require multiple treatments for complete stone clearance.
§Percutaneous nephrolithotomy may be the only option if the retrograde approach is not possible and SWL is contraindicated.
‖Open/laparoscopic surgery is limited to select cases in which PCNL cannot be performed or is contraindicated.

vessel clamping. Urine leak or urinoma is also a possible complication of anatrophic nephrolithotomy since the renal collecting system requires reconstruction after the stone is removed. Although serious complications are possible, these more invasive procedures can be accomplished safely and effectively in select cases.

Stone Factors

In order to choose the appropriate surgical treatment for nephrolithiasis, understanding of various stone factors or characteristics in addition to knowledge of treatment options is required. Stone disease of the kidney and/or ureter can be widely varied in presentation, appearance, shape, size, location, number, composition, and density. Likewise, there are several surgical options for treatment of stones within the kidney and the ureter. Thus, there is no single correct treatment option for most cases of urologic stone disease. Small differences in any single stone factor may significantly alter the clinical decision making. These various stone factors and how each factor might affect the selection of a surgical treatment option will be discussed in detail in this section (Table 27.2 for algorithm summary).

Urologic Stone Size

Perhaps the most commonly considered stone factor is size (diameter and volume). Renal stone size is important as it frequently dictates the location of the stone burden. Larger stones generally remain within the renal collecting system and are unlikely to migrate through an infundibulum or down the small-caliber ureter. Conversely, smaller renal stones may demonstrate more mobility by exiting a calyx and possibly travelling down the ureter, resulting in obstruction and renal colic. Especially for renal stones, size may play the most prominent role in determining surgical treatment. Larger stones are more likely to require secondary procedures to render the patient stone free, and therefore, factor into clinical decision making and patient counseling. In general, as the renal stone size increases, the number of surgical treatment options to render the patient stone-free decreases and the invasiveness increases.

Stone size is an extremely important factor in determining surgical treatment, and calculating volume is likely the most accurate assessment of renal stone burden. However, there are no official guidelines on measuring stone size to maintain uniformity. Among scientific literature, there is significant heterogeneity in methods of stone size measurement, which vary between one-, two-, and three-dimensional estimations.[21,22] In most studies and official panel guidelines, stone size is measured by the maximal linear measurement in the noncontrast CT scan axial images. Measurements in a single dimension are inherently inaccurate since the second and third dimensions of the stone are not considered. In a study of 151 stones measured on noncontrast CT scan with coronal reconstruction, there was a significant difference between axial versus coronal stone areas and largest axial versus coronal dimensions.[23] In the United Kingdom, 74% of radiologists and only 19% of urologists used electronic calipers on CT scans to measure linear stone dimensions.[24] The difficulty with measuring stone burdens in two and three dimensions is not only accurate stone measurements, but also the use of formulas to measure area and automated software for ellipsoid measurements of volume, respectively.[25] Stone volume is likely the most accurate estimate of nephrolithiasis burden, but the tools for uniform measurement are not yet widely available. Although not ideal, the largest linear measurement is used for the purposes of this chapter as used by the most recent panel guidelines regarding nephrolithiasis.

Stone Size >2 cm

The inverse relationship of stone size to the number of treatment options is likely best exemplified by renal stones measuring ≥2 cm. The recommended treatment options for nonstaghorn renal stones measuring ≥2 cm are generally limited to flexible URS with laser lithotripsy and PCNL. Shockwave lithotripsy in these cases is associated with low success and increased complications, such as steinstrasse.[26] Laparoscopic pyelolithotomy is also a surgical option for large stones localized to the renal pelvis. Overall, PCNL has demonstrated higher stone-free rates in a single treatment than retrograde URS for large stones. In a case–control study of 34 patients with renal stone burdens of 2–4 cm treated with flexible URS matched to similar cases treated with PCNL, Akman et al. reported that 91% of the PCNL cohort was stone free compared to 73.5% of the flexible URS cohort.[27] The operative time was also 20 minutes shorter in the PCNL cohort (38.7 minutes vs 58.2 minutes; p <0.0001), while the flexible URS cohort required a secondary procedure to achieve an approximate 88% stone-free rate. In a similar matched-pair analysis, the stone-free rate was 92.8% after a single PCNL versus 82.1% after a single flexible URS procedure with laser lithotripsy.[28] The operative time was ~25 minutes shorter in the PCNL cases (40.7 minutes vs 64.5 minutes; p <0.0001). At 3 months after stone treatment, stone-free rates determined by radiography of the kidneys, ureters, and bladder (KUB) were reported to have increased to 96.4% in the PCNL group and 92.8% in the retrograde URS group. In a meta-analysis of 460 renal units with a mean stone size of 2.5 cm treated with flexible URS and laser lithotripsy, Aboumarzouk et al. reported a 93.7% stone-free rate with an average of 1.6 procedures per patient.[29] The subgroup analysis of this meta-analysis demonstrated a lower stone-free rate of 84.6% for stones >3 cm compared to 95.7% stone-free rate for stones 2–3 cm (p = 0.01). The overall complication rate for flexible URS was 10.1% with a 5.3% major complication rate. Both flexible URS with laser lithotripsy and PCNL are effective surgical treatment options for nonstaghorn renal stones >2 cm. In the Clinical Research Office of Endourological Society (CROES) PCNL Global Study of 1,448 large solitary stone cases, PCNL demonstrated stone-free rates of 90.0%, 83.3%, and 84.1% for stone sizes of 2–3 cm, 3–4 cm, and 4–6 cm, respectively.[30] Higher rates of postoperative fever (17.9%) and blood transfusion (13.3%) were associated with stones >4 cm in size. Based on these results, this group concluded: "The significantly lower stone-free rate (for stones >4 cm) suggests that urologists are overly cautious when removing larger stones to avoid bleeding and thus, any damage that might compromise renal function or stone removal is inherently more difficult. Each would result in less rigorous removal of stone fragments." Thus, even with direct renal collecting access for efficient renal stone treatment, increasing stone sizes will be well treated with PCNL but may be accompanied by lower stone-free rates and more difficulty. However, given the frequently reported higher stone-free rates after a single procedure, PCNL is the preferred monotherapy option for treatment of large renal stone burdens without contraindications to this procedure.

Although there is a relatively higher degree of invasiveness compared to PCNL, laparoscopic pyelolithotomy (with or without robotic assistance) is also a viable option for treatment of large renal stones. A meta-analysis of seven non-randomized concurrent controlled trials of PCNL or laparoscopic pyelolithotomy for treatment of large renal pelvis stones in a total of 363 patients demonstrated similarly high stone-free rates between the procedures (odds ratio 0.33; 95% confidence interval 0.09–1.17).[31] Laparoscopic pyelolithotomy also demonstrated several benefits over PCNL, including 50.6 minutes shorter operative time, 0.66 days shorter length of stay, lower rate of postoperative fever, and less blood loss (but no difference in transfusions). Considering these advantages, laparoscopic pyelolithotomy is a good option for treatment of large renal pelvic stones, especially in cases where PCNL may be difficult or unsafe. These cases would include malrotated kidneys without posteriorly oriented calices, stenotic infundibula that would prevent access to the renal pelvis, or the presence of retrorenal structures, such as the spleen, colon, or liver (Figs. 27.1 and 27.2).

Shockwave lithotripsy has been used to treat renal stones measuring ≥2 cm. The limitations of SWL for large renal stone treatment are incomplete fragmentation, limited number of shockwaves that can be applied to the target stone, residual fragments, and significant risk of

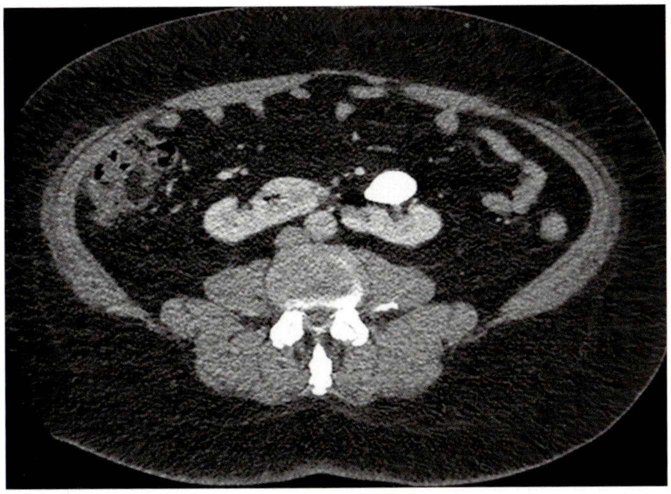

Fig. 27.1: Large renal pelvic stone in left moiety of a horseshoe kidney. Due to difficult access from percutaneous approach, laparoscopic pyelolithotomy was performed.

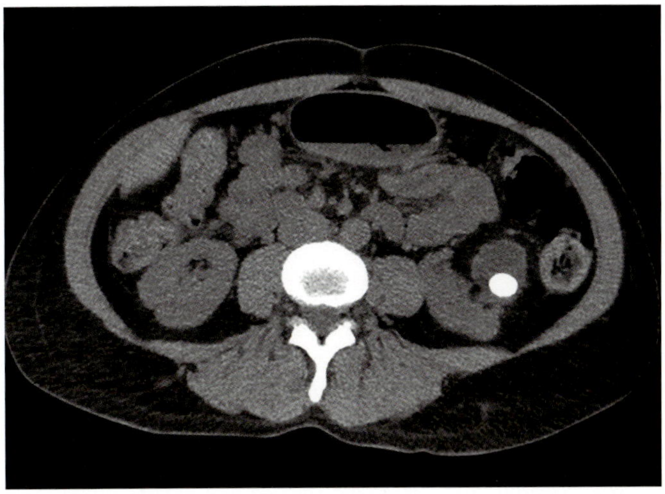

Fig. 27.2: Large renal pelvic stone in malrotated left kidney. Because of the lack of posteriorly oriented calices for percutaneous access, laparoscopic pyelolithotomy was performed.

steinstrasse with obstruction. The steinstrasse rate is ~4% overall but is 3.7 times higher after SWL for stones >2 cm.[32] Gleeson and Griffith reported on 199 large (≥3 cm) renal stones treated with SWL, 29 of which were solitary stones.[33] Among the large solitary kidney stones, SWL achieved only a 55.2% stone-free rate overall after 1.35 treatments per patient. Approximately 20.7% cases had >5 mm residual stone fragments. Among those with a solitary stone in the renal pelvis where stone fragments would presumably have the most direct exit route, the stone-free rate was only 70% with SWL monotherapy. Likewise, Murray et al. reported low stone-free rates with SWL monotherapy in 65 patients with renal stones measuring >3 cm.[34] At 3 months post-SWL, the overall success rate was only 27%. Although not necessarily contraindicated for the treatment of large renal stones, the poor success rate of SWL renders it a suboptimal treatment. For stones >2 cm, PCNL is the preferred treatment option. Flexible URS and laparoscopic pyelolithotomy are second-line treatment options, which in some cases may be preferred or necessary depending on the patient's anatomical and clinical factors.

Stone Size 1–2 cm

Although SWL is likely to be suboptimal monotherapy for large renal stone burdens, stones measuring <2 cm may be treated by several monotherapy options, including SWL. The reported success rates of SWL for stones 1–2 cm are varied. In a study of 3,241 cases of urolithiasis, 1,433 stones measuring 1–2 cm were successfully treated with SWL at a rate of 72.1%.[35] However, other large studies have demonstrated low stone-free rates despite more shockwaves per session, and a higher retreatment rate with increasing renal stone burden.[36] These success rates may be as low as 39.6% with retreatment rates as high as 76.2%. For ureteral stones >1 cm, the AUA/EAU Nephrolithiasis Panel ureteral calculi guidelines[7] report stone-free rates for the distal, mid-, and proximal ureter of 74%, 76%, and 68%, respectively, and designate the "recommendation" that SWL is an acceptable first-line treatment for these stones. With the varied success and retreatment rates for stones of this size, these stones may be more effectively treated with other modalities. However, there is no general consensus on a stone size limit for SWL treatment. Contributing to this lack of consensus are the multiple factors in addition to stone size, such as stone location, number, composition, and density. For solitary renal or ureteral stones in this size range (1–2 cm), SWL is a reasonable option. However, patients should be well educated on how the characteristics of their particular stone burden may affect the outcome and need for secondary procedures.

Ureteroscopy is the next level of invasiveness beyond SWL for the treatment of urolithiasis measuring 1–2 cm. For medium-sized ureteral stones, URS is the most frequently utilized option besides SWL. The AUA/EAU Nephrolithiasis Panel also analyzed studies on outcomes of ureteral stone treatment with URS, and designated URS as an acceptable first-line treatment for ureteral stones >1 cm based on high first-treatment stone-free rates and low complication rates.[7] The primary advantage of flexible URS is direct visualization of stone and subsequent treatment, which is particularly beneficial for radiolucent stones where fluoroscopic localization in SWL may not be possible. Direct visualization within the kidney also provides insight into the pathogenesis and specific location of the renal stone disease, such as the presence of Randall's plaques on papillae, calcifications within dilated ducts of Bellini, and other renal papillary changes. In a retrospective review comparing SWL, flexible URS, and PCNL for treatment of 1–2 cm radiolucent stones in 437 patients, flexible URS achieved a stone-free rate of 87% and required a secondary procedure in 8.7% of cases compared to a 66.5% stone-free rate and 21.9% secondary procedure rate for SWL patients.[37] The same factors that may affect SWL treatment (i.e. stone location, number, and density) may also affect URS, but the direct vision and maneuverability of the ureteroscope combined with auxiliary instruments, such as the holmium laser and stone retrieval baskets, provide advantages for treating larger stones with high success rates. The primary disadvantage with URS is postoperative ureteral stent-related pain. Although ureteral stent pain can be problematic, survey studies indicate that patients prefer familiarity with a procedure, choosing SWL again for future stone treatments despite lower stone-free rates and choosing URS again despite previous stent pain.[38] However, overall more SWL than URS patients would choose SWL again.[39] The importance of patient counseling was also emphasized by ~56% of patients relying on the physician's recommendation in cases where SWL or URS could be used.[38]

Frequently compared to flexible URS for treatment of medium-sized renal stones is PCNL. Percutaneous nephrolithotomy is both more invasive and more efficient owing to the short wide route into the kidney and simultaneous fragmentation/evacuation via larger instruments. Flexible URS is less invasive, but less efficient due to the small-caliber instruments and less direct access to the renal stone burden. In the same 437 patient study of 1–2 cm radiolucent stone treatment as previously described,[37] PCNL demonstrated a 91.4% stone-free rate and only 5.7% of patients required a secondary procedure. These positive results were somewhat tempered by significantly higher complication and transfusion rates compared to flexible URS. For special circumstances, such as large infection stones, ureteral stricture, urinary diversion, or UPJ obstruction, PCNL is a better option to access and treat an upper tract stone. Overall, for stones 1–2 cm in size, PCNL is more invasive but a good option. The access (i.e. retrograde versus antegrade) and need to remove all stone material (i.e. infection stone) should be considered when choosing between URS and PCNL for these stones.

In an attempt to decrease the invasiveness of PCNL while maintaining the advantage of direct, relatively large-caliber renal collecting system access, "microperc" or "miniperc" have been introduced. In miniperc, the nephrostomy tract is dilated only to 18–20 F compared to the conventional 30 F tract, but this requires specialized, smaller rigid instruments, which do not provide simultaneous fragmentation and evacuation. Generally, laser lithotripsy is required for stone fragmentation prior to using a stone evacuation device. Microperc is performed through a 3-channel 16-gauge needle, which utilizes irrigation, telescopic vision, and a holmium laser fiber through the respective channels. Microperc does not provide any stone fragment evacuation, but relies on spontaneous passage of resulting minute stone fragments. The very small-caliber access and telescopic vision also limit the ability of microperc to treat stones only in the path of its access (i.e. the corresponding renal calyx and potentially the renal pelvis). In a prospective, case–control study, 32 miniperc procedures were compared to 32 flexible URS procedures for the treatment of 1–2 cm solitary renal stones.[40] The stone-free rates at 4 weeks postoperatively for miniperc (100%) and flexible URS (97%) were similar; miniperc operative time was significantly shorter by a mean of 10 minutes, but required more pain medications postoperatively than flexible URS. In a similar randomized, controlled trial, 35 microperc procedures were compared to 35 flexible URS procedures for the treatment of 1-cm solitary renal stones.[41] The stone-free rates at 3 months postoperatively for microperc (97.1%) and flexible URS (94.3%) were similar; surgeon discomfort score was significantly higher in flexible URS, indicating more surgeon discomfort during the procedure. In a large study of the miniperc procedure consisting of 13,984 renal units with staghorn (31.5%), multiple (39.1%), or single large (29.4%) renal stones, the stone-free rate after the initial procedure was 78.6%, which increased after second look or auxiliary procedures to 89.9% and 94.8%, respectively.[42] Both miniperc and microperc have demonstrated promising results by striking a compromise between the advantages of both flexible URS and PCNL. However, renal stone treatment is frequently chosen based on its invasiveness or its stone-removal ability. Surgeons and patients alike may not desire a percutaneous procedure that would provide stone fragmentation without stone removal when another minimally invasive (i.e. URS) or noninvasive (i.e. SWL) procedure could provide the same benefit. Presently, the advantages of flexible

URS and conventional PCNL make these options the most viable for treatment of medium-sized renal stones.

In rare cases, open or laparoscopic pyelolithotomy or ureterolithotomy may be required for treatment of 1–2 cm renal or ureteral stones. Such procedures may be considered in cases where percutaneous access is difficult or impossible, such as ectopic kidney, unfavorable adjacent organ location, or malrotation; or in the case of ureteral stone associated with ureteral stricture where removal of the stone and strictured ureteral segment is performed. Since the vast majority of medium-sized stones are successfully treated with SWL, URS, or PCNL, the need for laparoscopic or open pyelolithotomy or ureterolithotomy is rare. If laparoscopic expertise is available, a laparoscopic approach instead of an open approach to these procedures is generally the best alternative unless the clinical scenario precludes it.

Stone Size <1 cm

The preferred surgical options for renal and ureteral stones <1 cm in size that require treatment are SWL and URS. For distal ureteral stones, URS is preferred as the bony pelvis often precludes definitive localization and targeting of the stone for SWL treatment. For ureteral stones <1 cm, the AUA/EAU Nephrolithiasis Panel ureteral calculi guidelines[7] report stone-free rates of SWL for the proximal, midureter, and distal ureter of 89%, 80%, and 80%, respectively, whereas the stone-free rates for URS are 80%, 91%, and 97%, respectively. For small renal stones, SWL may be effective but require multiple treatments. In a prospective series, for patients with a <1 cm solitary renal stone treated with SWL, there was an 85.9% stone-free rate and only an 8.8% failure rate, but a median of two treatments was required to achieve these results.[43] The average number of shocks was 3,787 with a 14 kV initial energy level, which was progressively increased to 20 kV. The progressively increasing energy level in the "ramping protocol" may play a role in the effectiveness of SWL in renal stones. In a prospective, randomized trial, Lambert et al. reported significantly higher stone-free rates (81% vs 48%) for patients treated with SWL for an average 8 mm renal stone who were randomized to an escalating energy strategy of 500 shocks at 14 kV, 1,000 shocks at 16 kV, and 1,000 shocks at 18 kV compared to a fixed energy strategy of 2,500 shocks at 18 kV.[44] Good stone fragmentation to enable spontaneous passage after SWL is better with an escalating energy strategy and is especially effective when concentrated on a small, solitary stone.

For treatment of small renal calculi with flexible URS, a systematic review and meta-analysis have shown a relative paucity of research comparing SWL and URS.[45] However, the weighted average stone-free rate from publications evaluating flexible ureterorenoscopy was ~88% in 140 patients.[46–48] There are clinical scenarios in which URS is preferred over SWL, including coagulopathy, pregnancy, morbid obesity, adjacent vascular calcifications, and large abdominal aortic aneurysms.

The use of more invasive procedures for small renal or ureteral calculi, such as PCNL or pyelolithotomy/ureterolithotomy, is limited. These procedures are generally restricted to special clinical scenarios, such as the use of percutaneous access and antegrade flexible URS for a small ureteral stone in a patient with lower urinary tract reconstruction or ureteral stricture preventing a retrograde approach or treatment of stones in ectopic/transplant kidneys. In these cases, a more invasive approach is often necessary to render the patient stone free.

Renal Stone Location and Conformation

Stone location and conformation are perhaps as important as stone size in determining treatment options. Stone location within the kidney and ureter differ based not only on the position on preoperative imaging (e.g. upper pole), but also on how direct the potential route to that location is for a treatment option. Other aspects of stone location to consider are whether resulting stone fragments will pass from the position postoperatively and how surrounding structures might affect treatment strategy. In addition, stone conformation has been shown to be the best outcome predictor for stone treatment other than stone size.[49] Thus, conformation, especially as it relates to large renal stones and staghorn calculi, is also a critical aspect to consider when determining treatment.

Renal Calyx Stones

Each renal calyx may vary in size, conformation, and number of papillae, but are connected to the renal pelvis by an infundibulum, which is frequently narrower than the calyx itself. In order for a renal calyx stone or stone fragment to pass, it must not only be small enough to pass through the UPJ and down the ureter, but also the infundibulum corresponding to its calyx. Thus, the renal calyx location is an additional aspect that should be considered regarding stone position and may affect the outcome of treatment.

For a stone in an upper pole renal calyx with normal anatomy, there are several options for treatment. The route to and from the renal collecting system outlet is relatively direct. Additionally, when the patient is in an upright position, the UPJ is in a dependent position in relation to upper pole calices. For small- and medium-sized upper pole renal stone burdens, treatment with SWL and flexible URS may benefit from these favorable characteristics for postoperative passage of resulting fragments. In relation to an interpolar calyx, the UPJ is typically in a less dependent position and the route between these two points is less direct compared to an upper pole calyx. However, the lower pole calyx is generally thought to be the least favorable position. From a lower pole calyx, a stone must exit through the infundibulum in a primarily upward direction in order to reach the renal pelvis before passing through the UPJ to leave the kidney. This path or trajectory from a lower pole calyx to the UPJ is known as the infundibulopelvic angle. An acute infundibulopelvic angle may portend less favorable outcomes for stone treatments such as SWL after which resulting stone fragments must pass spontaneously.[50] Infundibular length and width may also be factors to consider since long or narrow infundibula have been associated with decreased stone-free rates after SWL of lower pole calyx stones.[43]

These varying characteristics of upper, middle, and lower pole calices are demonstrated in the differences for stone-free and failure rates in SWL treatment of stones in these locations.[43, 51–54] In general, clearance of stone fragments after SWL is lower for lower pole stones than for upper pole and interpolar calyx stones. Success for SWL is usually highest for upper pole stones (stone-free rate range: 66–98%). Success of SWL in treatment of interpolar calyx stones varies but generally is better than that for lower pole stones. As may be expected, stone-free rates for lower pole stone treatment with SWL are not only lower than those for upper and interpolar stones, but also may be low overall. Despite patient's preference and short convalescence, SWL stone-free rates have been reported as low as 35%, even for small lower pole renal stones.[39]

Flexible URS may be a better option for lower pole stone treatment due to its ability to maneuver around the infundibulopelvic angle and remove stone material. Treatment with flexible URS is reported to have higher stone-free rates and requires fewer retreatments compared to SWL in lower pole renal stone treatment.[55] However, until recently, there have been few randomized controlled trials (RCTs) comparing flexible URS to SWL with regard to lower pole renal stone treatment, and meta-analyses report no significant difference in success rates between the two modalities.[18,45] In a recent RCT comparing SWL to flexible URS for treatment of small renal stones in 140 patients, Sener et al. report a 100% stone-free rate after flexible URS after a single treatment versus a 91.5% stone-free rate after a mean 2.7 treatments with SWL.[56] Conversely, PCNL has demonstrated better effectiveness of large lower pole renal stone treatment compared to SWL with a higher success rate for PCNL at 3 months (RR=0.39), fewer retreatments (RR = 1.81), fewer additional procedures (RR = 9.06), and a higher efficiency quotient.[18] For larger lower pole renal stones (>1 cm), flexible URS and PCNL are the best treatment options, especially considering the higher retreatment rates associated with SWL. The success of flexible URS depends on surgeon experience, equipment availability, patient anatomy, and stone size. One strategy to increase stone-free status with flexible URS for lower pole stones is relocation of a lower pole renal stone to a more favorable position, such as an upper pole calyx, prior to fragmentation/removal.[57] Relocation to an upper pole calyx will enable easier, more controlled laser fragmentation and stone removal by flexible URS. For a large lower pole renal stone burden, PCNL is a better option than flexible URS or SWL as stone-free rates are higher. The direct access, direct vision, and simultaneous fragmentation/evacuation afforded by PCNL make it the better option despite its invasiveness.

Renal Pelvis Stones

In normal renal collecting system anatomy, the renal pelvis is presumably the most ideal location for stone treatment. A renal pelvis stone is in close proximity to the UPJ. Other than normal anatomical narrowing of the UPJ, there are no other narrowings or acute angles to complicate the route a stone or instrument must traverse. These favorable anatomical features of the renal pelvis may play a role in improving treatment success for SWL. In a study of 438 patients treated with SWL, the stone-free rate for renal pelvic stones was 72.4%, which was significantly better than the overall stone-free rate of 65.1% or those of any of the renal calyx locations.[36] However, the stone-free rates declined markedly as stone size increased and resulted in need for retreatment for large proportion of the study population (78.1%). Although the passage route for resulting stone fragments may be favorable from the renal pelvis, the potential space surrounding the stone within the renal pelvis may be a disadvantage. If a renal pelvis is extra renal, is dilated, or is simply capacious, there is a potential for increased movement of the target stone during SWL.

Significant movement of the renal stone during SWL may lead to less efficient, less effective fragmentation. Yet, due to its noninvasiveness and decreased postoperative pain, a high rate of retreatment with SWL with resulting favorable stone-free rates may still result in greater rates of patient acceptance and shorter convalescence compared to other treatment modalities.[58]

The larger space of the renal pelvis compared to a calyx could also be a disadvantage in flexible URS where the stone may move significantly due to fluid irrigation or propulsion by laser energy. However, the direct vision of flexible URS allows for real-time tracking of the stone and subsequent stone fragments. Yet, for larger stones treated by PCNL, the renal pelvis may be ideal for stone treatment if the infundibulum corresponding to the entry calyx accommodates a rigid nephroscope, allowing access to the renal pelvis. In a comparison of renal pelvic stones measuring 1–2 cm treated by SWL, flexible URS, or PCNL in 149 patients, SWL achieved an 86% stone-free rate after multiple treatments compared to single-treatment stone-free rates of 91.4% and 98% for flexible URS and PCNL, respectively.[59] Slightly tempering the excellent success rate for PCNL was the 12% complication rate compared to the 7.6% and 6.3% complication rates for SWL and flexible URS, respectively. Overall, SWL may be a viable option for renal pelvis stone treatment, but retreatment may be required to achieve stone-free status. Conversely, flexible URS and PCNL may be better options for achieving stone-free status with a single treatment. This may be true especially with regard to PCNL for larger stone burdens, but the higher complication rate associated with PCNL should also be considered. Stone location must be considered in conjunction with stone size to determine the best treatment modality.

Given the potential complications associated with PCNL, some stone surgeons may advocate for laparoscopic pyelolithotomy. Whereas PCNL may require less operative time to treat a solitary, large renal pelvis stone and lead to a shorter hospital stay, laparoscopic pyelolithotomy patients may benefit from less bleeding and lower rates of postoperative fever.[31] As described previously, this meta-analysis of PCNL and laparoscopic pyelolithotomy studies demonstrates similar stone-free rates between these procedures, but is limited by a paucity of randomized, controlled trials. Given the high degree of technical difficulty in laparoscopic pyelolithotomy, such as intracorporeal suturing, this procedure is generally limited to more advanced laparoscopic surgeons. Thus, laparoscopic pyelolithotomy is generally recommended to be limited to patients with contraindications to PCNL.

Stone Conformation and Staghorn Renal Calculi

Renal stones that occupy multiple locations due to complex conformations pose a significant challenge compared to solitary nonstaghorn stones. Complex stones tend to be large, which will further complicate treatment and may narrow the surgical options. Notably, the terms "struvite" and "staghorn" are frequently used interchangeably due to the commonality of infection stone composition and conformation. However, there is no definitive standard for the use of the term "staghorn calculi." The AUA guidelines panel describes staghorn calculi as "branched stones that occupy a large portion of the collecting system. Typically, they fill the renal pelvis and branch into several or all of the calices."[60] Although many infection stones will have a staghorn configuration, not all staghorn calculi are the result of UTI and many staghorn stones have a noninfectious composition.[61] Additionally, there is no standard classification for "partial" and "complete" staghorn calculi, but complete staghorn stones are generally those that occupy the entire renal collecting system.

For complex renal stones, but especially in cases of complete staghorn renal calculi (Fig. 27.3), the complexity of treatment stems from both the large bulk of the stone burden and the challenge of obtaining access to all stone-containing areas of the collecting system. To address these challenges, the AUA Nephrolithiasis Guideline Panel developed guidelines for recommendations on the management of staghorn renal calculi.[60] According to these guidelines, for most patients with staghorn renal stones, functioning kidneys, and both amenable stone and body characteristics, PCNL is recommended as first-line treatment. This recommendation is based on one of the few RCTs, in which SWL monotherapy was compared to combined (initial) PCNL with SWL for treatment of complete staghorn renal calculi.[62] The combination of PCNL and SWL resulted in a significantly higher 74% stone-free rate compared to 22% for SWL monotherapy. Shockwave lithotripsy monotherapy also resulted in a significantly higher complication (especially, postoperative sepsis) and auxiliary procedure rates. These results also led to the same guidelines recommending against the use of SWL monotherapy for staghorn stones.

Due to the multiple infundibula and calices that may be occupied with stone in cases of staghorn renal calculi,

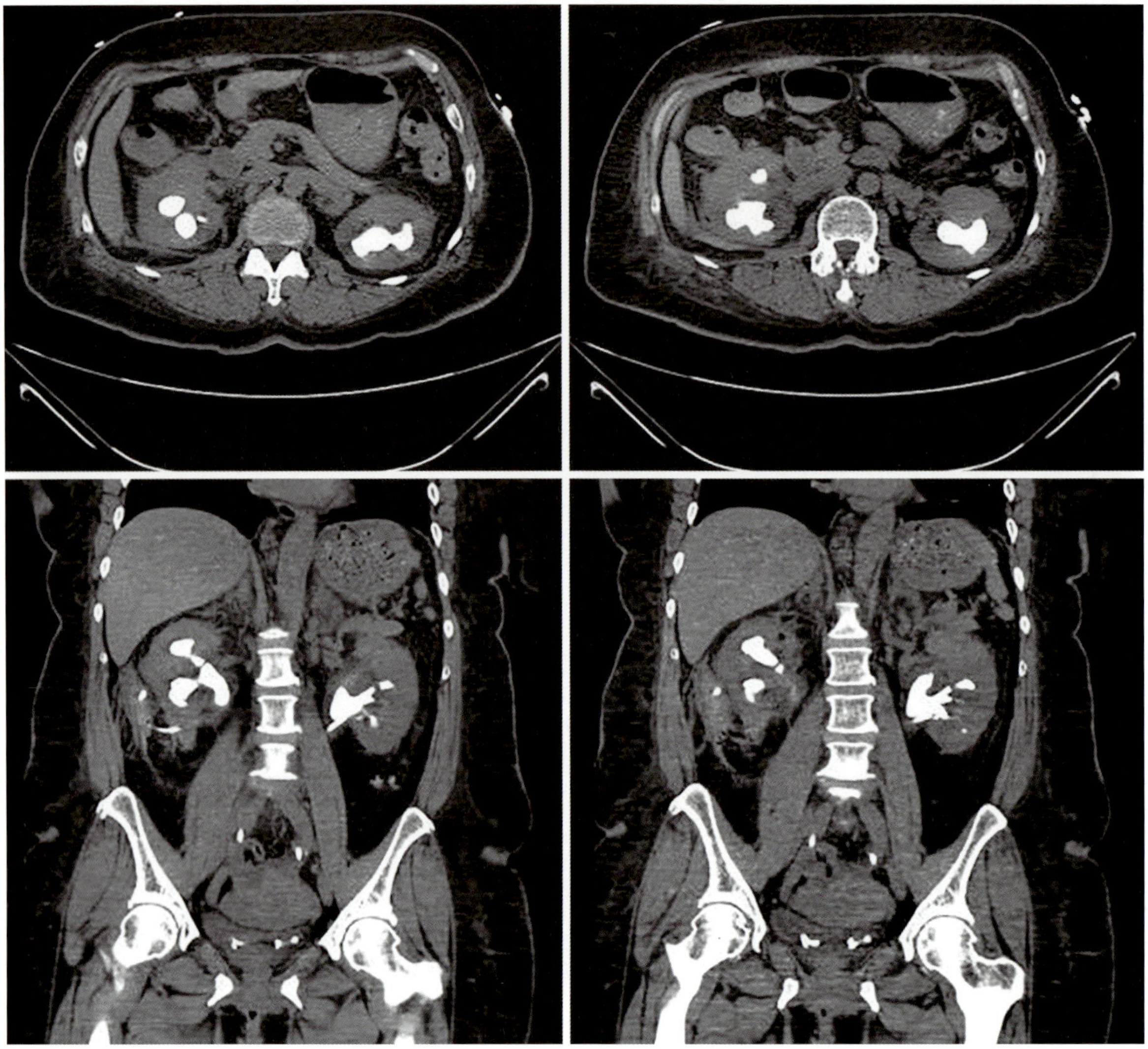

Fig. 27.3: Multipanel view of both axial and coronal noncontrast CT scan images showing bilateral complete staghorn calculi filling each renal collecting system. (CT: Computed tomography).

only a fraction of the stone burden may be accessible with rigid instruments through a single nephrostomy tract in PCNL; therefore, multiple access tracts may be required for stone clearance. Although multiple access tracts will allow use of rigid instruments in several stone-occupied areas and may lead to fewer overall procedures for stone clearance, creation of multiple access tracts may be associated with higher rates of postoperative sepsis and transfusion.[63,64] In order to avoid the potential morbidity of multiple access PCNL, "sandwich therapy" and combination procedures have been studied. Sandwich therapy for staghorn calculi treatment comprises primary debulking of the stone burden with PCNL (via single or multiple tracts) followed by further fragmentation with SWL, and if necessary, secondary/tertiary PCNL to remove residual stone burden. The stone-free rate reported for sandwich therapy was 63% at 1 month. This method, however, was also associated with long hospital admissions as well as high rates of transfusion and sepsis, especially in patients with struvite staghorn stones.[65] Conversely, combination therapy simultaneously combines PCNL with either antegrade or retrograde flexible URS/nephroscopy to provide access to as much stone or as many stone-occupied areas as possible in order to minimize the number of nephrostomy tracts created and procedures required to achieve stone clearance. Retrograde or antegrade flexible nephroscopy provides access to multiple areas of the collecting system to fragment stone with laser lithotripsy, followed by removal of stone fragments via the nephrostomy tract. This method utilizes the natural flow of the irrigant from the flexible nephroscope to flush stone fragments out of the corresponding calyx and toward the renal pelvis, where direct access has been established through the nephrostomy tract. When ureterorenoscopy is performed from a retrograde approach, the rigid nephroscope/instruments may be operated through the nephrostomy tract simultaneously. The main drawback with this approach, however, is that flexible ureterorenoscopy with the patient in the prone position can be technically challenging since the orientation of the collecting system will be completely reversed. In small studies, combination therapy for complete or partial staghorn calculi has resulted in reported stone-free rates up to 78% with a single procedure (via single percutaneous nephrostomy tract) and less estimated blood loss compared to multiple access PCNL.[66,67] Considering the direct access to more areas of the collecting system with rigid instruments, upper pole percutaneous nephrostomy access for PCNL may be especially effective in combination therapy.[68] However, the site-specific risks of upper pole access, such as pleural/thoracic violation, especially if the access is supracostal, must be considered. In the end, whether staghorn renal calculi are approached via single- or multiple-access PCNL, sandwich therapy, or combination therapy, percutaneous nephroscopy as the last procedure is recommended.[60] This recommendation is especially pertinent for patients with known struvite stones, since complete stone clearance is the only way to minimize stone recurrence.

Given the effectiveness of PCNL as monotherapy or in combination with flexible URS/nephroscopy and laser lithotripsy and the potential morbidity, "open surgery should not be used for most patients" with staghorn renal calculi.[60] In part, this recommendation was based upon reported differences in postoperative pain-medication requirements, hospital length of stay, and convalescence between laparoscopic and open surgical nephrectomy.[69] Reported series demonstrate that open anatrophic nephrolithotomy may achieve relatively good stone-free rates (80–85%) at the cost of lengthy hospital stays, relatively large estimated blood loss (325–500 mL), and slight worsening of renal function.[70,71] In a randomized, prospective comparison of 88 staghorn renal calculi treatment with open surgery (including pyelolithotomy, combined pyelo-/nephrolithotomy, anatrophic nephrolithotomy, and pyelocalicotomy) versus PCNL, the stone-free rates at 3 months postoperatively were similar (82% vs 74%).[72] Although the major postoperative complication rates were similar, open surgery was associated with a higher rate of intraoperative complications, longer operative time, longer hospital stay, and longer convalescence.

In order to decrease morbidity, procedures previously performed via an open approach are frequently attempted laparoscopically. Data associated with laparoscopic anatrophic nephrolithotomy for treatment of complex or staghorn renal calculi are generally limited to small case series ($\leq$10 patients) as first reports on developing techniques.[73-75] These case series do report similar operative times and complication rates to open surgery, but overall lower success rates. Likewise, procedures performed or attempted with conventional laparoscopy are frequently attempted with robotic assistance to decrease the technical difficulty of laparoscopy. Similar to laparoscopic anatrophic nephrolithotomy, robotic-assisted anatrophic nephrolithotomy data are limited to small introductory case series resulting in both stone-free and complication rates that have not been supported by further studies.[76,77] One significant disadvantage to consider is warm ischemia time, which could be prolonged in a difficult laparoscopic case and may lead to decreased postoperative renal function. Cold ischemia in laparoscopic anatrophic nephrolithotomy has been demonstrated,[76] but is not commonly utilized. Considering the high degree of technical difficulty and relative paucity of data, laparoscopic anatrophic nephrolithotomy (with or without robotic assistance) is a less desirable treatment option for complex or staghorn renal calculi, especially for surgeons with little training or experience in this area.

Renal Stone Number

The number of renal stones composing the stone burden to be treated should influence surgical treatment choice. If all other characteristics are equal between separate renal stone burdens, the number of stones for treatment may work in favor of the strengths of one treatment option in comparison to another procedure. In the end, when considering surgical treatment options, the degree of renal stone number is a matter of whether a solitary stone or multiple renal stones are to be treated.

If all stone characteristics are the same, treatment of a solitary renal stone will be less complex and result in better outcomes for all surgical modalities. Whether in SWL, URS with laser lithotripsy, or PCNL, a solitary renal stone is a single target for energy application during fragmentation. With regard to SWL, all shockwaves applied to the

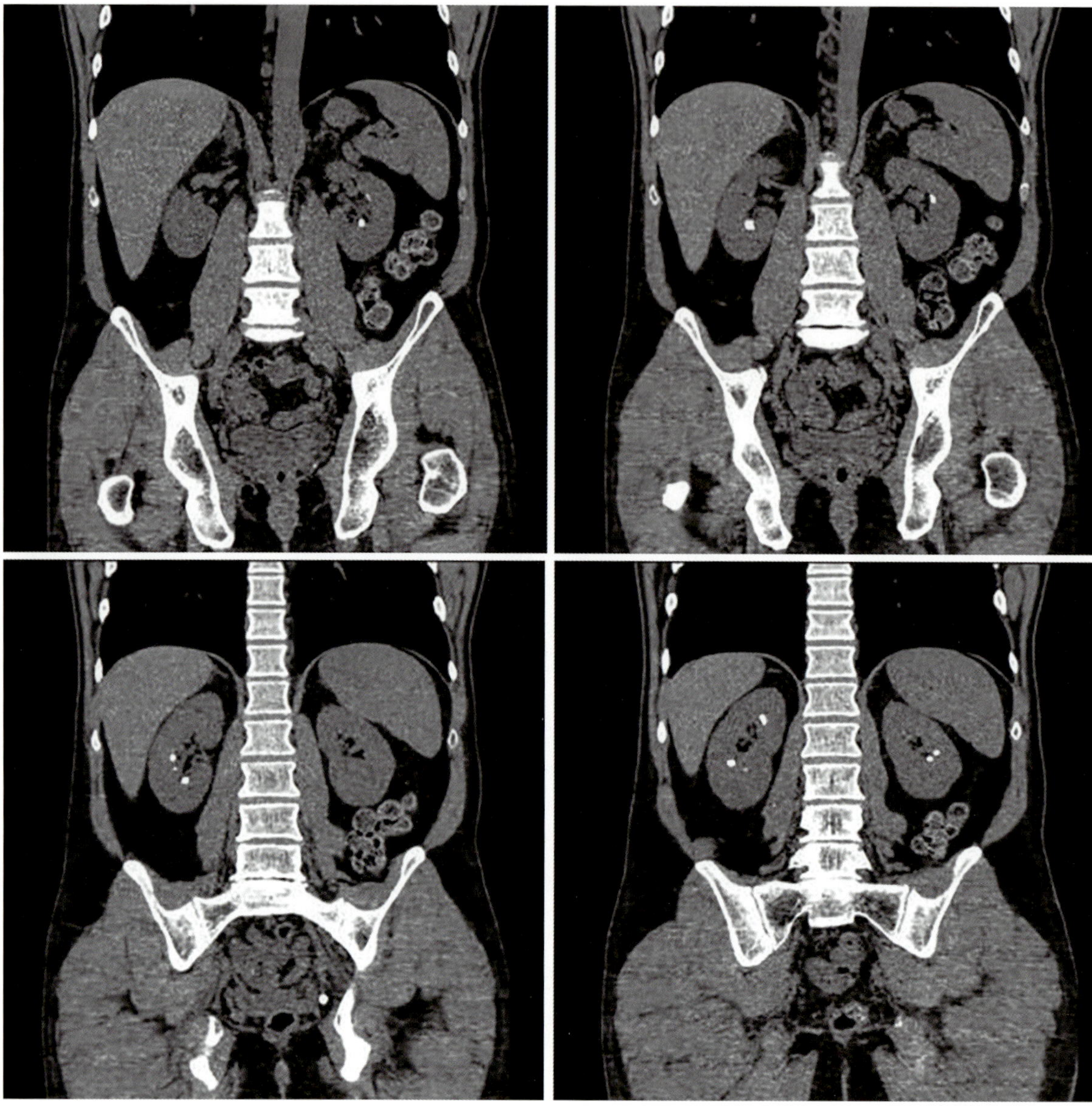

Fig. 27.4: Multipanel view of multiple small brushite renal stones bilaterally.

kidney ideally are applied to the target stone without concern for limiting the energy, aside from preventing renal injury. For URS and PCNL, direct visualization of a single stone's fragmentation and/or removal confirms treatment results. However, multiple renal stones may pose several problems with regard to surgical treatment or, at the very least, increase the difficulty of treatment. As opposed to a solitary stone, multiple renal stones will likely occupy several locations in the collecting system and have varying sizes (Fig. 27.4). Depending on the stone distribution throughout the collecting system (i.e., stones occupying many calices), a treatment option such as SWL may be limited since the energy cannot be focused on a central location to treat all of the stones simultaneously. Furthermore, in SWL, the total energy applied to a kidney must be limited, and therefore, divided between the stones, which may limit its ability to fragment multiple renal stones. In turn, inadequate fragmentation may lead to retreatment, complications, such as ureteral obstruction from steinstrasse, or both. Likewise, depending on the overall stone burden and anatomy, the approach for other commonly utilized procedures, such as URS and PCNL, may be affected. For widely distributed and small to medium-sized renal stones, flexible URS and laser lithotripsy may be advantageous since URS provides direct visualization of each stone for fragmentation and for removal. For larger stones in multiple locations, PCNL with flexible nephroscopy and laser lithotripsy may be the treatment of choice.

An important determinant for choosing a surgical stone treatment is the likelihood of success or complete stone removal, which can be difficult due to many factors. Novel scoring systems have been developed to quantify and standardize the complexity of PCNL in order to predict the postoperative stone-free and complication rates. The S.T.O.N.E. nephrolithometry scoring system is based on five variables of the stone burden seen on preoperative noncontrast CT scan corresponding to its acronym: stone size (S), tract length (T), obstruction (O), number of involved calices (N), and essence or density (E).[49] Guy's stone score is a grading system that grades stone complexity prior to PCNL based on stone number, location, conformation, and patient anatomy.[78] In addition to predicting PCNL success and complication rates, both scoring systems have demonstrated good inter-rater reliability and reproducibility.[79-81] A recent study by Labadie et al. retrospectively reviewed 246 patients who underwent PCNL and calculated the Guy's Stone Score, S.T.O.N. E. nephrolithometry, and CROES nephrolithometric nomogram based on preoperative CT imaging.[82] They found that all scoring systems and stone burden were equally predictive of stone-free status. The Guy's score and S.T.O.N. E. nephrolithometry were associated with estimated blood loss and length of hospital stay. Although many stones that could be rated may already be destined for PCNL, these scoring systems could provide significant benefit for patient counseling regarding treatment plan and expectations such as the need for secondary procedures or multiple percutaneous access.

Renal Stone Composition, Density, and Fragility

Stone composition and corresponding stone density are important aspects to consider when deciding upon surgical stone treatment. A patient's history of stone composition alone can dictate the choice of surgical stone treatment due to density, origin, or other factors. Consideration of stone composition and/or density most aptly applies to SWL, in part, because certain types of stones and the corresponding density lead to fragmentation resistance. Since there are limitations in the amount of shockwave energy that can be safely applied to a kidney and no direct visualization of stone fragmentation, SWL is not recommended for stones known to be resistant to fragmentation, such as cystine stones. Fragmentation-resistant stones treated with SWL could result in larger-than-desired stone pieces and lead to ureteral obstruction during passage (steinstrasse), increased retreatment rates, or both. Some stone types are not necessarily fragmentation resistant but may preclude SWL due to radiolucency, making targeting with fluoroscopy difficult. With regard to PCNL, the history of stone composition is significant when complete stone removal is crucial to prevent further stone formation (i.e. infection-related renal stones). In this section, the most important stone compositions and the potential relationships to surgical treatment options will be discussed.

Stone Composition

Stone composition is an important factor since there are varying degrees of difficulty in fragmentation regardless of treatment type, but especially for SWL.[83,84] Cystine and brushite stones are the most fragmentation resistant in SWL, followed by calcium oxalate monohydrate (Figs. 27.5A to D).[85] Stone compositions that are not particularly fragmentation resistant include calcium phosphate, uric acid, ammonium acid urate, medication (drug) stones, xanthine stones, matrix stones, calcium carbonate apatite, and magnesium ammonium phosphate (struvite). These stone compositions are generally amenable to fragmentation and removal via any surgical stone treatment. However, uric acid, ammonium acid urate, medication (drug) stones (especially protease inhibitors), xanthine stones, and matrix stones are typically radiolucent. Radiolucent renal stones may be difficult to localize and treat with SWL using fluoroscopy. Shockwave lithotripsy is also not recommended for renal stones with pathophysiology related to renal impairment, such as cystinuria, or brushite stone formers, since repeated SWL treatment could contribute to worsening renal function. Stone compositions related to or caused by recurrent/persistent UTI, which may include matrix, calcium carbonate apatite, and especially magnesium ammonium phosphate, require complete eradication of the stone burden to minimize recurrence. For large infection-related stone burdens, PCNL is recommended (discussed further later in this section). For patients without known previous stone composition to guide surgical treatment, consideration of past medical history and comorbid conditions may aid in the prediction of the likely stone composition to be treated. For example, patients who form stones following bariatric surgery are

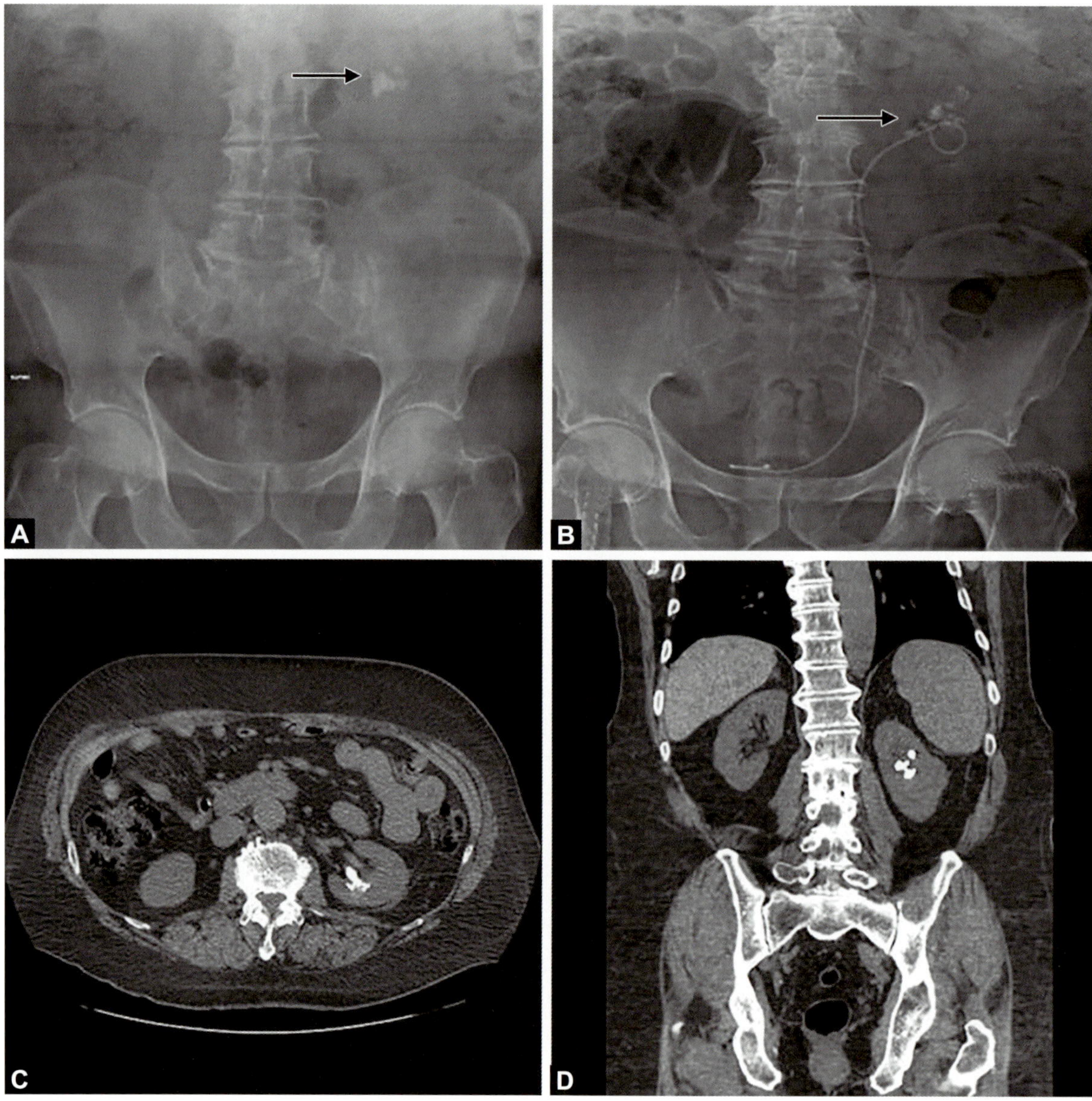

Figs. 27.5A to D: (A) Pre-SWL KUB image of large (>2 cm) calcium oxalate monohydrate stone indicated by an arrow. (B) Post-SWL KUB image demonstrating inadequate fragmentation (indicated by arrow) of large calcium oxalate monohydrate stone requiring indwelling ureteral stent due to stone obstruction at UPJ. (C) Post-SWL noncontrast CT axial and (D) coronal images demonstrating post-SWL residual stone burden measuring >900 HU and requiring URS secondary procedure. (SWL: Shockwave lithotripsy; KUB: Kidneys, ureters, and bladder; UPJ: Uretero-pelvic junction; URS: Ureteroscopy; CT: Computed tomography).

likely to be calcium oxalate stone formers due to enteric hyperoxaluria.

Stone Density and Fragility

Stone density and fragility are important in determining surgical treatment with regard to fragmentation and particularly SWL. Shockwave lithotripsy is not necessarily contraindicated for stones that are dense, but the increased likelihood for failure should be considered. Additionally, if SWL is attempted on these stone types and results in minimal or no fragmentation, repeat SWL is unlikely to achieve success. For patients without a known history of stone type or in those with a history of fragmentation-resistant stones but desiring SWL treatment, the possibility of success may be estimated on the basis of stone density appearance via Hounsfield units (HU) on CT scan. Stones with density range of ~900–1,200 HU or above on noncontrast CT scan have been shown to result in more shockwaves for fragmentation, less fragmentation overall, less stone clearance, and higher rates of retreatment after SWL (Figs. 27.5A to D).[86–88] Pure brushite stones have also been shown to be more resistant to SWL based on density, but fragility could not be determined on the basis of visible stone structure on CT scan.[89] Other stone compositions may have more or less fragmentation resistance based on internal structure organization and not necessarily on density. Calcium oxalate monohydrate stones studied with micro-CT imaging demonstrated more fragility with SWL when heterogeneity in the internal stone structure was present.[90] Stones with more homogeneous internal structures were more fragmentation resistant. Also, stone fragility did not correlate with Hounsfield units in this study. These are important considerations to minimize SWL treatment episodes, both with regard to inadequate stone clearance and potential recurrence. Patients with a history of stones that have been SWL resistant may be better treated with URS since even hard stones can be fragmented and have little resistance to holmium laser energy.[91] Additionally, numerous repeat SWL treatments may lead to long-term renal impairment, hypertension, and conversion to brushite stone composition.[92,93]

Cystine stones are generally thought to be SWL resistant and better treated with URS and holmium laser lithotripsy or PCNL (depending on the stone size and location). Cystine stones lead to much lower stone-free rates compared to other stone types treated with SWL.[94] The one caveat may be that cystine stones with "rough" morphology may be more susceptible to comminution by SWL. In vitro helical CT scans of "rough" cystine stones demonstrating internal structure with areas of low attenuation were 61% less SWL resistant than "smooth" cystine stones with homogeneous internal structure.[95] However, overall, inadequate treatment of cystine stones with SWL may compound upon the dilemma of frequent stone recurrence leading to increased frequency of surgical treatment. If repeated surgical treatments consist of SWL, previously described long-term sequelae of multiple SWL treatments are a concern. Similarly, any repeated surgical treatment increases the risk of long-term complications, including URS and holmium laser lithotripsy, and over time many procedures could increase the risk of developing a ureteral stricture. Yet, holmium laser energy under direct vision with URS will lead to more reliable stone fragmentation and, even if required repeatedly, will not contribute to further renal function deterioration. For larger cystine stone burdens, PCNL may be required. The hardness of cystine stones may be resistant to ultrasonic lithotripsy and may require pneumatic or holmium laser fragmentation.

Infection-related Renal Stones

Infection-related renal stones are generally composed of struvite, calcium carbonate apatite, matrix, or other compounds, which crystallize in an abnormally alkaline urinary environment produced by infection. The term "infection stone" comes from the association with UTI caused by urease-producing bacteria.[96] The main risk factors, such as physiologic/anatomic urinary tract obstruction, bladder dysfunction, urinary diversion/reconstruction, or foreign bodies (e.g. chronic urinary catheters or ureteral stents), promote urinary stasis or bacterial colonization/infection. Urease is produced by a variety of micro-organisms, the most important of which are *Proteus*, *Klebsiella*, *Pseudomonas*, and *Staphylococcus* but also include some atypical bacteria as well as yeast.[97] Theoretically, elimination of infection by any of these organisms would limit infection stone formation or subsequent growth. However, despite sterile urine after antibiotic treatment, bacteria generally remain viable within the interior of the kidney stone.[98] Thus, prolonged antibiotic treatment may cease UTI progression, but alone is unlikely to resolve the stone burden.

Due to the difficulty of complete renal stone sterilization, the goal of treatment is complete removal of the infected stone burden as recommended by the AUA Nephrolithiasis Guideline Panel, "especially when a struvite/calcium carbonate/apatite stone is present."[60] Thus, according to this panel, the standard for first-line treatment of most large-volume infection stone cases is PCNL. Other treatment options, including SWL and URS, do not result in stone-free rates sufficient to serve as first-line treatment or monotherapy for large infection stones. Open/laparoscopic surgery is limited to cases in which "the stone is not expected to be removed by a reasonable number of less invasive procedures," which does not apply to most patients.[60] Smaller infection stones may be treated with URS and stone basket extraction, but the risk of sepsis/systemic inflammatory response syndrome may be increased when working with pressurized irrigation, so a ureteral access sheath is recommended to keep intrarenal pressures low. Overall, the therapeutic goal is to remove all infected stone material since residual fragments, which likely still harbor bacteria, can act as a nidus for recurrence.[99]

CONCLUSION

There are many factors to consider in selecting the appropriate surgical treatment for nephrolithiasis. Each surgical modality has inherent advantages and disadvantages. However, various renal stone factors, such as size, location, conformation, number, composition, density, and fragility also influence treatment choice.

Stone size or volume is perhaps the most important "stone factor" determining treatment choice. Small stone size routinely has the most options for effective treatment since the smaller volume will likely lead to efficient treatment despite the procedure selected. Surgical treatment of small stones generally will be SWL or URS. Aside from special circumstances, PCNL is generally not a prominent option for small renal stones based on the invasiveness and associated complication risks. Likewise, open/laparoscopic procedures are rarely indicated for small stones. For medium-sized stones 1–2 cm, SWL and URS are primary options. For large stone burdens, PCNL is particularly suited for stone removal based on its direct access to the renal collecting system and efficient stone fragmentation/removal. Open/laparoscopic surgeries are recommended for select cases such as stones in ectopic kidneys.

Stone location may affect treatment choice with regard to SWL and PCNL more so than URS. Since stone resolution after SWL relies on fragment passage and PCNL utilizes large, rigid instruments, stone location is a critical consideration. Areas such as the calices in the upper pole and interpolar regions as well as the renal pelvis are favorable for fragment passage after SWL, and stone-free rates decrease for stones in the lower pole. For PCNL, a stone burden localized to a calyx corresponding to the percutaneous nephrostomy access and renal pelvis may be ideal. Staghorn or complex renal calculi may present the most likely scenario for open or laparoscopic surgical treatment. However, based on the effectiveness of PCNL and its variations, open or laparoscopic surgery is not recommended in most cases. Relocation of lower pole stones to the upper pole may improve stone-free rates for URS.

Stone number will also influence treatment choice. Flexible URS provides significant maneuverability to locate and treat stones distributed throughout the renal collecting system. A solitary stone is favorable for SWL or PCNL, but multiple stones or wide distribution throughout the renal collecting system will decrease the likelihood of complete stone removal with one treatment. Multiple stones, especially in a wide distribution, make open or laparoscopic surgery the least viable option for treatment.

Stone composition, density, and fragility are perhaps the least considered factors, but equally as important as other factors. Shockwave lithotripsy should be limited in patients with a known history of fragmentation-resistant stones. Repeat SWL may lead to long-term sequelae, such as renal dysfunction, hypertension, and conversion of stone formation to brushite composition. The ability of the holmium laser to break stones during URS is rather independent of stone composition or density; however, how well stone fragments or dusts may depend on composition and/or fragility. Stone composition is also an important consideration for patients with a history of recurrent UTI. Struvite stone, especially in large volume, should be treated with PCNL in order to removal all stone fragments. As per the AUA guidelines, complete eradication of struvite stone is indicated to minimize stone recurrence.

In the end, the primary surgical treatment options of SWL, URS, and PCNL are effective in treating the vast majority of nephrolithiasis cases. However, considering the renal stone factors in relationship to the strengths and weaknesses of these treatment modalities is important. Determining the optimal treatment with regard to these factors will not only maximize the effectiveness and minimize retreatment, but also limit associated complications.

REFERENCES

1. Stamatelou KK, Francis ME, Jones CA, et al. Time trends in reported prevalence of kidney stones in the United States: 1976–1994. Kidney Int. 2003;63:1817-23.
2. Pearle MS, Calhoun EA, Curhan GS. Urologic diseases in America project: urolithiasis. J Urol. 2005;173:848-57.
3. Hesse A, Brandle E, Wilbert D, et al. Study on the prevalence and incidence of urolithiasis in Germany comparing the years 1979 vs. 2000. Eur Urol. 2003;44:709-13.
4. Moe OW. Kidney stones: pathophysiology and medical management. Lancet. 2006;367:333-44.
5. Knoll T, Schubert AB, Fahlenkamp D, et al. Urolithiasis through the ages: Data on more than 200,000 urinary stone analyses. J Urol. 2011;185:1304-11.
6. Matlaga BR. Contemporary surgical management of upper urinary tract calculi. J Urol. 2009;181:2152-6.
7. Preminger GM, Tiselius HG, Assimos DG, et al. 2007 guideline for the management of ureteral calculi. J Urol. 2007;178:2418-34.
8. Neisius A, Wöllner J, Thomas C, et al. Treatment efficacy and outcomes using a third generation shockwave lithotripter. BJU Int. 2013;112:972-81.
9. Miller NL, Lingeman JE. Treatment of kidney stones: current lithotripsy devices are proving less effective in some cases. Nat Clin Pract Urol. 2006;3:236-7.
10. Albala DM, Siddiqui KM, Fulmer B, et al. Extracorporeal shock wave lithotripsy with a transportable electro-

hydraulic lithotripter: experience with >300 patients. BJU Int. 2005;96:603-7.
11. Dhar NB, Thornton J, Karafa MT, et al. A multivariate analysis of risk factors associated with subcapsular hematoma formation following electromagnetic shock wave lithotripsy. J Urol. 2004;172:2271-4.
12. Türk C, Knoll T, Petrik A, et al. (2013). Guidelines on Urolithiasis. [online] European Association of Urology. Available from www.uroweb.org.
13. Fedullo LM, Pollack HM, Banner MP, et al. The development of steinstrassen after ESWL: frequency, natural history, and radiologic management. AJR Am J Roentgenol. 1988;151:1145-7.
14. Schnabel MJ, Gierth M, Chaussy CG, et al. Incidence and risk factors of renal hematoma: a prospective study of 1,300 SWL treatments. Urolithiasis. 2014;42:247-53.
15. Janetschek G, Frauscher F, Knapp R, et al. New onset hypertension after extracorporeal shock wave lithotripsy: age related incidence and prediction by intrarenal resistive index. J Urol. 1997;158:346-51.
16. American Urological Association Education and Research, Inc. (2009). Current perspective on adverse effects in shock wave lithotripsy.[White paper]. [online] Available from http://www.auanet.org/education/guidelines/shock-wave-lithotripsy.cfm
17. Delvecchio FC, Auge BK, Brizuela RM, et al. Assessment of stricture formation with the ureteral access sheath. Urology. 2003;61(3):518-22.
18. Srisubat A, Potisat S, Lojanapiwat B, et al. Extracorporeal shock wave lithotripsy (ESWL) versus percutaneous nephrolithotomy (PCNL) or retrograde intrarenal surgery (RIRS) for kidney stones. Cochrane Database of Systematic Reviews 2014;(11):CD007044
19. De la Rosette JJ, Assimos D, Desai M, et al. The Clinical Research Office of the Endourological Society Percutaneous Nephrolithotomy Global Study: indications, complications, and outcomes in 5803 patients. J Endourol. 2011;25(1):11-7.
20. Michel MS, Trojan L, Rassweiler JJ. Complications in percutaneous nephrolithotomy. Eur Urol. 2007;51:899-906.
21. Hyams ES, Bruhn A, Lipkin M, et al. Heterogeneity in the reporting of disease characteristics and treatment outcomes in studies evaluating treatments for nephrolithiasis. J Endourol. 2010;24:1411-4.
22. Patel SR, Nakada SY. Quantification of preoperative stone burden for ureteroscopy and shock wave lithotripsy: current state and future recommendations. Urology. 2011;78:282-5.
23. Nadler RB, Stern JA, Kimm S, et al. Coronal imaging to assess urinary tract stone size. J Urol. 2004;172:962-4.
24. Kampa RJ, Ghani KR, Wahed S, et al. Size matters: a survey of how urinary-tract stones are measured in the UK. J Endourol. 2005;19:856-60.
25. Patel SR, Stanton P, Zelinski N, et al. Automated renal stone volume measurement by noncontrast computerized tomography is more reproducible than manual linear size measurement. J Urol. 2011;186:2275-9.
26. Madbouly K, Sheir KZ, Elsobky E, et al. Risk factors for the formation of a steinstrasse after extracorporeal shock wave lithotripsy: a statistical model. J Urol. 2002;167:1239-42.
27. Akman T, Binbay M, Ozgor F, et al. Comparison of percutaneous nephrolithotomy and retrograde flexible nephrolithotripsy for the management of 2–4 cm stones: a matched-pair analysis. BJU Int. 2011;109:1384-9.
28. Akman T, Binbay M, Ugurlu M, et al. Outcomes of retrograde intrarenal surgery compared with percutaneous nephrolithotomy in elderly patients with moderate-size kidney stones: a matched-pair analysis. J Endourol. 2012;26:625-9.
29. Aboumarzouk OM, Monga M, Kata SG, et al. Flexible ureteroscopy and laser lithotripsy for stones >2 cm: a systematic review and meta-analysis. J Endourol. 2012;26:1257-63.
30. Xue W, Pacik D, Boellard W, et al. Management of single large nonstaghorn renal stones in the CROES PCNL Global Study. J Urol. 2012;187:1293-7.
31. Wang X, Sheng L, Tongzu L, et al. Laparoscopic pyelolithotomy compared to percutaneous nephrolithotomy as surgical management for large renal pelvic calculi: a meta-analysis. J Urol. 2013;190:888-93.
32. Madbouly K, Sheir KZ, Elsobky E, et al. Risk factors for the formation of a steinstrasse after extracorporeal shock wave lithotripsy: a statistical model. J Urol. 2002;167:1239-42.
33. Gleeson MJ, Griffith DP. Extracorporeal shockwave lithotripsy monotherapy for large renal calculi. Br J Urol. 1989;64:329-32.
34. Murray MJ, Chandhoke PS, Berman CJ, et al. Outcome of extracorporeal shockwave lithotripsy monotherapy for large renal calculi: effect of stone and collecting system surface areas and cost-effectiveness of treatment. J Endourol. 1995;9:9-13.
35. Salem S, Mehrsai A, Zartab H, et al. Complications and outcomes following extracorporeal shock wave lithotripsy: a prospective study of 3,241 patients. Urol Res. 2010;38:135-42.
36. Khalil M. Which is more important in predicting the outcome of extracorporeal shockwave lithotripsy of solitary renal stones: stone location or stone burden? J Endourol. 2012;26:535-9.
37. Resorlu B, Unsal A, Ziypak T, et al. Comparison of retrograde intrarenal surgery, shockwave lithotripsy, and percutaneous nephrolithotomy for treatment of medium-sized radiolucent renal stones. World J Urol. 2012;31:1581-6.
38. Sarkissian C, Noble M, Li J, et al. Patient decision making for asymptomatic renal calculi: balancing benefit and risk. Urology. 2013;81:236-40.
39. Pearle MS, Lingeman JE, Leveillee R, et al. Prospective randomized trial comparing shock wave lithotripsy and ureteroscopy for lower pole caliceal calculi 1 cm or less. J Urol. 2008;179(5 Suppl):S69-73.
40. Sabnis RB, Jagtap J, Mishra S, et al. Treating renal calculi 1–2 cm in diameter with minipercutaneous or retrograde intrarenal surgery: a prospective comparative study. BJU Int. 2012;110:E346-9.
41. Sabnis RB, Ganesamoni R, Doshi A, et al. Micropercutaneous nephrolithotomy (microperc) vs retrograde intrarenal surgery for the management of small renal calculi: a randomized controlled trial. BJU Int. 2013;112:355-61.

42. Zeng G, Mai Z, Zhao Z, et al. Treatment of upper urinary calculi with Chinese minimally invasive percutaneous nephrolithotomy: a single-center experience with 12,482 consecutive patients over 20 years. Urolithiasis. 2013;41:225-9.
43. Turna B, Ekren F, Nazli O, et al. Comparative results of shockwave lithotripsy for renal calculi in upper, middle, and lower calices. J Endourol. 2007;21:951-6.
44. Lambert EH, Walsh R, Moreno MW, et al. Effect of escalating versus fixed voltage treatment on stone comminution and renal injury during extracorporeal shock wave lithotripsy: a prospective randomized trial. J Urol. 2010;183(2):580-4.
45. Matlaga BR, Jansen JP, Meckly LM, et al. Treatment of ureteral and renal stones: a systematic review and meta-analysis of randomized, controlled trials. J Urol. 2012;188:130-7.
46. Kourambas J, Delvecchio FC, Munver R, et al. Nitinol stone retrieval-assisted ureteroscopic management of lower pole renal calculi. Urology. 2000;56:935-9.
47. Kourambas J, Delvecchio FC, Preminger GM. Low-power holmium laser for the management of urinary tract calculi, structures, and tumors. J Endourol. 2001;15:529-32.
48. Irwin BH, Desai M. Ureteroscopic superiority to extracorporeal shockwave lithotripsy for the treatment of small-to-medium-sized intrarenal non-staghorn calculi. Urology. 2009;74:256-8.
49. Okhunov Z, Friedlander JI, George AK, et al. S.T.O.N.E. nephrolithometry: novel surgical classification system for kidney calculi. Urology. 2013;81:1154-9.
50. Ruggera L, Beltrami P, Ballario R, et al. Impact of anatomical pielocaliceal topography in the treatment of renal lower calyces stones with extracorporeal shock wave lithotripsy. Int J Urol. 2005;12:525-32.
51. Obek C, Onal B, Kanlay K, et al. The efficacy of extracorporeal shock wave lithotripsy for isolated lower pole calculi compared with isolated middle and upper caliceal calculi. J Urol. 2001;166:2081-5.
52. Lingeman JE, Seigel YI, Steele B, et al. Management of lower pole nephrolithiasis: a critical analysis. J Urol. 1994;151: 663-7.
53. Kosar A, Türkölmez K, Sarica K, et al. Calyceal stones: fate of shock wave therapy with respect to stone localization. Int Urol Nephrol. 1998;30;433-8.
54. Coz F, Orvieto M, Bustos M, et al. Extracorporeal shockwave lithotripsy of 2000 urinary calculi with the modulith SL-20: success and failure according to size and locations of stones. J Endourol. 2000;14:239-46.
55. El-Nahas AR, Ibrahim HM, Youssef RF, et al. Flexible ureterorenoscopy versus extracorporeal shock wave lithotripsy for treatment of lower pole stones of 10-20 mm. BJU Int. 2012;110:898-902.
56. Sener NC, Abdurrahim Imamoglu M, Bas O, et al. Prospective randomized trial comparing shock wave lithotripsy and flexible ureterorenoscopy for lower pole stones smaller than 1 cm. Urolithiasis. 2014;42(2):127-31.
57. Auge BK, Dahm P, Wu NZ, et al. Ureteroscopic management of lower-pole renal calculi: technique of calculus displacement. J Endourol. 2001;15:835-8.
58. Pearle MS, Lingeman JE, Leveillee R, et al. Prospective, randomized trial comparing shock wave lithotripsy and ureteroscopy for lower pole caliceal calculi 1 cm or less. J Urol. 2005;173:2005-9.
59. Bas O, Bakirtas H, Sener NC, et al. Comparison of shock wave lithotripsy, flexible ureterorenoscopy and percutaneous nephrolithotripsy on moderate size renal pelvis stones. Urolithiasis. 2014;42(2):115-20.
60. Preminger GM, Assimos DG, Lingeman JE, et al. Chapter 1: AUA guideline on management of staghorn calculi: diagnosis and treatment recommendations. J Urol. 2005;173:1991-2000.
61. Viprakasit DP, Sawyer MD, Herrell SD, et al. Changing composition of staghorn calculi. J Urol. 2011;186:2285-90.
62. Meretyk S, Gofrit ON, Gafni O, et al. Complete staghorn calculi: random prospective comparison between extracorporeal shock wave lithotripsy monotherapy and combined with percutaneous nephrostolithotomy. J Urol. 1997;157:780-6.
63. Akman T, Sari E, Binbay M, et al. Comparison of outcomes after percutaneous nephrolithotomy of staghorn calculi in those with single and multiple accesses. J Endourol. 2010;24:955-60.
64. Singla M, Srivastava A, Kapoor R, et al. Aggressive approach to staghorn calculi-safety and efficacy of multiple tracts percutaneous nephrolithotomy. Urology. 2008;71:1039-42.
65. Streem SB, Yost A, Dolmatch B. Combination "sandwich" therapy for extensive renal calculi in 100 consecutive patients: immediate, long-term and stratified results from a 10-year experience. J Urol. 1997;158:342-5.
66. Marguet CG, Springhart WP, Tan YH, et al. Simultaneous combined use of flexible ureteroscopy and percutaneous nephrolithotomy to reduce the number of access tracts in the management of complex renal calculi. BJU Int. 2005;96:1097-100.
67. Landman J, Venkatesh R, Lee DI, et al. Combined percutaneous and retrograde approach to staghorn calculi with application of the ureteral access sheath to facilitate percutaneous nephrolithotomy. J Urol. 2003;169:64-7.
68. Wong C, Leveillee RJ. Single upper-pole percutaneous access for treatment of ≥5 cm complex branched staghorn calculi: is shockwave lithotripsy necessary? J Endourol. 2002;16:477-81.
69. El-Galley R, Hood N, Young CJ, et al. Donor nephrectomy: a comparison of techniques and results of open, hand assisted and full laparoscopic nephrectomy. J Urol. 2004;171:40-3.
70. Morey AF, Nitahara KS, McAninch JW. Modified anatrophic nephrolithotomy for management of staghorn calculi: is renal function preserved? J Urol. 1999;162:670-3.
71. Melissourgos ND, Davilas EN, Fragoulis A, et al. Modified anatrophic nephrolithotomy for complete staghorn calculus disease—does it still have a place? Scand J Urol Nephrol. 2002;36:426-30.
72. Al-Kohlany KM, Shokeir AA, Mosbah A, et al. Treatment of complete staghorn stones: a prospective randomized comparison of open surgery versus percutaneous nephrolithotomy. J Urol. 2005;173:469-73.
73. Aminsharifi A, Hadian P, Boveiri K. Laparoscopic anatrophic nephrolithotomy for management of complete staghorn renal stone: clinical efficacy and intermediate-term functional outcome. J Endourol. 2013;27:573-8.

74. Giedelman C, Arriaga J, Carmona O, et al. Laparoscopic anatrophic nephrolithotomy: developments of the technique in the era of minimally invasive surgery. J Endourol. 2012;26:444-50.
75. Simforoosh N, Aminsharifi A, Tabibi A, et al. Laparoscopic anatrophic nephrolithotomy for managing large staghorn calculi. BJU Int. 2008;101:1293-6.
76. King SA, Klaassen Z, Madi R. Robot-assisted anatrophic nephrolithotomy: description of technique and early results. J Endourol. 2014;28:325-9.
77. Ghani KR, Rogers CG, Sood A, et al. Robot-assisted anatrophic nephrolithotomy with renal hypothermia for managing staghorn calculi. J Endourol. 2013;27:1393-8.
78. Thomas K, Smith NC, Hegarty N, et al. The Guy's stone score—grading the complexity of percutaneous nephrolithotomy procedures. Urology. 2011;78:277-81.
79. Okhunov Z, Helmy M, Perez-Lansac A, et al. Interobserver reliability and reproducibility of S.T.O.N.E. Nephrolithometry for renal calculi. J Endourol. 2013;27:1303-6.
80. Ingimarsson JP, Dagrosa LM, Hyams ES, et al. External validation of a preoperative renal stone grading system: reproducibility and inter-rater concordance of the Guy's stone score using preoperative computed tomography and rigorous postoperative stone-free criteria. Urology. 2014;83:45-9.
81. Vicentini FC, Marchini GS, Mazzucchi E, et al. Utility of the Guy's stone score based on computed tomographic scan findings for predicting percutaneous nephrolithotomy outcomes. Urology. 2014;83:1248-53.
82. Labadie K, Okhunov Z, Akhavein A, et al. Evaluation and comparison of urolithiasis scoring systems in percutaneous kidney stone surgery. J Urol. 2015;193(1):154-9.
83. Pearle MS. Shock-wave lithotripsy for renal calculi. N Engl J Med. 2012;367:50-7.
84. Dretler SP. Stone fragility—a new therapeutic distinction. J Urol. 1988;139:1124-7.
85. Saw KC, Lingeman JE. Lesson 20: management of calyceal calculi. AUA Update Ser. 1999;18:154-9.
86. Shah K, Kurien A, Mishra S, et al. Predicting effectiveness of extracorporeal shockwave lithotripsy by stone attenuation value. J Endourol. 2010;24:1169-73.
87. Ouzaid I, Al-qahtani S, Dominique S, et al. A 970 Hounsfield units (HU) threshold of kidney stone density on non-contrast computed tomography (NCCT) improves patients' selection for extracorporeal shockwave lithotripsy (ESWL): evidence from a prospective study. BJU Int. 2012;110:E438-42.
88. Foda K, Abdeldaeim H, Youssif M, et al. Calculating the number of shock waves, expulsion time, and optimum stone parameters based on noncontrast computerized tomography characteristics. Urology. 2013;82:1026-31.
89. Williams JC Jr, Hameed T, Jackson ME, et al. Fragility of brushite stones in shock wave lithotripsy: absence of correlation with computerized tomography visible structure. J Urol. 2012;188:996-1001.
90. Zarse CA, Hameed TA, Jackson ME, et al. CT visible internal stone structure, but not Hounsfield unit value, of calcium oxalate monohydrate (COM) calculi predicts lithotripsy fragility in vitro. Urol Res. 2007;35:201-6.
91. Wiener SV, Deters LA, Pais VM Jr. Effect of stone composition on operative time during ureteroscopic holmium:yttrium-aluminum-garnet laser lithotripsy with active fragment retrieval. Urology. 2012;80:790-4.
92. Smith LH, Drach G, Hall P, et al. National High Blood Pressure Education Program (NHBPEP) review paper on complications of shock wave lithotripsy for urinary calculi. Am J Med. 1991;91:635-41.
93. Krambeck AE, Handa SE, Evan AP, et al. Brushite stone disease as a consequence of lithotripsy? Urol Res. 2010;38:293-9.
94. Landau EH, Shenfeld OZ, Pode D, et al. Extracorporeal shock wave lithotripsy in prepubertal children: 22-year experience at a single institution with a single lithotripter. J Urol. 2009;182(4 Suppl):1835-9.
95. Kim SC, Burns EK, Lingeman JE, et al. Cystine calculi: correlation of CT-visible structure, CT number, and stone morphology with fragmentation by shock wave lithotripsy. Urol Res. 2007;35:319-24.
96. Hager BH, Magath TB. The etiology of encrusted cystitis with alkaline urine. JAMA. 1925;85:1352-5.
97. Healy KA, Ogan K. Pathophysiology and management of infectious staghorn calculi. Urol Clin North Am. 2007;34:363-74.
98. Nemoy NJ, Stamey TA. Surgical, bacteriological, and biochemical management of "infection stones." JAMA. 1971;215:1470-6.
99. Altunrende F, Tefekli A, Stein RJ, et al. Clinically insignificant residual fragments after percutaneous nephrolithotomy: medium-term follow-up. J Endourol. 2011;25:941-5.

CHAPTER

28

Preoperative Preparations for Stone Surgery

Daniel Schneider, William A Critchlow, Mitchell R Humphreys

INTRODUCTION

It has been estimated that 12% of American men and 6% of American women will have a stone episode in their lifetime.[1] The economic burden on society is substantial, with an estimated annual medical cost of $4.5 billion in the United States and $775 million in indirect costs for missed work.[2] Furthermore, the prevalence of stone disease appears to be on the rise, with the southeast United States being the most common location.[2,3] The treatment of stone disease has also made major advancements over the past 30 years, making endoscopic procedures easier, safer, and more effective for patients. This has led to an increase in procedures done for stone disease. Therefore, the preoperative evaluation and management thereof should be efficient and tailored to each individual nephrolithiasis patient. This chapter aims to provide the clinician with the tools necessary to appropriately evaluate and prepare the nephrolithiasis patient for surgery in order to avoid potential morbidities.

UNIQUE DEMOGRAPHICS OF STONE PATIENTS

In order to effectively manage newly diagnosed nephrolithiasis patients, their unique characteristics must be appreciated. The age at the time of diagnosis appears to vary between men and women. In men the incidence increases after the age of 20 and reaches its peak prior to age 60, whereas in women the peak incidence occurs in the late 20s and nadirs at around age 50.[3]

Previously described in the book are certain comorbid conditions that are more common in the nephrolithiasis population. For example, in children there is approximately a 50% incidence of obesity, hypertension, and diabetes in those who were admitted with stone disease compared to 25% of children admitted to the hospital for other conditions.[4] In the adult population, there are multiple comorbidities that are more prevalent in the nephrolithiasis population (Table 28.1). The medical complexity of this patient population is plainly evident.

Table 28.1: Comorbid conditions as independent risk factors for stone disease.[122–129]

Type II diabetes
Congestive heart failure
Corticosteroid use
End stage renal disease
Sarcoidosis
Obesity
Osteoporosis
Myeloproliferative disease
Inflammatory bowel disease
Hyperparathyroidism
Gastric bypass

PATIENT PRESENTATION WITH AN ACUTE URETERAL STONE EPISODE

The presentation of nephrolithiasis can vary greatly from a completely asymptomatic patient to the one with intractable pain, sepsis, irritative voiding symptoms, and hematuria. Even those patients who present with an asymptomatic stone are at considerable risk of becoming symptomatic in the future. Glowacki et al. performed a retrospective analysis on a cohort of 107 patients with asymptomatic renal pelvic stones, and during 32 months of followup 32% developed symptoms.[5]

It is important to recognize that there is a multitude of intra-abdominal conditions that can mimic the symptoms of acute renal colic; these include, but are not limited to, diverticulitis, appendicitis, herpes zoster, musculoskeletal pain, and pyelonephritis (Table 28.2). Therefore, the relevant questions asked should be designed to allow the clinician to elucidate the correct diagnosis or at least provide evidence to guide further evaluation.

Kidney stone pain typically initiates when the stone passes from the renal pelvis and obstructs the ureter, causing hydrodistention in the ureter and stretching of the

Table 28.2: Differential diagnosis for consideration of patient with symptoms of renal colic.[130–132]

System	*Differential diagnosis for renal colic*
Genitourinary	
	Pyelonephritis
	Cystitis
	Pelvic pain syndrome
	Hemorrhage
	Angiomyolipoma
	Renal neoplasms
	Testicular torsion
	Ovarian torsion
	Tubo-ovarian abscess
	Ruptured ovarian cyst
	Ectopic pregnancy
	Pelvic inflammatory disease
Integumentary	
	Appendicitis
	Diverticulitis
	Bowel obstruction
	Incarcerated hernia
	Enteritis
	Biliary colic
	Inflammatory bowel disease
	Volvulus
	Meckel's diverticulum
Musculoskeletal	
	Spondylolisthesis
	Foraminal stenosis
	Costochondritis of lower ribs
	Sacroiliitis
	Fibromyalgia
	Herpes zoster
Vascular	
	Ischemic colitis
	Mesenteric ischemia
	Aortic dissection

renal collecting system accompanied by an acute inflammatory response.[6] The pain is characterized as intermittent and sharp in nature. The location of pain largely depends on the location of the stone in the genitourinary (GU) system (Fig. 28.1). The pain can be referred and may be manifested anywhere along the distribution of the 12th

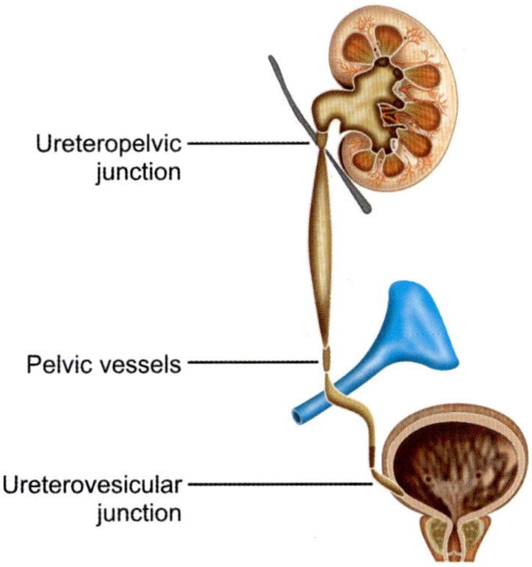

Fig. 28.1: Three most common anatomical locations for stone obstruction.

intercostal, ilioinguinal, iliohypogastric, or genitofemoral nerve depending on the location of the stone and obstruction. It should also be noted that as a stone approaches the ureterovesical junction, pain can be transmitted via the afferent fibers of the bladder and trigone, causing pain at the tip of the urethra, urinary frequency, urinary urgency, and dysuria and easily confusing the presentation with acute cystitis.

The duration of symptoms should also be ascertained as this can help to stratify certain patients for a trial of medical expulsive therapy (MET). It also provides important prognostic information to the physician regarding the potential damage to the upper urinary tracts. The data regarding obstruction-induced upper urinary tract damage come from the canine model, showing little to no renal recovery after 40 days of obstruction.[7]

The relevant history of a nephrolithiasis patient should be tailored around the acuity of the episode. Certain historical factors typically mandate intervention regardless of stone size. These include unremitting intractable pain requiring intravenous (IV) narcotics, inability to tolerate oral intake, symptoms of sepsis, a solitary kidney, or multiple readmissions to the hospital or emergency room.

Other elements important to the history include the number of previous stone episodes, stone composition, family history of nephrolithiasis or metabolic abnormalities, medications that predispose to nephrolithiasis (Table 28.3), and the number and type of previous interventions. If the patient has had extracorporeal shock wave lithotripsy (SWL), it is important to know the details of the procedure, such as the number of shocks and the need for

Table 28.3: Common medications associated with stone formation.[133,134]

Medication	*Type of stone*	*Mechanism of stone formation*	*Incidence of stone formation (%)*
Calcium and vitamin D	Calcium based	Absorptive hypercalcuria	NA
Vitamin C	Calcium oxalate	Oxalate production and excretion	NA
Topiramate	Calcium phosphate	Decreased hydrogen excretion of distal convoluted tubule leading to acquired distal RTA.	NA
Furosemide*	Calcium phosphate (nephrocalcinosis)	Ascending tubule calcium excretion	NA
Sulfonamides	N-acetyl-sulfamethoxazole	Drug metabolite crystallization	NA
Protease inhibitors (e.g. indinavir)	Drug salt	Precipitation and crystallization of medication in the nephron.	4
Acetazolamide	Calcium phosphate	Decreased hydrogen excretion of distal convoluted tubule leading to acquired distal RTA.	10
Triamterene	Triamterene salts	Drug crystal precipitation	0.4
Antibacterials	Drug salts	Drug crystal precipitation	NA
Laxatives	Ammonium urate	Ammoniagenesis	NA
Silicate-containing drugs	Amorphous silica	Drug crystal precipitation	NA
Guaifenesin	Beta-(2-methoxy-phenoxy)-lactic acid	Drug metabolite crystallization	0.05
Aluminum-containing drugs	Aluminum magnesium potassium urate	Drug crystal precipitation	NA
Allopurinol†	Oxypurinol	Drug crystal precipitation	NA

*Newborns predominantly.
†Only at doses ≥600 mg per day. (RTA: Renal tubular acidosis).

secondary procedures. This may provide empirical evidence that will guide future interventions. If the patient has had repeated ureteroscopic (URS) procedures, then ureteral strictures should be considered as a potential etiology of chronic colic or hydronephrosis. In the largest study looking at the stricture rate following URS, 11,885 patients were reviewed, showing a 0.3% risk of developing a ureteral stricture.[8] Imaging technology is an invaluable tool in the evaluation of nephrolithiasis patients.

Although drug-induced calculi are responsible for only 2% of nephrolithiasis, careful attention should be paid to the patient's current and past medication usage. The vast majority of drug-induced renal calculi are radiolucent on plain X-ray; therefore, the clinician needs to have a high index of suspicion when selecting the appropriate imaging modality to confirm the diagnosis.[9] Topiramate, an anticonvulsant, is one of the most commonly prescribed medications for migraine prevention but induces renal tubular acidosis (RTA), making it a familiar culprit for the induction of calcium phosphate stone disease.[10] This drug induces a two- to four-fold increase in stone formation by two separate mechanisms: (1) Inhibition of carbonic anhydrase leading to systemic acidosis and subsequent hypocitraturia, and (2) inhibition of hydrogen secretion in the distal nephron leading to a type 1 RTA presentation.[11]

A family history of nephrolithiasis can help predict metabolic abnormalities for a specific patient. In a dedicated study looking at the correlation of family history with the development of nephrolithiasis, Curhan et al. demonstrated that 12.8% of all stone patients had a positive family history of nephrolithiasis and that in those individuals who presented with a recurrent stone episode, the incidence was higher at 17.2% versus 6.4% of patients presenting with their initial stone event. They also demonstrated that if a person was <60 years old, a positive family history conferred a relative risk of 2.88 of developing nephrolithiasis compared to 1.74 in those older than 60 years.[12] When considering the family history, it is important to determine which family members (i.e. first vs second degree) had nephrolithiasis, as the risk of development has only been demonstrated in first-degree relatives.[13] The type of stone is also relevant as certain conditions (e.g. multiple

Table 28.4: Criteria for inflammatory response severity.[135]

Systemic inflammatory response syndrome	*Sepsis*	*Severe sepsis*	*Septic shock*	*Multiorgan dysfunction syndrome*
Two or more of the following: • Temperature >38° or <35° • Heart rate >90 bpm • WBCs >12,000 or <4,000 or >10% bands	SIRS with documented infection	Sepsis associated with decreased urine output or fluid responsive hypotension	Sepsis with hypotension refractory to fluid resuscitation	The previous with more than two organ systems failing with aggressive support

(SIRS: Systemic inflammatory response syndrome; WBC: White blood cell).

endocrine neoplasia type I, hyperparathyroidism, cystinuria, and primary hyperoxaluria) have a genetic predisposition to stone disease.

Physical examination provides essential information to the practitioner regarding the acuity of the stone event. Table 28.4 outlines the criteria of systemic inflammatory response versus sepsis versus septic shock that would indicate a critical patient and emergent need for intervention. The physical examination can also be used to rule out other potential etiologies of the presenting symptoms.

Serological evaluation and a comprehensive urine evaluation are paramount when evaluating the stone patient. At the bare minimum, a serological evaluation should include a basic metabolic panel and complete blood count with differential. The basic metabolic panel provides details of acute electrolyte abnormalities that may require attention. Serum creatinine, although informative about global renal function, may not help discern ongoing renal damage if the patient has a normal-functioning contralateral kidney. An acidotic patient with a low serum potassium can help draw attention to the possible presence or absence of RTA. Serum calcium, unless high (i.e. resorptive hypercalcuria), is not a very sensitive marker for a metabolic abnormality.[14] Blood urea nitrogen levels can discern the hydration status of the patient, and if not markedly elevated in the face of an elevated creatinine, they can suggest an obstructive renal etiology or possible secondary insensate loss due to emesis.

A careful examination of the urine sediment provides valuable data when evaluating a stone patient. The gross and microscopic examination of the urine can determine if blood is present and if there is evidence of infection. Specific gravity (SG) indicates the concentrating ability of the nephron and the hydration status of the patient (e.g. an SG of <1.008 is diluted and >1.020 is concentrated).[15] Urine pH usually mimics the acid base status of the patient except in those with an RTA. For example, in type 1 RTA, the patient will have a urine pH of >7.0, whereas in type 2 and type 4 RTA the urine pH is predominately acidic.

Microscopic hematuria is defined as having >3 red blood cells per high power field (RBCs/HPF).[16] Etiologies of false positives of hematuria on a dipstick include myoglobinuria and hemoglobinuria, and are distinguished via microscopy. False positives for hematuria under a microscope include menstrual bleeding and, in rare cases, gastrointestinal (GI) bleeding. The shape of the erythrocytes helps the surgeon to distinguish urinary tract bleeding from intrinsic renal hematuria. Glomerular bleeding typically demonstrates dysmorphic red blood cells and protein in the urine. Surgical or urologic bleeding typically has circular red blood cells and the absence of casts (Figs. 28.2A to C).[17] Nitrite and leukocyte esterase are both markers of infection in the urinary tract. Nitrite is never found naturally in the urine; therefore, when it is present, it is highly specific for a urinary tract infection (UTI). The sensitivity and specificity of nitrate for a UTI are 35–85% and 90%, respectively. Leucocyte esterase is a highly sensitive marker for an infection, but its specificity is lacking. The most specific marker of a bacterial infection of the urinary tract is the presence of bacteria on microscopy.[18] The typical conversion of the number of bacteria seen per HPF to colony-forming units (CFUs) is 1 per HPF equals 20,000 CFU.

Crystal observation in the urine can help determine the type of stone that a particular patient may possess. Figures 28.3A to D outline the typical shape of different stone crystals.

PATHOPHYSIOLOGY OF URINARY TRACT OBSTRUCTION

In addition to the symptomatology a patient experiences with acute urinary obstruction, there are physiological consequences from acute urinary blockage. In the first 5 hours of unilateral renal obstruction, there is a marked

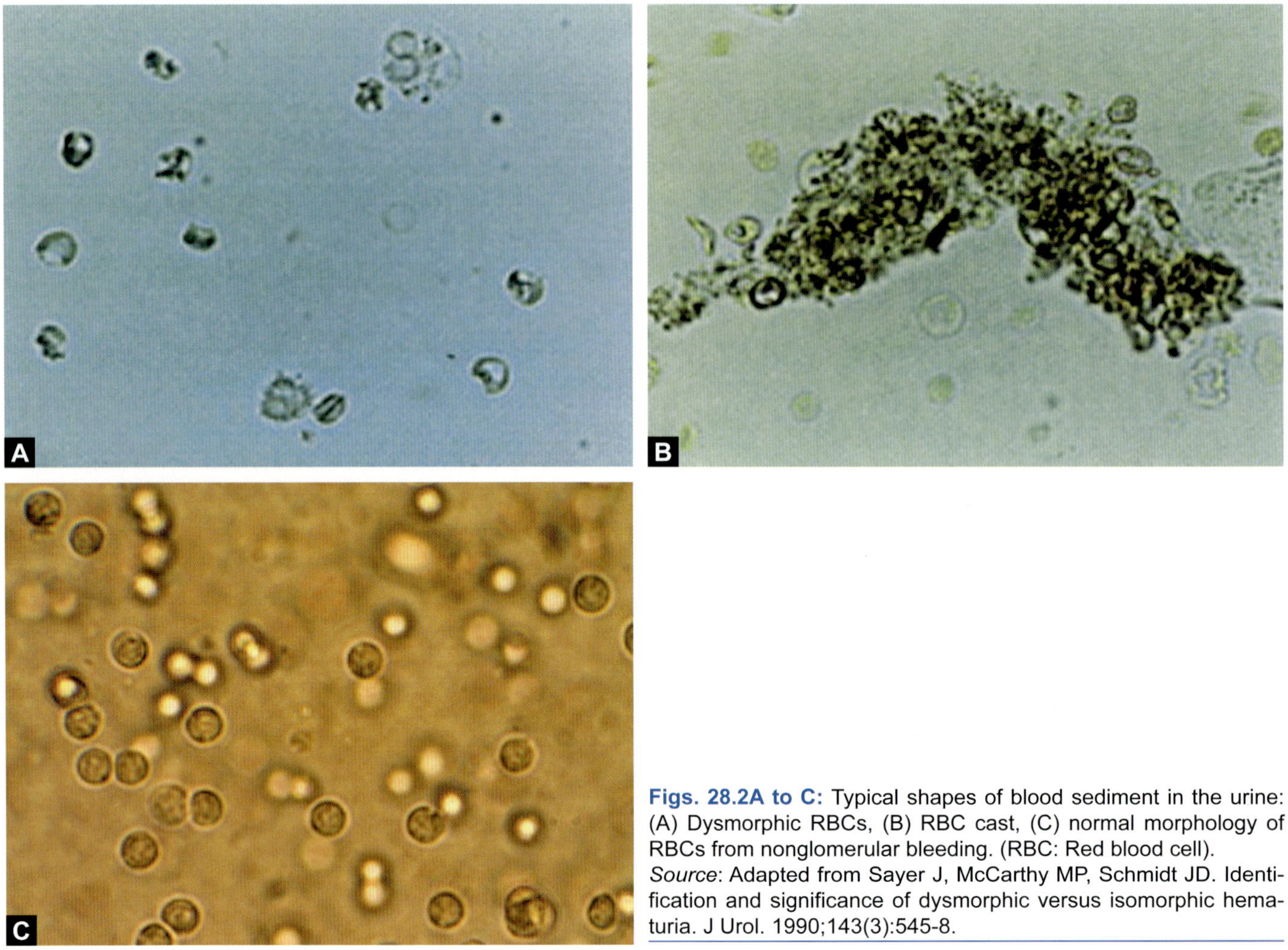

Figs. 28.2A to C: Typical shapes of blood sediment in the urine: (A) Dysmorphic RBCs, (B) RBC cast, (C) normal morphology of RBCs from nonglomerular bleeding. (RBC: Red blood cell).
Source: Adapted from Sayer J, McCarthy MP, Schmidt JD. Identification and significance of dysmorphic versus isomorphic hematuria. J Urol. 1990;143(3):545-8.

increase in renal blood flow (RBF) in an attempt to maintain glomerular filtration rate (GFR) on the affected side. After the initial hyperemic phase, RBF and GFR subsequently decline rapidly due to persistently elevated hydrostatic pressure. In the canine model, after 24 hours of obstruction, there is a 50% reduction in GFR on the affected side in a two-kidney model. In the contralateral unobstructed kidney, there is an increase in GFR and RBF secondary to an increase in prostaglandins.[19] In the situation of bilateral renal obstruction, ureteral pressures remains elevated for up to 24 hours, which leads to a markedly decreased GFR when compared to unilateral obstruction. There is also a more profound vasoconstriction of the renal vasculature, as described in Table 28.5.[20] The effects of ureteral obstruction on renal tubules are best demonstrated after the resolution of prolonged obstruction. The ability of the kidney to concentrate urine following the obstructive process can be severely impaired, leading to postobstructive diuresis. Postobstructive diuresis can be considered physiologic or pathologic, with the physiologic process being self-limited, lasting approximately 48 hours.[20,21] The mechanism involved in the pathologic variant is the loss of the medullary concentrating ability and subsequent loss of potassium, sodium, and water. Another proposed mechanism that plays a lesser role is the decreased expression of aquaporin channels.[21] If the obstruction persists, cellular death and fibrosis of the effected renal unit occurs, starting at day 4 and peaking at day 15.[22] This process is thought to be a result of the release of tumor necrosis factor alpha and angiotensin II.[23] Angiotensin is theorized as the initiator of fibrosis in the obstructed kidney. Previous studies have demonstrated that administration of angiotensin-converting enzyme (ACE) inhibitors has a protective effect against the formation of fibrosis via upregulating transforming growth factor beta.[23] Transforming growth factor beta leads to a proliferation of fibroblasts and collagen deposition.

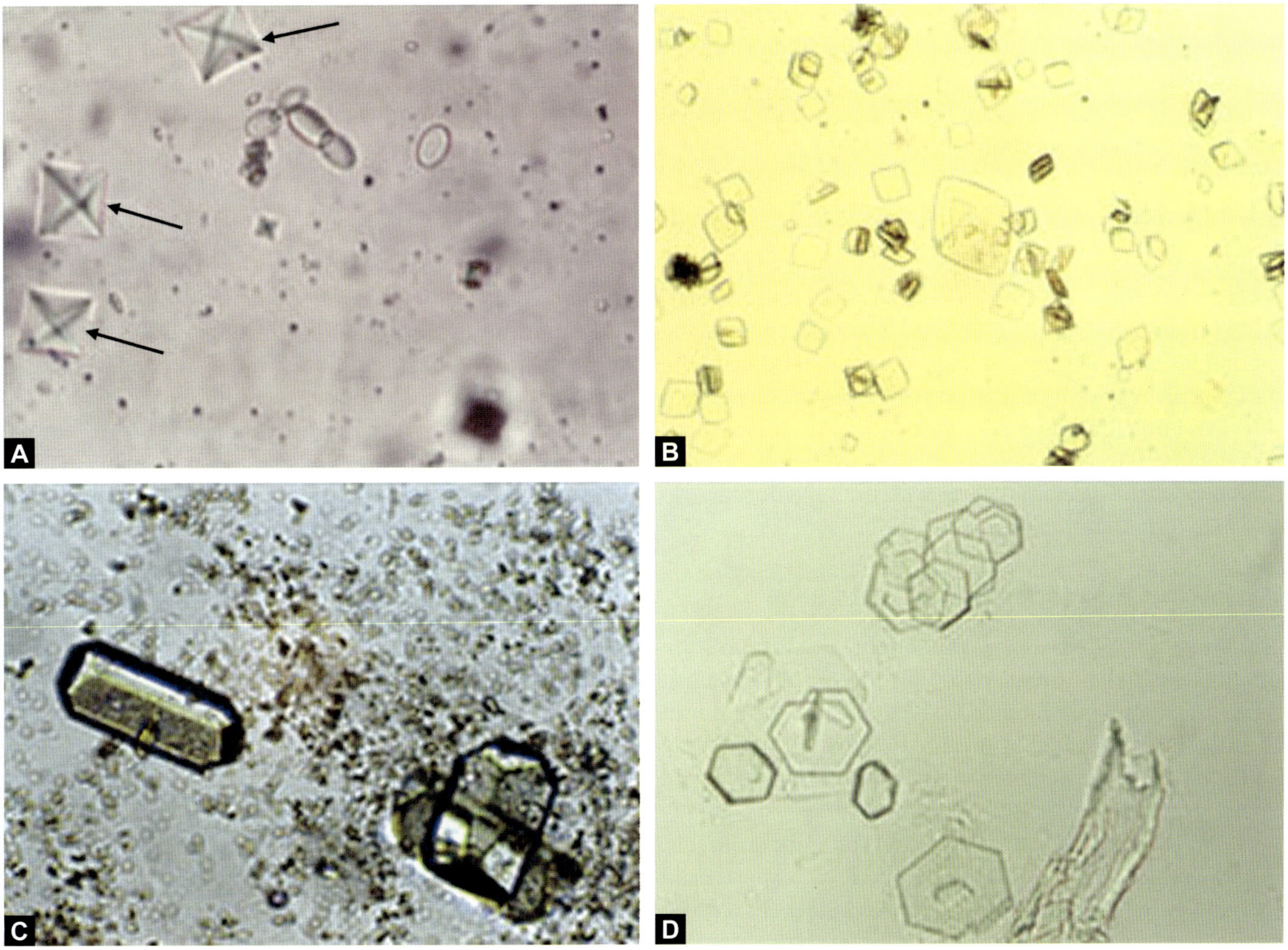

Figs. 28.3A to D: Crystal analysis of the different stone types: (A) Calcium oxalate, (B) triple phosphate, (C) uric acid, (D) cysteine.
Source: Adapted from Simerville JA, Maxted WC, Pahira JJ. Urinalysis: A comprehensive review. Am Fam Physician. 2005;71(6):1153-62.

Table 28.5: Effects of urinary obstruction on renal physiology.[136,137]

Urinary obstruction	*Renal blood flow*	*Renin release*	*Glomerular filtration rate*	*Volume status*
Unilateral renal obstruction	Initially markedly increased decreases rapidly with time	Increased initially	Initially preserved	Euvolemic
Bilateral urinary obstruction	Slightly increased initially	Unchanged initially increased with prolonged obstruction*	Decreased initially	Volume overload

*Greater than 24 hours.

Tumor necrosis factor alpha is an inflammatory mediator that activates caspases within the parenchyma of the kidney and leads to apoptosis and cell death.[23]

In the canine model, renal recovery after 2 weeks of obstruction shows that 70% of GFR could be preserved, versus only 30% at 4 weeks and no recovery after 6 weeks.[24]

The available studies in humans are difficult to interpret as it is hard to determine whether or not complete urinary obstruction was present and for how long the renal unit was obstructed. In a study by Lutaif et al. examining bilateral renal obstruction in cervical cancer patients, the prevailing risk factors that predicted poor renal recovery included duration of obstruction, renal parenchymal thickness, age, and baseline renal function.[24] Thus, the clinician should be aware of the possible consequences of renal obstruction and the potential long-term impact that may have on their nephrolithiasis patients.

IMAGING

Imaging is the cornerstone of the evaluation of nephrolithiasis patients and enables stratification into particular treatment strategies. There are a multitude of imaging modalities available, and a thorough understanding of the basic principles of each modality is necessary in order to select the right study for the right patient at any particular encounter. In the following section, each radiographic modality will be discussed along with the specific scenario in which they should be considered.

Radiation Exposure to Patients

The image obtained via conventional X-ray results from photons passing through tissue and being absorbed at different levels depending on tissue densities. The amount of radiation absorbed by a patient during an imaging episode has been calculated on the basis of the type of the imaging modality (Table 28.6). These values vary greatly between institutions, equipment, and different protocols. For reference, the average radiation level experienced by the general population in the United States in a given year is around 3 mSV. The amount of radiation that is considered "safe" is a controversial topic; however, multiple studies have demonstrated a clear correlation between cumulative levels of radiation exposure and the subsequent development of cancer. One study estimated that one in 470 women and 620 men would have a radiation-induced cancer from a single abdominal computed tomography (CT) scan with contrast.[25] Although the risk of cancer development may be low, one should be judicious and purposeful with imaging in nephrolithiasis patients who frequently have many imaging episodes over their lifetime.

Table 28.6: Amount of Sieverts absorbed radiation for different imaging modalities.[138]

Imaging modality	*Amount of radiation absorbed (effective dose)*
Baseline radiation exposure per year	1–3 mSv
Abdominal X-ray	0.1–1 mSv
Fluoroscopy	1 mSv/min
Abdominal CT without contrast	0.3–3 mSv
CT urogram	3–10 mSv
Intravenous pyelogram	1 mSv

(CT: Computed tomography).

Ultrasonography

This nonionizing imaging modality is generally well understood by most individuals. To become proficient with the utilization and interpretation of ultrasound imagery for stone patients, the practitioner must be well versed in the principles and the proper technique. With a working knowledge of ultrasonography, one can perform simple maneuvers that greatly enhance the image quality. Knowledge of ultrasonographic nomenclature is an important part of documentation. If a structure is hyperechoic, it is brighter than the surrounding tissues; if it is hypoechoic, it is darker; if it is isoechoic, it implies the same brightness as the surrounding tissues.

The basic principle of ultrasonographic imaging involves the generation of high-frequency mechanical waves that travel through a medium. Like all waves, they have a certain amplitude (e.g. peak to trough) and frequency (time from one peak to the next peak; Fig. 28.4). The medium into which the waves penetrate leads to a partial reflection of the wave back to the transducer, with the interface between different mediums causing the most apparent visual contrast. The transducer then creates electrical energy from the reflected wave, which is

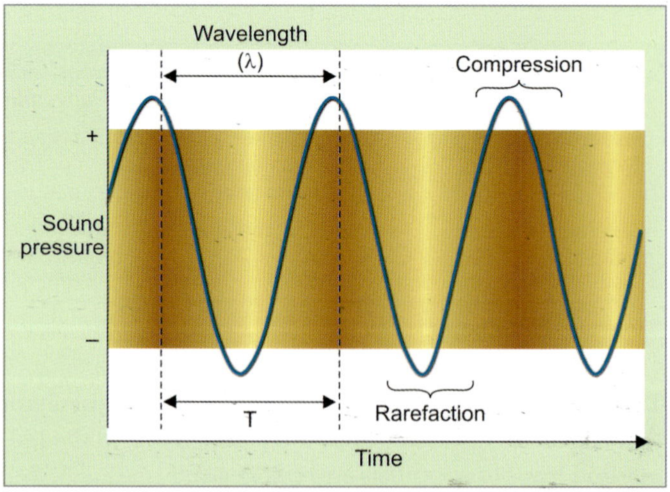

Fig. 28.4: Mechanism of ultrasonography. Source: Adapted with permission from Merritt CB. Physics of Ultrasound: Diagnostic Ultrasound, 3rd edition. St Louis, MO: Elsevier; 2005. p. 4.

Table 28.7: Recommended frequency for a given tissue examination with ultrasonography.[139]

Tissue type	Frequency (MHz)
Kidney	3–6
Bladder/pelvic	3.5–5
Prostate	8–10

Table 28.8: Average impedances of common tissue types in the retroperitoneum.[140]

Tissue	Impedance
Bone	3.8–7.4
Air	0.0004
Water (25°C)	1.48
Blood	1.67
Fat	1.40
Kidney	1.62
Muscle	1.70
Spleen	1.64
Liver	1.65

converted into an image. The amplitude of the reflected wave leads to a certain pixel value, with higher amplitudes giving a brighter image. The frequency of the transducer determines the depth of penetration, with higher-frequency wavelengths resulting in less tissue penetration but with more detail or resolution. There is a tradeoff between tissue penetration and resolution based on what frequency is selected. The optimum frequency for a given tissue type in the GU tract is demonstrated in Table 28.7.

As sound waves travel through tissue, their energy is scattered, absorbed, or reflected. The level at which a sound wave is reflected by a certain tissue type is referred to as impedance and is largely dependent on tissue density. For example, air and bone reflect most of the sound waves that interface with them, leading to an acoustic shadow. This shadow hampers the ability to see tissue and may also be observed when kidney stones are present. The impedance and density of different tissue types are described in Table 28.8. Given the dynamic nature of ultrasound imaging, it is very susceptible to artifacts or images that do not give all the relevant anatomic details. For example, when evaluating the renal parenchyma, a cyst may cause a phenomenon known as increase through transmission. Reverberation artifact results when there is a marked difference between tissue densities and the sound wave bounces between the two tissue types, leading to a perceived distance twice as far away. Another common artifact in ultrosonography is edging, where the sound waves hit a curvilinear surface, leading to a streak artifact on the recorder (Figs. 28.5A to D).[161]

Ultrasound also has several modes that can aid in anatomical detail and the directional flow of fluid in the body. Doppler ultrasound uses the principle that waves are reflected back at different velocities based on the velocity of the medium as it moves either toward or away from an object. This is frequently used to determine the blood flow of an organ. For the stone patient, determining the lack of urine flow from the ureteral orifice at the level of the bladder (ureteral jet) can indicate the presence of obstruction. The color assigned to a moving medium is typically red for when it moves toward to the transducer and blue if it is traveling away from the transducer (Fig. 28.6).[160]

A proper renal ultrasound can provide anatomic as well as functional information about the kidney. The transducer should be set to a value of 3.5–5.0 Hz depending on the body habitus of the individual, with the lower frequency better suited for heavier patients. Spatial compound imaging or B-mode imaging involves multiple ultrasound beams interrogating the same tissue region.[26] The advantage is that "noise" is cancelled out and a more crisp image is obtained. Another technological advancement is harmonic imaging in which two frequencies together cause more peaked sound waves and sharper echoes, thus minimizing the artifact.[27]

Rahmouni et al. described the phenomenon on color Doppler called the "twinkling" artifact. This is a process by which the sonographic waves are not only reflected by the surface of the stone but also by the internal chemical bonds within the stone, leading to an increase in pulse duration.[28] The reason for the internal reflections is that some stones form predominately by conglomeration of one or multiple pure crystalline structures. Lee et al. looked at 36 stones—20 renal and 16 ureteral stones—and showed that 83% of stones demonstrated twinkling artifacts.[29] Sorensen et al. compared B-mode imaging with color Doppler on renal stones that had been previously diagnosed via CT imaging. B mode imaging demonstrated a 71% sensitivity and a 48% specificity, whereas Doppler imaging had a 56% sensitivity and a 74% specificity. The authors concluded that the two ultrasound settings should be used concomitantly to improve the operating characteristics of ultrasound-detected nephrolithiasis.[30]

The sensitivity and specificity of ultrasonography depend on the stone location in the urinary tract. The

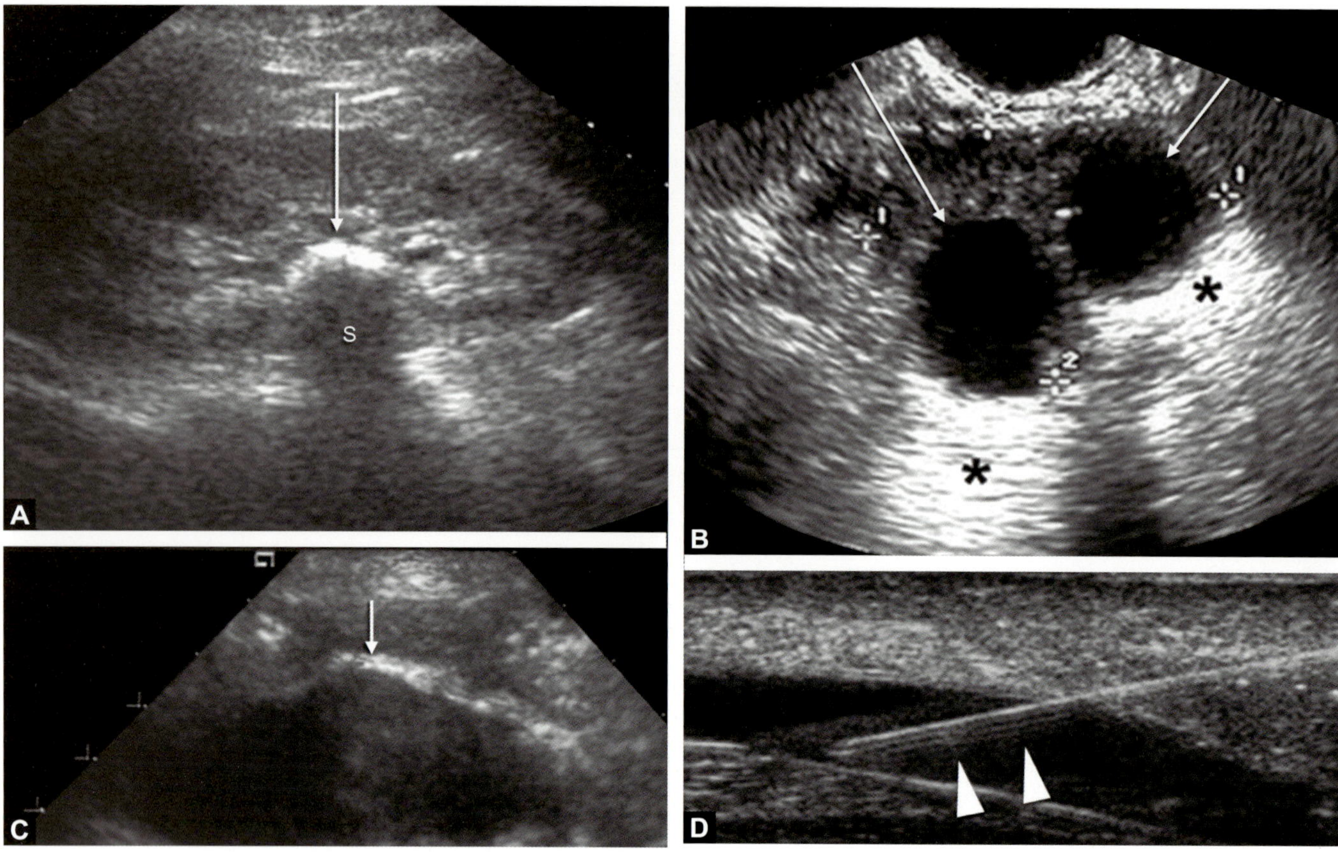

Figs. 28.5A to D: Different artifacts seen during ultrasonography. (A) Acoustic shadowing over a calcification in the renal pelvis. (B) Increased through transmission of simple renal cysts with increase echogenicity away from transducer. (C) Edging created between soft tissue and fluid-filled structure. (D) Reverberation artifact along curved liver edge.
(S: Shadow. * : The increased echogenicity mentioned in the note).
Source: Adopted from Kremkau FW, Taylor KJ. Artifacts in ultrasound imaging. J Ultrasound Med. 1986;5(4):227-37.

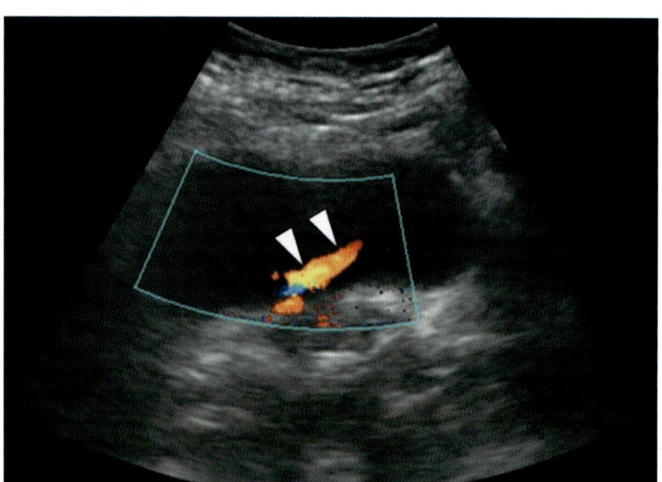

Fig. 28.6: Doppler ultrasound demonstrating a ureteral jet from right ureteral orifice.

operating characteristics of ultrasonography for ureteral stones were demonstrated in a comprehensive review of adult patients with a pooled sensitivity of 44.5%, a specificity of 93.8%, a positive predictive value of 92.6%, a negative predictive value of 49.5%, and an overall accuracy of 62.6%. For renal pelvic stones ultrasonography had a 44.7% sensitivity, a 87.5% specificity, a 77.9% positive predictive value, a 61.7% negative predictive value, and an 86.3% overall accuracy.[31] Ray et al. compared CT to ultrasound in regard to estimation of stone size in 71 stones; CT imaging found an average stone size of 7.4 ± 4.4 mm compared to 9.2 ± 4.6 mm, which was statistically significant. They concluded that ultrasound overestimates the size of most stones, and this is more pronounced for stones of ≤5 mm.[32]

In the pediatric population, a study by Palmer et al. that included 76 children demonstrated that ultrasound failed to identify 41% of patients with urolithiasis compared to a failure rate of 5% of patients with CT. They also showed that ultrasonography accuracy was highly variable depending on the stone's location, with a 90% accuracy rate in the kidney versus 75% with both a concomitant kidney and a ureteral stone, and only 38% accuracy for stones in the ureter alone.[33] Therefore, one should consider that ultrasound may be useful as an initial imaging modality but that definitive cross-sectional imaging should be considered if there is a high degree of suspicion despite a "negative" ultrasound examination.

In the pregnant population, ultrasound is utilized routinely in order to limit ionizing radiation exposure to the fetus. In pregnancy, the specificity of ultrasound is low given the natural dilation of the ureter from mechanical compression. If however, dilation of the ureter is seen below the pelvic vessels, then a distal ureteral stone should be suspected.[34] However, in a study looking at 96 pregnant women, ultrasound correctly identified only 43 stones. Burgess et al. determined that ultrasound had a sensitivity and a specificity of 54% and 78.6%, respectively, in the pregnant population.[35] In order to improve diagnostic accuracy, some authors have advocated the additional use of the RBF restrictive index (RI), which is not affected by the physiologic hydronephrosis of pregnancy. An RI value of 0.7 demonstrated a sensitivity of 45%, a specificity of 91%, and an accuracy of 87%; if a change in RI of just 0.06 is noted on subsequent imaging, the sensitivity, specificity, and accuracy became 95%, 100%, and 99%, respectively.[36] Ureteral jets, as mentioned earlier, have also been used to determine if ureteral obstruction is present. The standard technique is that the hydrated patient is observed for up to 15 minutes on each side for the presence or absence of a ureteral jet.[37] However, the literature has reported that there is asymmetry in only 62–68% of patients with obstructive calculi.[38] Additionally, it has been shown that as many as 15% of pregnant women will not have an ureteral jet who are asymptomatic with hydronephrosis without a stone.[38,39]

Intravenous Contrast

Prior to ordering a study utilizing iodinated contrast, one should have a working understanding of the medium itself, the adverse effects, risks, and the steps necessary to minimize those risks.

In CT, contrast agents contain predominantly iodine. It is placed in a variety of mediums, all of which have little to no radiopacity. The medium in which the iodine is found is what imparts the toxicity. Iodinated contrast agents come as high, medium, or low osmolar compounds as compared to serum (300 mOs/kg). Given that the carrier molecule is highly hydrophilic, it does not penetrate cellular membranes and thus is excreted very rapidly.[40]

The two biggest concerns with IV contrast agents include renal toxicity and allergic reactions. Allergic reactions to iodinated contrast are divided into minor, intermediate, and severe, and further subdivided into immediate versus delayed. These reactions are more common when using high-molecular-weight contrast agents, which is why most centers utilize a low-molecular-weight medium.[41] It is estimated that 3–8% of the US population has an allergy to contrast agents.[41] Risk factors for an allergy to contrast agents include a previous allergic response to iodinated contrast, a history of asthma or atopy, and anxiety disorders.[41] Minor reactions include flushing, itching, or emesis. These can be easily treated with histamine receptor blockers. More severe allergic reactions such as cardiovascular collapse, angioedema, and severe bronchospasm must be managed with epinephrine and supportive care.[42] Less commonly, iodinated contrast can cause cellular toxicity, hemolysis, and acute thyrotoxicosis; however, the occurrence of these reactions is extremely rare.

There have been multiple pretreatment algorithms proposed to lower the incidence of contrast-induced nephropathy. The best recognized is by the American College of Radiology. It requires the administration of 32 mg of methylprednisolone 12 and 2 hours prior to the study, followed by 50 mg of diphenhydramine 1 hour prior to the administration of contrast. This has been shown to lower the incidence of allergic reaction to 1.7%.[42,43]

Contrast-induced nephropathy is defined as a rise in serum creatinine of 0.5 mg/dL within 3 days of contrast instillation. The acute nephrolithiasis patient can have many of the risk factors for developing contrast-induced nephropathy, which include renal insufficiency and dehydration. Other risk factors include being on nonsteroidal anti-inflammatory drugs (NSAIDs), the extremes of age, and a cardiac ejection fraction of <40%.[44] Evidence-based pathways to prevent the development of contrast-induced nephropathy include aggressive pretest hydration, administration of sodium bicarbonate, N-acetyl cysteine, and the use of low-molecular-weight iodinated contrast agents.[45] The specific protocol used should be standardized at your institution with the guidance of your radiology colleagues.

Intravenous Pyelogram

Discussed here more for historical interest, the intravenous pyelogram (IVP) or excretory urogram has largely been replaced by cross-sectional CT imaging. Regardless, IVPs can provide valuable information about the level of urinary obstruction, renal function, and degree of upper obstruction while limiting radiation exposure. The technique involves a plain abdominal X-ray that confirms adequate positioning and the presence of any radiopaque calcifications. The patient then receives IV contrast, and additional images are obtained at defined intervals. The first image, called the nephrogenic phase, provides information about the function of the kidney. It can also provide gross information about perfusion deficits and the presence or absence of a delayed nephrogram. Repeat images are then obtained after additional time to provide contrast excretory information. During this excretory phase, hydronephrosis, filling defects, and aberrant anatomy can be visualized (Figs. 28.7A to D).[162] In certain cases, the IVP affords the ability to change patient positioning from supine to upright, which may help the surgeon to discern stones (which will retain their shape) from the layering pattern of milk of calcium. The limitation of this imaging modality is the time required to complete an examination and that CT scans can provide more information quicker, making IVP of historical interest or a specially ordered rare test.

Computed Tomography

Ever since its development in the late 1970s, CT has been a mainstay in the evaluation of nephrolithiasis patients. The image acquisition is based on similar principles to that of conventional radiography except that multiple images are taken in a systematic fashion as the beam and detector rotate around the patient. A computer can then reconstruct a three-dimensional image via spatial processing software if desired. Modern advances include multidetector CT scanners, low-dose CT scanners, and CT fluoroscopy. Most modern CT scanners are helical and utilize a spinning column of detectors in which a patient moves through at the speed of one breath.[46] On average, modern scanners can obtain a complete abdominal series in 10 seconds. The speed of a scan and the resolution are dependent on both the energy and the desired slice thickness (i.e. the smaller the slices the greater the radiation exposure).

For the acute renal colic patient, a helical CT scan is extremely sensitive and specific for diagnosing urolithiasis. When evaluating the sensitivity and specificity of CT scanners, most studies demonstrate >95% sensitivity and specificity for detecting nephrolithiasis.[47] Despite the overall accuracy of CT scans, certain aspects about a patient can obscure the diagnosis such as motion artifact and streak artifact (e.g. metallic joint precluding visualization of the distal ureter; Figs. 28.8A and B). Computed tomography scanners determine not only the presence of a stone but also the other relevant anatomic considerations and give the urologist an idea of stone density.

In keeping with the principal of minimizing lifetime exposure to ionizing radiation, there is a current trend to lower the radiation exposure by decreasing the energy of the scan in hopes of obtaining equivalent diagnostic accuracy. Conventional CT scans result in 8–16 mSV of exposure on average.[48] Most low-dose CT protocols expose the patient to <3.0 mSV, and some ultra-low-dose protocols have <1 mSV of radiation exposure.[49] In a meta-analysis evaluating only prospective randomized trials, Niemann et al. demonstrated a pooled sensitivity of 0.966 and a specificity of 0.949 with an accuracy of 99.32% when utilizing protocols with exposures averaging >3 mSV. The authors conclude that whenever possible, low-energy CT should be utilized in the evaluation of renal colic.[50]

Characteristics of a Stone on CT and Clinical Decision-making

Composition: Hounsfield units (HUs) are a quantitative standard to measure the relative radiodensity of an object on a CT scan. The HU scale is defined as the radiodensity (linear attenuation coefficient) of distilled water at standard pressure and temperature.[51] Not only can the HU help determine the stone type, but it can also aid in choosing the correct therapeutic intervention for a particular stone episode. Patel et al. prospectively evaluated 50 patients with renal pelvic stones (a mean size of 10.2 mm), and tried to determine a cutoff HU value in order to determine SWL success. They defined SWL success as either being stone free or having clinically insignificant residual fragments <4 mm at 1-month followup on CT imaging. The patients who had a successful treatment had a mean HU value of 715 ± 260 versus those who were not successful (1,196 ± 171). They determined that a cutoff value of 970 HU had the best operating characteristics for SWL.[52] Another study examined HU and the predictive value for success, and impact on operative time for ureteroscopy. A total of 212 procedures were examined, with no difference in HU in those patients who were and were not stone free at their 3-month follow-up. The authors did find that

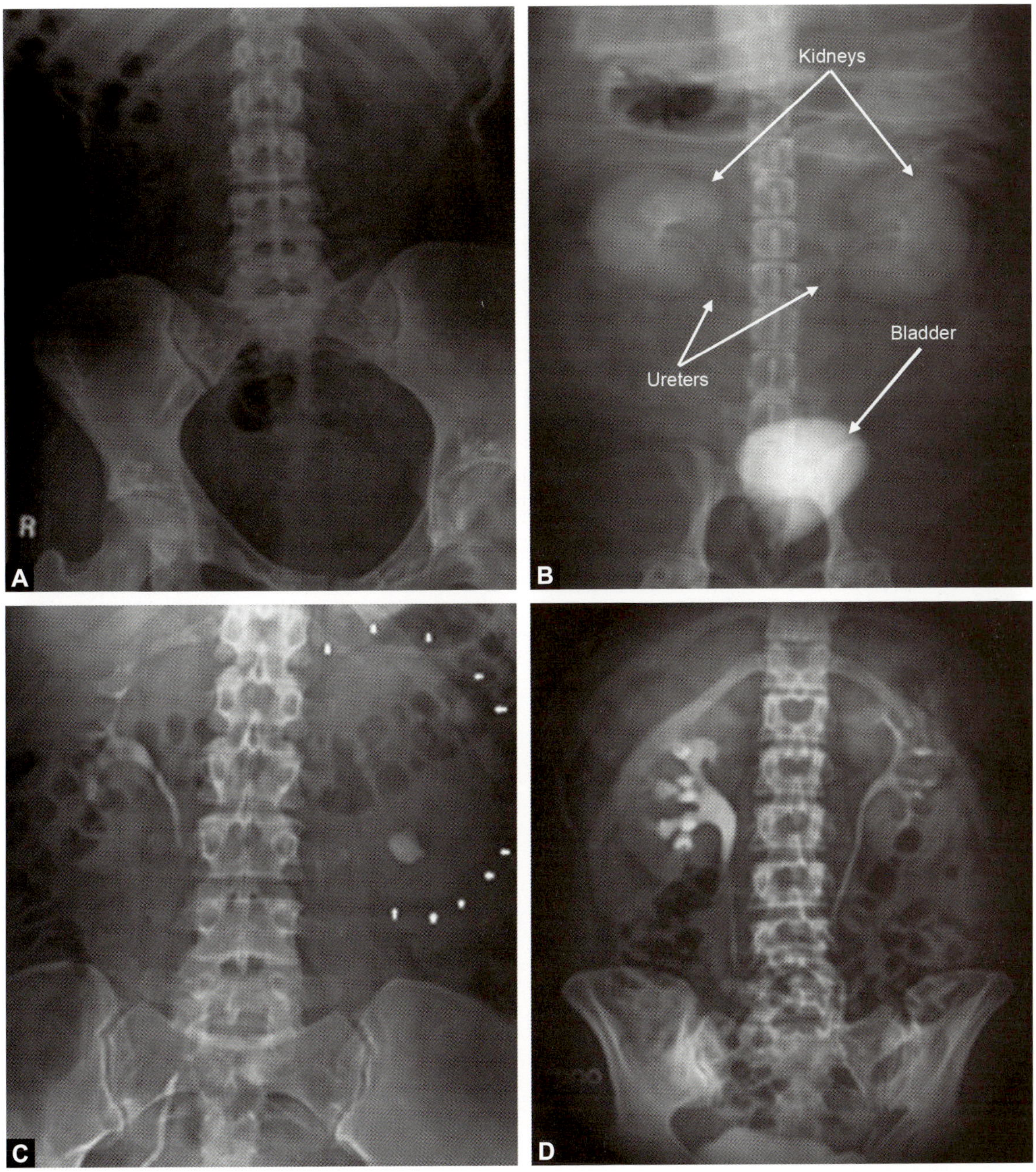

Figs. 28.7A to D: Intravenous pyelogram: (A) precontrast; (B) nephrogenic; (C) 10 minutes after contrast instillation demonstrating a delayed nephrogram on left; (D) excretory phase.
Source: Adapted with permission from Brenner BM, Chertow GM, Marsden PA, et al. Brenners and Rector's the Kidney, 9th edition, Chapter 27. Philadelphia, PA: Elsevier Saunders; 2012. pp. 930-1005.

fragmentation efficiency (defined as laser energy divided by stone size) was significantly less, the higher the HU or attenuation value.[53]

Determining stone composition based solely on standard CT is not possible. One study looked at 100 kidney stones that had been analyzed and tried to determine predictive HU ranges for different stone phenotypes. The authors noted a trend toward significance with calcium stones having an average HU density of 105 HU/mm, compared to 50 HU/mm and 53 HU/mm for uric acid and struvite stones, respectively.[54] Nakada et al. examined a similar question in which they compared HU and final stone

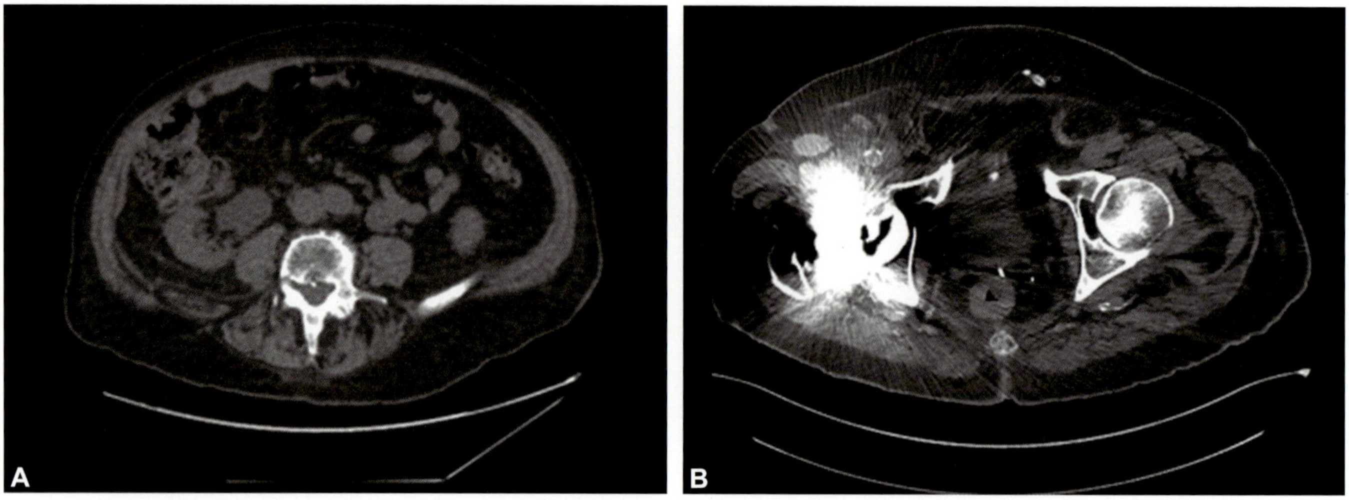

Figs. 28.8A and B: An 84-year-old with persistent hydronephrosis with a believed ureteral stricture found to have distal obstructive ureteral stone. (A) Proximal hydronephrosis. (B) Streak artifact inhibiting visualization of pelvic structures.

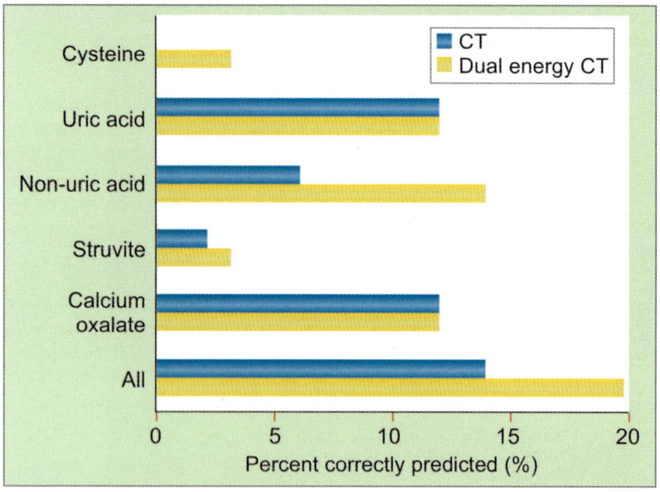

Fig. 28.9: Accuracy of dual-energy CT compared to conventional CT. (CT: Computed tomography).
Source: Adapted with permission from Wisenbaugh ES, Paden RG, Silva AC, et al. Dual-energy vs conventional computed tomography in determining stone composition. Urology. 2014;83(6):1243-7.

composition in patients who presented with acute renal colic. They were able to demonstrate a significant difference between uric acid and calcium-based stones only with HU densities of 344 ±152.5 versus 652 ± 490, respectively.[55]

Dual-energy CT (DECT) has shown promise to allow better discrimination of stone composition. This employs two different energy sources and two detectors, and calculates two separate HU for a given energy, typically 140 and 80 kilovolt peak (kV(p)); the difference between those values is used to determine stone composition. There are different types of DECT scanners available. One by Seimans (Malvern, PA) utilizes a dual-energy source with two X-ray tubes that work simultaneously at right angles to each other. A newer device by GE Healthcare (Milwaukee, WI) is referred to as a "fast kV-switching" device; it employs one X-ray tube that rapidly switches between 80 and 140 in 0.4 ms. A third device by Phillips Healthcare (Andover, MA) utilizes one X-ray tube and a dual-layer detector that absorbs low- and high-energy spectra and then reconstructs the images via integrated software.[56] Manglaviti et al. completed an in vivo study of 40 patients with 45 kidney and 4 ureteral stones of >5 mm in size. Dual-energy CT correctly identified all pure calcium oxalate, cysteine, and uric acid stones but misclassified stones of mixed composition (there were no pure calcium phosphate stones examined).[57] Wisenbaugh et al. compared DECT with conventional CT imaging by taking 27 stones of known composition and evaluating the operating characteristics of each one. Conventional CT accurately predicted the stone type in 52% of the specimens, compared to 74% with DECT. When comparing the two modalities' accuracy by stone type, DECT proved superior for nonuric acid calculi, most notably cysteine stones (Fig. 28.9).[56]

Nuclear Medicine Scans

Nuclear scintigraphy is a modality that can provide information regarding obstruction, differential renal function, and the presence or absence of parenchymal scarring. Scintigraphy has the ability to provide functional information about the kidney and drainage at a lower level of radiation exposure compared to IVP or CT urography.

Technetium 99 m mercaptoacetyl triglycine is one of the most common diuretic renal scans that is utilized in urology. This radiolabeled molecule is predominantly secreted by the renal tubules.[58] It is also highly bound to plasma proteins and, therefore, can be used to evaluate RBF. There are three phases depicted with this study: the initial flow phase, the renal phase, and the diuretic phase (Figs. 28.10A to C). The timing of diuretic administration should correlate to the maximum collecting system activity. During the diuretic phase, the presence of ureteral duplication and level of obstruction can also be ascertained. Figures 28.10A to C demonstrate abnormal diuretic curves.

Nuances of the test include asking the patient if they experience pain with the administration of the diuretic and having a Foley catheter in place to remove the possibility of a poorly compliant bladder or vesicoureteral reflux confounding the results. A limitation of the test is that 10% of the molecule is excreted by the liver; therefore, careful anatomic mapping is critical. Overall anatomic details with the test are poor. Furthermore, the technician must be well versed in determining the correct timing of diuretic administration and asking the patient about his or her perception of pain.

Indications for this imaging modality in a nephrolithiasis patient are limited. One such indication is reserved for those in whom differential renal function will change management. For example, if a particular nonfunctioning kidney is grossly involved with nephrolithiasis, a nephrectomy may be indicated. Another indication for scintigraphy in the stone patient would include poorly resolving hydronephrosis following stone management to rule out stricture disease. Furthermore, a diuretic scan could also prove helpful in the setting of a possible ureteropelvic obstruction in the face of nephrolithiasis to determine if additional procedures may be required at the time of stone treatment (Table 28.9).

WORKUP FOR COMPLEX STONE DISEASE

Staghorn Calculi

Staghorn calculi represent one end of the spectrum in the management of complex nephrolithiasis. The majority of staghorn calculi are composed of magnesium ammonium phosphate or struvite; however, cysteine, uric acid, and calcium oxalate stones can also form staghorn calculi. Viprakasit et al. retrospectively examined the composition of non-infectious staghorn calculi, with 55% being calcium phosphate, 21% being uric acid, 14% being calcium oxalate, and 10% being cysteine. They also noted that patients with metabolic stones had a lower complication rate compared to those with infection-based stones.[59] The biggest risk factors for developing struvite calculi include recurrent infections with urease-producing organisms and urinary stasis. The patient may be asymptomatic or, otherwise, compromised such as those with long-term indwelling Foley catheters, spinal cord injury, or those with significant metabolic or anatomic variants.[60]

The consequences of staghorn calculi have been well established. If left untreated, these calculi lead to progressive renal disfunction and mortality. Blandy and Singh demonstrated a 10-year mortality of 28% with conservatively managed staghorn calculi (n = 60) versus 7.2% in patients treated with surgery (n = 125).[60] Teichman et al. followed 177 patients and demonstrated a 31% renal deterioration rate in staghorn calculi patients. Renal deterioration was more common in those with solitary kidneys, previous stones, complete staghorns, and in the presence of a urinary diversion and neurogenic bladder (Table 28.10).[61] Koga et al. demonstrated in a cohort of 167 patients that, if left untreated, staghorn calculi lead to a 36% chronic renal failure rate.[62] The American Urological Association (AUA) published their recommendations in 2005 that all patients who can withstand surgical intervention with newly diagnosed staghorn calculi should be treated.[63]

Staghorn calculi are defined by multiple criteria. The traditional definition was any calculi or renal pelvic stone that extends into the renal calyces. The most widely accepted criteria for defining staghorn calculi were described by Di Silverio, who divided staghorn calculi into four groups (Table 28.11).[64] However, the majority of practical surgical decision making today revolves around determining the location and volume of the stone burden without the need for strict grading or classification.[65]

Asymptomatic Renal Stones

Patients who do not have symptoms from their nephrolithiasis represent a challenging treatment dilemma for the patient and the provider. The decision to treat largely depends on the size, number, and location of the patient's stone burden. Burgher et al. examined 300 patients with 3 years of follow-up, noting that 77% of the stones demonstrated progression (defined as the need for intervention, stone growth, or development of symptoms). If the calculi were >4 mm, there was a 26% increased likelihood that surgical intervention would be required.[66] Koh et al. provided a more recent review of 50 patients with 85 stones, an average size of 5.7 mm, and they found that the incidences of passage, progression in size, and need for intervention were 20%, 45.9%, and 7.1%, respectively.[67] One of the largest observation studies described 347 patients with asymptomatic stones over an average followup of 31 months. Stone events were defined as spontaneous passage with or without renal colic, stone growth, or the need for intervention. Average stone size was 4.39 mm, and 57% of stones were in the lower pole of the

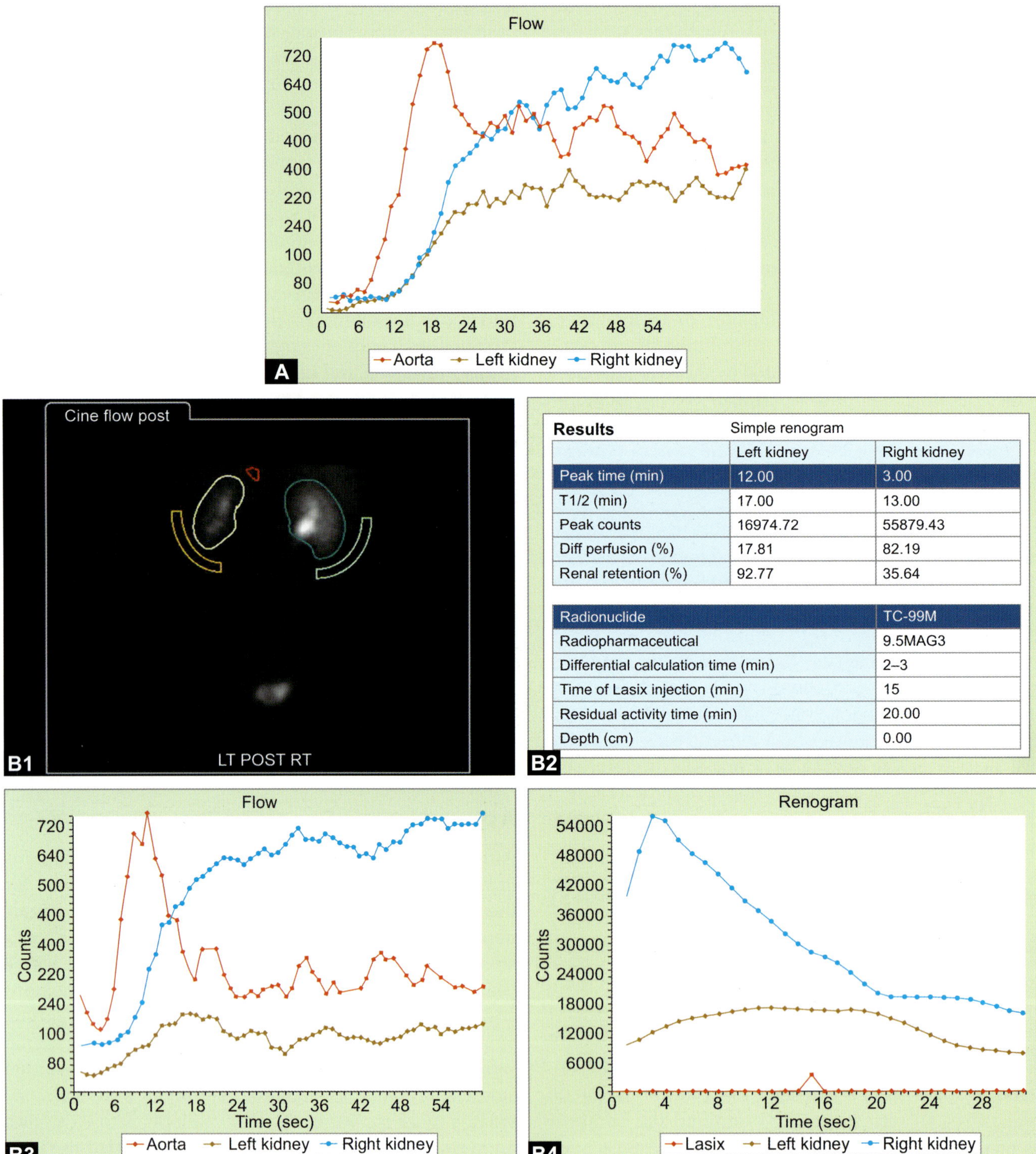

Results — Simple renogram

	Left kidney	Right kidney
Peak time (min)	12.00	3.00
T1/2 (min)	17.00	13.00
Peak counts	16974.72	55879.43
Diff perfusion (%)	17.81	82.19
Renal retention (%)	92.77	35.64

Radionuclide	TC-99M
Radiopharmaceutical	9.5MAG3
Differential calculation time (min)	2–3
Time of Lasix injection (min)	15
Residual activity time (min)	20.00
Depth (cm)	0.00

Figs. 28.10A and B

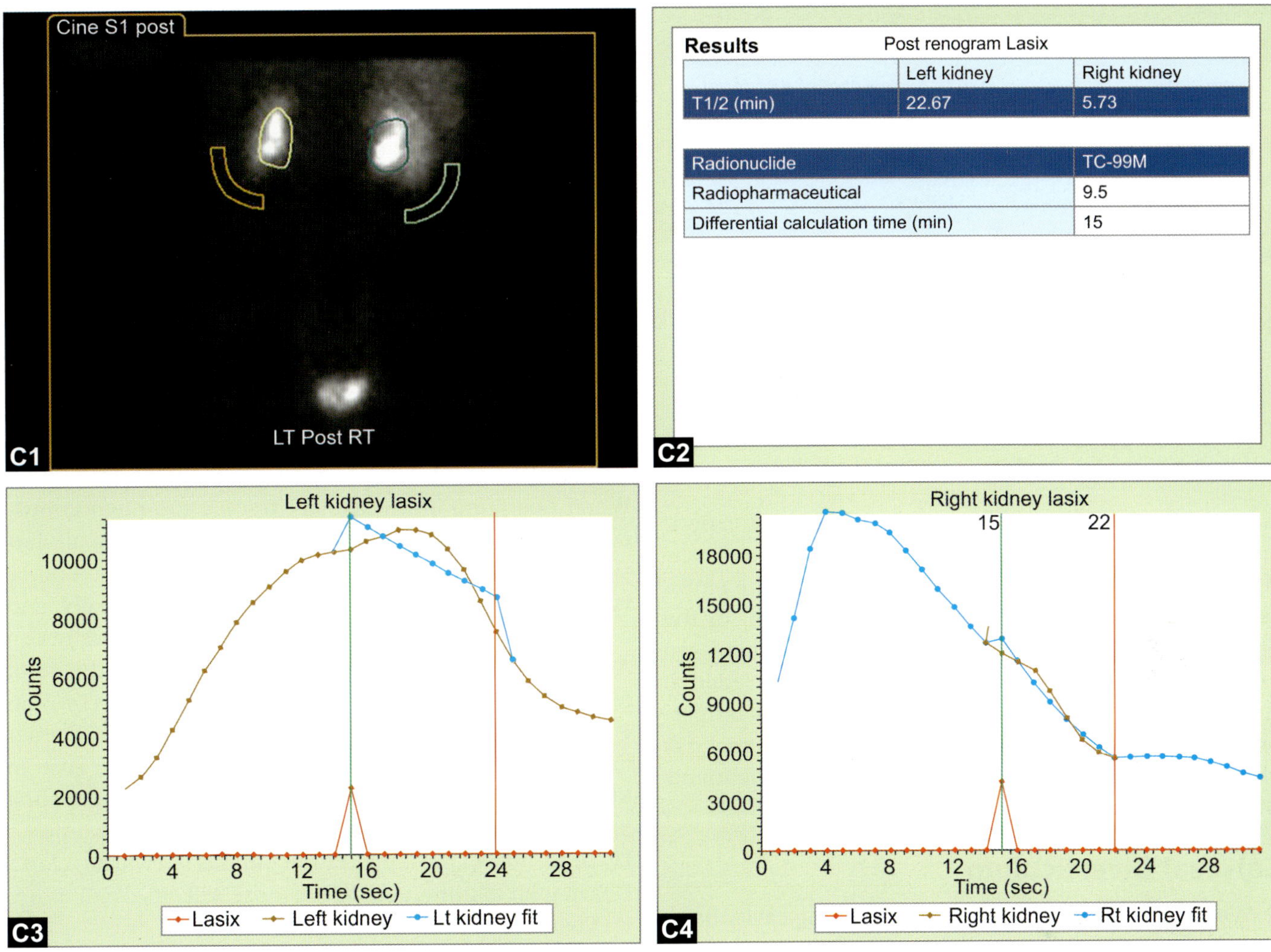

Figs. 28.10A to C: Diuretic renal scan in a patient with a known high-grade obstruction of the left renal unit. (A) Poor flow of radiotracer into left kidney. (B) Poor flow (bottom left) and uptake (bottom right) of radiotracer into left renal unit. (C) Prolonged T½ of 23 minutes in left kidney.

Table 28.9: Indications for diuretic renal scan in the stone patient.[141,142]

Indication	*Finding*	*Differential diagnosis*
Unresolving renal colic after definitive stone management	Pain present with administration of diuretic	Renal ptosis, loin pain hematuria, chronic pain
Persistent hydronephrosis after stone surgery	Increased *T½* time and pooling of radiolabeled markers	UPJ obstruction, ureteral stricture disease, vesicoureteral reflux
Unilateral recurrent stone burden in the setting of upper tract dilation	NA	Rule out anatomical obstruction
Questionable ureteral duplication with or without obstruction	Unilateral differential function	Higher incidence of ureteropelvic junction obstruction
Decreased parenchyma on the side of significant stone burden	Decreased renal blood flow and decreased contrast uptake on renal phase	NA
Followup after endopyelotomy or ureteral stricture lysis	Evaluate improvement in function and *T½* time	NA

(UPJ: Ureteropelvic junction).

Table 28.10: Risk factors for developing renal deterioration after treatment of staghorn calculi.[143]

Patient's characteristic	*Risk of development of renal deterioration (%)*
Previous stone	
Yes	50
No	14
Kidney status	
Solitary	67
Non	25
Stone burden	
Complete	42
Partial	0

kidney. Fifty four percent of their patient cohort experienced a stone-related event with 25% requiring an intervention, while 16% of the entire cohort visited the emergency room and 29% experienced stone growth. In the patients experiencing pain, 53% subsequently progressed to intervention. Unlike other studies, the authors failed to show a difference in stone-related events when comparing size and location.[68] These data demonstrate a real risk of stone progression and stone-related events in patients with stones that are currently asymptomatic.

Calyceal Diverticulum

A calyceal diverticulum is a urine-containing cavity lined with transitional urothelium that does not efficiently drain urine.[69] The most common type of diverticulum is one that communicates with a minor calyx in the upper pole of the kideny.[70] The incidence of calyceal diverticulum has been demonstrated to be 0.21–0.45% of the general population. Usually, they are not associated with symptoms, unless involved with stone disease. The prevalence of stone formation in these poorly draining systems has been shown to be as high as 9.5–39%, and they rarely allow spontaneous stone passage.[69,70] Management of stones in calyceal diverticulum has traditionally been through percutaneous nephrolithotomy (PCNL), but endoscopic advancements has made URS management an option. Shock wave lithotripsy has not been shown to be effective for this patient population secondary to poor stone clearance rates due to the poor drainage of the diverticulum.[71]

Nephrocalcinosis

Nephrocalcinosis is defined as calcifications in the renal parenchyma. The typical composition of this material is calcium phosphate. The presence of nephrocalcinosis can also be associated with glomerular injury and nephron fibrosis. The etiology of nephrocalcinosis can be a result of calcium-wasting diuretics, distal RTA, infectious, or idiopathic.[72] It is important to distinguish nephrocalcinosis from nephrolithiasis as the management of nephrocalcinosis is medical in nature. Cross-sectional imaging is required usually with contrast, or it may even require direct visual endoscopic examination as it is difficult to distinguish one from the other on plain radiography.[73]

INFECTIONS OF THE URINARY TRACT AND THE STONE PATIENT

Epidemiology of Urinary Tract Infections

When operating in the urinary tract, a thorough knowledge of infections of the GU system should be understood. Urinary tract infections account for 7 million office visits and 1 million emergency room visits annually, and account for $1.6 billion in annual medical expenditures.[74] Asymptomatic bacteria are present in ~1–3% of the adult female population, 25% of whom will develop a UTI within 1 year.[75] The frequency of UTIs largely depends on gender and age. In infants, the frequency is about 1–2%. Also in infancy, UTIs are much more common in boys for the first 3 months of life, then become more common in women.[76] Up to 40–50% of the female adult population will develop a UTI in their lifetime, and 20% of those will develop another UTI within the next 6 months.[75,77]

Urinary Tract Infections as a Risk Factor for Stones

A UTI is an inflammatory response to a foreign pathogen in the urinary system.[77] They are divided into complicated and uncomplicated infections based on patient factors (Table 28.12). Urinary tract infections can be further stratified as recurrent, meaning the original infection that was documented has resolved but recurred, versus a patient who has a persistent infection from the same organism. This is in contrast to asymptomatic bacteriuria, where there is the presence of bacteria in the urine that may be a result of contamination or colonization.[78] Pyelonephritis is divided into acute and chronic. Xanthogranulomatous pyelonephritis is a chronic destructive process of the parenchyma of the kidney that typically results from obstruction and infection and is commonly associated with nephrolithiasis.[79] The diagnosis and management of this condition will be discussed separately.

Table 28.11: Classification of staghorn calculi with associated radiographs.[144]

Group	*Characteristic*	*Radiographic image*
Group 1 (borderline)	Fills renal pelvis and branches into one calyx	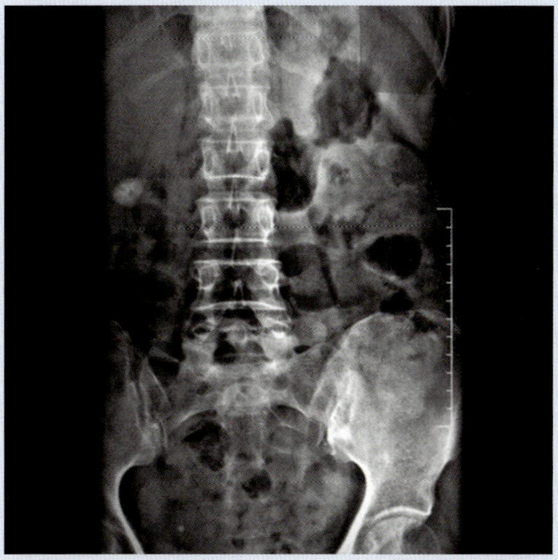
Group 2 (partial)	Fills renal pelvis and branches into the calyces <80% involvement	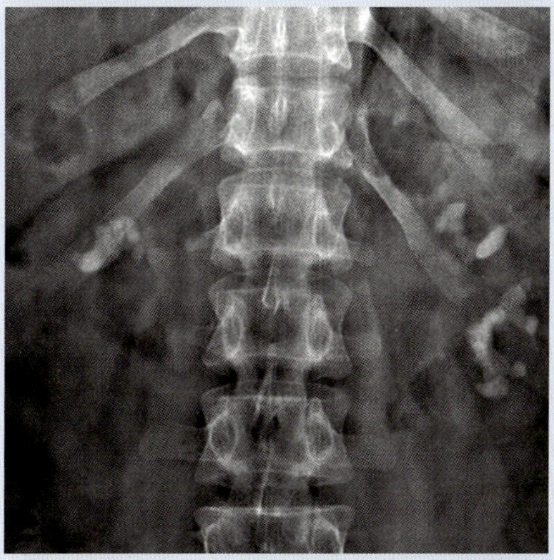
Group 3 (complete)	Fills >80% of collecting system	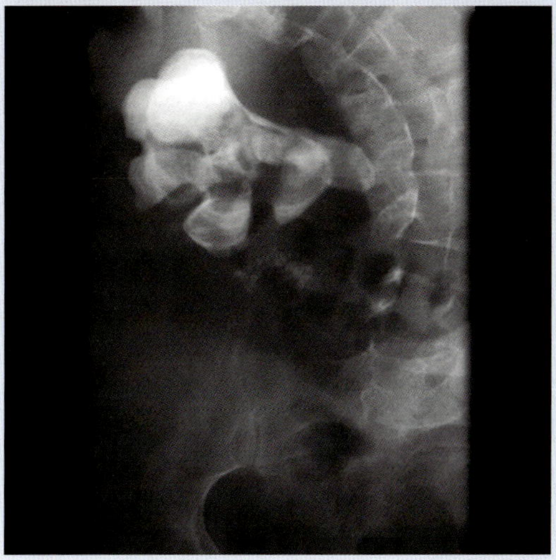

Contd...

Contd...

Group	Characteristic	Radiographic image
Group 4 (giant)	Fills a hugely dilated system completely	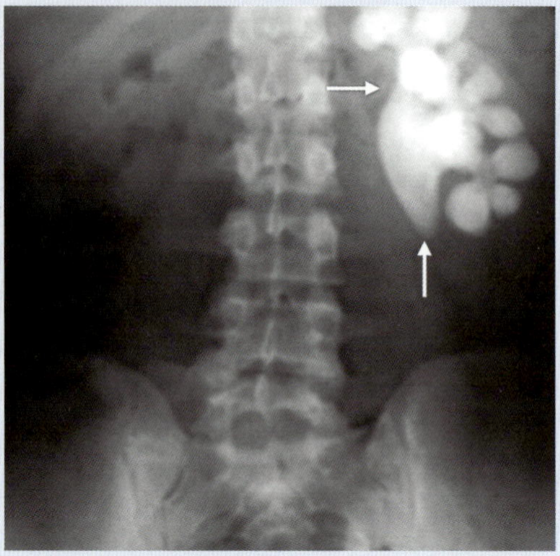

Table 28.12: Criteria for a complicated urinary tract infection.[145]

Criteria
Immunosuppressed
Anatomical variant in the urinary tract
Extrema of age
Foreign material in the urinary tract
Hospital acquired
Male gender
Presence of stones
Pregnancy

Diagnosis

Over 95% of UTIs are monobacterial, with *Escherichia coli* accounting for 80% of UTIs.[80,81] This pattern of infection greatly changes if a patient has recurrent infections or anatomical abnormalities. For example, in stone patients *Klebsiella*, staphylococcal species, *Proteus*, and pseudomonal species are more prevalent.[81]

Diagnosis largely depends on the patient's symptoms in conjunction with microscopic evaluation of the urine as well as the urine culture. Urine specimens are subject to contamination; therefore, the diagnostic accuracy is dependent on the mechanism of collection. For example, in a circumcised man, a midstream collection is rarely contaminated; therefore, a catheterized urine specimen is only indicated in a man if the patient has the inability to urinate. This is in stark contrast to women in which the paravaginal and introitus can easily contaminate the specimen. The easiest way to determine contamination is the presence of vaginal epithelial cells. Another way to statistically determine the presence of a UTI is by quantifying the bacterial load in the urine specimen. For example, even if there are 10^5 bacteria/mL in a clean-catch urine specimen in an asymptomatic woman, then there is only an 80% likelihood that this represents true bacteriuria and a confirmatory sample should be collected.[78] However, in asymptomatic men, a colony count of 10^3 in a midstream is >95% accurate for bacturia.[78] All nephrolithiasis patients should have a urine screen and, if positive, a culture should be performed with speciation and antibiotic sensitivities. This should be done even in the setting of a "contaminated" specimen as it will direct specific therapy to the patient, possibly preventing infectious complications during surgery.

Urinary Tract Infections and Stone Risk

Urease-producing organisms are known to initiate the formation of struvite and apatite. Struvite calculi only form if the urine pH is ≥7.2. A list of common urease-producing bacteria is given in Table 28.13. Another reason why infections may precipitate stone disease is the bacterial consumption of known stone-inhibiting substances such as citrate.[82] Chronic antibiotic use in the recurrently infected patient has been shown to decrease *Oxalobacter formigenes* in the bowel, thus increasing intestinal absorption of oxalate and the risk of subsequent nephrolithiasis.[83] Troxel et al. analyzed 35 calcium oxalate nephrolithiasis patients compared to nonstone formers and demonstrated that patients with stone disease were only colonized 26% of the time compared to 60% of controls with *O. formigenes*.[84]

Table 28.13: Common urease-producing organisms.[146]

Pathogen
Proteus
Staphylococcus aureus
Klebsiella
Providencia
Ureaplasma

Stone as a Risk Factor for Urinary Tract Infections

Stones cannot only be formed by bacteria, they can also harbor infection that is resistant to antibiotic therapy. No large epidemiological study has examined the concordance of nephrolithiasis complicated by UTI. The pathophysiology of UTI in the setting of stones likely is secondary to obstruction. As such, a patient may have a sterile bladder culture and still have infection above the level of obstruction. It is therefore imperative that cultures be obtained from the obstructed column of urine.[85] Watson et al. retrospectively examined 315 percutaneous nephrostomies; additional or different flora were found in 36.8% of patients, and 73% of them underwent a change in antibiotic or antifungal coverage.[86] What complicates antibiotic use in an obstructed renal unit is that RBF and subsequent antibiotic delivery to the affected side is impaired.[87] Efstathiou et al. performed a retrospective review demonstrating on multivariate analysis that the presence of nephrolithiasis was associated with antibiotic resistance.[88]

Common Antibiotics Side Effects and Indications

Prior to intervention, the goal of treatment is to completely remove the bacteria load or decrease the CFUs in the urinary tract in order to decrease the risk of developing bacteremia or sepsis during surgery. In order for an antimicrobial to be effective, it must reach the mean inhibitory concentration for a certain bacteria in the urine.[89] Tables 28.14 and 28.15 show common antimicrobials and the percentage that are excreted in the urine. In the absence of a complicated infection, recommended antibiotic choice in the setting of UTI of the upper and lower urinary tracts is shown in Table 28.16.[159]

Prophylaxis in the Urology Patient

The idea of prophylaxis centers on the idea of preventing the spread of bacteria from a procedure. The ideal timing of prophylaxis has been suggested to be ~30 minutes prior to the initiation of the procedure itself. The type of antibiotic largely depends on the type of procedure and the nature of bacterial contamination that is expected for a given procedure. Host factors should be considered when choosing antimicrobial prophylaxis, such as those that would impair the ability of a patient to fight off an opportunistic organism: immunosuppression, smoking, or anatomic abnormalities (i.e. ureteropelvic junction (UPJ) obstruction, ureteral stricture disease, urethral outlet obstruction, or bladder diverticulum). Furthermore, the presence of foreign bodies (e.g. pacemaker, heart valves, and orthopedic hardware) should be considered when determining the need of antibiotic prophylaxis. The best practice guidelines for antimicrobial prophylaxis are summarized in Table 28.17. Specific evidence for the requirements for the three most common stone procedures—ureteroscopy, PCNL, and SWL—is discussed below.

Table 28.14: Typical oral drugs, their respective time to peak serum level, and percentage excreted in the urine.[147]

Drug	*Time to peak serum level (h)*	*Excreted in urine (%)*
Ampicillin	2	42
Cephalexin	1.5	98
Ciprofloxacin	1.2	30
Levofloxacin	1.2	95
Nitrofurantoin	<2	42
TMP–SMX	2	55/50
Tetracycline	4	60

(TMP–SMX: Trimethoprim/sulfamethoxazole).

The incidence of bacteruria after SWL has been shown to be as high as 20%, whereas symptomatic UTI only occurs in 2–3% of patients undergoing SWL. This is further evidenced by the knowledge that 16–35% of stones harbor bacteria.[90] Ilker et al. performed a large trial that examined the benefit of preoperative antibiotics in patients undergoing SWL. Three hundred and eleven patients were randomized to either receive or not receive antibiotics; they found no difference between the groups as it pertained to the development of asymptomatic bacteruria or symptomatic UTIs after surgery.[91] However, a meta-analysis by Pearle and Roehrborn demonstrated that the rate of UTI after SWL was decreased to 2.1% from 5.7% with a single dose of prophylactic antibiotics in the setting of sterile preoperative urine cultures, translating to a relative risk of 0.45 in the antibiotic-treated group.[90] These data suggest that a single dose of trimethoprim/sulfamethoxazole (TMP–SMX) or a fluoroquinolone is indicated for patients undergoing SWL.

Table 28.15: Mechanism of action of oral antimicrobials, typical flora sensitivities, and common side effects/precautions.[148]

Drug	*Mechanism*	*Typical flora sensitivities*	*Adverse reactions /contraindications*
TMP–SMX	Blocks bacterial folate metabolism	*Streptococcal spp, staphylococcal spp, Enterobacter*. Not pseudomonal spp	Rash, photosensitivity, GI upset, Stevens Johnson's syndrome, hemolytic syndrome (immunosuppressed). Must avoid in all pregnant patients and with precaution in anticoagulated patients or AIDS patients
Quinolones	Blocks bacterial DNA gyrase	*Streptococcal spp, Staph spp*, most Gram negatives except *Pseudomonas*	Tendon rupture, photosensitivity, confusion, and mood disorder. Avoid in children and pregnancy, caution in patients on Coumadin therapy.
Beta lactams	Blocks the production of bacterial wall synthesis	Streptococcal spp, Enterococcal, *Escherichia coli*, and *Proteus spp*	Hypersensitivity reaction, GI effects. Only precaution is for those with a history of hypersensitivity.
Amoxicillin-clavulanic acid	Blocks bacterial wall synthesis and inhibits beta lactamase		
Nitrofurantoin	Blocks multiple bacterial enzymes	*Streptococcal spp, staphylococcal spp*, most *Enterobacter*. (Not *Serratia*, *Providencia* or *Acinetobacter*)	Hemolysis in G6PD, pulmonary fibrosis in setting of chronic use, neuropathy (more common if low GFR). Precaution in patient with decreased renal function.

(AIDS: Acquired immune deficiency syndrome; GI: Gastrointestinal; DNA: Deoxyribonucleic acid; GFR: Glomerular filtration rate).

Table 28.16: Recommendations for the treatment of urinary tract infections in the adult population.[148]

Acute pyelonephritis	*Oral agent*
Nonpregnant woman	
No urine Gram's stain available	Fluoroquinolone for 7 days
Gram-positive cocci in chains	Augmentin for 14 days
Gram-positive cocci in clusters	Linezolid or TMP–SMX for 14 days
Gram-negative bacilli	Fluoroquinolone for 7 days
Lower urinary symptoms	
Nonpregnant women	Fluoroquinolone for 3 days
Men	Fluoroquinolone or TMP–SMX for 7 days

(AUA: American Urological Association; TMP–SMX: Trimethoprim/sulfamethoxazole).

Ureteroscopy exposes the patient not only to bacteria that could be harbored in the kidney stone itself but also to the translocation of bacteria from the external genitalia into the urinary tract. Furthermore, if a ureteral access sheath (UAS) is not utilized, the pressure in the renal collecting system increases, thereby escalating the risk of bacteremia via pyelovenous or pyelosinus backflow. Auge et al. evaluated renal pelvic pressures in patients with or without a UAS; they determined that renal pelvic pressures was 15 mmHg when a UAS was used versus 60 mmHg when it was not used, again increasing theoretical fluid absorption.[92] Common skin flora includes *Staphylococcus aureus,* coagulase-negative staphylococcal species and group A streptococcal species. Conversely, common GU flora includes *E. coli, Proteus spp, Klebsiella spp,* and *Enterococcus.* The AUA advocates a preoperative fluoroquinolone or TMP–SMX; alternatives include amoxicillin–clavulanic acid, amino glycoside or a first- or second-generation cephalosporin. There are little data on antimicrobial prophylaxis in the URS patient population to date. Knopf et al. performed a randomized controlled trial looking at antibiotic prophylaxis in the setting of therapeutic URS in 113 patients; the antibiotic arm got a single dose of 250 mg Levaquin versus none in the control group. They found a 12.5% bacteriuria rate in the control arm versus 1.8% in the antibiotic arm; however, the development of a symptomatic UTI was similar in both groups.[93]

Percutaneous nephrolithotomy also exposes the patient to skin flora and GU flora, and also provides a direct conduit of bacteria or endotoxins directly into the circulatory system. Fourcade retrospectively reviewed 107 patients who did not receive perioperative antibiotics, 35% of whom developed asymptomatic bacteriuria and 10% of whom developed fever or sepsis.[94] Charton et al. did a randomized controlled trial looking at preoperative antimicrobials in 49 patients undergoing PCNL; although there was a trend toward increased asymptomatic bacteriuria (rate 12 % vs 5%), it failed to meet statistical significance.[95] The current recommendations from the AUA advocate for

Table 28.17: American Urological Association Guidelines for recommended antimicrobial prophylaxis for urologic procedures.[149]

Procedure	Prophylaxis indicated	Antimicrobial choice	Alternative antimicrobials
Cystoscopy with manipulation	All	TMP–SMX fluoroquinolone	Amoxicillin–clavulanate first/second-generation cephalosporin aminoglycoside
Ureteroscopy	All	TMP–SMX fluoroquinolone	Aminoglycoside, amoxicillin–clavulanate, first/second-generation cephalosporin
Percutaneous renal surgery	All	First-generation cephalosporin	Ampicillin–sulbactam fluoroquinolone
Extracorporeal shock wave lithotripsy	All	TMP–SMX fluoroquinolone	Amoxicillin–clavulanate first/second-generation cephalosporin aminoglycoside

(TMP–SMX: Trimethoprim/sulfamethoxazole).

antibiotic prophylaxis in this setting given the substantial theoretical risk to the patient. First-line antibiotics include a first- or second-generation cephalosporin, aminoglycoside, metronidazole, and clindamycin. Second-line antibiotics include ampicillin–sulbactam and ciprofloxacin. The current AUA guidelines for cystoscopy, extracorporeal shock wave lithotripsy (ESWL), URS, and PCNL are included in Table 28.17.

When choosing the correct antibiotic for a nephrolithiasis patient, the stone culture must also be considered. Mariappan et al. examined bladder cultures, renal pelvic urine cultures, and the culture from the fragmented stone for the purpose of trying to determine which would more accurately predict the development of systemic inflammatory response syndrome (SIRS). In 54 procedures, they determined that the renal pelvic culture better predicted the stone culture over a bladder culture. They also determined that the presence of an infected renal pelvic culture or infected stone was associated with a fourfold increase in the development of SIRS. [96] They concluded that these cultures should be a routine in the treatment of nephrolithiasis.

Special Circumstances

Asymptomatic Bacteriuria and Urologic Surgery

The incidence of asymptomatic bacteriuria depends largely on the risk factor profile of a given patient (Table 28.18).[97–99] The presence of bacteria in the urinary system increases the risk of infection of bacteria from the urinary tract. Therefore, every attempt should be made to clear the urinary tract of bacteria prior to surgery in the urinary tract or at least have the antimicrobial sensitivities should the patient develop a systemic infection. There have been few studies that have evaluated the specific question of endoscopic intervention in an infected field.

Antibiotic Coverage in Patients with Urinary Diversion

Urinary diversions are an independent risk factor for nephrolithiasis development. The proposed etiologies are stagnant urine and the presence of mucus and urease-splitting bacteria.[100] Furthermore, there are significant metabolic derangements, most notably systemic acidosis, that lead to hypercalciuria in patients with a urinary diversion.[100,101] Turk et al. retrospectively evaluated 94 cystectomy patients with 3 years of followup who either underwent the creation of an ileal conduit (IC) ($n = 54$) or a continent diversion ($n = 40$). Six patients (11%) developed upper urinary tract stones in the IC group compared to two patients (5%) in the continent diversion group.[102] Shimko et al. evaluated 1,057 patients who underwent a cystectomy and IC, 15.5-year median follow-up and noted that 15.3% of their patients developed nephrolithiasis, with the majority (87%) being upper tract calculi. Interestingly, of the patients who developed stones only 19.8% progressed to intervention.[103]

There are multiple types of urinary diversion, and bacteriuria or colonization is very common in all types due to the natural flora of the intestine and skin.[104] In a study prospectively looking at neobladder patients 4 years after their diversion, 50% of patients had a positive urinary culture. The type of bacteria in urinary conduits is largely dependent on the type of intestinal segment utilized. Ileum is the most common type of urinary diversion and 67–73% of the time is colonized with mixed bacterial growth patterns.[105] Typical bacteria seen with ileal diversions include *E. coli (12.5%), Klebsiella pneumoniae (8.9%), Staphylococcus*

Table 28.18: At-risk population and prevalence of asymptomatic bacteriuria.[150–155]

Patient demographic	*Asymptomatic bacteriuria risk (%)*
Adult women	5
Women >65 years	16
Institutionalized women >65 years	50*
Institutionalized men >65 years	30*
Diabetic women	9–27
Patient on self-intermittent catheterization	25–59
Renal transplant patients	51

epidermidis (8.9%), and *Enterococcus faecalis (10.7%).*[106] Very little research has been done on the appropriate preoperative antibiotic in the setting of urinary diversion. However, one would theorize that the antibiotic choice would have to include broad gram-positive and gram-negative coverages (e.g. piperacillin/tazobactam or an aminoglycoside plus metronidazole) to be effective.

Antibiotic Use in Pregnancy

The stone risk in a pregnant patient is similar to that of the general population.[107] Bacteriuria also appears to have the same incidence in this population.[108] The issue in pregnancy is that if bacteriuria is left untreated, some literature suggests at least a 20% rate of pyelonephritis versus 1–2% if treated.[109] Furthermore, certain antibiotics in the pregnant woman can have profound effects on the fetus. Table 28.19 provides a list of antibiotics that are safe to use in pregnancy along with the ones that are contraindicated and their associated birth defects.

Table 28.19: Antimicrobials and pregnancy.[156]

Antibiotic	*Contraindication*
Safe in pregnancy	
Beta lactams	
Macrolides	
Cephalosporins	
Fosfomycin	
Clindamycin	
Contraindication in pregnancy	
Trimethoprim	First trimester: It can cause neural tube defects via inhibition of folate metabolism.
Sulfonamides	Third trimester causes increased unbound bilirubin in the neonate leading to kernicterus.
Nitrofurantoin	Increased odds of cardiac defects
Aminoglycosides	During organogenesis, it can cause fetal ear damage.
Tetracyclines	Deposit in the developing enamel in teeth leading to discoloration. They also have been shown to inhibit bone growth.
Fluoroquinolones	Inhibit cartilage formation

SYMPTOM MANAGEMENT IN THE STONE PATIENT

Pain, nausea, and emesis are typically associated with the presentation of an acute stone event. The management of pain centers on three principles: (1) ureteral dilation, (2) decreasing ureteral inflammation, and (3) minimizing narcotic use. Traditional acute renal colic pain management strategies involve opioids. The problem is that it does nothing to address the cause of the pain, and it creates the potential for dependence, somnolence, and interference with activities of daily living. Other agents that have been utilized include NSAIDs. The proposed mechanism of action in this class of medications is that they lower GFR and subsequently lower the amount of urine production, which thereby lowers the frequency of peristaltic activity and lessens cellular swelling and pain.[110,111]

The common concern of these medications in the setting of an obstructive stone is that they have the potential to further compromise renal function and potentially increase the risk of surgical bleeding.[111] The patients who have been demonstrated to be at risk for acute kidney injury with the use of cyclo-oxygenase-2 inhibition include the following: those with systolic heart failure, patients on ACE inhibitors or loop diuretics, those with hepatic dysfunction or failure, and those with pre-existing renal impairment.[112] Holdgate and Pollock. performed a meta-analysis involving 20 trials and 1,613 patients and found that NSAIDs were more effective at lowering pain scores than opioids and were less likely to need "rescue" analgesia. Furthermore, in the trials looking at emesis there was a threefold increased rate of emesis in those who took opioids.[6] Therefore, NSAIDS have become the first-line therapy when treating a patient with acute renal colic. Table 28.20 provides a list of common NSAIDs and dosing.

Medical expulsive therapy aids in stone passage and lowers the incidence of renal colic. The theory behind the

Table 28.20: Commonly used nonsteroidal anti-inflammatory drugs and associated dosages.[157]

Drug	Dosage
Ketorolac	IV: 15–30 mg IV q 6–8 hours, maximum dose 120 mg per day
Diclofenac	PO: 18–35 mg PO q8 hours
Celecoxib	PO: 400 mg orally once plus one additional 200 mg dose the first day and maintenance 200 mg twice a day thereafter
Ibuprofen	200–400 orally every 4–6 hours, maximum 1,200 mg per day.

(IV: Intravenous; PO: By mouth).

Table 28.21: Commonly used alpha blockers and dosages.[158]

Drug	Mechanism of action	Dosage
Tamsulosin (Flomax)	Alpha-1A selective	0.4 mg PO QSH
Silodsin (Rapaflo)	Alpha-1A selective	8 mg PO qday
Alfuzosin (Uroxatral)	Nonselective	10 mg PO daily
Doxazosin (Cardura)	Nonselective	4 mg PO q am
Terazosin (Hytrin)	Nonselective	1 mg PO QSH titrate up to 10 mg

(PO: By mouth QSH: At bedtime).

efficacy of α blockade in the setting of acute renal colic is that it lowers ureteral peristaltic activity and decreases basal tone of the ureteral smooth muscle while lowering the pressure in the urinary bladder. These factors increase the stone passage rate and potentially lower pain associated with ureteral spasm.[113] In a prospective analysis looking at ureterovesicular nephrolithiasis, Dellabella et al. demonstrated that not only was tamsulosin more effective at achieving stone expulsion but it also lowered diclofenac usage and the need for hospitalization. This was despite the fact that the treatment group had a statistically large stone size.[114] Another study with 3,189 patients compared tamsulosin to nifedipine and found that there was a statistically significant reduction in pain medication use, time to stone passage, rate of stone passage, and side effect incidence in those treated with tamsulosin over nifedipine.[115] These data demonstrate that α-blocking therapy can be very effective in preventing hospitalization and narcotic requirement. Table 28.21 lists the available α antagonists and dosages. The AUA and European Association of Urology, when updating their guidelines regarding the medical management of stone disease, stated that stones of <10 mm in size should be given MET, which includes α-blocking agents.[116]

Another modality to alleviate renal colic, prevent systemic sepsis, and aid in the definitive management of nephrolithiasis involves decompression of the upper urinary tract with either a percutaneous nephrostomy tube or retrograde ureteral stent. The benefits of preoperative stenting include decreasing renal colic by relieving the obstruction, draining an infected field, and facilitating ureteral dilation for subsequent ureteroscopy. Pearle et al. evaluated ureteral stenting versus percutaneous nephrostomy tube placement and found no statistical difference in length of hospital stay or infectious outcomes.[117] Mokhmalji et al. prospectively evaluated 40 patients with obstructive urinary stones randomized to either a nephrostomy tube or a ureteral stent. They noted decreased analgesic use and duration of drainage, and procedural success rates were higher in the percutaneous nephrostomy tube group.[118] Chu et al. retrospectively looked at reoperation rates, stone clearance rates, and operative time with and without placement of a preoperative stent in 104 patients. They concluded that for a stone burden >1.0 cm, stenting decreased reoperation rates and operative time (93.3 vs 123.6 minutes) in the prestented versus nonstented cohorts, respectively.[119] Therefore, the acute management of an obstructed stone in the setting of infection must involve urgent decompression, realizing that the type of drainage may depend on available resources at the time.

In the pregnant population, upper tract decompression may delay definitive management until after delivery so as to not induce premature delivery or expose the fetus to ionizing radiation. Delakas et al. evaluated the safety of ultrasound-guided ureteral stent placement in pregnancy in 21 pregnant women. Overall, all women who were infected clinically improved within 24 hours and there were no major complications or premature deliveries as a result of ureteral stenting with ultrasound.[120] However, the use of ureteral stents in pregnancy is associated with a higher stent exchange rate secondary to hypercalcuria and stent encrustation, and some authors have advocated for primary ureteroscopy in the earlier trimesters to reduce anesthetic risk to the fetus.[121]

CONCLUSION

The goal in the evaluation and initial management of renal colic involves a careful history, medication review,

Flowchart. 28.1: Stepwise algorithm regarding the initial evaluation of a patient with renal colic.

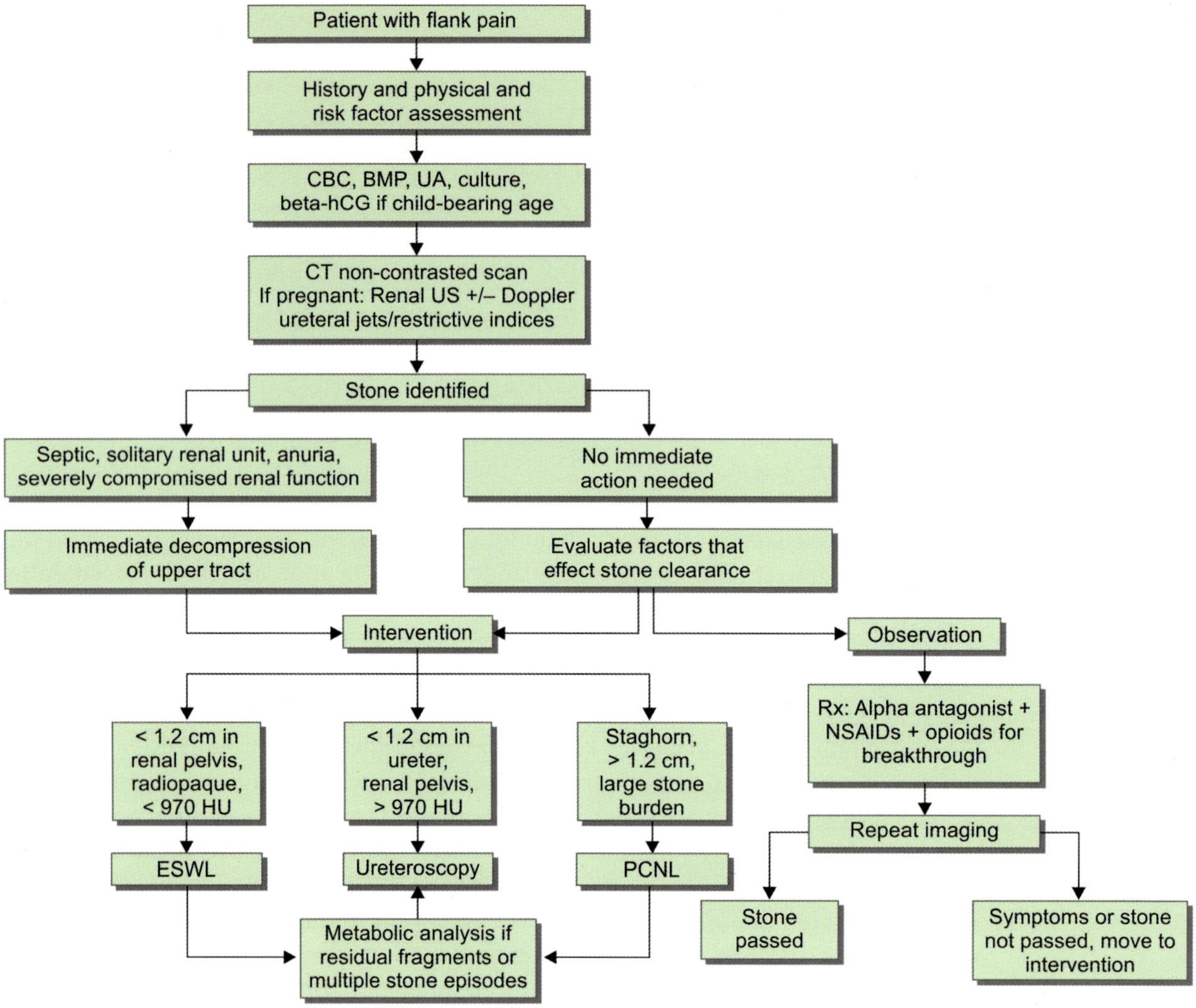

(CBC: Complete blood count; BMP: Basic metabolic panel; UA: Urinalysis CT: Computed tomography; hCG: Human chorionic gonadotropin; US: Ultrasound; HU: Hounsfield unit; NSAID: Nonsteroidal anti-inflammatory drug; ESWL: Extracorporeal shock wave lithotripsy; PCNL: Percutaneous nephrolithotomy).

symptom severity assessment, and judicious use of laboratories and imaging to establish the diagnosis and treatment plan. In the setting of pediatric patients and pregnancy, all efforts should be made to decrease ionizing radiation. Independent of the treatment modality, if bacteriuria is present, every effort should be made to clear the organism prior to therapy. The provider should be well versed in symptom management that reduces the use of opioid medications, which includes α-blocking therapy in conjunction with NSAIDs. Furthermore, the use of ureteral stents or renal drainage prior to definitive therapy may aid in the eventual surgical success rates and may be needed to temporize an infected patient. The management of renal colic in the preoperative setting should involve a stepwise approach that alleviates pain, accurately diagnoses nephrolithiasis, and does not delay either medical or surgical therapy. Flowchart 28.1 presents a general algorithm that may aid in the workup of a patient presenting with renal colic.

REFERENCES

1. Soucie JM, Coates RJ, McClellan W, et al. Relation between geographic variability in kidney stones prevalence and risk factors for stones. Am J Epidemiol. 1996;143(5):487-95.
2. Saigal CS, Joyce G, Timilsina AR. Direct and indirect costs of nephrolithiasis in an employed population: opportunity for disease management? Kidney Int. 2005;68(4):1808-14.
3. Curhan GC. Epidemiology of stone disease. Urol Clin North Am. 2007;34(3):287-93.

4. Schaeffer AJ, Feng Z, Trock BJ, et al. Medical comorbidities associated with pediatric kidney stone disease. Urology. 2011;77(1):195-9.
5. Glowacki LS, Beecroft ML, Cook RJ, et al. The natural history of asymptomatic urolithiasis. J Urol. 1992;147(2):319-21.
6. Holdgate A, Pollock T. Systematic review of the relative effi cacy of non-steroidal anti-inflammatory drugs and opioids in the treatment of acute renal colic. BMJ. 2004;328(7453):1401.
7. Vaughan ED Jr, Gillenwater JY. Recovery following complete chronic unilateral ureteral occlusion: functional, radiographic and pathologic alterations. J Urol. 1971;106(1):27-35.
8. de la Rosette J, Denstedt J, Geavlete P, et al. The Clinical Research Office of the Endourological Society Ureteroscopy Global Study: Indications, Complications, and Outcomes in 11,885 Patients. J Endourol. 2014;28(2):131-9.
9. Daudon M, Jungers P. Drug-induced renal calculi—Epidemiology, prevention and management. Drugs. 2004;64(3): 245-75.
10. Merck Frosst Canada Ltd. Crixivan (indinavir sulphate). Product monograph. Kirkland, QC, Canada: Merck Frost Canada and Co.; 1997.
11. Kuo RL, Moran ME, Kim DH, et al. Topiramate-induced nephrolithiasis. J Endourol. 2002;16(4):229-31.
12. Curhan GC, Willett WC, Rimm EB, et al. Family history and risk of kidney stones. J Am Soc Nephrol. 1997;8(10):1568-73.
13. Muslumanoglu AY, Binbay M, Yuruk E, et al. Updated epidemiologic study of urolithiasis in Turkey. I: Changing characteristics of urolithiasis. Urol Res. 2011;39(4):309-14.
14. Amaral LM, Queiroz DC, Marques TF, et al. Normocalcemic versus hypercalcemic primary hyperparathyroidism: more stone than bone? J Osteoporos. 2012;2012:128352.
15. Rowat A, Smith L, Graham C, et al. A pilot study to assess if urine specific gravity and urine colour charts are useful indicators of dehydration in acute stroke patients. J Adv Nurs. 2011;67(9):1976-83.
16. Grossfeld GD, Wolf JS, Litwan MS, et al. Asymptomatic microscopic hematuria in adults: summary of the AUA best practice policy recommendations. Am Fam Physician. 2001;63(6):1145-54.
17. Sayer J, McCarthy MP, Schmidt JD. Identification and significance of dysmorphic versus isomorphic hematuria. J Urol. 1990;143(3):545-8.
18. Pels RJ, Bor DH, Woolhandler S, et al. Dipstick urinalysis screening of asymptomatic adults for urinary tract disorders. II. Bacteriuria. J AMA. 1989;262(9):1221-4.
19. Vaughan ED, Marion D, Poppas DP, et al. Pathophysiology of unilateral ureteral obstruction: studies from Charlottesville to New York. J Urol. 2004;172(6 Pt 2):2563-9.
20. Dal Canton A, Corradi A, Stanziale R, et al. Glomerular hemodynamics before and after release of 24-hour bilateral ureteral obstruction. Kidney Int. 1980;17(7392422):491-6.
21. Jensen AM, Li C, Praetorius HA, et al. Angiotensin II mediates downregulation of aquaporin water channels and key renal sodium transporters in response to urinary tract obstruction. Am J Physiol Renal Physiol. 2006;291(5):F1021-32.
22. Misseri R, Rink RC, Meldrum DR, et al. Inflammatory mediators and growth factors in obstructive renal injury. J Surg Res. 2004;119(2):149-59.
23. Ishidoya S, Morrissey J, McCracken R, et al. Angiotensin II receptor antagonist ameliorates renal tubulointerstitial fibrosis caused by unilateral ureteral obstruction. Kidney Int. 1995;47(5):1285-94.
24. Lutaif NA, Yu L, Abdulkader RCRM. Factors influencing the non-recovery of renal function after the relief of urinary tract obstruction in women with cancer of cervix. Ren Fail. 2003;25(2):215-25.
25. Smith-Bindman R, Lipson J, Marcus R, et al. Radiation dose associated with common computed tomography examinations and the associated lifetime attributable risk of cancer. Arch Intern Med. 2009;169(22):2078-86.
26. Jespersen SK, Wilhjelm JE, Sillesen H. Multi-angle compound imaging. Ultrason Imaging. 1998;20(2):81-102.
27. Fakoya FA. Integrating ultrasound technology into teaching gross anatomy: point of order! Med Educ Online. 2013; 18:20888.
28. Rahmouni A, Bargoin R, Herment A, et al. Color Doppler twinkling artifact in hyperechoic regions. Radiology. 1996;199(1):269-71.
29. Lee JY, Kim SH, Cho JY, et al. Color and power Doppler twinkling artifacts from urinary stones: clinical observations and phantom studies. AJR Am J Roentgenol. 2001;176(6):1441-5.
30. Sorensen MD, Harper JD, Hsi RS, et al. B-mode ultrasound versus color Doppler twinkling artifact in detecting kidney stones. J Endourol. 2013;27(2):149-53.
31. Ulusan S, Koc Z, Tokmak N. Accuracy of sonography for detecting renal stone: comparison with CT. J Clin Ultrasound. 2007;35(5):256-61.
32. Ray AA, Ghiculete D, Pace KT, et al. Limitations to ultrasound in the detection and measurement of urinary tract calculi. Urology. 2010;76(2):295-300.
33. Palmer JS, Donaher ER, O'Riordan MA, et al. Diagnosis of pediatric urolithiasis: role of ultrasound and computerized tomography. J Urol. 2005;174(4 Pt 1):1413-6.
34. MacNeily AE, Goldenberg SL, Allen GJ, et al. Sonographic visualization of the ureter in pregnancy. J Urol. 1991;146(2): 298-301.
35. Burgess KL, Gettman MT, Rangel LJ, et al. Diagnosis of urolithiasis and rate of spontaneous passage during pregnancy. J Urol. 2011;186(6):2280-4.
36. Shokeir AA, Mahran MR, Abdulmaaboud M. Renal colic in pregnant women: role of renal resistive index. Urology. 2000;55(3):344-7.
37. Baker SM, Middleton WD. Color Doppler sonography of ureteral jets in normal volunteers: importance of the relative specific gravity of urine in the ureter and bladder. AJR Am J Roentgenol. 1992;159(4):773-5.
38. Wachsberg RH. Unilateral absence of ureteral jets in the third trimester of pregnancy: pitfall in color Doppler US diagnosis of urinary obstruction. Radiology. 1998;209(1):279-81.
39. Masselli G, Derme M, Laghi F, et al. Imaging of stone disease in pregnancy. Abdom Imaging. 2013;38(6):1409-14.
40. Bourin M, Jolliet P, Ballereau F. An overview of the clinical pharmacokinetics of X-ray contrast media. Clin Pharmacokinet. 1997;32(3):180-93.

41. Idee JM, Pines E, Prigent P, et al. Allergy-like reactions to iodinated contrast agents. A critical analysis. Fundam Clin Pharmacol. 2005;19(3):263-81.
42. Lasser EC, Berry CC, Mishkin MM, et al. Pretreatment with corticosteroids to prevent adverse reactions to nonionic contrast media. AJR Am J Roentgenol. 1994;162(3):523-6.
43. Morcos SK, Thomsen HS, Webb JA. Prevention of generalized reactions to contrast media: a consensus report and guidelines. Eur Radiol. 2001;11(9):1720-8.
44. Mehran R, Nikolsky E. Contrast-induced nephropathy: definition, epidemiology, and patients at risk. Kidney Int Suppl. 2006;69:S11-5.
45. Kelly AM, Dwamena B, Cronin P, et al. Meta-analysis: effectiveness of drugs for preventing contrast-induced nephropathy. Ann Intern Med. 2008;148(4):284-94.
46. Ptak THRJ, Novelline RA. Experience with a continuous, single-pass whole-body multidetector CT protocol for trauma: the three-minute multiple trauma CT scan. Emergency Radiol. 2001;8(5):250-6.
47. Ha M, MacDonald RD. Impact of CT scan in patients with first episode of suspected nephrolithiasis. J Emerg Med. 2004;27(3):225-31.
48. Cohnen M, Poll LJW, Puettmann C, et al. Effective doses in standard protocols for multi-slice CT scanning. Eur Radiol. 2003;13(5):1148-53.
49. Poletti PA, Platon A, Rutschmann OT, et al. Low-dose versus standard-dose CT protocol in patients with clinically suspected renal colic. AJR Am J Roentgenol. 2007;188(4):927-33.
50. Niemann T, Kollmann T, Bongartz G. Diagnostic performance of low-dose CT for the detection of urolithiasis: a meta-analysis. AJR Am J Roentgenol. 2008;191(2):396-401.
51. Feeman T. The Mathematics of Medical Imaging: A Beginner's Guide. New york: Springer; 2010.
52. Patel SR, Haleblian G, Zabbo A, et al. Hounsfield units on computed tomography predict calcium stone subtype composition. Urol Int. 2009;83(2):175-80.
53. Ito H, Kawahara T, Terao H, et al. Predictive value of attenuation coefficients measured as Hounsfield units on noncontrast computed tomography during flexible ureteroscopy with holmium laser lithotripsy: a single-center experience. J Endourol. 2012;26(9):1125-30.
54. Motley G, Dalrymple N, Keesling C, et al. Hounsfield unit density in the determination of urinary stone composition. Urology. 2001;58(2):170-3.
55. Nakada SY, Hoff DG, Attai S, et al. Determination of stone composition by noncontrast spiral computed tomography in the clinical setting. Urology. 2000;55(6):816-9.
56. Wisenbaugh ES, Paden RG, Silva AC, et al. Dual-energy vs conventional computed tomography in determining stone composition. Urology. 2014;83(6):1243-7.
57. Manglaviti G, Tresoldi S, Guerrer CS, et al. In vivo evaluation of the chemical composition of urinary stones using dual-energy CT. AJR Am J Roentgenol. 2011;197(1):W76-83.
58. Taylor A, Ziffer JA, Eshima D. Comparison of Tc-99m MAG3 and Tc-99m DTPA in renal transplant patients with impaired renal function. Clin Nucl Med. 1990;15(6):371-8.
59. Viprakasit DP, Sawyer MD, Herrell SD, et al. Changing composition of staghorn calculi. J Urol. 2011;186(6):2285-90.
60. Blandy JP, Singh M. The case for a more aggressive approach to staghorn stones. J Urol. 1976;115(5):505-6.
61. Teichman JM, Long RD, Hulbert JC. Long-term renal fate and prognosis after staghorn calculus management. J Urol. 1995;153(5):1403-7.
62. Koga S, Arakaki Y, Matsuoka M, et al. Staghorn calculi—long-term results of management. Br J Urol. 1991;68(2):122-4.
63. Preminger GM, Assimos DG, Lingeman JE, et al. Chapter 1: AUA guideline on management of staghorn calculi: diagnosis and treatment recommendations. J Urol. 2005;173(6):1991-2000.
64. Di Silverio F, Gallucci M, Alpi G. Staghorn calculi of the kidney: classification and therapy. Br J Urol. 1990;65(5):449-52.
65. Grasso M, Conlin M, Bagley D. Retrograde ureteropyeloscopic treatment of 2 cm. or greater upper urinary tract and minor Staghorn calculi. J Urol. 1998;160(2):346-51.
66. Burgher A, Beman M, Holtzman JL, et al. Progression of nephrolithiasis: long-term outcomes with observation of asymptomatic calculi. J Endourol. 2004;18(6):534-9.
67. Koh LT, Ng FC, Ng KK. Outcomes of long-term follow-up of patients with conservative management of asymptomatic renal calculi. BJU Int. 2012;109(4):622-5.
68. Kang HW, Lee SK, Kim WT, et al. Natural history of asymptomatic renal stones and prediction of stone related events. J Urol. 2013;189(5):1740-6.
69. Gross AJ, Herrmann TRW. Management of stones in calyceal diverticulum. Curr Opin Urol. 2007;17(2):136-40.
70. Ellis JH, Patterson SK, Sonda LP, et al. Stones and infection in renal caliceal diverticula: treatment with percutaneous procedures. AJR Am J Roentgenol. 1991;156(5):995-1000.
71. Canales B, Monga M. Surgical management of the calyceal diverticulum. Curr Opin Urol. 2003;13(3):255-60.
72. Semins MJ, Lang E, Matlaga BR. Nephrocalcinosis. J Urol. 2009;182(6):2910-1.
73. Cheidde L, Ajzen SA, Tamer Langen CH, et al. A critical appraisal of the radiological evaluation of nephrocalcinosis. Nephron Clin Pract. 2007;106(3):119-24.
74. Foxman B. Epidemiology of urinary tract infections: incidence, morbidity, and economic costs. Am J Med. 2002; 113(Suppl 1A):13.
75. Ronald AR, Pattullo AL. The natural history of urinary infection in adults. Med Clin North Am. 1991;75(2):299-312.
76. Zorc JJ, Kiddoo DA, Shaw KN. Diagnosis and management of pediatric urinary tract infections. Clin Microbiol Rev. 2005;18(2):417-22.
77. Nicolle LE. Uncomplicated urinary tract infection in adults including uncomplicated pyelonephritis. Urol Clin North Am. 2008;35(1):1-12.
78. Nicolle LE, Bradley S, Colgan R, et al. Infectious Diseases Society of America guidelines for the diagnosis and treatment of asymptomatic bacteriuria in adults. Clin Infect Dis. 2005;40(5):643-54.
79. Chuang CK, Lai MK, Chang PL, et al. Xanthogranulomatous pyelonephritis: experience in 36 cases. J Urol. 1992;147(2):333-6.
80. Ronald A. The etiology of urinary tract infection: traditional and emerging pathogens. Am J Med. 2002;113(Suppl 1A):19.

81. Ksycki MF, Namias N. Nosocomial urinary tract infection. Surg Clin North Am. 2009;89(2):475-81.
82. Edin-Liljegren A, Rodin L, Grenabo L, et al. The importance of glucose for the Escherichia coli mediated citrate depletion in synthetic and human urine. Scand J Urol Nephrol. 2001;35(2):106-11.
83. Siener R, Ebert D, Hesse A. Urinary oxalate excretion in female calcium oxalate stone formers with and without a history of recurrent urinary tract infections. Urol Res. 2001;29(4):245-8.
84. Troxel SA, Sidhu H, Kaul P, et al. Intestinal Oxalobacter formigenes colonization in calcium oxalate stone formers and its relation to urinary oxalate. J Endourol. 2003;17(3):173-6.
85. Brown PD. Management of urinary tract infections associated with nephrolithiasis. Curr Infect Dis Rep. 2010;12(6):450-4.
86. Watson RA, Esposito M, Richter F, et al. Percutaneous nephrostomy as adjunct management in advanced upper urinary tract infection. Urology. 1999;54(2):234-9.
87. Berger I, Wildhofen S, Lee A, et al. Emergency nephrectomy due to severe urosepsis: a retrospective, multicentre analysis of 65 cases. BJU Int. 2009;104(3):386-90.
88. Efstathiou SP, Pefanis AV, Tsioulos DI, et al. Acute pyelonephritis in adults: prediction of mortality and failure of treatment. Arch Intern Med. 2003;163(10):1206-12.
89. Rubin RH, Shapiro ED, Andriole VT, et al. Evaluation of new anti-infective drugs for the treatment of urinary tract infection. Infectious Diseases Society of America and the Food and Drug Administration. Clin Infect Dis. 1992;15 (Suppl 1): 216-27.
90. Pearle MS, Roehrborn CG. Antimicrobial prophylaxis prior to shock wave lithotripsy in patients with sterile urine before treatment: a meta-analysis and cost-effectiveness analysis. Urology. 1997;49(5):679-86.
91. Ilker Y, Turkeri LN, Korten V, et al. Antimicrobial prophylaxis in management of urinary tract stones by extracorporeal shock-wave lithotripsy: is it necessary? Urology. 1995;46(2):165-7.
92. Auge BK, Pietrow PK, Lallas CD, et al. Ureteral access sheath provides protection against elevated renal pressures during routine flexible ureteroscopic stone manipulation. J Endourol. 2004;18(1):33-6.
93. Knopf HJ, Graff HJ, Schulze H. Perioperative antibiotic prophylaxis in ureteroscopic stone removal. Eur Urol. 2003;44(1):115-8.
94. Fourcade RO. Antibiotic prophylaxis with cefotaxime in endoscopic extraction of upper urinary tract stones: a randomized study. The Cefotaxime Cooperative Group. J Antimicrob Chemother. 1990;26:77-83.
95. Charton M, Vallancien G, Veillon B, et al. Urinary tract infection in percutaneous surgery for renal calculi. J Urol. 1986;135(1):15-7.
96. Mariappan P, Smith G, Bariol SV, et al. Stone and pelvic urine culture and sensitivity are better than bladder urine as predictors of urosepsis following percutaneous nephrolithotomy: a prospective clinical study. J Urol. 2005;173(5):1610-4.
97. Raz R. Asymptomatic bacteriuria. Clinical significance and management. Int J Antimicrob Agents. 2003;22(Suppl 2):45-7.
98. Kasviki-Charvati P, Drolette-Kefakis B, Papanayiotou PC, et al. Turnover of bacteriuria in old age. Age Ageing. 1982;11(3):169-74.
99. Goya N, Tanabe K, Iguchi Y, et al. Prevalence of urinary tract infection during outpatient follow-up after renal transplantation. Infection. 1997;25(2):101-5.
100. Terai A, Arai Y, Kawakita M, et al. Effect of urinary intestinal diversion on urinary risk factors for urolithiasis. J Urol. 1995;153(1):37-41.
101. Beiko DT, Razvi H. Stones in urinary diversions: update on medical and surgical issues. Curr Opin Urol. 2002;12(4): 297-303.
102. Turk TMT, Koleski FC, Albala DM. Incidence of urolithiasis in cystectomy patients after intestinal conduit or continent urinary diversion. World J Urol. 1999;17(5):305-7.
103. Shimko MS, Tollefson MK, Umbreit EC, et al. Long-term complications of conduit urinary diversion. J Urol. 2011;185(2):562-7.
104. Wullt B, Agace W, Mansson W. Bladder, bowel and bugs—bacteriuria in patients with intestinal urinary diversion. World J Urol. 2004;22(3):186-95.
105. Hautmann RE, Abol-Enein H, Hafez K, et al. Urinary diversion. Urology. 2007;69(1 Suppl):17-49.
106. Wullt B, Holst E, Steven K, et al. Microbial flora in ileal and colonic neobladders. Eur Urol. 2004;45(2):233-9.
107. Hendricks SK, Ross SO, Krieger JN. An algorithm for diagnosis and therapy of management and complications of urolithiasis during pregnancy. Surg Gynecol Obstet. 1991;172(1): 49-54.
108. Fatima N, Ishrat S. Frequency and risk factors of asymptomatic bacteriuria during pregnancy. J Coll Physicians Surg Pak. 2006;16(4):273-5.
109. Smaill F. Asymptomatic bacteriuria in pregnancy. Best Pract Res Clin Obstet Gynaecol. 2007;21(3):439-50.
110. Teichman JMH. Clinical practice. Acute renal colic from ureteral calculus. N Engl J Med. 2004;350(7):684-93.
111. Brater DC. Effects of nonsteroidal anti-inflammatory drugs on renal function: focus on cyclooxygenase-2-selective inhibition. Am J Med. 1999;107(6A):70-71.
112. Ahmad SR, Kortepeter C, Brinker A, et al. Renal failure associated with the use of celecoxib and rofecoxib. Drug Saf. 2002;25(7):537-44.
113. Richardson CD, Donatucci CF, Page SO, et al. Pharmacology of tamsulosin: saturation-binding isotherms and competition analysis using cloned alpha 1-adrenergic receptor subtypes. Prostate. 1997;33(1):55-9.
114. Dellabella M, Milanese G, Muzzonigro G. Efficacy of tamsulosin in the medical management of juxtavesical ureteral stones. J Urol. 2003;170(6):2202-5.
115. Ye Z, Yang H, Li H, et al. A multicentre, prospective, randomized trial: comparative efficacy of tamsulosin and nifedipine in medical expulsive therapy for distal ureteric stones with renal colic. BJU Int. 2011;108(2):276-9.
116. Preminger GM, Tiselius H-G, Assimos DG, et al. 2007 Guideline for the management of ureteral calculi. Eur Urol. 2007;52(6):1610-31.
117. Pearle MS, Pierce HL, Miller GL, et al. Optimal method of urgent decompression of the collecting system for

obstruction and infection due to ureteral calculi. J Urol. 1998;160(4):1260-4.
118. Mokhmalji H, Braun PM, Martinez Portillo FJ, et al. Percutaneous nephrostomy versus ureteral stents for diversion of hydronephrosis caused by stones: a prospective, randomized clinical trial. J Urol. 2001;165(4):1088-92.
119. Chu L, Sternberg KM, Averch TD. Preoperative stenting decreases operative time and reoperative rates of ureteroscopy. J Endourol. 2011;25(5):751-4.
120. Delakas D, Karyotis I, Loumbakis P, et al. Ureteral drainage by double-J-catheters during pregnancy. Clin Exp Obstet Gynecol. 2000;27(3-4):200-2.
121. Semins MJ, Matlaga BR. Management of stone disease in pregnancy. Curr Opin Urol. 2010;20(2):174-7.
122. Domingos F, Serra A. Nephrolithiasis is associated with an increased prevalence of cardiovascular disease. Nephrol Dial Transplant. 2011;26(3):864-8.
123. Gillen DL, Coe FL, Worcester EM. Nephrolithiasis and increased blood pressure among females with high body mass index. Am J Kidney Dis. 2005;46(2):263-9.
124. Shekarriz B, Stoller ML. Uric acid nephrolithiasis: current concepts and controversies. J Urol. 2002;168(4 Pt 1):1307-14.
125. Nelson WK, Houghton SG, Milliner DS, et al. Enteric hyperoxaluria, nephrolithiasis, and oxalate nephropathy: potentially serious and unappreciated complications of Roux-en-Y gastric bypass. Surg Obes Relat Dis. 2005;1(5):481-5.
126. Ngo TC, Assimos DG. Uric acid nephrolithiasis: recent progress and future directions. Rev Urol. 2007;9(1):17-27.
127. Muther RS, McCarron DA, Bennett WM. Renal manifestations of sarcoidosis. Arch Intern Med. 1981;141(5):643-5.
128. Gelzayd EA, Breuer RI, Kirsner JB. Nephrolithiasis in inflammatory bowel disease. Am J Dig Dis. 1968;13(12):1027-34.
129. Romero V, Akpinar H, Assimos DG. Kidney stones: a global picture of prevalence, incidence, and associated risk factors. Rev Urol. 2010;12(2-3):86-96.
130. Portis AJ, Sundaram CP. Diagnosis and initial management of kidney stones. Am Fam Physician. 2001;63(7):1329-38.
131. Katz DS, Scheer M, Lumerman JH, et al. Alternative or additional diagnoses on unenhanced helical computed tomography for suspected renal colic: experience with 1000 consecutive examinations. Urology. 2000;56(1):53-7.
132. Seller R. Differential Diagnosis of Common Complaints. Philadelphia, PA: Elsevier; 2012.
133. Kuo RL, Moran ME, Kim DH, et al. Topiramate-induced nephrolithiasis. J Endourol. 2002;16(4):229-31.
134. Daudon M, Jungers P. Drug-induced renal calculi—Epidemiology, prevention and management. Drugs. 2004;64(3): 245-75.
135. Pittet D, Rangel-Frausto S, Li N, et al. Systemic inflammatory response syndrome, sepsis, severe sepsis and septic shock: incidence, morbidities and outcomes in surgical ICU patients. Intensive Care Med. 1995;21(4):302-9.
136. Vaughan ED, Marion D, Poppas DP, et al. Pathophysiology of unilateral ureteral obstruction: studies from Charlottesville to New York. J Urol. 2004;172(6 Pt 2):2563-9.
137. Dal Canton A, Corradi A, Stanziale R, et al. Glomerular hemodynamics before and after release of 24-hour bilateral ureteral obstruction. Kidney Int. 1980;17(4):491-6.
138. Lin EC. Radiation risk from medical imaging. Mayo Clin Proc. 2010;85(12):1142-6.
139. Chan V, Perlas A. Basics of ultrasound imaging. In: Narouze SN (Ed). Atlas of Ultrasound-Guided Procedures in Interventional Pain Management New York: Springer; 2011.
140. Chertin B, Fridmans A, Knizhnik M, et al. Does early detection of ureteropelvic junction obstruction improve surgical outcome in terms of renal function? J Urol. 1999;162(3 Pt 2):1037-40.
141. Dwivedi US, Goyal NK, Saxena V, et al. Xanthogranulomatous pyelonephritis: our experience with review of published reports. ANZ J Surg. 2006;76(11):1007-9.
142. LeRoy AJ. Diagnosis and treatment of nephrolithiasis: current perspectives. AJR Am J Roentgenol. 1994;163(6):1309-13.
143. Teichman JM, Long RD, Hulbert JC. Long-term renal fate and prognosis after staghorn calculus management. J Urol. 1995;153(5):1403-7.
144. Di Silverio F, Gallucci M, Alpi G. Staghorn calculi of the kidney: classification and therapy. Br J Urol. 1990;65(5):449-52.
145. Nicolle LE, AMMI Canada Guidelines Committee. Complicated urinary tract infection in adults. Can J Infect Dis Med Microbiol. 2005;16(6):349-60.
146. McLean RJ, Nickel JC, Cheng KJ, et al. The ecology and pathogenicity of urease-producing bacteria in the urinary tract. Crit Rev Microbiol. 1988;16(1):37-69.
147. Wein AJ, Kavoussi LR, Novick AC, et al. (Eds). Campell-Walsh Urology, 10th edition. Philadelphia, PA: Elsevier Sounders; 2012. pp. 257-326.
148. 13. Mandell, Douglas, and Bennett's Principles and Practice of Infectious Diseases, 7th Edition Edited by Gerald L. Mandell, John E. Bennett, and Raphael Dolin Philadelphia, PA: Churchill Livingstone Elsevier, 2009, Chapter 69; 2010. pp. 957-85.
149. Wolf JS, Bennett CJ, Dmochowski RR, et al. Best practice policy statement on urologic surgery antimicrobial prophylaxis. J Urol. 2008;179(4):1379-90.
150. Raz R. Asymptomatic bacteriuria. Clinical significance and management. Int J Antimicrob Agents. 2003;22(Suppl 2):45-7.
151. Kasviki-Charvati P, Drolette-Kefakis B, Papanayiotou PC, et al. Turnover of bacteriuria in old age. Age Ageing. 1982;11(3):169-74.
152. Goya N, Tanabe K, Iguchi Y, et al. Prevalence of urinary tract infection during outpatient follow-up after renal transplantation. Infection. 1997;25(2):101-5.
153. Fiorante S, Lopez-Medrano F, Lizasoain M, et al. Systematic screening and treatment of asymptomatic bacteriuria in renal transplant recipients. Kidney Int. 2010;78(8):774-81.
154. Wyndaele JJ. Complications of intermittent catheterization: their prevention and treatment. Spinal Cord. 2002;40(10): 536-41.
155. Nicolle LE, Bradley S, Colgan R, et al. Infectious Diseases Society of America guidelines for the diagnosis and

treatment of asymptomatic bacteriuria in adults. Clin Infect Dis. 2005;40(5):643-54.
156. Korzeniowski OM. Antibacterial agents in pregnancy. Infect Dis Clin North Am. 1995;9(3):639-51.
157. McCaffery M, Pasero C. Pain: Clinical Manual. St Louis, MO: Mosby; 1999.
158. Eri LM, Tveter KJ. Alpha-blockade in the treatment of symptomatic benign prostatic hyperplasia. J Urol. 1995;154(3):923-34.
159. Simerville JA, Maxted WC, Pahira JJ. Urinalysis: a comprehensive review. Am Fam Physician. 2005;71(6):1153-62.
160. Merritt CB. Physics of Ultrasound: Diagnostic Ultrasound,3rd edition. St Louis, MO: Elsevier; 2005. p. 4.
161. Kremkau FW, Taylor KJ. Artifacts in ultrasound imaging. J Ultrasound Med. 1986;5(4):227-37.
162. Brenner BM, Chertow GM, Marsden PA, et al. Brenners and Rector's the Kidney, 9th edition, Chapter 27. Philadelphia, PA: Elsevier Saunders; 2012. pp. 930-1005.

CHAPTER 29

Radiological Imaging of Nephrolithiasis: Emerging Technologies and Radiation Safety

Cynthia H McCollough, Joshua H Grimes

INTRODUCTION

Medical imaging plays an important role in the diagnosis and management of patients with nephrolithiasis. Stones as small as 1–2 mm can be detected and their position in the excretory system determined. Signs secondary to obstruction can also be visualized. Imaging of patients with suspected urinary stone disease has traditionally been performed with radiography of the kidney, ureter, and bladder, a procedure commonly referred to as a kidney, ureter and bladder (KUB) exam. Additionally, excretory urography, often referred to as intravenous urography (IVU), is a common radiographic examination. Both these exams are performed using traditional radiographic equipment. X-ray computed tomography (CT), performed without use of iodinated contrast media, has also been shown to be a sensitive and specific test for urinary stones and is considered the reference standard examination for the detection of urinary stones.[1-9] Ultrasonography (US) and magnetic resonance imaging (MRI), neither of which utilizes ionizing radiation, have varying degrees of utility in the imaging of patients with stone disease. Although they may be well suited for assessing secondary signs of nephrolithiasis, their ability to directly image the stone itself and give precise measurements of stone dimension is limited.

IMAGING MODALITIES USED IN NEPHROLITHIASIS

Radiographic Imaging

Radiography is the creation of a two-dimensional image from a three-dimensional object (namely, the patient). The procedure involves a source of radiation, the X-ray tube, and a radiation detector, which is either an X-ray sensitive film-screen combination, an X-ray sensitive phosphor plate, or another type of digital X-ray detector. The X-rays pass through the patient and are absorbed by different tissues within the patient, creating a shadow of the patient's anatomy on the detector. Only a small portion of the X-ray beam passes all the way through the patient without being absorbed, and these are the X-rays that are captured on the radiographic detector to form the radiographic image. Those X-rays that are absorbed within the patient contribute to the patient's radiation dose.

The most relevant radiographic examinations for suspected or known nephrolithiasis are the KUB and IVU. In an IVU exam, several KUB images are acquired in a time sequence, pre- and postadministration of iodinated contrast material, to follow the flow of contrast-enhanced urine through the excretory system. The acquired radiographic images, however, suffer from the superimposition of three-dimensional anatomy onto a two-dimensional image. This can obscure some stones, particularly small stones and/or uric acid (UA) stones. A technique used to mitigate this anatomical interference is linear or complex motion tomography, although this has largely been replaced by CT.

Computed Tomography

In 1975 American Alan Cormack and Briton Godfrey Hounsfield shared the Nobel Prize for the invention of X-ray CT. Computed tomography increased the sensitivity of X-ray imaging, particularly of small objects and objects having small differences in X-ray attenuation properties, by removing the superimposition of three-dimensional information. Linear or complex motion tomography, which partially mitigates this factor, is still limited to visualization of high-contrast structures such as bones, airways, and iodinated vessels, because the large area detectors used in radiography record a large percentage of scattered radiation, which decreases image contrast.

In the decades since the introduction of CT, the technology has advanced dramatically, such that *submillimeter* sections of anatomy can be imaged throughout an entire abdomen and pelvis within a matter of seconds. Computed tomography has been shown to be extremely sensitive and specific for the diagnosis of urinary stones,[1-9] and, when the cause of the patient's symptoms is not stones, studies have found CT can find the alternative diagnosis in 9–29% of cases.[3,4,10-14] Further, CT provides an accurate three-dimensional depiction of stones, allowing quantitative assessment of stone size and volume.[15]

Ultrasound

Ultrasound is considered particularly useful in the imaging of stone disease in children and pregnant women due to the desire to minimize exposure to ionizing radiation in these patient populations. There are limitations to ultrasound, however. Obese patients and those with large amounts of intra-abdominal air may be difficult to examine, and the quality of the examination varies tremendously with the experience of the sonographer. Recent studies of the sensitivity and specificity of ultrasound for stone diagnosis show improvement in clinical results, approaching that of CT.[16]

Magnetic Resonance Imaging

Magnetic resonance imaging studies are primarily used for imaging of hydrogen nuclei (protons). The lack of mobile hydrogen nuclei in urinary stones means that no signal can be generated from the stone itself. Thus, MRI detection of urinary stones is based on a signal void rather than signal from the stones themselves. These signal voids are most readily detected using a T2-weighted sequence, which result in a low signal from the stone and a high signal from the surrounding urine. Magnetic resonance imaging can be used to detect the secondary signs of obstruction and has been shown to be close in accuracy to CT for detecting the presence of ureteric obstruction.[17] Like ultrasound, MRI does not use ionizing radiation.

APPROPRIATENESS OF EACH IMAGING MODALITY

There are several considerations to take into account when choosing the most appropriate imaging study for the detection of urinary stones. These factors include whether the study is being performed for investigation of suspected nephrolithiasis or for follow-up evaluation after stone treatment. Furthermore, a patient's age and pregnancy status can factor into the decision. Computed tomography remains the most accurate method for detecting urinary stones, and in most patients it is the most appropriate radiological study to perform due to its ability to detect all stone types, accurately delineate stone size and location, identify the presence and degree of obstruction, and make alternative diagnoses in conditions that mimic renal colic.

According to the American College of Radiology Appropriateness Criteria for Acute Onset Flank Pain—Suspicion of Stone Disease,[18] a CT abdomen and pelvis exam without contrast is usually the most appropriate study. Ultrasound of the kidneys and bladder with Doppler and KUB, and MRI of the abdomen and pelvis with and without contrast, may also be appropriate. For patients with recurrent symptoms of stone disease, CT studies of the abdomen and pelvis without contrast are still appropriate. For this subset of patients, ultrasound of the kidneys and bladder with Doppler and a KUB is also an appropriate radiologic approach. A KUB, which is not usually appropriate for patients with suspected stone disease, may be appropriate for patients with recurrent symptoms of stone disease.

Despite its somewhat lower sensitivity, ultrasound is frequently the first-line study for detecting stones in children and pregnant patients with abdominal pain or colic. It has been suggested that MRI should be considered as a second-line test in pregnant patients if the ultrasound is nondiagnostic.[19] However, the risk to a fetus from a CT of the abdomen and pelvis is negligible, making it difficult to justify a more expensive and less sensitive imaging test of MRI over CT. If the results of an ultrasound (or MRI) are nondiagnostic in a child or pregnant patient with symptoms of urolithiasis, then CT should be performed for further evaluation, without concern about the negligible risk of the ionizing radiation, as will be discussed in the following section.

CONTROVERSIES REGARDING RADIATION SAFETY

Although CT has the highest sensitivity (95–96%) and specificity (98%) for stone detection of any imaging technique,[1-5] there remains concern regarding the use of CT in the diagnosis of stone disease, particularly in patients who are frequent stone formers. This is because there is a perception among some physicians and patients that the low doses of ionizing radiation associated with CT are dangerous. Based on this premise, a recent article in the *New England Journal of Medicine* suggests that the first-line imaging for suspected urinary stones should be ultrasound.[20] However, this perception is not consistent with data from numerous studies or with current consensus opinions from radiation protection organizations.

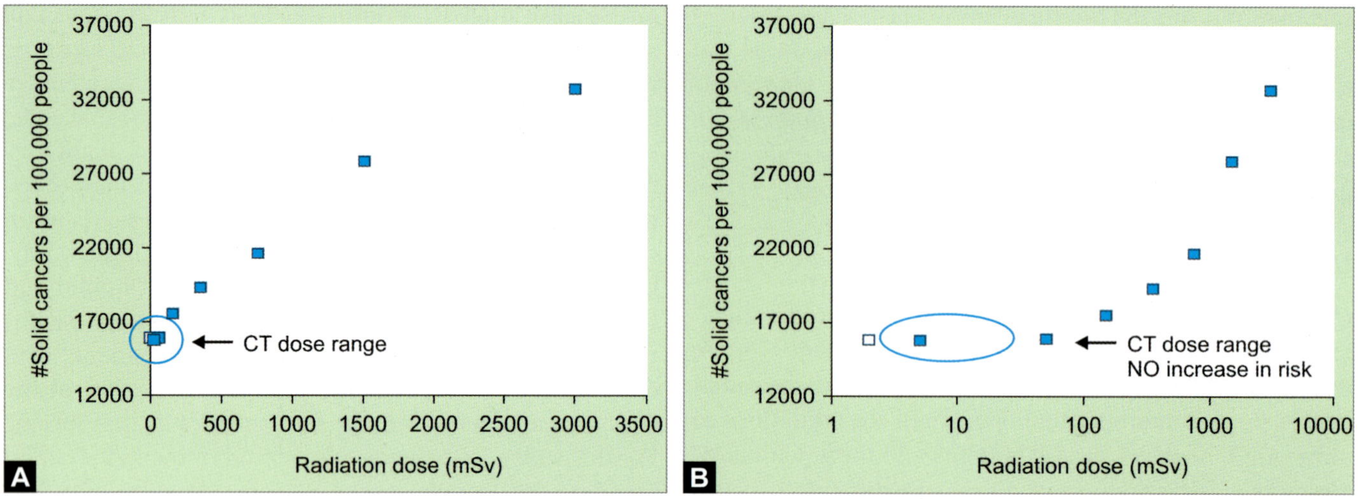

Figs. 29.1A and B: Dose–response curves from the atomic bombing survivors. Viewing both (A) linear and (B) logarithmic x-axis scales assists in visualizing that the cancer risk at low doses (i.e. <100 mSv) is not elevated, as it is above approximately 200 mSv. The white open square data point is the background cancer rate. The best model of the data estimates a threshold dose between 40 and 85 mSv.[23] (CT: Computed tomography).

Studies of medically exposed individuals and atomic bomb survivors have demonstrated an increased risk of cancer only for effective doses that exceed 100 mSv. This value is far greater than the dose levels used in CT imaging of the abdomen and pelvis, which is on the order of 5–10 mSv. The radiation dose from naturally occurring sources of radiation in our environment, such as cosmic rays and radon gas, ranges from 1 to 10 mSv in the United States, with an average of approximately 3 mSv per year. Thus, a CT examination of the abdomen and pelvis delivers a dose similar to background levels—levels at which there is no evidence of harm. In fact, states having the highest levels of radiation have the lowest cancer rates, and residents of regions with exceptionally high background radiation levels (100–260 mSv per year) have shown no increase in cancer risk relative to people living in areas with lower background dose levels.

Furthermore, individuals who were exposed to radiation as part of their occupation have been extensively studied in order to estimate the effects of low doses of radiation. The largest study of occupationally exposed individuals evaluated a cohort of approximately 500,000 individuals located in 15 countries.[21,22] These individuals received cumulative dose levels in the range of 30–60 mSv. No evidence of increased cancer risk has been found in these populations.

Analyses of cancer incidence and mortality in the atomic bomb survivors have not demonstrated any increased cancer risk from acute radiation exposures to doses below 100 mSv (Figs. 29.1A and B).[23] Because of the lack of evidence of long-term health effects from low doses of radiation, which are defined as doses below 100 mSv, radiation protection organizations have cautioned against ascribing risk to low-dose exposures. Indeed, any estimates of risk below 100 mSv are meaningless; the long-term effects are either too small to be observed or are nonexistent.[24] In their 2000 report to the United Nations General Assembly, the United Nations Scientific Committee on the Effects of Atomic Radiation noted that an increase in the incidence of health effects in populations cannot be attributed to exposure to radiation doses that are similar to background levels—that is, doses in the range of 1–10 mSv.[25] Thus, the premise on which the *New England Journal of Medicine* article advocates for use of ultrasound as a first-line imaging technique is questionable.[20]

In 2012 and 2013, respectively, publications from the United Kingdom and Australia suggested that children who received CT scans were at a higher risk for subsequent cancer.[26,27] Both of these studies, however, contained serious methodological flaws, the most egregious being the failure to take into account the clinical symptoms, signs, and comorbidities of the patients in the study. That is, the patient's underlying condition, rather than the CT scan itself, was not considered as a potential factor in the observed increase in cancers. Additionally, these studies lacked a control cohort, did not determine patient-specific doses, and yielded highly improbable results that were

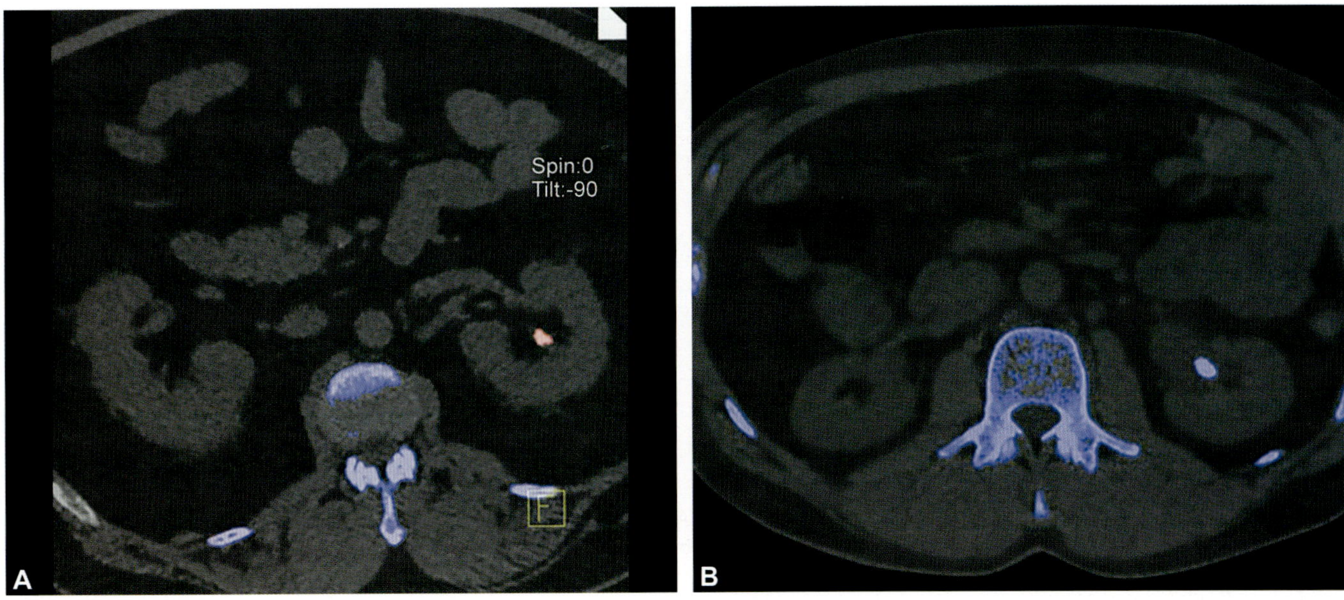

Figs. 29.2A and B: (A) Uric acid stone (colored in red) in a 67-year-old male and (B) nonuric acid stone (colored in blue) in a 45-year-old male. The color coding is automatically applied by the scanner software based on the CT numbers measured in the low- and high-energy images. (CT: Computed tomography).

inconsistent with the large body of literature on the biological effects of radiation in humans. A recent paper noted that when exam indicators were considered, no excess risk from CT was found.[28]

Because nephrolithiasis can be a chronic condition, with patients experiencing recurrent acute events, there is concern that although an individual CT scan may pose negligible risk, multiple CT scans accumulate risk and should be avoided. This belief assumes that the potential mechanism of damage is additive between exposures. In fact, they are completely independent events; the risk from a patient's 10th CT examination is no different than the risk from their first CT examination. The two events are statistically independent. Hence, the decision as to what imaging examination to order should be made based solely on the patient's current condition and symptoms, regardless of past exposure history.

NEW AND EMERGING CLINICAL APPLICATIONS

Dual-Energy CT

Since 2006, methods to determine urinary stone composition using dual-energy CT have been under development.[29-35] Differentiation of UA from other non-UA stones can be accomplished with dual-energy CT with nearly 100% sensitivity and specificity (Figs. 29.2A and B).[29,30,35] Differentiation between non-UA stone types, i.e. cystine, oxalate, or apatite, is difficult but has been demonstrated.[34,36] The differentiating power of dual-energy CT is improved when the X-ray energy spectra used in the dual-energy CT system are better separated.[32,37]

Low-Dose CT

Because of the high inherent contrast between stone material and soft tissue (stones are denser than tissue and calcium-containing stones stop X-rays more effectively than does tissue), the amount of radiation used to image stones need not be as high as that used for routine abdominopelvic CT. This is because the task of detecting the relatively bright stone material in a background of relatively gray soft tissue is easier than most other detection and characterization tasks in the abdomen and pelvis, such as the task of detecting liver metastases or diagnosing appendicitis.

A number of studies have demonstrated that detection sensitivity and specificity are not significantly changed when doses are reduced to approximately half of that used in routine abdominopelvic CT (Figs. 29.3A and B).[38-42] In other work, the ability to perform dual-energy CT at reduced dose levels has been evaluated.[43]

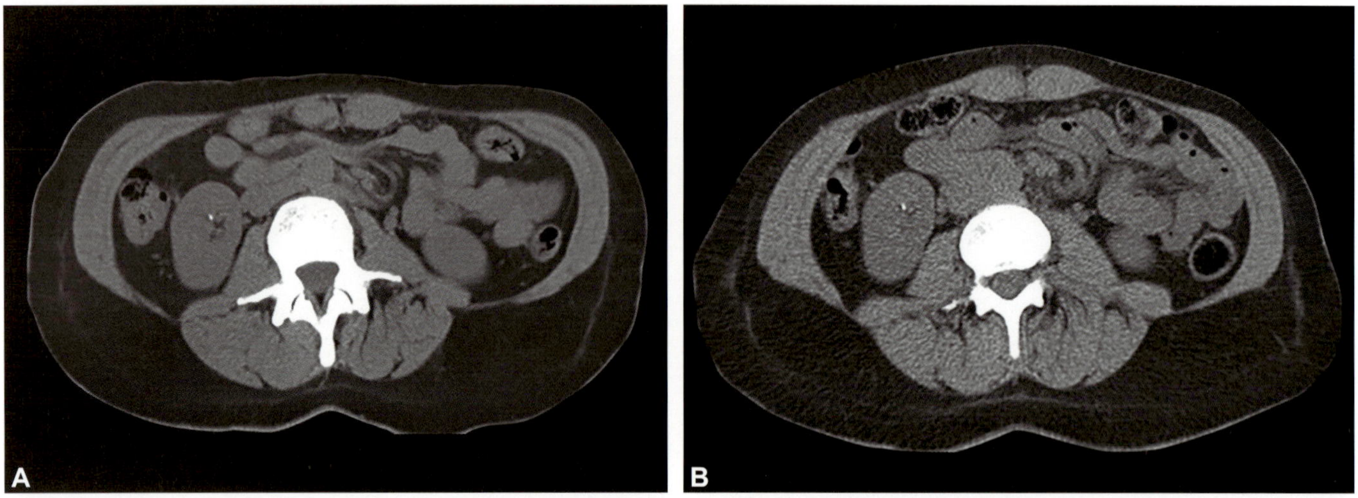

Figs. 29.3A and B: Images obtained in a 34-year-old male using (A) a full-dose routine abdomen scanning protocol and (B) only 42% of the full-dose level demonstrate that even for small stones, the increased noise of the low-dose scan does not interfere with stone visualization.

SUMMARY

Noninvasive detection and characterization of urinary stones plays an important role in the diagnosis and management of stone disease. X-ray CT plays a particularly significant role in this regard. The recent controversy regarding the safety of the radiation associated with CT neglects decades of research in radiation biology and radiation protection that do not support concerns regarding the low doses of ionizing radiation used in CT. Nonetheless, ongoing developments in CT technology continue to bring CT doses down to approximately annual background levels.

REFERENCES

1. Abramson S, Walders N, Applegate KE et al. Impact in the emergency department of unenhanced CT on diagnostic confidence and therapeutic efficacy in patients with suspected renal colic: a prospective survey. 2000 ARRS President's Award. American Roentgen Ray Society. Am J Roentgenol. 2000;175(6):1689-95.
2. Boridy IC, Kawashima A, Goldman SM et al. Acute ureterolithiasis: nonenhanced helical CT findings of perinephric edema for prediction of degree of ureteral obstruction. Radiology. 1999;213(3):663-7.
3. Katz DS, Lane MJ, Sommer FG. Unenhanced helical CT of ureteral stones: incidence of associated urinary tract findings. Am J Roentgenol. 1996;166(6):1319-22.
4. Smith RC, Verga M, McCarthy S et al. Diagnosis of acute flank pain: value of unenhanced helical CT. Am J Roentgenol. 1996;166(1):97-101.
5. Sourtzis S, Thibeau JF, Damry N et al. Radiologic investigation of renal colic: unenhanced helical CT compared with excretory urography. Am J Roentgenol. 1999;172(6):1491-4.
6. Chen MY, Zagoria RJ. Can noncontrast helical computed tomography replace intravenous urography for evaluation of patients with acute urinary tract colic? J Emerg Med. 1999;17(2):299-303.
7. Fielding JR, Steele G, Fox LA et al. Spiral computerized tomography in the evaluation of acute flank pain: a replacement for excretory urography. J Urol. 1997;157(6):2071-3.
8. Niall O, Russell J, MacGregor R et al. A comparison of noncontrast computerized tomography with excretory urography in the assessment of acute flank pain. J Urol. 1999;161(2):534-7.
9. Yilmaz S, Sindel T, Arslan G et al. Renal colic: comparison of spiral CT, US and IVU in the detection of ureteral calculi. Eur Radiol. 1998;8(2):212-7.
10. Eikefjord E, Askildsen JE, Rorvik J. Cost-effectiveness analysis (CEA) of intravenous urography (IVU) and unenhanced multidetector computed tomography (MDCT) for initial investigation of suspected acute ureterolithiasis. Acta Radiol. 2008;49(2):222-9.
11. Hoppe H, Studer R, Kessler TM et al. Alternate or additional findings to stone disease on unenhanced computerized tomography for acute flank pain can impact management. J Urol. 2006;175(5):1725-30.
12. Rucker CM, Menias CO, Bhalla S. Mimics of renal colic: alternative diagnoses at unenhanced helical CT. Radiographics. 2004;24(Suppl 1):S11-28.
13. Smith RC, Verga M, Dalrymple N et al. Acute ureteral obstruction: value of secondary signs of helical unenhanced CT. Am J Roentgenol. 1996;167(5):1109-13.
14. Takahashi N, Kawashima A, Ernst RD et al. Ureterolithiasis: can clinical outcome be predicted with unenhanced helical CT? Radiology. 1998;208(1):97-102.
15. Olcott EW, Sommer FG, Napel S. Accuracy of detection and measurement of renal calculi: in vitro comparison of three-dimensional spiral CT, radiography, and nephrotomography. Radiology. 1997;204(1):19-25.

16. Patlas M, Farkas A, Fisher D et al. Ultrasound vs CT for the detection of ureteric stones in patients with renal colic. Br J Radiol. 2001;74(886):901-4.
17. Regan F, Kuszyk B, Bohlman ME et al. Acute ureteric calculus obstruction: unenhanced spiral CT versus HASTE MR urography and abdominal radiograph. Br J Radiol. 2005;78(930):506-11.
18. American College of Radiology. Acute onset flank pain—suspicion of stone disease. 1995. (Accessed January 25, 2015) Available from https://acsearch.acr.org/docs/69362/Narrative/.
19. Masselli G, Derme M, Laghi F et al. Imaging of stone disease in pregnancy. Abdom Imaging. 2013;38(6):1409-14.
20. Smith-Bindman R, Aubin C, Bailitz J et al. Ultrasonography versus computed tomography for suspected nephrolithiasis. N Engl J Med. 2014;371(12):1100-10.
21. Cardis E, Vrijheid M, Blettner M et al. The 15-Country Collaborative Study of cancer risk among radiation workers in the nuclear industry: estimates of radiation-related cancer risks. Radiat Res. 2007;167(4):396-416.
22. Zablotska LB, Lane RS, Thompson PA. A reanalysis of cancer mortality in Canadian nuclear workers (1956–1994) based on revised exposure and cohort data. Br J Cancer. 2014;110(1):214-23.
23. Preston DL, Ron E, Tokuoka S et al. Solid cancer incidence in atomic bomb survivors: 1958–1998. Radiat Res. 2007;168(1):1-64.
24. Health Physics Society. Radiation risk in perspective: position statement of the Health Physics Society. 2010. (Accessed January 20, 2015) Available from http://hps.org/documents/risk_ps010-2.pdf.
25. United Nations Scientific Committee on the Effects of Atomic Radiation (UNSCEAR). Report of the United Nations Scientific Committee on the effects of atomic radiation. 2012 (Accessed January 21, 2015) [General Assembly Official Records, Sixty-seventh session, Supplement No. 46]. Available from http://daccess-dds-ny.un.org/doc/UNDOC/GEN/V12/553/85/PDF/V1255385.pdf?OpenElement.
26. Mathews JD, Forsythe AV, Brady Z et al. Cancer risk in 680,000 people exposed to computed tomography scans in childhood or adolescence: data linkage study of 11 million Australians. BMJ. 2013;346:f2360.
27. Pearce MS, Salotti JA, Little MP et al. Radiation exposure from CT scans in childhood and subsequent risk of leukaemia and brain tumours: a retrospective cohort study. Lancet. 2012;380(9840):499-505.
28. Journy N, Rehel JL, Ducou Le Pointe H et al. Are the studies on cancer risk from CT scans biased by indication? Elements of answer from a large-scale cohort study in France. Br J Cancer. 2015;112(1):185-93.
29. Graser A, Johnson TR, Bader M et al. Dual energy CT characterization of urinary calculi: initial in vitro and clinical experience. Invest Radiol. 2008;43(2):112-9.
30. Primak AN, Fletcher JG, Vrtiska TJ et al. Noninvasive differentiation of uric acid versus non-uric acid kidney stones using dual-energy CT. Acad Radiol. 2007;14(12):1441-7.
31. Stolzmann P, Kozomara M, Chuck N et al. In vivo identification of uric acid stones with dual-energy CT: diagnostic performance evaluation in patients. Abdom Imaging. 2010;35(5):629-35.
32. Stolzmann P, Leschka S, Scheffel H et al. Characterization of urinary stones with dual-energy CT: improved differentiation using a tin filter. Invest Radiol. 2010;45(1):1-6.
33. Matlaga BR, Kawamoto S, Fishman E. Dual source computed tomography: a novel technique to determine stone composition. Urology. 2008;72(5):1164-8.
34. Boll DT, Patil NA, Paulson EK et al. Renal stone assessment with dual-energy multidetector CT and advanced postprocessing techniques: improved characterization of renal stone composition—pilot study. Radiology. 2009;250(3):813-20.
35. Stolzmann P, Scheffel H, Rentsch K et al. Dual-energy computed tomography for the differentiation of uric acid stones: ex vivo performance evaluation. Urol Res. 2008;36(3-4):133-8.
36. Qu M, Ramirez-Giraldo JC, Leng S et al. Dual-energy dual-source CT with additional spectral filtration can improve the differentiation of non-uric acid renal stones: an ex vivo phantom study. Am J Roentgenol. 2011;196(6):1279-87.
37. Primak AN, Ramirez Giraldo JC, Liu X et al. Improved dual-energy material discrimination for dual-source CT by means of additional spectral filtration. Med Phys. 2009;36(4):1359-69.
38. Liu W, Esler SJ, Kenny BJ et al. Low-dose nonenhanced helical CT of renal colic: assessment of ureteric stone detection and measurement of effective dose equivalent. Radiology. 2000;215(1):51-4.
39. Spielmann AL, Heneghan JP, Lee LJ et al. Decreasing the radiation dose for renal stone CT: a feasibility study of single- and multidetector CT. Am J Roentgenol. 2002;178(5):1058-62.
40. Kulkarni NM, Uppot RN, Eisner BH et al. Radiation dose reduction at multidetector CT with adaptive statistical iterative reconstruction for evaluation of urolithiasis: how low can we go? Radiology. 2012;265(1):158-66.
41. McLaughlin PD, Murphy KP, Hayes SA et al. Non-contrast CT at comparable dose to an abdominal radiograph in patients with acute renal colic; impact of iterative reconstruction on image quality and diagnostic performance. Insights Imaging. 2014;5(2):217-30.
42. Winklehner A, Blume I, Winklhofer S et al. Iterative reconstructions versus filtered back-projection for urinary stone detection in low-dose CT. Acad Radiol. 2013;20(11):1429-35.
43. Thomas C, Patschan O, Ketelsen D et al. Dual-energy CT for the characterization of urinary calculi: in vitro and in vivo evaluation of a low-dose scanning protocol. Eur Radiol.2009;19(6):1553-9.

CHAPTER

30

Contemporary Outcomes for Shock Wave Lithotripsy, Ureteroscopy, and Percutaneous Nephrolithotomy

Yung-Khan Tan, Keng-Siang Png, Yew-Lam Chong, Michael YC Wong

Alice: Would you tell me, please, which way I ought to go from here?
The Cat: That depends a good deal on where you want to get to.
~Lewis Carroll, Alice in Wonderland

INTRODUCTION

The assessment of success after treatment of upper urinary tract stones is key information clinicians need to recommend treatment and counsel patients about expected outcomes. The discussion about success of treatment outcomes is, however, often confused by the lack of agreed-upon common language.

Stone-free rate (SFR) is a term that is easily understood but difficult to compare in the literature, as there is no uniformity in the choice of radiological assessment. With the introduction of shock wave lithotripsy (SWL), many patients could not achieve stone-free status and so the concept of clinically insignificant residual fragments was initially described as nonstruvite stone fragments that were 4 mm or less in size.[1] Hence, the term success rate was developed to include both patient groups with stone-free status and clinically insignificant residual fragments. Many authors also reported on the natural history of the "insignificant residual stone" using different size criteria and in heterogeneous patient groups. Literature on stone treatment outcomes rapidly became awash with different treatment endpoints that were difficult to compare, not only in SWL studies, but in ureteroscopy (URS) and percutaneous nephrolithotomy (PCNL) too. Regardless of SWL, URS, or PCNL, though, authors agreed that residual fragments lead to a 1-in-5 chance of regrowth of stone and a slightly <1-in-2 chance of an eventual need for intervention for a stone episode.[2-4]

Another measure of success relates to efficiency quotient (EQ) for SWL outcomes by Clayman, expressed as a percentage by taking into account the SFR divided by the sum of retreatment rate, auxiliary procedure rate, and one hundred. This proves to be a useful indicator when applied to all forms of endourology procedures as it takes into account the total procedure burden during the course of stone treatment. These methods of comparisons, while limited by the lack of standardization of terms, are still our most widely used measures of outcomes.

MANAGEMENT OF URETERAL STONES

In general, ureteral calculi of any size may result in obstruction and irreversible renal damage. For this reason, in patients with functioning renal units, ureteral calculi are always managed to ensure stone clearance with or without active surgical treatment. In determining whether a ureteral calculus may pass spontaneously, the single most important factor is the stone size. Stones measuring 5 mm or less have a high likelihood of spontaneous passage based on both historical and contemporary measurements.[5,6] Larger stones will require surgical treatment by one or more modalities. Shockwave lithotripsy and ureteroscopic laser lithotripsy are the two most common modalities used to treat ureteral stones. Less commonly, antegrade percutaneous lithotripsy or ureterolithotomy are used in select cases.

In determining the comparative efficacy of each of these modalities, it is best to divide ureteral stones into distal or proximal stones. Within each location, stone size will further determine the efficacy of each modality.

Contemporary Results with Proximal Ureteral Stones Based on Randomized Controlled Trials

Since the introduction of shockwave lithotripters in the 1980s, urologists have been treating proximal ureteral stones with SWL with great success. It was not until the development of narrow-caliber ureteroscopes that urologists had a viable alternative to the treatment of ureteral stones. However, initial ureteroscopes were still too large to reach proximal stones, leaving SWL the only minimally invasive modality for proximal ureteral stones. In the last decade, newer semirigid and flexible ureteroscopes have undergone tremendous technological advances such that stones in any part of the urinary tract can almost always be accessed by narrow-caliber flexible or semirigid ureteroscopes.

The comparative efficacy of URS versus SWL for proximal ureteral stones is still a topic of great debate. Few randomized studies had compared these two modalities of treatment. Salem randomized 200 patients with stones between 5 and 20 mm to be treated by SWL and semirigid URS.[7] Treatment outcomes were presented for stones measuring 10 mm or more and those <10 mm. The EQ was calculated to address the effect of repeat or auxiliary procedures. For stones 10 mm or greater, the initial SFR at 2 weeks was 60% for SWL compared to 88% for URS ($p > 0.05$). The EQ was lower at 0.43 for SWL compared to 0.79 for URS ($p < 0.05$). For stones <10 mm, SFR was 80% for SWL compared to 100% for URS ($p > 0.05$). The EQ was 0.70 and 0.88, respectively, which was not statistically significant.

There were four failures out of 88 patients who underwent URS for stones 10 mm or greater in the study by Salem et al. All four occurred in males, which illustrated the technical challenge in overcoming the psoas hump during semirigid URS in some well-built men. In two of these four cases, failure was due to the stone retropulsing into the kidney. The availability of modern flexible ureteroscopes and the numerous antiretropulsion devices has allowed the endourologist to effectively overcome these two common limitations of semirigid ureteroscope when treating proximal ureteral stones. These technical improvements over semirigid URS have further increased the efficacy of URS over SWL when treating larger proximal ureteral stones.

Contemporary Results with Distal Ureteral Stones Based on Randomized Controlled Trials

Distal ureteral stones have been treated more with URS compared to proximal stones due to easier accessibility with semirigid ureteroscopes. As a result, more randomized trials comparing SWL and URS are available for this group of stones. Three randomized trials were available that studied stones around the size of 5–15 mm (Table 30.1).[8-10] Both SWL and URS were highly effective in terms of SFRs at the end of the study period: 3 months in two of the studies and 43 days in the third study. The difference in efficacy between SWL and URS for distal stones was the shorter time to stone clearance for URS compared to SWL as demonstrated in one of the studies,[8] whereby 100% of stones <5 mm were stone free on the first postoperative day and by the eighth postoperative day for stones >5 mm. Retreatment rates were also higher in two of the studies in patients who underwent SWL. As in the case with contemporary practice, the latest study by Verze et al. left the decision for inserting a ureteric stent after URS

Table 30.1: Randomized trials in the management of distal ureteric stones.

	Stone size (mm)	*n*	*Study period*	*SFR*	*Retreatment*
Peschel et al.	2–16	80	Up to 43 days	<5 mm SWL: 17/20 patients URS: 100% >5 mm SWL: 19/20 patients URS: 100%	<5 mm SWL: 15% URS: 0% >5 mm SWL:5% URS: 0%
Pearle et al.	<15	200	Up to 3 months	SWL: 29/32 URS: 29/32	None in either group
Verze et al.	5–15	273	Up to 3 months	SWL: 92/7% URS: 94.85%	SWL: 44.8% URS: 7.75% *p<0.05

(SFR: Stone-free rate; SWL: Shock wave lithotripsy; URS: Ureteroscopy).

to the discretion of the surgeon, reducing the need for an office cystoscopy to remove the stent.[10]

A Dutch randomized study by Hendrikx et al. from three centers extended the inclusion criteria to extended midureteral and distal ureteral stones, defined as stones from the fifth transverse vertebral process and below.[11] A total of 156 patients underwent initial randomization, but 17 patients from the SWL group were switched to the URS group after initial randomization due to delay in SWL treatment. Overall SFRs after all retreatment and auxiliary procedures at 12 weeks were 51% for SWL (95% Cl 38–63%) and 91% for URS (95% Cl 82–96%). Patients could undergo either SWL or URS as retreatment in either arm. If we look at the success after the index treatment only, 45% of SWL patients required retreatment compared to 9% of URS patients.

Meta-analyses Comparing SWL and URS

Several meta-analyses were performed to create a decision algorithm between SWL and URS for the management of ureteral stones based on location and stone size. The American Urological Association (AUA)/European Association of Urology (EAU) 2007 meta-analysis classified stones according to stone size (more or less than 10 mm) and stone location (proximal, mid, and distal ureteral stones).[12] The most significant finding from this meta-analysis was in subanalysis of the proximal ureteral stone group. For proximal stones <10 mm, SWL was superior to URS (90% vs 80%), whereas for proximal stones >10 mm, the SFR for SWL dropped to 68% while URS was still maintained at 79%. For all other locations, SFR for URS was superior to SWL overall and in both size categories.

Matlaga and colleagues conducted an excellent meta-analysis comparing various modalities at various stone locations.[13] For distal ureteral stones, URS gave a greater SFR than SWL (pooled RR 1.55, 95% Cl 1.13–2.56) and lower retreatment rate (RR 0.14, 95% Cl 0.08–0.23). The study could not make any reasonable conclusion about the management of proximal ureteral stones.

The most recent Cochrane review in 2012 by Aboumarzouk and colleagues looked at radomized controlled trials (RCTs) conducted for ureteral stones comparing URS and SWL.[14] It indicated that SWL gave a lower SFR (RR 0.84, 95% Cl 0.73–0.96) and higher retreatment rates (RR 6.18, 95% Cl 3.68–10.38). The benefits of SWL were 57% less likely to require auxillary treatment (RR 0.43, 95% CI 0.25 to 0.74), fewer complications (RR 0.54, 95% Cl 0.33–0.88) and shorter length of hospital stay (MD –2.55 days, 95% Cl –3.24 to –1.86). The absence of results subcategorized according to stone location limits the application of this review to clinical practice.

These recent meta-analyses agreed on the superiority of URS over SWL in terms of SFR and retreatment rates, more so for distal ureteral stones than proximal stones. In the 2007 AUA/EAU meta-analysis, the superiority of URS was demonstrated in stones >10 mm but not in stones <10 mm.[12] Compared to the AUA 1997 guidelines, which did not favor URS as stones got larger, these contemporary data reflected the technological improvement in ureteroscopic treatment to enable the treatment of larger and more proximally located stones.

Medical Expulsion Therapy after SWL

The use of α-blockers to facilitate spontaneous passage of distal ureteral stones is widely practiced now. This effect has been applied to patients who had undergone SWL to facilitate passage of fragments. Several randomized trials had shown improved stone passage with α-blockers after SWL. A recent meta-analysis identified seven RCTs that studied the effect of medical expulsion therapy.[15] All seven trials used tamsulosin in their studies, which included 240 patients receiving the drug and 244 controls. The absolute risk increase of stone clearance was 16% (95% Cl 5–27%) in the tamsulosin group compared to controls. The rate of side effects experienced was 3% of patients who received tamsulosin.

Effect of Obstructed Stones on Efficacy of SWL

Ureteral obstruction results in changes to its peristaltic function, decreasing peristalsis, and decreased pressure. This may have an effect on stone passage. The effect of obstruction on SWL outcome is unclear. Delakas and colleagues have identified obstruction as a predictor for SWL failure in a regression analysis of 688 patients who underwent SWL.[16] Obstruction was categorized as only present or absent, and not the degree of obstruction. Seitz and colleagues retrospectively compared 130 patients according to four degrees of hydronephrosis caused by an obstructing proximal ureteral.[17] There was no difference among the four groups in time to stone clearance and failure rate. Demirbas et al. compared 165 patients with distal ureteral stones and also found no difference in stone-free status among four groups of patients with various degree of obstruction.[18]

Issue with Large Proximal Ureteral Stones

Large proximal ureteral stones are a controversial group to treat. Poor outcomes were obtained with either SWL or URS. Lee and colleagues randomized 42 patients with stones 15 mm or larger (mean length 17.6 mm vs 18.5 mm) to SWL or semirigid URS (22 vs 20).[19] After SWL monotherapy (mean sessions 1.7, range 1–4) the SFR was 63.6%. Only 31.8% were stone free after a single session of SWL. Eight out of the 22 (36.4%) SWL patients did not have remarkable fragmentation after the first session, of whom five (22.7%) underwent auxiliary procedures, including two URS and three open ureterolithotomy. In the URS arm, SFR after one session of URS was 35%. There were five cases of ureteral perforation, of which one required immediate open ureterolithotomy. The EQ for SWL and URS was 0.61 and 0.62, respectively.

The need for a more efficacious treatment had led to the use of antegrade techniques through a percutaneous approach as an alternative treatment option. Access can be obtained through a small-caliber sheath sufficient to manipulate a 16F flexible renoscope down the proximal ureter. If the stone is close to the ureteropelvic junction (UPJ), even smaller access can be used to allow a semirigid ureteroscope to reach the stone for laser lithotripsy to be carried out. When compared to semirigid URS in a randomized study (stone size 10–22 mm), PCNL using a semirigid ureteroscope through a 16F peel-away sheath had a higher SFR at discharge (95.3% vs 79.5%, p = 0.027) and at 1-month postprocedure (100% vs 86.4%, p = 0.026).[20] There was failure of access in one out of 44 (2.3%) PCNL and three out of 47 (6.8%) URS patients. All failures of access were converted to open ureterolithotomy. Percutaneous nephrolithotomy had a significantly longer time to normal activity (7.8 days vs 2.7 days, p = 0.001).

Laparoscopic ureterolithotomy has been advocated as another option of minimally invasive technique of stone clearance without the morbidity of traditional open ureterolithotomy. Ureterolithotomy gives a greater SFR after a single session compared to URS or SWL. Basiri and colleagues randomized 150 patients with stones >15 mm into semirigid URS, transperitoneal laparoscopic ureterolithotomy, and PCNL.[21] Stone-free rate at discharge for laparoscopic ureterolithotomy (88%) was significantly higher than URS (56%) and PCNL (64%). Urine leakage of >3 days occurred in 16% of patients with laparoscopic ureterolithotomy, but this could be due to the fact that not all the ureterotomies were closed primarily after stenting. Laparoscopic ureterolithotomy also had longer operative time and longer hospital stay compared to the other two modalities. Another smaller randomized study compared laparoscopic ureterolithotomy with SWL and semirigid URS for proximal ureteral stones >10 mm in 48 patients.[22] Laparoscopic ureterolithotomy had significantly higher SFR both at 1 week (93.3% vs 35.7% vs 50.0%) and 4 weeks (93.3% vs 35.7% vs 62.5%) after surgery compared to the other two modalities. Similar to the previous study, laparoscopic ureterolithotomy had longer hospital stay and also greater post-treatment pain requirement. In this study, the laparoscopic ureterolithotomy arm did not have any postoperative complication, including urine leakage.

MANAGEMENT OF RENAL STONES

A number of tools can be used to treat renal calculi. These include flexible ureteroscopes, SWL, and PCNL. Each set of instruments has been the beneficiary of continued technological advances and improved techniques such that outcomes from even 5 years ago may need to be revisited. For example, in the area of flexible ureteroscopes, there have been advances in imaging in the form of digital scopes, improved deflection, and smaller-diameter scopes that improve access to the kidney. The laser fibers used in association with ureteroscopes have also improved such that new fibers with atraumatic tips, like the Boston Scientific Accutrac fiber, can be inserted into fully deflected ureteroscopes with low risk of scope damage, improving options for in situ treatment of lower pole calculi. Newer baskets, like the Cook Medical N-gage basket and Bard Dimension basket, have also improved the surgeon's ability to extract renal calyceal stones. Similarly, there have been advances in SWL technology such that the newer machines have inline targeting and improved power-to-focal-zone ratios that may improve targeting and fragmentation, respectively. On the PCNL front, advances include the use of mini PCNL and now even micro PCNL, which may reduce tissue trauma and bleeding complications.

Just as in the ureter, treatment efficacies of the different modalities can broadly be divided by stone location and further subdivided by stone burden in these locations.

Stones in the Upper Pole, Midpole, and Renal Pelvis

The decision on treatment is often a balance of SFRs against the morbidity of the procedure. Unfortunately,

Table 30.2: Outcomes of SWL according to stone size and location.

	Upper calix	*Middle calix*	*Lower calix*	*Total*
Stone free				
<100 mm^2	19/19 (100)	23/26 (88.5)	10/12 (83.3)	52/57 (91.2)
100–200 mm^2	10/16 (62.5)	13/17 (76.5)	17/28 (60.7)	40/61 (65.5)
Total	29/35 (82.9)	36/43 (83.7)	27/40 (67.5)	92/118 (78)
Failure				
<100 mm^2	0/19	3/26 (11.5)	2/12 (16.7)	5/57 (8.8)
100–200 mm^2	6/16 (37.5)	4/17 (23.5)	11/28 (39.3)	21/61 (34.5)
Total	6/35 (17.1)	7/43 (16.3)	13/40 (32.5)	26/118 (22)

(SWL: Shock wave lithotripsy).
Source: With permission from Turna B, Ekren F, Nazli O, et al. Comparative results of shockwave lithotripsy for renal calculi in upper, middle, and lower calices. J Endourol. 2007;21:951-6.

there is a wide variation in outcomes. This variation may be attributed to different SWL machines with different shockwave characteristics and also the different protocols of shockwave therapy. The choice of imaging also plays a part in determining stone-free status. A computed tomography (CT) scan will obviously reveal more residual fragments as compared with a plain abdominal X-ray. Furthermore, definitions of "stone free" in the literature have ranged from totally stone free to the presence of stones <4 mm in size.

Overall, PCNL continues to achieve SFRs of 71–100%,[23-25] with contemporary studies showing an associated complication rate of up to 20%,[26,27] of which 50% were classified as Clavien 1 complications. Recently, the advent of mini PCNL has had similar SFRs for stones <3 cm in size and a lower complication rate. Pan et al. in their series of mini PCNL had a complication rate of 11.9%.[28]

Shock wave lithotripsy, on the other hand, has had widely varying success rates. Carlsson et al. in a randomized trial found an overall success rate of 77% for SWL versus 94% for PCNL at 1 month for stone size averaging 13 mm in diameter.[25] When analysis was done based on stone size, Obek et al. found a 66% SFR for stones <20 mm and 49% for stones >20 mm.[29] Furthermore, when stratified by location, SFRs at 3 months for SWL were 86–89% for renal pelvis stones, 71–83% for upper calyx, 73–84% for middle calyx, and 37–68% for lower calyx stones (Table 30.2).[29-31] Complication rates for SWL in renal stones range from 3.3% to 12.5%.[32-34]

Pan et al. in a retrospective review compared flexible URS versus mini PCNL for stones between 2 and 3 cm.[28] He found a SFR of 71.4% versus 96.6% favoring mini PCNL. In another reported series, Hussain et al. had a success rate of 58.3% after one treatment for renal stones 2–3 cm in size with flexible URS.[35]

In general, for stones >2 cm in these locations, PCNL continues to be the favored method of stone clearance.

For stones <2 cm in the mid and upper pole, there is continued debate about the best method of stone clearance. Current recommendations from the EAU guidelines on nephrolithiasis state that, in general, SWL would be the better option as flexible URS results are suboptimal when stones exceed 1.5 cm in size.[36] These recommendations are likely to change as results improve with flexible URS.

More recently, a retrospective review by Wiesenthal et al. that compared SWL to retrograde intrarenal surgery (RIRS) to PCNL for stones between 1 and 2 cm found SFRs of 60.4%, 87.8%, and 95.3%, respectively.[37] When SWL was repeated its success rate rose to 79.2% (Fig. 30.1). In this study, the stones in the SWL group were significantly larger than those in the RIRS group. The overall complication rates were 7.5%, 4.9%, and 14%, respectively, with most complications in all groups being Clavien 1 or 2. In a similar retrospective review by Resorlu et al. of 437 patients, success rates were 66.5%, 91.4%, and 87% for SWL, PCNL, and RIRS, respectively.[38] This was with attendant overall complication rates for the extracorporeal shock wave lithotripsy (ESWL), PCNL, and RIRS of 7.6%, 22.1%, and 10.9%, respectively. Hussain et al., in a retrospective review of their cases, found that RIRS treatment for stones <2 cm had a single treatment success rate of 96.5%.[35]

In general, for stones <2 cm both URS and SWL are viable modalities of treatment, with slightly higher complication rates in the URS group. Furthermore, it seems that in centers of excellence, URS achieves better SFRs compared to a single session of SWL.

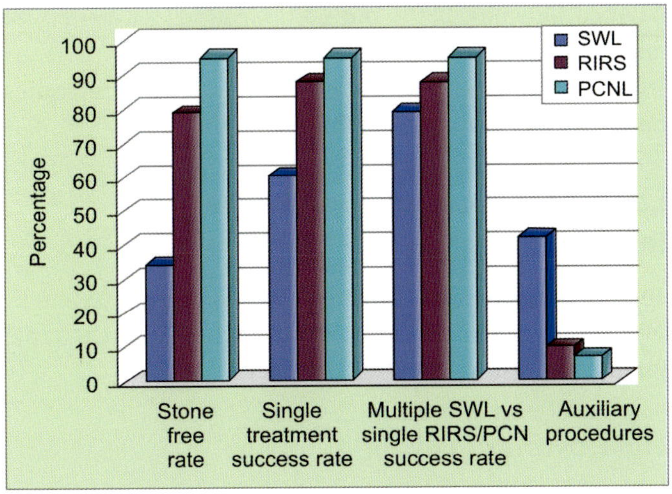

Fig. 30.1: Treatment outcomes across groups for 1–2 cm renal stones. (SWL: Shock wave lithotripsy; RIRS: Retrograde intrarenal surgery; PCNL: Percutaneous nephrolithotomy).
Source: Redrawn with permission from Wiesenthal JD, Ghiculete D, Dah RJ, et al. A comparison of treatment modalities for renal calculi between 100 and 300 mm^2: are shockwave lithotripsy, ureteroscopy, and percutaneous nephrolithotomy equivalent? J Endourol. 2011;25:481-5.

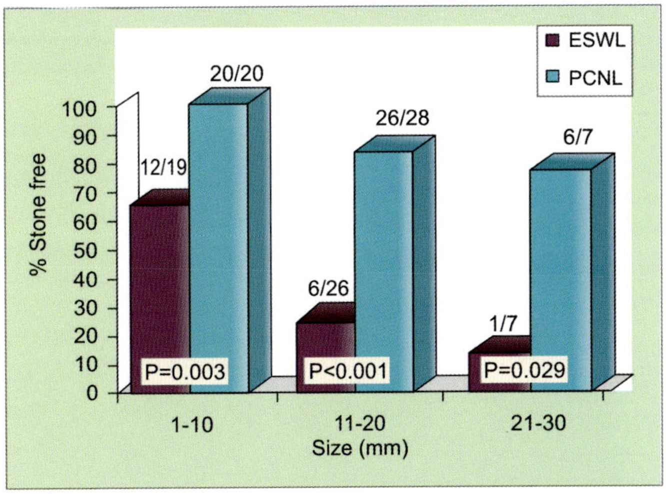

Fig. 30.2: Lower pole stone-free rates between ESWL and PCNL by stone size. (ESWL: Extracorporeal shock wave lithotripsy; PCNL: Percutaneous nephrolithotomy).
Source: Redrawn with permission from Albala DM, Assimos DG, Clayman RV, et al. Lower pole I: a prospective randomized trial of extracorporeal shock wave lithotripsy and percutaneous nephrostolithotomy for lower pole nephrolithiasis-initial results. J Urol. 2001;166:2072-80.

Lower Pole Stones

The lower pole of the renal collecting system presents a unique situation due to anatomical considerations and its dependent location. Two randomized trials from the lower pole study group attempted to address this. The first, by Albala et al., was a prospective randomized trial comparing SWL against PCNL.[30] One hundred and twenty eight patients were recruited with a mean stone size of 14.03 mm. The 3-month postoperative SFR overall was 95% for PCNL and 37% for SWL. In stones >10 mm, SWL achieved stone-free status in only 21% of patients. Furthermore, retreatment was required in 16% of the SWL group compared with 9% in the percutaneous group (Fig. 30.2).

As flexible URS became available, a follow-up randomized trial comparing SWL to flexible URS for stones in the lower pole <1 cm was performed. This randomized trial by Pearle et al. had better stone-clearance rates with flexible URS (50%) compared with SWL (35%), but this did not reach statistical significance.[39] This may have been a result of the small study size of 67 patients. Shock wave lithotripsy patients in this study also had better tolerance compared with patients from the flexible URS group.

In a Cochrane review, Srisubat et al. found that PCNL had the best SFRs for lower pole stones but also the highest morbidity compared with SWL.[40]

A retrospective review by Ozturk et al. for stones 10–20 mm in the lower pole found success rates of 94%, 76%, and 73% for PCNL, SWL, and flexible URS, respectively.[41] In another contemporary series of lower pole stones from 1 to 2 cm, the SFRs were 86.5% versus 67.7% for flexible URS and ESWL, respectively (Table 30.3).[34] There was no significant difference in terms of complications, comparisons between flexible URS and PCNL for lower pole stones by Bozkurt et al. found success rates of 92.8% for PCNL versus 89.2% for flexible URS in stones of 15–20 mm in size.[42] As expected, the PCNL group had a shorter operative time but longer hospital stay and was more likely to require transfusions. Unfortunately, due to the small study population none of the results reached significance.

In a series comparing flexible URS to mini PCNL for lower pole stones <15 mm, similar outcomes of around 88% were achieved with both groups not having any major complications, although the flexible URS group had shorter hospital stays while the miniPCNL group had shorter operating times.[43] What must be recognized is that most of the studies listed above are by tertiary institutions with excellent endourologists and the success and complication rates of PCNL and flexible URS may not be reflective of community practice.

A number of factors may make SWL less effective, including factors related to lower pelvicalyceal anatomy:

Table 30.3: Treatment and post-treatment data for patients who underwent treatment for single lower pole stone 10–20 mm.

Variable	F-URS 37 patients	ESWL 62 patients	P
Retreatment rate, *N* (%)	3 (8)	37 (59.7)	<0.001*
Complications, *N* (%)	5 (13.5)	3 (4.8)	0.146*
• Modified Clavien classification	4 (10.8)	2 (3.2)	
• Grade II	1 (2.7)	1 (1.6)	
• Grade IIIa	32 (86.5)	42 (67.7)	0.038†
SFR at 3 months, *N* (%)	4 (10.8)	10 (16)	0.595*
Secondary procedures, *N* (%)	3 (8)	0	
• ESWL	0	5 (8)	
• F-URS	1 (2.7)	5 (8)	
• PNL			0.018‡
Operative time (min)	73 (29)	92 (41)	
• Mean (SD)	40-190	40–135	
• Range			<0.001‡
Procedures per patient	1.1 (0.34)	2.2 (1.19)	
• Mean (SD)	1–2	1–5	
• Range			

*Fisher's exact text. †Chi-squared test. ‡test.
(F-URS: Flexible ureterorenoscopy; ESWL: Extracorporeal shock wave lithotripsy; SFR: Stone-free rate; PNL: Percutaneous nephrolithotomy; N: Number of patients).
Source: With permission from Ozturk U, Sener NC, Goktug HN, et al. Comparison of percutaneous nephrolithotomy, shock wave lithotripsy, and retrograde intrarenal surgery for lower pole renal calculi 10–20 mm. Urol Int. 2013;91(3):345-9.

steep infundibular-pelvic angle, longer calyx (>10 mm) or a narrow infundibulum (<5 mm).[44-46] Another factor is a shockwave-resistant stone. These are commonly calcium oxalate monohydrate, brushite, or cystine stones. A better quantification of stone resistance to shockwave is the Hounsfield units (HU) measured on CT scans. Ouzaid et al. found that a HU of 970 was a good cut-off for success in stone clearance with SWL, with a success rate of 96% for HU of <970 and 38% for HU >970.[47] In the presence of these negative factors, RIRS or PCNL may be a better option than SWL for stones <1.5 cm.

In general, stones >2 cm in the lower pole would be best managed with PCNL, which has consistently shown excellent SFRs in this location. For stones from 15 to 20 mm, flexible URS or PCNL are viable options with better SFRs with PCNL but lower complications with URS. Stones from 10 to 15 mm can be managed by all three modalities, although flexible URS may provide the best balance between SFRs and complications in centers of endourological excellence. For stones <10 mm, SWL or URS are viable options, with better stone-free outcomes for URS but fewer complications for SWL.

Laparoscopic and Open Surgery for Renal Stones

Today, where there is excellent results for the management of stones endoscopically, one may wonder if there is a role for laparoscopic or even open procedures.

Laparoscopic Pyelolithotomy

The indications of laparoscopic pyelolithotomy include failure of endoscopic procedures for the management of stone, complex staghorn stone disease, management of stones in ectopic kidneys, and lastly, when there is a need for a concomitant procedure like a pyeloplasty.[48]

Goel and Hemal in a retrospective review of a small cohort compared retroperitoneal pyelolithotomy to PCNL for renal stones 3 cm and larger and found that there was a 12.5% conversion to open for the laparoscopic group with increased operative time, hospital stay, and convalescence in the laparoscopic group.[49] In another retrospective review of laparoscopic transperitoneal pyelolithotomy to PCNL, Meria et al. found longer operative times for the laparoscopic group with a 12% conversion rate.[50] Thus, the laparoscopic approach should be limited to patients who have failed PCNL or are having concomitant procedures performed.

Laparoscopic Nephrolithotomy

Current indications for laparoscopic nephrolithotomy include ablation of diverticular mucosa for anteriorly located symptomatic calyceal diverticula with stones and the removal of staghorn calculi via an anatrophic nephrolithotomy. To date, there are only a few case reports of laparoscopic nephrolithotomy for calyceal stones.[51,52] Usually, these stones are toward the periphery with a thin parenchymal layer that would make localization and extraction easier. After the stone is extracted, the diverticuli are then fulgurized.

Laparoscopic Anatrophic Nephrolithotomy

Data are even sparser as to the efficacy and safety of this procedure. The largest series was published by Simforoosh et al., consisting of five patients.[53] Stone size averaged 5 cm and average operative time was 170 minutes with an average warm ischemia time of 32 minutes. There were no incidences of leakage or transfusion with two remnant stones of 8 mm and 6 mm and both were treated by SWL.

COMPLICATIONS IN PCNL

There are a number of possible complications related to PCNL. These include bleeding that may require transfusion or angioembolization; urinomas, infection that may lead to urosepsis; injury to the collecting system of the kidney; pleural injuries in upper pole punctures; and risk of injury to other organs, in particular the colon.

The Clinical Research Office of the Endourological Society (CROES) PCNL group looked at PCNL outcomes and complications over a year in a number of centers worldwide and found a complication rate of 20.5%, of which 4.1% were graded as Clavien 3 or 4 (Table 30.4).[54] There was a 5.7% incidence of hemorrhage requiring transfusion and a sepsis rate of 10.5%. This is in keeping with a review of the literature on PCNL, which found a 23.3% incidence of complications, with Clavien 3 and 4 complications making up 4.7% of the cases.[55] The incidences of important complications are listed in Table 30.5.

Mirheydar et al., looking at the American Nationwide Inpatient Sample database, found that higher comorbidities (Charlson comorbidity index ≥ 3) were the strongest factor on complications with an odds ratio of 2.2.[56] This is in keeping with Tefekli et al., who found that complications were 2.7 times more common in patients with diabetes mellitus (DM) and hypertension (HTN).[57]

In the same paper by Mirheydar et al., there has been an overall increase in complications from 14% to 19% for the period from 1998 to 2009. This rising complication rate could be attributable to the greater acceptance of PCNL in community practice where the number of cases treated by each physician may have been small. Opondo et al., using the same CROES database, found that complications were initially higher until 100–150 cases were achieved.[58]

Mini PCNL has been proposed as an alternative to PCNL that may reduce complications. A retrospective review of over 10,000 patients by Zeng et al. had a complication rate up to 18.5%, with a transfusion rate of up to 2.8% and embolization rate of 0.5%.[59] A prospective study by Li et al. found that surgical trauma (represented by tumor necrosis factor α, interleukin 6, interleukin 10, C-reactive protein) was similar in both groups, although the mini PCNL group had a lower transfusion rate of 1.1% versus 6.9%.[60]

Table 30.4: Distribution of perioperative complications of PCNL according to modified Clavien grading scores.

Clavien grading score	*Patients, n (%)*
0	4549 (79.5)
I	634 (11.1)
II	301 (5.3)
IIIa	134 (2.3)
IIIb	76 (1.3)
IVa	18 (0.3)
IVb	10 (0.2)
V	2 (0.03)

(PCNL: Percutaneous nephrolithotomy).
Source: With permission from de la Rosette J, Assimos D, Desai M, et al. The Clinical Research Office of the Endourological Society Percutaneous Nephrolithotomy Global Study: indications, complications, and outcomes in 5803 patients. J Endourol. 2011;25:11-7.

COMPLICATIONS IN URS

Serious complications are generally rare in contemporary URS. This is in great part due to improved surgical experience in the past two decades, smaller-caliber instruments, and the widespread use of safer intracorporeal holmium laser lithotripters.

Ureteral Perforation

This was a common complication in the early days of ureteroscopic lithotripsy, reported in up to 15% in older reports. Perforation occurs in a few scenarios. Older electrohydraulic lithotripters were associated with mucosal injury and perforation. An impacted stone causes thinning of the ureteral wall and subsequently increases the risk of perforation during lithotripsy. Ureteral perforation is recognized by a breach in the mucosa or the periureteral fat. The presence of a safety wire perforation can be managed in a conservative manner in most cases by insertion of a ureteral stent, accepting the possible late complication of stricture formation. Significant urine extravasation despite ureteral stenting will require further drainage with nephrostomy or operative intervention to repair the injury.

Newer ureteroscopes and greater surgical experience have markedly reduced perforation. A contemporary series found the incidence to be lower at 0–4%.[61]

Table 30.5: Important complications in PCNL and their rates.

Study	*Yr*	*n*	*Transfusion*	*Hemoglobin drop g/l*	*Embolization*	*Urinoma*	*Fever*	*Sepsis*	*Thoracic complication*	*Organ injury liver/spleen/ bowel*	*Death*
			%								
Holman et al.#	2002	150	5.3	1.7	0	NA	4.7	NA	0	0	0
Holman et al.	2002	300	4.7	1.4	0	NA	6.3	NA	0.7	1.7	0.3
Srivastava et al.	2005	1854	12.3	NA	1.5	NA	NA	NA	NA	NA	NA
Liatsikos et al.§	2005	100	45	NA	1	NA	NA	NA	1	NA	0
Osman et al.	2005	300	0	NA	0.3	0	32.1	NA	0	0	0
Tefekli et al.	2007	811	10.9	NA	0	NA	2.8	NA	0.3	0.3	0.3
El-Assmy et al.	2007	661	4.3	1.5	0.8	NA	NA	NA	0.15	0.3	0
El-Assmy et al.+	2007	612	2.1	1	0.3	NA	NA	NA	0.16	0.5	0
Michel et al.	2007	315	0	NA	NA	NA	32.1	NA	NA	0	0
Singh et al.*	2008	60	2	1.5	0	NA	0	NA	0	0	0.3
Wezeal et al.	2009	200	20	NA	NA	NA	NA	NA	NA	1	0
Resorlu	2010	192	5.6	1.6	0	NA	5.6	NA	1.1	0	0
After ESWL		86	5.7	1.5	0	NA	5.7	NA	0	0	0
After open surgery		132	6.1	1.8	0	NA	5.3	NA	0.7	0	0
Gupta et al.	2009	90	4.4	2.1	0	NA	15.6	NA	3.3	NA	NA
After open surgery		66	4.5	2.3	0	NA	12.1	NA	4.5	NA	NA
de la Rosette et al.	2011	5803	5.7	NA	NA	NA	10.5	NA	1.8	NA	0.03
Semins et al.$	2011	197	NA	NA	0	1	NA	N	11.6	0.5	0
Overall	–	11929	7	2.3	0.4	0.2	10.8	NA	1.5	0.4	0.05

(ESWL: Extracorporeal shock wave lithotripsy; PCNL: Percutaneous nephrolithotomy; NA: Not available).
Including bilateral percutaneous nephrolitholapaxy.
§ Staghorn stones only.
+ Access established by radiologist.
* Randomized controlled trials.
$ All patients with postoperative day 1 computed tomography scans.
Source: With permission from Seitz C, Desai M, Hacker A, et al. Incidence, prevention, and management of complications following percutaneous nephrolitholapaxy. Eur Urol. 2012;61:146-58.

Avulsion

This is a much-feared complication in URS. Fortunately, most series report it as a rare occurrence (<1% of cases). Avulsion can occur during advancing movements where the injury occurs below the tip of the ureteroscope unseen to the surgeon, or during withdrawal where the injury occurs proximal to the ureteroscope. Scenarios include overforceful advance of the ureteroscope, forced movement of a large calculus through a narrow ureter, and misuse of retrieval baskets or graspers during withdrawal. The first sign of an avulsion is the sudden loss of resistance, either during advancing or withdrawing of the ureteroscope. When the ureteroscope is withdrawn, a portion of ureter can be seen to be pulled out of the urethra. Frank extravasation with loss of smooth outline of ureteral lumen is seen on retrograde pyelography.

A delayed operative repair is preferred, and the affected kidney is immediately diverted with a nephrostomy. If only the distal segment of ureter is avulsed, leaving a viable proximal and midureter, reconstruction with a Boari flap may be considered. When the whole length of ureter is avulsed, reconstruction will require ileal ureter replacement or an autotransplant.

Stricture

This is probably the only long-term complication of URS. Contemporary series report late stricture formation occurring in 2–4%.[12] Older series report an incidence of up to 10%. Risk factors for stricture formation include an impacted stone that had eroded through the mucosal surface; ureteral perforation during URS; fragments remaining embedded in the submucosal tissue, causing fibrotic changes; and lithotripsy injury to the ureteral wall. Strictures can be a source of great morbidity, associated with multiple endoscopic procedures, stent-related symptoms and possibly surgical reconstruction. After determining the likely cause, site, and length of the stricture, endourological or surgical reconstruction techniques can be considered. Endourological techniques include balloon dilatation or ureterotomy. Unsuitable cases or those that had failed endourological techniques will require reconstructive surgery such as ureteroureterostomy, ureteroneocystostomy, psoas hitch, or Boari flap reconstruction.

Bleeding

Bleeding occurs due to mucosal tear or submucosal injury. When bleeding is brisk enough to obscure vision, it may be necessary to terminate the surgery and leave in a stent. In general, bleeding is extremely rare during uneventful URS with laser lithotripsy. Postoperative bleeding usually presents with gross hematuria, which clears out spontaneously most of the time. In severe cases, it may result in clot retention. Life-threatening hematoma from ureteral bleeding is rare and can be controlled by angiographic embolization.[62]

COMPLICATIONS IN SWL

Urinary Tract Infection

It is usual practice to obtain urine cultures before SWL and to treat any positive cultures before SWL. In the study conducted by Halachmi and associates, clinical urinary tract infections (UTIs) developed in 10.4% of patients; all of them successfully responded to antibiotics and intravenous fluids.[63] Ather et al. observed urosepsis in 7% of their cases.[64] In a meta-analysis by Pearle and Roehrborn of eight randomized prospective controlled trials of prophylaxis versus placebo or no prophylactic antibiotics before SWL, they demonstrated the superiority of prophylaxis over no treatment before SWL.[65] Urinary tract infection in these studies, however, was considered as a positive urine culture and not a febrile disease. In a retrospective review of 11,000 ESWL cases by Duvdevani et al., there was a 1.4% incidence of fever of >38°C in patients who did not receive antibiotic prophylaxis.[66] Patients in this cohort at risk of post-SWL sepsis were those with a percutaneous nephrostomy, ureteric stenting, previous UTI, or sepsis from the obstructing stone. This may indicate that selective use of prophylactic antibiotics may be more appropriate. In addition, special considerations should also be given to high-risk patient groups, which the AUA defines as advanced age, patients with anatomical anomalies of the urinary tract, those with poor nutritional status, chronic smokers, chronic steroid users, those with immunodeficiency, those with externalized catheters, and those with prolonged hospitalization.

Hemorrhage

The incidence of hemorrhage ranges from 0.5% to 1% on ultrasound[67] to 30% if CT or magnetic resonance imaging is used routinely for evaluation.[68] Dhar et al. reported that the incidence of hematoma and symptomatic hematoma following electromagnetic SWL was 4.1% and 0.7%, respectively.[69]

Furthermore, many hematomas are not picked up as it is often not routine practice to perform immediate post-SWL imaging unless there are signs of complications. Also, different shockwave machines with different energy sources, different shockwave settings, and number of shocks affect the incidence of hematomas.

Lee et al., in a review of 10,887 SWL cases, had a 0.32% incidence rate of renal hematoma. Patients with renal hematomas were then case matched, and it was found that hematomas were more common in patients with hypertension, a higher body mass index and larger stone size.[70]

The clinical signs often comprise severe renal colic, gross hematuria, uncontrollable flank pain, and hemodynamic instability. Management is usually supportive with analgesia and transfusions if there is hemodynamic instability. The most likely outcome is spontaneous radiographic resolution of the hematoma within 2 years without clinically evident adverse effects on blood pressure or renal function.[71]

Hypertension and Diabetes

Studies have shown acute nephron injury that can lead to renal scarring after SWL, but most seem to resolve over time.[72]

Janetschek et al. found that SWL was associated with an increased incidence of new-onset hypertension and increased resistive indexes, especially in older age-group patients.[73]

A number of studies, including two randomized trials, on hypertension after SWL did not show any differences in incidences of hypertension from the general population (8% vs 6%) in the near to short term.[74-76] Unfortunately, the follow-up periods of these studies do not address the issue of whether there are long-term detrimental effects on blood pressure.

In a recent retrospective review of patients who had undergone SWL with 19 years of follow-up, Segura's team found that there was an increased incidence of hypertension in patients who had received bilateral SWL and also an increased incidence of diabetes mellitus compared to controls.[77] Two subsequent retrospective reviews trying to answer the question of new-onset diabetes in patients who had undergone SWL did not show any link, but they were hampered by either too short a follow-up period or SWL conducted with lower than normal energy levels.[78,79]

In summary, caution should be advised in the use of SWL with regards to long-term complications of hypertension and diabetes. These changes are probably more likely to affect the elderly and may be dose dependent.

Steinstrasse

Overall, steinstrasse occurs in 1–4% of patients who undergo SWL. The occurrence rate increases to 5–10% of patients with large stones (>20 mm) and up to 40% of patients with partial or complete staghorn calculi. In the case of large calculi (>20 mm), stenting before SWL reduces the risk of obstruction and steinstrasse.[80,81]

Steps to Reduce Complications

According to the theory, treatment at a slower shockwave rate could decrease the incidence of renal injury while increasing the stone breakage efficacy.[82] This was shown in pigs that were treated with a first generation electrohydraulic Dornier HM3 lithotriptor at rate settings of 120, 60, and 30 pulses per minute. The pigs at the lowest rates had the smallest renal lesions.

A stepwise increase in shockwave power and employment of a pause is another treatment strategy to reduce renal injury.[83] Studies in pig models show that a 3-minute pause between doses had a significant impact on renal trauma. They were able to show a mean reduction of the SWL treatment lesion size from 4% to 0.5%.[84,85]

REFERENCES

1. Newman DM, Lingeman JE, Mertz JH, et al. Extracorporeal shock-wave lithotripsy. Urol Clin North Am. 1987;14:63-71.
2. Raman JD, Bagrodia A, Gupta A, et al. Natural history of residual fragments following percutaneous nephrostolithotomy. J Urol. 2009;181:1163-8.
3. Schatloff O, Lindner U, Ramon J, et al. Randomized trial of stone fragment active retrieval versus spontaneous passage during holmium laser lithotripsy for ureteral stones. J Urol. 2010;183:1031-5.
4. Streem SB, Yost A, Mascha E. Clinical implications of clinically insignificant store fragments after extracorporeal shock wave lithotripsy. J Urol. 1996;155:1186-90.
5. Ueno A, Kawamura T, Ogawa A, et al. Relation of spontaneous passage of ureteral calculi to size. Urology. 1977;10:544-6.
6. Coll DM, Varanelli MJ, Smith RC. Relationship of spontaneous passage of ureteral calculi to stone size and location as revealed by unenhanced helical CT. AJR Am J Roentgenol. 2002;178:101-3.
7. Salem HK. A prospective randomized study comparing shock wave lithotripsy and semirigid ureteroscopy for the management of proximal ureteral calculi. Urology. 2009;74:1216-21.
8. Peschel R, Janetschek G, Bartsch G. Extracorporeal shock wave lithotripsy versus ureteroscopy for distal ureteral calculi: a prospective randomized study. J Urol. 1999;162: 1909-12.
9. Pearle MS, Nadler R, Bercowsky E, et al. Prospective randomized trial comparing shock wave lithotripsy and

ureteroscopy for management of distal ureteral calculi. J Urol. 2001;166:1255-60.
10. Verze P, Imbimbo C, Cancelmo G, et al. Extracorporeal shockwave lithotripsy vs ureteroscopy as first-line therapy for patients with single, distal ureteric stones: a prospective randomized study. BJU Int. 2010;106:1748-52.
11. Hendrikx AJ, Strijbos WE, de Knijff DW, et al. Treatment for extended-mid and distal ureteral stones: SWL or ureteroscopy? Results of a multicenter study. J Endourol. 1999;13:727-33.
12. Preminger GM, Tiselius HG, Assimos DG, et al. 2007 Guideline for the management of ureteral calculi. J Urol. 2007;178(6):2418-34.
13. Matlaga BR, Jansen JP, Meckley LM, et al. Treatment of ureteral and renal stones: a systematic review and meta-analysis of randomized, controlled trials. J Urol. 2012;188:130-7.
14. Aboumarzouk OM, Kata SG, Keeley FX, et al. Extracorporeal shock wave lithotripsy (ESWL) versus ureteroscopic management for ureteric calculi. Cochrane Database Syst Rev. 2012;5:CD006029.
15. Zhu Y, Duijvesz D, Rovers MM, et al. Alpha-blockers to assist stone clearance after extracorporeal shock wave lithotripsy: a meta-analysis. BJU Int. 2010;106:256-61.
16. Delakas D, Karyotis I, Daskalopoulos G, et al. Independent predictors of failure of shockwave lithotripsy for ureteral stones employing a second-generation lithotripter. J Endourol. 2003;17:201-5.
17. Seitz C, Fajkovic H, Waldert M, et al. Extracorporeal shock wave lithotripsy in the treatment of proximal ureteral stones: does the presence and degree of hydronephrosis affect success? Eur Urol. 2006;49:378-83.
18. Demirbas M, Kose AC, Samli M, et al. Extracorporeal shockwave lithotripsy for solitary distal ureteral stones: does the degree of urinary obstruction affect success? J Endourol. 2004;18:237-40.
19. Lee YH, Tsai JY, Jiaan BP, et al. Prospective randomized trial comparing shock wave lithotripsy and ureteroscopic lithotripsy for management of large upper third ureteral stones. Urology. 2006;67:480-4; discussion 4.
20. Sun X, Xia S, Lu J, et al. Treatment of large impacted proximal ureteral stones: randomized comparison of percutaneous antegrade ureterolithotripsy versus retrograde ureterolithotripsy. J Endourol. 2008;22:913-7.
21. Basiri A, Simforoosh N, Ziaee A, et al. Retrograde, antegrade, and laparoscopic approaches for the management of large, proximal ureteral stones: a randomized clinical trial. J Endourol. 2008;22:2677-80.
22. Lopes Neto AC, Korkes F, Silva JL, 2nd, et al. Prospective randomized study of treatment of large proximal ureteral stones: extracorporeal shock wave lithotripsy versus ureterolithotripsy versus laparoscopy. J Urol. 2012;187:164-8.
23. Segura JW, Patterson DE, LeRoy AJ, et al. Percutaneous removal of kidney stones: review of 1,000 cases. J Urol. 1985;134:1077-81.
24. Osman M, Wendt-Nordahl G, Heger K, et al. Percutaneous nephrolithotomy with ultrasonography-guided renal access: experience from over 300 cases. BJU Int. 2005;96:875-8.
25. Carlsson P, Kinn AC, Tiselius HG, et al. Cost effectiveness of extracorporeal shock wave lithotripsy and percutaneous nephrolithotomy for medium-sized kidney stones. A randomised clinical trial. Scand J Urol Nephrol. 1992;26:257-63.
26. Xue W, Pacik D, Boellaard W, et al. Management of single large nonstaghorn renal stones in the CROES PCNL global study. J Urol. 2012;187:1293-7.
27. Labate G, Modi P, Timoney A, et al. The percutaneous nephrolithotomy global study: classification of complications. J Endourol. 2011;25:1275-80.
28. Pan J, Chen Q, Xue W, et al. RIRS versus mPCNL for single renal stone of 2–3 cm: clinical outcome and cost-effective analysis in Chinese medical setting. Urolithiasis. 2013;41:73-8.
29. Obek C, Onal B, Kantay K, et al. The efficacy of extracorporeal shock wave lithotripsy for isolated lower pole calculi compared with isolated middle and upper caliceal calculi. J Urol. 2001;166:2081-4; discussion 5.
30. Albala DM, Assimos DG, Clayman RV, et al. Lower pole I: a prospective randomized trial of extracorporeal shock wave lithotripsy and percutaneous nephrostolithotomy for lower pole nephrolithiasis-initial results. J Urol. 2001;166:2072-80.
31. Turna B, Ekren F, Nazli O, et al. Comparative results of shockwave lithotripsy for renal calculi in upper, middle, and lower calices. J Endourol. 2007;21:951-6.
32. Micali S, Sighinolfi MC, Grande M, et al. Dornier Lithotripter S 220 F EMSE: the first report of over 1000 treatments. Urology. 2009;74:1211-4.
33. Riedler I, Trummer H, Hebel P, et al. Outcome and safety of extracorporeal shock wave lithotripsy as first-line therapy of lower pole nephrolithiasis. Urol Int. 2003;71:350-4.
34. El-Nahas AR, Ibrahim HM, Youssef RF, et al. Flexible ureterorenoscopy versus extracorporeal shock wave lithotripsy for treatment of lower pole stones of 10–20 mm. BJU Int. 2012;110:898-902.
35. Hussain M, Acher P, Penev B, et al. Redefining the limits of flexible ureterorenoscopy. J Endourol. 2011;25:45-9.
36. Preminger GM, Tiselius HG, Assimos DG, et al. 2007 guideline for the management of ureteral calculi. J Urol. 2007;178:2418-34.
37. Wiesenthal JD, Ghiculete D, Dah RJ, et al. A comparison of treatment modalities for renal calculi between 100 and 300 mm^2: are shockwave lithotripsy, ureteroscopy, and percutaneous nephrolithotomy equivalent? J Endourol. 2011;25:481-5.
38. Resorlu B, Unsal A, Ziypak T, et al. Comparison of retrograde intrarenal surgery, shockwave lithotripsy, and percutaneous nephrolithotomy for treatment of medium-sized radiolucent renal stones. World J Urol. 2013;31:1581-6.
39. Pearle MS, Lingeman JE, Leveillee R, et al. Prospective, randomized trial comparing shock wave lithotripsy and ureteroscopy for lower pole caliceal calculi 1 cm or less. J Urol. 2005;173:2005-9.
40. Srisubat A, Potisat S, Lojanapiwat B, et al. Extracorporeal shock wave lithotripsy (ESWL) versus percutaneous nephrolithotomy (PCNL) or retrograde intrarenal surgery (RIRS) for kidney stones. Cochrane Database Syst Rev. 2009;7(4):CD007044. doi: 10.1002/14651858.CD007044.pub2.

41. Ozturk U, Sener NC, Goktug HN, et al. Comparison of percutaneous nephrolithotomy, shock wave lithotripsy, and retrograde intrarenal surgery for lower pole renal calculi 10–20 mm. Urol Int. 2013;91(3):345-9.
42. Bozkurt OF, Resorlu B, Yildiz Y, et al. Retrograde intrarenal surgery versus percutaneous nephrolithotomy in the management of lower-pole renal stones with a diameter of 15 to 20 mm. J Endourol. 2011;25:1131-5.
43. Kirac M, Bozkurt OF, Tunc L, et al. Comparison of retrograde intrarenal surgery and mini-percutaneous nephrolithotomy in management of lower-pole renal stones with a diameter of smaller than 15 mm. Urolithiasis. 2013;41:241-6.
44. Knoll T, Musial A, Trojan L, et al. Measurement of renal anatomy for prediction of lower-pole caliceal stone clearance: reproducibility of different parameters. J Endourol. 2003;17:447-51.
45. Ruggera L, Beltrami P, Ballario R, et al. Impact of anatomical pielocaliceal topography in the treatment of renal lower calyces stones with extracorporeal shock wave lithotripsy. Int J Urol. 2005;12:525-32.
46. Juan YS, Chuang SM, Wu WJ, et al. Impact of lower pole anatomy on stone clearance after shock wave lithotripsy. Kaohsiung J Med Sci. 2005;21:358-64.
47. Ouzaid I, Al-qahtani S, Dominique S, et al. A 970 Hounsfield units (HU) threshold of kidney stone density on non-contrast computed tomography (NCCT) improves patients' selection for extracorporeal shockwave lithotripsy (ESWL): evidence from a prospective study. BJU Int. 2012;110:E438-42.
48. Skolarikos A, Papatsoris AG, Albanis S, et al. Laparoscopic urinary stone surgery: an updated evidence-based review. Urol Res. 2010;38:337-44.
49. Goel A, Hemal AK. Evaluation of role of retroperitoneoscopic pyelolithotomy and its comparison with percutaneous nephrolithotripsy. Int Urol Nephrol. 2003;35:73-6.
50. Meria P, Milcent S, Desgrandchamps F, et al. Management of pelvic stones larger than 20 mm: laparoscopic transperitoneal pyelolithotomy or percutaneous nephrolithotomy? Urol Int. 2005;75:322-6.
51. Ruckle HC, Segura JW. Laparoscopic treatment of a stone-filled, caliceal diverticulum: a definitive, minimally invasive therapeutic option. J Urol. 1994;151:122-4.
52. Miller SD, Ng CS, Streem SB, et al. Laparoscopic management of caliceal diverticular calculi. J Urol. 2002;167:1248-52.
53. Simforoosh N, Aminsharifi A, Tabibi A, et al. Laparoscopic anatrophic nephrolithotomy for managing large staghorn calculi. BJU Int. 2008;101:1293-6.
54. de la Rosette J, Assimos D, Desai M, et al. The Clinical Research Office of the Endourological Society Percutaneous Nephrolithotomy Global Study: indications, complications, and outcomes in 5803 patients. J Endourol. 2011;25:11-7.
55. Seitz C, Desai M, Hacker A, et al. Incidence, prevention, and management of complications following percutaneous nephrolitholapaxy. Eur Urol. 2012;61:146-58.
56. Mirheydar HS, Palazzi KL, Derweesh IH, et al. Percutaneous nephrolithotomy use is increasing in the United States: an analysis of trends and complications. J Endourol. 2013;27:979-83.
57. Tefekli A, Kurtoglu H, Tepeler K, et al. Does the metabolic syndrome or its components affect the outcome of percutaneous nephrolithotomy? J Endourol. 2008;22:35-40.
58. Opondo D, Tefekli A, Esen T, et al. Impact of case volumes on the outcomes of percutaneous nephrolithotomy. Eur Urol. 2012;62:1181-7.
59. Zeng G, Zhao Z, Wan S, et al. Minimally invasive percutaneous nephrolithotomy for simple and complex renal caliceal stones: a comparative analysis of more than 10,000 cases. J Endourol. 2013;27:1203-8.
60. Li LY, Gao X, Yang M, et al. Does a smaller tract in percutaneous nephrolithotomy contribute to less invasiveness? A prospective comparative study. Urology. 2010;75:56-61.
61. Geavlete P, Georgescu D, Nita G, et al. Complications of 2735 retrograde semirigid ureteroscopy procedures: a single-center experience. J Endourol. 2006;20:179-85.
62. Kase DJ, Crystal KS, Naidich JB, et al. Embolization to control iatrogenic ureteral hemorrhage: a case report. J Urol. 1994;151:420-1.
63. Halachmi S, Nagar M, Golan S, et al. Extracorporeal shock wave lithotripsy for large ureteral stones using HM3 lithotriptor. J Urol. 2006;176:1449-52; discussion 52.
64. Ather MH, Paryani J, Memon A, et al. A 10-year experience of managing ureteric calculi: changing trends towards endourological intervention—is there a role for open surgery? BJU Int. 2001;88:173-7.
65. Pearle MS, Roehrborn CG. Antimicrobial prophylaxis prior to shock wave lithotripsy in patients with sterile urine before treatment: a meta-analysis and cost-effectiveness analysis. Urology. 1997;49:679-86.
66. Duvdevani M, Lorber G, Gofrit ON, et al. Fever after shock-wave lithotripsy—risk factors and indications for prophylactic antimicrobial treatment. J Endourol. 2010;24:277-81.
67. Skolarikos A, Alivizatos G, de la Rosette J. Extracorporeal shock wave lithotripsy 25 years later: complications and their prevention. Eur Urol. 2006;50:981-90; discussion 90.
68. Salem S, Mehrsai A, Zartab H, et al. Complications and outcomes following extracorporeal shock wave lithotripsy: a prospective study of 3,241 patients. Urol Res. 2010;38:135-42.
69. Dhar NB, Thornton J, Karafa MT, et al. A multivariate analysis of risk factors associated with subcapsular hematoma formation following electromagnetic shock wave lithotripsy. J Urol. 2004;172:2271-4.
70. Lee HY, Yang YH, Shen JT, et al. Risk factors survey for extracorporeal shockwave lithotripsy-induced renal hematoma. J Endourol. 2013;27:763-7.
71. Krishnamurthi V, Streem SB. Long-term radiographic and functional outcome of extracorporeal shock wave lithotripsy induced perirenal hematomas. J Urol. 1995;154:1673-5.
72. Evan AP, Willis LR, Lingeman JE, et al. Renal trauma and the risk of long-term complications in shock wave lithotripsy. Nephron. 1998;78:1-8.
73. Janetschek G, Frauscher F, Knapp R, et al. New onset hypertension after extracorporeal shock wave lithotripsy: age related incidence and prediction by intrarenal resistive index. J Urol. 1997;158:346-51.
74. Lingeman JE, Woods JR, Toth PD. Blood pressure changes following extracorporeal shock wave lithotripsy and other

forms of treatment for nephrolithiasis. JAMA. 1990;263: 1789-94.
75. Jewett MA, Bombardier C, Logan AG, et al. A randomized controlled trial to assess the incidence of new onset hypertension in patients after shock wave lithotripsy for asymptomatic renal calculi. J Urol. 1998;160:1241-3.
76. Elves AW, Tilling K, Menezes P, et al. Early observations of the effect of extracorporeal shockwave lithotripsy on blood pressure: a prospective randomized control clinical trial. BJU Int. 2000;85:611-5.
77. Krambeck AE, Gettman MT, Rohlinger AL, et al. Diabetes mellitus and hypertension associated with shock wave lithotripsy of renal and proximal ureteral stones at 19 years of followup. J Urol. 2006;175:1742-7.
78. Makhlouf AA, Thorner D, Ugarte R, et al. Shock wave lithotripsy not associated with development of diabetes mellitus at 6 years of follow-up. Urology. 2009;73:4-8; discussion.
79. Sato Y, Tanda H, Kato S, et al. Shock wave lithotripsy for renal stones is not associated with hypertension and diabetes mellitus. Urology. 2008;71:586-91; discussion 91-2.
80. Madbouly K, Sheir KZ, Elsobky E, et al. Risk factors for the formation of a steinstrasse after extracorporeal shock wave lithotripsy: a statistical model. J Urol. 2002;167:1239-42.
81. Bierkens AF, Hendrikx AJ, Lemmens WA, et al. Extracorporeal shock wave lithotripsy for large renal calculi: the role of ureteral stents. A randomized trial. J Urol. 1991;145:699-702.
82. Evan AP, McAteer JA, Connors BA, et al. Renal injury during shock wave lithotripsy is significantly reduced by slowing the rate of shock wave delivery. BJU Int. 2007;100:624-7; discussion 7-8.
83. McAteer JA, Evan AP, Williams JC, Jr., et al. Treatment protocols to reduce renal injury during shock wave lithotripsy. Curr Opin Urol. 2009;19:192-5.
84. Connors BA, Evan AP, Blomgren PM, et al. Effect of initial shock wave voltage on shock wave lithotripsy-induced lesion size during step-wise voltage ramping. BJU Int. 2009;103:104-7.
85. Handa RK, Bailey MR, Paun M, et al. Pretreatment with low-energy shock waves induces renal vasoconstriction during standard shock wave lithotripsy (SWL): a treatment protocol known to reduce SWL-induced renal injury. BJU Int. 2009;103:1270-4.

CHAPTER

31 Shock Wave Lithotripsy in Management of Stones

Michelle Jo Semins, Brian R Matlaga

INTRODUCTION

Shock wave lithotripsy (SWL) permanently transformed the management of kidney stones with its introduction in 1980. Earlier periods required invasive, open surgical procedures with lengthy hospitalizations for removal of upper urinary tract stones. Shock wave lithotripsy revolutionized the standard treatment of proximal ureteral and renal calculi by allowing for a noninvasive, outpatient, low-morbidity alternative. It quickly became extensively utilized, and although ureteroscopy is gaining popularity with its recent advances, SWL is still the most commonly used treatment option today.[1-3]

Over the past three-and-a-half decades, SWL technology has undergone significant transformations. Shock wave lithotripsy success rates have varied with these changes, leading experts to generate a well-defined range of uses for the technology to better optimize the results and reduce failures. Although SWL is noninvasive with low morbidity, it does have its unique set of complications.

In this chapter, we discuss the progression of the field to the contemporary instrumentation of SWL today. We also discuss the range of uses of SWL and its limitations, with a focus on how to maximize success rates. Relative and absolute clinical contraindications of SWL are addressed and selected based on poor response to therapy or increased risk for morbidity. We conclude the chapter with a thorough review of surgical complications specific to SWL in the treatment of kidney stones.

CONTEMPORARY INSTRUMENTS

Since its introduction in 1980, SWL has undergone significant evolution over the last three and a half decades. The Dornier Human Model 3 (HM3) Lithotripter was the first machine approved and used in the United States. It is the benchmark by which all current devices are compared. Although the first-generation machines were exciting because they revolutionized the treatment of upper urinary tract stones secondary to their noninvasive nature, several limitations were quickly noticed. Efficacy varied based on stone burden, location, and composition. Additionally, the machines were large, awkward, and fixed. Lastly, concern over potential damage to the kidney from the technology ensued. With these constraints came significant modification to the technology in the effort to make the practice more convenient, effective, and safer. Advances in instrumentation have included changes in the size of the lithotripter, the source of the shock wave, coupling mechanisms, imaging modality used, focal zone width, and pressure delivered. With these changes, through the different generations of devices, came hopes to make the technology available to everyone with improved success rates and lower complication rates. Many of the device parameters that have evolved have succeeded in increasing the transportability of the machines; however, their effects on efficacy are variable. Efficacy has been show to vary between lithotripters.[4-8] Many of these parameters can be controlled to maximize stone fragmentation. Herein, we discuss the evolution of the lithotripter technology, contemporary instrumentation, and strategies to optimize SWL with the modern machines.

The first-generation machine was quite large, occupying a good portion of an operating room, built-in, and not transportable. The cumbersome nature of the machine and the immobility of the technology limited access to a number of providers and patients. Therefore, one of the first changes made to the next-generation lithotripter was scaling down the size of the machine with the hopes of increasing utilization of the technology. One reason for the excessive size was the coupling mechanism used. With the Dornier HM3, the patient was immersed into a large water bath with the degassed water serving as an acoustic medium for the shock waves to travel from electrode to stone. In order to reduce the size of the machine and allow transportability, the coupling mechanism also had to adapt. After complete water bath came partial water bath, and the most modern lithotripters have dry treatment heads, which do not require water as a medium for coupling at all. This change allowed for the miniaturization of the machine. With dry treatment heads, the patient is coupled to the device using either gel or oil and placed up against the head. Although the transition to the new dry treatment head allows for improved access of the technology due to the increased mobility of the units, it unfortunately can have a negative impact on the efficacy of the treatment. Whereas the water bath was degassed, allowing for near-perfect coupling, air bubbles form in the newer coupling agents used, which leads to a loss of energy as the shock waves travel through the medium. This loss of energy of the shock wave on its way to the stone from the lithotripter decreases the success rate of SWL. A study by Pishchalnikov et al. demonstrated that as little as 2% of air pockets in the medium can diminish calculus fragmentation by 20–40%.[9] Repositioning the patient during SWL contributes to creation of the air pockets and causes decoupling and recoupling during the procedure, diminishing the energy of the shock waves and thus decreasing stone breakage. Ideally, there would be a way to monitor the connection between the patient and the treatment head during the procedure, but currently this is not available. The same groups that demonstrated the effect of the air pockets on the efficacy of SWL also described methods to minimize the creation of them.[10] Squirt bottle dispensing and hand application is associated with coupling degradation. They showed that applying the gel as a mound in a large volume from the stock jug produces the lowest measurement of air bubbles. Additionally, rather than manually spreading the gel on the patient's skin, it is best to allow the medium to naturally spread on its own as the patient and the treatment head come into contact with each other. Following this principle can minimize the negative impact of the dry treatment head and allow for the benefit of its smaller size. Live-monitoring of coupling and new coupling techniques are ideal targets for future research.

An additional modern development of the coupling mechanism is the creation of two treatment heads. Dual-head lithotripters trigger shock waves from separate sources along two paths to target the stone and can discharge simultaneously or in alternating mode. This design could potentially augment stone breakage and decrease procedure time.[11-14] Concern for potential increased tissue injury with this dual-head apparatus has not been borne out in porcine studies evaluating for renal damage.[15,16]

Imaging and stone targeting capabilities have also evolved with the different generation machines. Traditionally, biplanar fluoroscopy was exclusively used with the lithotripters; now ultrasound has been incorporated into different apparatus designs. The combination of ultrasound with fluoroscopy allows for active, continuous feedback without the use of radiation. This is beneficial to the patient, physician, and operating room staff. It also allows for targeting of radiolucent stones, which are not visualized by fluoroscopy unless a retrograde pyelogram is performed. Its use is limited as a sole modality, given its limitations targeting ureteral stones and difficulty with visualization in obese patients. Additionally, advanced training is required to perform ultrasonography.

Shock wave source has evolved over time as well. There are three types of shock wave generators: electrohydraulic, electromagnetic, and piezoelectric. Piezoelectric was a generator that was in use only briefly as treatment outcomes were inferior to the other devices.[17] The technique was based on firing of a capacitor through a collection of piezoceramic elements situated on a reflector, which resulted in generation of a shock wave by nonlinear propagation.[18] The original shock wave generator used to treat kidney stones was electrohydraulic. The HM3 Dornier lithotripter used this technology as a shock wave source, and many lithotripters still do. These machines are based on spark gap technology. Once fully charged, a capacitor fires and creates an explosion at the spark gap electrode. This burst causes the water between the electrodes to evaporate, and the energy created generates a spherical shock wave. The shock wave then encounters an ellipsoid reflector that focuses the wave. The electrodes in this electrohydraulic technology can only produce a set number of shock waves before eroding and requiring replacement.[18,19] As the electrodes erode, the shock waves produced are unpredictable and erratic, directly affecting efficacy. Although more modern electrodes have a longer life span and increased consistency because of encapsulation and self-advancing technology, the limitation of this technology, with variability and electrode replacement requirements, led to a movement to design a more durable and reliable technology. The result was the manufacturing of the electromagnetic shock wave generator. Similar to the electrohydraulic lithotripters, a capacitor discharges, but instead of creating a burst at a spark gap, a magnetic field is created. The basis of this technology is the presence of a coil. There are variable constructs of electromagnetic lithotripters. The coil present is either around a cylinder, on the inside plane of a spherical cap, or on a flat exterior with an overlying conductive membrane.[19] The magnetic field produced causes repulsion of a membrane, resulting in the generation of a shock wave. It is focused from origination or with a parabolic reflector or acoustic lens. Electromagnetic generators last for millions of shock waves versus only several thousand offered by the electrohydraulic technology.[19]

Regardless of the generator used, all lithotripters have a focal zone. The focal zone, the area where the acoustic pressure is highest, surrounds the focal point, which is where the shock wave is directed. Over the last three and a half decades, the focal zone parameters and the acoustic pressures have transformed from machine to machine. The goal is to make certain the target remains in the focal zone, nearest the focal point as possible, while limiting the surrounding effects on the kidney and other adjacent organs. A broad focal zone is more likely to keep the stone in the region of highest acoustic pressure, the treatment zone, but it is also more likely to increase neighboring tissue effect as well, and induce more discomfort. The pain occurs at the skin site of shock wave entry. The more narrow the entry site at the skin, the more pressure is directed at one place, and the more pain is sensed. This can be modified by opening or closing the lithotripter aperture, with a closed aperture associated with a wider focal zone and narrow entry site. If the stone travels outside of the focal zone, it is not receiving a dose of energy with each shock wave discharge, but some tissue is receiving that energy with each pulse. With these principles in mind, the different generations of lithotripters evolved with varying focal zone widths and acoustic pressures to optimize stone fragmentation and minimize nearby tissue injury. The first modification was narrowing the focal zone and increasing the acoustic pressures in the hope of treating the stone with higher pressures and affecting less surrounding tissue. Later-generation devices had maximal focal zones of 5 mm compared to the zone of 15 by 60 mm that the Dornier HM3 had.[18] Efficacy was quickly noticed to be inferior for these newer-generation lithotripters. The focal zone was too narrow to keep the target within it at all times, as stone location would travel outside the focal zone with respiratory motion. With fewer pulses reaching the stone, fragmentation was compromised. In addition, tissue injury was greater because the acoustic pressures in the focal zone were much higher than the original machine, increasing the risk for kidney injury and hematoma.[20,21] One way to minimize the risk of tissue injury and potentially improve stone breakage as well is by "ramping-up" the energy voltage of the device.[21,22] Studies have demonstrated that pretreating with 100–200 shock waves at a lower energy (i.e. 12 kV) results in less kidney damage as a measure of functional renal volume lesions size.[23] A porcine model suggested that the ramping-up process with a 3–4-minute pause is more important than the actual voltage used as the lesion size was significantly reduced with priming doses of 12, 18, and 24 kV.[24,25] A vasoconstrictive process is believed to be responsible for this protective effect, as administration of dopamine was shown to block the beneficial outcome.[26]

The most modern machines are distinguished from one another based on their peak pressure and focal zone size, or they allow for adjustment of these parameters by the practitioner, with in vitro research showing that lower pressures with broader focal zones may be most optimal.[21,27-30] The shape of the focal zone can vary as well, with most lithotripters producing a cigar-shaped region. To get the full power of shear and tensile stress, the focal zone should be wider than the stone.

One way to optimize the narrower focal zone in many modern lithotripters, without modifying the design of the lithotripter further, is by administering full general anesthesia. This allows for greater respiratory control of rate and volume and less variation of kidney motion, increasing the likelihood of the target stone staying within the focal zone. The newer machines were designed in the hope of allowing for no anesthesia or mild sedation versus general anesthesia, making the procedure even less invasive than it already is. However, this was achieved by widening the aperture as discussed previously, decreasing the skin entry site size but resulting in a narrower focal width. This narrow focal width negatively impacts stone fragmentation and may even increase tissue injury with the higher pressures used.[21] Higher stone-free rates using general endotracheal anesthesia versus intravenous sedation have been reported by two clinical studies, with 78–87% success rate versus 51–55%, respectively.[31,32]

All contemporary machines also allow control of shock wave rate delivery and the total number of shock waves discharged. A slow rate can potentially decrease vascular injury. A rate of 60 shocks per minute versus 120 was shown to reduce lesion size as measured by functional renal volume, similar to the ramping-up protocols discussed previously.[33,34] A slow rate can not only reduce renal injury, it can also improve treatment outcome.[33,35-39] One meta-analysis of randomized controlled trials showed 60 shock waves per minute to be the ideal rate at which to deliver energy to the stone and effect breakage.[40] This was compared to both 90 and 120 shocks per minute. Cavitation is hypothesized to be responsible for this effect, with the bubbles created from each energy wave building up and sheltering the effect of each subsequent wave. The slower the rate, the more time the bubbles have to dissipate, the less shielding, and the more effective the energy from each wave. This does, of course, increase treatment time, as the number of shock waves to be delivered is usually predetermined. The fewest number of shock waves needed to fragment the stone should be used to minimize injury; however, it remains challenging to know what this number is, and most patients are generally overtreated, in the hope of a successful outcome and no necessity for further procedures. How to determine the optimal number of shock waves or when the stone is satisfactorily fragmented is an excellent area for future research.

There are many areas of the shock wave discipline that are a target of current and future research. Given its noninvasive nature, it is a highly desirable field to improve upon and develop. Although imaging with both ultrasound and fluoroscopy is now available to target the stone, there are currently no methods for active feedback despite the ability to live-monitor, to halt delivery of a shock if the stone is out of the focal zone.[18] A mechanism by which a shock wave is created and administered only if the calculus is within the treatment zone is a desirable area for future research. Despite the ability to continuously monitor the stone, there remains no way to discern when the stone is satisfactorily fragmented, often resulting in treatment with additional, unnecessary energy waves. This is an area for potential improvement whether current imaging modalities are modified or whether alternative imaging modalities are developed or incorporated into the shock wave technology.[18] An additional area for future research is the dual-pulse technology. Two pulses can be delivered from separate treatment heads or in tandem from a single treatment head.[12,41-43] The clinical effect of such technology is not officially known, but initial experimental results are promising and theoretically treatment time could be reduced. The effect on the kidney with this technology has been assessed, and it has been found to be safe. Further research is needed.[15,16]

Future research should aim to improve results further while minimizing complications. Broadening the range of use should also be a focus of future research, as there are currently many stone patients who do not respond well to SWL, with high failure rates if used. Shock wave source, focal zone, acoustic output, voltage used, imaging modalities, focusing techniques, and coupling are all areas amenable to modification and may be the key to achieving better results. Lastly, technician and operator experience is also important for success.

RANGE OF USES

Shock wave lithotripsy has a wide range of uses for nephrolithiasis and still accounts for over 50% of kidney stone cases performed in the United States today, although it may be declining.[1-3] Shock wave lithotripsy is used often for kidney stones and, per the current American Urological Association (AUA) guidelines for management of ureteral calculi, it is still a primary treatment modality for the management of these stones if surgical therapy is needed.[44] Shock wave lithotripsy can be used in both adult and pediatric patients and may be more successful in children, with some evidence that they pass fragments more readily.[44]

Technically, SWL could be used for any urinary calculus; however, the success rate decreases and the complication rate increases for certain clinical situations. Since 1980 when it was first introduced, the success rate for SWL has decreased. This is for a multitude of reasons, including the aforementioned changes in equipment as well as the nonselective use of the technology by urologists. Herein, we discuss the range of uses urologists should consider when treating a urinary calculus with SWL to maximize success and realize limitations.

Before even considering selection criterion, several patient features influence the decision to proceed with SWL. There are both absolute and relative contraindications. Patients with a bleeding diathesis or uncorrected coagulopathy should not undergo SWL, given the increased complication risk of bleeding. Shock wave lithotripsy is also contraindicated in patients with severe skeletal malformations or deformities.[45] Shock wave lithotripsy should not be used in pregnant patients or for stones in the mid and distal ureter in females of childbearing age.[44] In young, nonpregnant women there is a theoretical risk of injury to the ovaries and unfertilized eggs; although this has not been scientifically confirmed, many practices require written acknowledgment of this potential risk should the patient still desire this therapy, and other institutions will not offer it to this population.[46,47] There have been reports of accidental use of SWL in pregnant patients with good outcomes, but it still remains contraindicated given the theoretical risk of spontaneous abortion, placental abruption, and intrauterine growth retardation that exists. Shock wave lithotripsy can also affect male fertility, although this has been shown to be only temporary.[48]

If there are no contraindications, there is a large amount of literature on controllable parameters that can affect the treatment outcome of SWL. Although SWL can be theoretically used for any stone, anywhere, and many patients opt for the noninvasive technology, more selective use of the procedure will maximize the success rate and minimize the complications. Both patient- and stone-specific factors are considered for optimal case selection.

Obesity is associated with a poor outcome for SWL. Positioning of patients with high body mass index (BMI) to target the stone is challenging, and the excess adipose tissue subsequently dampens the energy from the shock wave as it travels to the focus.[49] Of more importance as an outcome predictor than actual BMI may be skin-to-stone distance (SSD) as measured on computed tomography.[50] Several groups have reported stone-free rates to be significantly lower when SSD is >9 or 10 cm.[50,51] Although abdominal compression and an extended shock wave blast-path can be used to potentially improve results, the use of SWL in obese patients can be problematic.[52]

Renal anatomy of a patient as well is important. Ectopic renal units such as pelvic kidneys and horseshoe kidneys can be treated with SWL but may have a lower success rate. One report of SWL in horseshoe kidneys revealed a 31% stone-free rate over a 16-year experience, in addition to an increased need for secondary procedures and more shock waves needed per session.[53] Similarly, another report of SWL in 14 pelvic kidneys revealed a stone-free rate of 57% at 3 months.[54]

Patient anatomy further becomes important if the patient has an obstruction distal to the offending stone, such as a second more distal stone or a stricture. Shock wave lithotripsy is not advised in this circumstance as stone passage is unlikely. Significant hydronephrosis is associated with a lower stone-free rate. Additionally, SWL should not be used if infection and obstruction are present together, as the procedure could induce a dangerous urosepsis.[44] Urine culture is also always recommended as part of the preoperative evaluation.

Although the mechanism is not completely understood, outcomes have also been shown to be poorer with renal insufficiency.[55] Also, with theoretical risk of tissue injury secondary to SWL, it may be best to choose a different treatment modality should renal insufficiency be present.

In addition to patient-specific factors that limit the range of use, there are also critical stone features that can make SWL less than ideal. Specifically, stone size and number, composition, density, and location all play a role in the success rate of SWL. As stone size increases over 2 cm, there is a higher failure rate and a higher incidence of complications such as steinstrasse or partial obstruction and need for secondary procedures, limiting the use of SWL for these patients.[56-59] Given the results for stones over 2 cm, it is not surprising that the presence of a staghorn calculus is also associated with a poor outcome when SWL is used. Shock wave lithotripsy monotherapy for staghorn calculi is associated with a high chance for residual stone, need for multiple procedures, and increased procedure-specific complications, including acute loss of kidney, pain, bleeding, infection, and steinstrasse.[60] The 2005 AUA's Nephrolithiasis Guideline Panel recommends against the use of SWL as monotherapy for these patients, with the overall stone-free rate being only 54%.[60] Exceptions would be small stone burden and pediatric patients. Also, if the decision is made to proceed with SWL monotherapy in these special circumstances, drainage should be undertaken prior to the procedure with either stent or nephrostomy tube to help prevent obstruction and sepsis and to assist with passage of stone pieces. Although SWL is not the preferred choice for staghorn monotherapy, it can be used as an adjunct to other therapies to initially treat the large stone burden. For example, a residual fragment <2 cm following percutaneous nephrolithotomy is amenable to SWL. Also, if there are multiple stones within the kidney, energy cannot be realistically administered to all of them in one session, particularly if they are dispersed throughout the entire organ. Clinical scenarios with multiple stones present in the targeted kidney may best be treated with another procedure such as ureteroscopy, where the clearance rate may be higher with fewer sessions.

How easily a stone will fracture by SWL is directly related to its crystalline structure, which can be easily anticipated if its composition is known (i.e. in a recurrent stone former or via crystals present on urinalysis). Stone fragility can also be predicted by density as measured in Hounsfield units (HU) on preoperative axial imaging. Both brushite and cystine stones are relatively resistant to SWL.[61] The stone-free rate for brushite stones has been shown to be only 11% with multiple sessions needed and a 65% success rate, defined as residual fragments ≤4 mm.[62] Both Hockley and colleagues and Kachel and associates reported low stone-free rates for cystine stones undergoing SWL, particularly if >2 cm.[63,64] Chow and Streem confirmed these findings and suggested only small stone size is acceptable for SWL therapy.[65] AUA guidelines state that SWL monotherapy is not acceptable for staghorn calculi of cystine composition.[60] Calcium oxalate monohydrate also typically responds very poorly to SWL.[61] Lastly, matrix stones, with an internal structure of mostly (65%) organic matter, do not fracture well with SWL and are best treated with ureteroscopy or percutaneous nephrolithotomy.[66]

If stone composition is not known, the density of the calculus as measured by HU on preoperative axial imaging can predict stone fragility and response to SWL.[67] Joseph and associates found a significantly reduced stone-free rate of 54.5% for calculi >1,000 HU.[68] In contradistinction, if stones were <500 HU they found a 100% success rate, and for stones between 500 and 1,000 HU, the clearance rate was 85.7%. Gupta and collaborators found that HU predicted stone clearance by SWL better than stone size alone.[69] They found that over 70% of patients with calculus density over 750 HU needed three or more SWL sessions for only a 65% clearance rate, whereas if the stone was <750 HU, 80% needed three or fewer treatments.

Lastly, stone location influences outcome of SWL. Lower pole calculi, as one could imagine secondary to gravity, are most difficult to attain stone-free status with SWL, even if fragmentation occurs. Lower pole I was a study performed by Albala and collaborators comparing success rates for lower pole calculi treated with SWL or percutaneous nephrolithotomy.[70] This prospective, multi-center, randomized-controlled trial revealed a stone-free rate of 95% for PCNL versus 37% for SWL at 3 months post-operatively for lower pole stones. Combining two stone features, location and size, more strongly predicts treatment outcome. The stone-free rate for calculi in the lower pole was 63% (12/19) if <1 cm versus 14% (1/7) if >2 cm.[70] This study was followed by another prospective, multi-center, randomized-controlled trial, lower pole II, utilizing size as a criteria (<1 cm) and comparing ureteroscopy to SWL for lower pole stones.[71] There was no statistically significant difference between the two techniques, although there was a trend favoring ureteroscopy.

Ureteral location is also considered when choosing surgical technique. Shock wave lithotripsy of distal ureteral calculi, in addition to being contraindicated in young females of childbearing potential, is associated with lower success. The guidelines for the management of ureteral calculi pooled data on SWL outcomes, and their meta-analysis published in 2007 revealed an 82% stone-free rate in the proximal ureter, reporting on 41 studies with 6,428 patients; 73% stone-free rate in the mid ureter, reporting on 31 studies in 1,607 patients; and 74% stone-free rate in the distal ureter, reporting on 50 studies in 6,981 patients.[44] Stone-free rates were higher for each location when stone size was <1 cm.

An additional anatomic factor that can alter the success rate for treatment of lower pole calculi with SWL is infundibulopelvic angle and infundibular width and length. Elbahnasy and colleagues evaluated intrinsic renal anatomy using intravenous pyelogram features.[72] They found that a wide angle or short length with a broad width (regardless of angle) was associated with a higher success rate for SWL. As expected, upper pole, renal pelvic, and ureteropelvic junction stones have the highest success rates among stones treated with SWL when evaluating location.[73]

Calyceal diverticula are a unique clinical scenario that is controversial when discussing the appropriateness of SWL. With the neck of the diverticulum being classically quite narrow, it can be very challenging to fragment the stone enough to get clearance of all or any of the pieces. One study revealed a stone-free rate of only 21%.[74] However, despite the low clearance rate, many patients (60%) were still symptom free, although the mechanism to explain this is not known. Further study is needed to confirm this as follow-up was of a short duration. Patient selection may be key in this subgroup, with good visualization of the ostium on preoperative imaging, the diverticula filling with contrast, and stone size being small. Streem and Yost demonstrated good success rates for calyceal diverticular stones when these features were present.[75] Nonetheless, caution should be exercised when using SWL as a monotherapy for calyceal diverticular stones. It may be better used in adjunct with another technique such as ureteroscopy, with dilation of the diverticular neck following fragmentation with SWL.

Although the features discussed help predict outcome and are a general guideline for the range of use of SWL, realistically, many patients still desire an attempt with SWL, even if they are not the ideal candidate, because of its noninvasive nature. Patients will accept a risk of failed treatment and need for a secondary procedure, knowing no instrumentation will be necessary with the first attempt.

COMPLICATIONS

Shock wave lithotripsy is desirable because of its noninvasive nature and its overall minimal morbidity. Complication rate is overall low and major events are rare. However, SWL does carry its own unique risks. Most unfavorable consequences that occur are acute, minor, and self-limited. There are also some adverse outcomes associated with SWL that uncommonly may lead to more chronic issues. Herein, we review both acute and chronic complications that can occur secondary to SWL.

In 2009, a Task Force from the AUA published an up-to-date perspective on the complications associated with the SWL.[76] Their goals were to establish the safety of the procedure, determine the significance of any long-term consequences, weigh the risks and benefits of SWL, and inform the urologic community of these findings. They concluded that, overall, SWL is safe and effective; however, as with any surgical procedure, some risk is present and adverse events will occur. Research has revealed several strategies to minimize risk and maximize success, and the task force encouraged ongoing investigation to continue improvement of the technology. De la Rosette's group also reported in 2006 on their evaluation of 3,937 abstracts and 220 papers. They deemed SWL to be a safe stone treatment method when following the recommended range of uses and recognizing the limitations of the procedure.[77]

Some basic acute complications of SWL are well known and acceptable given the noninvasive nature of the procedure. Once the stone is fragmented, the pieces must travel out of the urinary tract in order to achieve a successful outcome. This can be associated with pain, which is initially managed with analgesics and has been estimated to occur in 40% of patients.[78] In circumstances where the acute renal colic is not controlled, admission to the hospital or a secondary procedure with stent placement and/or ureteroscopy may be necessary. Also requiring further intervention with an additional procedure is acute obstruction associated with a fragment too large to pass or signs of infection, such as fever. Steinstrasse, or "street of stones," is a unique, less common complication that consists of all stone fragments passing into the ureter simultaneously and obstructing the flow of urine, typically resulting in significant renal colic. Sometimes these pieces will pass on their own with conservative management, but drainage may be necessary with stent or nephrostomy tube and/or subsequent ureteroscopy. Steinstrasse happens 1–4% of the time, but is more common when treating a larger stone, occurring in up to 10% of cases with stones >2 cm and in up to 40% with staghorn stones.[45] Although stents can be placed to try to prevent this for larger stones, routine stenting is not recommended for routine SWL. Whether failure requiring subsequent procedures is also considered a complication, this can be reduced by applying the principles discussed in "Range of Uses" in the previous section. Retreatment is necessary in up to 37% of patients.[78]

Acute tissue damage from the shock wave energy with subsequent injury to the kidney is also a unique complication of SWL that has been shown to be dose-dependent with regard to the number of shocks and energy settings used.[20,26,76,79-81] This has been demonstrated extensively in numerous animal studies, with specific concern for vascular changes and injury seen.[80,82-84] Both shear with vessel rupture and cavitation have been identified as possible mechanisms for the vascular damage.[85-88] As discussed previously, ramping-up with a pretreatment protocol and a several-minute pause has been shown to reduce lesion size as measured by functional renal volume in animal studies, as has a slow treatment rate.[23-25,33,34] Clinically, vascular changes and injury can translate to intraparenchymal hemorrhage, subcapsular hematoma, and perinephric bleeding.[89-92] As mentioned earlier, anticoagulation and bleeding diatheses are contraindications to SWL, and bleeding complications will likely occur if these patients undergo the procedure. Not all bleeding is clinically detected, and many hematomas are incidentally diagnosed if imaging is performed. Symptomatic bleeding occurs in <1% of patients, whereas incidental detection on imaging raises the incidence to 25%.[93] Parenchymal bleeding is generally not able to be detected radiographically. If the patient is hemodynamically stable, bleeding and hematomas are managed conservatively and most resolve. Major bleeding is quite rare, but if it occurs, could result in the need for blood transfusion, acute renal failure, or, theoretically, loss of a kidney. Several studies identified risk factors for SWL-induced subcapsular hematoma.[92,93] Age is one risk factor, with the incidence of hematoma doubling every 10 years. Additionally, clinically significant hematomas have increased with the newer machines, with a current rate of 3–12%.[94] This is thought to be secondary to the higher pressures administered by contemporary machines. Gross hematuria is quite common and happens in over 30% of patients.[78]

Infection is also a potential complication from SWL, as it is with any surgical intervention; however, the rate is so low that no perioperative antibiotics are recommended by the AUA unless bacteriuria or an infected stone is present. If infection does occur, it could range from a low-grade bladder infection with minor symptoms to sepsis requiring intensive care. Symptomatic bacteriuria has been shown to occur in up to 10% of patients after SWL.[78] The rate of sepsis is <1% in standard SWL.[95] Sepsis is higher when treating a staghorn stone at 2.7%, and bacteremia after SWL can occur in up to 14% of cases.[56,77,95] Other predisposing factors for infection are pre-existing urinary infection, infected stones, multiple calculi, history of infections, obstruction, and urinary instrumentation at the time of SWL.[77]

Although bleeding, infection, pain, and the need for secondary procedures are the most common immediate complications, less common acute adverse events have been reported. Ferroni et al. reported renal vein thrombus in a young female with no evidence of hypercoagulability, resulting in pulmonary embolus and subsequent need for anticoagulation.[96] The final outcome for this patient was renal atrophy and complete loss of ipsilateral kidney function. Other incidences of venous thrombosis have been reported but associated with hypercoagulable states.[77]

Adjacent organ injury is rare, but can occur. Acute pancreatitis and injury to the liver, spleen, and lung have all been reported.[97] Theoretically, organomegaly could increase this risk, so we would advise against the use of SWL in these patients. Gastrointestinal injury to stomach, colon, bile duct, and small intestine, including erosion, ulcer, perforation, anastomotic dehiscence, and bleeding, have also been reported in patients undergoing SWL.[77,98] Psoas abscess has also been reported.[78] Arterial aneurysm is a relative contraindication for SWL as rupture has been reported following the procedure; although there is not literature supporting a causative effect, with other reasonable treatment options available, SWL is generally avoided in these patients.[99] Routine anesthesia risks are also present with the possibility of cardiovascular and stroke complications in susceptible patients. Cardiac arrhythmias can occur as well and are decreased by using gated SWL.[100] Lastly, development of antiglomerular basement membrane disease after SWL has also been reported.[101]

In addition to acute complications from SWL, there may also be chronic side effects. These potential long-term consequences are not as well understood as acute injury and are often hotly debated. Reports of new-onset hypertension have been made since the introduction of the technology in 1980.[76,102] Multiple studies over the years have found an association between SWL and high blood pressure, and age may be an independent risk factor.[76,102-105] A more recent population-based cohort did not reveal an association between SWL and new-onset hypertension.[106] Although it remains quite controversial and the mechanism is not known, this repeated link is cause for concern and needs further study, ideally with a long-term, prospective, randomized trial.

More well established is scar formation following SWL. This has been shown in both animal and human studies. Dose-dependent fibrosis and scarring have been shown to occur after SWL in dogs, pigs, and rabbits.[82,107] Radiographic proof with single photon emission computed tomography of human scarring has also been demonstrated after SWL, with decreased radiolabel uptake corresponding to areas larger than the focal zone when compared to preoperative imaging.[108] Despite the tissue injury demonstrated in animal studies and the scarring demonstrated in humans with short-term reduction of glomerular filtration rate, long-term renal insufficiency has not been demonstrated and is not reported in the literature.

More recently, attention has been given to the potential formation of diabetes mellitus following SWL. Krambeck et al. recently reported an increase in the incidence of new-onset diabetes mellitus following treatment with SWL using the Dornier HM3 lithotripter in 1985, based on a survey and 288 respondents.[102] These results remained true even after controlling for obesity; however, there were many issues with their study design and the study must be interpreted with caution. Several subsequent studies did not show a relationship between the development of diabetes mellitus and SWL; however, the methodology was also flawed in these studies, leaving the question still unanswered.[109,110] A more recent population-based cohort study showed no association between SWL and diabetes mellitus.[106] Although it may simply be that diabetes is associated with kidney stones in general and not necessarily related to SWL, this area still needs further research.

As discussed here, SWL is quite safe overall with a low complication rate. Common complications are of minimal severity, and major adverse effects are rare. Benefits overall outweigh risks, but it is important to be aware of the potential risks discussed, manage them appropriately should they occur, and take action to prevent them by following the general guidelines, realizing the limitations of the technology, and optimizing the outcome by properly selecting patients.

REFERENCES

1. Scales CD Jr, Krupski TL, Curtis LH, et al. Urologic Diseases of America Project. Practice variation in the surgical management of urinary lithiasis. J Urol. 2011;186(1):146-50.
2. Kerbl K, Rehman J, Landman J, et al. Current management of urolithiasis. J Endourol. 2002;16(5):281-8.
3. Pearle MS, Calhoun EA, Curhan GC. Urologic Diseases of America Project. Urologic diseases in America project: urolithiasis. J Urol. 2005;173(3):848-57.
4. Bierkans AF, Hendrikx AJ, de Kort VJ, et al. Efficacy of second generation lithotriptors: a multi-center comparative study of 2,206 extracorporeal shock wave lithotripsy treatment

with the Siemens Lihtostar, Dornier HM4, Wolf Piezolith 2300, Direx Tripter X-1, and Breakstone lithotriptors. J Urol. 1992;148(3 Pt 2):1052.
5. Zehnder P, Roth B, Birkhauser F, et al. A prospective randomised trial comparing the modified HM3 with the MODULITH SLX-F2 lithotripter. Eur Urol. 2011;59(4):637-44.
6. Chan SL, Stothers L, Rowley A, et al. A prospective trial comparing the efficacy and complications of the modified Dornier HM3 and MFL 5000 lithotriptors for solitary renal calculi. J Urol. 1995;153(6):1794-97.
7. Portis AJ, Yan Y, Pattaras JG, et al. Matched pair analysis of shock wave lithotripsy effectiveness for comparison of lithotriptors. J Urol. 2003;169(1):58-62.
8. Hoag CC, Taylor WN, Rowley VA. The efficacy of the Dornier Doli S lithotripter for renal stones. Can J Urol. 2006; 13(6):3358-63.
9. Pishchalnikov YA, Neucks JS, VonDerHaar Jn, et al. Air pockets trapped during routine coupling in dry head lithotripsy can significantly decrease the delivery of shock wave energy. J Urol. 2006;176:2706-10.
10. Neucks JS, Pishchalnikov YA, Zancanaro AJ, et al. Improved acoustic coupling for shock wave lithotripsy. Urol Res. 2008; 36:61-6.
11. Sheir KZ, Elhalwagy SM, Abo-Elghar ME, et al. Evaluation of a synchronous twin-pulse technique for shock wave lithotripsy: a prospective randomized study of effectiveness and safety in comparison to standard single-pulse technique. BJU Int 2007;101(11):1420-5.
12. Lingeman JE, MCAteer JA, Gnessin E, et al. Shock wave lithotripsy: Advances in technology and technique. Nat Rev Urol. 2009;6:660-70.
13. Sokolov DL, Bailey MR, Crum LA. Dual-pulse lithotripter accelerates stone fragmentation and reduces cell lysis in Vitro. Ultrasound Med Biol. 2003;29:1045-52.
14. Sokolov DL, Bailey MR, Crum LA. Use of a dual-pulse lithotripter to generate a localized and intensified cavitation field. J Acoustic Soc Am. 2001;110:1685-95.
15. Handa RK, McAteer JA, Evan AP, et al. Assessment of renal injury with a clinical dual head lithotriptor delivering 240 shock waves per minute. J Urol. 2009;181:884-9.
16. Handa RK, McAteer JA, Willis LR, et al. Dual-head lithotripsy in synchronous mode: Acute effect on renal function and-morphology in the pig. BJU Int. 2007;99(5):1134-42.
17. Ng CF, McLornan L, Thompson TJ, et al. Comparison of 2 generations of piezoelecric lithotriptors using matched pair analysis. J Urol. 2004;172(5 Pt 1):1887-91.
18. Cleveland RO, McAteer JA. The Physics of Shock Wave Lithotripsy. In: Smith AD, Badlani G, Bagley (eds). Smith's Textbook of Endourology. 2nd ed. Hamilton, ON, Canada: BC Decker, 2007: 317-332.
19. Lingeman JE, Beiko DT, Cleveland RO, et al. Stone Technology: Shock Wave and Intracorporeal Lithotripsy. In: Denstedt JD, Khoury S (eds). Stone Disease. Paris: Health Publications, 2008: 85-135.
20. Connors BA, Evan AP, Willis LR, et al. The effect of discharge voltage on renal injury and impairment caused by lithotripsy in the pig. J Am Soc Nephrol. 2000;112:310-8.
21. McAteer JA, Bailey MR, Williams JC Jr, et al. Strategies for improved shock wave lithotripsy. Minerva Urol Nefrol. 2005;574:271-87.
22. Zhou Y, Cocks FH, Preminger GM, et al. The effect of treatment strategy on stone comminution efficiency in shock wave lithotripsy. J Urol. 2004;1721:349-54.
23. Willis LR, Evan AP, Connors BA, et al. Prevention of lithotripsy-induced renal injury by pretreating kidneys with low-energy shock waves. J Am Soc Nephrol. 2006;173:663-73.
24. Connors BA, Evan AP, Blomgren PM, et al. Effect of initial shock wave voltage on shock wave lithotripsy-induced lesion size during step-wise voltage ramping. Br J Urol Int. 2009;103: 104-7.
25. McAteer JA, Evan AP, Williams JC Jr, et al. Treatment protocols to reduce renal injury during shock wave lithotripsy. Curr Opin Urol. 2009;19:192-5.
26. Willis LR, Evan AP, Connors BA, et al. Shockwave lithotripsy: dose-related effects on renal structure, hemodynamics, and tubular function. J Endourol. 2005;191:90-101.
27. Sapozhnikov OA, Maxwell AD, MacConaghy B, et al. A mechanistic analysis of stone fracture in lithotripsy. J Acoust Soc Am. 2007;1212:1190-202.
28. Cleveland RO, Sapozhnikov OA. Modeling elastic wave propagation in kidney stones with application to shock wave lithotripsy. J Acoust Soc Am. 2005;1184:2667-76.
29. Eisenmenger W, Du XX, Tang C, et al. The first clinical results of "Wide-focus And Low-Pressure" ESWL. Ultrasound Med Biol. 2002;28:769-74.
30. Evan AP, McAteer JA, Connors BA, et al. Independent assessment of a wide-focus, low-pressure electromagnetic lithotripter: absence of renal bioeffects in the pig. BJU Int. 2008;101(3):382-8.
31. Sorenson C, Chandhoke P, Moore M, et al. Comparison of intravenous sedation versus general anesthesia on the efficacy of the Doli 50 lithotriptor. J Urol. 2002;1681:35-7.
32. Eichel L, Batzold P, Erturk E. Operator experience and adequate anesthesia improve treatment outcome with third-generation lithotripters. J Endourol. 2001;157:671-3.
33. Evan AP, McAteer JA, Connors BA, et al. Renal injury during shock wave lithotripsy is significantly reduced by slowing the rate of shock wave delivery. BJU Int. 2007;100(3):624-7.
34. Connors BA, Evan AP, Blomgren PM, et al. Extracorporeal shock wave lithotripsy at 60 shock waves/min reduces renal injury in a porcine model. BJU Int. 2009;104(7):1004-8.
35. Madbouly K, El-Tiraifi AM, Seida M, et al. Slow versus fast shock wave lithotripsy rate for urolithiasis: a prospective randomized study. J Urol. 2005;2005(173):1.
36. Yilmaz E, Batislam E, Basar M, et al. Optimal frequency in extracorporeal shock wave lithotripsy: prospective randomized study. Urology. 2005;66(6):1160-4.
37. Pace KT, Ghiculete D, Harju M, et al. Shock wave lithotripsy at 60 or 120 shocks per minute: a randomized, double-blind trial. J Urol. 2005;174(2):595-9.
38. Chacko J, Moore M, Sankey N, et al. Does a slower treatment rate impact the efficacy of extracorporeal shock wave lithotripsy for solitary kidney or ureteral stones? J Urol. 2006;175(4):1370-3.

39. Kato Y, Yamaguchi S, Hori J, et al. Improvement of stone comminution by slow delivery rate of shock waves in extracorporeal lithotripsy. Int J Urol. 2006;13(12):1461-5.
40. Semins MJ, Trock BJ, Matlaga BR. The effect of shock wave rate on the outcome of shock wave lithotripsy: a meta-analysis. J Urol. 2008;179(1):1954-97.
41. Fernandez F, Fernandez G, Loske AM. Treatment time reduction: using tandem shockwaves for lithotripsy: an in vivo study. J Endourol. 2009;23:1247-53.
42. Zhou Y, Cocks FH, Preminger GM, et al. Innovations in shock wave lithotripsy technology: Updates in experimental studies. J Urol. 2004;172:1892-8.
43. Xi X, Zhong P. Improvement of stone fragmentation during shock-wave lithotripsy using a combined EH/PEAA shock-wave generator-in-vitro experiments. Ultrasound Med Biol. 2000;26:457-67.
44. Preminger GM, Tiselius HG, Assimos D, et al. Guideline for the management of ureteral calculi. J Urol. 2007;178(6): 2418-34.
45. D'Addessi A, Vittori M, Racioppi M, et al. Complications of extracorporeal shock wave lithotripsy for urinary stones: to know and to manage them - A review. Scientific World Journal. 2012;2012:1-6.
46. Carol PR, Shi RY. Genetic toxicity of high energy shockwaves: assessment using the induction of mutations or micronuclei in Chinese hamster ovary. J Urol. 1986;135:292.
47. Vieweg J, Weber HM, Miller K, et al. Female fertility following extracorporeal shock wave lithotripsy of distal ureteral calculi. J Urol. 1992;148:1007.
48. Gulum M, Yeni E, Kocyigit A, et al. Sperm DNA damage and seminal oxidative status after shock-wave lithotripsy for distal ureteral stones. Fertil Steril. 2011;96(5):1087-90.
49. Pareek G, Armenakas NA, Panagopoulos G, et al. Extracorporeal shock wave lithotripsy success based on body mass index and Hounsfield units. Urology. 2005;651:33-6.
50. Pareek G, Hedican SP, Lee FT Jr, et al. Shock wave lithotripsy success determined by skin-to-stone distance on computed tomograpy. Urology. 2005;665:941-4.
51. Perks AE, Schuler TD, Lee J, et al. Stone attenuation and skin-to-stone distance on computed tomography predicts for stone fragmentation by shock wave lithotripsy. Urology. 2008;724:765-9.
52. Thomas R, Cass AS. Extracorporeal shock wave lithotripsy in morbidly obese patients. J Urol. 1993;1501:30-2.
53. Viola D, Anagnostou T, Thompson TJ, et al. Sixteen years of experience with stone management in horseshoe kidneys. Urol Int. 2007;783:214-8.
54. Tunc L, Tokgoz H, Tan MO, et al. Stones in anomalous kidneys: results of treatment by shock wave lithotripsy in 150 patients. Int J Urol. 2004;1110:831-6.
55. Hung SF, Chung SD, Wang SM, et al. Chronic kidney disease affects the stone-free rate after extracorporeal shock wave lithotripsy for proximal ureteric stones. BJU Int. 2010;105(8):1162-7.
56. Lingeman JE, Coury TA, Newman DM, et al. Comparison of results and morbidity of percutaneous nephrostolithotomy and extracorporeal shock wave lithotripsy. J Urol. 1987;138(3):485-90.
57. Egilmez T, Tekin MI, Gonen M, et al. Efficacy and safety of a new-generation shockwave lithotripsy machine in the treatment of single renal or ureteral stones: experience with 2670 patients. J Endourol. 2007;21(1):23-7.
58. Galvin DJ, Pearle MS. The contemporary management of renal and ureteric calculi. BJU Int. 2006;986:1283-8.
59. Abe T, Akakura K, Kawaguchi M, et al. Outcomes of shock-wave lithotripsy for upper urinary-tract stones: a large-scale study at a single institution. J Endourol. 2005;19(7):768-73.
60. Preminger GM, Assimos D, Lingeman JE, et al. AUA Nephrolithiasis Guideline Panel. Chapter 1: AUA guideline on management of staghorn calculi: diagnosis and treatment recommendations. J Urol. 2005;173(6):1991-2000.
61. Williams JC Jr, Saw KC, Paterson RF, et al. Variability of renal stone fragility in shock wave lithotripsy. Urology. 2003;61(6): 1092-6.
62. Klee LW, Brito CG, Lingeman JE. The clinical implications of brushite calculi. J Urol. 1991;145(4):715-8.
63. Hockley NM, Lingeman JE, Hutchinson CL. Relative efficacy of extracorporeal shock wave lithotripsy and percutaneous nephrolithotomy in the management of cystine calculi. J Endourol. 1989;2:273-85.
64. Kachel TA, Vijan SR, Dretler SP. Endourological experience with cystine calculi and a treatment algorithm. J Urol. 1991;145(1):25-8.
65. Chow GK, Streem SB. Contemporary urological intervention for cystinuric patients: immediate and long-term impact and implications. J Urol. 1998;160(2):344-5.
66. Bani-Hani AH, Segura JW, Leroy AJ. Urinary matrix calculi: our experience at a single institution. J Urol 2005;173(1): 120-3.
67. Saw KC, McAteer JA, Fineberg NS, et al. Calcium stone fragility is predicted by helical CT attenuation values. J Endourol. 2000;14(6):471-4.
68. Joseph P, Mandal AK, Singh SK, et al. Computerized tomography attenuation value of renal calculus: can it predict successful fragmentation of the calculus by extracorporeal shock wave lithotripsy? A Preliminary study. J Urol. 2002;167(5):1968-71.
69. Gupta NP, Ansari MS, Kesarvani P, et al. Role of computed tomography with no contrast medium enhancement in predicting the outcome of extracorporeal shock wave lithotripsy for urinary calculi. BJU Int. 2005;95(0):1285-8.
70. Albala DM, Assimos DG, Clayman RV, et al. Lower pole I: a prospective randomized trial of extracorporeal shock wave lithotripsy and percutaneous nephrolithotomy for lower pole nephrolithiasis-initial results. J Urol. 2001;166(6):2072-80.
71. Pearle MS, Lingeman JE, Leveilee RJ, et al. Prospective randomized trial comparing shock wave lithotripsy and ureteroscopy for lower pole caliceal calculi 1cm or less. J Urol 2005;173(6):2005-9.
72. Elbahnasy AM, Shalhav AL, Hoenig DM, et al. Lower caliceal stone clearance after shock wave lithotripsy or ureteroscopy: the impact of lower pole radiographic anatomy. J Urol. 1998;159(3):676-82.
73. Weld KJ, Montiglio C, Morris MS, et al. Shock wave lithotripsy success for renal stones based on patient and stone computed tomography characteristics. Urology. 2007;706:1043-6.

74. Turna B, Raza A, Moussa SA, et al. Management of calyceal diverticular stones with extracorporeal shock wave lithotripsy and percutaneous nephrolithotomy: long-term outcome. BJU Int. 2007;100(1):151-6.
75. Streem SB, Yost A. Treatment of caliceal diverticular calculi with extracorporeal shock wave lithotripsy: patient selection and extended followup. J Urol. 1992;148(3 Pt 2):1043-6.
76. Lingeman JE, McAteer JA, Assimos DG, et al. Current Perspective on Adverse Effects in Shock Wave Lithotripsy. American Urological Association Education and Research Inc. 2009.
77. Skolarikos A, Alivizatos G, de la Rosette J. Extracorporeal shock wave lithotripsy 25 years later: complications and Their Prevention. EAU. 2006;50:981-90.
78. Salem S, Mehrsai A, Zartab H, et al. Complications and outcomes following extracorporeal shock wave lithotripsy: a prospective study of 3,241 patients. Urol Res. 2010;38:135-42.
79. Connors BA, Evan AP, Blomgren PM, et al. Reducing shock number dramatically decreases lesion size in a juvenile kidney model. J Endourol. 2006;20(9):607-11.
80. Evan AP, Willis LR, Lingeman JE, et al. Renal trauma and the risk of long-term complications in shock wave lithotripsy. Nephron. 1998;78(1):1-8.
81. McAteer JA, Evan AP. The acute and long-term adverse effects of shock wave lithotripsy. Semin Nephrol. 2008;28(2):200-13.
82. Newman R, Hackett R, Senior D, et al. Pathological effects of ESWL on canine renal tissue. Urology. 1987;29(2):194-200.
83. Shao Y, Connors BA, Evan AP, et al. Morphological changes induced in the pig kidney by extracorporeal shock wave lithotripsy: nephron injury. Anat Rec A Discov Mol Cell Evol Biol. 2003;275(1):979-89.
84. Willis LR, Evan AP, Connors BA, et al. Relationship between kidney size, renal injury, and renal impairment induced by shock wave lithotripsy. J Am Soc Nephrol. 1999;10(8):1753-62.
85. Zhong P, Zhou Y, Zhu S. Dynamics of bubble oscillation in constrained media and mechanisms of vessel rupture in SWL. Ultrasound Med Biol. 2001;27(1):119-34.
86. Zhong P, Cioanta J, Zhu S, et al. Effects of tissue constraint on shock wave-induced bubble expansion in vivo. J Acoust Soc Am. 1998;104(5):3126-9.
87. Matlaga BR, McAteer JA, Connors BA, et al. Potential for cavitation-mediated tissue damage in shockwave lithotripsy. J Endourol. 2008;22(1):121-6.
88. Evan AP, Willis LR, McAteer JA, et al. Kidney damage and renal functional changes are minimized by waveform control that suppresses cavitation in shock wave lithotripsy. J Urol. 2002;168(4 pt 1):1556-62.
89. Krishnamurthi V, Streem SB. Long-term radiographic and functional outcome of extracorporeal shock wave lithotripsy induced perirenal hematomas. J Urol. 1995;154:1673-5.
90. Maziak DE, Ralph-Edwards A, Deitel M, et al. Massive perirenal and intra-abdominal bleeding after shock-wave lithotripsy: case report. Can J Surg. 1994;37(4):329-32.
91. Knapp PM, Kulb TB, Lingeman JE, et al. Extracorporeal shock wave lithotripsy-induced perirenal hematomas. J Urol. 1988;139(4):700-3.
92. Newman DM, Saltzman B. Idenitifying risk factors in development of clinically significant post-shock-wave lithotripsy subcapsular hematomas. Urology. 1991;38(1):35-8.
93. Dhar NB, Thornton J, Karafa MT, et al. A multivariate analysis of risk factors associated with subcapsular hematoma formation following electromagnetic shock wave lithotripsy. J Urol. 2004;172(6):2271-4.
94. Krambeck AE. Bioeffects of shock wave lithotripsy: an update. AUA News. 2014;February:24.
95. Muller-Mattheis VGO, Schmale D, Seewald M, et al. Bacteremia during extracorporeal shock wave lithotripsy of renal calculi. J Urol 1991;146(3):733-6.
96. Ferroni MC, Turner RM, Semins MJ. Acute renal vein thrombus and renal atrophy following shock wave lithotripsy: a unique complication. Can J Urol. 2014;21(1):7151-3.
97. Abe H, Nisimura T, Osawa S, et al. Acute pancreatitis caused by extracorporeal shock wave lithotripsy for bilateral renal pelvic calculi. Int J Urol 2000;7(2):65-8.
98. Maker V, Layke J. Gastrointestinal injury secondary to extracorporeal shock wave lithotripsy: a review of the literature since its inception. J Am Coll Surg. 2004;198:128-35.
99. Tse GH, Qazi HA, Halsall AK, et al. Shockwave lithotripsy: arterial aneurysm and vascular complications. J Endourol. 2011;25(3):403-11.
100. Zanetti G, Ostini F, Montanari E, et al. Cardiac dysrhythmias induced by extracorporeal shockwave lithotripsy. J Endourol. 1999;13(6):409-12.
101. Xenocostas A, Jothy S, Collins B, et al. Anti-glomerular basement membrane glomerulonephritis after extracorporeal shockwavelithotripsy. Am J Kidney Dis. 1999;33(1): 128-32.
102. Krambeck AE, Gettman MT, Rohlinger AL, et al. Diabetes mellitus and hypertension associated with shock wave lithotripsy of renal and proximal ureteral stones at 19 years of follow-up. J Urol. 2006;175(5):1742-7.
103. Jewett MAS, Bombardier C, Logan AG. A randomized controlled trial to assess the incidence of new onset hypertension in patients after shock wave lithotripsy for asymptomatic renal calculi. J Urol. 1998;160:1241.
104. Janetschek G, Frauscher F, Knapp R, et al. New onset hypertension after extracorporeal shock wave lithotripsy: age related incidence and prediction by intrarenal resistive index. J Urol. 1997;158:346.
105. Elves AWS, Tilling K, Menezes P. Early observations of the effect of extracorporeal shockwave lithotripsy on blood pressure: a prospective randomized control clinical trial. BJU Int. 2000;85:611.
106. de Cogain M, Krambeck AE, Rule AD, et al. Shock wave lithotripsy and diabetes mellitus: a population based cohort study. Urology. 2012;79(2):298-302.
107. Morris MS, Hussmann DA, Wilson WT. Temporal effects of shock wave lithotripsy. J Urol. 1991;145:881.
108. Lechevallier E, Siles S, Ortega MC. Comparison by SPECT of renal scars after extracorporeal shock wave lithotripsy and percutaneous nephrolithotomy. J Endourol. 1993;7: 465.
109. Makhlouf AA, Thorner D, Ugarte R. Shock wave lithotripsy not associated with development of diabetes mellitus at 6 years of follow-up. Urology. 2009;73:4.
110. Sato Y, Tanda H, Kato S. Shock wave lithotripsy for renal stones is not associated with hypertension and diabetes mellitus. Urology. 2008;71:586.

CHAPTER

32 Ureteroscopy in the Management of Stones

Fernando Cabrera, Michael Lipkin, Glenn M Preminger

INTRODUCTION

Ureteroscopy (URS) has quickly evolved to become one of the most common procedures performed by urologists. Advances in technology, including improved fiberoptics and optical chips, have allowed for the development of smaller, safer, and more efficient instruments with improved high-definition optics. Additional devices, including ureteral access sheaths (UASs), intracorporeal lithotripters, and stone retrieval devices, have also been developed to facilitate stone fragmentation and removal. This chapter will consist of a comprehensive review regarding URS for the treatment of nephrolithiasis.

HISTORY AND DEVELOPMENT

Blind extraction of ureteral stones was initially reported by Gustav Kolisher.[1] He described passing a metal-tipped catheter into the ureteral orifice to inject viscous oil to displace stones.[1] As technology improved, so did techniques and equipment used for the treatment of renal and ureteral stones. Hugh Hampton Young performed the first unplanned URS and pyeloscopy in 1929. While performing cystoscopy on a patient with posterior urethral valves, he was able to advance the pediatric cystoscope into a dilated ureter to the level of the renal pelvis and intrarenal collecting system.[2] Ureteroscopes were then developed using the knowledge and techniques evolved from regular rigid cystoscopy. Curtiss and Hirschowitz combined their knowledge of fiberoptics and physics to create the first flexible endoscope in 1957. They fused optical glass rods together into small fibers to allow individual movement. Finally, they used another layer of glass material with a low refractive index over the fused fibers that would allow light to travel to the distal end of the endoscope. This principle was called total internal reflectance, and was a breakthrough for modern endoscopy in 1957.[3]

The first flexible ureteroscopes, although described 10 years earlier than rigid ureteroscopes, lacked the aid of irrigation channels and deflection mechanisms. Marshall performed the first flexible URS and renoscopy in 1964 by passing the ureteroscope in a retrograde fashion through a ureterotomy.[4] In the past three decades, multiple advancements have allowed active deflection and improved optics. Recent flexible scopes have been introduced with up to 270° of primary deflection. The recent development of complementary metal oxide semiconductor (CMOS) chips has allowed for the design of ureteroscopes with significantly improved resolution and color reproduction as compared with traditional fiberoptic flexible ureteroscopes.[5]

The first rigid ureteroscopes were developed in the late 1970s and used a large rod lens that evolved from pediatric cystoscopes.[6] Modern rigid or semirigid ureteroscopes are smaller and more flexible thanks to the use of fiberoptics.

The development of intracorporeal lithotripsy devices has also been essential for the advancement of the field of endourology. In 1955, Yutkin used a spark plug to develop a powerful shock wave to fragment stones in a liquid environment. This technology was then refined in the late 1970s into a 9-Fr flexible probe that could be passed through a cystoscope or ureteroscope to treat nephrolithiasis.[128] These advances have paved the way for more modern intracorporeal lithotripsy.

INDICATIONS FOR URETEROSCOPY

Increasing miniaturization of ureteroscopes and improvements in intracorporeal lithotripsy and stone manipulation have decreased the morbidity of URS. These advances have allowed for the treatment of stones ureteroscopically independent of stone location, stone size, and stone composition. The indication to treat ureteral and renal stones is multifactorial and depends on stone and patient factors.

Stone Location

Ureteral Stones

Ureteral stones are a common cause of patient morbidity and are usually associated with renal colic and obstruction.

Table 32.1: Indications for the treatment of ureteral stones.

Stone factors	*Patient factors*
Location	Persistent pain despite adequate analgesic medication
Stone size	Renal insufficiency (renal failure, bilateral obstruction, or solitary kidney)
Stone composition: Ca Ox, brushite, cystine	Persistent obstruction
	Social situation of the patient (pilots or business travel)

There are clear indications for treatment of ureteral stones, including intractable pain, infection, severe obstruction with worsening renal function, and a stone that is unlikely to pass or has failed spontaneous passage. Also, patients who are not candidates for conservative management (pilots) should undergo treatment. Table 32.1 lists the current indications for the treatment of ureteral stones according to the American Association of Urology (AUA) and European Association of Urology (EAU) guidelines.[7,8]

Historically, shock wave lithotripsy (SWL) was the procedure of choice for proximal ureteral stones. According to the AUA guidelines in 1997, SWL was first-line therapy for stones <1 cm in the proximal ureter with an 83% stone-free rate (SFR). The historical suboptimal success of URS for proximal ureteral stones reflected the inability to reach stones in the proximal ureter and safely remove fragments. In addition, retropulsion of the stones into the kidney was a significant limitation due to lack of flexible instrumentation.[9] With recent advancements in semirigid, flexible URS, and intracorporeal lithotripsy, the outcomes of treatment of proximal stones are similar to treatment of distal ureteral stones. The distinction between outcomes is less dependent on location in the ureter and more dependent on other factors like stone size.[10,11] Hyams et al. recently published a prospective, multi-institutional cohort study of patients undergoing flexible URS for proximal ureteral stones <2 cm in size. Using rigid criteria for postoperative assessment of SFRs, they demonstrated a 95% SFR, associated with low morbidity and complication rates.

Currently, SWL and URS are the most common modalities for the treatment of ureteral stones. In 2007 AUA/EAU guidelines on ureteral stones presented a meta-analysis that suggested that both URS and SWL are first-line therapy for the treatment of ureteral stones. They reported that for distal ureteral stones URS had better SFRs (94%) compared to SWL (74%).[12] The two procedures had a comparable SFR for the treatment of proximal ureteral stones, just over 80% for both procedures. However, the meta-analysis showed that these studies were generally small, reported the outcomes of semirigid rather than flexible technology, and used variable types of lithotripsy techniques and different methods to assess postoperative SFRs. Regardless, patients might still prefer SWL over URS since it is a less invasive modality and by historical data, URS has a higher ureteral stricture rate.[13] The Cochrane Collaboration recently published a meta-analysis comparing SWL and URS for the treatment of ureteral stones.[14] They included seven randomized trials for a total of 1,205 patients. Ureteroscopic removal was associated with significantly improved SFRs. Auxiliary procedures were higher in the URS group, since more patients require ureteral stents after URS. Minor complications were also higher in the URS, including rates of urinary tract infections (UTIs). Although they report an increase in hospital stay in the URS group, most ureteroscopic cases performed in the United States are ambulatory. Although they report more morbidity in the URS group, all the cases were performed with a rigid ureteroscope, which could be associated with higher complications compared to a flexible ureteroscope. Recent cost analysis has determined that SWL is less cost effective than URS, since patients may require more than one procedure to clear their stones.[15]

A recent study by the Clinical Research Office of the Endourology Society Ureteroscopy Global Study Group compared the differences in outcomes after URS for different ureteral stone locations.[16] They reviewed 9,681 patients who underwent URS and compared outcomes for different stone location. They found excellent SFRs for distal and midureteral stones, with close to 90% SFRs. They found lower SFRs for proximal ureteral stones (85%). Low intraoperative and postoperative complication rates were reported, although long-term follow-up was not available in this study.

Renal Calculi

Regardless of treatment approach, renal stones should be treated in the presence of obstruction and a history of infected stones. Patients with renal colic, loss of renal function, or stone growth might benefit from treatment. Table 32.2 shows the indications for retrograde intrarenal stone surgery according to the recent EAU guidelines.[8]

Selection of specific treatment modality depends on stone size, stone location, and composition (i.e. staghorn vs nonstaghorn calculus). Patient characteristics, including the use of anticoagulants, anatomic variations, and to

Table 32.2: Indications for ureteroscopy for renal stones.

Stone factors	*Patient factors*
Stone growth, obstruction caused by stones	Symptomatic stones (renal colic, hematuria)
Stones in high-risk patients for stone formation (cystinuria)	Patient preference
Stones >15 mm, stones <15 mm if observation is not the option of choice	Comorbidities
Stone composition: Ca Ox, brushite, cysteine	Social situation of the patient (pilots or business travel)
Infection	Immunocompromised patients

some degree patient preference, influence management decision. Until recently most renal stones were treated with SWL or percutaneous nephrolithotomy (PNL) alone. Now flexible URS allows easy access to virtually every part of the upper collecting system. The development of new devices, including access sheaths, baskets, and lasers, has allowed for an expanding role of URS for the treatment of intrarenal stones.

Recent guidelines suggest SWL, URS, and PNL, either alone or in combination, as viable treatment options for 1–2 cm renal stones.[8] They recommend SWL as first-line option for renal stones 1–2 cm in size. The exception to this is stones located in the lower pole calix in which URS achieves better SFRs and lower retreatment rates.[17] The dependent nature of the lower pole, including a long lower infundibulum and acute angle of the calix, has been hypothesized as the reason for decreased SFR after SWL for lower pole stones in earlier series.[18] In a randomized controlled trial performed in 2005, patients with lower pole stones were randomized to retrograde intrarenal surgery (RIRS) or SWL. The authors did not find a significant difference for the two modalities when treating smaller lower pole stones and reported that SWL was associated with less morbidity.[13] In a more recent study, Koo and his group performed a retrospective study that compared SWL versus flexible URS in the treatment of lower pole renal calculi; they found similar SFRs but that SWL was more cost effective.[19]

Current guidelines recommend PNL as first-line treatment for renal stones >2 cm in size. Despite its high success rate, PNL is still associated with significant complications including urinary extravasation, bleeding requiring transfusion, visceral injury, and pleural effusion. The term RIRS refers to the ureteroscopic treatment of intrarenal renal calculi, including renal pelvic or caliceal stones. Currently, RIRS is considered second-line treatment unless a contraindication exists for PNL, in which case SWL or URS would be performed.[20]

Recent advances in RIRS have allowed safe and effective treatment of intrarenal stones. A recent meta-analysis comparing PNL, URS, and mini-PNL reported significantly higher stone-free and complication rates for the PNL group. The URS group had less complications overall and better SFRs than mini-PNL.[21]

Stone Size

The EAU, AUA, and Japanese guidelines suggest that SWL and URS are acceptable first-line options for managing ureteral stones <2 cm in size.[8,12,22] Although SWL has a high success rate for solitary, small, proximal ureteral stones, efficiency is decreased for larger impacted proximal ureteral stones. Wu et al. in 2005 assessed 220 patients treated with URS or SWL for proximal ureteral stones. Overall stone rates for SWL and URS were 63.9% and 83.2%, respectively. Patients treated for upper ureteral stones of >1 cm achieved a SFR of 35%. In this study, URS for proximal ureteral stones of >1 cm was associated with a SFR of 76.8%.[23]

In selected patients, URS and RIRS might be a reasonable option for larger stone burdens. One group recently reported on their outcomes of 145 patients with large (>2 cm) proximal ureteral and renal stones treated with RIRS.[24] They included 164 stone burdens with a mean stone size of 29 mm and performed 1.6 procedures for each stone burden. They demonstrated 97% and 94% for proximal ureter and renal pelvis stones, respectively. They observed lower stone-clearance rates in lower pole and staghorn stones with 83% and 81%, respectively. The major indications for RIRS in this series were a failed prior PNL, morbid obesity, and patient preference. They reported no intraoperative complications and did not mention any postoperative complications.

For the management of larger renal stones (>2 cm), several trials have been performed comparing RIRS and PNL. The outcomes associated with PNL (SFRs) are better than RIRS, but the complication rates with PNL tend to be higher, although some studies found this difference not statistically significant.[25] Retrograde intrarenal surgery is less invasive than PNL, which is an advantage; however, it often requires staged procedures to treat these large stones.[26] In patients with a contraindication to PNL, such as irreversible coagulopathy, RIRS offers a viable alternative in treating these large stones.

A recent meta-analysis that compared RIRS, standard PNL, and micro-PNL extracted data from 10 studies, including two randomized controlled trials.[21] In the study standard, PNL was associated with higher SFR, a higher complication rate, and a larger drop in hematocrit. Compared to standard PNL, RIRS was associated with a shorter hospital stay and no difference was found in terms of operative times and auxiliary procedures.

Retrograde intrarenal surgery can achieve satisfactory outcomes for larger intrarenal stones of >2 cm. Tepeler et al. performed a matched paired analysis of 34 patients treated with RIRS for stones between 2 and 4 cm who were then compared to PNL.[27] Mean stone size for both groups was 270 mm^2. Stone-free rates with one session were 73.5% and 91.2% for RIRS and PNL, respectively. Although patients undergoing PNL had a better SFR, they also had a higher complication rate and need for blood transfusions.

Stone Composition

The composition of renal stones has been shown to be a predictor for the success of SWL.[28] Cystine and calcium oxalate monohydrate stones produce large fragments that can be difficult to fragment or pass from the collecting system when treated with SWL.[29] In vitro fragmentation of different stone compositions has been shown to vary with the holmium:YAG (Ho:YAG) laser. Calcium oxalate stones tend to be more resistant to produce craters and usually require more energy to fragment.[30] In clinical terms, stone composition has been shown to have little effect on operating times for ureteroscopic lithotripsy using the Ho:YAG laser.[31] Therefore, these types of stones tend to be more resistant to SWL and should be treated with URS or PNL.

Cystine stone formers have a high rate of stone recurrence and undergo multiple surgical procedures to treat their stones. Therefore, a minimally invasive approach with URS is preferable to conserve renal function.[32] There are minimal data regarding RIRS for the treatment of struvite stones. Retrograde intrarenal surgery for struvite stones is usually reserved for patients who are not candidates for more invasive surgical options. In the absence of active infection and stone matrix, Grasso et al. reported a 76% SFR with a single procedure and a 91% SFR after a staged procedure for smaller struvite stones.

Patient Factors

Obesity

In contrast to SWL, URS has been shown to be equally efficacious in terms of SFRs in normal, overweight, and obese patients.[33] Regarding morbidity, Preminger et al. found no difference in obese patients treated for ureteral stones and found the ureteroscopic approach preferable for those without an excessively large stone burden.[12]

Anticoagulation

For patients who are taking pharmacologic anticoagulation, it is preferable to discontinue these agents prior to URS. For patients who cannot safely discontinue these agents or who have an inherent coagulopathy, URS with laser lithotripsy has been shown to be effective and safe.[34] The electrohydraulic lithotripter should be avoided due to possible increase in bleeding risk.[35] Turna et al. published a match pair analysis comparing patients who had undergone flexible URS while anticoagulated and those who were not. In either arm, none of the procedures were aborted and there was no difference in SFRs and intraoperative or postoperative complications, including postoperative hemorrhage and thromboembolic events.[36]

Anatomic Deformity

Patients with anatomic deformities are not uncommon in the pediatric urologic population. These patients can usually have a neurogenic bladder, spinal deformities, and limb contractures that can limit surgical stone retrieval. In these cases, the use of spreader bars and flexible instruments, including the flexible cystoscope, ureteroscope, and access sheaths, is advantageous.

Colangelo and colleagues reported a series of pediatric patients with spinal hardware and spinal deformities with ureteral stones treated with URS.[37] Although they reported a decreased SFR and a higher complication rate, this is likely due to a larger median stone size and immobility in this cohort.

Cost

Multiple studies have performed analyses to determine the cost efficiency of different ureteral stone treatment modalities. Lotan and Wolf reviewed their series of patients with ureteral stones and found the initial SWL treatment to be more expensive than URS. This difference increased when adding the additional costs of complications and retreatment in the SWL group.[38,39] In a recent published retrospective series, URS was found to be more cost effective than SWL for the treatment of renal stones of <1.5 cm.[15]

CONTRAINDICATIONS

There is no absolute contraindications for URS, but patients with an active infection/UTI should be treated appropriately prior to treatment to avoid bacteremia and sepsis. Some relative contraindications include a large stone burden and struvite stone with matrix. Conditions that alter renal and collecting system anatomy, preventing safe access to the stone, might be considered relative contraindications as well in selected patients. Anatomic anomalies, including ureteral stricture, previous ureteral reimplantation, urinary diversion, caliceal diverticulum, and transureteroureterostomy, may make accessing the ureter and kidney more challenging endoscopically.

PREOPERATIVE PREPARATION

An appropriate clinical history and physical examination should complement additional laboratory workup prior to deciding on treatment modality. Additionally, upper tract imaging is necessary to identify stone location, burden, and any anatomic anomalies. A history of prior urologic surgery or gynecologic pelvic surgery, malignancies or radiation should be inquired. Previous endourologic manipulation, including a history of ureteral strictures, is important for assessment. Please refer to Chapter 32 for preoperative preparations for stone surgery.

Patient Expectations

Patients with symptomatic nephrolithiasis or ureteral stones who elect for treatment of their stones should have a clear understanding of all treatment options and related risks. For URS they should understand the risk of inability to access or eliminate the stone, requiring additional or staged procedures. They should also be counseled on possible intraoperative and postoperative complication risks. Patients should also understand the possibility of requiring a temporary ureteral stent following URS. Following the URS they should have a clear understanding of how long they will have the stent and clear plans for its removal. Stents can be removed by pulling on an attached string or cystoscopically. Stent-related symptoms, as well as appropriate interventions to alleviate symptoms, should be clearly explained to the patient.

Imaging

Imaging plays an important role in the diagnosis and management of nephrolithiasis. Prior to selecting the treatment modality, imaging is used to determine the stone location, burden, and composition. Plain abdominal radiography [kidneys, ureters, and bladder (KUB)], renal ultrasound (US) and/or noncontrast computed tomography (NCCT) can be used in the initial diagnosis of suspected nephrolithiasis. Other modalities performed include intravenous pyelogram (IVP), digital tomosynthesis (tomos), and magnetic resonance imaging.

Noncontrast computed tomography has become the first-line imaging modality for the evaluation of patients with nephrolithiasis due to its high sensitivity and specificity of 96% and 98%, respectively.[40,41] Noncontrast computed tomography also allows identification of other possible pathology, gives adequate anatomy data, and identifies the presence of hydronephrosis, perinephric stranding, and other renal pathology. It also allows for evaluation of other causes of flank pain. Additional pathologic conditions have been found in up to 47% of patients undergoing NCCT.[42]

Ultrasound, unlike NCCT, is inexpensive and not associated with radiation exposure to the patient. Sensitivities and specificities for evaluating renal stones vary from 29% to 81% and 82% to 90%.[43,44] Ultrasound is less useful for identifying ureteral stones compared to renal stones, especially for smaller stones <4 mm in size and in heavier patients.[45]

Historically, IVP and KUB were considered the standard for evaluation of renal colic and urolithiasis. Intravenous pyelogram is useful for evaluating renal anatomy, filling defects, and pelvicaliectasis. The sensitivities and specificities for IVP are lower when compared to NCCT at 85% and 90%, respectively. The limitations of IVP compared to NCCT are the use of intravenous (IV) contrast and the potential for adverse reactions. The sensitivity and specificity of plain KUB are poor when compared to NCCT and US; ranges are 45–58% sensitive and 69–77% specific. The use of US and KUB in combination greatly increases sensitivity and specificity in the detection of ureteral stones.[46]

Antibiotic Prophylaxis

The purpose of antibiotic prophylaxis prior to URS is to prevent infectious complications. There are limited data recommending antibiotic use prior to URS in low-risk patients. According to the EAU panel on antibiotic prophylaxis, antibiotic prophylaxis should be stratified according to patient risk factors. This assessment includes patient comorbidities and special risk factors that increase the bacterial load in the patient. Some factors that may increase the bacterial load include urinary obstruction, external catheter, indwelling stents, and a recent or prolonged hospitalization. URS cases should be distinguished between low-risk procedures, including diagnostic procedures and distal ureteral stones, and high-risk procedures, including larger, impacted, more proximal stones. Low-risk procedures should only undergo a single dose of prophylaxis when patients are high risk. Antibiotics for diagnostic URS include second-generation cephalosporins or *trimethoprim*-sulfamethoxazole (TMP/SMX). For distal ureteral stones, second- and third-generation cephalosporin, TMP/SMX, fluoroquinolones, or aminopenicillin/β-lactamase inhibitors can be used. For higher-risk procedures, including URS for proximal, intrarenal, or impacted stones, all patients should receive a short course of prophylactic antibiotics with second- or third-generation cephalosporin, TMP/SMX, *fluoroquinolones*, or aminopenicillin/β-lactamase inhibitor.

The current AUA best practice statement recommends a short course of prophylaxis for <24 hours for all patients undergoing URS. They recommend a *fluoroquinolone* or TMP/SMX as first-line agents and aminopenicillin/β-lactamase inhibitor, second- or third-generation cephalosporin, and an aminoglycoside with or without ampicillin as second-line agents.

A urine chemistry or urine culture is recommended prior to ureteroscopic stone surgery, and patients with an active infection should be treated appropriately. Patients who are considered at high risk for infectious complications, such as those with indwelling catheters, recurrent UTIs, large stone burden, who are immunocompromised, and those with neurologic deficits, can be placed on culture-specific antibiotics prior to their surgery. The length and benefit of extended preprocedure antibiotics is controversial, but in general positive urine cultures are often treated with 1 week of culture-specific antibiotics. For those at risk with a negative culture, consideration can be given to starting an oral antibiotic such as nitrofurantoin 1 week prior to their procedure.

A recent online survey was sent to the members of the Endourological Society, querying the duration of antibiotics prior to uncomplicated URS. Most respondents reported giving a single perioperative dose to patients with a negative urine culture (71%). In patients with positive cultures, there were more heterogeneous responses. In the presence of positive culture prior to URS, 13% preferred a single perioperative dose and >50% treated for >4 days.[47]

Room Setup and Patient Positioning

Room setup and patient positioning are key components to successful outcomes during URS. Like many endoscopic and laparoscopic procedures, URS tends to require maximum space and multiple instruments. Room ergonomics are important for adequate staff and equipment flow. Adequate patient positioning allows the surgeon to access key structures. Any misbalance in setup or positioning can translate into suboptimal outcomes, positional injuries for patients, and potential injury to the surgeon.[48]

Room Setup

Room setup for URS should start with the initial blueprints of the operating room. Close communication between the architect, construction manager, surgeon, and operating room (OR) staff is essential. Adequate design includes a wide OR gate for the stretcher, C-arm, and equipment entry and exit. A central drainage system, hanging thin-monitor screens, and an electronic work station are ideal.[49] A scheme for an ideal room setup for URS is shown in Figure 32.1.

Anesthesia should set up at the head of the operating table. The Genito-Urinary (GU) operating table should be radiolucent, capable of sliding forward and back, have a detachable lower leg, and be capable of supporting stirrups for lithotomy. We recommend an adjustable IV pole with pressure bags or "level 1 rapid infuser"; see Figure 32.2 for irrigation.

An endoscopic video tower or boom is positioned at the patient's left side. The C-arm or fluoroscopic unit will enter usually from the left or where it does not interfere with other equipment. A laser source is positioned to the patient's lower right, and a laser fiber is secured using a damp towel, avoiding unwanted pulling and contamination. The monitor screen should ideally hang from the ceiling and be adjustable. An endoscopic tower can also supply a thin-panel monitor that can be adjustable for URS (Fig. 32.3). A large back table is key for proper organization and should be capable of supporting a large array of endoscopes while preventing clutter (Fig. 32.4).

Additionally, X-ray lead gowns with thyroid shields must be available for all personnel.

Prior to the start of surgery, it is our practice to communicate with the OR staff preparing the room. We discuss any particular situation regarding the case that might vary from the standard and any special instrument request that might be needed in the room.

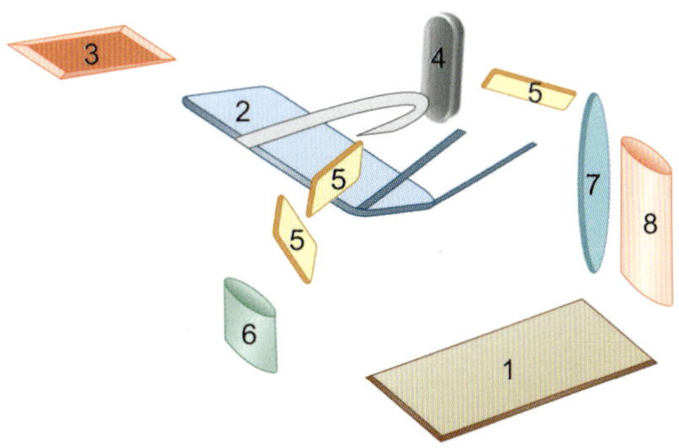

Fig. 32.1: Ureteroscopy room setup scheme.

1. Table for cystoscopy, ureteroscope, and other surgical instruments: This is the main working operating room table that will hold most sterile working instruments.
2. Genitourinary (GU) imaging ready, operating table: The patient will be positioned in a radiolucent table, which will allow for standard lithotomy positioning.
3. Anesthesia boom: The anesthesiologist and his equipment will be positioned near the head of the patient. An anesthesia boom increases room flexibility by allowing anesthesia and surgical equipment to be separate.
4. Mobile C-arm or fixed fluoroscopy unit: The C-shaped (X-ray source) can move under patient and can swivel horizontally, vertically and around. The fixed fluoroscopy unit is fixed and stationary. They both provide real time X-ray images during surgery.
5. Monitor screens: Surgical endoscopic video is displayed on flat panel typically mounted, either on booms, carts, wall or ceiling mounts.
6. Laser source: Lithotripsy energy source typically holmium laser.
7. IV pole or level 1: Irrigation unit, with pressure calibrating device and warmer.
8. Endoscopy boom or tower: Endoscopic equipment supported on a boom.

Patient Positioning

The standard positioning for URS involves a dorsal lithotomy or "low" lithotomy position. Correct lithotomy placement is ideal for adequate access and to prevent positional injury. Prior to positioning, the patient has sequential compression stockings placed on the lower calves. The patient is then moved down and the footrest of the table is removed. Both legs are placed simultaneously in adequately padded stirrups. It is important that the knee and the hip achieve a 90° angle; also, the ipsilateral shoulder, knee, and toe should be aligned (Fig. 32.5). Complications of positioning are discussed later in this chapter.

The arm ipsilateral to the C-arm is tucked and the *contralateral* arm can be left in a traditional arm board. The genital and lower abdomen is then prepped with either betadine or chlorhexidine.

Irrigation

Irrigation during URS is essential for proper visualization. Normal saline (0.9% NaCl) is used for all of our ureteroscopies in which the holmium laser is used. The saline is warmed to body temperature before use to prevent hypothermia. This can also be achieved via the level 1 rapid infuser (Smiths Medical). We recommend using pressurized irrigation from 100 to 200 mm Hg during the ureteroscopic portion of the case. Pressure should be used with caution, especially when performing URS without an access sheath. Alternatively, hand-controlled pressure irrigation can be used. A number of devices exist to allow for

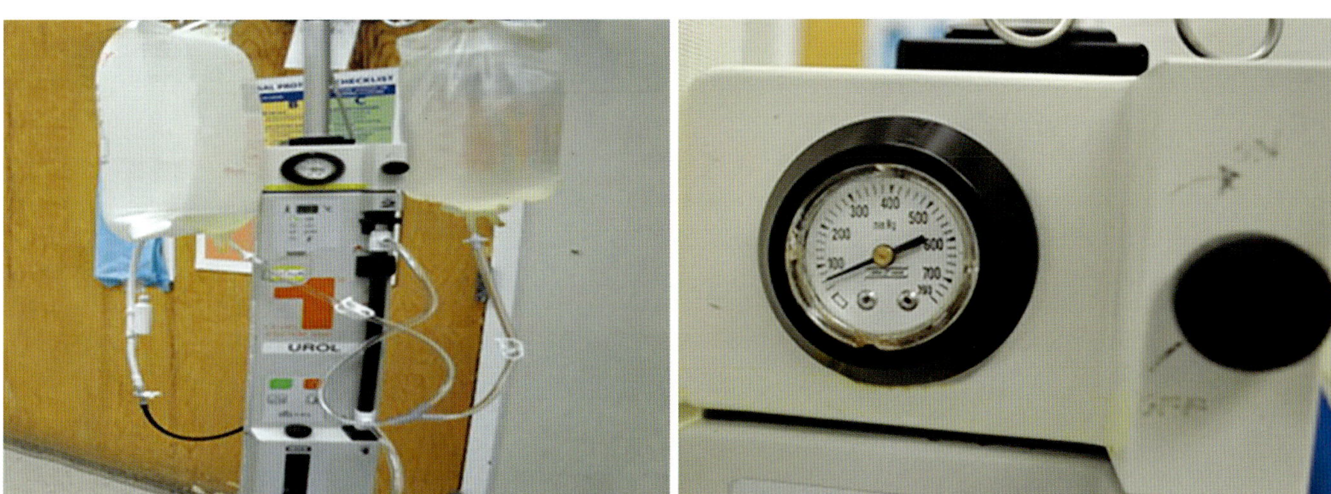

Fig. 32.2: Irrigation set up, including level infuser, warmer and pressure gauge.

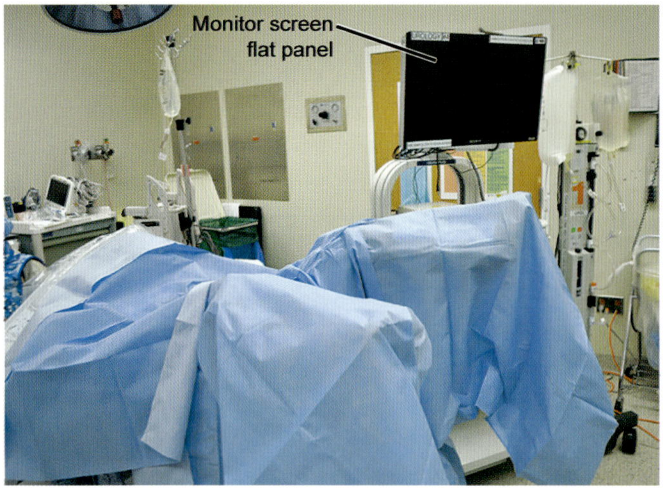

Fig. 32.3: Monitor screen: surgical endoscopic video is displayed on flat panel.

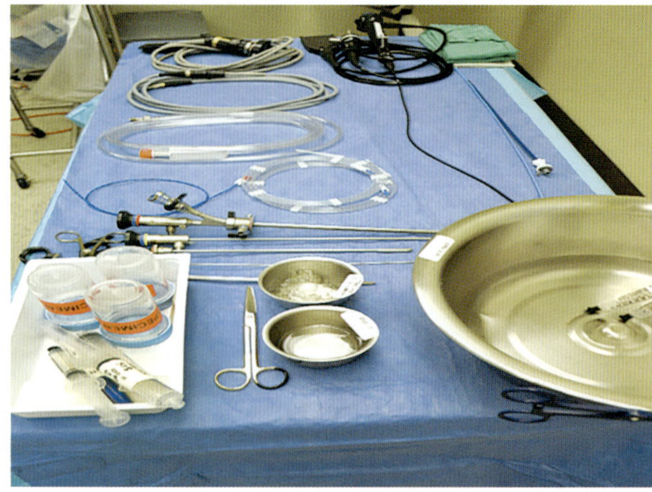

Fig. 32.4: Large table for cystoscopy, ureteroscope, and other surgical instruments.

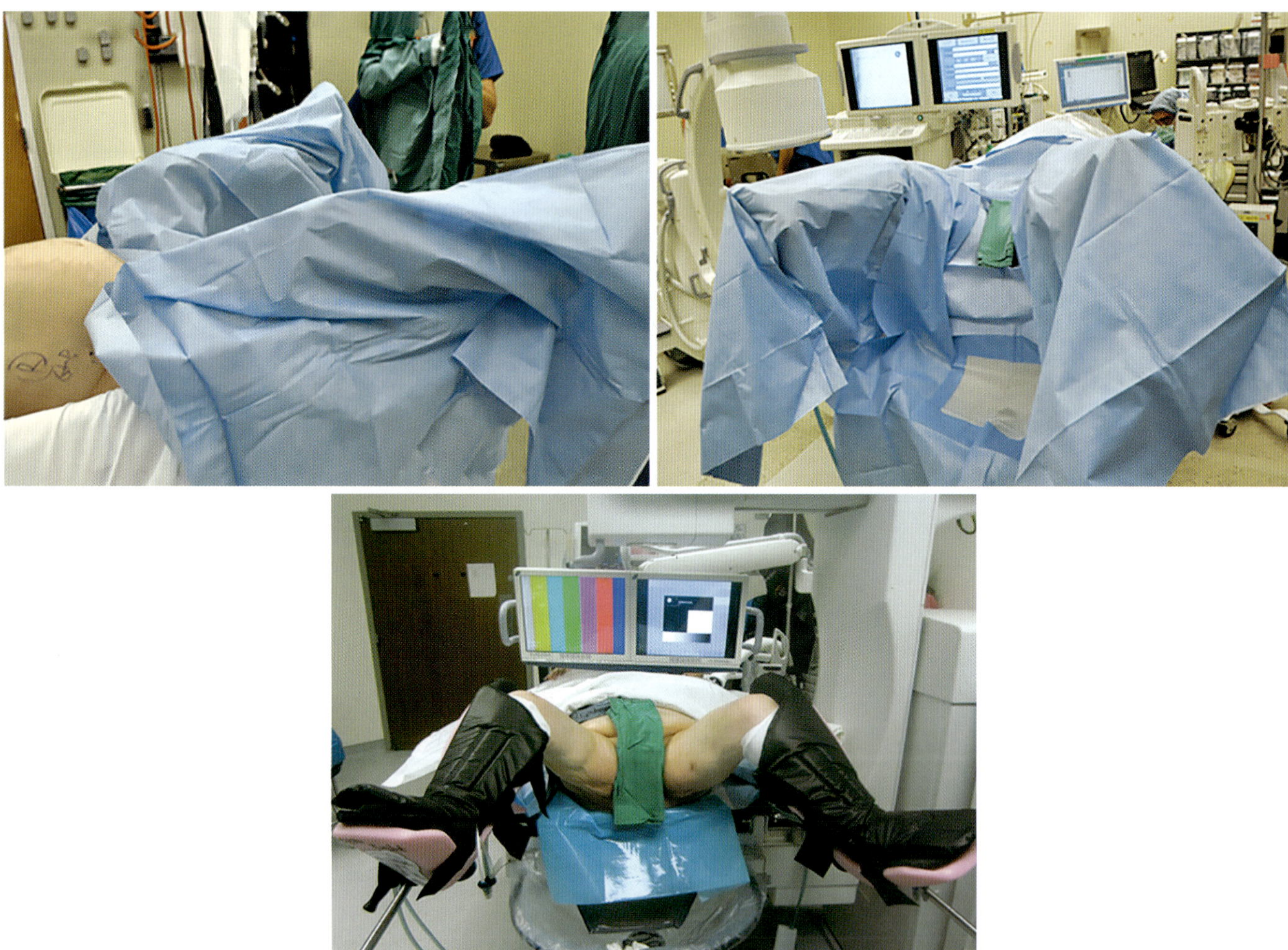

Fig. 32.5: Adequate positioned and padded patient in dorsal lithotomy.

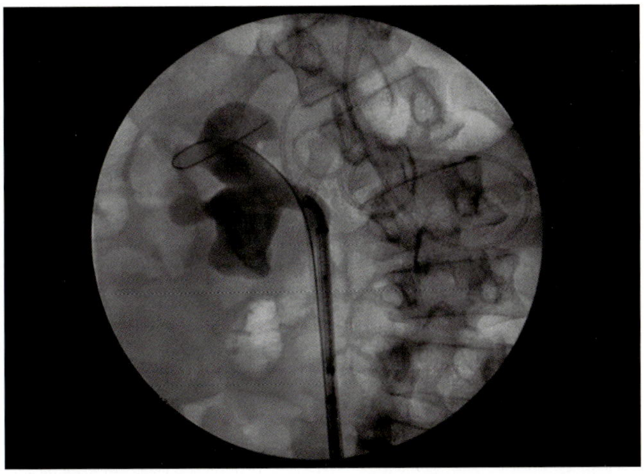

Fig. 32.6: Fluoroscopic imaging during flexible ureteroscopy. Retrograde pyelogram performed opacifies renal collecting system and serves as road map delineating collecting system anatomy.

hand-controlled irrigation such as the Single Action Pumping System (Boston Scientific Corp, Marlborough, MA).

Intraoperative Imaging for Ureteroscopy

The urologist should be trained to be able to look at both the endoscopic and fluoroscopic images during URS. A proper retrograde pyelogram (RPG) is essential to delineate renal and collecting system anatomy, and it is used as a "road map" prior to any URS (Fig. 32.6).

Judicious use of fluoroscopic X-ray is recommended to reduce exposure to the patient, surgeon and OR staff. The principle of "as low as reasonably possible" should be employed. This principle is based on techniques that lower radiation exposure while using fluoroscopy, including collimation, spot fluoroscopy, decreasing the distance between patient and image intensifier, and last image hold.[50,51] The image intensifier should be set above the patient.

A C-arm is preferable to a fixed table fluoroscopy unit, since it is portable and easily moved. We have shown in a simulated URS model that the fixed table is associated with up to 10 times the amount of radiation exposure compared to a C-arm. This is likely due to a fixed radiation source.[52] Also, patients who are obese should be aware of an increase in radiation exposure from fluoroscopy due to an larger exposed area.[53]

Anesthesia

Smaller ureteroscopes and flexible instruments have decreased the anesthetic requirements and allowed ureteroscopies to be performed on an outpatient basis. Sedation and analgesia have been used successfully in patients undergoing URS with high stone-free rates, especially for distal ureteral stones.[54] For larger, complex, proximal ureteral, and renal stones, a general anesthetic with paralysis is recommended. This will minimize diaphragmatic movement and allow successful stone removal.

INTRAOPERATIVE INSTRUMENTS, TECHNOLOGY AND TECHNIQUE

Access Technique

Access to the ureter begins by performing urethroscopy and gaining access into the bladder. After a thorough inspection of the bladder for lesions or urolithiasis, the ureteral orifices are identified. Once the correct ureteral orifice is located, a guidewire is gently passed into the bladder and stabilized with an open-ended ureteral catheter. The catheter is then advanced into the distal ureter and a RPG is performed to delineate ureteral and renal anatomy. The wire is then advanced into the collecting system under fluoroscopic guidance and the ureteral catheter removed.

Safety Guidewire

The use of a 0.035 or 0.038 guidewire is the standard since it secures access, straightens the ureter, and provides orientation during URS. It gives the urologist the ability to place a ureteral stent at any time during the procedure. During semirigid URS, a second wire is sometimes needed in order to advance the ureteroscope past narrow sections in the ureter, including the ureteral orifice and iliac vessels (Fig. 32.7). The safety wire opens the ureter, while the scope is advanced in between both wires in a "railroad" technique.

Ureteral Dilation

In cases where the ureteroscope is unable to be advanced up the ureter to the location of the stone, placing a ureteral stent, and returning to the operating room in 1 to 2 weeks is a reasonable option. Alternatively, ureteral dilation can be performed. Dilation of the distal ureter and ureteral orifice is sometimes required prior to passage of an ureteroscope. An 8 out of 10 coaxial catheter is sometimes used to dilate the UO, but uses shearing forces in the UO and distal ureter, which can cause injury to the ureter. In some cases, dilation can be accomplished visually by passing a semirigid ureteroscope up the distal ureter under vision,

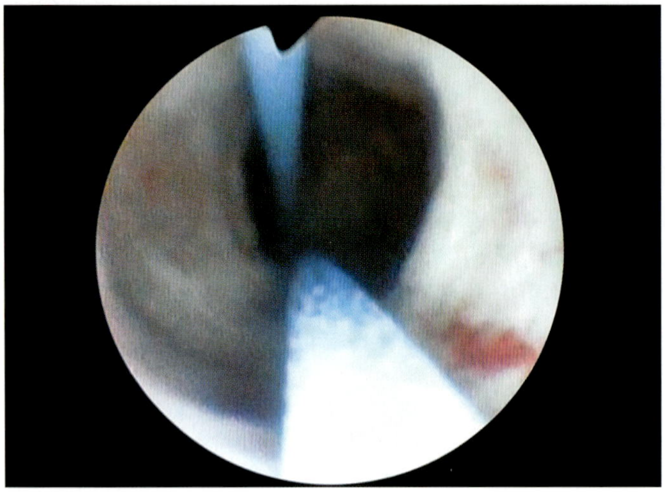

Fig. 32.7: Second wire during semirigid ureteroscopy helps to navigate narrow aspects of the ureter.

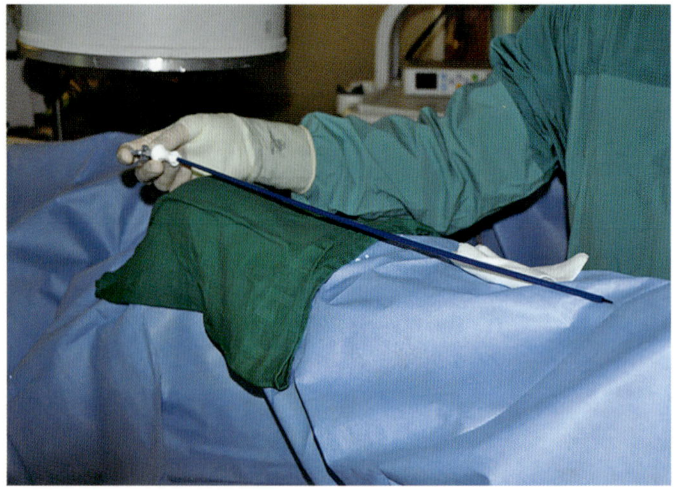

Fig. 32.8: Ureteral access sheath.

particularly in cases with narrow ureteral orifices or intramural ureters.

It is our preference to perform balloon dilation since it provides gradual, controlled inflation and produces even radial forces. Additionally, it produces a waist defect that identifies the narrow portion. We prefer an 18-Fr, 4- or 10-cm balloon, inflated up to 15–16 atm, using the Encore (Boston Scientific Corp, Marlborough, MA) inflator device. The balloon is then advanced via the guidewire and the narrow defect is positioned in between radiopaque markers of the balloon using *fluoroscopy*. Dilute contrast is used to fill the balloon and to identify dilation using fluoroscopy. If the waist persists, multiple dilations from proximal to distal might be necessary. One needs to be cautious in cases of ureteral stones and steinstrasse, since balloon dilation of the location of the stone can cause ureteral wall trauma.

In a contemporary review, balloon dilation of the ureter prior to endoscopic treatment of stone disease was associated with a high success rate and few complications.[55] In this series of 151 patients, an 18-Fr/10-cm ureteral balloon dilator was used in all cases. The authors reported an intraoperative complication rate of 5%. The balloon failure rate was 6%. The rate of ureteral stricture formation was 1% with a median follow-up of 12 months. They report that balloon dilation might prevent a secondary procedure associated with prestenting, thereby reducing additional costs.[55]

If attempts at ureteral balloon dilation fail, it is our practice to prestent the patient and return for definitive URS in 1–2 weeks.

Preoperative Stent

Preoperative ureteral stent placement involves placement of a ureteral stent prior to definite stone therapy to allow passive dilation of the ureter. Routine ureteral stent placement is usually not necessary prior to URS. It should be considered in complex cases with a large stone burden since it has been associated with good SFRs and few complications.[56] Kawahara et al. achieved a 72% SFR in a prestented group compared to a 55% SFR in a nonstented group. This is likely due to an increase in successful access sheath placement in the prestented group.

A recent series determined a cost benefit of prestenting patients with stone burdens of >1 cm undergoing URS. The authors report a cost benefit of $10,100 in prestented patients in this cohort. They also report that an increase in cost in prestenting for stone burdens of <1 cm.[57]

Ureteral Access Sheaths

A UAS is useful for treatment of proximal ureteral and intrarenal stones since it permits easy in-and-out access using a flexible ureteroscope (Fig. 32.8). Multiple passages allow for more efficient stone removal while protecting the lower ureter from trauma. Ureteral access sheaths are available in a variety of sizes ranging from 10/12 Fr to 14/16 Fr. It is our current practice to use the UAS routinely during ureteroscopic treatment of renal and upper ureteral calculi.

In a randomized trial of 62 ureteroscopic procedures, use of a UAS was associated with lower operative times and associated costs. There were no significant differences in postoperative symptoms, early complication rates, or stone-free status between the two groups.[58] Delvecchio et al. reviewed 150 URS cases using a UAS followed for 11 months and found a 1.4% injury risk and only one ureteral stricture on follow-up imaging.[59]

Lower renal pelvic pressures have been demonstrated while using a UAS, which might be beneficial in reducing infectious complications, particularly when treating suspected infectious stone.[60]

In addition to facilitating ureteroscopic access, reducing costs, and lowering intrarenal pressures, the use of a UAS has been shown to improve SFRs. A series of 256 ureteroscopic procedures in which 67% underwent UAS placement resulted in improved SFR in the UAS group (79%) compared to the non-UAS group (67%).[61]

In cases, where UAS is difficult and resistance is encountered, either balloon dilation of ureter can be attempted. Alternatively, attempts can be made to advance the flexible ureteroscope over a wire without the use of an access sheath. If this is unsuccessful, consideration should be given to placement of a ureteral stent to allow the ureter to passively dilate and the procedure can be staged. A recent prospective visual evaluation of the ureter after UAS reported a 46% ureteral injury rate and severe injury involving smooth muscle layers in 13% of cases. Patients who had been prestented were associated with less severe ureteral injuries.[62] The authors did not report any follow-up data regarding the clinical significance of these visually identified ureteral injuries.

Technique

Semirigid Ureteroscopy

The procedure starts by passing the ureteroscope under vision through the urethra alongside the safety guidewire up to the bladder. It is important to keep the male urethra on stretch while passing the ureteroscope (Fig. 32.9). The ureter is carefully engaged with the wire at the 12-o'clock position tenting up the ureteral orifice. Alternatively, a second wire can be passed into the ureter and the scope positioned between the two wires (*see* Fig. 32.7). A "railroad" technique allows placement of the scope in between the wires and will open the ureteral lumen. Another alternative is to place a second wire through the semirigid ureteroscope and advance the scope over the wire under vision.

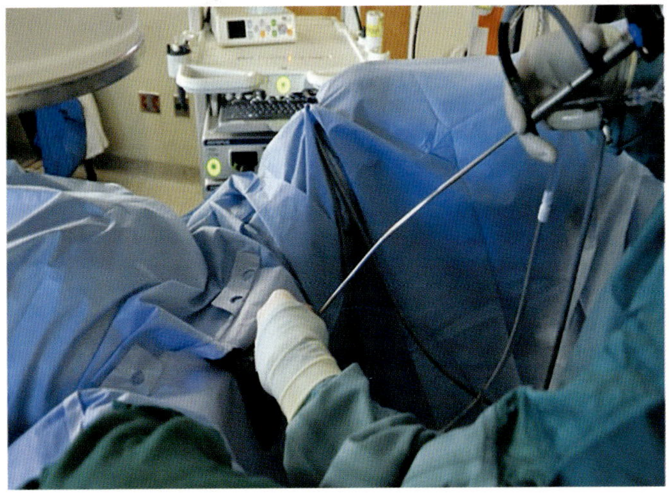

Fig. 32.9: Passing a semirigid ureteroscope into the bladder via the male urethra.

As the ureteroscope is advanced in the ureter, fluoroscopy should be used to identify the position and orientation of the scope if there is difficulty advancing the scope. Causes for having difficulty advancing the ureteroscope include a full bladder, a tight ureteral orifice or distal ureter, a large prostatic medial lobe, and intrinsic or extrinsic compression of the ureter. For longer procedures, we sometimes place a small 10-Fr red rubber catheter into the bladder to allow continuous drainage of the bladder.

Flexible Ureteroscopy

A second guidewire that serves as a safety wire is placed into the kidney as well. Fluoroscopy should be used to confirm that both wires are coiled within the renal pelvis. It is our practice to place a 12–14-Fr access prior to flexible URS. The access sheath is advanced over a wire under fluoroscopic guidance into the proximal ureter. If resistance is encountered, we often dilate the distal ureter using the inner 12-Fr sheath. If this is unsuccessful, balloon dilation of the UO usually allows safe placement of the UAS. It is important to monitor UAS placement using fluoroscopy (Fig. 32.10). The flexible ureteroscope is then passed into the proximal ureter and kidney. Alternatively, if a UAS is not used, the ureteroscope is passed over one of the wires up into the kidney under fluoroscopic guidance. Once the ureteroscope has been placed in the collecting system, the working guidewire can be removed. It is our routine to keep the safety guidewire coiled within the renal pelvis *at all times*.

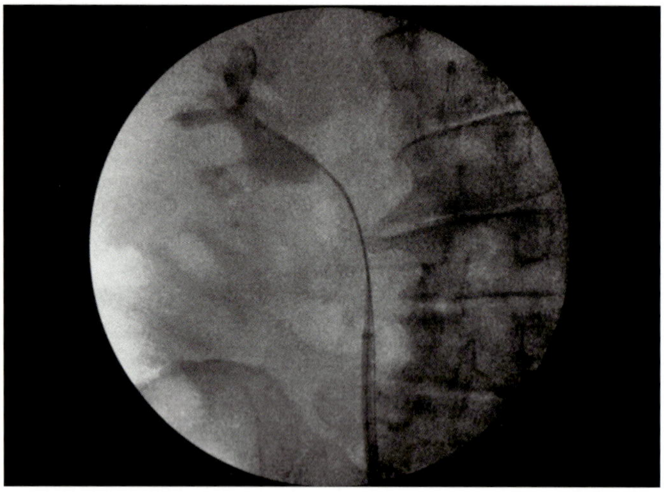

Fig. 32.10: Fluoroscopic imaging during ureteroscopy, shows retrograde placement of ureteral access sheath along guidewire.

Instrumentation

Semirigid Ureteroscopy

Modern rigid ureteroscopes use fiberoptic technology, which allows some flexibility of the scope. Scope diameters range from 6.9 to 9.4 Fr and have one or more working channels. The advantage of having two separate working channels is the minimal impact on irrigant flow during insertion of instruments. Most eyepieces are in line with the shaft, but older ureteroscopes used an offset eyepiece to allow passage of rigid instruments. The distal shaft of the ureteroscope is smaller than the midshaft and the tip is usually beveled to minimize trauma.

Flexible Ureteroscopy

The flexible ureteroscope has evolved significantly over the last two decades. Progress in technology has allowed miniaturized scopes currently from 7 to 10 Fr, with active deflection and a working/irrigation channel. These scopes have the ability to survey the entire collecting system.

Factors to consider when selecting a flexible ureteroscope should include cost, durability, flexibility, working channel/irrigation flow, size, optics, and digital versus fiberoptic. Flexible ureteroscopes are highly expensive and range from $15,000 to $25,000. It is important to consider the durability and cost of repair when selecting a flexible ureteroscope. In a study from Landman et al. comparing fiberoptic scopes, each scope repair ranges from $3,495 to $5,900 and usually repairs are needed every 9–25 cases, depending on the scope used. According to the study, the American Cystoscope Makers, Inc. (ACMI) DUR-8 was the most durable, requiring repair after 25 cases and averaging a total cost of $38,600 after 100 cases.[63]

The conventional fiberoptic flexible scopes, still widely used in clinical practice, offer a maximal active tip deflection of 170°/120°, loss of maximal active tip deflection and irrigation flow after inserting instruments into the working channel. This often prevents successful stone removal from the kidney despite possible stone access with the empty scope.[64] The light cord and camera are usually separate and need to be attached to the scope. It is common to have a honeycomb picture, which needs to be adjusted and focused.

A new generation of flexible fiberoptic ureteroscopes has been introduced in recent years. They offer better deflection and a stiffer shaft, making them more durable.[65] New-generation scopes allow for more flexibility with active deflection that ranges from 180° to 270°. This allows access to every calyx, especially the lower pole, but is limited when placing instruments through the working channel. Irrigation is also affected when placing instruments through the scope. Irrigation pressure has been shown to decrease from 20% to 25% when placing a 1.9-Fr stone basket.[66]

New digital flexible ureteroscopes use a chip-miniaturization technology that allows placement of a complementary metal oxide semiconductor (CMOS) or charge-coupled device (CCD) chip at the tip of the flexible ureteroscope ("chip on a stick"). This allows for larger working channels, and stronger and durable deflection cables. The digital platform allows the highest degree of image fidelity, resolution, and enhancement (Fig. 32.11). In a comparison study between the Olympus URF-V digital scope and the URF-P3 fiberoptic scope, the URF-V was found to have up to three times better resolution, improved color reproducibility, and a larger image size.[5] In a retrospective clinical comparison, Binbay et al. compared outcomes using the ACMI DUR-D (digital) versus the Storz Flex-X2 (fiberoptic).[67] Similar SFRs were noted for both scopes, but decreased OR times were reported with the digital scope. Disadvantages of the digital scopes are the larger size and high costs.

INTRACORPOREAL LITHOTRIPTERS

Rigid Lithotripters

Ballistic/Pneumatic

The Swiss lithoclast (Electro Medical Systems) was the original pneumatic lithotrite. It consists of a rigid probe with a small metal projectile at its tip, which is propelled

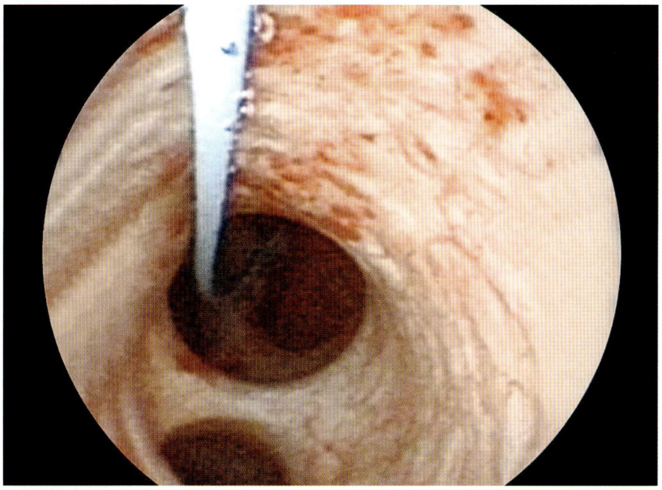

Fig. 32.11: Digital flexible ureteroscopy showing high-resolution images of the upper pole calices.

by controlled bursts of compressed air at 12 cycles per second. The probe needs direct contact with the stone for fragmentation. *Electrokinetic* lithotripters or EKLs are ballistic lithotripters that utilize a rheostat and an electricoil, which vibrates up to 30 cycles/second. In a randomized controlled trial comparing the Swiss Lithoclast and EKL Olympus (Keymed), there was no difference in SFRs, OR duration, or retropulsion with both lithotrites.[68] Recently, more mobile, cordless, and less bulky lithotrites have been developed, including the EKL Swiss LithoBreaker (EMS) and the pneumatic StoneBreaker (Cook). In an in vitro ureteral model, ureteroscopic stone fragmentation was compared while using the LithoBreaker (EKL), StoneBreaker, and holmium laser fiber.[69] Stone fragmentation times were comparable between the EKL and StoneBreaker at 1.6 minutes and 2.4 minutes, respectively. Both showed significantly decreased times compared to the holmium laser (5.1 minutes). Rane et al. reported on 48 *ureteroscopic* stone fragmentations treated using the StoneBreaker with a mean stone size of 1.1 cm. All patients were rendered stone free on postoperative KUB with a mean of nine shocks. Also, retropulsion and ureteral trauma were minimal. They reported no complications following fragmentation, but report no long-term data.[70]

The main advantage of pneumatic lithotripters includes a low risk of ureteral trauma and perforation compared to electrohydraulic lithotripsy (EHL) and its low cost.[71] The disadvantage of this group is that it uses a rigid probe and loses power if the probe is bent.[72] Pneumatic devices also produce large >4 mm residual stones fragments and a high retropulsion rate in dilated ureters.[72] The use of pneumatic lithotripters is limited to the treatment of ureteral stones using a semirigid or rigid ureteroscope.

Ultrasonic Lithotripsy

Ultrasonic lithotripsy works by agitating a piezoceramic plate, which resonates and generates sound waves at around 23,000–27,000 Hz. The sound waves are transmitted along a rigid steel probe and into the stone. It is used more commonly during cystolitholapaxy and PNL. Ultrasonic lithotripsy in the ureter requires a large 11.5-Fr ureteroscope with a 4.5-Fr hollow probe. Ureteral dilation may be needed to advance the large probe into the ureter. Its main advantage is its suction device, which can remove stone fragments. In practice it has been shown to be safe and achieves good stone clearance, even for distal steinstrasse.[73] It is not frequently used during URS due to its rigid probe, the need for ureteral dilation and heat generation. As with the pneumatic lithotripter, bending of the probe results in loss of energy and possible breakage.

Flexible Probes

Electrohydraulic Lithotripsy

Electrohydraulic lithotripsy consists of an underwater sparkplug that generates a shockwave, which creates a cavitation bubble at the tip of the probe. The oscillation of this cavitation bubble fragments the stone on contact.[74] The probes are durable and reusable. The EHL probe is also cheaper and more flexible than standard laser fibers.[75] Its disadvantage is mainly its poor margin of safety. It carries the highest risk of ureteral injury of all the intracorporeal lithotripters, including a high risk of ureteral perforation for impacted stones.[76] Weaker fragmentation, larger stone fragments, and increased stone retropulsion also limit its contemporary use.[77]

Laser

A laser consists of light energy transmitted in a concentrated manner. For intracorporeal lithotripsy, pulsed laser energy is used since it generates a bubble that fragments the stone and dissipates heat. The first available lithotripsy laser was the Coumarin pulsed-dye laser. The available fiber was 200 um and was used in semirigid and flexible URS. Results with the dye laser were adequate except for harder stones, including cystine and calcium oxalate monohydrate.[78] Another disadvantage was the high cost of the fiber and maintenance of the laser.

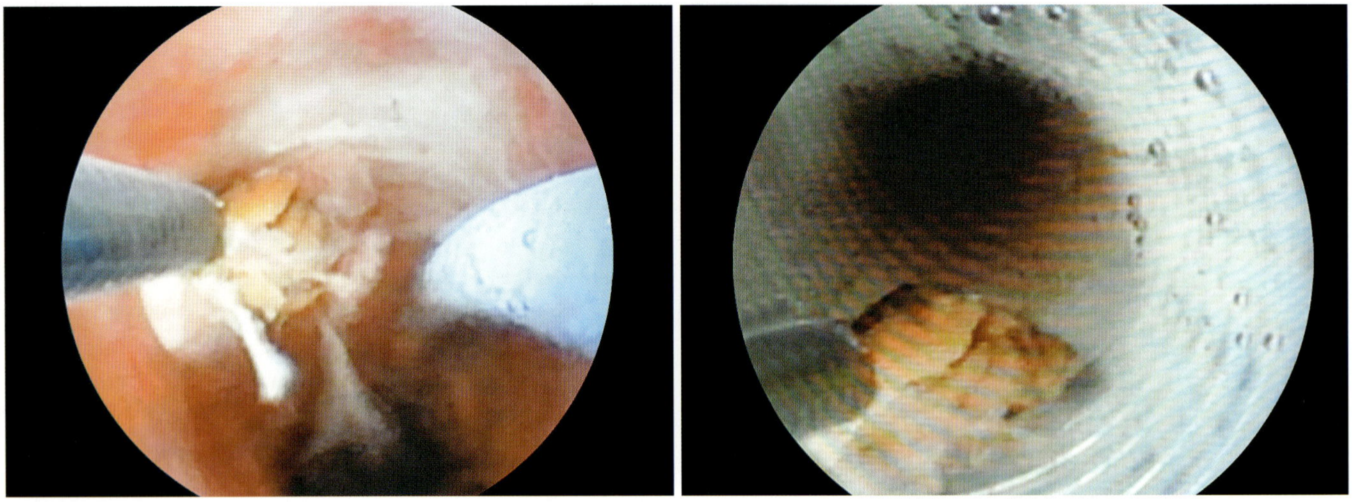

Fig. 32.12: Stone removal using a zero-tip nitinol basket.

The development of the Ho:YAG laser has set the standard for laser lithotrites due to its monochromatic and unidirectional properties. The laser generates a cavitation bubble that creates a shockwave that vaporizes the stone. The probe has been shown to be safer than the EHL since the site of fragmentation ranges from 0.5 mm to 1.0 mm in depth.[79] The laser fares well with multiple stone compositions, including harder stones. It also creates smaller stone fragments and produces less retropulsion. Lower energy settings of 0.2 J and high frequency (20–40 Hz) have shown adequate stone fragmentation, but resulted in smaller stone fragments and less stone retropulsion.[80] The major disadvantage of the Ho:YAG is the high cost of the laser and fibers.

The laser can be used in both semirigid and flexible ureteroscopes. In flexible ureteroscopes, smaller laser fibers should be used to minimize the impact on irrigation flow and deflection of the scope. In an ex vivo model, the DUR-8 flexible ureteroscope (ACMI) was evaluated to determine alterations in deflection caused by a 200-μm and 365-μm holmium laser fiber. Loss of maximal downward deflection was 43° with the 200-μm laser fiber and 365-μm laser fiber, compared to <6° with a 1.6 F EHL probe.[81] Larger fibers have been shown to decrease scope irrigation flow from 45% to 80% while using a 200 μm and 365 μm, respectively.[82]

When performing lithotripsy, care must be taken to avoid direct contact with tissue as well as any wires or other instruments. Both wires and baskets can be damaged from contact with the laser.[83] The laser fiber is capable of penetrating and damaging the flexible ureteroscope lining when the fiber is advanced while the scope is deflected. Smaller fibers advanced with a straight scope has been shown to extend the life of the flexible ureteroscope.[84]

Recently, ball tip laser fibers have been designed to minimize damage to the inner working channels. Although there have not been studies demonstrating decreased damage, investigations have shown that it requires significantly less force to insert a ball tip laser fiber through a deflected working channel compared to a standard flat tip fiber, thereby minimizing the likelihood of the ureteroscope wreaking channel damage.[85]

Safety eyewear is essential to prevent possible corneal laser absorption causing cataracts or corneal burns. Corneal absorption occurs when the retina is within 10 cm of the operating laser fiber. Access to the OR should be restricted to essential personnel and warning signs should be placed on the doors, since the laser has been shown to reflect and scatter.[86]

Stone Retrieval Devices

Baskets

A stone basket serves the purpose of stone retrieval. It consists of a handle, a wire, a sheath, and the basket (Fig. 32.12). The handle allows control of the basket by pulling it out and returning it inside the sheath. Multiple shapes, sizes, and configuration are available, including tipless or zero-tip baskets that minimize urothelium damage during stone manipulation. Basket composition also varies from steel to nitinol alloy, the latter providing strength, flexibility, and memory. The basket shape varies, including spherical and elliptical shapes. Some baskets contain flat wire, which can traumatize tissue if rotated. We prefer a 1.9-Fr zero-tip nitinol basket with cylindrical wires.

Despite improvement in flexible ureteroscopes, the use of stone basket continues to reduce irrigation flow, affecting visualization during stone extraction. A recent study compared differences irrigation flow while using a 1.9-Fr basket. An approximately 80% reduction in irrigation flow has been shown while using a zero-tip 1.9-Fr basket (Boston Scientific) with the URF/P-5 (Olympus), DUR-D (ACMI), and Flex-X2 (Storz) scopes.[66]

Wires

Guidewires are essential tools for the urologist performing URS. They serve to guide safe entry and exit into the collecting system. Most guidewires used during URS vary from 145 to 150 cm long and 0.035 or 0.038 in. We typically use a 0.038 in "floppy tip" nitinol combination wire as our safety and working wire. In cases where it is difficult to gain access to the upper ureter, such as a ureteral kink, tortuosity, impacted stone, or ureteral stricture, it is advantageous to use a hydrophilic guidewire with an angled tip. The hydrophilic wire should be wet prior to use in order to activate the polymer. Once the wire is advanced into the kidney, a catheter can be advanced over it and it can be exchanged for a different working wire. The Amplatz Super Stiff wire (Boston Scientific Corp, Marlborough, MA) is sometimes used if more stiffness is needed since it is more resistant to buckling or kinking due to a greater intrinsic rigidity. It has a steel core. It can also be used to straighten out a tortuous ureter.

Antiretropulsion Devices

Stone retropulsion is a common problem, which has been reported in up to 15% of distal and close to 50% of proximal ureteral stones.[87,88] Migrated stones may result in increased operative times, radiation exposure, and secondary procedures, including the need to convert to flexible URS. Migrated stones can become symptomatic, which can lead to additional patient morbidity and healthcare costs.[129]

Several devices have been engineered to address the problem of retropulsion using mechanical or gel-based obstruction. The Escape (Boston Scientific Corp, Marlborough, MA) is a zero-tip nitinol stone retrieval basket that includes a Y adapter that allows simultaneous laser lithotripsy while engaging a stone with the basket. Limitations includes basket wire damage from laser lithotripsy.[89] The

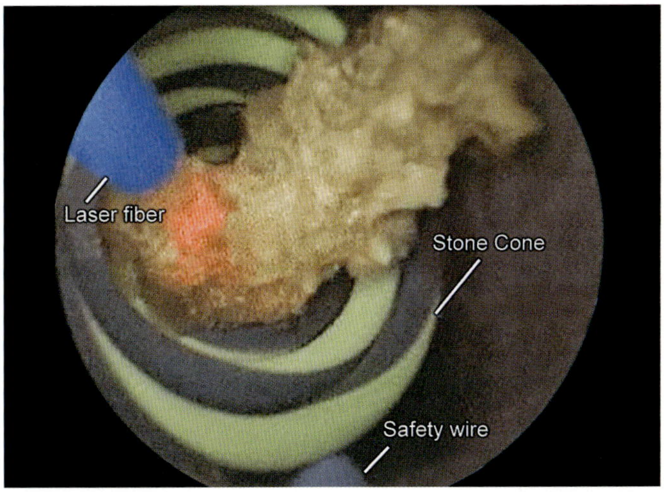

Fig. 32.13: Example of an activated Stone Cone while performing laser lithotripsy in the distal ureter.

Stone Cone (Boston Scientific Corp, Marlborough, MA) consists of a stainless steel wire wound with a strand of nitinol and is baked in a mold to produce a spiral form at the distal tip. During introduction, the coil lies straight inside the carrying catheter. Advancing the double strand wire beyond the tip deploys the cone (Fig. 32.13).

Paradillis et al. randomized patients undergoing URS to Stone Cone and standard basket. He reported a significant decrease in residual stones and auxiliary procedures in the group treated with the Stone Cone.[90] The NTrap (Cook Urological, Bloomington, IN) consists of a shaft with a wire mesh net composed of tightly woven nitinol wires that is placed proximal to the stone.

BackStop (Boston Scientific Corp, Marlborough, MA) is a water-soluble biocompatible polymer with reverse thermosensitive properties. It exists as a liquid at temperatures below 16°C and as a soft but injectable gel at room temperature, which then transitions to a viscous gel at body temperature. In a randomized controlled trial by Rane et al., BackStop was efficient in prevention of stone migration, but failed to show a significant difference in regard to SFRs.[91] In a comparative randomized controlled trial of Ntrap, Stone Cone, and no device, Farahat and colleagues reported significantly lower SFRs, auxiliary procedures, and stone migration with the Stone Cone compared to Ntrap and the control. A recent cost decision analysis reported that antiretropulsive devices become cost effective at a 6.3% retropulsion rate. In this study by Ursiny et al., the reported retropulsion rate was 16.3% versus 1.9% when using an antiretropulsion device. The average savings per case when using these devices was found to be $568.[92]

POSTOPERATIVE CONSIDERATIONS

Postoperative Stenting

Routine placement of a ureteral stent is not necessary after an uncomplicated URS. Nabi et al. performed a meta-analysis to determine if there was a benefit to routine stenting after URS. They found an increase in lower urinary tract symptoms and worsened quality of life in the stented patients compared to the nonstented group. There was no significant difference in postoperative requirement for analgesia, UTIs, SFR, and ureteric strictures in the two groups. There was a nonsignificant reduction in unplanned visits in the nonstented group.

A risk analysis performed for patients following URS was performed by Matani et al., which showed an 11% risk of emergent stent placement within 24 hours of discharge from their URS.[93,94] In our practice we leave a double J ureteral stent with a string for 3–5 days in most patients. For complicated cases, with retained stones, infection, or ureteral or collecting system injury, we place an indwelling double J ureteral stent for 2–4 weeks. Having an indwelling ureteral stents for >15 days was associated with worsened renal colic and febrile complications.[95]

We routinely place a ureteral stent after using a UAS. Animal models have shown persistent ureteral edema after dilation persistent for up to 96 hours.[96] In a recent series of patients who underwent URS with a UAS, unstented patients had more unplanned encounters for pain (26% vs 4%).[97]

α-Blockers have been shown to improve stent-related symptoms after URS. In a double-blind, randomized, controlled trial of Alfuzosin versus placebo, there was a significant decrease in lower urinary tract symptoms and mean pain score. There was also an improvement in the quality of life in the α-blocker group.[98] Stent colic following removal of a ureteral stent can occur in >50% of patients. A recent double-blind, placebo-controlled trial showed significant benefit of a one-time dose of nonsteroidal anti-inflammatory drug (NSAID; Rofecoxib) prior to stent removal.[99]

Residual Stones

Residual stones after URS are common when using strict CT criteria. Close to 40% of patients undergoing ureteroscopic lithotripsy have residual stones based on strict CT criteria, and up to 50% of these had a stone of >1 cm.[100] Residual stones after URS should be followed closely since they can serve as a nidus for infection, grow over time, and become symptomatic.[101] The incidence of residual stones can be reduced by actively retrieving stone fragments with a nitinol basket, before placing a ureteral stent.

Postoperative Imaging

Postoperative imaging after URS is warranted to evaluate for stone clearance and the resolution of obstruction. It is also important for the detection of unanticipated new obstruction from a ureteral stricture. Although postoperative strictures rates are low, they usually are difficult to predict. Weizer et al. reviewed a series of 188 asymptomatic patients post-URS and found a 3.7% obstruction rate. They reported that up to 23% of patients with hydronephrosis after URS will not present with any symptoms.[102]

Following URS and intact stone removal, a renal US to evaluate for obstruction is sufficient. In cases where stone fragmentation is performed, a KUB and US are used to evaluate for residual stones and for hydronephrosis. Patients with radiolucent stones, postoperative symptoms, or hydronephrosis on postoperative US should undergo a NCCT.[103] In our practice, we perform a renal US and digital tomosynthesis or KUB 8 weeks after URS.

Routine imaging with KUB/US after URS has been shown cost effective when compared to selective imaging based on symptoms. A recent cost analysis showed a $130 increase between selective versus routine imaging. This small cost increase is justified due to the morbidity of silent obstruction with possible kidney loss.[104]

TIPS AND TRICKS

Herein, we describe scenarios that can often present challenges during an endourologic case, along with various methods and approaches to overcome them.

BPH/Median Lobe

In the case of a significantly enlarged prostate, a severely hypertrophic median lobe can present a significant challenge to even access the bladder lumen prior to gaining access to the ureter.

- Employ a 70° lens to directly view the obstacle path from the verumontanum.
- Rotate a rigid cystoscope 180° to use the rounded/beveled beak to retract the middle lobe.
- Obtain access to the bladder using a flexible cystoscope.
- Use a narrower instrument, such as a rigid or semirigid ureteroscope or finally a flexible ureteroscope.

- Use an angled-tip guidewire to gain wire access to the lumen.
- If anticipated, and the patient has significant symptoms due to outlet obstruction, perform a simultaneous or staged pre-URS transurethral resection of the prostate.
- Obtain percutaneous access and perform antegrade guidewire passage.

Narrowed Ureteral Orifice

In the setting of a ureteral orifice that cannot be intubated with a ureteroscope, the general principle is to use successively smaller instruments for access and attempt to minimize invasiveness. Avoid blind access or aggressive force.

- Start with a smaller semirigid ureteroscope alongside the safety guidewire.
- Insert a semirigid ureteroscope over a second wire, or with a sensor wire protruding from the working channel as a guide.
- Vary the degree of bladder distention. An emptied bladder may allow relaxation of the transmural portion of the ureter.
- Gentle serial dilation with an access sheath. Serial dilation can be performed with the 8/10 coaxial ureteral dilators. Recommend placement of ureteral stent after ureteral dilation.
- Balloon dilation of the ureteral orifice. The ureteral balloon is passed using fluoroscopy and cystoscopic view into the ureteral orifice. Proper dilation is confirmed by fluoroscopy. Ureteral stenting is recommended following balloon dilation.
- Place a ureteral stent and return to the operating room in 1–2 weeks to allow for passive dilation of the ureter.

Ureteral Kinks: Wire Access

Tortuosity within the ureter can present a significant obstacle toward ensuring access and a safety wire from the urethra to the renal pelvis. The first step is to obtain wire access across the area of interest. Extreme care must be taken not to puncture the ureteral wall.

- Pass the area with a hydrophilic guidewire.
- Pass with an angled-tip wire.
- Guide the wire with an angled-tip catheter or angiocatheter.
- If the patient is prepared and secured, place the table in steep *Trendelenburg*.
- Inflate a balloon distal to kink and apply gentle traction under fluoroscopy.

Ureteral Kinks: Instrument Access

Once wire access is obtained across a ureteral kink, the ureter can be attempted to be straightened to allow passage of instruments.

- Pass a ureteral catheter over the access wire; gently pull the wire and catheter back to uncoil the kink.
- Pass the obturator of an access sheath over the access wire.
- Use a dual wire introducer to pass a second wire across the kink, allowing use of the second wire to manipulate the ureter.
- Once the ureter is straightened, keep a superstiff wire in place as a safety wire.
- If the ureter cannot be safely straightened, place a ureteral stent and perform surveillance with serial X-rays in the outpatient setting.

Impacted Stone

Once the wire coils distal to the stone and the impacted stone is identified, perform an adequate RPG.

- Place a ureteral catheter a few millimeters distal to the stone.
- Advance a sensor wire, if not successful.
- Keep the ureteral catheter in place; use an angle hydrophilic wire, using a torque device, which allows precise rotation of the wire. If successful, advance the ureteral catheter over the glide into the renal pelvis and perform a RPG to confirm position.
- If unsuccessful, keep the wire in place distal to the stone, remove the ureteral catheter, and place an angled hydrophilic catheter and advance just distal to the stone, then attempt to advance wire and catheter past the stone. If successful, perform a RPG and exchange for sensor wire. If unsuccessful, consider a percutaneous approach or URS to attempt passage of wire under vision if comfortable doing so.
- Place sensor wire just distal to the stone, advance the ureteroscope into the ureter to identify the stone, and attempt to pass wire in between the ureteral wall and the stone. Be careful not to perforate the ureter and have a low threshold to stop and return for antegrade approach. Do not attempt laser lithotripsy without a safety wire, which can result in disorientation and ureteral perforation.

Impacted Basket

After engaging a stone in the kidney or ureter, the basket is impacted and does not return with your scope.

- Do not attempt to forcefully pull on the basket, which could lead to ureteral avulsion.
- With scissors, cut the wire near the baskets handle, so the handle is free.
- Remove the ureteroscope from the patient as you push and pull the wire of the basket, keeping the basket inside the patient.
- Replace the ureteroscope to find the impacted basket and stone.
- Perform laser lithotripsy of the stone, taking care not to cut the basket wires.
- After the stone is completely fragmented, attempt to gently pull the basket out with the ureteroscope. If unsuccessful, consider a percutaneous approach.

Lower Pole Stone

The lower pole stone is a classic problem for retrograde intrarenal surgery. Although modern flexible ureteroscopes allow access to the lower pole, challenges still exist, such as the loss of maneuverability with instruments within the working channel, and the risk of damage to the working channel when passing instruments through a deflected ureteroscope.

- When positioning following induction with anesthesia, position the patient prone, and tilt the table head-down at least 20°, which will allow gravity to assist in displacement of the stone in a more favorable location during the operation.[105]
- If the stone is not impacted, extract it from the lower pole with a basket and place within a more favorable location within an upper or upper lateral calcyx.[106]
- If the stone is impacted or the target is a lesion needing biopsy or fulguration, use instruments designed to reduce trauma to the working channel (ball tip laser fiber and nitinol baskets) when the instrument is deflected.

COMPLICATIONS

As with any interventional procedure, there is potential for complications from URS of which both the provider and patient must be aware. The overall risk of side effects and complications has been reported to range from 9% to 25%.[9,12,59,107-110]

Hematuria

Hematuria is a common and typically benign complication from URS and typically results from localized trauma to the urothelium, causing bleeding. This is usually self-limiting. Persistent hematuria has been reported to occur at a rate of 2.04%.[107] If significant enough to form clots, this can cause obstruction of the ureter or the urethra. Caution should be used in this setting, and it should be approached in the same fashion as clot retention from any other cause in the acute setting.

However, gross hematuria following URS may be an indication of the development of a ureteral-iliac artery fistula. This is a rare complication with a predisposition toward patients with prior pelvic surgery, radiation, arterial prosthetic grafts, or indwelling ureteral stents.[111] If the suspicion is high or if pulsatile flow is observed from the ureter during cystoscopy, workup includes angiography and possible placement of an endovascular stent. If the diagnosis is confirmed during cystoscopy, it may be advantageous to place a ureteral catheter, which can be manipulated during angiography.[111] More complex situations may require more invasive intervention such as ureteral diversion, direct artery repair, or arterial bypass.

Stent Pain/Renal Colic

Stent colic is one of the major reasons that practitioners avoid routine stenting after URS. It has been demonstrated in two meta-analyses that for uncomplicated URS, a ureteral stent can be omitted.[94,112] Ureteral edema or spasm following URS or even removal of a ureteral stent may cause renal colic and temporary obstruction, which can be severe. In a large series of 2,735 ureteroscopic procedures evaluated in which 67% underwent stent placement, the rate of renal colic was 2.23%.[107] If the colic is severe, further evaluation with imaging is warranted.

During complicated URS with ureteral edema or significant manipulation, a ureteral stent should be placed. Patients can have a wide range of experience due to an indwelling stent, from minimal symptoms to having a large impact on quality of life. A randomized, double-blind, placebo-controlled trial demonstrated improvement of urinary frequency, urgency, and urge incontinence, as well as overall patient satisfaction with an α-blocker (Alfuzosin) in the setting of a multilength stent placed after pneumatic lithotripsy.[98] A randomized, double-blind, placebo-controlled trial demonstrated improvement in severe pain following stent removal with the use of Rofecoxib.[99] Although this medication was removed from the market due to concerns for cardiac toxicity, this effect may be seen with other NSAIDs. It is our practice to routinely provide patients who had undergone URS with a short course of a selective α-blocker and, if there is adequate renal function, NSAIDs for the relief and prevention of postprocedural renal colic both with and without an indwelling ureteral stent.

UTI/Sepsis

Rates of fever or sepsis have been reported to be from 1.13% to 4%.[12,107] There is currently no consensus among practicing endourologists with regard to antibiotic prophylaxis. In high-risk patients who have had previous sepsis or colonization of multidrug-resistant organisms, a more aggressive perioperative antibiotic regimen may be warranted. Regimens in use today for these patients range from several days of preoperative antibiotics, either in the outpatient or inpatient setting, to standard perioperative regimens. If oral regimens are not available, a peripherally inserted central catheter can be utilized.

Steinstrasse

During URS for the treatment of nephrolithiasis, the management of stone fragments remains a controversial one. The primary point of debate is whether to dust or "popcorn" stones to fragments of minimal size (typically less than the diameter of a guidewire), or attempt basket retrieval of all fragments to render the patient truly stone free.

Steinstrasse has been reported in up to 2% of patients undergoing URS for proximal ureteral stones.[12] Although typically benign and amenable to medical expulsive therapy, these fragments have the potential to cause ureteral colic, obstruction, and urosepsis. Asymptomatic patients have been demonstrated to have stone-clearance rates of 60–80%, making them amenable to observation.[113-115] Patients with bilateral steinstrasse, a solitary kidney, severe symptoms, or infected hydronephrosis typically require ureteral stent placement, percutaneous nephrostomy drainage, and/or repeat URS with lithotripsy or fragment retrieval. Interestingly, patients managed with percutaneous nephrostomy drainage alone have been observed to successfully pass all fragments in 75% of cases.[116] During observation, or following urinary diversion, intervention may be necessary if the steinstrasse does not resolve within 3–4 weeks.[117] In addition to repeat URS, extracorporeal shockwave lithotripsy of the leading fragment has been reported to have a high success rate in patients who had a primary shockwave lithotripsy.[118] Finally, PNL may be considered if significant renal stone burden remains.

Ureteral Injury

Injury to the ureter during URS results from direct trauma in the form of perforation or creation of a false passage. Rates of occurrence have been reported to be 0.65–6%.[12,107,119] Primarily, these occur from the passage of instruments or wires, forceful manipulation of a stone, direct delivery of energy during lithotripsy, and ureteral dilation, either by serial axial dilation with an access sheath/obturator, or balloon dilation. Among lithotrites, EHL carries a high risk of perforation. It is also possible to ensnare the ureter when manipulating a stone with a wire basket, inadvertently causing a perforation.

Care should always be taken when advancing instruments or wires, and advancement of blunt or firm tipped implements without wire guidance should be avoided. These injuries have been associated with increased OR time, which may be indicative of an increasingly difficult ureteroscopic procedure.[120] It is important for the urologist to be cognizant of attempting increasingly aggressive maneuvers during a difficult procedure. Rather than risk escalating the potential injury and potentially producing a catastrophic outcome, it may be in the patient's best interest to stop the procedure, place a ureteral stent, and return for a staged procedure.

If a ureteral perforation or false passage is identified, the procedure should be terminated and a ureteral stent should be placed at the completion of the procedure to facilitate healing. Duration of stent placement should be for 4–6 weeks. Prophylactic antibiotics should be considered if there is concern for extravasation and formation of a urinoma. If severe enough, an imaging test with antegrade or retrograde luminal contrast may be considered prior to removal of the stent. Following stent removal, upper tract imaging such as a pyelogram, US, or renal scan should be performed to ensure healing and adequate drainage and monitor for stricture formation.

Ureteral Avulsion

Complete or partial avulsion of the ureter is a dreaded complication of URS. Fortunately, this is typically very rare. Recent reviews have reported a rate of up to 0.16%.[107,119,121] The mechanism for this injury is typically aggressive instrument removal and the aggressive manipulation of a large or impacted stone. Avulsion in the caudal/distal direction typically presents as an intussuscepted portion of ureter extending into the bladder lumen from the location of the orifice, or removal of a portion of the ureter from the patient when removing instruments. Avulsion in the cephalad/proximal direction can be observed as a complete, circumferential loss of ureteral mucosa during URS.

Prevention lies within proper endourologic technique and the avoidance of blind manipulation of grasping implements and baskets. Basket retrieval of stone fragments should be only performed under direct vision and with extreme care. The endourologist should continually evaluate the size of the stone relative to the luminal diameter during active manipulation.

Management involves urgent urinary diversion with percutaneous nephrostomy tube. In the case of extravasation, urinomas can be drained percutaneously. Exploration will be necessary to determine the extent of ureteral injury. The subsequent repair will depend highly on the location and extent of injury. Distal injuries may be amenable to ureteral reimplantation with a psoas hitch or Boari flap. More proximal or extensive injuries may require an ileal ureter interposition or renal autotransplantation to account for loss of ureteral length. A nephrectomy should be considered with care, as the risk of recurrent stone disease and the potential for chronic loss of renal function need to be considered. Finally, a transureteroureterostomy is generally contraindicated in the presence of stone disease.

Submucosal Stone/Lost Stone

Infrequently, a stone or fragment can be displaced to a submucosal location. This has been reported to occur at a rate of 0.18%.[107] This finding typically occurs when a perforation injury is induced, and irrigation or direct manipulation displaces the stone out of the luminal space. Laser excision of the submucosa and stent placement should be performed. These patients should be carefully monitored due to an increased risk of stricture formation.

If the stone has been pushed beyond the submucosa and resides completely outside of the collecting system, it should be left alone. Attempted retrieval may induce significant extravasation and exacerbation of the ureteral perforation. Once identified, a ureteral stent should be placed. Antibiotics should be considered if a risk of infection exists in order to prevent abscess formation. As with a submucosal stone, these patients should be monitored carefully for stricture formation. Lastly, these patients must be counseled appropriately so that future providers do not mistake the displaced stone for an active ureteral calculus.

Collateral Injury

Injury beyond the ureter is a rare but undesirable complication, as these injuries are less amenable to correction with simple ureteral stenting as is typical of most ureteral injury. The type of or potential for injury depends on the anatomic location of nearby organs and structures and the instrument with which the injury occurs. The recipient of collateral injury can be classified by location along the ureter. At the UPJ, the great vessels are medial, and the renal vessels lie anterior and posterior. The abdominal ureter is adjacent to the great vessels medially and the gonadal vessels and bowel anteriorly. The urologist must be very cognizant of the iliac vessels as the ureter drapes directly over them at the pelvic brim. Within the pelvis, the ureter is in close proximity to the internal iliac vessels, which lie laterally. Finally, at the ureterovesical junction the inferior vesicle artery lies laterally. Injuries to these structures may require endovascular or general surgery consultation and risk fistula formation.

Ureteral Stricture

Stricture formation is multifactorial, with both procedure-related and patient-related influences. An overall stricture rate of 1.4–4% has been reported.[12,59] It has been observed that impacted stones are associated with as high as 24% stricture formation at the site of impaction despite successful endourologic management of the stone.[122] Patients at risk for reduced ureteral perfusion, such as those with a history of prior ureteral surgery, abdominal or pelvic radiation, or trauma, may be at higher risk for formation of stricture.

Management of the stricture will ultimately require balloon dilation, endoureterotomy, or open/laparoscopic repair. In kidneys that have been demonstrated to have poor or no function, a nephrectomy should be considered.

Renal Unit Loss

Silent obstruction, the insidious manifestation of a stricture, has been reported to occur at a frequency of 2.9%.[102] This asymptomatic ureteral obstruction will result in renal unit loss if it remains undetected. Therefore, the authors strongly recommend routine postoperative imaging for patient who have undergone URS. These patients will require relief of the obstruction and definitive repair in order to minimize the potential for loss of renal function.

FUTURE OF URETEROSCOPY

Since the introduction of the modern ureteroscope, we have seen significant development and maturation of technology. However, there continues to be a need for further improvements in current technology. It is this need that will drive continued innovation.

The further miniaturization of retrograde instruments is necessary. Reducing the size of working implements that are used within the working channel of a ureteroscope will minimize the loss of irrigation pressure and loss of ureteroscope flexibility. Reducing the diameter of ureteroscopes will reduce collateral tissue trauma, allow for the use of smaller access sheaths, and minimize the need for balloon dilation, all of which will aid in minimizing collateral tissue trauma and thereby reduce the number of needed interventions and anesthesia, improve patient recovery rates and reduce postoperative pain.

Although the da Vinci robot is not without its disadvantages, it is safe to say that it has revolutionized laparoscopic urology. At many academic centers, the robotic-assisted laparoscopic prostatectomy has become the modus operandi for the surgical treatment of prostate cancer. Similarly, the application of robotic technology to endoscopy has the potential to facilitate various procedures. This new technology may improve surgical precision and solve many ergonomic problems for the practicing urologist. Similar to the da Vinci, users may have to overcome a greater learning curve and also justify the inherently greater cost of equipment and support infrastructure. The Roboflex Avicenna is a framework that allows for robotic-assisted flexible URS. The main advantages are the reduction of ergonomic problems common in standard URS. Other potential advantages are precise, fine movements in the ureter and safe insertion of the laser fiber. In a series of 82 patients, the Roboflex Avicenna allowed for complete fragmentation in 79 cases.[123]

Continued improvements in lithotrites are needed. In addition to miniaturization, more durable laser fibers are needed to be able to deliver a greater amount of energy while minimizing degradation of the tip. This is becoming more important as urologists are able to tackle larger intrarenal stones than previously thought possible.[124] Additionally, designs meant to reduce ureteroscope trauma are needed, such as the ball tip of the TracTip laser fiber (Boston Scientific, Natick, MA, USA). It has been observed that a significant cause of ureteroscope repair is working channel damage due to simple instrument insertion or extraction.[125]

There continues to be a need for improved stone fragment retrieval. The removal of fragments during retrograde surgery remains a challenge. Current basket technology is not very efficient and is prone to material fatigue from repeated use and subsequent basket failure. Finally, these baskets are not efficient at removal of smaller stone fragments. Although these stone fragments typically will pass on their own, they risk causing renal colic or even retention within the renal collecting system, acting as a nidus for future stone formation. An innovative retrieval method of these smaller stones would be a welcome addition.

Better strategies for management of stent symptoms are needed. Significant morbidity can occur from stent colic and can have a large impact on quality of life. Design improvements such as the Polaris Loop (Boston Scientific, Natick, MA) should continue to be explored.[126] Pharmacotherapy for stent discomfort warrants further exploration. These improvements would reduce the cost of stent morbidity from time lost from work, unplanned visits to healthcare providers and costs of adjunctive pain medications used to reduce symptoms.

Finally, as we continue in an age of cost and environmental consciousness and social sustainability, the cost of devices and the reusability of parts need to be strongly considered. The expense of ureteroscopes, necessary associated equipment, and costs for repair can be a major burden for providers. The significant costs and infrastructure necessary for URS present a significant barrier to the use of this technique in low-resource environments. The cost of ancillary ureteroscope equipment is also significant. In fact, it has been suggested that the cost of disposables may exceed that of ureteroscope purchase and maintenance for retrograde flexible ureteroscopic lithotripsy.[127] Further development of recyclable devices has potential advantages with regard to cost and environmental friendliness. However, the challenge of effective sterilization between patients and instrument resilience to the sterilization process needs to be overcome. Within the heart of the matter lies the reality that stone and collecting system disease affects people worldwide and improving access, whether by better, cheaper, or more sustainable technology, remains the ultimate future direction of URS.

REFERENCES

1. Murphy LJT, Desnos E. The History of Urology. Springfield, IL: Thomas; 1972.
2. Young HH, McKay RW. Congenital valvular obstruction of the prostatic urethra. Surg Gynecol Obstet. 1929;48:509.

3. Hirschowitz BI, Peters CW, Curtiss LE. Preliminary report on a long fiberscope for examination of stomach and duodenum. Med Bull (Ann Arbor). 1957;23(5):178-80.
4. Marshall VF. Fiber optics in urology. J Urol. 1964;91:110-4.
5. Zilberman DE, Lipkin ME, Ferrandino MN, et al. The digital flexible ureteroscope: in vitro assessment of optical characteristics. J Endourol. 2011;25(3):519-22.
6. Goodman TM. Ureteroscopy with pediatric cystoscope in adults. Urology. 1977;9(4):394.
7. Preminger GM, Tiselius HG, Assimos DG, et al. 2007 Guideline for the management of ureteral calculi. Eur Urol. 2007;52(6):1610-31.
8. Türk C, Knoll T, Petrik A, et al. Guidelines on Urolithiasis. European Association of Urology; 2014. Available from http://www.uroweb.org/gls/pdf/22%20Urolithiasis_LR.pdf:0-104, 2016.
9. Segura JW, Preminger GM, Assimos DG, et al. Ureteral Stones Clinical Guidelines Panel summary report on the management of ureteral calculi. The American Urological Association. J Urol. 1997;158(5):1915-21.
10. Yaycioglu O, Guvel S, Kilinc F, et al. Results with 7.5 F versus 10 F rigid ureteroscopes in treatment of ureteral calculi. Urology. 2004;64(4):643-6; discussion 6-7.
11. Hyams E, Monga M, Pearle M, et al. A prospective, multi-institutional study of flexible ureteroscopy for proximal ureteral stones smaller than 2 cm. J Urol. 2015;193(1):165-9.
12. Preminger GM, Tiselius HG, Assimos DG, et al. 2007 Guideline for the management of ureteral calculi. J Urol. 2007;178(6):2418-34.
13. Pearle MS, Lingeman JE, Leveillee R, et al. Prospective, randomized trial comparing shock wave lithotripsy and ureteroscopy for lower pole caliceal calculi 1 cm or less. J Urol. 2005;173(6):2005-9.
14. Aboumarzouk OM, Kata SG, Keeley FX, et al. Extracorporeal shock wave lithotripsy (ESWL) versus ureteroscopic management for ureteric calculi. Cochrane Database Syst Rev. 2012;5:Cd006029.
15. Cone EB, Eisner BH, Ursiny M, et al. Cost-effectiveness comparison of renal calculi treated with ureteroscopic laser lithotripsy versus shockwave lithotripsy. J Endourol. 2014;28(6):639-43.
16. Perez Castro E, Osther PJ, Jinga V, et al. Differences in ureteroscopic stone treatment and outcomes for distal, mid-, proximal, or multiple ureteral locations: the Clinical Research Office of the Endourological Society ureteroscopy global study. Eur Urol. 2014;66(1):102-9.
17. Kumar A, Kumar N, Vasudeva P, et al. A prospective, randomized comparison of shock wave lithotripsy, retrograde intrarenal surgery and miniperc for treatment of 1 to 2 cm radiolucent lower calyceal renal calculi: a single center experience. J Urol. 2015;193(1):160-4.
18. Tiselius HG, Ackermann D, Alken P, et al. Guidelines on urolithiasis. Eur Urol. 2001;40(4):362-71.
19. Koo V, Young M, Thompson T, et al. Cost-effectiveness and efficiency of shockwave lithotripsy vs flexible ureteroscopic holmium:yttrium-aluminium-garnet laser lithotripsy in the treatment of lower pole renal calculi. BJU Int. 2011;108(11):1913-6.
20. Wen CC, Nakada SY. Treatment selection and outcomes: renal calculi. Urol Clin North Am. 2007;34(3):409-19.
21. De S, Autorino R, Kim FJ, et al. Percutaneous nephrolithotomy versus retrograde intrarenal surgery: a systematic review and meta-analysis. Eur Urol. 2015:67(1):125-37.
22. Mugiya S. Guidelines on urolithiasis: update of diagnosis and treatment. Hinyokika Kiyo. 2012;58(12):703-6.
23. Wu CF, Chen CS, Lin WY, et al. Therapeutic options for proximal ureter stone: extracorporeal shock wave lithotripsy versus semirigid ureterorenoscope with holmium:yttrium-aluminum-garnet laser lithotripsy. Urology. 2005;65(6):1075-9.
24. Cohen J, Cohen S, Grasso M. Ureteropyeloscopic treatment of large, complex intrarenal and proximal ureteral calculi. BJU Int. 2013;111(3 Pt B):E127-31.
25. Bryniarski P, Paradysz A, Zyczkowski M, et al. A randomized controlled study to analyze the safety and efficacy of percutaneous nephrolithotripsy and retrograde intrarenal surgery in the management of renal stones more than 2 cm in diameter. J Endourol. 2012;26(1):52-7.
26. Ricchiuti DJ, Smaldone MC, Jacobs BL, et al. Staged retrograde endoscopic lithotripsy as alternative to PCNL in select patients with large renal calculi. J Endourol. 2007;21(12):1421-4.
27. Tepeler A, Akman T, Silay MS, et al. Comparison of intrarenal pelvic pressure during micro-percutaneous nephrolithotomy and conventional percutaneous nephrolithotomy. Urolithiasis. 2014;42(3):275-9.
28. Salem HK. A prospective randomized study comparing shock wave lithotripsy and semirigid ureteroscopy for the management of proximal ureteral calculi. Urology. 2009;74(6):1216-21.
29. Pittomvils G, Vandeursen H, Wevers M, et al. The influence of internal stone structure upon the fracture behaviour of urinary calculi. Ultrasound Med Biol. 1994;20(8):803-10.
30. Teichman JM, Vassar GJ, Glickman RD. Holmium:yttrium-aluminum-garnet lithotripsy efficiency varies with stone composition. Urology. 1998;52(3):392-7.
31. Wiener SV, Deters LA, Pais VM, Jr. Effect of stone composition on operative time during ureteroscopic holmium:yttrium-aluminum-garnet laser lithotripsy with active fragment retrieval. Urology. 2012;80(4):790-4.
32. Assimos DG, Leslie SW, Ng C, et al. The impact of cystinuria on renal function. J Urol. 2002;168(1):27-30.
33. Natalin R, Xavier K, Okeke Z, et al. Impact of obesity on ureteroscopic laser lithotripsy of urinary tract calculi. Int Braz J Urol. 2009;35(1):36-41; discussion-2.
34. Grasso M, Chalik Y. Principles and applications of laser lithotripsy: experience with the holmium laser lithotrite. J Clin Laser Med Surg. 1998;16(1):3-7.
35. Watterson JD, Girvan AR, Cook AJ, et al. Safety and efficacy of holmium:YAG laser lithotripsy in patients with bleeding diatheses. J Urol. 2002;168(2):442-5.
36. Turna B, Stein RJ, Smaldone MC, et al. Safety and efficacy of flexible ureterorenoscopy and holmium:YAG lithotripsy for intrarenal stones in anticoagulated cases. J Urol. 2008;179(4):1415-9.

37. Colangelo CJ, Kaplan G, Palazzi K, et al. Ureteroscopy in pediatric patients with spinal abnormalities. J Endourol. 2013;27(5):545-8.
38. Lotan Y, Gettman MT, Roehrborn CG, et al. Management of ureteral calculi: a cost comparison and decision making analysis. J Urol. 2002;167(4):1621-9.
39. Wolf JS, Jr., Carroll PR, Stoller ML. Cost-effectiveness v patient preference in the choice of treatment for distal ureteral calculi: a literature-based decision analysis. J Endourol. 1995;9(3):243-8.
40. Ahn SH, Mayo-Smith WW, Murphy BL, et al. Acute non-traumatic abdominal pain in adult patients: abdominal radiography compared with CT evaluation. Radiology. 2002;225(1):159-64.
41. Vieweg J, Teh C, Freed K, et al. Unenhanced helical computerized tomography for the evaluation of patients with acute flank pain. J Urol. 1998;160(3 Pt 1):679-84.
42. Hoppe H, Studer R, Kessler TM, et al. Alternate or additional findings to stone disease on unenhanced computerized tomography for acute flank pain can impact management. J Urol. 2006;175(5):1725-30; discussion 30.
43. Fowler KA, Locken JA, Duchesne JH, et al. US for detecting renal calculi with nonenhanced CT as a reference standard. Radiology. 2002;222(1):109-13.
44. Ulusan S, Koc Z, Tokmak N. Accuracy of sonography for detecting renal stone: comparison with CT. J Clin Ultrasound. 2007;35(5):256-61.
45. Pichler R, Skradski V, Aigner F, et al. In young adults with a low body mass index ultrasonography is sufficient as a diagnostic tool for ureteric stones. BJU Int. 2012;109(5):770-4.
46. Mitterberger M, Pinggera GM, Pallwein L, et al. Plain abdominal radiography with transabdominal native tissue harmonic imaging ultrasonography vs unenhanced computed tomography in renal colic. BJU Int. 2007;100(4):887-90.
47. Youssef R, Shin R, Cabrera F, et al. Antimicrobial utilization prior to endourological surgery for urolithiasis: endourological society survey results. In: World Congress of Endourology 2014; 2014. p. MP09-16.
48. Wong SW, Smith R, Crowe P. Optimizing the operating theatre environment. ANZ J Surg. 2010;80(12):917-24.
49. Sabnis RB, Mishra S, Sharma R, et al. Preoperative planning and designing of a fluorocompatible endourology operating room. J Endourol. 2009;23(10):1579-85.
50. Yang RM, Morgan T, Bellman GC. Radiation protection during percutaneous nephrolithotomy: a new urologic surgery radiation shield. J Endourol. 2002;16(10):727-31.
51. Cabrera F, Preminger GM, Lipkin ME. As low as reasonably achievable: methods for reducing radiation exposure during the management of renal and ureteral stones. Indian J Urol. 2014;30(1):55-9.
52. Cabrera F, Shin R, Nguyen G, et al. Increased radiation exposure from fluoroscopy with fixed table versus portable C-arm. J Urol. 2014; 191(4):e1-958:MP12-1.
53. Cabrera F, Shin R, Nguyen G, et al. Increased radiation exposure during ureteroscopy in the obese patient. J Urol. 2014; 191(4):e1-958:MP73-05.
54. Rao MP, Kumar S, Dutta B, et al. Safety and efficacy of ureteroscopic lithotripsy for ureteral calculi under sedoanalgesia—a prospective study. Int Urol Nephrol. 2005;37(2):219-24.
55. Kuntz N, Neisius A, Tsivian M, et al. Balloon dilation of the ureter: a contemporary review of outcomes and complications. J Endourol. 2013;27:A402.
56. Rubenstein RA, Zhao LC, Loeb S, et al. Prestenting improves ureteroscopic stone-free rates. J Endourol. 2007;21(11):1277-80.
57. Chu L, Farris CA, Corcoran AT, et al. Preoperative stent placement decreases cost of ureteroscopy. Urology. 2011;78(2):309-13.
58. Kourambas J, Byrne RR, Preminger GM. Does a ureteral access sheath facilitate ureteroscopy? J Urol. 2001;165(3):789-93.
59. Delvecchio FC, Auge BK, Brizuela RM, et al. Assessment of stricture formation with the ureteral access sheath. Urology. 2003;61(3):518-22; discussion 22.
60. Rehman J, Monga M, Landman J, et al. Characterization of intrapelvic pressure during ureteropyeloscopy with ureteral access sheaths. Urology. 2003;61(4):713-8.
61. L'Esperance J O, Ekeruo WO, Scales CD, Jr., et al. Effect of ureteral access sheath on stone-free rates in patients undergoing ureteroscopic management of renal calculi. Urology. 2005;66(2):252-5.
62. Traxer O, Thomas A. Prospective evaluation and classification of ureteral wall injuries resulting from insertion of a ureteral access sheath during retrograde intrarenal surgery. J Urol. 2013;189(2):580-4.
63. Landman J, Lee DI, Lee C, et al. Evaluation of overall costs of currently available small flexible ureteroscopes. Urology. 2003;62(2):218-22.
64. Afane JS, Olweny EO, Bercowsky E, et al. Flexible ureteroscopes: a single center evaluation of the durability and function of the new endoscopes smaller than 9 Fr. J Urol. 2000;164(4):1164-8.
65. Traxer O, Dubosq F, Jamali K, et al. New-generation flexible ureterorenoscopes are more durable than previous ones. Urology. 2006;68(2):276-9; discussion 80-1.
66. Kruck S, Anastasiadis AG, Gakis G, et al. Flow matters: irrigation flow differs in flexible ureteroscopes of the newest generation. Urol Res. 2011;39(6):483-6.
67. Binbay M, Yuruk E, Akman T, et al. Is there a difference in outcomes between digital and fiberoptic flexible ureterorenoscopy procedures? J Endourol. 2010;24(12):1929-34.
68. Menezes P, Kumar PV, Timoney AG. A randomized trial comparing lithoclast with an electrokinetic lithotripter in the management of ureteric stones. BJU Int. 2000;85(1):22-5.
69. Wang AJ, Baldwin GT, Gabriel JC, et al. In-vitro assessment of a new portable ballistic lithotripter with percutaneous and ureteroscopic models. J Endourol. 2012;26(11):1500-5.
70. Rane A, Kommu SS, Kandaswamy SV, et al. Initial clinical evaluation of a new pneumatic intracorporeal lithotripter. BJU Int. 2007;100(3):629-32.
71. Piergiovanni M, Desgrandchamps F, Cochand-Priollet B, et al. Ureteral and bladder lesions after ballistic, ultrasonic, electrohydraulic, or laser lithotripsy. J Endourol. 1994;8(4):293-9.
72. Knispel HH, Klan R, Heicappell R, et al. Pneumatic lithotripsy applied through deflected working channel of miniureteroscope: results in 143 patients. J Endourol. 1998;12(6):513-5.

73. Segura JW. Intracorporeal lithotripsy. AUA Update Ser. 1999;18:66-71.
74. Zhong P, Tong HL, Cocks FH, et al. Transient oscillation of cavitation bubbles near stone surface during electrohydraulic lithotripsy. J Endourol. 1997;11(1):55-61.
75. Poon M, Beaghler M, Baldwin D. Flexible endoscope deflectability: changes using a variety of working instruments and laser fibers. J Endourol. 1997;11(4):247-9.
76. Hofbauer J, Hobarth K, Marberger M. Electrohydraulic versus pneumatic disintegration in the treatment of ureteral stones: a randomized, prospective trial. J Urol. 1995;153(3 Pt 1): 623-5.
77. Teichman JM, Rao RD, Rogenes VJ, et al. Ureteroscopic management of ureteral calculi: electrohydraulic versus holmium:YAG lithotripsy. J Urol. 1997;158(4):1357-61.
78. Bhatta KM, Prien EL, Jr, Dretler SP. Cystine calculi—rough and smooth: a new clinical distinction. J Urol. 1989;142(4):937-40.
79. Wollin TA, Denstedt JD. The holmium laser in urology. J Clin Laser Med Surg. 1998;16(1):13-20.
80. Sea J, Jonat LM, Chew BH, et al. Optimal power settings for Holmium:YAG lithotripsy. J Urol. 2012;187(3):914-9.
81. Lobik L, Lopez-Pujals A, Leveillee RJ. Variables affecting deflection of a new third-generation flexible ureteropyeloscope (DUR-8 elite). J Endourol. 2003;17(9):733-6.
82. Abdelshehid C, Ahlering MT, Chou D, et al. Comparison of flexible ureteroscopes: deflection, irrigant flow and optical characteristics. J Urol. 2005;173(6):2017-21.
83. Lane BR, Singh D, Meraney A, et al. Novel endourologic applications for holmium laser. Urology. 2005;65(5):991-3.
84. Pietrow PK, Auge BK, Delvecchio FC, et al. Techniques to maximize flexible ureteroscope longevity. Urology. 2002;60(5):784-8.
85. Shin R, Fernando C, Shami C, et al. Ball-tip holmium laser fiber may reduce flexible ureteroscope damage. J Urol. 2014;191(4):e1-958.
86. Scarpa RM, De Lisa A, Porru D, et al. Holmium:YAG laser ureterolithotripsy. Eur Urol. 1999;35(3):233-8.
87. Chow GK, Patterson DE, Blute ML, et al. Ureteroscopy: effect of technology and technique on clinical practice. J Urol. 2003;170(1):99-102.
88. Eisner BH, Dretler SP. Use of the Stone Cone for prevention of calculus retropulsion during holmium:YAG laser lithotripsy: case series and review of the literature. Urol Int. 2009;82(3):356-60.
89. Kesler SS, Pierre SA, Brison DI, et al. Use of the escape nitinol stone retrieval basket facilitates fragmentation and extraction of ureteral and renal calculi: a pilot study. J Endourol. 2008;22(6):1213-7.
90. Pardalidis NP, Papatsoris AG, Kosmaoglou EV. Prevention of retrograde calculus migration with the Stone Cone. Urol Res. 2005;33(1):61-4.
91. Rane A, Bradoo A, Rao P, et al. The use of a novel reverse thermosensitive polymer to prevent ureteral stone retropulsion during intracorporeal lithotripsy: a randomized, controlled trial. J Urol. 2010;183(4):1417-21.
92. Ursiny M, Eisner BH. Cost-effectiveness of anti-retropulsion devices for ureteroscopic lithotripsy. J Urol. 2013;189(5):1762-6.
93. Matani YS, Al-Ghazo MA, Al-azab RS, et al. Emergency double-J stent insertion following uncomplicated ureteroscopy: risk-factor analysis and recommendations. Int Braz J Urol. 2013;39(2):203-8.
94. Nabi G, Cook J, N'Dow J, et al. Outcomes of stenting after uncomplicated ureteroscopy: systematic review and meta-analysis. BMJ. 2007;334(7593):572.
95. Shigemura K, Yasufuku T, Yamanaka K, et al. How long should double J stent be kept in after ureteroscopic lithotripsy? Urol Res. 2012;40(4):373-6.
96. Boddy SA, Nimmon CC, Jones S, et al. Acute ureteric dilatation for ureteroscopy. An experimental study. Br J Urol. 1988;61(1):27-31.
97. Torricelli FC, De S, Hinck B, et al. Flexible ureteroscopy with a ureteral access sheath: when to stent? Urology. 2014; 83(2):278-81.
98. Nazim SM, Ather MH. Alpha-blockers impact stent-related symptoms: a randomized, double-blind, placebo-controlled trial. J Endourol. 2012;26(9):1237-41.
99. Tadros NN, Bland L, Legg E, et al. A single dose of a non-steroidal anti-inflammatory drug (NSAID) prevents severe pain after ureteric stent removal: a prospective, randomised, double-blind, placebo-controlled trial. BJU Int. 2013;111(1):101-5.
100. Rippel CA, Nikkel L, Lin YK, et al. Residual fragments following ureteroscopic lithotripsy: incidence and predictors on postoperative computerized tomography. J Urol. 2012; 188(6):2246-51.
101. Candau C, Saussine C, Lang H, et al. Natural history of residual renal stone fragments after ESWL. Eur Urol. 2000; 37(1):18-22.
102. Weizer AZ, Auge BK, Silverstein AD, et al. Routine postoperative imaging is important after ureteroscopic stone manipulation. J Urol. 2002;168(1):46-50.
103. Fulgham PF, Assimos DG, Pearle MS, et al. Clinical effectiveness protocols for imaging in the management of ureteral calculous disease: AUA technology assessment. J Urol. 2013;189(4):1203-13.
104. Sutherland TN, Pearle MS, Lotan Y. How much is a kidney worth? Cost-effectiveness of routine imaging after ureteroscopy to prevent silent obstruction. J Urol. 2013;189(6): 2136-41.
105. Bercowsky E, Shalhav AL, Elbahnasy AM, et al. The effect of patient position on intrarenal anatomy. J Endourol. 1999;13(4):257-60.
106. Auge BK, Dahm P, Wu NZ, et al. Ureteroscopic management of lower-pole renal calculi: technique of calculus displacement. J Endourol. 2001;15(8):835-8.
107. Geavlete P, Georgescu D, Nita G, et al. Complications of 2735 retrograde semirigid ureteroscopy procedures: a single-center experience. J Endourol. 2006;20(3):179-85.
108. Stern JM, Yiee J, Park S. Safety and efficacy of ureteral access sheaths. J Endourol. 2007;21(2):119-23.
109. Matlaga BR, Lingeman JE. Surgical management of stones: new technology. Adv Chronic Kidney Dis. 2009;16(1):60-4.
110. Monga M, Beeman WW. Advanced intrarenal ureteroscopic procedures. Urol Clin North Am. 2004;31(1):129-35.

111. Malgor RD, Oderich GS, Andrews JC, et al. Evolution from open surgical to endovascular treatment of ureteral-iliac artery fistula. J Vasc Surg. 2012;55(4):1072-80.
112. Makarov DV, Trock BJ, Allaf ME, et al. The effect of ureteral stent placement on post-ureteroscopy complications: a meta-analysis. Urology. 2008;71(5):796-800.
113. Fedullo LM, Pollack HM, Banner MP, et al. The development of steinstrassen after ESWL: frequency, natural history, and radiologic management. AJR Am J Roentgenol. 1988;151(6):1145-7.
114. Preminger GM, Kettelhut MC, Elkins SL, et al. Ureteral stenting during extracorporeal shock wave lithotripsy: help or hindrance? J Urol. 1989;142(1):32-6.
115. Kim SC, Oh CH, Moon YT, et al. Treatment of steinstrasse with repeat extracorporeal shock wave lithotripsy: experience with piezoelectric lithotriptor. J Urol. 1991;145(3):489-91.
116. Coptcoat MJ, Webb DR, Kellet MJ, et al. The steinstrasse: a legacy of extracorporeal lithotripsy? Eur Urol. 1988;14(2):93-5.
117. Coptcoat MJ, Webb DR, Kellett MJ, et al. The treatment of 100 consecutive patients with ureteral calculi in a British stone center. J Urol. 1987;137(6):1122-3.
118. Sulaiman MN, Buchholz NP, Clark PB. The role of ureteral stent placement in the prevention of steinstrasse. J Endourol. 1999;13(3):151-5.
119. Tepeler A, Resorlu B, Sahin T, et al. Categorization of intraoperative ureteroscopy complications using modified Satava classification system. World J Urol. 2014;32(1):131-6.
120. Schuster TG, Hollenbeck BK, Faerber GJ, et al. Ureteroscopic treatment of lower pole calculi: comparison of lithotripsy in situ and after displacement. J Urol. 2002;168(1):43-5.
121. Krambeck AE, Murat FJ, Gettman MT, et al. The evolution of ureteroscopy: a modern single-institution series. Mayo Clin Proc. 2006;81(4):468-73.
122. Roberts WW, Cadeddu JA, Micali S, et al. Ureteral stricture formation after removal of impacted calculi. J Urol. 1998;159(3):723-6.
123. Saglam R, Muslumanoglu AY, Tokatli Z, et al. A new robot for flexible ureteroscopy: development and early clinical results (Ideal Stage 1-2b). Eur Urol. 2014;66(6):1092-100.
124. Palmero JL, Castello A, Miralles J, et al. Results of retrograde intrarenal surgery in the treatment of renal stones greater than 2 cm. Actas Urol Esp. 2014;38(4):257-62.
125. Sung JC, Springhart WP, Marguet CG, et al. Location and etiology of flexible and semirigid ureteroscope damage. Urology. 2005;66(5):958-63.
126. Kawahara T, Ito H, Terao H, et al. Changing to a loop-type ureteral stent decreases patients' stent-related symptoms. Urol Res. 2012;40(6):763-7.
127. Gurbuz C, Atis G, Arikan O, et al. The cost analysis of flexible ureteroscopic lithotripsy in 302 cases. Urolithiasis. 2014; 42(2):155-8.
128. Raney AM. Electrohydranlic ureterolithotripsy. Urology. 1978;12:284.
129. Eisner BH, Pengune W, Stoller ML. Use of an antiretropulsion device to prevent stone retropulsion significantly increases the efficiency of pneumatic lithotripsy: an in vitro study. BJU Int. 2009;104(6):858-61.

CHAPTER

33

Percutaneous Nephrolithotomy in Management of Stones: Present Role, Approaches, Outcomes and Complications

Arvind P Ganpule, Mohan Kumar, Mahesh Desai

INTRODUCTION

Percutaneous nephrolithotomy (PCNL) is the procedure of choice for treatment of renal calculi. Since it was described in the eighties it has undergone evolution with regards to choice of access, method of dilatation and the energy source used for fragmentation of the stone. The various complications that can be encountered include bleeding, infection and residual stones.

With the advent of newer techniques such as extracorporeal shockwave lithotripsy (ESWL) and flexible ureteroscopy (FURS) there has been a paradigm shift in the indications for PCNL where only larger stones used to be treated by PCNL. With the rapid development in optics and stone fragmentation device we can now treat even small stones with methods such as miniPCNL and micro-PCNL with minimal morbidity and good stone clearance.

In this chapter, we allude to the various approaches for gaining percutaneous access to the pelvicalyceal system, complications and newer concepts in percutaneous surgery.

PRESENT ROLE OF PERCUTANEOUS NEPHROLITHOTOMY

The factors which determine the indications for percutaneous nephrolithotomy include stone factors (stone size, stone composition, stone location), patient factors (habitus, renal anomalies), failure of other treatment modalities (ESWL, flexible ureteroscopy). The usual indications for PCNL are stones >20 mm^2, staghorn, partial staghorn calculi. The contraindications for PCNL include UTI, pregnancy and coagulation abnormalities.[1]

Percutaneous nephrolithotomy (PCNL) is the treatment of choice for large stone. It attains stone free rates of up to 95% as it offers direct removal of stone fragments through the nephrostomy tract. For stones of <2 cm in size the treatment algorithm becomes more complicated because of multiple variables involved. American Urological Association (AUA) guidelines recommend PCNL as a treatment of choice for staghorn calculi. PCNL should be the recommended modality for staghorn calculi as clearance rates are three times that of ESWL. The following are the treatment options in staghorn calculi:-

1. Percutaneous nephrolithotomy should be the first treatment utilized for most patients (Level 2 evidence).
2. Extracorporeal Shock Wave Lithotripsy (ESWL) should not be used as the preferred treatment modality for staghorn stones.
3. Open surgery should be recommended only if the stones are not expected to be removed in a reasonable number of stages.
4. Nephrectomy should be considered in nonfunctioning kidneys.

To summarize, PCNL is the first choice for staghorn calculi.[1] Open surgery is desirable in the situation when expertise is not available wherein the stone can be cleared in reasonable number of stages and tracts. Nephrectomy should be considered for nonfunctioning kidneys.

Role of PCNL in Large Stones

Larger stones of the lower pole are best managed by PCNL as a first treatment option irrespective to the lower pole anatomy. Treatment of lower polar stones should be guided by the diameter of the stone. Data from meta-analysis suggests that larger lower polar stones have lower clearance rates and higher retreatment rates[2] (level 1 evidence). A large multicenter prospective randomized trial comparing PCNL with ESWL showed PCNL to have a significantly higher stone free rate (91%) compared to ESWL (21%), in addition the need for ancillary procedures and retreatment rates were higher for ESWL as compared to PCNL (level 1 evidence).[3] While considering the stone location, the calyceal stone burden is the most important factor in predicting the clearance.

Calyceal diverticulum is nonsecretory urothelium lined compartments in communication with the renal collecting system. Asymptomatic stones in the diverticulum may be left alone; however, stones causing pain, hematuria

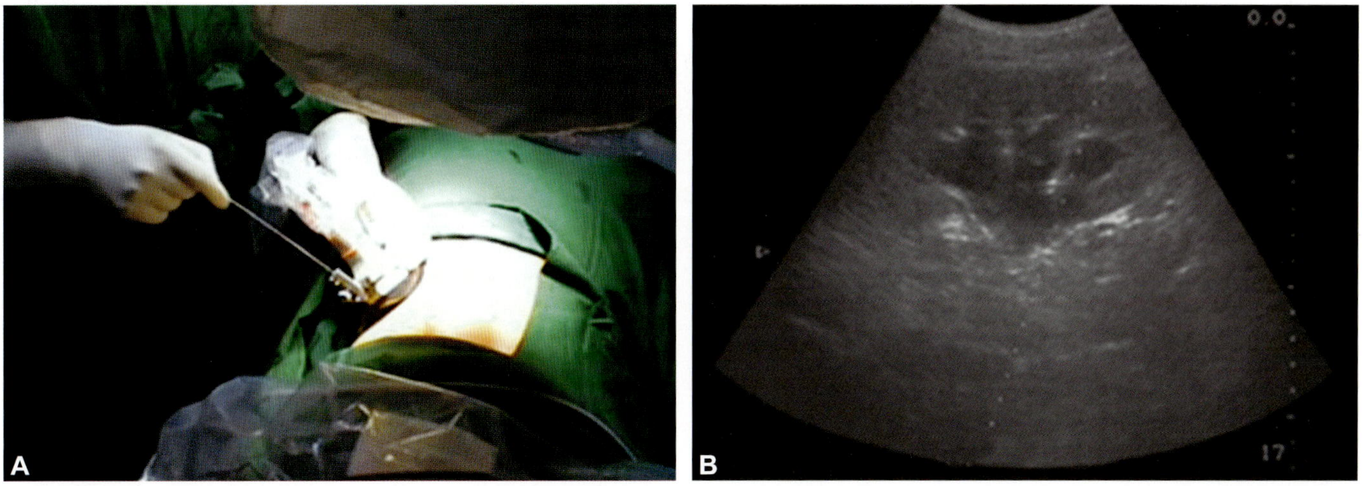

Figs. 33.1A and B: USG Ultrasound guided puncture. (A) The procedure of USG-guided puncture. (B) USG showing needle tip in PCS. (USG: Ultrasound sonography test; PCS: Pelvicalyceal system).

and infection should be treated. PCNL offers better stone free rates. Although there have been no randomized trials comparing laparoscopy with PCNL and ureteroscopy. PCNL is considered to be a gold standard in management of calyceal diverticular stones. In comparison to ESWL, PCNL has higher stone free rates with similar recurrence rates and complication rates.[4] The stone free rates for PCNL range from 85 to 93%, the added advantage of PCNL include it provides excellent access for obliteration of the diverticular sac.[5]

Stone composition and the fragility is a "key" factor in determining the modality of treatment to be choosen. The composition of the stone is an important factor for predicting the success rates of renal calculi. Specific stone compositions have different clearance rates because of the varying fragility of stones. Cystine stones are harder to fragment; hence cystine stones larger than 15 mm should not be treated with ESWL. PCNL would be a good option in these patients. The measurement of stone density with noncontrast computed tomography (NCCT) helps in predicting success rates of ESWL and the need for PCNL. Stones with > 1000 Hounsfield units (HU) show poor results with ESWL. Struvite stones are best dealt with using PCNL.

THE APPROACH

Position for Gaining Access

Supine or Prone PCNL

In conventional PCNL prone position is best suited because posterior calyx can be directly accessed in this position and bowel can be avoided. Supine PCNL has the advantages of combined antegrade and retrograde approaches without change in position and this position is best suited for patients with comorbidities. The Barts modification of Valdivia position uses both X-ray and USG in combination.[5,6]

Choice of Access

Ultrasound-guided access: The ultrasound access has advantages such as no radiation and it is safe in pregnancy but it has a learning curve and not all steps can easily be done with ultrasound. We requie fluoroscopy in the later stages such as dilatation.

Technique

The 3 Mhz or 5 Mhz probe is used usually with a puncture attachment (Fig. 33.1A). The path of the needle is given by the dotted line on the USG screen (Fig. 33.1B). An echo-tip needle helps in better visualization of needle in USG. The kidney should be scanned posterior to anterior. The posterior calyx is seen first and puncture is done when the calyx, infundibulum and pelvis are all seen. In a perfect puncture the needle is seen throughout the course and there is egress of urine on removing the stillette.

Fluoroscopic-guided Puncture

Fluoroscopic-guided puncture has the advantage of gaining access through the posterior calyx as it can be clearly seen as an end on calyx. But the disadvantage is that the

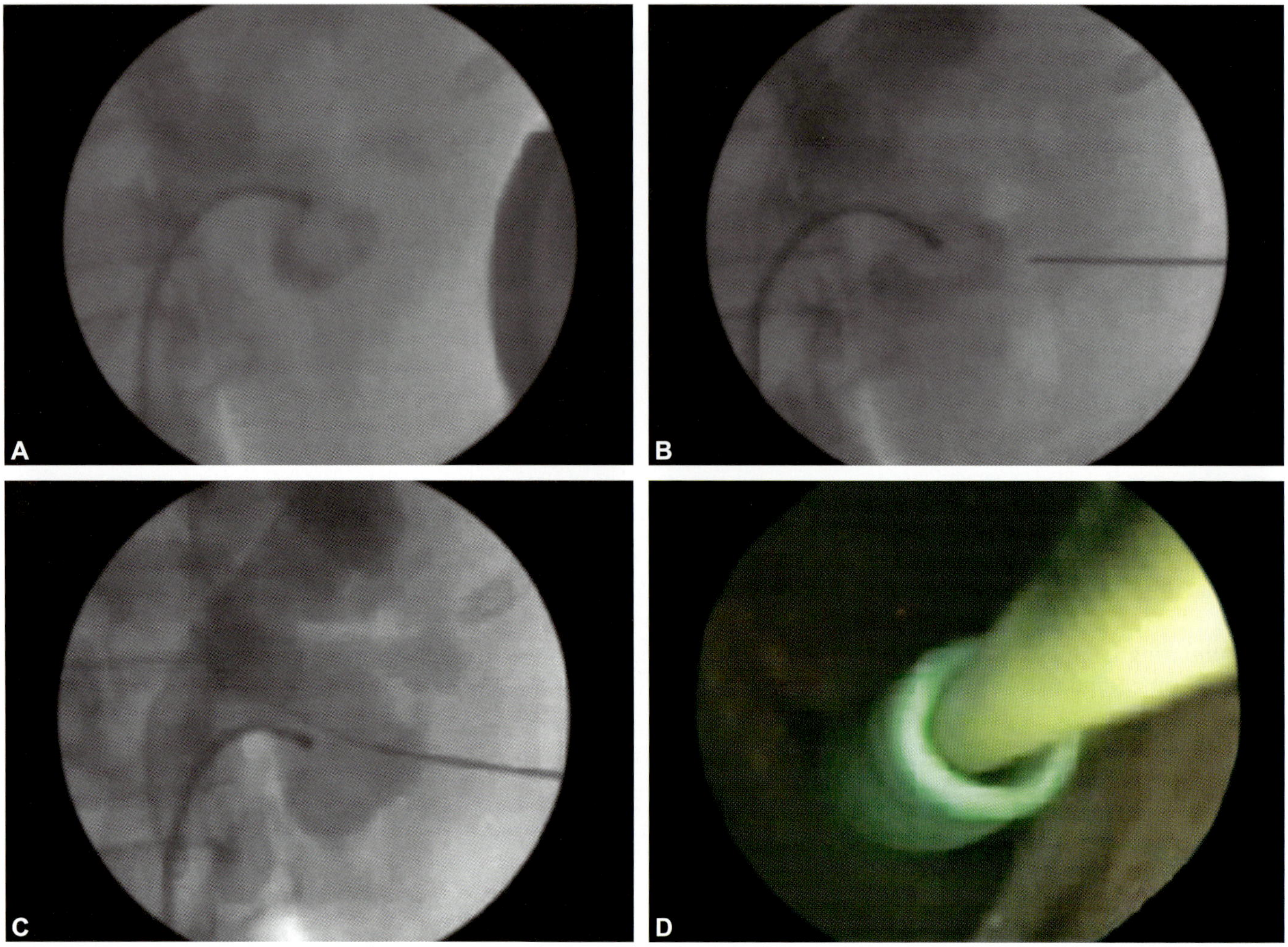

Figs. 33.2A to D: Endoscopic-guided puncture. (A) Flexible ureteroscope in the system. (B) Flexible ureteroscope with the puncture needle. (C) Flexible ureteroscope with the guidewire in the PCS through percutaneous puncture. (D) Endoscopic view of Amplatz sheath with the guidewire. (PCS: Pelvicalyceal system).

risk of radiation exposure is high and the chance of bowel and other viscera injury is more in fluoro-guided puncture than in USG.

In the triangulation technique the C-arm is placed over the patient in the vertical position. A retrograde pyelogram is obtained, and the skin over the desired calyx is marked. The C-arm is then rotated 30° toward the surgeon for an end-on view of the posterior group of calyces. The skin site over the calyx is marked lateral to the first site. Move in a vertical line inferiorly until a site 1–2 cm below the 12th rib is reached. This third site is marked and serves as the site of needle entry. From this point, the needle is advanced to the junction of the vertical plane and the 30° plane. Access is achieved at the junction of all three axes.[7]

Endoscopic Guided Renal Access (EGA)

Technique

In this technique we use a flexible ureteroscope to identify the ideal calyx for puncture (Fig. 33.2A). A flexible ureteroscope is advanced into the pelvicalyceal system (Fig. 33.2B) and the calyx entry is confirmed seeing the tip of the needle entry into the concerned calyx (Fig. 33.2C). After the gidewire is inserted the other steps of dilatation can either be done by fluoro guidance or direct endoscopic guidance (Fig. 33.2D).

In a study the endoscopic guided access (EGA)[8] was compared with fluoroscopic guided puncture (FGA). EGA had shorter fluoroscopy time (3.2 vs 16.8 minutes, $P < .001$)

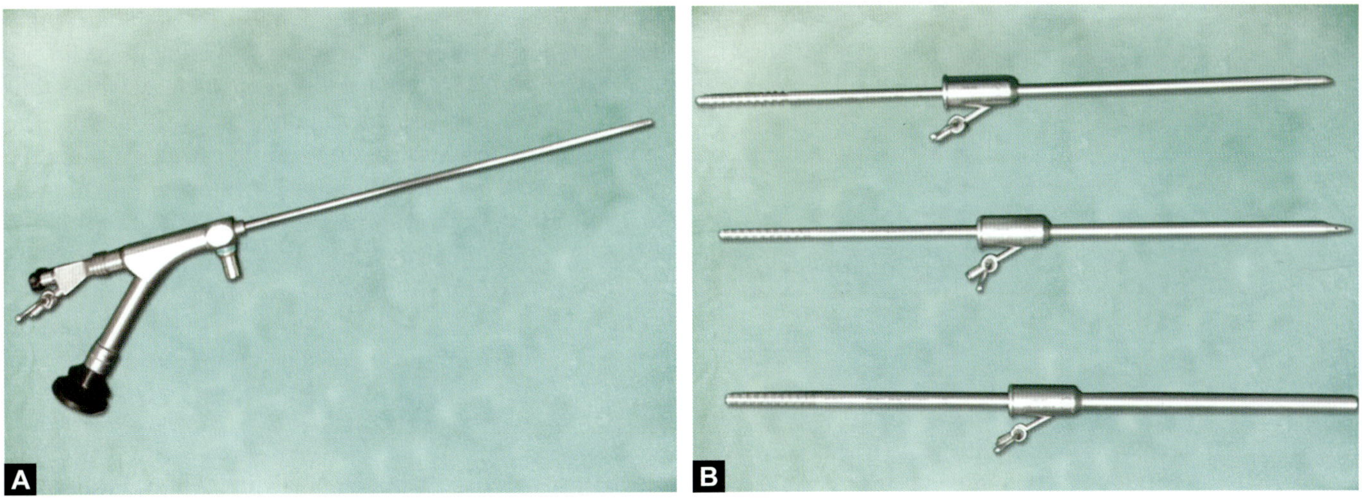

Figs. 33.3A and B: Miniperc. (A) Miniperc 12-Fr telescope. (B) Miniperc sheaths: 20, 16, and 12 Fr.

and lower access number (1.03 vs 1.22 $P = .002$). Fluoroscopy time was longer for FGA than for EGA after adjusting for BMI, staghorn stones, and access number ($P < .001$). No significant difference was noted in change in hemoglobin, blood transfusion rate, operative time, or intraoperative complications between groups. The authors concluded that EGA is safe and effective and leads to decreased fluoroscopy time, decreased need for multiple accesses, and decreased risk of early termination of the procedure or need for secondary procedures. These findings need to be validated in large multicenter comparative trials.

Multiperc PCNL

The preoperative CT IVU helps in deciding the primary calyx of puncture through which the majority of the stone bulk is to be cleared, stones situated in separate calyces and which are unlikely to be cleared through the primary tract are also identified. Once the patient is placed in prone position a ultrasound examination is done to identify the primary calyx of puncture. A guidewire is passed in the ureter, following which access is gained in the proposed secondary tracts. Once all the desired access has been gained and the guidewires are in position, the primary tract is dilated. It is imperative that the tract should not be dilated at the outset as this would lead to extravasation and subsequent difficulty. The operating time is limited to ninety minutes because it has been shown in number of studies of the risk of fluid absorption with prolonged surgery. If it is decided that the procedure is to be staged the 14 Fr malecot tubes are inserted in the secondary access tracts. These serve the dual purpose of achieving mature tracts and providing a conduit for subsequent intervention. The primary tracts are dilated up to 26 Fr while the secondary tracts are dilated till 20 Fr.[9]

The points in favor of multitract PCNL are that it has the ability to clear stones without increasing the cost of instrumentation. In addition the argument is that the person who can create a primary tract can very well create additional tracts without additional learning curve. The multitract PCNL also does not depend on anatomy such as infundibular stenosis.

Single Tract with Use of Flexible Instrumentation

This technique involves creation of a strategic tract which clears majority of stones. Once the bulk is cleared, stones present in inaccessible calyces are approached with flexible instruments.[10] The downside of this approach is additional cost for instrumentation.

NEWER CONCEPTS IN PERCUTANEOUS SURGERY

Miniperc

In Miniperc the sheath size is not more than 20 Fr. Although miniperc was originally devised for pediatric population[11] it has been extensively used in adults due to its advantages such as reduced blood loss, improved recovery with comparable stone clearance rates.

In miniperc the scopes used range from 8–16 Fr. (Fig. 33.3A) and the tract size varies from 12 Fr to 20 Fr (Fig. 33.3B). We can use all the modalities of energy such as

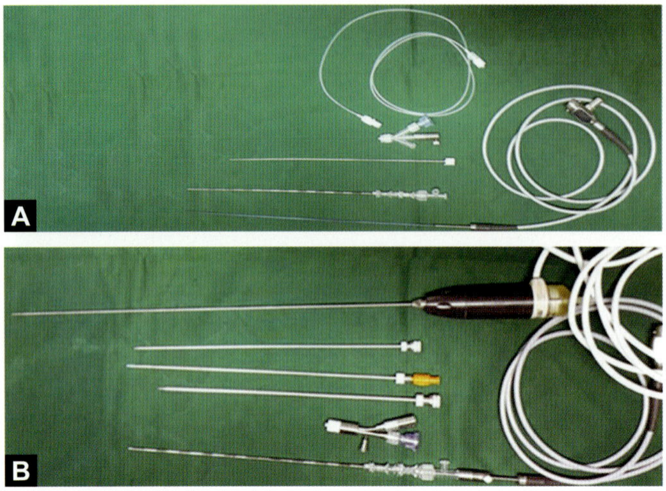

Figs. 33.4A and B: Microperc. (A) Microperc assembly showing the all-seeing needle, adapter, and flexible telescope. (B) Sheaths of various sizes with lithoclast.

laser lithoclast etc. Miniperc[12] is best used for stones ranging from 1 cm to 2.5 cm.

Mishra et al.[12] demonstrated that miniperc has comparable stone clearance rates with standard PCNL and also has an advantage decreased blood loss and early recovery. Mishra et al.[12] noted that miniperc has a drawback of lengthy operative time. Reasons for the same might be due to diminished intraoperative field visibility, the need for fragmentation by laser into very small stones suitable for ureteroscopic graspers and/or baskets, and the small sheath.

Microperc

Microperc still pushes the limit of miniaturization in PCNL. Microperc uses 16 G needle (Fig. 33.4A) and stones refragmented through the same needle with the help of needloscope and laser.

Technique of Microperc

In lithotomy position under general anesthesia (GA) ureteric catheter is inserted under fluoro guidance. The ureteric catheter is fixed to a urethral catheter and the patient is turned to prone position. Then saline is injected to dilate the PCS and USG or fluoro guided puncture done with 16 G all seeing needle. After appropriate calyceal access, a three-way connector is attached to the needle. This connects saline irrigation tube, a 'Touhy Borst' adapter to allow 272 μm laser fiber and a 0.9 mm flexible microperc telescope (Fig. 33.4A). Saline irrigation is carried out using a mechanical pump with foot pedal control. Saline irrigation is kept to a minimum, which is just enough for proper vision. Generally, intermittent saline irrigation with a flow rate of 100 mL/min provides good vision without increasing intrarenal pressures. The ureteric catheter drains the pelvicalyceal system continuously. Intermittent manual suction through the ureteric catheter further reduces the intrarenal pressure. The stone is completely fragmented with laser. Ureteric catheter is removed along with Foley catheter in first post-operative day. Patient is discharged in first postoperative day if there is no complication.

Modifications in Microperc

Since the microperc needle is of narrow caliber, it can bend if it is manipulated inside the pelvicalyceal system. Moreover, there is a theoretical risk of parenchymal tear if there is excessive intrarenal manipulation. In order to overcome these problems, an 8 Fr metallic sheath has been developed (Fig. 33.4B). This so-called "mini-microperc" sheath allows the attachment of the same three-way connector with accessories as in standard microperc. The sheath allows intrarenal manipulations from one calyx to another. Another important advantage of mini-microperc is the ability to insert a 1.6 mm ultrasonic lithotripter, which can fragment and suck the fragments out of the kidney. The microperc telescope has a 0.9 mm working diameter with 10,000 pixel resolution.

Current Role of Microperc

Microperc is still in its early stages of development. It is currently used to manage single renal calculus or multiple renal calculi, which can be accessed with a single puncture and cumulative diameter of less than 1.5 cm in diameter. Though it can be used in intermediate sized calculi, it is preferable to use mini-microperc so that the fragments can be removed from pelvicalyceal system. It can be safely used in the pediatric age group. In a comparative study done by Sabnis et al[13] it was proved that Microperc is a safe and effective alternative to retrograde intrarenal surgery (RIRS) for the management of small renal calculi and has similar stone clearance and complication rates when Compared to RIRS.

Ultraminiperc

The Armamentarium

A Mini nephroscope and a novel working sheath (Fig. 33.5A) are utilized. One of the special basic instruments

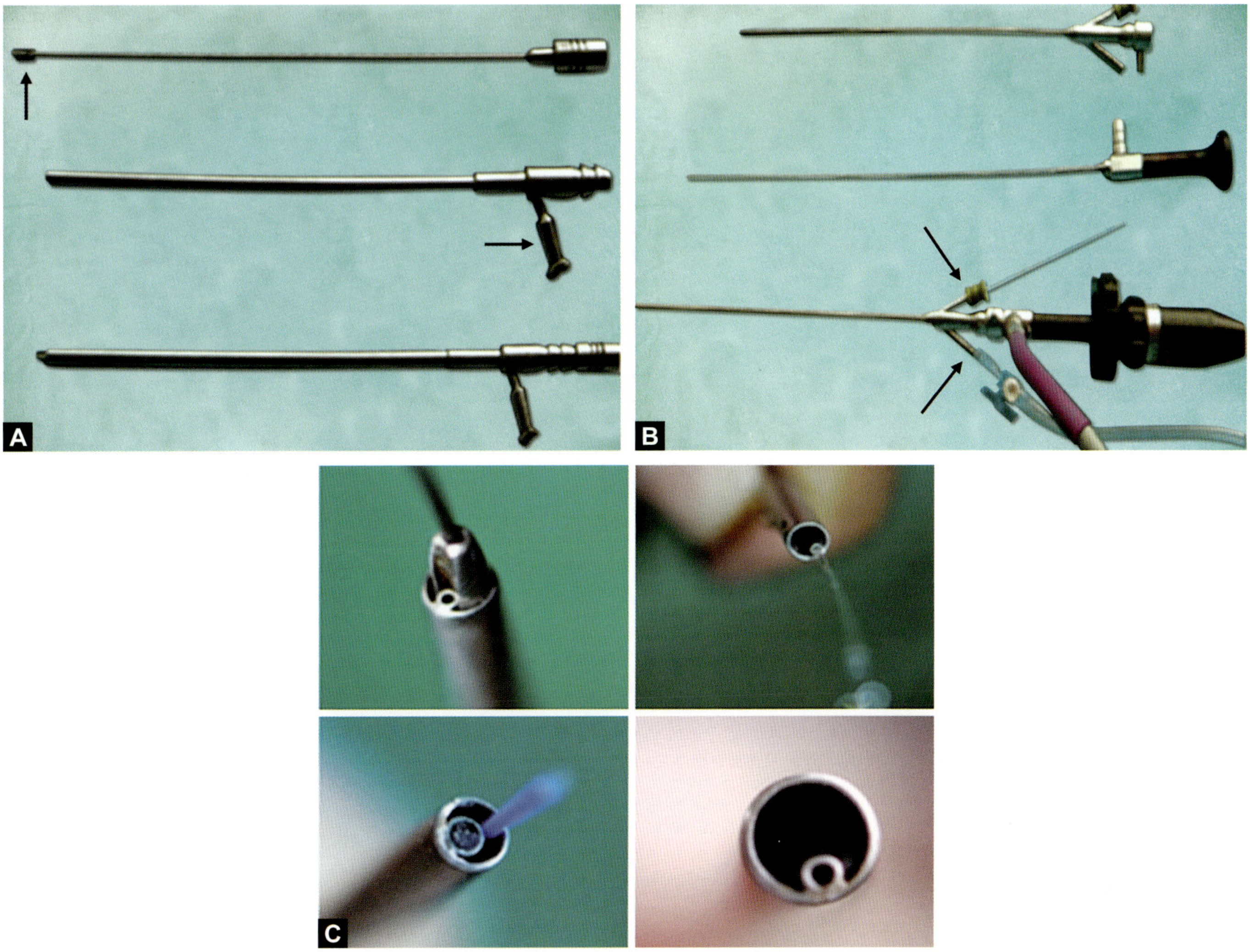

Figs. 33.5A to C: Ultra-miniperc. (A) The working metal sheath and its obturator. (B) Spatial location of the fine tube, obturator, guidewire, and laser fiber, and water jet out from inner fine tube. (C) Mininephroscope assembled with a 3.5-Fr telescope and a 6-Fr demountable telescope (inner) sheath. The 3.5-Fr telescope passes through the central channel. Irrigation connection and laser fiber are each attached to one side port. Optics are connected to a zoom ocular and light adapter.
Source: Desai JD, Zeng G, Zhao Z, et al. A novel technique of ultra-mini-percutaneous nephrolithotomy: introduction and an initial experience for treatment of upper urinary calculi less than 2 cm. Biomed Res Int. 2013;2013:490793.

set of the ultra miniperc (UMP) is an 11 Fr or 13 Fr metal sheath with an integrated side port. It has a housed 1mm diameter of inner fine tube (LUT-GmbH, Germany). There is a channel from the inner fine tube to the side port, and the side port can attach a syringe to produce a water jet. The metal sheath can be matched with an obturator inside itself. The obturator is beveled with a side groove in the distal end, so the guidewire can pass through the obturator (Fig. 33.5B). Another special basic instrument is a 3.5 Fr telescope with a 6 Fr demountable telescope sheath (LUT-GmbH, Germany), and the telescope sheath has two side ports. The assembled 6 Fr telescope is used for visualization. One side port of the telescope sheath is connected to an irrigation pump for irrigation and the other side port is used to pass the laser fiber. Optics is connected via a zoom ocular and light adapter to a standard endoscopic camera system (Fig. 33.5C).

UMP Technique

After anesthesia, and patient in prone position, fluoroscopy or USG guided percutaneous puncture is made followed by passage of an 18-gauge needle (Cook Incorporated, Bloomington, IN, USA). The puncture is confirmed

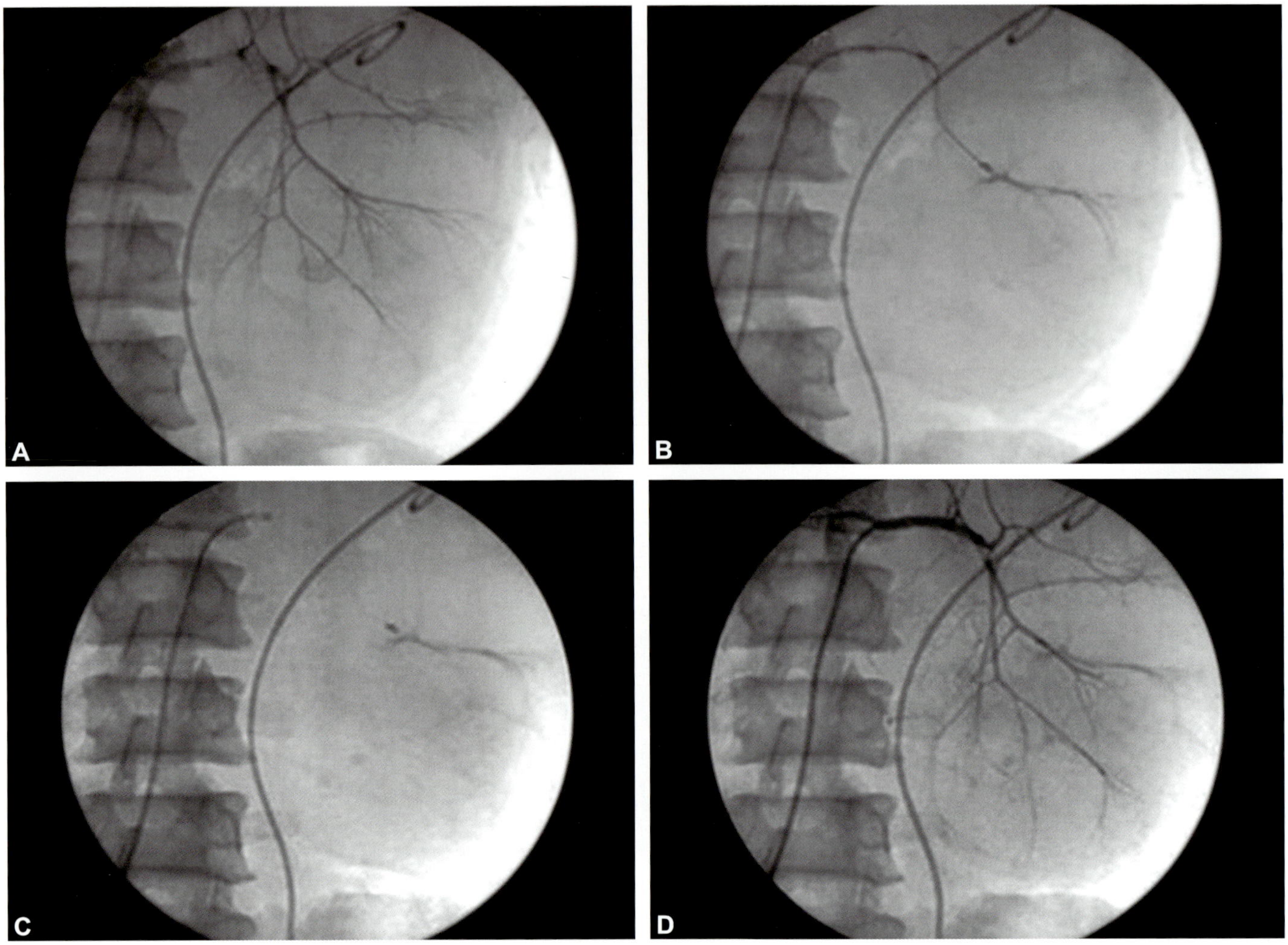

Figs. 33.6A to D: Angioembolization of the lower segmental branch of the renal artery post PCNL bleed. (A) Delineation of arterial anatomy. (B) Coils are advanced over guidewire. (C) Coils in place. (D) Angiogram with coils in place.
(PCNL: Percutaneous nephrolithotomy).

by flow of urine from the needle and by injecting contrast and seeing whether the PCS is visualized. A guidewire is then inserted into renal collecting system or down the ureter through the needle sheath (Fig. 33.6A) under fluoroscopic guidance and the needle is withdrawn. Then, the working sheath assembled with an obturator is gradually advanced over the guidewire to an appropriate location in the desire calyx. Next, the obturator is removed, and the sheath is still placed as a working sheath. Subsequently, the assembled 6 Fr telescope is inserted to the working metal sheath to inspect the collecting system.

The calculus is then fragmented by laser under direct visualization. In the UMP procedure the authors found 100~150 mm Hg pressure to be adequate to maintain vision.[14]

iPad-Guided PCNL

In iPad-assisted navigation, three-dimensional (3D) 'augmented virtual reality' can display all the relevant anatomical details. Limited vision, which is a disadvantage of USG nkp-guided puncture is negated by this method. The iPad takes the picture of the puncture site and it is assessed with the help of a software which syncs these images with the preloaded CT images and sends back the feed to the Ipad. The exact overlay of real and virtual markers allows a 'virtual insight' into the patient and thus gain access.[15]

New Concepts in Staghorn Classification

Staghorns are historically defined as branched calculi. The literature is not consistent as regards the classification of these stones thus it becomes challenging to compare the literature. A number of classifications have been proposed in this regard. They can be broadly classified as

(a) Morphological classification
(b) Anatomical classification
(c) Stone burden classification[16]

Recently with the addition of CT in the armamentarium of the urologist a number of classifications have been described.

Stone Classification

Staghorn Morphometry Classification

Staghorn morphometry" is the measurement of staghorn stone volumetric burden distribution in the collecting system. It helps in prediction of number of tracts and stages in which a stone can be cleared. [17] This can be done by means of a software which uses the CT scan images to analyze the data (3D-DOCTOR™; Able Software Corp., USA). The software works by extracting object boundaries using 3D image segmentation functions, and creating 3D surface volume rendering for visualization, object measurement, and quantitative analysis.

Complications

The study, conducted by the Clinical Research of the Endourological Society (CROES)[18], utilized the modified Clavien system for reporting complications. The majority of complications were minor. Minor complications include fever and nephrostomy leak.[19] Major complications occur during either access creation or at the time of stone removal.

Related to Access

Pleura

The pleura might be injured more during supracostal access than infracostal.[18,20] We usually use infracostal approach for routine access unless special indications such as requirement of upper pole access.

Liver and Spleen

Injury to the liver during PCNL is rare . In such cases the main worry is injury to intrahepatic vasculature. In such a situation of liver injury if vascular injury is ruled out then the nephrostomy tube should be remove, and the kidney should be decompressed by either stent or ureteric catheterization . This prevents retrobiliary fistula. In case of severe bleeding angioembolization has to be done.

Splenic injury is also a rare during PCNL . The injury is suspected intraoperatively when there is hemodynamic instability with no visible bleeding. If there is uncontrollable hemorrhage then splenectomy might be indicated in those cases.

Colon

Injury to colon, can occur in 0.2% to 1% of PCNL patients.[21,22] It is more common in patients with previous bowel surgery and also left side access.[23, 24] Colonic injury can be diagnosed intraoperatively if the colon is enhancing after contrast injection. Postoperative diagnosis can be made by CT or nephrostomogram. The symptoms in the postoperative period are fever, ileus, pain and feces or gas from PCN tube. It is treated with antibiotics and bowel rest and preferably a drain placement if necessary.

Duodenum and Jejunum

Duodenal and jejunal injury is extremely uncommon in PCNL. The diagnosis is made by CT scan. Mostly treated by open exploration. Conservative management in form of bowel rest , with or without percutaneous duodenal and kidney drainage can also be done.

Related to Stone Removal

Infection and Urosepsis

Mild fever post PCNL occurs in about one third of the patients, but incidence of sepsis is much lower, in patients treated with appropriate perioperative antibiotics. Sepsis can be prevented if appropriate antibiotic is used preoperatively combined with intraoperative use of low pressure irrigation along with postoperative nephrostomy.

Intravascular Fluid Overload

Intravascular fluid overload occurs if the surgery is prolonged or in case of use of high pressure irrigation, hypotonic solutions, or intraoperative vascular injury. These can be prevented by understanding the risks and by practicing good surgical techniques.[25]

Extravasation of Fluid

Extravasation occurs because of injury to the PCS (pelvi calyceal system). If it is identified in the postoperative period, it can be managed conservatively or can be aspirated under USG guidance if symptomatic or leading to any other complications.

Post Percutaneous Nephrolithotomy Bleeding

Post PCNL bleeding is the most dreaded complication following PCNL. A perfect puncture is a" key" to avoid post PCNL bleeding. Most of post PCNL bleeds subside with conservative management in form of bed rest and close monitoring and transfusion if required. Superselective angioembolization (SAE) (Figs. 33.6A to D) is a efficacious and safe method of controlling post PCNL bleeding. Success rates of SAE exceed 80%. Pseudoaneurysm is commonly responsible for post PCNL bleeding. Jain V et al[26] demonstrated that the risk factors for failure of SAE are multiple punctures and greater than 2 bleeding sites identified during renal angiography. Significant number of patients experience post infarction syndrome in varying degree of severity after SAE.

CONCLUSION

The size of tract has gone from standard PCNL to mini to ultra mini to micro. Even in the era of RIRS and ESWL PCNL had stood forte with its own innovations and improvements and will be the most important companion to the urologist in tackling stone disease.

REFERENCES

1. Preminger GM, Assimos DG, Lingeman JE et al Nephrolithiasis guideline panel Chapter 1 AUA guideline on management of staghorn calculi: Diagnosis and treatment recommendation J Urol 2005;173(6):1991-2000.
2. Lingeman JE, Siegel YI, Steele B. Management of lower pole nephrolithiasis. J Urol 2005; 173:469-73.
3. Albala DM, Assimos DG, Clayman RV et al. A prospective randomized trial of extracorporeal shock wave lithotripsy and percutaneous nephrostlithotomy for lower pole nephrolithiasis. J Urol 2001:166:2072-80.
4. Turna B, Raza A, Moussa S, et al. Management of calyceal diverticular stones with extracorporeal shock wave lithotripsy and percutaneous nephrolithotomy; long term outcome. BJU Int 2007;100:151-6.
5. Yanbo Wang, Yan Wang, Yunming Yao, et al. Prone versus Modified supine position in percutaneous nephrolithotomy: a prospective randomized study. Int J Med Sci 2013; 10(11):1518-23.
6. Valdivia JG, Scarpa RM, Duvdevani N. et al. Supine versus prone position during percutaneous nephrolithotomy: a report from the clinical research office of the endourological society percutaneous nephrolithotomy global Study. J Endourol. 2011;25:1619-25.
7. Stuart Wolf J. Percutaneous approaches to upper urinary tract collecting system, Campbell Walsh Urology 10th ed. Saunders Elsevier 2011. P1334.
8. Isac W, Rizkala E, Liu X, et al. Endoscopic-guided versus fluoroscopic-guided renal access for percutaneous nephrolithotomy: a comparative analysis. 2013;81(2):251-6.
9. Ganpule AP, Desai MR. Management of staghorn calculus multiple tract versus single tract percutaneous nephrolithotomy. Cur. Opin Urol 2008,18(2) 220-3.
10. Williams SK, Leveille RJ Managemnt of staghorn calculus: single puncture with judicious use of the flexible nephroscope. Curr Opin Urol 2008;18:224-228.
11. Helal M, Black T, Lockhart J, et al. The Hickman peel-away sheath: alternative for pediatric percutaneous nephrolithotomy. J Endourol. 1997;11:171–2.
12. Mishra S, Sharma R, Garg C, . Prospective comparative study of miniperc and standard PCNL for treatment of 1 to 2 cm size renal stone. BJU Int. 2011;108(6):896-9.
13. Sabnis RB, Ganesamoni R, Doshi A, et al. Micropercutaneous nephrolithotomy (microperc) vs retrograde intrarenal surgery for the management of small renal calculi: a randomized controlled trial. BJU Int. 2013;112(3):355-61.
14. Desai JD,Zeng G,Zhao Z et al. A novel technique of ultra-mini-percutaneous nephrolithotomy: introduction and an initial experience for treatment of upper urinary calculi less than 2 cm. Biomed Res Int. 2013; 2013: 490793
15. Müller M, Rassweiler MC, Klein J et al. Mobile augmented reality for computer-assisted percutaneous nephrolithotomy. Int J Comput Assist Radiol Surg. 2013;8(4):663-75.
16. Mishra S, Bhattu AS, Sabnis RB, et al. Staghorn classification: Platform for morphometry assessment. Ind J Urol 2014; 30(1):80-83.
17. Mishra S, Sabnis RB, Desai M. Staghorn morphometry: a new tool for clinical classification and prediction model for percutaneous nephrolithotomy monotherapy. J. Endourol 2012;26(1):6-14.
18. Tefekli A, van Rees Vellinga S, de la Rosette J. The CRORES percutaneous nephrolithotomy final study: Global report. J Endourol. 2012;26(12):1536-9.
19. Shin TS, Cho HJ, Hong SH, et al. Complications of percutaneous nephrolithotomy classified by the modified clavien grading system: a single center's experience over 16 Years. Korean J Urol. 2011;52:769-75
20. Shaban A, Kodera A, El Ghoneimy MN, et al. Safety and efficacy of supracostal access in percutaneous renal surgery. J Endourol. 2008;22:29-34.
21. El-Nahas AR, Shokeir AA, El-Assmy AM, et al. Colonic perforation during percutaneous nephrolithotomy: study of risk factors. Urology. 2006;67:937-41.
22. Mousavi-Bahar SH, Mehrabi S, Moslemi MK. Percutaneous nephrolithotomy complications in 671 consecutive patients: a single-center experience. Urol. J 2011;8:271-6.
23. El-Nahas AR, Shokeir AA, El-Assmy AM, et al. Colonic perforation during percutaneous nephrolithotomy: study of risk factors. Urology. 2006;67:937-41.
24. Michel MS, Trojan L, Rassweiler JJ. Complications in percutaneous nephrolithotomy. Eur Urol 2007;51:899-906; discussion 906.
25. Kukreja R, Desai M, Patel S, et al. Factors affecting blood loss during percutaneous nephrolithotomy: prospective study. J Endourol 2004;18:715-22.
26. Jain V, Ganpule A, Vyas J, et al. Management of non-neoplastic renal hemorrhage by transarterial embolization. Urology. 2009;74(3):522-6.

CHAPTER

34 Special Considerations in Ureteroscopy

Mitra R de Cógáin, Amy E Krambeck

INTRODUCTION

Ureteroscopy is one of the most frequently utilized techniques to diagnose and treat upper tract urolithiasis and urothelial tumors. Certain patient circumstances, such as pregnancy or a history of urinary diversion, or anatomical abnormalities, such as a calyceal diverticulum, renal anomalies, or previous genitourinary surgeries, may require modification of surgical technique to achieve the end goal of ureteroscopy. This chapter addresses how to best approach various unusual situations that the urologist may encounter in planned ureteroscopic procedures.

URINARY DIVERSION

When patients require urinary diversion, either for malignant or nonmalignant conditions necessitating cystectomy, bowel segments, typically ileum or colon, are utilized. Regardless of the type of urinary diversions, whether it be ileal or colon conduit, ileal neobladder, Indiana pouch, or other type of diversion, metabolic derangements including hypercalciuria, hyperoxaluria, and acidosis may occur. Such metabolic derangements increase the risk for urolithiasis development in patients with urinary diversion above that of the general population.[1-3] In fact, stones have been reported in up to 15% of diversion patients.[2,4,5] Anatomical changes that cause urinary stasis and the risk of urinary tract infections with urea-splitting bacteria may further contribute to the increased stone risk in this group.[2,4] The most commonly reported stone types in patients with urinary diversion are struvite and calcium phosphate.[6,7] Furthermore, if the cystectomy was performed for urothelial carcinoma, the patient is at an increased risk (from 1% in low-risk patients up to 20–25% in high-risk patients) for the development of upper tract urothelial cancer.[8] Thus, patients with urinary diversion have a reasonable risk of requiring upper tract endoscopic access for treatment of either stones or tumor. Various methods of treating the upper urinary tract have been described in this patient population, including shock wave lithotripsy (SWL), percutaneous nephrolithotomy (PCNL)/tumor ablation, and ureteroscopy. Of these procedures, ureteroscopy is the only technique that mandates modification of the procedure to accomplish the task at hand, whereas SWL and PCNL can typically be performed in the standard fashion.

It is exceedingly important to obtain perioperative urine cultures prior to upper urinary tract manipulation in patients with bowel diversion. Chronic bacterial colonization of the bowel segment can lead to symptomatic urinary tract infections and increase the risk of perioperative sepsis. It is our clinical practice to prescribe 1 week of culture-specific antibiotic therapy and periprocedural intravenous (IV) antibiotic therapy prior to ureteroscopy in patients with urinary diversion. If the upper tracts cannot be accessed in a retrograde fashion, but the uretero-bowel anastomosis freely refluxes, the surgeon can consider converting to a percutaneous procedure using fluoroscopic guidance or ultrasound guidance and then performing an anterograde ureteroscopic procedure. As per current guidelines, patients undergo a follow-up KUB (kidneys, ureters, and bladder) and renal ultrasound 4–6 weeks following their anterograde ureteroscopy via urinary diversion.

Ileal Conduit

In multiple studies, ureteroscopy via an ileal conduit has been shown to be safe and effective. However, stone-free rates have varied widely across reports. In a small, early retrospective study by Wolf and Stoller, the authors reported successful ureteroscopic stone removal in all three of their patients undergoing trans-stomal ureteroscopy, whereas Cass et al. described success in 75% (six of eight attempts) of attempted ureteroscopy via an ileal conduit for treatment of residual stones after SWL.[6,7] Subsequently, in a study by Hyams et al. in 2009, upper tract access with ureteroscopy via stoma was gained successfully in 11 of 15 patients (73%).[9] However, in a recent study by Hertzig et al.

only three of nine patients (33%) were able to successfully have their upper tract stone treated ureteroscopically. Inability to identify the ureteral orifices or to gain access to the orifice was the reason for failure in four of the six unsuccessful cases. Of note, this study was a retrospective review spanning nearly 30 years, and the authors conclude that success with current equipment and techniques available should surpass their reported rates. Thus, understanding of the anatomy following creation of an ileal conduit and optimization of operative conditions is imperative to achieve the highest chance of success.

In the creation of an ileal conduit, with the stoma located in the most common location in the right lower quadrant, the left ureter is passed behind the sigmoid mesentery, and typically the left ureteroileal anastomosis lies at the more proximal end of the conduit whereas the right is located slightly more distally.[10] Classically, the anastomoses are located at the lateral aspect of the conduit, although other sites may be selected on the basis of the lie of the conduit. Familiarity with this anatomy should significantly improve the ability of the surgeon to gain access to the upper tract of concern. Typically, navigation of an ileal conduit is technically easier than with other types of urinary diversion, as there is no afferent limb.[11]

To perform ureteroscopy in a patient with an ileal conduit, the patient is positioned in the supine position. Our current technique includes the use of a flexible cystoscope with gravity irrigation to navigate the length of the ileal conduit down to the most proximal end. Once the end of the conduit is identified, the cystoscope is withdrawn toward the skin to identify the ureteral orifices. A sensor wire is advanced proximally to the level of the renal pelvis. If the sensor wire does not advance easily into the ureteral orifice due to an acute angle, then an angled glidewire with a 6-Fr ureteral catheter is used. Once the glidewire is advanced successfully into the renal pelvis, the 6-Fr catheter is then advanced over the wire and used to exchange the glidewire for a sensor wire. Next, a limited retrograde pyelogram and a second sensor safety wire are placed with the aid of a 10-Fr dual lumen catheter. Then, a 12/14-Fr ureteral access sheath is placed, and ureteroscopy is carried out in the standard fashion, with the aid of pressurized irrigant to ensure optimal visualization.

If access to the most proximal end of the conduit is difficult to gain, a wire may be used to provide a guide for cystoscope advancement. Furthermore, if the ureteral orifices cannot be easily identified, indigo carmine or methylene blue may be administered intravenously to help with ureteral localization as blue starts to efflux from the ureter. Another option is to perform a preoperative or intraoperative loopogram. If the anastomoses are freely refluxing, contrast may enter the upper tracts freely, again helping the surgeon to identify their location. If the conduit is markedly long or there are other stomal issues, such as retraction, stenosis, or herniation, retrograde ureteroscopy can be considerably more difficult. However, the use of a flexible cystoscope and wire guidance can generally overcome many anatomic conduit concerns. We recommend using combination wires such as the sensor wire (Boston Scientific) with both a flexible tip and firm length to minimize trauma to the conduit. However, on occasion, a stiffer wire, such as the super stiff (Boston Scientific) or ultra-stiff (Cook), may be necessary if the conduit or ureters are very redundant, making navigation difficult. The stiffer wire may help the conduit or ureter to straighten, providing easier accessibility. Once the ureteroscopic task at hand (lithotripsy, ureteral biopsy, etc.) is accomplished, the patient may be left with an indwelling single J stent, cut appropriately to traverse the conduit, and lie easily in the stoma appliance. Care should be taken not to cut the stent too short to avoid retraction into the stoma. The surgeon may elect to leave the stent indwelling if access was difficult and a repeat procedure is planned, or to remove the stent at an appointed time if no further procedures are indicated. Furthermore, in freely refluxing systems, the requirement for a stent may be lower, as these ureters tend to be quite dilated and thus allow more ready passage of debris and blood clot.

Neobladder

Ureteroscopy via an orthotopic neobladder may at first appear more routine than ureteroscopy per ileal conduit, as access to the diversion is accomplished per urethra.[12] However, once access to the diversion is gained, the same issues described above with anatomic variation after bowel diversion are encountered. Several series have been reported, establishing ureteroscopy via ilea neobladder as a safe approach to upper tract pathology management. Nelson et al. performed ureteroscopy successfully in 10 of 13 attempted renal units (77%) with 3 failures due to the inability to visualize or access the ureter.[13] The authors discuss that a thorough understanding of the bowel diversion anatomy and judicious use of fluoroscopy with contrast are necessary to optimize the likelihood of obtaining access to the upper tracts. Hyams et al. also described their experience with neobladder ureteroscopy.[9] They were able to gain access in 9 of 10 attempts (90%). In a recent neobladder series from our institution, which also included one Indiana pouch patient, anterograde ureteroscopy was successful in 10 of 17 attempts (59%) over the study period, but with improvements in technique had increased to 75% in the last 5 years. There were no complications related to the ureteroscopic procedure in the series.[12]

As previously mentioned, knowledge of the type of orthotopic diversion and the location of the ureteral orifices is of the utmost importance in optimizing the likelihood of success. In the construction of an ileal neobladder, a partially detubularized segment is folded into a U shape to create the near-spherical reservoir, whereas a small tubularized segment is used as an afferent limb. This afferent limb is where the ureteroileal anastomosis is performed. Typically, the ureters are located near the antimesenteric border, and the right ureter is located 1 cm distal to the left.

Patients are prepped in the dorsal lithotomy position, and flexible cystoscopy using gravity irrigation is performed per urethra. Initial navigation of the neobladder is performed to access the afferent limb, which is usually near the 9–12-o'clock position. A sensor wire is advanced into the afferent limb and can be used to guide the cystoscope into the limb, as the path may be tortuous and difficult to access. If the afferent limb or neobladder is long or capacious, the flexible cystoscope may not provide adequate length to inspect for the ureteral orifices. If such conditions are encountered, first try draining all fluid from the neobladder and re-evaluate with minimal irrigation. If the neobladder continues to be too long or capacious for the flexible cystoscope to identify the ureteral orifices, then a flexible ureteroscope can be employed. To utilize a flexible ureteroscope, a sensor wire is advanced up the afferent limb fluoroscopically. A dual-lumen catheter is then used to inject contrast to confirm location and to place a second wire. An access sheath is advanced over the second wire into the afferent limb. With the access sheath in place, pressurized irrigant may be employed to improve visualization through the ureteroscope and access sheath and ultimately identify the ureteral orifices. Indigo carmine administration may also help with the identification of the ureteral orifices, and if the anastomoses reflux, a neobladder cystogram, particularly of the afferent limb, may help the surgeon to provide further useful anatomic information about the ureteroileal anastomosis location. Once the scope has been advanced into the afferent limb, careful inspection should be performed to identify the ureteral orifices. A sensor wire is advanced through the scope under fluoroscopic guidance to the level of the renal pelvis.

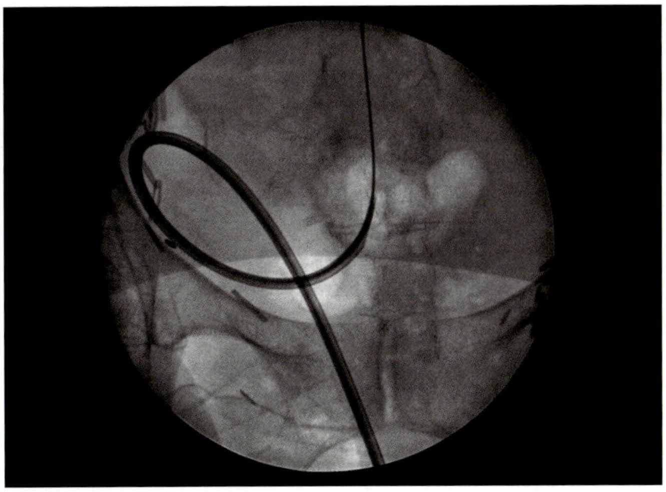

Fig. 34.1: A 6/10-Fr dual-lumen catheter advanced over a superstiff wire and utilized to place a safety wire via the afferent limb of the neobladder to the level of the renal pelvis.

If the ureteral orifice can be seen but not easily accessed due to angulation, an angled hydrophilic wire may be useful. A ureteral catheter is then used to exchange the wire for a superstiff wire, which can help the surgeon to provide a more direct access through a torturous ureter and afferent limb. A 6/10-Fr dual-lumen catheter is then used to place a safety wire up the ureter (Fig. 34.1). A ureteral access sheath is then placed to the level of the renal pelvis, and ureteroscopy is carried out in the standard fashion, with the aid of pressurized irrigant to ensure optimal visualization. If a ureteral stent is required, an 8.5-Fr single J stent may be used, with the straight tail left long in the neobladder to allow for cystoscopic removal in the office.

In using the techniques described, the urologist can have confidence in embarking on the challenges faced in ureteroscopy following urinary diversion. In general, fluoroscopy and the use of multiple scopes and wires can safely establish access to the upper tract in ileal conduits and continent urinary diversions. It is important to recognize, however, that if the procedure is not proceeding in an acceptable manner and the urinary conduit is at risk for injury, it is appropriate to terminate the procedure and instead perform ureteroscopy through an antegrade approach either by fluoroscopic- or ultrasound-guided percutaneous renal access.

CALYCEAL DIVERTICULA

A calyceal diverticulum is a urothelial-lined, urine-containing congenital defect of the renal parenchyma that communicates with the intrarenal collecting system, and may be confused with a renal cyst or dilated calyx.[14,15] The incidence of a calyceal diverticulum is reported to be up to 0.45% in adult patients, although the true prevalence may be an underestimation as the majority of diverticula are asymptomatic.[16] The diverticula may be classified into two subgroups: type 1, which describes a diverticulum in a polar location, off of a minor calyx (typically upper pole); and type 2, which is found near the renal pelvis or a major calyx, in a central location. Between 10% and 50% of calyceal diverticula may contain stones, which can cause symptoms.[17,18] The diagnosis is typically made with the aid of contrast imaging [computed tomography (CT) urogram or intravenous pyelogram (IVP)]; this demonstrates a fluid-filled structure that does not pool contrast on initial excretory images, in contrast to infundibular stenosis (the most common differential diagnosis), which fills on initial excretory imaging. If the diverticulum contains a stone, then that stone will appear to be isolated from the intrarenal collecting system.[14] If the patient is symptomatic from a stone-containing diverticulum, with pain, hematuria, recurrent infections, or other complaints, then intervention is warranted. However, if the patient is asymptomatic, no intervention is required.

Once the diagnosis is made and the patient elects to proceed with intervention, various treatment options must be discussed, namely, laparoscopic stone removal and diverticulectomy, SWL, PCNL, and ureteroscopy.[14,15,19,20] Historically, open stone removal and marsupialization of the diverticulum was utilized, but this technique has been ousted in favor of more minimally invasive techniques.[14] Percutaneous nephrolithotomy and laparoscopic stone removal provide the highest stone clearance rates, but these techniques are more invasive and technically difficult. The relatively small diverticulum may be difficult to identify and access if located anteriorly or near the renal hilum. Furthermore, PCNL and laparoscopic approaches lead to overnight hospitalization at least and have a number of potential complications, including sepsis, bleeding, and injury to surrounding organs.[18] Shockwave lithotripsy is capable of fragmenting the target calculus; however, clearance of the fragments is difficult if not impossible in many cases due to narrow necks connecting the diverticulum to the collecting system.[15] In a recent review article, Canales and Monga state that SWL should only be performed in a select group of patients who have a large, easily targeted stone in a diverticulum with a wide neck, to allow for appropriate stone passage.

Fuchs and colleagues first reported the use of flexible ureteroscopy for treatment of a stone-containing calyceal diverticulum.[21] Although that group initially had technical difficulties owing to the poor deflection of the ureteroscope, subsequent series with more advanced ureteroscopes have had limited problems with diverticulum access.[14] Ureteroscopy has since been reported as a feasible option for treatment, with stone-free rates ranging from 19% to 58% in more recent studies.[22,23] However, despite the lower stone-free rates achieved, given the minimally invasive nature of this approach, ureteroscopic management may be favored by both patients and urologists alike. If ureteroscopic management of a stone-containing diverticulum is undertaken, the goals should be twofold, including treatment of the stone and then ablation of the calyceal diverticulum and its communication to the collecting system.[15] Although in the past the primary goal was to achieve a stone-free state, current recommendations focus on treating the diverticulum as well, to decrease the likelihood for repeat symptoms or recurrent stone disease.

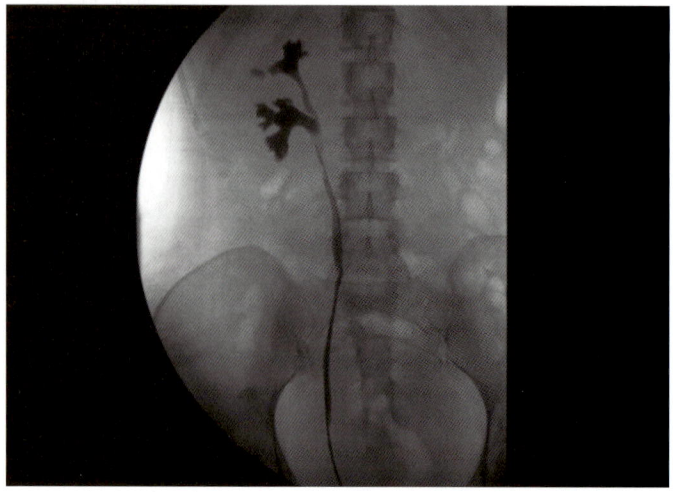

Fig. 34.2: A retrograde pyelogram is performed in this patient with a calyceal diverticulum. The narrow-necked diverticulum can be seen emanating from the upper pole of this bifid collecting system.

Ureteroscopy is initially performed in the standard fashion. The patient is placed in the dorsal lithotomy position for the procedure. A retrograde pyelogram (which may opacify the diverticulum) is obtained via a ureteral catheter or using a 6/10-Fr dual-lumen catheter, and two flexible-tip guidewires are placed into the intrarenal collecting system (Fig. 34.2). A 12/14-Fr access sheath is advanced over the working wire to a level just distal to the ureteropelvic junction (UPJ), and the flexible ureteroscope is introduced through the access sheath. Careful inspection of the intrarenal collecting system is carried out, with the aid of fluoroscopy, to identify the diverticular neck.

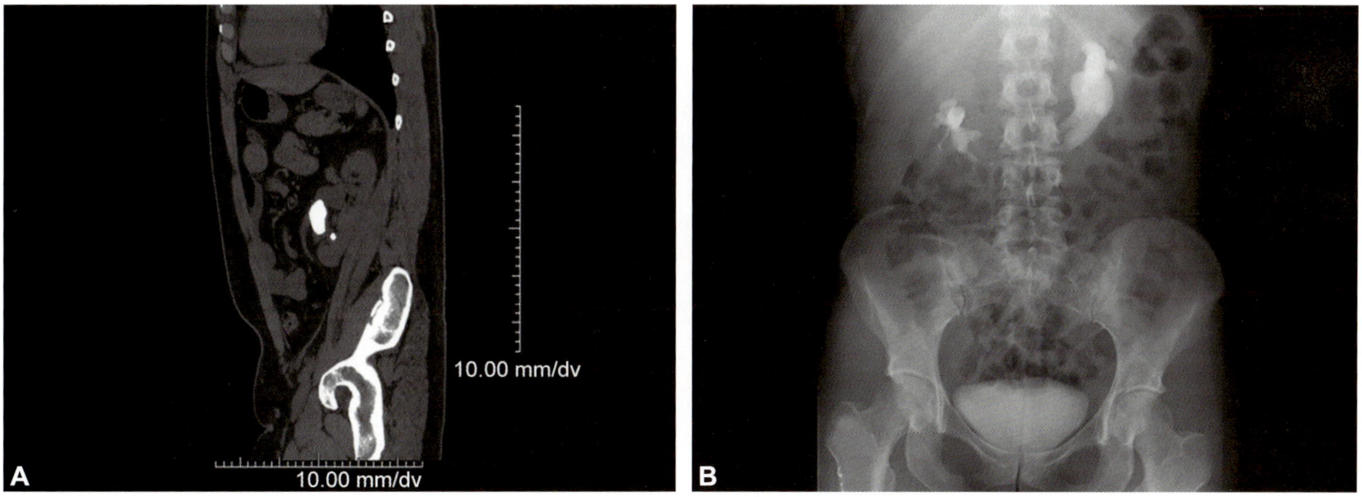

Figs. 34.3A and B: A noncontrast enhanced CT (coronal view) demonstrates (A) a large stone at the inferior aspect of this horseshoe kidney and (B) the topogram images demonstrate the abnormal lie of the intrarenal collecting system, with calyceal structures that point in a more posteromedial direction, with the upper poles angled out laterally.
(CT: Computed tomography).

A wire is then advanced into the diverticulum, and the neck incised using a holmium laser or a small balloon dilator to allow access of the flexible ureteroscope. If incision is performed, the flow through the ureteroscope should be stopped and the area to be incised should be inspected for pulsation. Do not incise an area of urothelium with active pulsation, as there is most likely vasculature in the vicinity. Once entry is gained into the diverticulum, laser lithotripsy and basket stone extraction of every fragment are performed. After stone extraction, the diverticulum is fulgurated using the holmium laser or a Bugbee electrode, to allow the cavity to collapse. If the surgeon has difficulty locating the diverticulum during ureteroscopy, injection of indigo carmine and subsequent washing of the intrarenal collecting system, then observation of blue efflux from the diverticular neck, may be helpful. Following this procedure, a ureteral stent should be left in place to allow for easy passage of blood clots that may result from gaining entry into the diverticulum and also to allow for any potential infected urine contained within the diverticulum to drain easily.

HORSESHOE KIDNEY

Horseshoe kidney is the most common renal anomaly, occurring in 1 of 400–800 patients.[24-27] The horseshoe fusion abnormality of the lower poles occurs as the kidneys ascend during fetal development and result in a single renal unit. The horseshoe kidney is often lower in location than standard kidneys due to limited renal ascent from the pelvis by the inferior mesenteric artery. Because of the fusion and limited ascent, the horseshoe kidney is malrotated, resulting in calyceal structures that point in a more posteromedial direction, with the upper poles angled out laterally (Figs. 34.3A and B). The ureters, which may be quite tortuous, are also deviated anteriorly over the isthmus of the kidney and typically have a high insertion at the renal pelvis. The resulting urinary stasis may lead to a higher likelihood for stone formation in these patients; in fact, up to 20% of horseshoe kidney patients suffer from urolithiasis.[28] However, urinary stasis is not the only predisposing factor contributing to stone formation in patients with horseshoe kidneys, as underlying metabolic disease appears to be prevalent in this patient population.[29-31] One study described 59% of horseshoe kidney patients as having an underlying metabolic abnormality that may predispose them to stone formation.[32] Evans and Resnick also found metabolic abnormalities in 75% of their stone-forming horseshoe kidney patients, and Raj et al.[33] report that in 11 patients with horseshoe kidneys and stones, all patients had at least one metabolic abnormality and, on average, each patient had 2.7 metabolic abnormalities, leading to a predilection for stones. The vascular structures supplying the kidney are also highly variable, and, thus, any procedure requiring retroperitoneal or transperitoneal access to the kidney can be quite difficult. Thus, urolithiasis in a horseshoe kidney can prove a difficult treatment dilemma, owing primarily to the variable and challenging anatomy. Innervation to the horseshoe kidney is the same as in the orthotopically located kidney; thus, presenting symptoms of renal colic are generally quite similar. However, atypical abdominal pain or isolated nausea and emesis may also indicate urolithiasis in a horseshoe kidney, due to the abnormal anatomic location.[26]

The most appropriate treatment modality must be selected on the basis of the patient's anatomy with consideration for the aberrant vascular structures and the stone characteristics, including stone volume, location, and accessibility. Shock wave lithotripsy has been employed frequently in treatment of urolithiasis in a horseshoe kidney. A recent study by Ray et al. looked at 41 patients undergoing SWL in this patient population.[34] They found that after a single treatment, 26.2% of patients were stone free at 2 weeks, whereas 72.7% of patients required an ancillary procedure, either repeat SWL, PCNL, or ureteroscopy, for treatment of their stone at 3 months of follow-up. In evaluating predictors for success, the authors note that greater stone burden, larger body mass index, and upper calyceal location may predict SWL treatment failure in horseshoe kidneys. Percutaneous nephrolithotomy has also been extensively evaluated in this patient population. Symons and colleagues comment that PCNL is generally thought to be a safe and effective treatment option for urolithiasis in the horseshoe kidney.[24] However, again anatomic limitations leading to the inability of the nephroscope to access certain areas of the collecting system, including the lower calyces or the isthmus, or the inability to access the collecting system percutaneously due to anterior lie of calyces may limit the applicability of this technique. Laparoscopic or open pyelolithotomy can also be considered in patients with extremely challenging anatomy or very large stones that cannot be easily managed percutaneously.[24] The final treatment option available to patients for stone treatment is ureteroscopic stone extraction. Ureteroscopy is typically performed for patients who have a relatively small stone burden or stones that would be difficult to access with the other aforementioned techniques. Ureteroscopy is an attractive intervention in the horseshoe kidney, as in general it can be performed with little morbidity, is safe in anticoagulated patients, and avoids many of the pitfalls associated with the variable anatomy of the horseshoe kidney. One pitfall of ureteroscopy is that access of lower pole calyces may not be possible due to the high insertion of the ureter and extreme angle of deflection necessary to reach the lower pole of the horseshoe kidney.

Molimard et al. reported on the use of flexible ureteroscopy for stone treatment in a horseshoe kidney in 2010.[28] Staged ureteroscopy was required in 41.2% (7/15) of patients and was associated with a larger stone burden (average stone burden was 1.6 cm, range 7–35 cm). The mean operative time of each procedure was 92 minutes. The authors report no ureteroscopic complications, and 88.2% (15/17) of patients were stone free following their final ureteroscopic intervention. Atis et al. also evaluated their success with ureteroscopy in horseshoe kidneys following PCNL or SWL failure.[35] They found that 70% (14/20) of patients with a mean stone size of 17.8 ± 4.5 mm were stone free following a single ureteroscopic intervention, and 6 patients required subsequent SWL therapy. This group reported a minor complication rate (Clavien I or II) of 25%. Furthermore, in a study, Weizer et al. were able to achieve a stone-free state in 75% of their patients with either a pelvic or a horseshoe kidney, and none of their patients required repeat intervention at their last stone follow-up.[36] Thus, in an appropriately selected patient population, ureteroscopy appears to be a safe and viable option, with a high stone-free rate, although this may require multiple surgical procedures to achieve.

When patients and their surgeons decide to proceed with ureteroscopy in a horseshoe kidney, thorough understanding of the anatomy, potential pitfalls, and complications is imperative to ensure that a safe procedure with optimal results is performed. Standard positioning in the dorsal lithotomy position is performed. Rigid cystoscopy should demonstrate orthotopic ureteral orifices. A retrograde pyelogram of the collecting system of interest is obtained via a ureteral catheter or using a 6/10-Fr dual-lumen catheter, and two flexible-tip guidewires are placed into the intrarenal collecting system. An access sheath is advanced over the working wire. This step is imperative to the success of the operation, as the access sheath can help the surgeon to straighten the course of a very tortuous ureter.[36] Flexible ureteroscopy can then be carried out with the aid of pressurized irrigation. As the ureter may be shorter than those associated with orthotopically located kidneys, the use of a shorter access sheath, especially in women, should be considered. Careful attention should be paid to the positioning of the access sheath, as the anteriorly directed renal pelvis may be more susceptible to trauma and perforation. Once access is gained to the intrarenal collecting system, stones in the lower pole may be difficult due to the extreme angle of the lower pole calyces as previously described. Often, a nitinol basket or other flexible grasping device can be used to reposition lower pole stones to the upper pole, allowing for easier access and laser lithotripsy. Once successful stone fragmentation is performed, removal of all possible stone fragments should be undertaken, as again, due to the high insertion of the ureter, they may be less likely to pass spontaneously.[26] A ureteral stent can be placed as indicated, at the discretion of the operating surgeon. The UPJ in horseshoe kidney patients may be somewhat tight, and thus the urologist should strongly consider ureteral stent placement at the conclusion of the procedure. The techniques described can also be extrapolated to pelvic and other anomalously located kidneys.

URETERAL REIMPLANTATION

Vesicoureteral reflux (VUR) occurs in 30% of children with a febrile urinary tract infection and is one of the most common pediatric urologic maladies.[37-39] Although conservative management of VUR has become more in vogue in recent years, high-grade reflux, reflux associated with breakthrough urinary tract infections, or deterioration in renal function is often surgically treated. Endoscopic management of reflux, including procedures such as Deflux injection, does not significantly impede the ability of the urologist to gain ureteroscopic access to the upper urinary tract as necessary. However, ureteroscopy following surgical trans- or extravesical reimplantation can prove to be challenging for the endoscopist. Little information about the incidence of urolithiasis in reflux patients following surgical correction exists. In our experience, patients with a history of VUR as a child do appear to have a high likelihood of recurrent stone disease if they are in fact stone formers, but it is unknown whether the actual incidence of urolithiasis is increased in this patient population.

All ureteral reimplantation techniques have the potential to alter ureteral anatomy such that standard instruments, including ureteroscopic access sheaths and ureteroscopes, cannot be accommodated. One particularly difficult case to approach is ureteroscopy following a Cohen cross-trigonal ureteral reimplantation.[38,39] This transvesical reimplantation technique, which is preferred in situations where ureteral orifices are quite lateral and concern for persistent reflux exists, involves creation of a long, submucosal tunnel across the trigone, with the ureter reimplanted just cephalad to the contralateral ureteral orifice.[40] The Glenn-Anderson ureteral advancement technique is another commonly performed transvesical procedure that involves creation of a submucosal tunnel on the ipsilateral side of interest, allowing the surgeon to relocate the ureteral orifice in a more distal location, near the bladder neck. The Politano-Leadbetter procedure is an intraextravesical procedure, which involves the extravesical mobilization of the ureter and transvesical reimplantation, with creation of a more distal ureteral orifice on the ipsilateral side and a longer submucosal tunnel. Other transvesical approaches exist; however, the three techniques mentioned are those most often performed. Extravesical approaches, such as the Lich-Gregoir or the Barry procedure, also involve lengthening the submucosal tunnel; however, the approach is via the muscular layers of the bladder, working from the outside inward. The ureteral orifice position may be adjusted, as in the Barry technique, or the submucosal tunnel simply lengthened, as in the Lich-Gregoir procedure. Whichever of these techniques is performed, it is important for the urologist evaluating the patient for upper tract disease to be aware of the previous surgical procedure and, if possible, have detailed knowledge of which surgical procedure was performed. Krambeck et al. published a study of 24 patients who required management of urolithiasis following either a Cohen cross-trigonal or Glenn-Anderson ureteroneocystostomy.[41] They described a higher failure rate of minimally invasive procedures for upper tract stones, including ureteroscopy following a cross-trigonal reimplant, whereas ureteroscopy was successful in all (4/4) patients who underwent ureteroscopic stone management following a Glenn-Anderson procedure. In fact, the majority of patients who had previously undergone a Cohen procedure and had a stone procedure performed required either an upfront PCNL or PCNL following failure of SWL or ureteroscopy (57.4%, 4/7), and no patient in that group was successfully managed ureteroscopically. Detailed knowledge of the patient's altered anatomy will allow for the most efficient approach to ureteroscopic intervention to be taken.

If the patient underwent a ureteral reimplantation technique where the ureteral orifices remained at or near their congenital location, often the approach to ureteroscopic intervention is similar to the standard approach. However, if a significant alteration of anatomy is performed, the surgeon must modify the operative approach to access the orifices. In fact, one strong criticism of the Cohen cross-trigonal reimplantation technique is the difficulty in gaining retrograde access to the upper urinary tract.[38] Initially, standard procedures are carried out. Rigid cystoscopy is performed to identify the ureteral orifices. Although attempts to cannulate the ureteral orifice may be made with a standard sensor wire, often it is difficult to advance the wire due to angulation of the ureter as it traverses the extended intramural tunnel. An angled glidewire used with or without an angled cobra angiographic catheter may allow easier access to the ureter. Wallis et al. state that the use of a combination of an angled glide wire and a cobra angiographic catheter allows for the wire to be passed up to an angle of 120° from the cystoscope.[38] Once the glidewire is negotiated into the proximal ureter, the catheter can be advanced over this, and the glidewire exchanged for a standard sensor wire, or, alternatively, a superstiff working wire, which may straighten the ureter and allow for easier working channels. A retrograde pyelogram of the collecting system of interest is obtained via a ureteral catheter or using a 10-Fr dual-lumen catheter, and two guidewires are placed into the intrarenal collecting system. An access sheath is advanced over the working wire. In some cases, the ureteral orifice or intramural portion of the ureter may be tight, and balloon dilation of the ureteral orifice or serial ureteral dilation can be carried out to accommodate passage of the access sheath. Ureteroscopic intervention is subsequently carried out in the standard fashion. A ureteral stent may be placed at the discretion of the operating surgeon and should be strongly considered, especially with trauma to the neoureteral orifice or dilation of the distal ureter. If safe access cannot be achieved in a retrograde fashion, then an anterograde procedure (PCNL or ureteroscopy) should be considered. A novel technique was reported by Santarosa et al., whereby access to the reimplanted ureter following a Cohen cross-trigonal procedure was gained using transvesical percutaneous access, and this method should also be considered if standard retrograde access is not possible.[42] Shock wave lithotripsy can also be considered, however, if a real risk of persistent distal ureteral stones exists, due to the tight, typically small caliber of the tunneled reimplanted distal ureter.

RENAL TRANSPLANTATION

Urolithiasis is reported to occur in up to 1% of renal transplant patients.[43-46] These stones may form de novo in transplanted kidneys or result from transplantation of a stone-containing kidney (donor-gifted stones).[43] Multiple factors that contribute to de novo stone formation in transplant patients have been reported, including the presence of a more alkaline urine following transplantation, as well as other underlying metabolic abnormalities (hypercalciuria, hypophosphatemia, and hyperuricosuria) or comorbid conditions (secondary or tertiary hyperparathyroidism due to chronic kidney disease, gout, or previous urinary diversion).[43,47] The immunocompromised state of the transplant recipient on immune-modulating medications may also predispose them to recurrent urinary tract infections, potentially leading to alkalinization of the urine.[26] Furthermore, cyclosporine A, which is a commonly administered immunosuppressant used in transplant patients, may cause hyperuricosuria, and steroids may lead to hypercalciuria.[26,48] The most commonly reported stone type in the renal transplant patient population is calcium oxalate; however, other stone compositions have been reported.[49]

Transplantation of a stone-producing kidney has gained wider acceptance over the past couple of years. Previously, this was a relative contraindication, with the underlying reasoning that stone formers are likely to have recurrent stone diseases and measures should be taken to preserve their renal function.[43] However, more recently, multiple studies have demonstrated the efficacious management of urolithiasis in transplant allografts. Lu et al. described percutaneous stone management soon after transplantation of kidneys with pre-existing stones, and Rashid et al. describe ex vivo ureteroscopic stone extraction of pre-existing nephrolithiasis prior to transplantation.[50,51] Torrecilla et al. were able to successfully manage 18 kidney or ureteral stones during or following renal transplantation, and they argue that urolithiasis should not be a reason to refuse a renal allograft.[52] Since the overall incidence of urolithiasis is increasing in the general population, we will likely see a parallel increase in stone disease in renal transplant patients.[53]

The management of urolithiasis after renal transplantation can be challenging, as the allograft typically lies in the iliac fossa with a short tortuous ureter, generally implanted near the bladder dome. Even diagnosis may prove difficult, as the pelvic location of the kidney may impact the ability to visualize the stone on KUB or renal ultrasound.[46] Typically, a noncontrast CT is the best imaging modality to diagnose stones in renal transplant patients.[26] Despite difficulties with treatment and diagnosis, intervention in transplant patients with stones is of the utmost importance. The transplanted kidney is a functional solitary kidney that is denervated. Obstruction can be completely asymptomatic and can result in significant renal dysfunction.[26] Patients may present late, with atypical signs such as vague abdominal pain, decreased urine output, or worsening renal function.[26]

Despite the unusual anatomy of a transplant kidney, virtually all standard treatment options for urolithiasis are possible in transplant patients, including medical expulsive therapy, SWL, PCNL, ureteroscopy, and open or laparoscopic stone removal. In the case of obstruction associated with infection, nephrostomy tube placement with subsequent intervention is preferred due to issues with reliable stent placement in this population.[54] Conservative management appears safe for stones of <4 mm, as the reported spontaneous passage rate is between 38% and 60%.[55,56] In fact, because of the short course of the ureter and its dilated nature, spontaneous passage may occur more readily than with a native kidney. However, spontaneous passage may be a less than ideal option in a patient with a solitary renal unit, due to concerns over intermittent obstruction and potential renal dysfunction. Shock wave lithotripsy has been successfully performed in transplant patients; however, the necessity for repeat treatments in the solitary renal units, along with the unpredictability associated with relying on stone passage following SWL, may make this modality less than optimal. Li et al. reported success in treatment of seven stone-transplant patients with repeated low-dose SWL, for stones ranging in size from 0.4 to 1.1 cm.[57] Challacombe et al. also successfully treated 13 transplant patients with SWL; however, 7 of these (53.8%) required an ancillary procedure, such as a stent, nephrostomy tube, or repeat SWL.[43]

Multiple studies have evaluated the use of PCNL in the transplant patient. Krambeck et al. found that in 13 patients undergoing PCNL in a renal transplant, 10 patients were rendered stone free after their initial procedure (76.9%), whereas 3 patients (23.1%) required repeat procedures for stone clearance, with few perioperative complications reported.[58] Although this is a feasible option for stone treatment in transplant patients, it does require passage through the allograft parenchyma to obtain access, which has the potential to result in parenchymal damage. Open or laparoscopic stone surgery may also be performed, although, as with urolithiasis in native kidneys, there are rare indications for such invasive procedures.

The final treatment option available for treatment of transplant urolithiasis is ureteroscopic stone extraction. Ureteroscopy may be attractive because of the ability to treat obstruction rapidly, with minimal risk to the kidney parenchyma and overall renal function. Hyams et al. evaluated their ability to ureteroscopically treat upper tract urolithiasis in 12 patients.[48] Retrograde ureteroscopy was successful in seven patients, whereas five patients underwent an anterograde procedure. The average stone size treated was 0.8 cm (range 0.4–1.5 cm). Stone-free status was obtained in 91.6% (11/12) of patients, with 2 reported complications of an encrusted stent and a nephrocutaneous fistula occurring in the anterograde group. The authors conclude that ureteroscopy is safe and effective in renal transplant recipients, especially for a smaller stone burden than what would typically be approached with PCNL. Furthermore, they state that with the development of smaller ureteroscopes with improved active deflection, the transplant kidney can be thoroughly investigated and treated.

Although ureteroscopic stone extraction is an enticing treatment option, execution of the procedure may be difficult due to the altered ureteral and renal anatomies. As mentioned, improvements in equipment have helped push ureteroscopic intervention to the forefront in transplant patients, but certain anatomical factors must be overcome in order to achieve successful stone clearance. The patient is positioned in dorsal lithotomy. Rigid cystoscopy will typically demonstrate the transplant ureteral orifice near the bladder dome. Often, it is difficult to gain access to the ureter, and so a cobra angiographic catheter may be used to aid in wire positioning. This may be the most troublesome portion of the procedure. An angled hydrophilic wire used in tandem with the cobra catheter may also be helpful. Once access to the transplant ureter is gained, a retrograde pyelogram of the collecting system of interest is obtained via a ureteral catheter or using a 6/10-Fr dual-lumen catheter, and two flexible tip guide wires are placed into the intrarenal collecting system. An access sheath is advanced over the working wire. Typically, the access sheath required for transplant kidneys is much shorter than the standard access sheath due to the kidney's pelvic location. Flexible ureteroscopy can then be carried out with the aid of pressurized irrigation. Laser lithotripsy and basket stone extraction are then carried out in the standard fashion. A ureteral stent should be left in place postprocedure since the transplant kidney is a functional, solitary unit.

PREGNANCY

The incidence of stones in pregnancy is reported to be up to twice that in nonpregnant, comparable patients. In fact, kidney stones or flank pain are thought to be the most common nonobstetric reason for pregnant patients to get admitted to the hospital. Anatomic changes, such as the physiologic hydronephrosis of pregnancy, may make stones more readily passable into the proximal ureter and then cause obstruction distally as the ureter narrows in the pelvis.[59,60] Furthermore, changes to urinary constituents that occur during pregnancy may make patients more likely to form stones. During pregnancy, total body vascular volume increases, causing an increase in renal plasma flow. Urine volume is increased parallel to the elevated renal plasma flow; however, if significant nausea and vomiting are present, dehydration may cause decreased urine volume. Glomerular filtration rate subsequently increases by 30–50%, in turn, resulting in a significant increase in urinary sodium, citrate, uric acid, magnesium, calcium, and urinary glycoproteins.[61] The increase in promoters of stone formation is thought to be counteracted somewhat by the inhibitors that are excreted at higher amounts (citrate, magnesium, and glycoproteins); however, higher levels of urinary citrate may alkalinize the urine, leading to a higher likelihood for calcium phosphate stone formation.[60,62] Furthermore, hypercalciuria increases as a patient's pregnancy progresses due to the placental production of vitamin D, leading to an absorptive hypercalciuria.[60] This elevated calcium load causes not only an increased calcium delivery to the kidney, but also, in turn, low parathyroid hormone, resulting in a further decreased reabsorption of calcium by the kidney. The net effect of all of the aforementioned changes in urinary constituents accounts for the rapid encrustation of stents or nephrostomy tubes seen in pregnancy and may also account for more rapid stone formation during pregnancy in patients who are predisposed.[63]

Urolithiasis during pregnancy can be a difficult and challenging condition for the patient and the physician from both a diagnostic and a treatment standpoint. Because of concerns of fetal exposure to radiation, the choice of investigatory studies in pregnant women is somewhat limited. The most often employed first imaging modality is ultrasound, as this does not expose the fetus to radiation but still has the power to diagnose ureteral obstruction, and sometimes a stone (Fig. 34.4). Both retroperitoneal and endovaginal ultrasound views should be obtained whenever there is concern for an obstructing ureteral calculus, assessing for hydronephrosis, the stone, or the presence or absence of a ureteral jet. Hydronephrosis seen on ultrasound is not diagnostic, however, as up to 90% of women in their third trimester demonstrate nonobstructive hydronephrosis, especially on the right-hand side, due to the dextrorotation of the gravid uterus.[64,65] Because of the fact that physiologic hydronephrosis is primarily caused by a mass effect of the uterus, it should not occur below the pelvic brim on either the right or the left side.[64,65] Although distinguishing physiologic hydronephrosis from hydronephrosis secondary to obstruction

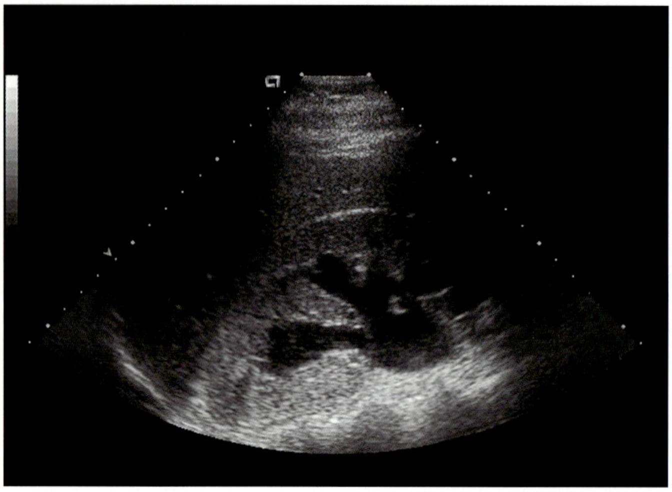

Fig. 34.4: A retroperitoneal ultrasound image in a pregnant woman with flank pain demonstrates right-sided hydronephrosis.

can be difficult, dilation of pelvic ureter, severe left-sided hydronephrosis, and the absence of a ureteral jet suggest obstruction.[66,67] In fact, the lack of a ureteral jet may be observed in >60% of patients with urolithiasis when endovaginal ultrasound is employed.[68] However, endovaginal ultrasound views should not be performed if the patient has preterm premature rupture of membranes or prolapsed membranes.[67] An experienced ultrasonographer may also be able to identify a distinct ureteral stone, with posterior acoustic shadowing.

In some instances, ultrasound imaging is nondiagnostic, and the patient and the physician are faced with the dilemma of possibly taking the patient for an unnecessary procedure or proceeding with some sort of diagnostic study requiring radiation exposure. Historically, an abdominal X-ray of the KUB or IVP was performed in a pregnant patient who had a nondiagnostic ultrasound; currently, with the recent availability of low-dose CT; these less-detailed studies have fallen out of favor. The American Congress of Obstetricians and Gynecologists (ACOG) guidelines state that X-ray exposure carries some potential risks to the developing fetus, including teratogenesis, carcinogenesis, and genetic mutations, with the risk being highest during the first trimester, specifically 8–15 weeks' gestation. However, if imaging is necessary in the best interest to the mother, it can be carried out safely if total fetal exposure during pregnancy is <50 mGy.[69] In fact, no reports of fetal malformation have been reported with radiation exposure <150 mGy. Thus, performing a CT (range 2–14 mGy) in the appropriately selected patient

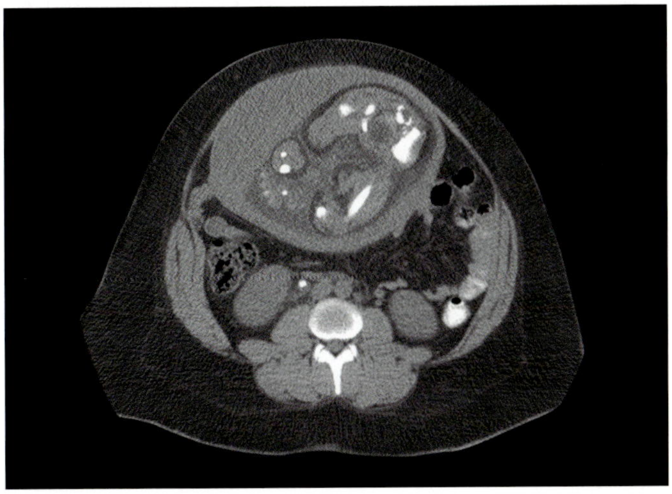

Fig. 34.5: A low-dose CT performed in a pregnant woman demonstrates a gravid uterus and a right-sided ureteral calculus. (CT: Computed tomography).

should have a small risk of fetal complications (Fig. 34.5). In a study by White et al. CT was found to have the best positive predictive value of all imaging studies (96%) for suspected urolithiasis in pregnancy.[70] Thus, the most recent imaging guidelines from the American Urological Association (AUA) recommend a low-dose noncontrast CT as the second study of choice for imaging pregnant women with possible urolithiasis. Of note, ACOG guidelines state that IV contrast is unlikely to cause harm, but should be used only if the benefit outweighs the risk, as these agents have not been studied in humans and may potentially induce neonatal hypothyroidism.[71] In summary, if imaging with radiation exposure is required to provide the best possible care for the pregnant patient, then it may be performed with the lowest exposure achievable to accomplish the goal at hand.

Magnetic resonance imaging (MRI) has also been described as a second-line imaging modality for pregnant women since it does not require ionizing radiation. However, MRI is not ideal for imaging stones, as they are seen as a void in the final films and not a discrete, identifiable calculus, and the studies tend to take a long time to perform. However, half-Fourier single shot turbo spin echo MRI has decreased imaging time and does not require IV contrast, and T2-weighting allows for excellent imaging of fluid-filled structures such as the genitourinary tract.[72] One study by Mulkins et al. evaluated the use of MRI in nine pregnant patients with stone symptoms and a negative ultrasound. In eight of the nine patients (88%), MRI was able to definitively demonstrate the presence or absence of a stone.[73] Therefore, although MRI is not as sensitive as CT, the AUA imaging guidelines recommend MRI as the second-line imaging modality in the first trimester of pregnancy when ultrasound imaging has failed, thereby providing cross-sectional imaging whereas limiting radiation exposure to the fetus during organogenesis.[74]

Once the diagnosis of ureteral obstruction is made, the patient, her obstetrical team, and the urologist must determine a plan of care. Because of the risk of any procedure to the patient and her fetus, the first-line therapy is expectant management, as the majority of patients will pass their stones with conservative management.[75] Conservative management is considered a failure if the patient has persistent pain despite pain medication, intractable nausea and vomiting, worsening renal function, or signs of infection. If conservative management fails, the historic standard interventional treatment for urolithiasis or ureteral obstruction in pregnancy was urinary tract drainage with either an indwelling nephrostomy tube or ureteral stents. Temporary renal drainage is an attractive option as ureteral stenting and percutaneous nephrostomy tube placement can often be performed under local anesthetic or conscious sedation. However, these temporizing measures are less than ideal, as they cause significant discomfort during pregnancy, in addition to the necessity for more frequent exchanges (every 4–6 weeks) due to worsening encrustation, which can occur during pregnancy.[76,77]

Because of the pitfalls of temporizing measures, treatment has shifted toward definitive stone management during pregnancy. In one study, 42.1% of patients treated with temporary ureteral stent placement (8/19) required early induction of labor at a mean of 38.3 weeks of pregnancy due to stent-related discomfort, and 10.9% (2/19) of patients went into premature labor within 24 hours of stent placement.[75] Pregnant patients are not candidates for shockwave lithotripsy, as it has been suggested to potentially cause fetal growth retardation, nor is PCNL advised, as use of the ultrasonic lithotripter may cause untoward damage to the fetal inner ear structures. Furthermore, the prone positioning required for PCNL and use of extensive fluoroscopy is not advised with a gravid uterus. Recently, ureteroscopic intervention has garnered support as a primary treatment option, by limiting the overall duration of pain and the number of procedures. Ulvik et al. first reported performing ureteroscopy in 24 pregnant women in 1995 and described no complications.[78]

Since Ulvik's first series, multiple subsequent small ureteroscopic series have been safely performed in

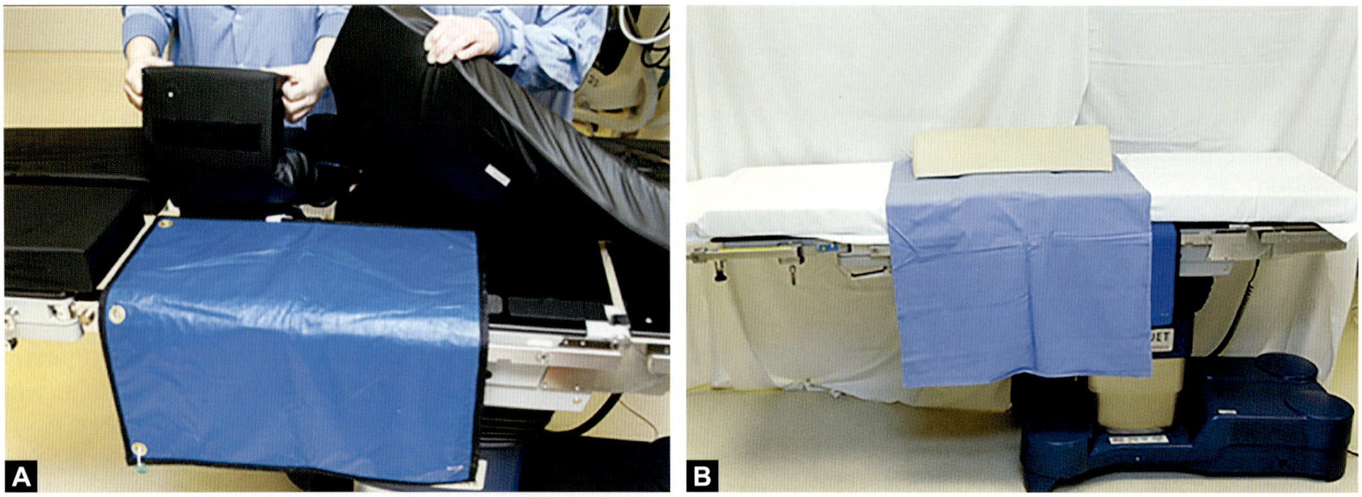

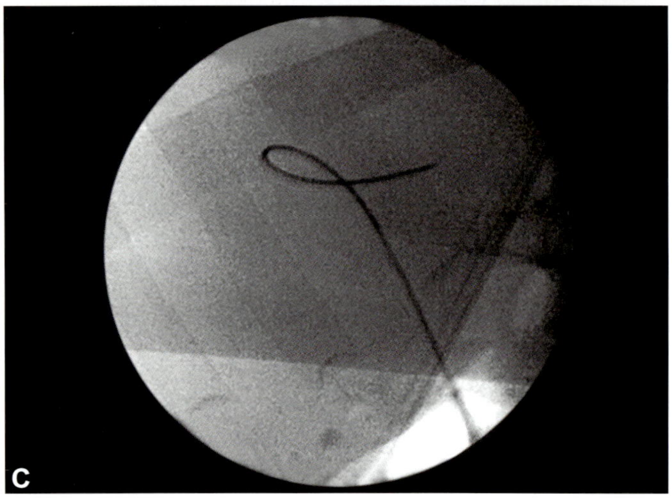

Figs. 34.6A to C: Important technical and positioning points are demonstrated here. (A) A lead shield is placed between the X-ray source and the fetus, (B) a foam wedge is used to accomplish the modified lithotomy position, and (C) low-dose pulsed fluoroscopy is used, with the image coned in to avoid undue radiation exposure to the fetus.

pregnant patients. Semins et al. performed a meta-analysis of 14 ureteroscopic studies in the pregnant patients and found that the rate of urologic complications in these patients was no greater than that in the nonpregnant patients.[79] With regard to obstetric complications, a recent study from five high-volume endourology institutions focused on obstetric complications in 46 patients undergoing ureteroscopic stone removal during pregnancy.[80] The study found two (4.3%) obstetric complications, both premature contractions in the third trimester, with one resulting in uncomplicated premature delivery at 33 weeks' gestational age. Thus, ureteroscopy performed during pregnancy is associated with a low likelihood of ureteroscopic and obstetric complications. Song et al. performed a retrospective review of 54 pregnant patients with urolithiasis, of whom 17 underwent double J ureteral stent placement, 16 had percutaneous nephrostomy tubes inserted, and 21 underwent ureteroscopy for definitive stone treatment.[81] The authors found that patients undergoing upfront ureteroscopic stone extraction experienced the fewest complications, further highlighting the benefit of definitive management in the pregnant patient.

Ureteroscopy performed in a pregnant patient is quite similar to that in a nonpregnant individual; however, modification of positioning, fluoroscopic imaging, and potentially the time spent to manage a stone must all be appropriately made. Optimal positioning during pregnancy is in the left lateral decubitus position, to decrease compression of the inferior vena cava. Thus, in preparation for ureteroscopy, the patient is placed in a modified dorsal lithotomy position with a foam wedge under the right side (Figs. 34.6A to C). A lead shield can be placed under the contralateral side of the abdomen, from the midline lateral. Low-dose pulsed imaging mode should be used with a fluoroscopic C-arm, with the image coned in onto the renal unit of interest. Although optimally the C-arm should be positioned exactly over the kidney, if there is any question, the fluoroscopy technician should start superiorly (toward the patient's chest) and work inferiorly, to limit radiation exposure to the fetus. Fluoroscopy should only be performed with an under-table source C-arm to limit radiation scatter. Fluoroscopy should be kept to a bare minimum; we recommend only two spot films if at all possible, one to image the wire in the intrarenal collecting system and the other to confirm the position of the ureteral stent proximal curl in the renal pelvis. Stents should be placed under direct vision, not fluoroscopically, again to decrease the amount of radiation exposure. First, rigid cystoscopy is performed and a ureteral wire is placed into the kidney. Semirigid ureteroscopy is then performed to evaluate for a distal ureteral stone. If a stone is encountered, it can be fragmented using the holmium laser and basket stone extraction performed as necessary. Then, flexible ureteroscopy can be performed to evaluate the proximal ureter and intrarenal collecting system. Typically, the ureters are quite dilated during pregnancy and ureteroscopy can be successfully performed without ureteral dilation. No clear guidelines exist regarding the use of temporary stenting in pregnancy; however, we choose to take a conservative approach and place a short-term (48 hours) ureteral stent in all pregnant ureteroscopic patients. If no ureteral injury is identified and all stone fragments are removed, the stent can be left on a dangle and removed at the discretion of the urologist.[82]

As described, ureteroscopy in the pregnant patient appears to be safe and efficacious when appropriate steps are taken to minimize maternal and fetal complications. It is imperative that the patient and her healthcare team discuss all risks involved prior to proceeding with any surgical intervention. However, when done appropriately, ureteroscopic intervention during pregnancy can be performed with excellent results.

CONCLUSION

With the advent of new, more easily deflectable ureteroscopes and improved ancillary equipment, ureteroscopic management of urolithiasis and upper tract urothelial disease is possible in a variety of patient situations, with various comorbid conditions. Ureteroscopy is safe and effective in the anomalous kidney, anatomic renal malformations, following urinary diversion, ureteral reimplantation, and in pregnancy. The operating surgeon, however, must have a thorough understanding of the patient's variant anatomy in order to accomplish the goal at hand safely and effectively. Furthermore, a wide range of equipment and steady supply of patience are beneficial to the success of the ureteroscopic procedure.

REFERENCES

1. Hall MC, Koch MO, McDougal WS. Metabolic consequences of urinary diversion through intestinal segments. Urol Clin North Am. 1991;18:725-35.
2. Terai A, Arai Y, Kawakita M, et al. Effect of urinary intestinal diversion on urinary risk factors for urolithiasis. J Urol. 1995;153:37-41.
3. Steiner MS, Morton RA. Nutritional and gastrointestinal complications of the use of bowel segments in the lower urinary tract. Urol Clin North Am. 1991;18:743-54.
4. Hertzig LL, Iwaszko MR, Rangel LJ, et al. Urolithiasis after ileal conduit urinary diversion: a comparison of minimally invasive therapies. J Urol. 2013;189(6):2152-7.
5. Shimko MS, Tollefson MK, Umbreit EC, et al. Long-term complications of conduit urinary diversion. J Urol. 2011;185: 562-7.
6. Wolf JS, Stoller ML. Management of upper tract calculi in patients with tubularized urinary diversions. J Urol. 1991;145:266-9.
7. Cass AS, Lee JY, Aliabadi H. Extracorporeal shock wave lithotripsy and endoscopic management of renal calculi with urinary diversions. J Urol. 1992;148:1123-5.
8. Sternberg IA, Keren Paz GE, Chen LY, et al. Upper tract imaging surveillance is not effective in diagnosing upper tract recurrence in patients followed for nonmuscle invasive bladder cancer. J Urol. 2013;190(4):1187-91.
9. Hyams ES, Winer AG, Shah O. Retrograde ureteral and renal access in patients with urinary diversion. Urology. 2009;74:47-50.
10. Scherr DS, Barocas DA. Ileal conduit. In: Smith JA, Howards SS, Preminger GM, et al. (Eds). Hinman's Atlas of Urologic Surgery, 3rd edition, Chapter 96. Philadelphia, PA: Saunders Elsevier; 2012. pp. 615-28.
11. Okhunov Z, Duty B, Smith AD, et al. Management of urolithiasis in patients after urinary diversions. BJU Int. 2011;108(3):330-6.
12. Rivera ME, Krambeck AE. Retrograde ureteroscopy via a continent urinary diversion: surgical techniques and common pitfalls. J Endourol. 2014;28(7):763-6.
13. Nelson CP, Wolf JS Jr, Montie JE, et al. Retrograde ureteroscopy in patients with orthotopic ileal neobladder urinary diversion. J Urol. 2003;170:107-10.
14. Sejiny M, Al-Qahtani S, Elhaous A, et al. Efficacy of flexible ureterorenoscopy with holmium laser in the management of stone-bearing caliceal diverticula. J Endourol. 2010;24(6):961-7.
15. Canales B, Monga M. Surgical management of the calyceal diverticulum. Curr Opin Urol. 2003;13:255-60.
16. Timmons JW, Malek RS, Hattery RR, et al. Caliceal diverticulum. J Urol. 1975;114:6-9.

17. Middleton AW, Pfister RC. Stone-containing pyelocaliceal diverticulum: embryogenic, anatomic, radiologic and clinical characteristics. J Urol. 1974;111:2-6.
18. Jones JA, Lingeman JE, Steidle CP, et al. The roles of extracorporeal shock wave lithotripsy and percutaneous nephrostolithotomy in the management of pyelocaliceal diverticula. J Urol. 1991;146:724-7.
19. Monga M, Smith R, Ferral H, et al. Percutaneous ablation of caliceal diverticulum: long-term followup. J Urol. 2000;163:28-32.
20. Gross AJ, Herrmann TR. Management of stones in calyceal diverticulum. Curr Opin Urol. 2007;17:136-40.
21. Fuchs GI, Fuchs AM. Flexible endoscopy of the upper urinary tract new minimally invasive treatment approach. Urologe A. 1990;29:313-20.
22. AugeBK, Munver R, Kourambas J, et al. Endoscopic management of symptomatic caliceal diverticula: a retrospective comparison of percutaneous nephrolithotripsy and ureteroscopy. J Endourol. 2002;16:557-63.
23. Batter SJ, Dretler SP. Ureterorenoscopic approach to the symptomatic caliceal diverticulum. J Urol. 1997;158:709-13.
24. Symons SJ, Ramachandran A, Kurien A, et al. Urolithiasis in the horseshoe kidney: a single-centre experience. BJU Int. 2008;102(11):1676-80.
25. Weizer AZ, Silverstein AD, Auge BK, et al. Determining the incidence of horseshoe kidney from radiographic data at a single institution. J Urol. 2003;170:1722-6.
26. Tan YK, Cha DY, Gupta M. Management of stones in abnormal situations. Urol Clin North Am. 2013;40(1):79-97.
27. Raj GV, Auge BK, Weizer AZ, et al. Percutaneous management of calculi within horseshoe kidneys. J Urol. 2003;170(1):48-51.
28. Molimard B, Al-Qahtani S, Lakmichi A, et al. Flexible ureterorenoscopy with holmium laser in horseshoe kidneys. Urology. 2010;76(6):1334-7.
29. Evans WP, Resnick MI. Horseshoe kidney and urolithiasis. J Urol. 1981;125:620-1.
30. Mottola A, Selli C, Carini M, et al. Lithiasis in horseshoe kidney. Acta Urol Belg. 1984;52:355-60.
31. Gambaro G, Fabris A, Puliatta D, et al. Lithiasis in cystic kidney disease and malformations of the urinary tract. Urol Res. 2006;34:102-7.
32. Collado Serra A, Parada Moreno R, Rousaud Barón F, et al. Current management of calculi in horseshoe kidneys. Scand J Urol Nephrol. 2000;34(2):114-8.
33. Raj GV, Auge BK, Assimos D, et al. Metabolic abnormalities associated with renal calculi in patients with horseshoe kidneys. J Endourol. 2004;18:157-61.
34. Ray AA, Ghiculete D, D'A Honey RJ, et al. Shockwave lithotripsy in patients with horseshoe kidney: determinants of success. J Endourol. 2011;25(3):487-93.
35. Atis G, Resorlu B, Gurbuz C, et al. Retrograde intrarenal surgery in patients with horseshoe kidneys. Urolithiasis. 2013;41(1):79-83.
36. Weizer AZ, Springhart WP, Ekeruo WO, et al. Ureteroscopic management of renal calculi in anomalous kidneys. Urology. 2005;65(2):265-9.
37. Baek M, Kim KD. Current surgical management of vesicoureteral reflux. Korean J Urol. 2013;54(11):732-7.
38. Wallis MC, Brown DH, Jayanthi VR, et al. A novel technique for ureteral catheterization and/or retrograde ureteroscopy after cross-trigonal ureteral reimplantation. J Urol. 2003;170(4):1664-6.
39. Lusuardi L, Hruby S, Jeschke S, et al. A new technique for retrograde flexible ureteroscopy after Cohen cross-trigonal ureteral reimplantation. Urol Int. 2011;87(3):260-2.
40. Pope J, Makari J. Ureteroneocystostomy. In: Smith JA, Howards SS, Preminger GM, et al. (Eds). Hinman's Atlas of Urologic Surgery, 3rd edition, Chapter 111. Philadelphia, PA: Saunders Elsevier; 2012. pp. 711-26.
41. Krambeck AE, Gettman MT, BaniHani AH, et al. Management of nephrolithiasis after Cohen cross-trigonal and Glenn–Anderson advancement ureteroneocystostomy. J Urol. 2007;177(1):174-8.
42. Santarosa RP, Hensle TW, Shabsigh R. Percutaneous transvesical ureteroscopy for removal of distal ureteral stone in reimplanted ureter. Urology. 1993;42(3):313-6.
43. Challacombe B, Dasgupta P, Tiptaft R, et al. Multimodal management of urolithiasis in renal transplantation. BJU Int. 2005;96(3):385-9.
44. Rattiazzi LC, Simmons RL, Markland C, et al. Calculi complicating renal transplantation into ileal conduits. Urology. 1975;5:29-31.
45. Mundy AR, Podesta ML, Bewick M. The urological complications of 1000 renal transplants. Br J Urol. 1981;53:397-402.
46. Rhee BK, Bretan PN Jr, Stoller ML. Urolithiasis in renal and combined pancreas/renal transplant recipients. J Urol. 1999;161:1458-62.
47. Harper JM, Samuell CT, Hallson PC, et al. Risk factors for calculus formation in patients with renal transplants. Br J Urol. 1994;74(2):147-50.
48. Hyams E, Marien T, Bruhn A, et al. Ureteroscopy for transplant lithiasis. J Endourol. 2012;26(7):819-22.
49. Stravodimos KG, Adamis S, Tyritzis S, et al. Renal transplant lithiasis: analysis of our series and review of the literature. J Endourol. 2012;26:38-44.
50. Lu HF, Shekarriz B, Stoller ML. Donor gifted allograft urolithiasis: early percutaneous management. Urology. 2002;59:25-7.
51. Rashid MG, Konnak JW, Wolf JS Jr, et al. Ex vivo ureteroscopic treatment of calculi in donor kidneys at renal transplantation. J Urol. 2004;171:58-60.
52. Torrecilla Ortiz C, Gonzalez-Satue C, Riera CL, et al. [Incidence and treatment of urinary lithiasis in renal transplantation]. Actas Urol Esp. 2001;25:357-63.
53. Pearle MS, Calhoun EA, Curhan GC. Urologic diseases in America project: urolithiasis. J Urol. 2005;173(3):848-57.
54. Wong KA, Olsburgh J. Management of stones in renal transplant. Curr Opin Urol. 2013;23(2):175.
55. Devasia A, Chacko N, Gnanaraj L, et al. Stone-bearing livedonor kidneys for transplantation. BJU Int. 2005;95:394-7.
56. Ho K, Chow G. Prevalence and early outcome of donor graft lithiasis in living renal transplants at the Mayo Clinic. J Urol. 2005;173:439-41.
57. Li SD, Wang QT, Chen WG. Treatment of urinary lithiasis following kidney transplantation with extracorporeal shockwave lithotripsy. Chin Med J. 2011;124:1431-4.

58. Krambeck AE, Leroy AJ, Patterson DE, et al. Percutaneous nephrolithotomy success in the transplant kidney. J Urol. 2008;180(6):2545-9.
59. Parulkar BG, Hopkins TB, Wollin MR, et al. Renal colic during pregnancy: a case for conservative treatment. J Urol. 1998;159:365-8.
60. Coe FL, Parks JH, Lindheimer MD. Nephrolithiasis during pregnancy. N Engl J Med. 1978;298:324-6.
61. Smith CL, Kristensen C, Davis M, et al. An evaluation of the physicochemical risk of renal stone disease during pregnancy. Clin Nephrol. 2001;55:205-11.
62. Matlaga BR, Lingeman JE. Surgical management of upper urinary tract calculi. In: Wein AJ, Kavoussi LR, Novick AC, et al. (Eds). Campbell-Walsh Urology, 10th edition, Chapter 48. Philadelphia, PA: Saunders Elsevier; 2012. pp. 1357-410.
63. McAleer SJ, Loughlin KR. Nephrolithiasis and pregnancy. Curr Opin Urol. 2004;14:123-7.
64. Biyani CS, Joyce AD. Urolithiasis in pregnancy. I: pathophysiology, fetal considerations and diagnosis. BJU Int. 2002;89:811-8.
65. Charalambous S, Fotas A, Rizk DE. Urolithiasis in pregnancy. Int Urogynecol J. 2009;20:1133-6.
66. Shokeir AA, Mahran MR, Abdulmaaboud M. Renal colic in pregnant women: role of resistive index. Urology. 2000;55:344-7.
67. Vallurapalli K, Krambeck AE, Atwell T. Pearls and pitfalls in sonographic imaging of urolithiasis in pregnancy. Ultrasound Q. 2013;29:51-9.
68. Sheafor DH, Hertzberg BS, Freed KS, et al. Nonenhanced helical CT and US in the emergency evaluation of patients with renal colic: prospective comparison. Radiology. 2000;217:792-7.
69. Berlin L. Radiation exposure to the pregnant patient. AJR Am J Roentgenol. 1996;167:1377-7.
70. White WM, Johnson EB, Site EB, Et al. Predictive Value Current imging modalities for the detection of urolithiasis during pregnancy: a multicenter, longitudinal study. J Urol. 2013;189:931-4
71. ACOG Committee on Obstetric Practice. ACOG Committee Opinion. Number 299, September 2004 (replaces No. 158, September 1995). Guidelines for diagnostic imaging during pregnancy. Obstet Gynecol. 2004;104:647-51.
72. Spencer JA, Chahal R, Kelly A, et al. Evaluation of painful hydronephrosis in pregnancy: magnetic resonance urographic patterns in physiological dilatation versus calculous obstruction. J Urol. 2004;171:256-60.
73. Mulkins JK, Semins MJ, Hyams ES, et al. Half Fourier single-shot turbo spin-echo magnetic resonance urography for the evaluation of suspected renal colic in pregnancy. Urology. 2012;79:1252-5.
74. Fulgham PF, Assimos DG, Pearle MS, et al. AUA Technology Assessment. J Urol. 2012;189:1203-13.
75. Burgess KL, Gettman MT, Rangel LJ, et al. Diagnosis of uro lithiasis and rate of spontaneous passage during pregnancy. J Urol. 2011;186:2280-4.
76. Kavoussi LR, Albala DM, Basler JW, et al. Percutaneous management of urolithiasis during pregnancy. J Urol. 1992;148:1069-71.
77. Loughlin KR, Bailey RB. Internal ureteral stents for conservative management of ureteral calculi during pregnancy. N Engl J Med. 1986;315:1647-9.
78. Ulvik NM, Bakke A, Høisaeter PA. Ureteroscopy in pregnancy. J Urol. 1995;154:1660-3.
79. Semins MJ, Trock BJ, Matlaga BR. The safety of ureteroscopy during pregnancy: a systematic review and meta-analysis. J Urol. 2009;181(1):139-43.
80. Johnson EB, Krambeck AE, White WM, et al. Obstetric complications of ureteroscopy during pregnancy. J Urol. 2012;188:151-4.
81. Song Y, Fei X, Song Y. Diagnosis and operative intervention for problematic ureteral calculi during pregnancy. Int J Gynaecol Obstet. 2013;12:115-8.
82. Preminger GM, Tiselius HG, Assimos DG, et al. 2007 Guideline for the management of ureteral calculi. Eur Urol. 2007;52:1610-31.

CHAPTER

35

Role of Laparoscopic, Robotic Assisted and Open Surgery in Management of Urolithiasis

Amit Bhattu, Mihir M Desai

INTRODUCTION

Over the past 3 decades, the introduction and refinement of endourologic techniques such as surgical treatment percutaneous nephrolithotomy (PCNL), semirigid and flexible ureteroscopy, and shock wave lithotripsy (SWL) has resulted in a dramatic change in the surgical treatment of urolithiasis. In the current era, open surgical techniques may still have a limited indication for managing urolithiasis, as defined by guidelines from the American Urological Association and European Association of Urology.[1-3] The use of a minimally invasive laparoscopic approach may reduce the morbidity and serve as an attractive alternative to open surgery. The robotic platform may increase the reproducibility and reduce the learning curve as compared to the somewhat technically challenging laparoscopic approach.

Currently in the United States of America, only approximately 2% of surgeries done for nephrolithiasis in Medicare patients use an open approach.[4] Similarly, only 1–5% of surgeries for nephrolithiasis are done by open approach across the globe.[5]

INDICATIONS FOR OPEN SURGERY FOR UROLITHIASIS[6]

The contemporary indications for open surgery in existing guidelines are summarized in Table 35.1.

1. *Complex renal stone disease:* Complex and large stones that may require an impractically high number of endourological or SWL procedures may be treated by open surgery. Examples include large staghorn calculi with multiple branches, very large renal pelvic or ureteral calculi. This indication obviously depends on the availability of endourologic expertise and instrumentation resources and is left to the discretion of the surgeon.
2. *Failures of endourological and SWL treatment:* Failure of endourological and SWL treatment or inability to clear the stone in a reasonable number of sessions may be an indication for open surgery. What is defined as a "reasonable number" of endourological sessions is very subjective, and with advances in technology and expertise this indication is shrinking.
3. *Anatomical abnormalities:* Abnormalities such as pelviureteric junction obstruction, calyceal diverticulum, infundibular stenosis, and ureteric stricture can complicate and predispose to complex and recurrent stone formation. As such, the goal of treatment in most instances includes correction of the associated abnormality at the time of stone removal. Although in many such instances endourological interventions such as endopyelotomy or laser infundibulotomy may treat these anatomic abnormalities, and surgical reconstruction such as pyeloplasty may provide a superior outcome and should be preferred.
4. *Comorbidities:* Severe medical or anatomic comorbid conditions may preclude multistage procedures and multiple anesthetics that may be required for complex stone treatment by endourological means. Open surgery may allow the maximal stone clearance in a single sitting and may be indicated in highly select patients with severe comorbidities.
5. *Nephrectomy:* Urolithiasis may lead to loss of renal function, recurrent infection and occasionally xanthogranulomatous pyelonephritis, and squamous or urothelial carcinoma. Nephrectomy is the best option in these situations via either an open or a laparoscopic approach. Rarely, focal destruction may be amenable to partial or heminephrectomy.
6. *Patient's preference for open surgery:* Occasionally some patients may prefer a single treatment session via an open approach to multiple endoscopic interventions.

ROLE OF LAPAROSCOPIC AND ROBOTIC SURGERY

Over the past 2 decades, there has been an exponential increase in the use of laparoscopy and more recently

Table 35.1: AUA–EAU consensus panel guidelines for management of ureteric stones as related to open surgery.

Open ureterolithotomy	• Rarely necessary for management of urolithiasis • When open surgery is necessary for other simultaneous pathology • To be combined with reconstructive surgery for ureteric pathology
Laparoscopic ureterolithotomy	• To be preferred over open ureterolithotomy in cases of failed SWL or ureteroscopy for multiple, large or impacted ureteric stones
AUA guidelines for management of staghorn stones pertinent to open surgery[2]	
Recommendations for indexed patient	• PCNL should be the main line of management • If multimodal treatment is considered, then the PCNL should be the last completing procedure for most patients • Open procedure should not be used for most patients
Options for indexed patients	• Open procedure can be considered for those patients in whom the stone burden is so large that clearance would not be possible with reasonable number of endourological procedures the anatomical malformation • Obesity that precludes the use of endourological interventions
Recommendations for nonindex patients	• Laparoscopic or open nephrectomy for patients with stone laden poorly functioning kidneys
EAU guidelines for management of urolithiasis[3]	
Recommendation	*Level of evidence (LE)*
• Laparoscopic or open surgery for stones in which endourological or SWL techniques have failed or are unlikely to be successful	4
• Whenever expertise is available then the laparoscopic approach should be preferred over the open approach except in conditions with complex anatomy or stone characteristics where laparoscopy may not be possible or successful	4
• Laparoscopy should be considered for ureterolithotomy for large and/or impacted urolithiasis in which ureteroscopy or SWL has failed or is unlikely to be successful	2

(AUA: American Urological Association; EUA: Egyptian Urological Association; PCNL: Percutaneous nephrolithotomy; SWL: Shock wave lithotripsy).

Source: Preminger GM, Tiselius HG, Assimos DG, et al. EAU/AUA Nephrolithiasis Guideline Panel. J Urol. 2007;178(6):2418-34.

robotic-assisted surgery for various urologic conditions, ablative and reconstructive. The indications of these minimally invasive approaches for treating urolithiasis should be identical to those of open surgery mentioned earlier and therefore also be infrequent. Even though they are minimally invasive compared to open surgery, they are still more invasive than endourological approaches that continue to remain the gold standard. The introduction of robotic assistance may increase the use of minimally invasive approaches, especially when reconstruction is required.

Laparoscopic and Robotic Pyelolithotomy

Gaur et al. published the initial five cases of retroperitoneal laparoscopic pyelolithotomy for stones not amenable to SWL and PCNL.[7] The retroperitoneal approach prevents peritoneal contamination in these often-infected kidneys. Additionally, it also offers a more direct approach to the renal pelvis that is posterior to the hilar vessels. Sinha et al. reported 20 retroperitoneal laparoscopic pyelolithotomy for stones ranging from only 1.6 cm to 5 cm. The pelvis was not closed in the initial 14 patients, and 2 patients developed urinary leak. Open conversion was required in four cases.[8] The reported stone-free rates with laparoscopic pyelolithotomy ranged from 71% to 100% and the need for open conversion is 0–27%.[9,10] These data show inferior outcomes for stone size that should be amenable to an endourologic or SWL approach.

Al-Hunayan et al. compared retroperitoneal laparoscopic pyelolithotomy (N = 55) and PCNL (N = 55) for solitary renal pelvic stones. Both groups were comparable in terms of blood loss, transfusion rate, hospital stay, and stone-free rates. Mean operative time in the laparoscopic group was longer, and one patient required conversion to open pyelolithotomy for uncontrolled bleeding.[11] Another study compared laparoscopic pyelolithotomy versus PCNL for pelvic stones >2 cm. The laparoscopic approach was equivalent to PCNL in terms of hospital stay, transfusion rate, and complication rate. However, the laparoscopic approach was associated with shorter operative time, less blood loss, and a higher stone-free rate (98% vs. 90%) compared to PCNL.[12] In contrast, Meria et al. reported on 32 patients with pelvic stone >2 cm randomized into transperitoneal laparoscopic pyelolithotomy (N = 16) and PCNL (N = 16). The stone-free rate was 88% and 82% with the laparoscopic and percutaneous approaches, respectively (P = 0.08). The operative time, urine leakage rate, and conversion to open surgery were higher with the laparoscopic approach, and so the authors recommended PCNL as the standard of care for uncomplicated renal pelvic stone.[13]

Robotic assistance may reduce the learning curve of laparoscopic surgery, especially with intracorporeal suturing. Badani and colleagues reported a case series of robotic pyelolithotomy in 12 partial and 1 complete staghorn calculi. All procedures were successfully completed without conversion to laparoscopy or open surgery. Complete stone-free status could be achieved in all partial staghorn stones but the solitary complete staghorn in this report had residual stones. Mean operative time was 158 minutes, and mean console time was 108 minutes. Mean estimated blood loss was 100 mL, and no patient required transfusion.[14]

Hemal et al. reported data on 50 patients who underwent robotic-assisted surgery for management of upper urinary tract urolithiasis. These included 29 patients undergoing pyeloplasty with pyelolithotomy and eight patients undergoing pyelolithotomy alone. Complete stone clearance was achieved in 93.1% of the patients. Open conversion was required in one case, and one patient required selective renal angioembolization for postoperative hematuria. They concluded that the robotic approach was superior and provided a specific advantage in reconstructive work in view of better control, dexterity, and precision.[15]

These studies suggest that laparoscopic or robotic pyelolithotomy may be used for select patients with a large single pelvic stone. Since laparoscopic and robotic pyelolithotomy avoid entry through the renal parenchyma, uncomplicated cases should have a lower risk of bleeding compared to PCNL where the risk of bleeding is likely proportional to the number and caliber of percutaneous tracts. Thus, laparoscopic and robotic pyelolithotomy may be a useful option in patients at higher risk of bleeding or in patients who refuse blood transfusion.

Laparoscopic and Robotic Anatrophic Nephrolithotomy

The technical feasibility of laparoscopic anatrophic nephrolithotomy (LAN) in the porcine model was first reported by Kaouk et al.[16] followed by the initial clinical report by Deger et al. in 2004.[17] Simforoosh and colleagues published their experience of five cases of LAN for complex branched calculi with an average stone size of 53 mm.[18] They used complete hilar clamping using laparoscopic bulldog clamps. An incision was made over the Brodel's line and stones were removed. The nephrotomy was suture repaired with laparoscopic free-hand suturing using Hem-o-lok clips as pledgets on the renal cortex. An intraoperative ultrasound probe was used in the last two patients to evaluate the residual calculi. No patient developed infundibular stenosis in subsequent imaging, and two patients had small residual calculi. The authors concluded that the technique is effective but recommended a study with larger numbers.

Giedelman et al. published a series of 12 patients who underwent LAN for a mean stone size of 53 mm.[19] On postoperative imaging, 37% patients had residual calculi. Mean warm ischemia time was 20.8 minutes, and blood loss was 315 mL. One patient required angioembolization for a renal arteriovenous fistula associated with hematuria. The authors recommended this single-stage, minimally invasive technique for large complex renal stones, which would otherwise require multiple tracts and stages with PCNL for clearance.

Aminsharifi and coworkers published a series of 10 patients who underwent transperitoneal LAN for mean renal stone size of 67.3 mm.[20] The mean warm ischemia time was 33 minutes. One patient required splenectomy in the immediate postoperative period for a splenic laceration. Over a mean follow-up of 11.9 months, the average reduction in GFR was 14.5% in the treated renal unit on dimercaptosuccinic acid renogram. The overall stone-free rate was 80% in this series. Similarly, Zhou et al. performed transperitoneal LAN in 11 patients. Mean stone size was 52 mm, complete stone clearance was achieved in 10 patients, and mean warm ischemia time was 31 minutes.[21]

Menon and coworkers reported a series of three patients who underwent robotic-assisted anatrophic nephrolithotomy (RANL) for staghorn stones with mean stone volume of 12888 mm^3.[22] Renal hypothermia was achieved by inserting ice slush through a GelPOINT Device (Applied Medical). Core renal parenchymal temperature was <9°C, and mean cold ischemia time was 30 minutes. There were no complications, and two patients had residual stones measuring 13 mm and 9 mm, respectively. King et al. reported a series of seven patients (five with complete staghorn calculi) who underwent RANL without renal hypothermia.[23] Mean warm ischemia was 35 minutes. Complete clearance was achieved in two patients, and the remaining five patients had residual calculi estimated to account for <10% of the baseline stone burden.

Most reports of robotic and LAN are retrospective case series in very limited number of patients; there are no data regarding the comparative efficacy of laparoscopic/robotic anatrophic nephrolithotomy with standard endourologic techniques.

Laparoscopic and Robotic Ureterolithotomy

Wickham performed the first retroperitoneoscopic ureterolithotomy in 1979.[24] Kumar et al. reported 110 patients with >2 cm calculus in the upper ureter randomized into laparoscopic ureterolithotomy (LU) versus ureteroscopy and pneumatic lithotripsy. Overall, the stone-free rate at 3 months was 100% versus 76% with LU and ureteroscopy, respectively ($P = 0.02$). Additionally, LU was associated with a lower retreatment rate (0% vs 8%, $P = 0.01$), auxiliary procedure rate (0% vs 26%, $P = 0.001$), and complication rate (12% vs 26%, $P = 0.001$).[25]

A prospective randomized controlled trial comparing LU and open ureterolithotomy suggested that LU is associated with the same stone-free rate as open ureterolithotomy but is associated with lesser pain and analgesic requirement and shorter convalescence and hospital stay.[26]

A prospective randomized controlled trial comparing LU with ureteroscopy and PCNL for upper ureteric stones >1 cm showed that LU was associated with a stone-free rate at discharge of 88% compared to 56% with ureteroscopy and 64% with PCNL ($P = 0.001$ and 0.005).[27] The operative time was 128, 94, and 43 minutes with LU, PCNL, and ureteroscopy, respectively. In the LU group two procedures were converted to open surgery because of stones lost in the peritoneal cavity after extraction from the ureter that could not be localized laparoscopically. Another prospective randomized study comparing LU, SWL, and ureteroscopy for proximal urolithiasis showed that LU was associated with the highest stone-free status in a single session and lowest retreatment rates. However, LU is associated with longer operative time and hospital stay and greater analgesic requirements.[28]

Even though these studies suggest a potential advantage of LU over ureteroscopy, several issues need to be kept in mind. First, endourologic arms in these studies used semirigid endoscopy and in many instances pneumatic lithotripsy. These studies should ideally be repeated using modern flexible endoscopy and laser lithotripsy. Second, the laparoscopic/robotic approaches should be restricted to large (ideally >2 cm) calculi only.

From a technical standpoint, LU can be performed by the retroperitoneal or transperitoneal approach. The advantages of the retroperitoneal approach include direct ureteral access without the need for bowel mobilization and avoiding peritoneal contamination. The retroperitoneal approach is limited by working space and access to only the proximal ureter. Bove et al. compared the transperitoneal and retroperitoneal approach for LU at two different centers.[29] They found that the time required for identifying the ureter, ureterotomy closure and total operative time was longer in retroperitoneal group compared to the transperitoneal group. Thus, for surgeons learning laparoscopy the transperitoneal approach is preferred, but for experts the choice of approach should be left to the individual surgeon's discretion.

The issue of stenting the ureter or closing of ureterotomy is controversial. Urine leak occurs in 0–20% and ureteral strictures in 1.4–5.2% of patients after LU.[30,31] Technical factors that may help reduce ureteral strictures include a short transverse incision, using a cold knife in place of diathermy and milking the stone into a proximal dilated area to avoid making the ureterotomy at the site of impaction.[31] Few studies suggested increased stricture rates after suturing ureterotomy.[30-32] Providing adequate drainage in the form of stenting is likely to prevent urinary leakage. A challenging technical problem during LU is inability to locate the stone and stone migration that may result in a need for open conversion to palpate the stone. Vessel loops or atraumatic clamps may be used above and below the stone to avoid this issue.

Robotic assistance has been used for performing ureterolithotomy with the aim of reducing the technical skills for suturing.[33] However, another study claimed no substantial advantage of robotic assistance over standard laparoscopy for ureterolithotomy.[15]

Laparoscopic and Robotic Approach for Urolithiasis and Concomitant Procedures

The laparoscopic and robotic approaches are particularly attractive if there is an associated pathology such as ureteral or ureteropelvic strictures or calyceal diverticuli that require simultaneous correction. Several authors have reported on simultaneous stone extraction and laparoscopic/robotic pyeloplasty. Larger pelvic stones can be grasped and extracted easily. Smaller calyceal stones may be more challenging and may require the use of flexible endoscopy through a laparoscopic port and basketting.[34]

Combined Use of Laparoscopic or Robotic Approach with Endourological Approach for Urolithiasis

Laparoscopic visualization has been used to guide percutaneous access during PCNL in pelvic ectopic kidneys.[35] This approach allows retraction of the bowel overlying the kidney and avoids bowel injury during percutaneous access. It also allows for the closure of nephrotomy, which may reduce bleeding from the tract. As mentioned earlier, patients with multiple renal calculi with ureteropelvic junction obstruction may require the use of flexible ureterorenoscopy through the laparoscopic ports for retrieval of calyceal stones.

Lost Stones during Laparoscopic and Robotic Procedures

One potential problem with laparoscopic and robotic urinary stone removal is the risk of retained stone fragments in the peritoneal or retroperitoneal space. This is more common when removing struvite stones, which tend to be friable and get crushed during grasping and extraction. Such stones, especially struvite, may lead to intraperitoneal, pelvic, or abdominal wall abscess formation. Several technical maneuvers that may help prevent this complication include the use of a laparoscopic spoon and immediate placement of the stone fragments into a laparoscopic retrieval bag or on a gauze placed intra-abdominally.

CONCLUSION

Endourological techniques such as ureteroscopy, PCNL, and SWL are the gold standard for treatment of the vast majority of urolithiasis. The need for open surgery is restricted to the few select patients in whom stone size and complexity would require an impractical number of endourologic interventions, if endourologic interventions have failed, or an associated pathology may have better success with open repair. Laparoscopic and robotic interventions may reduce the morbidity of open surgery but should be used for precisely similar indications. Larger prospective comparative studies are needed to assess whether the indications for laparoscopic and robotic approaches for stone disease can be expanded.

REFERENCES

1. Preminger GM, Tiselius HG, Assimos DG, et al. EAU/AUA Nephrolithiasis Guideline Panel. J Urol. 2007;178(6):2418-34.
2. Preminger GM, Assimos DG, Lingeman JE, et al. AUA Nephrolithiasis Guideline Panel). Chapter 1: AUA guideline on management of staghorn calculi: diagnosis and treatment recommendations. J Urol. 2005;173(6):1991-2000.
3. Türk C, Knoll T, Petrik A, et al. EAU Guidelines on urolithiasis updated in 2014.
4. Kerbl K, Rehman J, Landman J et al. Current management of urolithiasis: progress or regress? J Endourol. 2002;16:281-8.
5. Alivizatos G, Skolarikos A.Is there still a role for open surgery in management of renal stones? Curr Opin Urol. 2006;16: 106-11
6. Paik M, Resnick M. Is there a role for open stone surgery? In: Resnick M (Ed.). Urolithiasis. Urol Clin North Am. 2000;27(2):323-31.
7. Gaur DD, Agarwal DK, Purohit KC. Retroperitoneal laparoscopic pyelolithotomy. J Urol. 1994;151:927-9.
8. Sinha R, Sharma N. Retroperitoneal laparoscopic management of urolithiasis. J Laparoendosc Adv Surg Tech A. 1997;7(2):95-8.
9. Hemal AK, Goel A, Kumar M, et al. Evaluation of laparoscopic retroperitoneal surgery in urinary stone disease. J Endourol. 2001;15(7):701-5.
10. Nambirajan T, Jeschke S, Albqami N, et al. Role of laparoscopy in management of renal stones: single-center experience and review of literature. J Endourol. 2005;19(3):353-9.
11. Al-Hunayan A, Khalil M, Hassabo M, et al. Management of solitary renal pelvic stone: laparoscopic retroperitoneal pyelolithotomy versus percutaneous nephrolithotomy. J Endourol. 2011;25(6):975-8.
12. Sheng Li, Liu TZ, Wang XH, et al. Randomized controlled trial comparing retroperitoneal laparoscopic pyelolithotomy versus percutaneous nephrolithotomy for the treatment of large renal pelvic calculi: a pilot study. J Endourol. 2014;28(8): 946-50.
13. Meria P, Milcent S, Desgrandchamps F, et al. Management of pelvic stones larger than 20 mm: laparoscopic transperitoneal pyelolithotomy or percutaneous nephrolithotomy? Urol Int. 2005;75:322-6.
14. Badani KK, Hemal AK, Fumo M, et al. Robotic extended pyelolithotomy for treatment of renal calculi: a feasibility study. World J Urol. 2006;24(2):198-201.
15. Hemal AK, Nayyar R, Gupta NP, et al. Experience with robotic assisted laparoscopic surgery in upper tract urolithiasis. Can J Urol. 2010;17(4):5299-305.
16. Kaouk JH, Gill IS, Desai MM. Laparoscopic anatrophic nephrolithotomy: feasibility study in a chronic porcine model. J Urol. 2003;169(2):691-6.
17. Deger S, Tuellmann M, Schoenberger B, et al. Laparoscopic anatrophic nephrolithotomy. Scand J Urol Nephrol. 2004;38(3):263-5.
18. Simforoosh N, Aminsharifi A, Tabibi A, et al. Laparoscopic anatrophic nephrolithotomy for managing large staghorn calculi. BJU Int. 2008;101(10):1293-6.

19. Giedelman C, Arriaga J, Carmona O, et al. Laparoscopic anatrophic nephrolithotomy: developments of the technique in the era of minimally invasive surgery. J Endourol. 2012;26(5):444-50.
20. Aminsharifi A, Hadian P, Boveiri K. Laparoscopic anatrophic nephrolithotomy for management of complete staghorn renal stone: clinical efficacy and intermediate-term functional outcome. J Endourol. 2013;27(5):573-8.
21. Zhou L, Xuan Q, Wu B, et al. Retroperitoneal laparoscopic anatrophic nephrolithotomy for large staghorn calculi. Int J Urol. 2011;18(2):126-9.
22. Ghani KR, Rogers CG, Sood A, et al. Robot-assisted anatrophic nephrolithotomy with renal hypothermia for managing staghorn calculi. J Endourol. 2013;27(11):1393-8.
23. King SA, Klaassen Z, Madi R. Robot-assisted anatrophic nephrolithotomy: description of technique and early results. J Endourol. 2014;28(3):325-9.
24. Wickham JE. The surgical treatment of renal lithiasis. In: Wickham JE (Ed). Urinary Calculous Disease. Edinburgh: Churchill Livingstone; 1979. pp.145-98.
25. Kumar A, Vasudeva P, Nanda B, et al. A prospective randomized comparison between laparoscopic ureterolithotomy and semirigid ureteroscopy for upper urolithiasis >2 cm: a single-center experience. J Endourol. 2015;29(11):1248-52.
26. Garg M, Singh V, Sinha RJ, et al. Prospective randomized comparison of open versus transperitoneal laparoscopic ureterolithotomy: experience of a single center from Northern India. Curr Urol. 2013;7(2):83-9.
27. Basiri A, Simforoosh N, Ziaee A, et al. Retrograde, antegrade, and laparoscopic approaches for the management of large, proximal urolithiasis: a randomized clinical trial. J Endourol. 2008;22(12):2677-80.
28. Lopes Neto AC, Korkes F, Silva JL 2nd, et al. Prospective randomized study of treatment of large proximal urolithiasis: extracorporeal shock wave lithotripsy versus ureterolithotripsy versus laparoscopy. J Urol. 2012;187(1):164-8.
29. Bove P, Micali S, Miano R, et al. Laparoscopic ureterolithotomy: a comparison between the transperitoneal and the retroperitoneal approach during the learning curve. J Endourol. 2009;23(6):953-7.
30. Gaur DD, Trivedi S, Prabhudesai MR, et al. Laparoscopic ureterotomy: technical considerations and long-term follow-up. BJU Int. 2002;89(4):339-43.
31. Kijvikai K, Patcharatrakul S. Laparoscopic ureterolithotomy: its role and some controversial technical considerations. Int J Urol. 2006;13(3):206-10.
32. Keeley FX, Gialas I, Pillai M, et al. Laparoscopic ureterolithotomy: the Edinburgh experience. BJU Int. 1999;84(7):765-9.
33. Dogra PN, Regmi SK, Singh P, et al. Lower urolithiasis revisited: expanding the horizons of robotics. Urology. 2013;82(1):95-9.
34. Salvado JA, Guzman S, Trucco CA, et al. Laparoscopic pyelolithotomy: optimizing surgical technique. J Endourol. 2009;23(4):575-8.
35. Eshghi AM, Roth JS, Smith AD. Percutaneous transperitoneal approach to a pelvic kidney for endourological removal of staghorn calculus. J Urol. 1985;134(3):525-7.

CHAPTER

36 Surgical Management of Stones in Children

Stephen Scott Sparks, Craig A Peters

INTRODUCTION

Although pediatric stone disease is known to be a global problem and is endemic to certain developing countries, it has traditionally been seen infrequently in more developed/Western nations. If left untreated or incompletely treated, stones can be associated with the development of various related disease processes such as infection, hypertension, and end-stage renal disease. In 1999, an estimated 18.4 per 100,000 pediatric hospital admissions in the United States were attributed to urolithiasis.[1] Since that time, the incidence has risen dramatically and now accounts for ~57 per 100,000 in 2008.[2] Though we see a definite rise in the incidence of pediatric urolithiasis in the literature, there is a lack of epidemiologic data in this population.[3] Etiology of stones impacts treatment and varies widely by geographic location. For example, in developing nations, bladder stones are the most common form of urolithiasis and are typically composed of uric acid and ammonium acid urate. This finding is strongly suggestive of a dietary source, which is further supported with decreasing incidence as these countries develop.[4] In European countries, there is a higher incidence of struvite stones (magnesium ammonium phosphate) and they are more likely to be associated with infection and abnormal urinary tract anatomy. In the United States, however, calculi related to infection or uric acid are relatively rare in children and calcium stones predominate.[5,6]

Treatment modalities for urinary stone disease are similar to the adult population and vary widely. Current options for treatment of stones range from noninvasive medical therapy to major open surgical approaches, although there is a trend toward less invasive approaches. The particular treatment modality that is employed is determined based on a variety of factors, including stone size, location, and composition. Other factors that influence this decision are patient size/age and the anatomy of the urinary tract.

In order to assess patients with suspected stones, imaging modalities that can diagnose and ideally help delineate stones as well as define the anatomy of the urinary tract are also varied. Although computed tomography (CT) imaging has traditionally been used preferentially (and still is in the adult population), the amount of radiation associated with a typical CT has caused concern among most pediatric urologists. This has led most to move away from its use in routine cases. Whenever possible, ultrasound imaging with judicious use of plain films is employed for diagnosis.

The goal of treatment is to provide stone-free status safely, while minimizing invasiveness and anesthesia time. Nonsurgical treatment in children is effective and appropriate for certain stones, even in the acute setting,[7] and especially with the introduction of medical expulsive therapy is particularly useful for smaller or more distally located stones. Open or endoscopic surgical treatment of stones is typically reserved for larger stones or those that fail to pass. There are currently little evidence-based data relating to selection of individual surgical techniques, although many studies have demonstrated the safety and efficacy of the various treatment modalities, even in infants.[8,9] The ultimate treatment should be based on stone and patient factors as well as the preference of the surgeon.

EPIDEMIOLOGY

Stone disease in children has traditionally been seen as a rare entity in developed countries in the Western hemisphere. Adult data describe an incidence of urolithiasis of 1.5%,[10] with about 12% of men and 5% of women developing a kidney stone at some point in their life.[11] In the pediatric population, it is much less common, accounting for only ~2% of all patients with stone disease in some older series.[1] More recent reports are, however, showing an increasing incidence. VanDervoort et al. demonstrated a nearly fivefold increase in the incidence of urolithiasis at their institution over a 10- to 11-year period (1994–2005).[3] Routh et al. were able to demonstrate an increase in the incidence over multiple institutions through the Pediatric Health Information System database.[2] They found that the number of stone cases per hospital per year increased from 13.9 to 32.6 between 1999 and 2008, for an adjusted annual increase of 10.6%. Some of this increase may be attributable to better reporting, improved ability to diagnose stones in this population, or changing referral patterns, but this is felt to be unlikely to account for such a large change.

Many theories for the rising incidence of pediatric urolithiasis have been put forth, but there is no definitive reason for the trend. Changes in diet and physical activity may account for the rise, but so far, no studies have been able to demonstrate this definitively. Obesity and elevated body mass index have certainly been shown to increase stone incidence in the adult population,[12,13] but, so far, studies do not confirm obesity as a risk factor for the development of stone disease in the pediatric population.[14]

Stone disease is more commonly seen in Caucasians, and this seems to hold true in the pediatric population as well.[15] It is, however, seen in children of all ages.[16] Boys are more often diagnosed with urolithiasis during the first 10 years of their life, whereas girls are more often seen with stone disease in the second decade of their life.[17]

Stone composition in children can be very different from that seen in adults. This difference, however, diminishes as the age of the child increases, i.e. stone composition in teenagers is very similar to that of adults. A large study by Gabrielsen et al.[18] demonstrated that in the United States calcium was present in 89.2% and that oxalate composition increased with age, whereas magnesium ammonium phosphate and ammonium acid urate stones decreased in incidence with age. In addition, they were able to show that stones related to infection (magnesium ammonium phosphate and ammonium acid urate) were more common in women, whereas uric acid stones were more commonly seen in men. Uric acid stones account for ~3–10% of all calculi.[19] Overall, despite the difference in composition seen with age and gender, ~75% of pediatric urolithiasis is composed of calcium oxalate.

PRESENTATION

Although the typical constellation of incapacitating flank pain and hematuria associated with passage of a stone is seen more commonly in adults, children present with more subtle findings that may require a high degree of suspicion to diagnose promptly. In addition to the subtlety of presenting symptoms in children, a considerable variation with age may be observed. This is most notable in younger children, who may have more nonspecific symptoms, whereas adolescents tend to present with classic renal colic. Children may present with nausea, vomiting, or fever without overt pain. In infants, urinary calculi may present as a urinary tract infection (UTI), gross or microscopic hematuria, and nonspecific or diffuse abdominal pain that may mimic colic.[20] Hematuria may be present in any age group and should always raise suspicion for calculi, although it may be encountered in children with hypercalciuria, hyperoxaluria, and other metabolic disorders without obvious urolithiasis.[21] Also, although microscopic and/or macroscopic hematuria can be seen in 30–90% of children with urolithiasis, it is important to remember that there is a significant number of children without this sign.[22]

When a child presents with a stone episode, a pediatric urologist should be consulted to aid in further evaluation and treatment. Surgical management of urolithiasis has dramatically evolved in the past few decades, although the evaluation of these patients has remained relatively stable. Clinically, symptoms often dictate the urgency with which surgical intervention is considered. Patients with symptoms indicating obstruction, such as intractable pain or nausea, often require prompt surgical intervention. Urinary tract infections or associated signs and symptoms, especially fever or an elevated white blood cell count, are indication for more rapid surgical management (Flowchart 36.1).

EVALUATION

As with any condition, the evaluation of a patient suspected of having urolithiasis begins with a thorough history and physical examination. During this portion of the evaluation, particular attention should be paid to medications (current and past), concurrent illnesses and medical conditions, diet (especially a ketogenic diet,[23] which is common to children with significant seizure history), and family history of stones or conditions associated with stones. These areas are of particular interest in younger patients as they will more frequently be noted to have a metabolic issue or family history than older children (teenagers), who are more likely to have stones related to dehydration, etc.

The physical examination should of course attempt to better characterize and localize the symptoms, but as previously noted, children may not demonstrate typical patterns of pain and a high index of suspicion is required.

Laboratory Evaluation

In the acute setting, laboratory evaluation is used to determine the acuity of the stone and to help guide treatment.

Flowchart 36.1: Algorithm for evaluation and initial management of the child presenting with acute flank pain with or without nausea, vomiting, and hematuria.

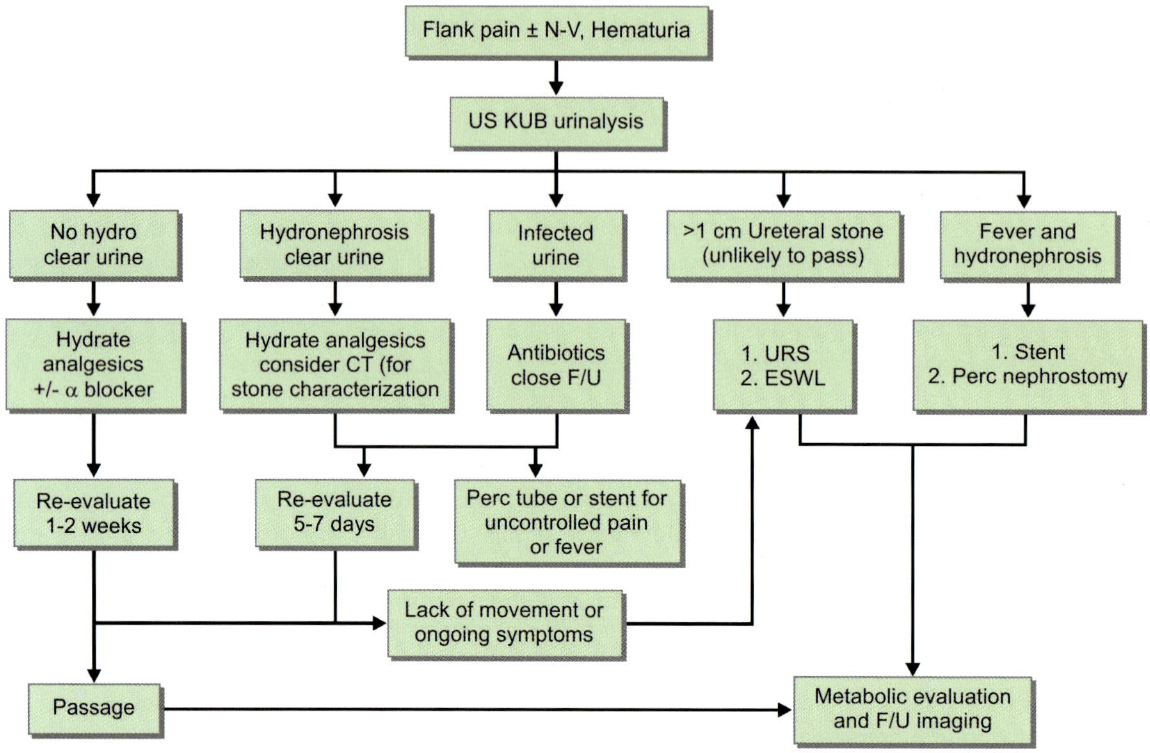

Source: Modified from Hwang K, Mason MD, Peters CA. Clinical practice: surgical approaches to urolithiasis in children. Eur J Pediatr. 2011;170:681-8. (US: Ultrasound; KUB: Kidney, ureters, and bladder; CT: Computed tomography; URS: Ureteroscopy; ESWL: Extracorporeal shock wave lithotripsy).

As part of the initial workup, children should have routine urine laboratories—urinalysis as well as urine culture and sensitivity—to identify hematuria (which may be useful in diagnosis) or a UTI. Urinary tract infection may complicate treatment and should be noted prior to any surgical management. Serum laboratories at initial workup should include complete blood count and a basic metabolic panel, which should include electrolytes, blood urea nitrogen (BUN), and creatinine. These tests can help determine the acuity of the patient and help decide between urgent operative intervention and observation/trial of passage. Significantly elevated creatinine and white blood count (especially in a patient who is febrile or in intractable pain) are typically signs that the patient should be taken for urgent surgical intervention.

Metabolic workup for stones is an invaluable part of the evaluation of the stone patient, especially in children, and can even be used to help distinguish the stone composition when a specimen is not available for analysis.[24] Significant differences in metabolic evaluations between normal children and those who form stones have been demonstrated.[25] The metabolic evaluation for children is the same as in adults: 24-hour urine for pH, volume, calcium, sodium, citrate, uric acid, creatinine, oxalate, and cysteine. Although supersaturation data are frequently utilized and are extremely helpful to determine stone composition,[26] it is important to remember that adult reference ranges are not applicable to children.[27] Also, normal reference ranges for calcium, oxalate, and citrate, when referenced to creatinine, are higher in children than adults.[28] Serum laboratories also used for the metabolic workup of urolithiasis include electrolytes, BUN, creatinine, calcium, phosphorus, magnesium, and parathyroid hormone.

Major metabolic causes in children need to be suspected in certain contexts. The infant with multiple bilateral stones may have primary hyperoxaluria type 1; the young adolescent presenting with large stone burden must be evaluated for cystinuria (Fig. 36.1); children with severe developmental delays and self-abuse with a uric acid stone may have Lesch-Nyhan syndrome. Former

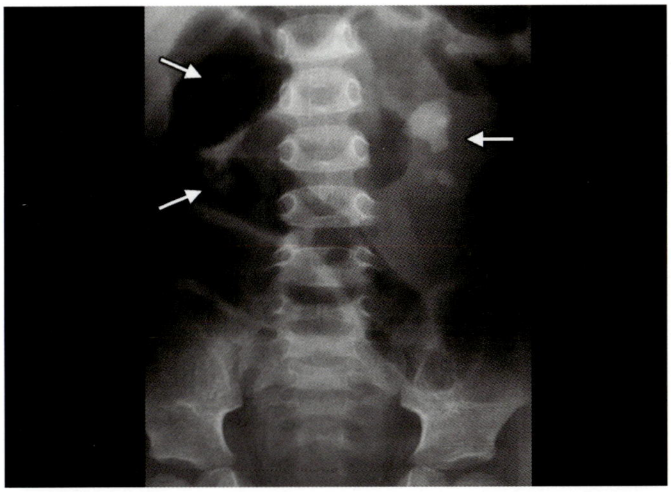

Fig. 36.1: Kidney, ureters, and bladder of a young teen with bilateral cystine stones at initial presentation. There is a partial staghorn on the left and multiple stones in the right renal calyces (arrows). Such stones presentations will require multiple staged interventions in most cases.

premature infants may be seen to have multiple small calculi bordering on a nephrocalcinosis picture due to prior diuretic therapy. These will usually resolve spontaneously.

The metabolic workup to determine the etiology of stones should ideally be performed once the patient is stone free. This will help reduce the risk of false-positive findings and will mitigate confounding factors.

Imaging

The workup of children with suspected stones differs from that of adults. Although noncontrast CT scan is typically considered the gold standard for the workup of acute abdominal pain in adults because of its ability to quickly and accurately diagnose stones,[29] it is typically avoided in the pediatric population given the radiation used. Review of the medical literature suggests that even doses of radiation associated with CT scan, while generally considered low in the adult population, can be associated with an increased risk of cancer in children—as much as 1 fatal cancer for every 1,000 CT scans performed in young children.[30] For this reason, CT scan is generally avoided except in rare circumstances where diagnosis cannot otherwise be made such as in the evaluation of small, radiolucent uric acid stones.[31] Computed tomography imaging, however, can be of particular value in treatment planning and assessing stone burden (Figs. 36.2A to C).

Renal/bladder ultrasound and plain films of the kidney, ureters, and bladder (KUB) are primarily used as the favored diagnostic modalities in children (Fig. 36.3). Diagnosis of stones can be confidently made using these tests in ~90% of children with suspected urolithiasis.[32] Recent innovations using color Doppler in addition to traditional grayscale ultrasonography have been able to diagnose stones in up to 99.6% of patients.[33]

Other modalities that may be useful in limited circumstances are intravenous urography (IVU) or voiding cystourethrogram. The use of IVU was previously considered the gold standard for diagnosis of stones in both children and adults; however, with the widespread availability of CT scan in adults and improved ultrasound resolution in children as well as radiation concerns in this population, it is less commonly used now.

MANAGEMENT

Urolithiasis in a pediatric patient presents a unique challenge, and management must be customized for each individual. The introduction of extracorporeal shock wave lithotripsy (SWL) in the early 1980s revolutionized the treatment of calculi in children.[34] This modality soon became the treatment of choice for most upper tract stones because of its safety, efficacy, and ease of use. Recent progress in enhancement and modification of modern endoscopic equipment has yielded more options for treatment, and subsequent access to the urinary tract has expanded. There are currently multiple surgical options available to the urologist for the management of calculi, including extracorporeal SWL, percutaneous nephrolithotomy (PCNL), ureteroscopy (URS), laparoscopic and robotic-assisted pyelolithotomy, and open surgery.

Stone composition influences the effectiveness of lithotripsy via a percutaneous, endoscopic, or extracorporeal approach. Although it is frequently unknown for patients with a first stone episode, the pretreatment knowledge of stone composition allows for a more efficient and appropriate surgical decision and treatment. Cystine stones, being very hard, are resistant to extracorporeal SWL and may require a percutaneous or even an open surgical extraction. Calcium oxalate monohydrate stones may also be difficult to fragment with SWL and produce large obstructing fragments (Figs. 36.4A and B). In addition, laser settings may need to be altered from typical levels to adequately fragment these stones. Uric acid and calcium oxalate dihydrate stones are the most fragile, while calcium phosphate and magnesium ammonium

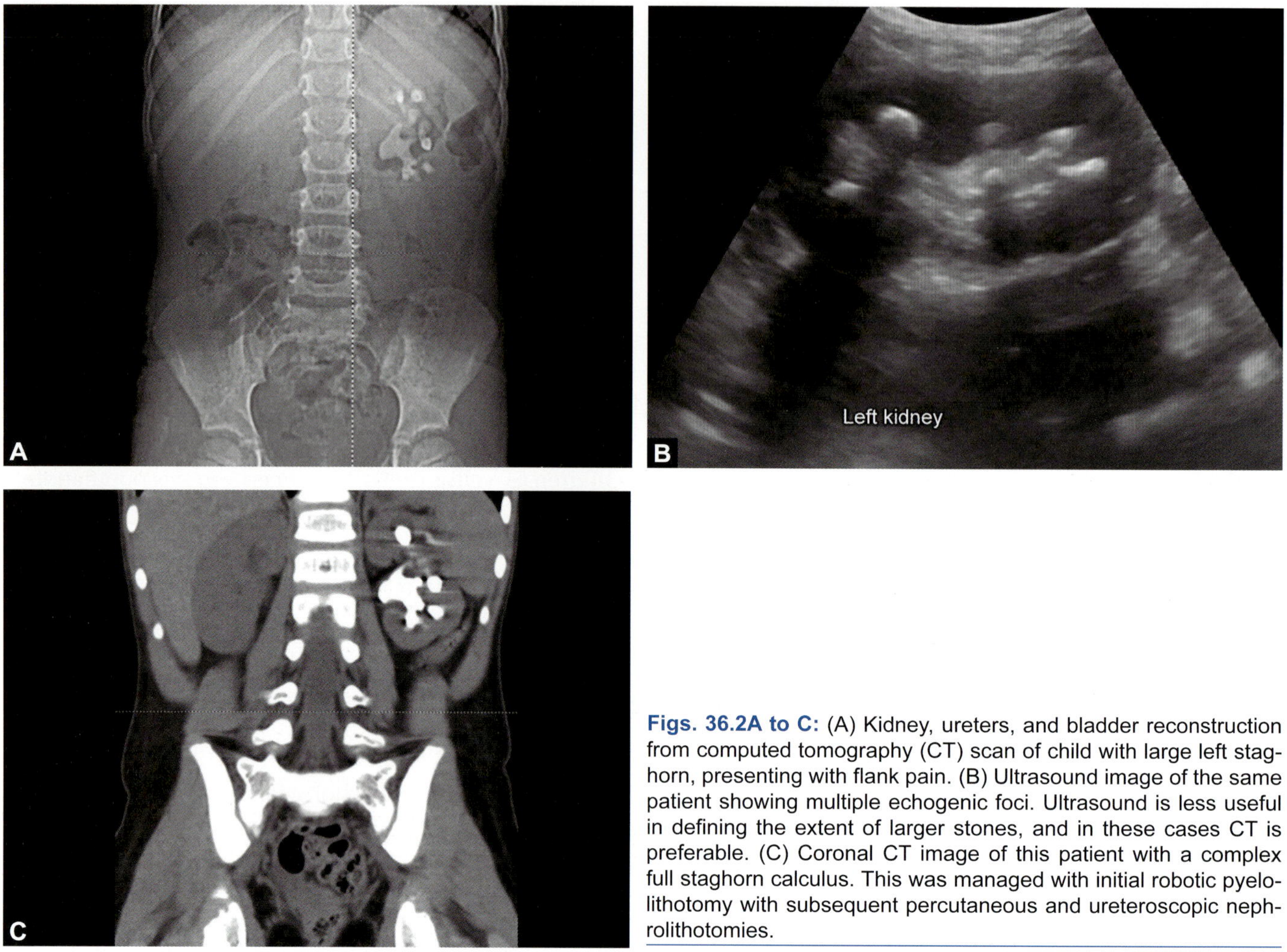

Figs. 36.2A to C: (A) Kidney, ureters, and bladder reconstruction from computed tomography (CT) scan of child with large left staghorn, presenting with flank pain. (B) Ultrasound image of the same patient showing multiple echogenic foci. Ultrasound is less useful in defining the extent of larger stones, and in these cases CT is preferable. (C) Coronal CT image of this patient with a complex full staghorn calculus. This was managed with initial robotic pyelolithotomy with subsequent percutaneous and ureteroscopic nephrolithotomies.

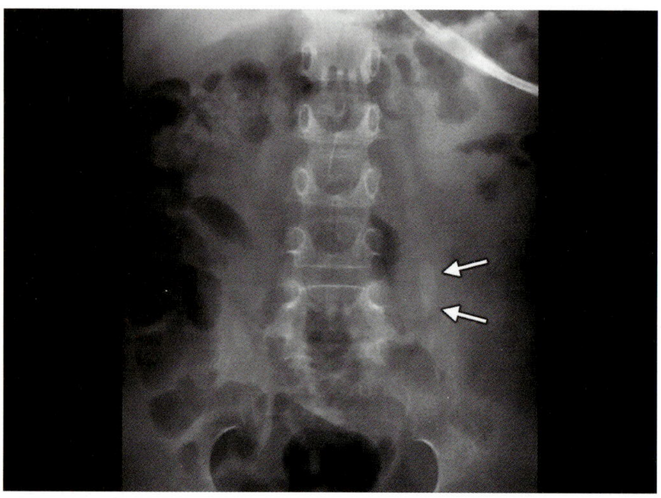

Fig. 36.3: Kidney, ureters, and bladder showing midureteral stone (arrows) presenting with flank pain and hematuria.

phosphate stones are less responsive to fragmentation.[35,36] Although the location and size of the stone may not be an absolute indication for surgical intervention, these factors certainly play a crucial role in choosing a surgical technique. The efficacy of each surgical approach varies greatly depending on the location of the stone, particularly when addressing upper versus lower tract.

Another consideration is the presence of anatomic abnormalities such as ureteropelvic junction (UPJ) obstruction and calyceal diverticula. These conditions present unique challenges and can many times require multimodal therapy. In addition, patients who have undergone previous urological surgeries, such as ureteral reimplantation and urinary diversion, often require special consideration.

Fortunately, up to 50% of children with urinary calculi will pass the stones spontaneously.[37] This statistic also

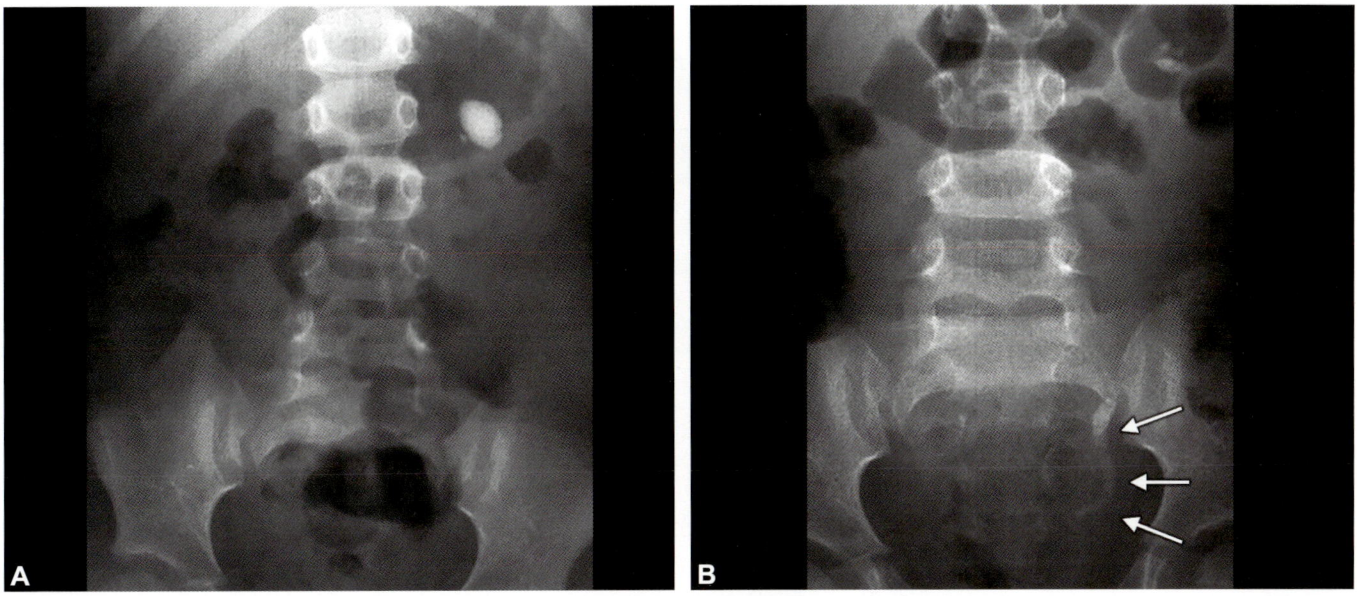

Figs. 36.4A and B: (A) Kidney, ureters, and bladder of a 6-year-old boy with left renal pelvic stone at time of treatment with extracorporeal shock wave lithotripsy (SWL). The stone appears particularly dense and was subsequently found to be calcium oxalate monohydrate. (B) Kidney, ureters, and bladder of this boy at 1 week post-SWL with an obstructing steinstrasse (arrows). He was completely asymptomatic and required ureteral stent placement with dislodgment of the lead stone fragments.

reinforces the importance of nonoperative management. Previously, only analgesia and fluid support were utilized in children, but now other pharmacological agents are available and are being more frequently utilized in children.

Acute Medical Management

The hallmark of medical management of all patients with urolithiasis is pain control. The treatment of children is no different, and adequate analgesia is required to give the patient the appropriate time to pass the calculus. Various medications are used to this end. In the acute setting, intravenous (IV) narcotics and nonsteroidal anti-inflammatory drugs are helpful to attain pain control and may be reasonable to continue in the short-term during observation as an inpatient. Also, IV fluid should be instituted upon initial evaluation to replace fluids as well as to facilitate stone expulsion from the urinary tract. More frequently, however, oral medications are used on an outpatient basis during a trial of passage. In children, non-narcotic agents such as acetaminophen and ibuprofen are used as first choice, although they will often not provide adequate pain control. Oral narcotic agents may be added to these medications to obtain pain relief.

More recently, expulsive medical therapy has been utilized safely in children. Alpha blockers are the most widely used ones and work by relaxing the smooth muscle of the intramural ureters and decreasing the frequency and force of peristalsis, which allows urine and stones to pass through more easily. Although no studies have specifically looked at the efficacy of α-blockers for stone passage in children, they have been demonstrated to increase success of stone passage and decrease time to passage in adults.[38,39] In addition, tamsulosin, which is the most widely used α-blocker currently on the market, has been demonstrated to be safe in the pediatric population.[40]

Calcium channel blockers have also been used as expulsive therapy for stones in adults, but no studies of safety or efficacy have been done in children. These medications suppress distal ureteral smooth muscle contraction and decrease ureteral spasm to facilitate stone passage. Nonsteroidal anti-inflammatory drugs and corticosteroids have been used to facilitate stone passage by decreasing ureteral wall edema.

Surgical Management (Flowchart 36.2)

Shock Wave Lithotripsy

Although there are various machines, all models function similarly. The stone is fragmented by generating and precisely focusing shock wave energy at the stone, and the resulting pieces are passed through the urinary tract.

Flowchart 36.2: Algorithm for surgical management of the child with a renal pelvic stone.

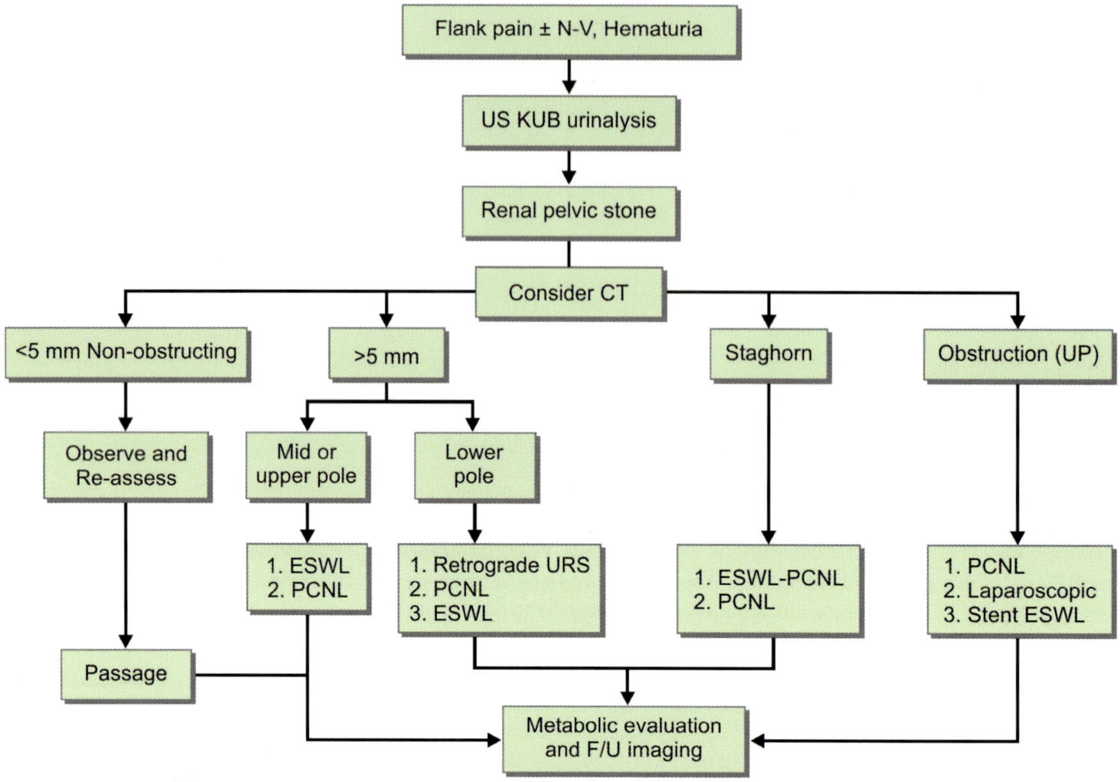

Source: Modified from Hwang K, Mason MD, Peters CA. Clinical practice: surgical approaches to urolithiasis in children. Eur J Pediatr. 2011;170:681-8. (US: Ultrasound; KUB: Kidney, ureters, and bladder; CT: Computed tomography; UPJ: Ureteropelvic junction; ESWL: Extracorporeal shock wave lithotripsy; PCNL: Percutaneous nephrolithotomy).

Children typically are placed under general anesthesia to limit stone movement and repeated repositioning. Shock wave lithotripsy with the Dornier HM3 lithotripter (Dornier Medical Systems, Kennesaw, GA, USA) has been clinically available since the mid-1980s and has successfully been used to treat upper tract stones in children.[41] Although experience in the pediatric population is limited in comparison, initial series reported complication, stone-free, and safety rates similar to those in adults.[42] Complications are relatively minimal and range in severity from hematuria and ecchymosis to obstruction and sepsis.

In treating renal stones, important variables including stone burden and renal anatomy are crucial in selecting the most effective treatment modality. Surgeons' preference, however, remains an extremely important factor as well. There is good evidence that SWL is considered safe and effective for small upper tract stones and even for stones up to 15 mm, with success rates approaching 75–80%.[43,44] Stone-free rates of up to 98% at 3 months postoperatively have been demonstrated in some series with stones as large as 2.5 cm.[45] For many surgeons, SWL remains the first-line treatment for small upper tract stones. Although the most effective management for large lower pole stones has yet to be determined, SWL failure and relatively high retreatment rates (≥40%)[46] tend to suggest that this may not be the ideal treatment for lower pole stones. A recent review has shown SWL performed with portable lithotripters to be of limited value in children with complex urological conditions. Children with pre-existing urological abnormalities experienced a stone-free rate of as low as 12.5%.[47] Most children do not require preoperative stenting, even for large stones, since children are typically able to pass proportionately larger fragments than adults.[48]

Staghorn calculi are those stones that fill the majority of the renal collecting system and are typically composed of struvite and associated with UTI with protease splitting organisms.[49] Although complete staghorn calculi are fairly rare in children, they pose a unique challenge. Traditionally, SWL monotherapy success rates are poor; however, the stone-free rates in children are surprisingly much higher.[69] Taking into account the disadvantages of the need for ureteral stenting and multiple sessions, SWL monotherapy is considered an acceptable treatment option in children due to the higher stone-free rates (~80%).[50] As opposed to other renal calculi, it may be beneficial to stent children with staghorns prior to SWL to facilitate fragment passage.[1]

Proximal ureteral stones can be treated with SWL and, in some series, have achieved comparable success rates to renal stones, although ureteral stenting to aid in localization of the stone as well as stone clearance is more often recommended. Mid to lower ureteral stones should be approached with caution when considering SWL therapy due to the potential for injury to reproductive organs,[51] as well as the difficulty in visualization of the stone overlying the pelvic bones. Another consideration for ureteral stones in children is difficult visualization due to constipation.

Even though the US Food and Drug Administration has not formally endorsed its use in children, SWL is considered to be safe and efficacious, and even young children and infants can be treated safely.[9]

Ureteroscopy

Ureteroscopy was first reported on a child in 1929[52] but did not become more accepted until 1988 when Ritchey reported on a technique for the treatment of urolithiasis.[53] The safety and efficacy of endoscopic treatment in management of urinary stones in children has been greatly improved with advances of endoscopic equipment and the adoption of the holmium:Yttrium Aluminum Garnet (YAG) laser. Ureteroscopy is ideally suited for removal or fragmentation of distal ureteral stones. Its use has, however, been broadened and it is now frequently the treatment of choice for management of upper tract stones. This modality can be especially useful for stones that are resistant to SWL or cannot be visualized for SWL.

Adoption of techniques used commonly in adults has made the pediatric ureter and kidney more accessible for endoscopic examination. In particular, the use of a ureteral access sheath as well as balloon or sequential coaxial ureteral orifice dilation may be required in many children to attain access to the ureter and kidney.[54] These techniques have engendered caution regarding possible ischemic stricture formation and development of vesicoureteral reflux, but the incidence of these sequelae is quite low.[55] With the advent of smaller ureteroscopes and improved optics, ureteral dilation is actually used quite infrequently.[56]

Routine ureteral stenting is performed with significant variability among pediatric urologists, and no definitive recommendations exist regarding its use. Preoperative stenting is sometimes required to dilate the ureter temporarily if initial access to the ureter cannot be done safely. Even in cases where access to the ureter is possible, a surgeon may choose to stent if an access sheath is necessary in order to prepare the ureter for placement of the sheath. Preoperative stenting is widely accepted, although it does require an additional anesthetic session for children. Postoperative stenting is controversial. The decision to place a stent postoperatively is dependent on the experience of the surgeon and other factors, which may include the length of the procedure, number of passes with the instrument, and degree of visible ureteral trauma or edema at the conclusion of the procedure. Although stenting may prevent postoperative obstruction, facilitate passage of small residual stones, and aid in the recovery of minor trauma to the ureter, children can experience significant discomfort from the stents.

A significant benefit of URS is that it can be used in a wide variety of scenarios. Good success rates have been demonstrated in patients with stones throughout the urinary tract, including the lower pole calyces.[69] It can also be used successfully in children with anatomic abnormalities or who have undergone previous urologic reconstructive procedures.

Significant complications from URS are rare. More frequently, minor postoperative issues such as hematuria and UTIs are encountered and require treatments ranging from observation to antibiotic administration. More severe complications, including ureteral perforation and later stricture formation, typically require further intervention. Simple perforation can often be successfully managed with a temporary stent. Fortunately, more significant tears and avulsions are rarely encountered.

Percutaneous Nephrolithotomy

The introduction of percutaneous techniques in approaching renal stones in the late 1970s revolutionized treatment for large stone burdens. Prior to this, all large stones required open surgical techniques, which conferred significant morbidity and mortality. It was not until the late 1990s that special instrumentation was adapted for children,[57] and now it is an established approach in children with proven safety and efficacy as monotherapy as well as in combination with other modalities, especially SWL.

There is no current consensus, but relative indications for PCNL parallel those in adults, including large stone burden (>15 mm) and failure of previous surgery. Stone-free rates range from 68 to 95% and can be improved with the use of multiple tracts as well as a staged approach, where percutaneous access is obtained initially, and then through the mature tract the stone is fragmented a few days later.[58,59] Because increased tract size has been directly correlated with increased complications such as bleeding and renal damage, it is generally accepted that the smallest sheath that will provide safe and effective access to the stone should be used. To increase the safety of this procedure for even small children, various techniques have been used with significant success, including utilization of a 15-Fr peel-away sheath[60] and the 11-Fr miniperc.[61] Complications include intraoperative bleeding requiring transfusion, injury to pelvicalyceal system, and hydrothorax, as well as fever and sepsis.

Historically, lower pole access to the collecting system via a subcostal puncture was viewed as the safest approach. However, when performed by experienced and skilled endourologists, supracostal access to the upper pole of the kidney can be accomplished with a high degree of safety and efficacy.[62] Several series have shown that multiple percutaneous sites can increase the success rate of the procedure and have not been shown to increase transfusion rates. Placement of a postoperative stent or nephrostomy tube varies among series and is determined by the experience of the surgeon.

In the unusual child with prior urinary tract reconstruction including the ureters, antegrade ureteroscopy may be the most direct approach to the stone. With reimplanted, tapered, or re-routed (e.g. transureteroureterostomy (TUU)) ureters, retrograde access may be both difficult and potentially injurious. In such cases, midpole percutaneous access with antegrade ureteroscopic access to the stone can be quite effective and efficient. The ureter proximal to the stone is usually dilated and retrieval can be straightforward. Although TUU is often considered high risk, it is a very effective means to complex reconstruction. An obstructing stone, however, can create bilateral obstruction if distal to the anastomosis. A single-sided percutaneous nephrostomy relieves both kidneys and can be used for definitive stone removal.

Laparoscopic and Robotic-assisted Pyelolithotomy

The role of laparoscopy in the treatment of urolithiasis in children continues to evolve. There is very little evidence in the literature to support routine use of this modality due to limited number of patients, although there are clearly scenarios where it can be of use. Laparoscopic pyelolithotomy in children who previously failed PCNL has been described in multiple series with no noted major complications.[63,64]

In adults, laparoscopy and robotic-assisted laparoscopy have been used successfully for the simultaneous treatment of UPJ obstruction and large calculi, but this approach has been explored in children only recently. Lee et al. described their experience of robotic-assisted laparoscopic pyelolithotomy with five procedures consisting of four patients with refractory cystine staghorn calculi and one child with concurrent UPJ obstruction.[65] Four of these procedures were completed robotically, with one case requiring conversion to an open procedure. This technique may also be of use in children with anatomic considerations that make access via more traditional techniques more difficult, such as ectopic kidneys.[66] Further studies are needed to determine if shorter operative times are achievable and if these procedures can be completed safely in children. It seems likely, however, that laparoscopic and robotic-assisted laparoscopic procedures will be reserved for children with more complex anatomy or stones that are refractory to other treatments (Figs. 36.5A to C).

Open Surgical Management of Urolithiasis

Management of urolithiasis in children has undergone dramatic changes. The need for the open approach to stone management has waned significantly, especially with the introduction and widespread use of minimally invasive modalities.[67] These technological advancements have made open surgical management increasingly rare.

Even bladder calculi that previously required open surgical removal via a suprapubic cystolithotomy are now amenable to endoscopic management.[68] Endoscopic treatment of bladder calculi is possible; however, there is some controversy surrounding this approach when used after lower urinary tract reconstruction. Particularly in patients with augmented bladder or continent reservoirs, it can be extremely difficult to clear all stone fragments endoscopically. If the bladder or reservoir can only be accessed via a continent catheterizable channel, the risk of injury to the continence mechanism must be considered. In some cases, with multiple or large stones, open removal of the intact stones seems preferable to creating numerous fragments that may act as the nidus for future stones.

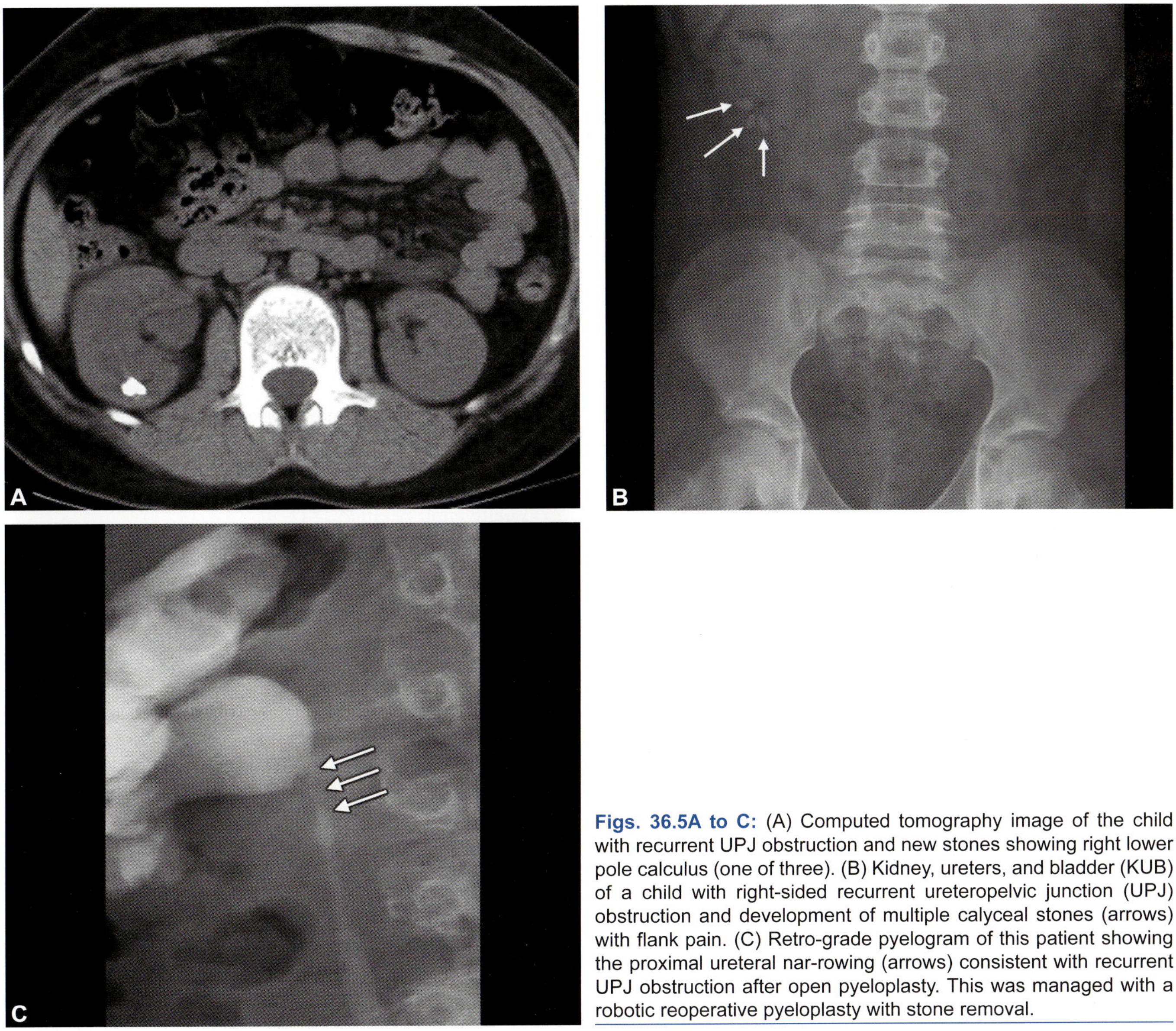

Figs. 36.5A to C: (A) Computed tomography image of the child with recurrent UPJ obstruction and new stones showing right lower pole calculus (one of three). (B) Kidney, ureters, and bladder (KUB) of a child with right-sided recurrent ureteropelvic junction (UPJ) obstruction and development of multiple calyceal stones (arrows) with flank pain. (C) Retro-grade pyelogram of this patient showing the proximal ureteral nar-rowing (arrows) consistent with recurrent UPJ obstruction after open pyeloplasty. This was managed with a robotic reoperative pyeloplasty with stone removal.

Open surgical approaches of upper tract urolithiasis are even less frequently employed than in cases involving the lower urinary tract. This approach is rarely needed, even with large-burden staghorn calculi. If concomitant open reconstruction is needed, however, open removal is reasonable.

CONCLUSION

Urolithiasis in children is of diverse etiology requiring carefully planned, customized diagnostic and management strategies. Although many similarities can exist between adult and pediatric stone disease, the key differences can offer management challenges. Research continues to better define the risk factors for developing stone disease, as does the improvement in diagnostic capability. With current technical sophistication in SWL, endoscopic, and percutaneous and laparoscopic techniques, the reality of a safe, effective, and minimally invasive treatment for all cases of pediatric urolithiasis is becoming more attainable. Even in children with complex anatomy or prior surgical reconstruction, endoscopic techniques remain the first-line treatment with a high likelihood of success.

REFERENCES

1. Stapleton FB. Nephrolithiasis in children. Pediatr Rev. 1989;11(1):21-30.
2. Routh J, Graham D, Nelson C. Epidemiological trends in pediatric urolithiasis at United States freestanding pediatric hospitals. J Urol. 2010;184(3):1100-5.
3. VanDervoort K, Wiesen J, Frank R, et al. Urolithiasis in pediatric patients: a single center study of incidence, clinical presentation and outcome. J Urol. 2007;177(6):2300-5.
4. Rizvi SA, Naqvi SA, Hussain Z, et al. Pediatric urolithiasis: developing nation perspectives. J Urol. 2002;168(4 Pt 1): 1522-5.
5. Bartosh SM. Medical management of pediatric stone disease. Urol Clin North Am. 2004;31(3):575-87; x-xi.
6. Sarica K. Pediatric urolithiasis: etiology, specific pathogenesis and medical treatment. Urol Res. 2006;34(2):96-101.
7. Kaya M, Boleken ME, Soran M, et al. Acute renal failure due to bilateral uric acid lithiasis in infants. Urol Res. 2007;35(3):119-22.
8. Smaldone MC, Cannon GM Jr, Wu HY, et al. Is ureteroscopy first line treatment for pediatric stone disease? J Urol. 2007;178(5):2128-31; discussion 2131.
9. Wadhwa P, Aron M, Bal CS, et al. Critical prospective appraisal of renal morphology and function in children undergoing shockwave lithotripsy and percutaneous nephrolithotomy. J Endourol. 2007;21(9):961-6.
10. Persaud AC, Stevenson MD, McMahon DR, et al. Pediatric urolithiasis: clinical predictors in the emergency department. Pediatrics. 2009;124:888-94.
11. Coe FL, Evan A, Worcester E. Kidney stone disease. J Clin Invest. 2005;115:2598-608.
12. Taylor EN, Stampfer MJ, Curhan GC. Obesity, weight gain, and the risk of kidney stones. J Am Med Assoc. 2005;293: 455-62.
13. Semins MJ, Shore AD, Makary MA, et al. The association of increasing body mass index and kidney stone disease. J Urol. 2010;183:571-5.
14. Roddy JT, Ghousheh AI, Christensen MA, et al. Metabolic evaluation of urolithiasis and obesity in a midwestern pediatric population. J Urol. 2013;191(3):771-6.
15. Remzi D, Bakkaloglu MA, Erkan I, et al. Pediatric urolithiasis. Turk J Pediatr. 1984;26:43-9.
16. Alon US. Nephrocalcinosis. Curr Opin Pediatr. 1997;9:160-5.
17. Novak TE, Lakshmanan Y, Trock BJ, et al. Sex Prevalence of pediatric kidney stone disease in the United States: an epidemiologic investigation. Urology. 2009;74(1):104-7.
18. Gabrielsen JS, Laciak RJ, Frank EL, et al. Pediatric urinary stone composition in the United States. J Urol. 2012;187(6):2182-7.
19. Steele BT, Lowe P, Rance CP, et al. Urinary tract calculi in children. Int J Pediatr Nephrol. 1983;4(1):47-52.
20. Gearhart JP, Herzberg GZ, Jeffs RD. Childhood urolithiasis: experiences and advances. Pediatrics. 1991;87:445-50.
21. Milliner DS, Murphy ME. Urolithiasis in pediatric patients. Mayo Clin Proc. 1993;68(3):241-8.
22. Stapleton FB. Current approaches to pediatric stone disease. AUA Update Ser. 2000;19:314.
23. Paul E, Conant KD, Dunne IE, et al. Urolithiasis on the ketogenic diet with concurrent topiramate or zonisamide therapy. Epilepsy Res. 2010;90(1-2):151-6.
24. Torricelli FC, De S, Liu X, et al. Can 24-hour urine stone risk profiles predict urinary stone composition? J Endourol. 2014;28(6):735-8.
25. DeFoor W, Asplin J, Jackson E, et al. Urinary metabolic evaluations in normal and stone forming children. J Urol. 2006;176(4 Pt 2):1793-6.
26. Asplin J, Parks J, Lingeman J, et al. Supersaturation and stone composition in a network of dispersed treatment sites. J Urol. 1998;159:1821-5.
27. Battino BS, DeFoor W, Coe F, et al. Metabolic evaluation of children with urolithiasis: are adult references for supersaturation appropriate? J Urol. 2002;168:2568-71.
28. DeFoor W, Asplin J, Jackson C, et al. Results of a prospective trial to compare normal urine supersaturation in children and adults. J Urol. 2005;174:1708-10.
29. Chen MY, Zagoria RJ, Saunders HS, et al. Trends in the use of unenhanced helical CT for acute urinary colic. AJR Am J Roentgenol. 1999;173:1447-50.
30. Rice HE, Frush DP, Farmer D, et al. Review of radiation risks from computed tomography: essentials for the pediatric surgeon. APSA Education Committee. J Pediatr Surg. 2007;42(4):603-7.
31. Resnick MI, Kursh ED, Cohen AM. Use of computerized tomography in the delineation of uric acid calculi. J Urol. 1984;131(1):9-10.
32. Johnson E, Faerber G, Roberts W, et al. Are stone protocol computed tomography scans mandatory for children with suspected urinary calculi? Urology. 2011;78:662-6.
33. Elnagar M, Alsobky E. 2181 Value of ultrasound, KUB, and urinalysis in diagnosis of renal colic due to ureteral stones. J Urol. 2012;187(4, Suppl): e879-80.
34. Chaussy C, Schmiedt E, Jocham D, et al. First clinical experience with extracorporeally induced destruction of kidney stones by shock waves. J Urol. 1982;127(3):417-20.
35. Fuchs G, Miller K, Rassweiler J, et al. Extracorporeal shockwave lithotripsy: one-year experience with the Dornier lithotripter. Eur Urol. 1985;11(3):145-9.
36. Wu HY, Docimo SG. Surgical management of children with urolithiasis. Urol Clin North Am. 2004;31(3):589-94; xi.
37. Pietrow PK, Pope JC 4th, Adams MC, et al. Clinical outcome of pediatric stone disease. J Urol. 2002;167(2 Pt 1):670-3.
38. Cervenakov I, Fillo J, Mardiak J, et al. Speedy elimination of ureterolithiasis in lower part of ureters with the alpha 1-blocker tamsulosin. Int Urol Nephrol. 2002;34(1):25-9.
39. Dellabella M, Milanese G, Muzzonigro G. Efficacy of tamsulosin in the medical management of juxtavesical ureteral stones. J Urol. 2003;170:2202-5.
40. VanderBrink B, Gitlin J, Toro S, et al. Effect of tamsulosin on systemic blood pressure and nonneurogenic dysfunctional voiding in children. J Urol. 2009;181:817-22.
41. Kramolowsky EV, Willoughby BL, Loening SA. Extracorporeal shock wave lithotripsy in children. J Urol. 1987;137(5):939-41.
42. Newman DM, Coury T, Lingeman JE, et al. Extracorporeal shock wave lithotripsy experience in children. J Urol. 1986;136(1 Pt 2):238-40.

43. Ather MH, Noor MA. Does size and site matter for renal stones up to 30-mm in size in children treated by extracorporeal lithotripsy? Urology. 2003;61(1):212-5; discussion 215.
44. Elsobky E, Sheir KZ, Madbouly K, et al. Extracorporeal shock wave lithotripsy in children: experience using two second-generation lithotripters. BJU Int. 2000;86(7):851-6.
45. Netto N, Longo J, Ikonomidis J, et al. Extracorporeal shock wave lithotripsy in children. J Urol. 2002;167:2164-6.
46. Onal B, Demirkesen O, Tansu N, et al. The impact of caliceal pelvic anatomy on stone clearance after shock wave lithotripsy for pediatric lower pole stones. J Urol. 2004;172(3):1082-6.
47. Nelson CP, Diamond DA, Cendron M, et al. Extracorporeal shock wave lithotripsy in pediatric patients using a late generation portable lithotriptor: experience at Children's Hospital Boston. J Urol. 2008;180(4 Suppl):1865-8.
48. Mobley T, Myers D, Jenkins J, et al. Effects of stents on lithotripsy of renal calculi: treatment results with 18,825 calculi using the lithostar lithotripter. J Urol. 1989;152:53-6.
49. Segura JW, Preminger GM, Assimos DG, et al. Nephrolithiasis Clinical Guidelines Panel summary report on the management of staghorn calculi. The American Urological Association Nephrolithiasis Clinical Guidelines Panel. J Urol. 1994;151(6):1648-51.
50. Al-Busaidy SS, Prem AR, Medhat M. Pediatric staghorn calculi: the role of extracorporeal shock wave lithotripsy monotherapy with special reference to ureteral stenting. J Urol. 2003;169(2):629-33.
51. Basar MM, Samli MM, Erbil M, et al. Early effects of extracorporeal shock-wave lithotripsy exposure on testicular sperm morphology. Scand J Urol Nephrol. 2004;38(1):38-41.
52. Young H, McKay R. Congenital valvular obstruction of the prostatic urethra. Surg Gynecol Obstet. 1929;48:509-11.
53. Ritchey M, Patterson D, Kelalis P, et al. A case of pediatric ureteroscopic lithotripsy. J Urol. 1988;139:1272-4.
54. Uygun I, Okur MH, Aydogdu B, et al. Efficacy and safety of endoscopic laser lithotripsy for urinary stone treatment in children. Urol Res. 2012;40(6):751-5.
55. Schuster TG, Russell KY, Bloom DA, et al. Ureteroscopy for the treatment of urolithiasis in children. J Urol. 2002;167(4):1813; discussion 1815-6.
56. Herndon CD, Viamonte L, Joseph DB. Ureteroscopy in children: is there a need for ureteral dilation and postoperative stenting? J Pediatr Urol. 2006;2(4):290-3.
57. Jackman SV, Docimo SG, Cadeddu JA, et al. The "mini-perc" technique: a less invasive alternative to percutaneous nephrolithotomy. World J Urol. 1998;16(6):371-4.
58. Badawy H, Salama A, Eissa M, et al. Percutaneous management of renal calculi: experience with percutaneous nephrolithotomy in 60 children. J Urol. 1999;162(5):1710-3.
59. Salah MA, Toth C, Khan AM, et al. Percutaneous nephrolithotomy in children: experience with 138 cases in a developing country. World J Urol. 2004;22(4):277-80.
60. Helal M, Black T, Lockhart J, et al. The Hickman peel-away sheath: alternative for pediatric percutaneous nephrolithotomy. J Endourol. 1997;11:171-2.
61. Jackman S, Hedican S, Peters C, et al. Percutaneous nephrolithotomy in infants and school aged children: experience with a new technique. Urology. 1998;52:697-700.
62. El-Nahas AR, Shokeir AA, El-Kenawy MR, et al. Safety and efficacy of supracostal percutaneous nephrolithotomy in pediatric patients. J Urol. 2008;180(2):676-80.
63. Casale P, Grady RW, Joyner BD, et al. Transperitoneal laparoscopic pyelolithotomy after failed percutaneous access in the pediatric patient. J Urol. 2004;172(2):680-3; discussion 683.
64. Nambirajan T, Jeschke S, Albqami N, et al. Role of laparoscopy in management of renal stones: single center experience and review of literature. J Endourol. 2005;19(3):353-9.
65. Lee RS, Passerotti CC, Cendron M, et al. Early results of robot assisted laparoscopic lithotomy in adolescents. J Urol. 2007;177(6):2306-9; discussion 2309-10.
66. Kamat N, Khandelwal P. Laparoscopic pyelolithotomy—a technique for the management of stones in the ectopic pelvic kidney. Int J Urol. 2004;11(7):581-4.
67. Paik ML, Wainstein MA, Spirnak JP, et al. Current indications for open stone surgery in the treatment of renal and ureteral calculi. J Urol. 1998;159(2):374-8; discussion 378-9.
68. Fragoso AC, Valla JS, Steyaert H, et al. Minimal access surgery in the management of pediatric urolithiasis. J Pediatr Urol. 2009;5(1):42-6.
69. Smaldone MC, Corcoran AT, Docimo SG, et al. Endourological management of pediatric stone disease: present status. J Urol. 2009;181(1):17-28.
70. Hwang K, Mason MD, Peters CA. Clinical practice: surgical approaches to urolithiasis in children. Eur J Pediatr. 2011;170:681-8.

Index

Page numbers followed by *b* refer to box, *f* refer to figure, and *t* refer to table

G

H

I

J

S

V

W

X

Y

Z